D1605484

Handbook of Research Methods in Cardiovascular Behavioral Medicine

THE PLENUM SERIES IN BEHAVIORAL PSYCHOPHYSIOLOGY AND MEDICINE

Series Editor:
William J. Ray, *Pennsylvania State University, University Park, Pennsylvania*

BIOLOGICAL BARRIERS IN BEHAVIORAL MEDICINE
Edited by Wolfgang Linden

HANDBOOK OF RESEARCH METHODS IN CARDIOVASCULAR
BEHAVIORAL MEDICINE
Edited by Neil Schneiderman, Stephen M. Weiss, and Peter G. Kaufmann

PHYSIOLOGY AND BEHAVIOR THERAPY
Conceptual Guidelines for the Clinician
James G. Hollandsworth, Jr.

Handbook of Research Methods in Cardiovascular Behavioral Medicine

Edited by

Neil Schneiderman
University of Miami
Coral Gables, Florida

Stephen M. Weiss
and
Peter G. Kaufmann
National Heart, Lung, and Blood Institute
Bethesda, Maryland

Plenum Press • New York and London

Library of Congress Cataloging in Publication Data

Handbook of research methods in cardiovascular behavioral medicine / edited by Neil
Schneiderman, Stephen M. Weiss, and Peter Kaufmann.
       p.   cm.—(Plenum series in behavioral psychophysiology and medicine)
    Includes bibliographies and index.
    ISBN 0-306-42960-8
    1. Cardiovascular system—Diseases—Psychosomatic aspects—Research—Methodology.
2. Medicine and psychology—Research—Methodology. 3. Medicine, Psychosomatic—
Research—Methodology. 4. Patient monitoring. I. Schneiderman, Neil. II. Weiss, Stephen M.
III. Kaufmann, Peter (Peter G).) IV. Series.
    [DNLM: 1. Behavioral Medicine. 2. Cardiovascular System—physiology. 3. Research—
methods. WG 100 H2358]
RC669.H28   1989
616.1'208—dc19
DNLM/DLC   89-3705
for Library of Congress   CIP

© 1989 Plenum Press, New York
A Division of Plenum Publishing Corporation
233 Spring Street, New York, N.Y. 10013

Printed in the United States of America

Contributors

Erling A. Anderson, Departments of Anesthesia and Internal Medicine, Cardiovascular and Clinical Research Centers, University of Iowa College of Medicine, Iowa City, Iowa 52242

Norman B. Anderson, Department of Psychiatry, Duke University Medical School, and Geriatric Research, Education, and Clinical Center, Veterans Administration Medical Center, Durham, North Carolina 27710

Steven A. Atlas, Cardiovascular Center and Department of Medicine, Cornell University Medical College, New York, New York 10021

Garth Bissette, Laboratory of Psychoneuroendocrinology, Department of Psychiatry, Duke University Medical Center, Durham, North Carolina 27710

Seymour G. Blank, Department of Medicine, Cardiovascular Center, The New York Hospital–Cornell Medical Center, New York, New York 10021

Charles S. Carver, Department of Psychology, University of Miami, Coral Gables, Florida 33124

Margaret A. Chesney, Department of Epidemiology, School of Medicine, University of California at San Francisco, San Francisco, California 94143

L. A. Clark, AT&T Bell Laboratories, Murray Hill, New Jersey 07974

Theodore M. Dembroski, Department of Psychology, University of Maryland Baltimore County, Catonsville, Maryland 21228

L. Denby, AT&T Bell Laboratories, Murray Hill, New Jersey 07974

Vincent DeQuattro, Department of Medicine, University of Southern California School of Medicine, Los Angeles, California 90007

Joel E. Dimsdale, Department of Psychiatry, University of California, San Diego Medical Center, San Diego, California 92103

E. D. Dunlap, Division of Endocrinology and Metabolism, Veterans Administration Medical Center, Louisville, Kentucky 40202

Bonita Falkner, Department of Pediatrics, Hahnemann University, Philadelphia, Pennsylvania 19102

Gregory A. Harshfield, Department of Pediatrics, University of Tennessee, Memphis, Tennessee 38103

Larry V. Hedges, Department of Education, University of Chicago, Chicago, Illinois 60637

Alan S. Hollister, Departments of Medicine and Pharmacology, Vanderbilt University Medical Center, Nashville, Tennessee 37232

B. Kent Houston, Department of Psychology, University of Kansas, Lawrence, Kansas 66045

Chun Hwang, Hypertension Center, Department of Medicine, Charles R. Drew Postgraduate Medical School, Los Angeles, California 90059

Gail H. Ironson, Department of Psychiatry and Behavioral Sciences, Stanford University Medical Center, Stanford, California 94305

Theodore Jacob, Division of Family Studies, University of Arizona, Tucson, Arizona 85721

Stevo Julius, Division of Hypertension, Department of Internal Medicine, University of Michigan Medical Center, Ann Arbor, Michigan 48109-0356

Jay R. Kaplan, Department of Comparative Medicine, Bowman Gray School of Medicine, Wake Forest University, Winston-Salem, North Carolina 27109

Alfred L. Kasprowicz, Department of Psychology, University of Pittsburgh, Pittsburgh, Pennsylvania 15260

Peter G. Kaufmann, Behavioral Medicine Branch, National Heart, Lung, and Blood Institute, Bethesda, Maryland 20892

Paul Kligfield, Division of Cardiology, Department of Medicine, The New York Hospital–Cornell Medical Center, New York, New York 10021

George F. Koob, Division of Preclinical Neuroscience and Endocrinology, Research Institute of Scripps Clinic, La Jolla, California 92037

David S. Krantz, Department of Medical Psychology, Uniformed Services University of the Health Sciences, Bethesda, Maryland 20814

Cynthia M. Kuhn, Department of Pharmacology, Duke University Medical Center, Durham, North Carolina 27710

Lewis H. Kuller, Department of Epidemiology, University of Pittsburgh, Graduate School of Public Health, Pittsburgh, Pennsylvania 15261

John H. Laragh, Cardiovascular Center and Department of Medicine, Cornell University Medical College, New York, New York 10021

Kevin T. Larkin, Department of Psychology, West Virginia University, Morgantown, West Virginia 26506

Debora De-Ping Lee, Department of Medicine, University of Southern California School of Medicine, Los Angeles, California 90007

Kathleen C. Light, Departments of Psychiatry and Physiology, University of North Carolina at Chapel Hill, Chapel Hill, North Carolina 27599

William R. Lovallo, Behavioral Sciences Laboratories, Veterans Administration Medical Center and University of Oklahoma Health Sciences Center, Oklahoma City, Oklahoma 73104

Stephen B. Manuck, Department of Psychology, University of Pittsburgh, Pittsburgh, Pennsylvania 15260

Allyn L. Mark, Departments of Anesthesia and Internal Medicine, Cardiovascular and Clinical Research Centers, University of Iowa College of Medicine, Iowa City, Iowa 52242

Karen A. Matthews, Department of Psychiatry, Western Psychiatric Institute and Clinic, Pittsburgh, Pennsylvania 15213

Philip M. McCabe, Behavioral Medicine Research Center, Department of Psychology, University of Miami, Coral Gables, Florida 33124

Mikhail Menshikov, Myasnikov Institute of the All-Union Cardiological Research Center, Moscow, U.S.S.R.

Scott M. Monroe, Department of Psychology, University of Pittsburgh, Pittsburgh, Pennsylvania 15260

Larry R. Muenz, SRA Technologies, Inc., 4700 King Street, Alexandria, Virginia, 22302

Yelena Parfyonova, Myasnikov Institute of the All-Union Cardiological Research Center, Moscow, U.S.S.R.

M. A. Pfeifer, Division of Endocrinology and Metabolism, Veterans Administration Medical Center, Louisville, Kentucky 40202

Thomas G. Pickering, Department of Medicine, Cardiovascular Center, The New York Hospital–Cornell Medical Center, New York, New York 10021

Gwendolyn A. Pincomb, Behavioral Sciences Laboratories, Veterans Administration Medical Center and University of Oklahoma Health Sciences Center, Oklahoma City, Oklahoma 73104

D. Pregibon, AT&T Bell Laboratories, Murray Hill, New Jersey 07974

Jeffrey Ratliff-Crain, Department of Medical Psychology, Uniformed Services University of the Health Sciences, Bethesda, Maryland 20814

William J. Ray, Department of Psychology, Pennsylvania State University, University Park, Pennsylvania 16802

David Robertson, Departments of Medicine and Pharmacology, Vanderbilt University Medical Center, Nashville, Tennessee 37232

Robert F. Rushmer, Center for Bioengineering, University of Washington, Seattle, Washington 98105

Patrice G. Saab, Department of Psychology, University of Miami, Coral Gables, Florida 33124

Vikas Saini, Cardiovascular Laboratories, Harvard University School of Public Health, Boston, Massachusetts 02115

Neil Schneiderman, Behavioral Medicine Research Center, Department of Psychology, University of Miami, Coral Gables, Florida 33124

Jean E. Sealey, Cardiovascular Center and Department of Medicine, Cornell University Medical College, New York, New York 10021

Jerome E. Singer, Department of Medical Psychology, Uniformed Services University of the Health Sciences, Bethesda, Maryland 20814

Jay S. Skyler, Departments of Medicine, Pediatrics, and Psychology, University of Miami, Miami, Florida 33101

Michael J Strube, Department of Psychology, Washington University, St. Louis, Missouri 63130

Daniel L. Tennenbaum, Department of Psychology, Kent State University, Kent, Ohio 44242

Lawrence F. Van Egeren, Department of Psychiatry, Michigan State University, East Lansing, Michigan 48824

Richard L. Verrier, Department of Cardiology, Tufts University Medical School, Boston, Massachusetts 02115, and Department of Pharmacology, Georgetown University Medical Center, Washington, D.C. 20007

Myron H. Weinberger, Department of Medicine, Indiana University School of Medicine, Indianapolis, Indiana 46223

Redford B. Williams, Department of Psychiatry, Duke University Medical Center, Durham, North Carolina 27710

Michael F. Wilson, ACOS for Research, Veterans Administration Medical Center and University of Oklahoma Health Sciences Center, Oklahoma City, Oklahoma 73104

Michael G. Ziegler, Department of Medicine, University of California, San Diego Medical Center, San Diego, California 92103

Preface

Cardiovascular disease continues to be the number one source of morbidity and mortality in our country. Despite a 35% reduction since 1964, these diseases, particularly coronary heart disease (CHD), claim nearly 1,000,000 lives each year in the United States (Havlik & Feinleib, 1979).

The Framingham study, among others, has identified three major risk factors implicated in the development of CHD: smoking, elevated serum cholesterol, and high blood pressure (Castelli *et al.*, 1986). Given that these factors account for less than 50% of the variance associated with CHD (Jenkins, 1976), it has become obvious that additional risk factors must be identified if further progress is to be made in disease prevention and control.

During the past twenty years, health researchers have given increased attention to behavioral, psychosocial, and environmental variables as potential contributors to the spectrum of risk factors. Initial studies focused on the *association* of various personality types, behavior patterns, and life events (stressors) with the prevalence of CHD, hypertension, and sudden cardiac death. Although these studies produced somewhat equivocal results, there appeared to be sufficient positive findings to warrant continued investigation. Yet investigators from the various disciplines engaged in independent research on these topics were somewhat stymied as to how best to proceed.

Approximately ten years ago, a small group of distinguished health scientists gathered to share their collective frustrations with the seeming inability of the biomedical and behavioral science communities to come to terms more effectively with the diversity of variables related to prevention and control of chronic diseases. From these and subsequent discussions, the concept of "behav-ioral medicine" was developed and shaped into the following definition:

> Behavioral medicine is the interdisciplinary field concerned with the development and integration of behavioral and biomedical science knowledge and techniques relevant to the understanding of health and illness and the application of this knowledge and these techniques to prevention, diagnosis, treatment and rehabilitation. (Schwartz & Weiss, 1978)

This concept of "biobehavioral" collaboration challenged scientists and clinicians of many disciplines to consider how they might more effectively develop diagnostic, treatment, and prevention strategies by merging their perspectives to address simultaneously, among others, behavioral, psychosocial, genetic, physiological, biochemical, and cellular factors, i.e., to attempt to address the problem at *all* levels at which it presented itself (Schwartz, 1981).

Three related principles guided their formulations:

1. Behavioral/psychological factors might have an *interactive* as well as an independent contribution to disease processes.
2. Demonstrating an association between behavior and disease state would not in itself be sufficient; one would also have to ultimately identify mechanisms of action to understand the causal relationships between behavioral and disease processes as well as to develop specific strategies of intervention and prevention.
3. Advances in noninvasive, nonintrusive bioinstrumentation have permitted simultaneous, continuous measurement of physiological and biochemical responses to psychological/environmental challenge. Such opportunities would

allow us to assess the *range* of such responses as well as "resting state" values.

With respect to cardiovascular behavioral medicine, the first principle extends the multifactorial perspective to include *interaction* among putative risk factors that may produce an effect in addition to, and perhaps qualitatively as well as quantitatively different from, the independent contribution of such factors. For example, although diet and psychosocial stressors are reputed to exert independent effects on the development of atherosclerosis, the combination of these factors produces a synergistic response that is greater than the additive contributions. Traditional research designs have preferred single-factor independent variables, but the complexity of biobehavioral studies requires factorial designs that also assess the unique properties associated with combining variables across different system levels (see, e.g., Schwartz, 1981). Thus, the interactive as well as the independent contributions of implicated risk factors must be understood before the "mosaic" of factors responsible for the development and progression of the cardiovascular diseases can be fully comprehended.

Another issue that needs to be understood is how biobehavioral variables influence susceptibility to (or protection from) disease (Smith, Galosy, & Weiss, 1981). Epidemiological and clinical investigations have effectively established associations between putative risk factors and disease occurrence and progression. Those studies addressing behavioral variables as potential contributors have also produced encouraging findings. Recent advances in bioinstrumentation now permit simultaneous and continuous measurements of behavioral, physiological, and biochemical processes, which provide the critical gateway to exploring mechanisms of action (Herd, Gotto, Kaufmann, & Weiss, 1984). Such studies provide the basis for understanding *how* behavioral factors, independently and in conjunction with other risk factors, influence the physiological and biochemical processes that, over time, render one susceptible to (or protected from) disease.

In cardiovascular behavioral medicine, the various regulatory processes and systems appear particularly responsive to neural input involving both central and peripheral influences. A better understanding of such mediating factors will permit increasingly sophisticated investigations of behavioral–neural–cardiovascular interactions. Again, one must include interaction with biological variables to capture the synergistic potential inherent in such multifactorial paradigms.

The third related principle addresses the ability of our newly developed biotechnology to assess *biobehavioral* interactions in response to behavioral/environmental challenge.

Until recently, the lack of such technology limited us to "resting state" measurements of the state of the organism. From such measurements, epidemiological studies established associations with *presumed* processes. Now we are gradually acquiring the capability to measure the processes directly in the presence of the behavioral or environmental perturbations that may influence these processes in health- or disease-enhancing directions (Matthews *et al.*, 1986).

Understanding the physiological/biochemical reactivity of the organism to acute laboratory stressors will provide a theoretical basis for extrapolation to a chronic system disregulation as a precursor contributor to disease. Noninvasive, nonintrusive ambulatory field monitoring will provide additional "snapshot" information that will further support the validity of such extrapolations. The continued development of sophisticated bioinstrumentation will provide the means to better understand the intricacies of biobehavioral interactions and their impact on health.

It is essential that our theoretical formulations keep pace with technological developments, lest we become too technology-driven, constantly compiling data in search of explanatory principles rather than systematically testing experimental hypotheses. It is also essential that our measurement strategies incorporate similar levels of sophistication and comparable procedures to establish a credible data base for these theoretical formulations.

Finally, the experimental design and statistical analyses performed should be appropriate to the complexity of the issues under investigation. In reviewing the "state of science" in cardiovascular behavioral medicine research, it became obvious that the multiplicity of standards of measurement, the inconsistency of types of measures taken across studies, and the variations in design and analysis made it extremely difficult to develop a cohesive picture of exactly what was known—and what was needed to advance the field. These variations also produced inconsistencies in results by investigators ostensibly concerned with the same phenomena, a circumstance that created credibility problems for this area of science as well as confusion among the investigators themselves.

In discussing these problems with respected scientists in the field, the idea of developing a handbook as a "gold standard" for measurement, design, and analysis strategies was conceived. On the one hand, such a resource would undoubtedly resolve many of the concerns noted above. On the other hand, how could individual authors, replete with their own biases and predilections, reflect the consensus of the field on the myriad topics to be covered in such a handbook? One could foresee editorial chaos in trying to ensure balanced expositions by having two or three reviewers for each chapter independently offering their assessments, opinions, and requested modifications. The prospect of multiplying this scenario by the 42 chapters of the handbook gave the senior editors serious pause. Into this context was born the idea of an "editorial conference," in which each chapter author, selected on the basis of prominence in the field, would be prepared to have his or her work simultaneously reviewed by five or six colleagues. The "peer review" concept, cornerstone of the NIH system of scientific merit review, was modified to provide direct written and oral feedback to each author from primary, secondary, and tertiary reviewers, followed by discussion chaired by the section editor. In this way, all contributions to this handbook received the benefit of both independent and consensus review during an intensive three-day meeting, cosponsored by the National Heart, Lung and Blood Institute and the University of Miami. Parenthetically, chapter authors felt the process was constructive as well as instructive, and provided them with information they would not have been likely to receive by the more traditional review process.

This handbook is divided into six sections, each of which covers a different methodological domain. In some instances, the material in a given chapter could also have been included in another section, in which case editorial considerations usually determined its final assignment.

Assessment of cardiovascular function, a major consideration in behavioral medicine and psychophysiological research, is covered in Section I. Many tests that formerly required invasive procedures can now be performed noninvasively, including complex hemodynamic measures. As cardiovascular performance often depends on effective functioning of other systems, this section also includes techniques for measuring renal and autonomic nervous system function that are likely to be of interest in studies of human subjects. In many instances, it is also important to understand the mechanisms that underlie changes in cardiovascular regulation, and whether these are due to changes on the input side, such as transmitters, hormones, or receptors, or on the output side, such as myocardial contractility. Section II of the handbook, therefore, deals with laboratory assays for electrolytes, catecholamines, the renin–angiotensin–aldosterone system, corticotropin-releasing factor, vasopressin, atrial natriuretic peptide, and other neuroactive peptides that may be relevant to behavioral research, particularly in relation to stress.

Most inferences drawn from laboratory experiments ultimately must be tested in a field setting. Obtaining reliable and valid measures from ambulatory subjects often requires procedures that are specifically adapted to situations in which far less control can be exerted over extraneous variables. Thus, Section III deals with measurement of a variety of parameters of cardiovascular function, including on-line electrocardiographic analysis, which enables one to relate specific life events to episodes of transient myocardial ischemia. For those concerned with urine and blood chemistry, this section also discusses special problems related to the drawing and preserving of specimens from ambulatory subjects.

Section IV deals with laboratory procedures and tasks that provoke cardiovascular reactions in the subject. Many of the procedures are especially valuable in studies of cardiovascular reactivity, for which numerous approaches have been devised by different investigators. The nature of these tasks differs along several dimensions, with important influences on the systems activated, the psychological effects on the subjects, and the social context in which they occur. All of these act against a background of individual differences, which are addressed in the chapters in Section V concerning psychometric assessment of the individual.

Finally, Section VI deals with research design and statistical analysis. Obviously, this section is not intended to be a comprehensive treatise on the subject, but it does provide, for example, an introduction to power calculations, considerations for the design and execution of clinical trials, and metaanalysis, subjects not usually addressed in one source.

Many of the methodologies covered in this volume make use of recent technological advances which in turn open the way for new research opportunities. It is this feature of the handbook— combined with the breadth of material selected to cover the full range of research methodologies in cardiovascular behavioral medicine and written by experts in their fields—that may ultimately be of greatest interest to experienced investigators and graduate students alike.

NEIL SCHNEIDERMAN
STEPHEN M. WEISS
PETER G. KAUFMANN

References

Castelli, W. P., Garrison, R. J., Wilson, P. W. F., Abbott, R. D., Kalousdian, S., & Kannel, W. B. (1986). Incidence of coronary heart disease and lipoprotein cholesterol levels: The Framingham Study. *Journal of the American Medical Association, 256,* 2835–2838.

Havlik, R., & Feinleib, M. (Eds.). (1979). Proceedings of the conference on the decline in coronary heart disease mortality. NIH Publ. No. 1 79-1610.

Herd, A. J., Gotto, A. M., Kaufmann, P. G., & Weiss, S. M. (Eds.). (1984). Cardiovascular Instrumentation. Proceedings of the Working Conference on Applicability of New Technology to Biobehavioral Research. NIH Publ. No. 84-1654.

Jenkins, C. D. (1976). Recent evidence supporting psychologic and social risk factors for coronary disease. *New England Journal of Medicine, 294,* 987–94, 1033–38.

Matthews, K., Weiss, S. M., Detre, T., Manuck, S., Falkner, D., Dembroski, T., & Williams, R. (Eds.). (1986). *Handbook of stress reactivity and cardiovascular disease.* New York: Wiley.

Schwartz, G. E. (1981). A systems analysis of psychobiology and behavior therapy: Implications for behavioral medicine. *Psychotherapy and Psychosomatics, 36,* 159–184.

Schwartz, G. E., & Weiss, S. M. (1978). Behavioral medicine revisited: An amended definition. *Journal of Behavioral Medicine, 1,* 249–251.

Smith, O. A., Galosy, R. A., & Weiss, S. M. (Eds.). (1981). *Circulation, neurobiology and behavior.* New York: Academic Press.

Contents

Cardiovascular Measurement in Behavioral Medicine Research

Section Editor: William R. Lovallo

The purpose of this unit of the handbook is to describe a variety of techniques for measuring cardiovascular, renal, and autonomic nervous system functions likely to be sampled in studies of human subjects participating in behavioral medicine and psychophysiological research.

The organization and content of these chapters is based on two guiding principles. The first is that the study of a given physiological function vis-à-vis ongoing behaviors, emotional states, or personality traits must proceed from an understanding of the complex biological context surrounding that function. Many studies in the field attempt to relate a physiological parameter to a behavioral or emotional concomitant, and thus a strong temptation exists to view the physiological data as a simple expression of the ongoing emotional or behavioral process. This approach may lead the investigator to lose sight of the fact that the heart rate, as one example, reflects the primary cardiac function of maintaining blood supply to the body. In view of this fact, the extent to which heart rate may reflect behavioral or emotional states is limited by necessity.

William R. Lovallo • Behavioral Sciences Laboratories, Veterans Administration Medical Center and University of Oklahoma Health Sciences Center, Oklahoma City, Oklahoma 73104.

The second consideration in interpreting data presumed to reflect the behavioral–physiological interplay is to be aware of the degree to which a physiological function is itself controlled or controlling and how directly it may be capable of paralleling ongoing behavior processes. For example, blood pressure is often used to estimate the physiological response to a variety of behavioral manipulations. An increase in pressure is usually viewed as reflecting a state of stress or increased arousal, although it is in fact an outcome of the operation of at least two controlling parameters, cardiac output and systemic vascular resistance, which in turn are each influenced by multiple factors. A given level of, or change in, blood pressure may thus mean different things at different times and is not subject to a unitary mechanistic interpretation. Along the same lines, systolic and diastolic pressures are often viewed as equivalent reflections of stress-related arousal such that increases in both pressures are expected as arousal level increases. In fact, they are each influenced differently during responses to challenge. For example, increased β-adrenergically mediated activity may increase systolic pressure due to increased cardiac activity while simultaneously producing a slight drop or an attenuated increase in diastolic pressure, reflecting vasodilation due to the influence of β receptors in the arteries of the skeletal muscles.

These considerations alert us to beware of construing simple physiological ''indices'' as reflecting behavioral or emotional states, and they alert us to be cautious in interpreting different physiological parameters as though they were equivalent reflections of such states. They alert us to be wary of interpreting change in a given direction to reflect a state of ''activation'' or ''stress.'' These points have been raised effectively by Obrist (1981, pp. 1–7).

This section of the handbook is therefore intended to present a biologically based orientation to problems of measurement in behavioral studies of cardiovascular function. The choice of what physiological response to measure and the interpretation of changes in activity should proceed from an appreciation of the multiple determinants of that function and of its role in the system.

A further set of considerations may be useful in comparing and choosing among alternative methods. Experience indicates that behaviorally focused research is best conducted using minimally obtrusive techniques. The question then arises, which measurement method is best? The following factors should be considered: safety, degree of intrusiveness on the behavioral situation, cost, repeatability, and duration of recording. For many methods of measurement, the most accurate, ''gold standard'' method comes up short on most of these points, particularly if the method is highly invasive.

Two major issues then apply in the final choice of any technique. The first issue is the extent to which the method directly measures a known physical quantity reflecting a physiological function, and second, how accurately it does so. Most methods, however invasive, rely on a model relating the physiological function in question to the output of the measuring system by means of a more or less well-known physical relationship. Some methods have well-known relationships based on physical principles. Measurement of blood pressure via a mercury manometer is one example in which the height of the mercury column in relation to the Korotkoff sounds directly reflects pressure within the artery, and hence has a one-to-one-relationship with the underlying blood pressure. Most methods employ less well-known or more imprecise models. For example, photoplethysmographic estimations of pulsatile skin blood flow rely on applying some numerical interpretation to an analogue wave form using a model having certain assumptions about the physical, and hence, physiological causes of the changes in light level reaching the sensor. The presumed relationship between the wave form and the original physiological process is the basis of our interpretation of the meaning of the wave form. Obviously, the stronger the model and the better known the physical relationship, the stronger is the inference about the underlying function.

The second issue concerns the accuracy of the method. In fact, two questions arise here. How well does the mean of a set of measurements target the underlying process being measured (validity)? Second, how well do successive measurement attempts approximate each other (reliability)? A method with a known, consistent direction and degree of deviation may be preferred over one that is more accurate in the long run but that has a wider dispersion and hence is less reliable. Accuracy and reliability must therefore be considered in the context of the researcher's goals.

Bearing these considerations in mind and with the philosophical orientation expressed above, we proceed with our discussion of specific measurement techniques. In order to reinforce the importance of placing each candidate dependent variable in its systemic context, this section of the handbook opens in Chapter 1 with a concise review of the cardiovascular system by Dr. Robert Rushmer, who addresses the higher-order integrative controls to which this system is subject as well as the renal system with which it interacts. Following this introduction, Wilson, Lovallo, and Pincomb in Chapter 2 review a variety of current methods for measuring the activity of the heart, including its electrical activity, structural and functional characteristics, contractile state, and volume output. This review should introduce a variety of possible methods suitable to different purposes. Chapter 3 by Saini and Verrier presents a detailed review of methods to assess normal and abnormal electrical conduction of the myocardium during behavioral manipulations. This very informative approach to studying behavioral–cardiovascular interactions should find wider application as the methodology becomes better understood and the technology becomes more readily available.

The next two chapters deal with measuring the activity of the vascular tree. In Chapter 4, Pickering and Blank provide a focused review of blood pressure measurement techniques, their relative strengths and weaknesses, and special problems of measurement in elderly and obese adults. Chapter 5 by Anderson discusses Doppler and plethysmographic techniques to determine arterial flow and techniques to measure venous tone.

The final three chapters in this section present methodologies for measuring functions which are noncardiovascular but which interact importantly with that sytem. In Chapter 6, Dunlap and Pfeifer discuss techniques for inferring the degree and type of activity of the cardiovascular portion of the autonomic nervous system. Chapter 7 by Anderson and Mark deals with the related issue of measuring sympathetic nervous influence on the blood vessels of the muscles and skin using the direct recording technique of microneurography. This technique could well find useful applications in studies designed to assess changes in skeletal muscle activity related to preparation for motor activity, induction of the defense reaction, fear, or anger, among others. Finally, in Chapter 8, Falkner discusses measurement of fluid volume regulation by the renal system. It is included here because no consideration of cardiovascular function can be considered complete without a recognition of the importance of fluid volume. While the cardiovascular system is responsible for flow and distribution of blood, the renal system plays the intimately related role of regulating the volume of blood available to the heart and blood vessels. Measurement of renal function will play an increasingly significant role in evaluation of behavioral–physiological interactions in studies of precursors of hypertension or other states in which volume regulation interacts with cardiovascular function.

The chapters in this section should be viewed as brief presentations of specialized measurement techniques. They are intended as introductions only, and the researcher wishing to apply any one of them should examine the references related to that particular method. Finally, many methods require considerable skill in their technical application, and their use in research is advisable only after a period of hands-on training with an already-skilled practitioner.

Reference

Obrist, P. (1981). *Cardiovascular psychophysiology: A perspective*. New York: Plenum Press.

CHAPTER 1

Structure and Function of the Cardiovascular System

Robert F. Rushmer

Introduction

Growing interest in behavioral medicine has focused attention on the function and control of the cardiovascular system, partly because of its involuntary responsiveness to emotional and stressful situations. The external manifestations of cardiovascular responses provide objective indications of the changing psychological status of normal subjects and patients. An expanding array of noninvasive techniques open opportunities for new and exciting research regarding the potential roles of psychological and behavioral factors in the development of dysfunction and disease. Current concepts of cardiovascular psychophysiology have been presented in a comprehensive overview edited by Obrist (1981).

The cardiovascular system must be capable of adapting rapidly and effectively to changing requirements to enable the relatively small blood volume to serve the vital needs of the millions of cells in the various organs of the human body.

Living cells survive, function, and thrive only in stable chemical and physical environments from which they can easily extract the essential nutrients and oxygen while eliminating toxic waste products

Robert F. Rushmer • Center for Bioengineering, University of Washington, Seattle, Washington 98105.

derived from their metabolic activities. Primitive, single-celled organisms originated in the oceans where they were surrounded by large volumes of fluid with relatively stable composition and temperature. Their essential nutrients derived from these fluids by a process of diffusion resulting from the universal tendency for substances dissolved or suspended in a liquid to move from regions of higher concentration to regions of lower concentration. Each specific substance moves at a rate determined by its concentration gradient, i.e., the difference in concentration over a specified distance. Metabolic activity depletes the intracellular concentration of nutrient materials and oxygen which are replaced by diffusion from outside the cell at rates dependent on the concentration gradient for each. Similarly, waste products accumulate within the cell and diffuse outward through the cell membrane into the surrounding fluid and beyond. Obviously, increased metabolic activity produces faster utilization of nutrients, steeper concentration gradients, and accelerated diffusion into and out of the cells.

The movement of molecules by simple diffusion (without mixing) occurs extremely slowly along shallow concentration gradients (e.g., over long distances). For example, a cylinder of tissue cells 1 cm in diameter, suddenly exposed to 100% oxygen, would become 90% saturated with oxygen in about 2 h. In contrast, a single cell only 7 μm in diameter would be 90% saturated in about 0.0054 s. For this reason, organisms consisting of large cell masses have developed various intricate mechanisms for maintaining relatively constant the film of fluid immediately surrounding each cell. Some simple organisms move through the fluid, others pump fluid in and out of hollow interiors. In large and complex organisms with specialized tissues and organs having widely varying levels of activity, highly adaptable circulatory systems have developed expressly for the purpose of conveying a specialized fluid (i.e., blood) into the immediate vicinity of each cell in the body. The layer of fluid just outside each cell represents a small sample of a tropical ocean continuously maintained at nearly constant composition by flow of arterial blood into networks of capillaries widely distributed in immediate proximity to all the body cells. The capillaries are only about 0.017 mm in diameter and bring circulating blood to within about 0.1 mm from most cells. Their combined length would amount to 60,000 miles. The capillary networks present an enormous surface area to the tissues so that only about 5 liters of blood can serve the body of a 170-kg person.

The many different functions of tissues require different and widely varying blood flow rates under various conditions. An extreme example is the transition from rest to vigorous exercise during which the blood flow through large muscle masses increases many fold in response to their greatly increased metabolic activity and energy release. At the same time, blood flow to the skin is increased to dissipate heat. Despite curtailed blood flow through inactive tissues, the total blood flow through the systemic circulation is increased and the pumping action of the heart is both accelerated and enhanced instantaneously or even in anticipation of exertion. Diverse, integrated patterns of response occur automatically under many different circumstances induced by neural and hormonal controls.

These involuntary control systems respond to various emotional or psychological stresses by cardiovascular responses such as blushing, pallor, rapid pulse, fainting, or "palpitations" of the heart. More subtle, reliable, and reproducible indicators of psychophysiological status can be derived by objective physical and chemical measurements of appropriate cardiovascular variables. Recent technical advances provide new and exciting opportunities to monitor performance of the heart, changes in blood pressure, variations of blood flowing through easily accessible tissues, alterations in blood volume, and changing concentrations of many crucial chemical constituents of blood and body fluids. This book is designed to present a broad spectrum of modern methods available to explore human psychobiology.

General Characteristics of the Cardiovascular System

The function and control of the human circulatory system are so complex that they defy comprehension. The fundamental functions of its component parts can be more readily visualized in terms of a simple, basic hydraulic model as illustrated in Figure 1. A common configuration is driven by a piston pump, powered by an external source of energy. The pumping chamber fills from an adjacent reservoir as the piston withdraws during the filling phase. At the end of the filling phase, the inlet valves close and fluid is propelled through opened outlet valves into a rigid pipe. An adjacent chamber contains air which is compressed by the rising pressure and cushions the violent impulse that would otherwise occur during the ejection phase. The compressed air also serves to store energy, sustaining the driving pressure while the pumping cylinder is refilling. If the repetition rate of the pump is set so that each successive ejection occurs while the pressure in the outflow channels is still falling, a pulsatory inflow is converted in a fluctuating but continuous outflow through the exchanger.

Control valves are situated at the entrance of each of the many parallel channels. These valves can be adjusted to manipulate the distribution of flow through alternate channels in the exchanger. The resistance offered by these valves determines

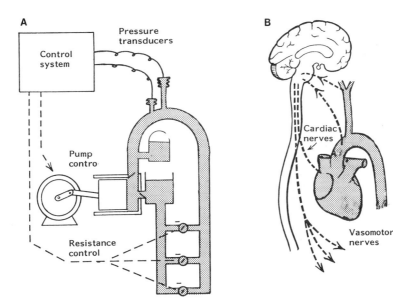

Figure 1. (A) Cardiovascular function and control are illustrated by a simple hydraulic model. A pulsatile pump propels fluid through a distribution system with a high driving pressure maintained by a feedback control system with input from pressure sensors and output to both the pump and the valves controlling outflow. (B) The human circulatory system has corresponding features and similar functions. From Rushmer (1976); reprinted by permission of Saunders.

the rate of outflow through the various parallel channels. If some of the control valves are opened wider so that the total resistance is lowered, the pumping rate must be correspondingly increased to avoid a drop in the driving pressure. The balance between the inflow and outflow of the high-pressure distribution system is maintained so long as the mean driving pressure remains constant. A control system for maintaining the driving pressure within a narrow range is illustrated in Figure 1. Pressure sensors transmit signals to a ''black box'' control system that automatically regulates the output of the pump (cycle rate) and at the same time adjusts the outflow valves to maintain a constant average driving pressure in the system.

Corresponding components can be identified in the human cardiovascular system. The left ventricle serves as the pump, forcibly ejecting blood into the aortic arch having walls rich in elastic fibers. The elastic expansion of the aortic wall serves to dampen violent pressure surges as does the compression chamber in the mechanical model.

Pressure sensors (baroreceptors) in the walls of the aorta and the carotid artery transmit impulses to the central nervous system at frequencies related to the fluctuating arterial pressure. The signals are processed within the nervous system and deliver efferent impulses along the autonomic nerves (vagus and sympathetic) distributed to heart and peripheral circulation. The hormones released at their nerve terminals influence heart rate, the vigor of cardiac contraction, and adjust the resistance to flow through terminal arterioles and precapillary sphincters in the myriad microcirculatory beds in all parts of the body. The actions of these neural control mechanisms are supplemented by circulating hormones acting generally throughout the system. In addition, local controls of blood flow through capillary networks are manifest by accumulating metabolic products in active tissues, which produce vasodilation by relaxing tension in the smooth muscle cuffs in arterioles and precapillary sphincters.

This greatly simplified portrayal of the human cardiovascular system provides some insight into the basic mechanisms by which it serves a vital role in supplying the widely varying demands of the many tissues and organs of the human organism. The driving pressure required to preserve the function of the brain is assured by reflexly curtailing flow through nonessential organs when the total demands of the body exceed the capacity of the heart to increase its output.

The complex mechanisms maintaining systemic arterial pressure and adjusting the distribution of blood flow to the widely varying demands of the tissues and organs are only one of many different control systems. Obvious examples are the integrated responses to changes in posture, exercise, or environmental temperature. Not so obvious are the multitude of control mechanisms which maintain the chemical composition and physical characteristics of the blood and body fluids. For example, the total quantity of body fluids is maintained within remarkably narrow limits despite wide variations in the intake of fluids and foods and continually changing outputs of liquids through many different channels, including bowels, bladder, lungs, and skin. Even more remarkable is the fact that the chemical and cellular composition of the blood is maintained within narrow limits despite the continually changing input–output relationships of dissolved gases, electrolytes, small organic molecules, proteins, hormones, blood cells, and the many products of metabolism.

The various constituents of the blood and body fluids must be independently regulated since their sources and ultimate fates are all different. During the past half-century, our understanding of control mechanisms has been expanding at a prodigious rate with respect to the several organs (i.e., lungs, liver, gastrointestinal tract, kidneys) involved in maintaining the appropriate input–output relations of the various chemical and cellular species. However, great gaps persist regarding the integration and control of these processes by neural and hormonal mechanisms. The emerging discipline of behavioral medicine is envisioned as a means of addressing some of the overriding influences of the higher levels of the nervous system on organ functions in health and disease. These considerations extend to the significance and clinical relevance of health habits, life-styles, environmental stresses,

and social pressures as they affect the health and well-being of people in today's world.

Technical Specifications for the Cardiovascular System

The intricacy and complexity of the human cardiovascular system is brought into sharp perspective by listing some of the essential features that would be contained in engineering specifications for developing an artificial counterpart. The human cardiovascular system must conform to the following essential features, among many others:

1. The circulatory system must develop and maintain remarkably constant the chemical and cellular composition of arterial blood within very narrow ranges by replacing oxygen, electrolytes, small organic molecules, proteins, hormones, and cells as they are utilized or eliminated.
2. This specialized fluid must be delivered from a single source to the immediate vicinity of each of the millions of body cells through a successively branching system leading to millions of capillaries smaller than human hairs.
3. Appropriate pressure gradients must be maintained from arteries to veins through capillary networks at all levels from head to toe despite widely varying flow rates required to meet the changing requirements of various organs.
4. The volume flow of blood through each tissue must be regulated independently in accordance with its specific function and level of activity.
5. General and local control mechanisms must promptly respond to changing levels of activity in diverse organs while maintaining adequate perfusion of vital organs and supporting essential functions of the organism as a whole.
6. The capacity of the venous reservoir system must accommodate changes in blood volume

and its distribution during changes from supine and standing positions or from rest to exercise.

7. Neurohumoral control mechanisms must be capable of rapidly inducing appropriate patterns of circulatory adjustment to conditions such as exercise and changes in posture, environmental conditions, or psychological stresses.

Structure and Function of the Heart

The specifications listed above can be met only by components of a system endowed with most remarkable structural and functional characteristics. For example, the normal heart contracts around 70 times per minute, more than 30,000,000 times a year for 70 years or even more. It functions without interruption for maintenance or repair and rarely rests longer than a second or two at most. Its ignition system is represented by a specialized pacemaker under exquisitely precise neural control. If the pacemaker fails to function for a very few seconds, a new pacemaker site automatically takes over. Indeed, virtually any site in the heart muscle can assume the role of pacemaker or source of extra beats.

The normal heart ejects liquid more forcefully and reaches peak velocity faster than the best mechanical pump. In all respects, the most advanced of the available artificial hearts are crude, primitive, and inept substitutes for the normal human heart. Similarly, the arteries, capillary networks, venous system, and lungs all display functional characteristics that defy duplication in any manmade substitute.

The simultaneous contraction of the myocardial bundles in the walls of the two ventricles develops the pressures necessary to force the blood through the systemic and pulmonary circuits. The thin-walled right ventricle ejects blood into the low-pressure, low-resistance pulmonary circuit in the lungs. The powerful, thick-walled left ventricle impels blood under high pressure into the high-resistance systemic vascular tree that serves the remainder of the body. The walls of the two ventri-

cles are comprised of sheets and bundles of myocardial fibers complexly intertwined something like the windings of a turban. On the external or epicardial surface, the fibers generally spiral from the base toward the apex of the heart where they undergo an abrupt twist and continue to spiral back toward the base of the heart on the inner or endocardial surface. In the wall of the left ventricle, a thick cuff of muscle fibers encircles the chamber, interposed between the inner and outer spiral layers. It serves as the powerful constrictor of the cavity capable of ejecting blood into the aorta at very high peak velocities (see Figure 3).

Myocardial Mechanics

Experimental studies of myocardial samples have consistently demonstrated that their contractile tension develops rapidly and is well sustained if they are prevented from shortening, the so-called isometric contraction. In general, greater contractile tension is generated if the relaxed bundles of fibers are lengthened over their functional range before stimulating contraction. When myocardial bundles contract to move a load, their maximum rate of shortening occurs immediately after the onset and contractile tension falls off rapidly as shortening proceeds (Sonnenblick, 1962). These properties of isolated strips of myocardium are clearly represented in the characteristics of left ventricular ejection.

The left ventricular configuration and the properties of its myocardial bundles are well suited to the task of forcefully propelling blood against the high pressures in the aorta. In contrast, the right ventricular chamber is roughly crescent shaped in cross section, enclosed between the relatively thin free wall and the thick interventricular septum. Its internal surface area is large because its shape resembles a pocket. It functions like a bellows and is capable of propelling large volumes through the low-resistance vasculature of the lungs with pressures about one-fifth of the systemic circulation (Rushmer, 1976). The atria and their adjacent large central veins serve as immediately accessible reservoirs of blood for rapid filling of the ventricular chambers during each diastolic interval.

Each ventricle is equipped with inlet and outlet valves so strong and flexible that they close and seal against high pressures without backward leak. The roots of these valves are attached to fibrous rings that insulate the ventricles from the corresponding atrial chambers during their excitation.

Excitation of the Heart

The functional properties of the heart are dependent on the unique characteristics of heart muscle (myocardium). Myocardial cells are striated and have contractile mechanisms like those of skeletal muscles. However, myocardial cells are not activated by nerves but instead are excited by the spread of excitation from one cell to its contiguous neighbors. Myocardial cells are cylindrical in shape with branchings joined end-to-end to produce a dense meshwork. This syncytial arrangement of branching fibers provides uninterrupted pathways from any site in the atria or in the ventricles to all other contiguous parts of the same chamber.

The excitability of myocardial fibers is dependent on the existence of electrical potentials across the cell membranes. In common with all living cells, the concentrations of electrolytes (particularly sodium and potassium) are distinctly different inside the cell membrane as opposed to those in the extracellular fluid (see Figure 6). This separation of ions functions like a battery and produces an electrical potential of about −90 mV. If this membrane potential is reduced below a specific threshold level, the membrane permeability to ions abruptly changes and the membrane potential rises rapidly, briefly overshooting the zero potential level (Figure 2A). Following the peak, the membrane potential exhibits a plateau and then rapidly returns to the stable polarized resting condition. The myocardial fibers contract during the plateau while the membranes remains depolarized. When the membrane potential returns to the stable resting level, the myocardial fibers relax.

Sinoatrial Node: The Pacemaker of the Heart

A club-shaped collection of specialized myocardial cells, called the sinoatrial (S-A) node, is located in the wall of the right atrium near the point of entrance of the systemic veins (Figure 2D). These spindle-shaped cells normally serve as the "pacemaker" of the heart, originating successive

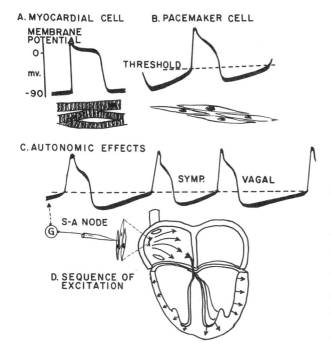

Figure 2. (A) Myocardial cells are excited to contract during a prolonged action potential that spreads to adjacent cells of the branching syncytial network. (B) In pacemaker cells, the resting membrane potential spontaneously rises to reach threshold and activates an action potential that invades contiguous myocardial fibers. (C) Autonomic nerves influence heart rate by modifying the slope of the resting membrane potential. (D) Waves of excitation originating at the S-A node spread throughout the atrial walls and through special conducting bundles to activate the right and left ventricles.

waves of excitation which rapidly envelop the walls of the right and left atria and then invade the two ventricles. In contrast to the stable resting potential of the typical myocardial cells, the specialized cells in the S-A node exhibit a spontaneous rise in membrane potential toward the threshold level and initiate the next wave of excitation (Figure 2B). The structure, function, and control of the sinus node are presented in great detail in a book devoted to this single subject (Bonke, 1978).

Autonomic Regulation of Heart Rate

The interval between successive heart beats is determined normally by the rate at which the membrane potential of an S-A nodal cell rises to cross the threshold level. The rate at which the membrane potential of these cells moves toward threshold is influenced by the action of sympathetic and parasympathetic (vagus) nerve endings, concentrated in or near the S-A node (Figure 2C). Acetylcholine discharged by vagus nerve endings decreases the rate of rise of the membrane potential, increases the interval between beats, and slows the heart rate. Conversely, sympathetic nerve discharges cause the S-A nodal membrane potentials to rise more steeply toward the threshold and quicken the heart rate. This reciprocal innervation of the heart by the autonomic nerves provides rapid responses of the heart rate, often within the interval of a single cardiac cycle. Sympathetic stimulation which accelerates the heart rate also enhances the functional performance of myocardium as discussed below and in subsequent sections.

Because the cells of the heart are arranged in a branching syncytium, a wave of excitation in one cell will spread to all adjacent fibers, rapidly invading the walls of both atria. The wave of excitation spreads so rapidly that all the myocardial cells in both atrial chamber walls contract almost simultaneously (Figure 2).

Excitation of the Ventricles

Fibrous rings connect the atria with the ventricles and block the spread of excitation into the ventricles except by way of a specialized bundle of conducting tissue. At the upper end is the atrioventricular (A-V) node, which is located in the partition between the two atria and serves as a kind of one-way gateway to the ventricles. A common bundle of rapidly conducting fibers passes across the connective tissue barrier and into the interventricular septum at velocities of about 1 m/s (Figure 2D). This common bundle divides into two main bundle branches that are distributed over the endocardial surfaces of the two ventricles. Terminal branches extend into the wall of the ventricles, particularly in the thick-walled left ventricle. The spread of excitation along the rapidly conducting fibers activates the full thickness of the two ventricular chambers and induces coordinated contraction of these main pumping chambers.

Sequence of Events during Typical Cardiac Cycles

The importance of this normal pattern of contractions is illustrated by the fact that abnormal sequences of excitation produce contractions that are neither as forceful nor as complete as normal beats (see also Chapter 3).

The pattern of excitation described above proscribes an optimal time sequence for the cardiac cycle. During the diastolic interval, blood gushes into each ventricle from the corresponding atrium and the large central veins during early diastole. At normal or slow heart rates, the latter part of diastolic filling slows or plateaus. Atrial contraction propels an additional increment of blood into the ventricle, producing eddy currents that help to bring the open inlet valves into apposition. Synchronous excitation of the ventricular walls produces almost simultaneous contraction of the two ventricles with both inlet and outlet valves closed. Although no blood is ejected at this time, the long axis of the left ventricle shortens and its powerful cuff of muscle is stretched just before it begins to contract. Contractile tension in the left ventricular myocardium abruptly elevates the intraventricular pressure to reach and exceed the pressure at the root of the aorta. The brief interval during which all four cardiac valves are closed is commonly called the isometric contraction because the myocardial fibers develop tension but do not eject blood from the chambers until the aortic and pulmonary valves open. The maximum tension development and the most rapid ejection of blood occur immediately after the onset of ventricular contraction producing an initial impulse of great power particularly in the left ventricle.

Initial Ventricular Impulse

The power cuff of the left ventricle is excited to contract just as its myocardium is stretched. During the phase of isometric contraction, left ventricular pressure rises extremely steeply until it exceeds the pressure in the aorta and the aortic valve opens (Figure 3). The sudden overshoot of ventricular pressure over aortic pressure represents a steep pressure gradient providing a powerful impulse to the ejection velocity. During this initial impulse, ejection velocity rises precipitously to a sharp peak in early systole (Rushmer, 1964, 1976). This steep upward slope in ejection velocity denotes rapid rate of change of velocity or acceleration (dV/dt) of the blood. Thus, the forceful ventricular ejection accelerates the blood flow into the elastic aortic root at rates of 3000 cm/s per s to rapidly reach peak velocities of some 200 cm/s during the initial phase of systolic contraction (Spencer and Greiss, 1962; Noble, Trenchard, & Guz, 1966).

After reaching its peak, the outflow velocity rapidly declines. In other words, the velocity of blood flow in the aorta rapidly diminishes because the myocardial contractile tension falls off and the blood is carried forward by its own momentum. This sequence of events indicates that the initial impulse of ventricular contraction more closely resembles striking a piston with a mallet than a sustained milking action or clenching of a fist.

It is common experience that the heart pounds with excitement or fear. Indeed, the impulse of each heart beat shakes the entire body as can be directly observed by standing on a sensitive scale and noting the oscillations synchronous with each heart beat. The displacement of the body in synchrony with the heart beat was the basis for the development of a device designed to record the recoil of the body from the acceleration induced by the contracting ventricles (e.g., the ballistocardiograph).

Factors Affecting Output of the Heart

The output of the heart per minute (cardiac output) is determined by the heart rate (the number of beats per minute) and the stroke volume (the quantity of blood ejected during ventricular contractions). The stroke volume represents the difference between the ventricular volume at the end of the filling period (end-diastolic volume) and the volume of blood remaining in the ventricular chamber at the end of its contraction (end-systolic volume).

All of these ventricular volumes are subject to change under various circumstances. For example, the end-diastolic volume depends on the filling pressure (central venous pressure) and the distensibility of the ventricular walls plus the increment added by atrial contraction. The ejection fraction is the proportion of the end-diastolic volume ejected during ventricular contractions. The end-systolic volume (and the ejection fraction) are greatly influenced by a wide variety of factors, including the length of the myocardial fibers (diastolic volume), the tension developed and sustained in the contracting myocardial walls, the rate of myocardial

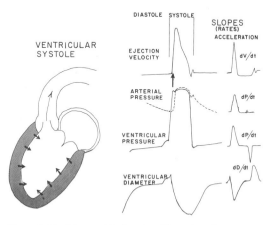

Figure 3. The left ventricle functions like an impulse generator, characterized by a precipitous rise in ventricular pressure which overshoots the aortic pressure and rapidly accelerates outflow to a peak velocity in early systole. Performance of the ventricle is best expressed by the rate of change of velocity (acceleration, dV/dt), rate of change of pressure (dP/dt), or rate of change of diameter (dD/dt).

shortening, and the impedance to ejection offered by the pressure in the arterial channels.

As all of these factors are subject to change under various conditions, efforts at describing and measuring the overall performance of the heart have proved to be extremely complicated and confusing. For example, changes in the functioning of the heart during exercise, stimulation of sympathetic nerves, or injection of catecholamines (e.g., epinephrine) produce many and varied effects on the pressures, dimensions, and flow rates in and near the ventricular chambers. It is obvious that the ventricles beat more forcefully or more vigorously under these conditions but appropriate criteria for these changes in function have remained controversial.

The Concept of Contractility

The term *contractility* is generally employed to cover the changes in ventricular performance that cannot be attributed to length of the myocardial fibers as influenced by diastolic filling pressure (preload) or by impedance to ejection imposed by the arterial pressure (afterload). A variety of criteria have been proposed as indicators of contractility, including rate of rise of ventricular or arterial pressure (dP/dt), ejection fraction, maximal velocity of myocardial shortening (V_{max}), peak flow

velocities, and acceleration at the root of the aorta among many others. Direct recordings of the relevent dimensions, pressures, flow rates, and derived variables have demonstrated that sympathetic stimulation of the heart produces profound effects on many different aspects of ventricular function.

Autonomic Influences on Cardiac Contraction

The effects of sympathetic stimulation on ventricular performance are illustrated in Figure 4. They include faster heart rate, shorter systolic and diastolic intervals, higher peak ventricular pressures, and steeper upslope and downslope (dP/dt) along with more forceful ejection with greater acceleration to higher peak outflow velocities, earlier deceleration, shorter ejection period, with little or no increase in stroke volume. The ventricular dimensions often display a smaller diastolic volume, more complete systolic ejection, and larger ejection fraction. Conversely, stimulation of vagus nerves to the heart is now believed to have a depressive effect on the heart rate and on ventricular performance (see Levy and Martin, 1984).

There is growing conviction that such dynamic indicators of cardiac performance as those in Figure 4 are valuable additions to more traditional measures such as stroke volume, cardiac output, and systemic arterial pressure (Lambert, Nichols,

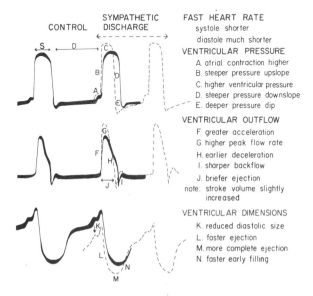

Figure 4. Sympathetic stimulation induces profound effects on left ventricular pressures, outflow, and dimensions, characterized by steeper slopes or rates of change of flow, velocity, pressure, or diameter as well as shorter systolic intervals and smaller diastolic and systolic dimensions. These dynamic changes in ventricular function are all implicit in the expression "increased contractility." From Rushmer (1976); reprinted by permission of Saunders.

& Pepine, 1983; Levy, Targett, Bardou, & McIlroy, 1985).

Dynamic Indicators of Ventricular Performance

The outflow acceleration, peak flow velocity,
rate of change of pressures (dP/dt), or rate of
change of ventricular dimensions (i.e., dD/dt) are
greatly exaggerated by sympathetic nerve stimulation and circulating catecholamines (Rushmer,
1976). Since the left ventricle normally functions
as an impulse generator, its performance is more
accurately represented by the dynamic properties
listed in Figure 3 than by the systolic pressure,
stroke volume or cardiac output.

Comprehensive analysis of cardiac function employing continuously recording sensors in intact
animals has helped to specify the kinds of measurements which would be most useful in monitoring changing ventricular performance in human
subjects and patients (see Chapter 2, this volume).
Newly developed ultrasonic flow sensing devices
can detect outflow velocity and acceleration in humans by placing a transducer at the sternal notch
(Huntsman *et al.*, 1983; Bennett, Barclay, Davis,
Mannering, & Mehta, 1984). The noninvasive
monitoring of this key aspect of ventricular performance is becoming widespread in its acceptance
and application to clinical research and management.

The Arterial Distribution System

The arterial tree serves both as a highly branched
distribution system and as a pressure reservoir to
maintain during diastole the driving pressure required to propel blood through the multitude of
microcirculatory beds and back to the heart through
the venous system. For this purpose, arterial perfusion pressure normally fluctuates between 120 and
80 mm Hg at heart level.

The level of systematic arterial pressure is ultimately determined by the balance between the cardiac output and the total peripheral resistance to
outflow through the terminal arterioles, precapillary sphincters, and capillary networks. An uncom-

pensated reduction in either the output from the
heart or the total peripheral resistance necessarily
results in a fall in blood pressure.

Arterial blood pressure may be elevated either
acutely or chronically but is reflexly prevented
from falling below some critical level of about
60/40 mm Hg lest perfusion of the brain be insufficient to sustain consciousness or the functional
integrity of vital organs be jeopardized.

The periodic contraction of the ventricles produces widely fluctuating pressure pulses in the arterial system which are partially dampened by the
resilience of the arterial walls. During the diastolic
period while the relaxed ventricles are filling,
blood flows out of the arterial system through the
terminal arterioles and myriad microcirculatory
beds.

Arterial Pressure Pulses

The vigorous contraction of the left ventricle
abruptly impels a bolus of blood through the aortic
valve, precipitously elevating the arterial pressure
in the aortic arch. The inertia of the long columns
of blood in the arteries prevents instantaneous acceleration along their length. Instead, the stroke
volume initially piles up in the elastic arch of the
aorta, increasing the tension in the walls. This localized increase in tension propels blood forward
into the next section which in turn is stretched. By
this mechanism, a pulse of pressure (and flow)
travels rapidly along the aorta to the peripheral
arterial channels at about 1 m/s.

Distortion of the Arterial Pulse Wave

The leading edge of this arterial pulse wave is
reflected backward from branch points while the
main body of the pulse wave is still advancing. For
this reason, the arterial pulse wave in peripheral
arteries ascends more rapidly to a higher peak than
at the root of the aorta. This distortion of the arterial pressure pulse is reminiscent of the peaking
of an advancing oceanic wave as it encounters a
wave reflected from a breakwater. The two waves
summate to produce steeper slopes to higher peak
values.

Factors Affecting the Arterial Pulse Pressure

When the peak systolic pressure is 120 mm Hg and the diastolic pressure is 80 mm Hg, the different between the two is 40 mm Hg and is called the pulse pressure. The peak arterial or systolic pressure is elevated by numerous factors including larger stroke volumes, more rapid ejection, or reduced arterial elasticity. The diastolic pressure is influenced by the stroke volume or heart rate (diastolic interval) but reflects most notably the changes in the total peripheral vascular resistance as it is influenced by the vasomotor control of sphincters leading to microcirculations in the various tissues and organs of the body. The regulation of blood flow through the microcirculations in tissues with widely varying requirements is vested in diverse local mechanisms that adapt the caliber of terminal resistance vessels to the level of activity of the individual tissue or organ (see Granger, Borders, Meininger, Goodman, & Barnes, 1983).

When several different organs are active simultaneously, the reduction in peripheral resistance could precipitate a fall in the arterial perfusion pressure unless there is a concomitant increase in the output of the heart and/or an overriding vasoconstriction in active or nonessential tissues. For this purpose, generalized neurohumoral controls act to maintain the systemic arterial pressure and the blood flow through vital organs (i.e., brain and heart) which otherwise could sustain permanent damage by lowered arterial blood pressure and inadequate perfusion.

Peripheral Vascular Control Mechanisms

The quantity of blood flowing through vascular beds within the different tissues of the body depends on the pressure gradient from arteries to veins and on the caliber of the sites of controlled resistance at the terminal arterioles and precapillary sphincters. The metabolic requirements of the various tissues are extremely diverse and variable. For example, the metabolism of the brain is remarkably constant and the cerebral vascular bed is remarkably insensitive to any vasomotor influences (with the possible exception of carbon dioxide). In contrast, blood flow to skeletal muscle or skin is strongly influenced by neural, hormonal, and chemical influences.

Local Vascular Control Mechanisms

Tissues with widely varying levels of metabolic activity generally exhibit a diversity of local control mechanisms which automatically sustain the blood flow in the face of changes in perfusion pressure or adjust the blood flow to the functional requirements of the local tissue cells. As examples, skeletal muscle, myocardium, and skin exhibit profound vasodilation after release of temporary restriction or interruption of blood flow for a few minutes. This response, commonly called "reactive hyperemia," is an example of an intrinsic, automatic regulatory mechanism modulating blood flow in accordance with changing metabolic requirements of specialized tissues.

Blood flow in skeletal muscle at rest is rather modest (e.g., 5 ml/min per 100 g of tissue) but may increase 10- to 15-fold with intense physical exercise primarily through action of chemical vasodilators from increased metabolic activity (Figure 5). Potential mechanisms for vasodilation in skeletal muscle include:

1. Inhibition of sympathetic vasoconstriction.
2. Activation of sympathetic vasodilator system.
3. Circulating L-epinephrine acting on β receptors.
4. Increased carbon dioxide, diminished oxygen tension.
5. Autoregulation:
   a. Metabolic: Related to level of functional activity.
   b. Myogenic: Intrinsic responses of smooth muscle.

Myogenic Autoregulation

The maintenance of cellular environments of tissue cells under widely varying levels of func-

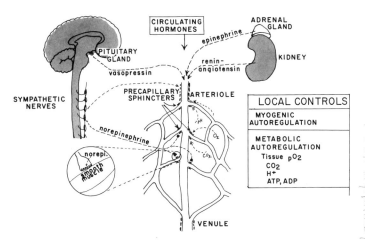

Figure 5. The control of blood flow and its distribution through typical capillary networks is vested in smooth muscle cuffs surrounding the terminal arterioles and precapillary sphincters. Flow through the capillary networks is influenced by sympathetic nerves, circulating hormones, and local control mechanisms.

tional activity is generally believed to depend on intrinsic feedback responses affecting the terminal arterioles and precapillary sphincters within individual microcirculatory networks. For example, many tissues of the body exhibit responses that tend to sustain perfusion rates in the face of experimentally induced changes in arterial pressure, venous pressure, arterial oxygen tension, or metabolic activity. Such autoregulation can be demonstrated in tissues lacking neural or hormonal influences or even in organs removed from the body and perfused by artificial means. It is commonly ascribed to a natural tendency for vascular smooth muscle cells in terminal resistance vessels to contract when stretched by elevated internal pressure or to relax when the perfusion pressure is lowered.

Metabolic Autoregulation

The multitude of mechanisms that modulate blood flow in response to increased metabolic activity are most apparent in the case of vigorously contracting skeletal muscle. Specifically, the tone of microvascular smooth muscle is affected by the levels of oxygen tension and carbon dioxide in the surrounding tissue. Actively contracting muscles deplete the oxygen and elevate the carbon dioxide levels in the tissue fluid that bathes both the muscle fibers and the adjacent microcirculatory channels (Figure 5). The vasodilation produced by these

factors may be supplemented by other chemical vasodilator influences such as acid radicals, ADP, and possibly other factors that have not been fully elucidated. This imposing array of metabolically related mechanisms is believed to be effective in those tissues that exhibit reactive hyperemia in response to temporary interruption of their blood flow, notably heart muscle, certain abdominal organs, and skin. Regulation of blood flow through skin involves some additional mechanisms, including changes in ambient temperature, release of histamine from physical damage to tissues, as well as expressions of emotions such as blushing or pallor. The ready accessibility of skin for study renders the diversity of control mechanisms particularly relevant to psychobiological investigations.

Interaction between Myogenic and Metabolic Controls

Myogenic and metabolic control mechanisms may act synergistically when reduced perfusion is accompanied by falling oxygen tensions (i.e., diminished perfusion pressure). Conversely, increased intravascular tension may be accompanied by diminished capillary flow during venous obstruction. Under these conditions, the myogenic influence would induce constriction but the metabolic mechanisms would promote vasodilation. The resultant changes in blood flow would indicate which mechanism was dominant under a particular set of circumstances.

Remote Control of Peripheral Vessels

Neural control of the peripheral circulation is exerted by the sympathetic nerves that originate in the intermediolateral cell column of the spinal cord and are distributed widely to the vasculature of the various organs of the body (Figure 5).

Neural Control Mechanisms

Sympathetic nerve terminals are located very near the surface of vascular smooth muscle cells in arterioles, precapillary sphincters, and venules (see Figure 5, insert). In these terminals, norepinephrine is synthesized from tyrosine and encapsulated in tiny vesicles which are released into the intervening gap to initiate contraction by binding to specialized α receptors on the smooth muscle cell surface (Greenberg, Curro, & Tanaka, 1983). The rate of norepinephrine release is determined by the rate of arrival of impulses along the nerve fiber.

Stimulation of sympathetic nerves at rates of about 6 impulses/s releases quantities of norepinephrine sufficient to reduce capillary blood flow to about a quarter of control values. Active constriction of precapillary sphincters blocks flow into some capillaries and reduces the proportion of capillaries through which blood is actively flowing. Sympathetic vasoconstrictor fibers are distributed to many areas of the body including skin, striated muscles, and abdominal viscera.

Sympathetic vasodilation has been described in experimental animals through release of acetylcholine to produce increased blood flow in skin and striated muscle. Its existence in humans remains debatable.

Hormonal Effects on Peripheral Vessels

The adrenal glands, posterior pituitary, and the kidneys are the principal sources of hormones involved in circulatory regulation. Norepinephrine released into the blood by the adrenal glands produces patterns of response similar to the effects of stimulating sympathetic adrenergic nerves producing constriction of arterioles, precapillary sphincters, venules, and small veins (Figure 5). Epinephrine has a similar action in most organs but also has a powerful vasodilator action in skeletal muscle and myocardium. The demonstration that epinephrine can induce vasoconstriction or vasodilation led Ahlquist (1958) to postulate two different receptor sites: α receptors in vascular smooth muscle in skin, skeletal muscle, myocardium, and abdominal organs respond by constriction to epinephrine, norepinephrine, and related catecholamines; β receptors respond to similar stimulation by vasodilation, accelerated heart rate, and more forceful cardiac contraction and vasodilation in skeletal muscle and coronary circulation. Isoproterenol is a synthetic product that mimics the action of epinephrine on the β receptors (Granger et al., 1983).

Paradoxical Effects of Circulating Norepinephrine

The direct effects of norepinephrine released by sympathetic nerve endings in the heart are increased heart rate and more poweful contractions. Circulating norepinephrine has such a profound vasoconstrictor action that the arterial blood pressure is elevated. Pressoreceptor reflexes activate such great vagal discharge that the heart rate slows, masking the direct effect of the norepinephrine on the pacemaker cells.

Renal Factors in Vascular Control

The kidneys are also ascribed a role in vascular control through the elaboration of a hormone called renin when the renal blood flow is diminished. Renin combines with a plasma protein circulating in the blood to form angiotensin, which produces elevation of arterial blood pressure through increased total peripheral resistance. Indirectly, renin is believed to act on the adjacent adrenal gland to release a hormone called aldosterone acting on the kidney to increase blood volume through retention of salt and water (Figure 5).

Body Fluid Volume and Distribution

More than half of the body weight of humans is due to water. Specifically, an average person weighing 70 kg contains about 40 liters of water of which more than half (60%) is located within cells (intracellular fluid). The extracellular fluid amounts to about 10 liters (located in the interstitial spaces between cells or in body cavities) and about 5 liters of blood containing 3 liters of plasma and 2 liters of cells, primarily red blood cells (see Figure 6).

Chemical Composition of Body Fluids

The chemical composition of the fluids inside cells differs greatly from that immediately outside the membranes that enclose the cellular protoplasm. In addition to the many organic compounds involved in the structure and metabolism of cells, intracellular fluid has relatively high concentrations of certain ions (i.e., potassium; magnesium, and phosphate). In contrast, the extracellular fluid contains much greater concentrations of sodium, chloride, and bicarbonate (HCO₃). Such differences in ionic concentration across the cell membrane are the result of active transport of ions, particularly sodium, across the membrane against steep concentration gradients. The disparity in ionic composition on opposite sides of the cell membrane is characteristic of living cells and is responsible for the electrical potentials essential for excitability of some of them (i.e., nerves and muscles).

The cell membranes are semipermeable so that differences in total concentration of the various ions and molecules are equalized by powerful osmotic attraction that impels water to move from regions of higher concentration to regions of lower concentration across such membranes.

The cell membranes are obviously very effective in inhibiting the movement of some ions and actively transporting others to maintain the wide discrepancies between the composition of the fluids inside and outside the cells. On the other hand, the capillary walls which separate the blood from the interstitial fluid are comprised of delicate tubes of endothelial cells which are very permeable to water, electrolytes, oxygen, carbon dioxide, and small organic molecules. The relatively uninhibited movement of these materials between the blood and tissue spaces is essential for the prompt and effective transport of nutrients and waste products to preserve the cellular environment in all the tissues of the body. The hydraulic pressure required to propel blood through the capillaries and back to the heart is sufficient to rapidly deplete the blood vascular system of its free fluid were it not for the osmotic attraction of the proteins in the blood.

Fluid Balance at the Capillary Walls

The hydrodynamic conditions at the capillary walls vary greatly in different tissues under various

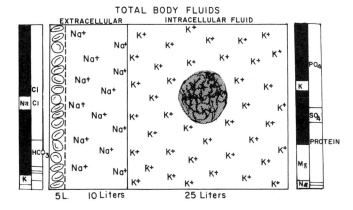

Figure 6. The volumes and chemical composition of the fluids within body cells are contrasted with the extracellular fluids which are composed of the fluids between cells, in body cavities, and the blood plasma. Strictly speaking, the fluid in blood cells is intracellular, a distinction not included in this diagram.

conditions but a typical capillary at heart level is generally illustrated as having an internal pressure of about 35 mm Hg at the arteriolar end and at or near venous pressure (i.e., 10 mm Hg) at the venule. Tissue pressure outside capillaries is difficult to measure but is generally considered to be less than 10 mm Hg. Thus, the pressure that propels the blood through the capillary would also propel the fluid through the capillary wall into tissue spaces along its entire length were it not for the osmotic pressure of the proteins in the blood. The permeability of the capillary wall does not extend to large molecules like the albumin and globulins in the blood plasma. These proteins are largely retained within the capillary and exert an osmotic attraction for water in the range of around 25 mm Hg. This colloid osmotic pressure opposes capillary pressures that promote outward movement of water into the tissues. Thus, the osmotic attraction of plasma proteins acts to maintain the blood volume.

This balance of forces across the capillary walls is often portrayed as an outward migration of water at the arteriolar end of the capillary and an inward movement of water at the venous end where the colloid osmotic pressure exceeds the effective capillary pressure. This simplistic view of capillary fluid balance at heart level in resting tissues neglects the conceptual problems that arise when arterioles dilate and elevate capillary pressure to steepen the gradient and accelerate flow. Even more troublesome is the maintenance of capillary fluid balance in dependent portions of the body in erect humans where a venous pressure as great as 80 mm Hg greatly exceeds colloid osmotic pressure. Under such conditions, water escapes from the capillaries into the tissues and is returned to the circulation by way of the lymphatic system.

Such a brief discussion of this complicated subject neglects nuances and details that are beyond the scope of the present discussion. Suffice it to say that the blood volume is maintained within remarkably narrow limits despite many and varied circumstances that would appear to threaten its stability. Since the blood is the transport medium for all the substances that enter or leave the tissues, it is intimately involved in the maintenance of the total body fluids and their distribution among the various regions, organs, and tissues. In general, the osmotic attraction of electrolytes is so great that water inevitably follows the movement of those ions that appear in greatest concentration. As indicated in Figure 6, sodium and chloride are the dominant ions in the extracellular fluids and regulation of sodium content by the kidney is a crucial element in the renal regulation of body fluid volumes.

Input–Output Balance of Body Fluids

The quantity of fluids, salts, and nutrients ingested is extremely varied, depending on such factors as individual habits, cultural differences, and environmental conditions. The intake of foods, salts, and fluids is intermittent during the day and changes with the seasons and in accordance with individual preferences or drives. At the same time, corresponding substances leave the body at widely varying rates from the intestinal tract, lungs, skin, and kidneys. The primary role of the kidneys is to excrete urine having such volume and composition that the total body fluids and their chemical composition remain within remarkably narrow limits over extended periods of times.

Function of the Kidneys

The kidneys are paired organs situated on either side of the aorta and each comprised of about 1 million nephrons emptying into collecting tubules as schematically illustrated in Figure 7. Each nephron consists of a glomerulus containing a tiny network of parallel capillaries within a cuplike structure called Bowman's capsule. These glomerular capillaries are extremely permeable to the filtration of water and solutes from the blood into Bowman's capsule. The glomerular filtrate passes through a long and tortuous ductile system that leads ultimately to a collecting tubule and finally to the urinary tract.

To accomplish its crucial function, a very large fraction (i.e., 20%) of the total resting cardiac output flows through the multitude of glomerular capillaries (see Figure 7A). The glomerular vessels are equipped with smooth muscle cuffs at both the entrance and exit of the glomerular vessels. Thus,

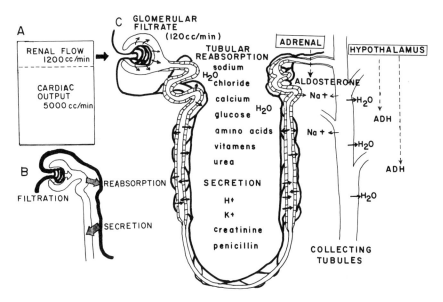

Figure 7. (A) In maintaining the volume and composition of the body fluids, the kidneys are perfused by a massive blood flow (about 20% of the total resting cardiac output). Each minute, a filtrate of about 120 cm³/min enters the nephron units. (C) Most of the water and solutes are selectively reabsorbed during passage through the tubules to provide a urine volume of about 1 cm³/min. Certain excess or toxic materials are actively secreted into the tubular fluid for excretion.

both the efferent and afferent vessels of the glomerulus are sites of controlled vascular resistance. The renal circulation exhibits a remarkable degree of autoregulation such that the blood flow through the kidney remains remarkably stable in the face of either elevation or lowering of the systemic arterial blood pressure. In addition, sustained obstruction to renal blood flow impels the kidneys to produce elaborated renin, which converts a circulating precursor into angiotensin, which in turn produces vasoconstriction and elevates arterial pressure.

The controlled resistance at both the entrance and exit from the glomerulus also functions to to maintain the volume of fluid filtering into the glomerulus at around 120 cm³/min. As the glomerular filtrate progresses along the tubules of each nephron, most of the water and solutes are reabsorbed into a second capillary network that accompanies each tubule. By this means, essential ingredients, such as glucose or amino acids, are restored to the blood. Superfluous solutes, toxic substances, and certain metabolic products such as urea are excreted either by the process of reabsorp-

tion or by active secretion back into the blood by the tubular cells (see Figure 7B). The most prominent examples of substances which are reabsorbed or secreted are enumerated in Figure 7C.

Control over the excretion of sodium and related electrolytes is largely vested in the action of aldosterone, a hormone produced by the adrenal glands in response to changes in the composition of extracellular fluids. The major action of aldosterone occurs at the distal convolution of the tubules just before entrance into the collecting tubule (see Figure 7C).

The kidneys are capable of excreting either large quantities of dilute urine or small quantities of highly concentrated urine depending on the water intake, among other things. The final adjustment in the excreted volume occurs in the collecting tubule under the influence of an antidiuretic hormone (ADH) excreted by cells in the hypothalamus at the base of the brain. It is generally conceded that sensors responsive to changes in the osmotic concentrations of extracellular fluids initiate the release of this important control mechanism.

The magnitude and diversity of renal function are illustrated by the fact that about 1 cm³ of urine is formed each minute from a filtrate of 120 cm³/min derived from a renal blood flow of about 1200 cm³/min. In the process, the total quantity of many different substances in the body fluids is controlled within narrow limits by a complex process that deals individually with a great diversity of solutes. This challenging objective involves intrinsic renal mechanisms under the influence of external neural and humoral regulatory mechanisms.

Neural Origins of Cardiovascular Responses

The autonomic nervous system plays prominent roles in many aspects of cardiovascular control. The parasympathetic nervous system acts through the vagus nerves to slow heart rate but has little direct influence on the peripheral vascular system. Conversely, the sympathetic nervous system acts to accelerate heart rate, enhance the force of cardiac contraction, and can produce patterns of peripheral vascular responses that are appropriate for vigorous exertion. Since some of these reactions may emerge in anticipation of exercise, the central nervous system is the logical site of their origin. The hypothalamus has long been recognized as an important source of neural outflow through the intermediolateral cell columns of the spinal cord out to the sympathetic chain and its widespread distribution.

In search of the origins of integrated patterns of cardiovascular responses, stimulation of selected sites in the hypothalmus elicited cardiovascular responses that closely resembled those recorded during spontaneous exercise by experimental animals (Smith, Rushmer, & Lasher, 1960). In some instances, running movements of the legs were produced by the same stimuli that induced the cardiovascular responses. The cardiovascular responses to psychological or emotional stimuli clearly establish the brain as an important source of integrated patterns of autonomic discharge. A great deal of interest and effort focused on identifying the neural pathways and connections between the higher levels of the brain and the outflow to the sympathetic nervous system (Rushmer & Smith, 1959).

Cardiovascular responses that would be expected to accompany severe emotional displays of rage, anger, or defense have been obtained by stimulating particular sites in the amydala. The cardiovascular response includes fast heart rate, increased arterial pressure, vasoconstriction in the kidneys, intestines, and skin, and vasodilation in skeletal muscles.

Hypothalamic Areas Controlling Emotional Responses

Using an operationally defined conditioned emotional response in conjunction with a variety of recording techniques to monitor cardiovascular response in unanesthetized animals, Stebbins and Smith (1964) demonstrated patterns of responses associated with emotion that could be reproduced repeatedly. The same cardiovascular response could be elicited by electrical stimulation of the medial portion of the lateral hypothalamus. Discrete destruction of this area led to complete disappearance of the previously observed response when the animals were again retested for the conditioned emotional response. The anatomical site(s) which produced these effects was designated *hypothalamic area controlling emotional responses* (Smith & DeVito, 1984). This area projects directly and indirectly on the sympathetic outflow to the cardiovascular system. The demonstration of direct connections to the sympathetic outflow suggests a very precise and specific output stemming from higher centers of the nervous system.

Summary

The cardiovascular system is known to respond in diverse ways to both physiological and psychological stresses. Initiation of most of these responses stems from the central nervous system acting through the autonomic nervous system, primarily the sympathetic outflow to the heart and sites of peripheral resistance in the peripheral vessels. The circulatory manifestations which accompany changes in psychological state have been the central focus of investigations exploring behavioral responses. In recent years, many and varied new technologies have emerged that provide new opportunities to monitor changes in human cardiovascular parameters more or less continuously without discomfort or hazard. The emergence of such technologies promises to greatly extend the tools available for research in psychobiology. This book is intended to illuminate and elucidate these modern techniques and their potential utilization in behavioral research.

References

Ahlquist, R. P. (1958). Adrenergic drugs. In V. A. Drill (Ed.), *Pharmacology in medicine*. New York: MacGraw–Hill.

Bennett, E. D., Barclay, S. A., Davis, A. L., Mannering, D., & Mehta, N. (1984). Ascending aortic blood velocity and acceleration using Doppler ultrasound in the assessment of left ventricular function. *Cardiovascular Research, 18,* 632–638.

Bonke, F. I. M. (1978). *The sinus node: Structure, function and clinical relevance*. The Hague: Nijhoff Medicine Division.

Granger, H. J., Borders, J. L., Meininger, G. A., Goodman, A. H., & Barnes, G. E. (1983). Microcirculatory control systems. In N. A. Mortillaro (Ed.), *The physiology and pharmacology of the microcirculation* (Vol. 1). New York: Academic Press.

Greenberg, S., Curro, F. A., & Tanaka, T. P. (1983). Regulation of vascular smooth muscle in the microcirculation. In N. A. Mortillaro (Ed.), *The physiology and pharmacology of the microcirculation*. New York: Academic Press.

Huntsman, L. L., Stewart, D. K., Barnes, S. R., Franklin, S.

B., Colocousis, J. S., & Hessel, E. A. (1983). Noninvasive Doppler determination of cardiac output in man: Clinical validation. *Circulation 67,* 593–602.

Lambert, C. R., Jr., Nichols, W. W., & Pepine, C. J. (1983). Indices of ventricular contractile state: Comparative sensitivity and specificity. *American Heart Journal, 106,* 136–144.

Levy, B., Targett, R. C., Bardou, A., & McIlroy, M. B. (1985). Quantitative ascending aortic Doppler blood velocity in normal human subjects. *Cardiovascular Research, 19,* 383–393.

Levy, M. N., & Martin, P. J. (1984). Parasympathetic control of the heart. In W. C. Randall (Ed.), *Nervous control of cardiac function*. London: Oxford University Press.

Noble, M. I. M., Trenchard, D., & Guz, A. (1966). Left ventricular ejection in conscious dogs: Measurement and significance of maximal acceleration of the blood from the left ventricle. *Circulation Research, 19,* 139–147.

Obrist, P. A. (1981). *Cardiovascular psychophysiology: A perspective*. New York: Plenum Press.

Rushmer, R. F. (1964). Initial ventricular impulse; a potential key to cardiac evaluation. *Circulation, 29,* 268–283.

Rushmer, R. F. (1976). *Cardiovascular dynamics* (4th ed.) Philadelphia: Saunders.

Rushmer, R. F., & Smith, O. A. (1959). Cardiac control. *Physiological Reviews, 39,* 41–68.

Smith, O. A., & DeVito, J. L. (1984). Central neural integration for the control of autonomic responses associated with emotion. *Annual Review of Neuroscience, 7,* 43–65.

Smith, O. A., Rushmer, R. F., & Lasher, E. P. (1960). Similarity of cardiovascular responses to exercise and to diencephalic stimulation. *American Journal of Physiology, 198,* 1139–1142.

Sonnenblick, E. H. (1962). Force–velocity relations in mammalian heart muscle. *American Journal of Physiology, 202,* 931–939.

Spencer, M.P., & Greiss, F.C. (1962). Dynamics of ventricular ejection. *Circulation Research, 10,* 274–279.

Stebbins, W. C., & Smith, O. A. (1964). Cardiovascular concomitants of the conditioned emotional response in the monkey. *Science, 144,* 881–883.

CHAPTER 2

Noninvasive Measurement of Cardiac Functions

Michael F. Wilson, William R. Lovallo, and Gwendolyn A. Pincomb

Introduction

The preceding chapter summarized the physiology of the cardiovascular system and suggested avenues, especially neural and hormonal mechanisms, through which behavioral or psychological factors might influence its regulation. The focus of this chapter will be to describe methodologies for observing changes in cardiac function which are particularly suitable for behavioral studies in humans due to their low risk, noninvasiveness, and for some methodologies, their unobtrusiveness.

Techniques for measuring cardiac function may be organized according to the cardiac function measured. These are: (1) the rate and rhythm of cardiac activity; (2) the specific events within the cardiac cycle and their inter- or intrarelationships; (3) the quantification of cardiac output and related cardiac volumes; and (4) the estimation of changes in cardiac contractility. In practice, the major methods described in this chapter may yield data about several different cardiac variables which may be applicable to one or more categories; and frequently more than one method can be used to obtain information about a particular variable. Thus, the specific measurements or variables within each category, possible applications to behavioral studies, and relevant techniques for measuring these variables will be briefly summarized. The remainder of the chapter provides an intensive examination of four major methods which have significant potential as tools for exploring how behavioral manipulations may alter cardiac function: electrocardiography, echocardiography, nuclear cardiography, and impedance cardiography.

Cardiac Function

Rate and Rhythm

Heart rate (HR; the number of ventricular contractions within a given time interval) is designated in beats per minute (bpm) with normal adult resting rates ranging from 60 to 100 bpm and a tremendous reserve capacity to more than triple these rates during challenge. HR is highly sensitive to behavioral manipulations including changes in posture or emotional state, engagement in psychomotor or cognitive tasks, the performance of phys-

Michael F. Wilson • ACOS for Research, Veterans Administration Medical Center and University of Oklahoma Health Sciences Center, Oklahoma City, Oklahoma 73104. *William R. Lovallo and Gwendolyn A. Pincomb* • Behavioral Sciences Laboratories, Veterans Administration Medical Center and University of Oklahoma Health Sciences Center, Oklahoma City, Oklahoma 73104.

ical exercise, and eating. Determinants of resting HR and HR response include gender, age, physical conditioning, constitutional reactivity, cardiovascular disease risk, and perhaps many other psychological/behavioral factors. Also, HR is an essential component in the regulation of cardiac output and blood pressure.

Periodic normal fluctuations in HR which are entrained to respiratory cycles are called sinus arrhythmias; and these are characterized by acceleration during inspiration and deceleration during expiration. The magnitude, frequency, and phase relationship of these respiratory-induced changes reflect complex interactions between reflex mechanisms and centrally integrated vagal stimulation. Sinus arrhythmias tend to become less pronounced with increasing age and more prominent when respiration or blood pressure is increased. Newer techniques employing spectral analysis of sinus arrhythmias may reveal that they are sensitive to a variety of individual difference factors and behavioral manipulations.

Various abnormal fluctuations in cardiac rhythm may occur, some of which have clinical significance. Diagnostic evaluation of these arrhythmias generally requires information about electrical activity throughout the cardiac cycle and not simply HR. Central sympathetic and parasympathetic activity play significant roles in determining whether underlying physiological preconditions result in the expression of arrhythmias. Arrhythmogenic mechanisms and their regulation are described more thoroughly in Chapter 3 (this volume). With respect to measurement considerations, it is important to note that behavioral manipulations may influence the occurrence and frequency of arrhythmias; these abnormal cardiac cycles may be accompanied by aberrant changes in HR and other measures of cardiac function, especially cardiac volumes and contractility. These changes are usually transient, but depending on the sampling procedure used, they may result in a significant source of artifact unless the arrhythmias are themselves a focus of investigation.

Heart rate and rhythm are among the simplest cardiac functions commonly measured. HR can be counted during manual palpation of the pulse, but automated techniques have the advantages of unobtrusiveness, greater precision, and the ability to obtain continuous beat-to-beat information that can even be precisely time-locked to behavioral manipulations. These automated techniques are varied, but all rely on measuring some physical manifestation of each beat and include: oscillometric measurement of pressure fluctuations, plethysmography, and phonocardiography, as well as the four major methodologies discussed in this chapter (see Table 1). Electrocardiography provides the most information about alterations in cardiac rhythm.

Cardiac Cycle

Each cardiac cycle involves a complex orchestration of electrical events, and mechanical events reflected by hemodynamic changes in pressure, volume, and flow, and valve action. The temporal relationships between these events are depicted in Figure 1. With the exception of atrial, ventricular, and aortic pressures, all of these functions can be examined noninvasively. The applicable techniques are listed in Table 1. The ability to record specific events within the cardiac cycle is crucial to obtaining measurements of cardiac volumes and contractility.

Cardiac Output and Volumes

Cardiac output (CO) is a measurement of the volume of blood ejected by the heart over a given period of time. Physiologically, this value represents the goal of complex regulatory processes to maintain the blood supply at a level appropriate for the prevailing physical and behavioral conditions. Along with vascular resistance, CO is a major determinant of blood pressure values. Resting adult values for CO are about 5 liter/min and there is a reserve capacity of as much as 25 liters/min.

CO is directly determined by three important cardiac volumes each of which can yield important information about cardiac function. Left ventricular end-diastolic volume (LVEDV) is the amount of blood present in the left ventricle after the mitral valve closes and before ejection occurs. LVEDV is sensitive to changes in diastolic filling

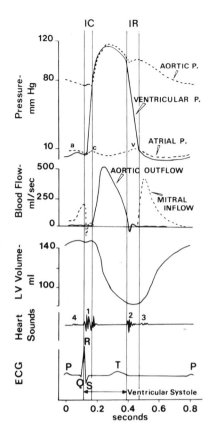

Figure 1. Events of the cardiac cycle for the left heart are expressed in terms of pressures (aortic, ventricular, and atrial), flows (aortic and mitral), left ventricular volume, heart sounds, and the electrocardiogram.

Table 1. *Common Noninvasive Methods of Measurement*

Events	ECG	Echo	Nuclear	ZCG
Electrical	Direct			
Heart sounds				Direct[a]
Pressures[b]		Indirect		
Cardiac volumes		Indirect	Direct	
Cardiac output		Direct	Direct	Indirect
Valve motion	Indirect	Direct		Indirect

[a]Certain impedance applications include direct phonocardiographic recording of heart sounds.
[b]Direct pressure measurement requires invasive techniques beyond the scope of this chapter. Aortic pressures, systolic, diastolic, and mean, are well estimated by the cuff method.

which may be influenced by HR, posture, venous compliance, pulmonary resistance, and other factors. Left ventricular end-systolic volume (LVESV) is the amount of blood remaining in the left ventricle following ejection after the aortic valve closes and before reopening of the mitral valve initiates a new diastolic filling period. LVESV is sensitive to changes in preload conditions reflected in LVEDV, to cardiac contractility, and to afterload conditions related to the opposing pressure of blood in the aorta and peripheral circulation. Stroke volume (SV) is the amount of blood ejected (in milliliters) during a single cardiac cycle and is determined by the difference between LVEDV and LVESV (SV = LVEDV − LVESV). By convention, CO is designated as a volume per minute and obtained from the formula CO(liters/min) = SV(ml) × HR(bpm)/1000. The comparability of these volumes across individuals may be enhanced by controlling for body surface area (BSA) based on the formula BSA (m^2) = height$^{0.725}$ (cm) × weight$^{0.425}$ (kg) × (0.007184). CO and SV are commonly expressed as cardiac index (CI = CO/BSA) and stroke volume index (SVI = SV/BSA).

Until recently, CO and other related cardiac volumes could not be estimated reliably without invasive procedures. The most accurate method is generally agreed to be based on the Fick principle which relates oxygen consumption and delivery to blood flow. Somewhat less accurate but commonly used procedures are based on the principle of indicator or thermal dilution (Berne & Levy, 1972, pp. 178–182). Each of these methods involves some sources of estimation error, but their most serious limitation involves their invasive nature and associated risks of injury and infection. Discomfort and anxiety associated with the procedure can require medication or produce confounding influences in cardiovascular regulation which may interact with changes related to behavioral manipulations. Also, the impact of fluid for the dilution procedures may itself produce transient artifacts in cardiac functions. Thus, these techniques have limited direct application to cardiovascular behavioral research.

Measurement of CO by indirect Fick and measurement of mixed venous PCO_2 is a noninvasive method that has regained popularity for use in the exercise laboratory (Jones, 1982). This method of respiratory gas analysis owes its renaissance to advances in physical detectors and rapid processing of data. Two approaches are being used: (1) rebreathing from a bag with low CO_2 concentration, and (2) equilibration using a bag with high concentration of CO_2 in oxygen. Reproducibility is within $\pm 20\%$ at rest and improves at higher cardiac outputs, e.g., during exercise. These determinations are intermittent and moderately obtrusive; therefore, we have not given them an indepth discussion.

The availability of newer, noninvasive methods for assessment of cardiac parameters represents a major technological advancement for behavioral investigations concerning cardiovascular regulation. Not very many years ago (less than one to two decades), the four measurement techniques to be discussed in depth in this chapter would be limited to the electrocardiogram. Echocardiography and nuclear cardiac imaging are very recent developments for clinical noninvasive cardiac assessment. Both are well suited for behavioral medicine and research where quantitative cardiac and/or myocardial assessments are part of the experimental design. The use of impedance cardiography for cardiovascular behavioral research was pioneered in our research laboratories with great success. Table 1 summarizes the methodologies which yield information based on various volume or flow relationships.

Myocardial Contractility

Myocardial contractility is a dynamic concept which expresses the state of cardiac performance that is independent from loading conditions, i.e., preload measured by end-diastolic volume, afterload which is a function of aortic blood pressure, and HR. Under constant loading conditions an augmentation of cardiac performance indicates increased contractility (positive inotropic effect), and a depression of cardiac performance a decreased contractility (negative inotropic effect). In the intact cardiovascular system, contractility is an important factor in regulating SV, CO, and arterial blood pressure. Contractility indices which have been used in humans are listed below.

1. Pressure-related index (dP/dt) is derived from the development (or increase) in left ventricular pressure (mm Hg) over time (s) after closing of the mitral valve. This index, which is influenced by afterload, cannot be obtained directly without invasive instrumentation using cardiac catheterization.

2. Systolic time intervals (PEP and LVET) can be derived from noninvasive measurements for intervals within the cardiac cycle (Lewis, Rittgers, Forester, & Boudoulas, 1977). Preejection period (PEP) represents the time during which the left ventricle is contracting isovolumetrically prior to ejection. Left ventricular ejection time (LVET) represents the period during which the aortic valve is open. The ratio (PEP/LVET) has been used to partially control for preload and afterload conditions. The best methods for systolic time interval measurements are: (a) impedance, (b) Doppler, and (c) the carotid pulse/heart sound technique. The electrocardiogram is used in each as a timing device.

3. Volume-related indices (ESV and EF) can be derived noninvasively from estimation of the volumes of blood in the left or right ventricle before and after ejection. End-systolic volume (ESV) and ejection fraction (EF = SV/EDV) have been used extensively for clinical and research applications. However, both are influenced by loading conditions. Nuclear cardiac blood pool imaging using multiple gated acquisition (MUGA) is the standard for left ventricular ejection fraction (LVEF). When directly calibrated, it is also the most accurate noninvasive method for ventricular volumes at rest and with bicycle exercise.

4. Flow-related indices can be derived noninvasively from changes in blood flow through the aorta or the thoracic cavity (Rushmer, Watson, Harding, & Baker, 1963). The Heather index of contractility (HI) is based on ejection acceleration and is obtained by impedance cardiography. Doppler measurements of aortic flow velocity and acceleration are sensitive parameters for detecting changes in ventricular systolic function. These indices are influenced inversely by changes in ar-

terial blood pressure. The most accurate measure of aortic flow, velocity, and acceleration is with Doppler echo. Nuclear techniques are equally as precise for determination of CO. Impedance is an excellent low-cost method for evaluating CO and contractility.

5. The systolic pressure/volume ratio (SBP/LVESV) can be derived noninvasively by nuclear ventriculographic estimations of LVESV and simultaneous measurements of systolic blood pressure. This recently developed index of contractility shows promise for more widespread clinical and research applications because of its apparent relative insensitivity to loading conditions (Sagawa, Sanagawa, & Naughan, 1985). Quantitative nuclear ventriculography is the most accurate and reproducible noninvasive method for this assessment of ventricular contractility at rest and also during maximum exertion (Wilson, Sung, Thadani, Brackett, & Burow, 1985).

Access to Equipment

Availability of this highly sophisticated instrumentation, such as echocardiography and nuclear imaging techniques, and the skill to properly interpret the data will often depend on an effective liaison and working relationship between the behavioral scientist and cardiologist. Electrocardiography at rest, with ambulatory electrocardiographic (Holter) monitoring, and during exercise stress are performed many times daily by the cardiologist in the Heart Station. Echocardiography (M-mode, 2-D, and Doppler) are standard clinical cardiology procedures; these modalities are rapidly advancing in technical development under the influence and auspices of clinical research. At most academic institutions, nuclear cardiac imaging is located within Nuclear Medicine, but it is usually highly dependent on interactions with nuclear medicine-trained cardiologists for the "cutting-edge" nuclear cardiac research and development. Cost factors, ease of use, and relative merits of one method compared to another will vary depending on local developments among institutions. These various considerations are discussed in more detail under the individual sections.

Measurement Technique

Electrocardiography

Description of Technique

Physical Parameter Measured. The electrocardiogram (ECG) is a graphical recording of cardiac electrical currents measured as voltages (potentials) from the body surface by conducting electrodes attached to a galvanometer, an amplifier, and recording system. The electrocardiographic potentials are inscribed on paper moving at a constant speed so that both the sequence and the frequency (HR) of cardiac excitation can be determined (Goldberger & Goldberger, 1981).

The normal ECG sequence consists of a P wave, QRS complex, T wave, and often a U wave (Figure 2). The times between these waves are called the PR and ST segments. Two intervals of importance to ECG interpretation are the QT and the R–R intervals. Each normal heart beat begins with electrical activation (excitation) of pacemaker cells in the sinus node located in the upper portion of the right atrium near its junction with the superior vena cava (see Chapter 1). This excitation spreads into the right and left atria where it is recorded from the body surface as the P wave. When the electrical activity is coursing through the specialized conduction tissue between the atrial and ventricular myocardial chambers, it is "silent" and not de-

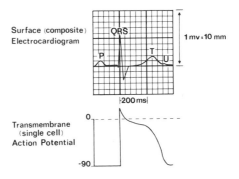

Figure 2. (Top) Composite surface electrocardiogram with major waveforms (P, QRS, T, U), shown at standard recording speed (25 mm/s) and calibration (1 mV = 10 mm). (Bottom) Transmembrane action potential from a single ventricular myocardial cell showing that the duration of activation is similar to the QT interval (onset of QRS to end of T wave).

tected from the body surface, and the isoelectric PR segment is inscribed. The QRS complex represents spread of the active wave of excitation into the ventricles and the sequential depolarization of left and right ventricular myocardial cell membranes. The ST segment located between the end of the QRS complex and the beginning of the T wave is normally isoelectric. The ST segment represents the duration of time between completion of depolarization and beginning of repolarization of ventricular myocardial cell membranes. The point of junction between the QRS complex and the ST segment is known as the J point. The T wave is the wave of ventricular repolarization (recovery). The U wave is an ''afterpotential'' wave which follows the T wave and is normally of low amplitude. The QT interval describes the duration of electrical systole and is measured from the beginning of the QRS complex to the end of the T wave. The QT interval varies inversely with HR and therefore a corrected QT interval (QT_c) may be calculated (Manion, Whitsett, & Wilson, 1980). The R–R interval represents one cardiac cycle and thus is a reciprocal function of HR.

The electrical activity of the heart, recorded from the body surface as the ECG, is brought about through a repetitive sequence of excitation and recovery of cardiac cell membranes which is coupled by reversible changes in membrane electrochemical characteristics and ionic currents to the intracellular contractile machinery (Rushmer & Guntheroth, 1976). Thus, the electrical events precede and initiate the mechanical events of the cardiac cycle (see Figure 1). It is for this reason that the electrocardiograph is so valuable as a timing device in the noninvasive measurement of cardiac functions.

Theory of Technique. Techniques for recording and interpreting the ECG are based on a composite picture brought together from the following three types of information:

1. Electrophysiology of myocardial fibers.
2. Sequence of excitation (depolarization) and recovery (repolarization) of the heart.
3. An understanding of volume conductor theory.

Membrane potentials in resting myocardial fibers and in other excitable cells (nerve, skeletal and smooth muscle) are produced by active processes requiring metabolic energy. These active processes cause a separation of ions across the cell membrane which is semipermeable or selectively permeable; thus, the cell membrane functions as an electrical insulating barrier with a selective and variable resistance to passage by the major ions, e.g., sodium, potassium, and calcium. Separation of charges (ions) by an insulator (cell membrane) is in essence a battery which maintains a potential difference between the positive and negative poles. The charge separation and selective permeabilities at rest are such that K^+ ions leak out, causing the inside to be negative to the outside. This resting membrane potential (voltage) is on the order of magnitude of 0.1 V. That this is true for each ''patch'' of cell membrane can be determined by placing microelectrodes into a resting myocardial fiber.

Excitation (depolarization) recorded as an action potential (Figure 2) is both an active and a passive process. In a ''patch'' of membrane, the active process is the selective opening of ionic membrane channels which permits the passive flow of the selected ions across the membrane down their electrochemical gradients. On excitation, Na^+ ions enter the cell rapidly through membrane channels, causing the transmembrane potential difference to fall to zero and even overshoot (inside is transiently positive). In other excitable tissue (nerve, skeletal muscle), this process also recovers fairly rapidly; however, in cardiac muscle the rapid and short-lived inward Na^+ current is followed by a slow and prolonged inward Ca^{2+} ion current which accounts for the plateau of the cardiac cell action potential. At this time the cell interior and exterior are nearly equipotential. Recovery of the cellular transmembrane potential difference (inside negative) occurs with a decrease of Ca^{2+} permeability and increase of K^+ permeability.

The sequence of excitation begins with sinus node pacemaker cells which spontaneously depolarize (see Figure 2 of Chapter 1). From this initial source, excitation spreads (is conducted) over the atria, into the specialized conducting tissue connecting the atrial and ventricular myocardium and then into and through the ventricular muscle mass. Conduction velocity of the cell membrane electrical currents moving along myocardial fibers is dependent on fiber size. Larger fibers have greater currents and faster velocities. Excitation moves across myocardial tissue as a front creating at any moment in time a demarcation line between excited and resting myocardial membrane. This demarcation line of excitation invading resting tissue is described as a *dipole* with a positive leading edge (head) and a negative trailing edge (tail). The excitation dipole describes a vector which has: (1) polarity, positive head and negative tail, (2) direction, from excited to resting myocardium, and (3) magnitude, which depends on the amount of tissue undergoing excitation at a given moment.

The body fluids are volume conductors since biological cells are immersed in a surrounding volume of salinity consisting of water and salts (ions) similar to the oceans. The potential differences which are recorded at the body surface as the ECG result from electrical currents flowing through the volume conductor. The current source, considered to be the dipole, is the demarcation line or front between excited and resting myocardium. If the excitation dipole is approaching the recording electrode a positive (upward) potential is inscribed and when it is moving away a negative potential is recorded. Current density, and potential, decrease with increasing distance from the current source. The magnitude of the current source is proportional to the amount of myocardial membrane undergoing depolarization at a given moment in time, i.e., the size of the demarcation line or excitation dipole. An indifferent électrode connected to one side of the galvanometer and an ''exploring electrode'' to the other side are used to record surface potentials from the volume conductor.

The surface ECG is different from the monophasic membrane action potential of an individual myocardial fiber (see Figure 2). The surface ECG records the moving boundaries of excitation (P wave for atria and QRS for ventricles) and recovery (T wave for ventricles). Electrocardiographic recording may also be obtained by intracardiac catheters with bipolar electrodes at the tip of the catheter. These recordings are called electrograms

(atrial, His bundle, or ventricular). The cardiac electrogram, like the surface ECG, records multicellular activity within a volume conductor, but being much closer to the current source they have larger potentials which reflect only the immediately adjacent activity.

Specific Application

Placement of Sensors. The standard 12-lead clinical ECG is recorded by arrays of electrodes connected to the two ECG galvanometer inputs by a switching knob. There are two types of extremity (limb) lead systems, bipolar and unipolar, with 3 leads each plus a 6-lead unipolar chest or precordial system. The bipolar limb leads (I, II, III) and the unipolar limb leads (aVR, aVL, aVF) are recorded by means of electrodes placed on the limbs. The unipolar precordial (chest) leads (V_1, V_2, V_3, V_4, V_5, V_6) are recorded from electrodes placed at specified locations on the chest wall (see Figure 3).

To record the extremity leads, the patient is connected to the electrocardiograph by placing electrodes on the arms and legs. The right leg electrode is connected to ground. Traditionally, the electrodes are placed at the wrist and ankles away from large skeletal muscle masses to reduce artifacts from noncardiac biopotentials. The electrical activity of the heart is transmitted through the torso to the extremities via the volume conductor medium (extracellular fluid). An electrode placed at the wrist or ankle will record essentially the same voltage pattern as the shoulder or hip, respectively. The bipolar extremity leads (I, II, III) record the difference in potential (voltage) between electrodes placed on two extremities. Lead I is the difference in voltage between the left arm (LA) minus the right arm (RA). Lead II is the difference in voltage between the left leg (LL) minus the RA. Lead III is the difference in voltage between the LL minus the left arm (LA). This was the arrangement by which Einthoven, the Dutch physician who invented the electrocardiograph, hooked up his patients. He also represented the bipolar leads I, II, and III as a triangle (Figure 3). Because of the lead arrangement, voltages for the bipolar extremity leads have the following relationship: Lead I + Lead III = Lead II.

unipolar extremity leads are summed, they should equal zero.

The ECG extremity leads, both bipolar and unipolar, characterize the electrical activity of the heart in the frontal plane. Their potentials may be described as vectors with orientation, magnitude, and polarity which are projected onto a schematic hexaxial lead diagram representing the frontal plane in relation to the subject's torso. The precordial (chest) leads have the exploring electrode placed in each of six locations along a horizontal plane of the chest and the indifferent electrode as the central terminal of Wilson comprised of the three extremity leads connected through 5000-ohm resistors to the single terminal point (Wilson *et al.*, 1944). The precordial leads then represent vectors in a horizontal plane. Use of vector concepts to assist electrocardiographic interpretation has greatly improved the value of the electrocardiogram as both a diagnostic and an analytical tool.

Recording Requirements. Concerns of frequency response, optimal damping, balancing of the recording stylus or pen, proper grounding for artifact-free tracings and patient safety, and calibration of the electrocardiographic instrument to maintain standard amplification of signals are all important to recording of interpretable ECGs. The instruments should have a frequency response of 50 Hz or greater. For balancing, modern instruments are resistor–condenser coupled from the patient to the input amplifiers with a time constant of 3 s. This restores the stylus or recording pen to the center point of the tracing relatively quickly. A properly grounded instrument is free from 60-cycle noise and stray extraneous currents. For standardized calibration, the gain of the amplifier should be set so that the calibration signal of 1 mV deflects the baseline signal by 10 mm.

The ECG paper is scored into 1-mm squares. Every fifth line is heavier on both the horizontal and vertical axes. The paper moves at a standard speed of 25 mm/s. Therefore, each millimeter of ECG tracing horizontally equals 0.04 s (40 ms) and each heavier line (5 mm) equals 0.20 s (200 ms). Calculation of HR from the ECG is achieved by either of two simple methods provided there is a regular rhythm. The easiest method is to count the

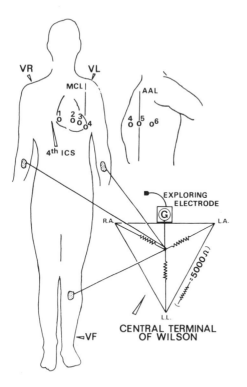

Figure 3. Central terminal of Wilson with extremity and chest lead positions. For accurate unipolar electrocardiographic recordings, a stable indifferent electrode is required. This is accomplished by connecting all three extremity leads to a central terminal and then through 5000-ohm resistors to one pole of the galvanometer; the other pole being attached to the exploring electrode. G, galvanometer; R.A., right arm; L.A., left arm; L.L., left leg; MCL, midclavicular line; ICS, intercostal space; AAL, anterior axillary line.

The unipolar extremity leads measure cardiac potentials from an exploring electrode placed on one limb versus a central terminal which represents the other two limbs combined through an electrical resistance network (Goldberger, 1953). The exploring electrode is electronically augmented. This arrangement is called the augmented unipolar limb lead (Figure 3). They are designated as aVR, aVL, and aFV, which represent the placement of the exploring electrode on the right arm or shoulder, left arm or shoulder, and left foot or hip, respectively. Just as the bipolar limb leads are related to Einthoven's equation, so are the unipolar leads; they are related as follows: aVR + aVL + aVF = 0. This means that when the voltages in the three number of large squares (0.2 s) for an R–R interval and divide the number into 300. For example, if there are three large squares, the HR is 100 bpm. The second simple method is to count the number of small squares over an R–R interval and divide into 1500. When the HR is irregular, an average rate can be determined by counting the number of cycles over 6 s and multiplying the number by 10. The ECG paper has a time mark every 3 s. Normal HR at rest is between 60 and 100 bpm. A rate slower than 60 bpm is called bradycardia and a rate faster than 100 bpm is called trachycardia.

Measurement Considerations

Validity. Electrocardiography has developed over the past 50 years into a primary diagnostic tool that is considered essential to the clinical cardiac examination. The actual recording of the ECG is simple, noninvasive, unobtrusive, and safe. (As with all electrical recording instruments, the electrocardiograph must undergo a safety check for proper isolation before clinical use.)

Important clinical characteristics determined by the electrocardiograph include: (1) rhythm and conduction abnormalities, (2) hypertrophy and/or enlargement of the left or right ventricle or atria, (3) ischemia, recent and old myocardial infarction, (4) electrolyte disturbances, and (5) numerous other special features.

Reliability. Accuracy of the electrocardiograph is greatest for the interpretation of rhythm and conduction abnormalities. A cardiology arrhythmia subspecialty consisting of invasive electrophysiology and noninvasive ambulatory ECG (Holter) monitoring with the use of 24-h tape-recorded ECGs and equipment for rapid scanning of the 24 h of electrocardiographic tracings has evolved. The electrocardiograph is quite reliable, with relatively high accuracy and nearly identical tracings (reproducibility) recorded with a stable condition (e.g., normal tracing, ventricular hypertrophy, old myocardial infarction, and stable arrhythmias), or a typical pattern of evolution with a progressive change in condition, such as a recent myocardial infarction.

Sources of Artifact. The electrocardiograph is subject to both electrical and motion artifacts. The instrument needs to be correctly grounded and coupled to the patient. Motion artifacts can be mistaken for ectopic beats (arrhythmia) including even ventricular tachycardia; therefore, awareness and attention to detail is important as increasingly ambulatory ECG recordings are employed.

Considerations for Data Collection

Conditions for Optimal Recording. The best recordings are achieved with the subject reclining quietly in an environment free from strong electrical fields, e.g., created by electric motors. Nevertheless, clinically reliable ECG tracings are routinely obtained during the treadmill exercise test and with Holter monitoring. One of us (M.F.W.) has recorded the ECG from racehorses in full gallop using a telemetry system and pocket transmitter.

Because the electrocardiograph is a highly accurate means to detect and record cardiac activation, and therefore the rate and rhythm of the heart, it is commonly used as a triggering device for other cardiac instruments, e.g., the nuclear camera, pacemakers, cardiovertors, and defibrillators.

Limitations on Use. The clinical electrocardiograph has enjoyed a wide use and varied applications for measurement of cardiac electrophysiology from the body surface. Electrodes attached to a lead wire are often swallowed for recording an esophageal lead to improve interpretation and diagnosis of supraventricular tachycardias by closer approximation of the exploring electrode to the atria.

Future Prospects

Electrocardiography is a fully mature discipline with broad applications to clinical medicine and to cardiovascular behavioral research. The use of ambulatory electrocardiographic techniques in behavioral research has hardly been tapped. Computer-assisted signal averaging and autocorrelation techniques are expanding the use and value of the electrocardiograph to detect underlying electrophysiological disturbances which carry a high risk for sudden cardiac death.

Echocardiography

Since its introduction into clinical cardiology two decades ago, echocardiography has expanded remarkably so that it is now available in all large- and most medium-sized hospitals, and in many clinics and physicians' offices. Its use to evaluate both functional and structural features of the heart has made a major impact in the clinical cardiac exam. The advantages of echocardiography are that the technique is completely safe, relatively inexpensive, and can readily furnish qualitative and quantitative data of heart chamber size and wall motion, movements of heart valves, and assessment of blood flow including forward (cardiac output) and backward (regurgitant flow) across heart valves. The method is the "gold standard" for detecting the presence of pericardial effusion and intracardiac thrombi (clots). A disadvantage for behavioral studies is that echocardiographic sensors used in standard practice are hand-held; the standard technique thus lacks the element of unobtrusiveness (Feigenbaum, 1976).

Description of Technique

Physical Parameter Measured. Echocardiography employs high-frequency, low-intensity sound waves (ultrasound) to display cardiac structure and function. This noninvasive diagnostic procedure has been particularly valuable for visualization and characterization of cardiac valvular function and abnormalities. However, its applicability is much broader and includes the feature of being able to measure both acute and chronic changes in heart function and chamber sizes. Acute time-related changes can be recorded either as visual images on recording devices (paper, film, video) or in some cases as on-line numerical data. The three principal types of data acquisition and presentation are: (1) M-mode, (2) two-dimensional (2-D), and (3) Doppler echocardiography. Each has its special features, advantages, and disadvantages. Echocardiography today is a sophisticated diagnostic imaging tool with no known hazard to the subject (Cohn & Wynne, 1982).

Ultrasound comprises frequencies greater than 20,000 Hz; these frequencies are above the audible range of the human ear. The ultrasound instruments used for cardiac diagnostic purposes have frequencies above 2 MHz. Sound with a frequency of 2 MHz has echoes that can be resolved into distinct images for detecting interfaces of 1 mm separation. Several features make ultrasound useful as a diagnostic imaging tool: the beam is more easily directed than is one of lower frequency, it obeys physical laws of reflection and refraction, and it is reflected by objects of small size. The principal disadvantage is that ultrasound propagates poorly through air. Therefore, the transducer must have direct contact with the skin, and parts of the body such as the lungs are difficult to examine.

Theory of Technique. Sound waves produce vibrations in a medium consisting of alternating compressions and rarefactions. Physical characteristics are described in terms of a cycle, wavelength, velocity, and frequency. A cycle (c) is the sequence of one compression and one rarefaction. The wavelength (λ) is the distance (d) from the onset of one cycle to the next (λ = d/c). Sound wave velocity (v) is defined as the distance traversed per second (v = d/s). The frequency of sound waves is measured in cycles per second (f = c/s). Therefore, the velocity is equal to the frequency times the wavelength (v = f $\times$ λ). For a given medium, frequency and velocity are inversely related. The velocity of sound varies with density and elastic properties of the medium, being faster through a dense medium such as bone. The velocity through soft tissue at body temperature is 1540 m/s.

The concept of acoustic impedance is of particular importance to the use of ultrasound. Acoustic impedance is defined as the product of velocity and density in a medium. The ease with which ultrasound travels through a medium is directly related to density and inversely to acoustic impedance. For example, muscle is slightly more dense than blood and therefore has a lower acoustic impedance. Ultrasound travels poorly through air which is of low density and high acoustic impedance. When a beam is directed through a medium, it travels in a straight line until it strikes a boundary or interface which has a different acoustic impedance. At this interface a portion of the ultrasound energy is reflected back toward the source and the remainder continues until it strikes the next interface.

The amount of sound reflected and therefore the intensity of the echo signal depends on the degree of acoustic impedance mismatch at the boundary and on the angle between the beam and the particular interface. The strongest echoes are formed with greater acoustic mismatch and when the angle is more nearly perpendicular. Higher-frequency ultrasound is reflected from smaller interfaces which results in greater resolution and greater energy absorption, thus less penetration. Ultrasound frequency commonly used in adult echocardiography is 2.25 MHz, whereas in pediatrics the need for penetration is lower and frequencies up to 5 MHz can be used, which results in improved resolution.

Specific Application

Placement of Sensors. Ultrasonic transducers contain piezoelectric crystals that both generate the ultrasonic signals and receive the echoes from the tissue reflective interfaces. The signals are focused into ultrasonic beams which are emitted as sound pulses of approximately 1 μs duration and these pulses are repeated every millisecond. The brief burst of 1 μs of ultrasound energy sent into the body 1000 times/s will occupy 1 ms; the remaining 999 ms is available for "listening" and receiving the echoes. This configuration of the input signals accomplishes two useful purposes: (1) There is very little energy transmitted into the tissue by this pulsed technique as compared to diathermy, for example, which uses continuous sound waves of much greater magnitude to generate heat. (2) The pulse train frequency of 1000 pulses/s is fast enough to record all cardiac mechanical events in a smooth, flicker-free motion display.

Recording Requirements. For a quality echocardiographic exam, considerable training and skill is required which includes knowledge of cardiac structure and function, anatomical relationships within the thorax, and an understanding of the instrumentation controls. The ultrasound transducer/sensor is hand-held against the chest in a pool of bubble-free gel for good acoustic cou-

pling. The location and direction of the transducer depend on: (1) which type of data acquisition is being used—M-mode, 2-D, or Doppler, (2) the information desired, and (3) the acoustic "window" available for examination.

M-mode. The standard M-mode echocardiographic exam consists of four cross-sectional views of the heart structures visualized as the ultrasonic beam is sequentially directed from the cardiac apex to the base. The transducer is placed (hand-held) over the precordium just to the left of the sternum in an intercostal space and tilted slightly to obtain the desired views as shown in Figures 4 and 5. This technique presents an "ice-pick" view of the heart with the vertical axis representing distance from the transducer and the horizontal axis being time displayed on an oscilloscope or moving strip chart recorder.

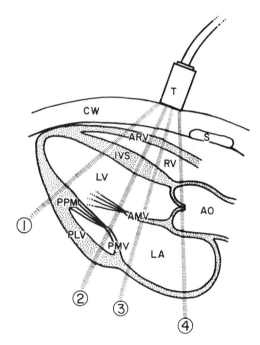

Figure 4. A cross section of the heart showing the structures through which the ultrasonic beam passes as it is directed from the apex toward the base of the heart. CW, chest wall; T, transducer; S, sternum; ARV, anterior right ventricular wall; RV, right ventricular cavity; IVS, interventricular septum; LV, left ventricle; PPM, posterior papillary muscle; PLV, posterior left ventricular wall; AMV, anterior mitral valve; PMV, posterior mitral valve; AO, aorta; LA, left atrium. From Feigenbaum (1972); reprinted by permission.

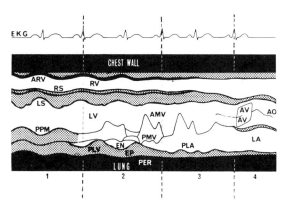

Figure 5. Diagrammatic representation of the echocardiogram as the transducer is directed from the apex (position 1) to the base of the heart (position 4). The areas between the dashed lines correspond to the transducer positions as depicted in Figure 4. EN, endocardium of the left ventricle; EP, epicardium of the left ventricle; PER, pericardium; PLA, posterior left atrial wall. The other abbreviations are explained in Figure 4. From Feigenbaum (1972); reprinted by permission.

2-D. In two-dimensional echocardiography, the 2-D transducer records a cross-sectional image along a tomographic plane. These 2-D slices or planes are then displayed in motion pictures. This gives a much improved visual presentation of cardiac structure and function. Imaging of the heart is performed in three principal planes: parasternal long axis, parasternal short axis, and the apical two- or four-chamber view. The 2-D transducer is positioned over the left fourth intercostal space for the parasternal view with a 90° rotation between long and short axis, and at the cardiac apex for the view in the apical plane. Other views are also employed for diagnostic purposes. Both M-mode and 2-D echocardiographic exams assess: valve function, cardiac chamber dimensions and wall motion, wall thickness, presence of atrial or ventricular thrombi (clots) and of pericardial effusion (fluid). The 2-D technique is substantially better at quantifying valvular impairment, and at identifying atrial or ventricular septal defects, regional wall motion impairment, ventricular thrombi, and aneurysms.

Doppler. Doppler echocardiography employs a different principle than the M-mode and 2-D transit time concept. This technique utilizes the shift in frequency that occurs from rebounding sound waves reflected from moving objects or interfaces to record velocity and direction of movement (Baker, Rubenstein, & Lorch, 1977). The "Doppler effect," first described in 1842, states that certain properties of light and sound waves depend on the relative motion of the observer and the wave source (White, 1982). The pitch or frequency of an approaching wave source is increased and of a receding wave source is decreased in proportion to relative velocity. This technique has developed major instrumentation for astronomy, for sonar detection of underwater objects, and more recently for medical diagnosis relating to cardiac and peripheral blood flow. Reliable information about flow velocities through the heart is now available using the noninvasive Doppler technology. Clinical applications include: (1) measurement of blood flow and cardiac output, (2) detection and measurement of valvular regurgitation and cardiac shunts, (3) assessment of ventricular function, and (4) identification of peripheral blood flow characteristics in the evaluation of vascular disease (Kisslo, Adams, & Mark, 1986). In addition to important information about the patterns of normal and abnormal blood flow, Doppler echocardiography also provides clinically useful estimates of intrathoracic and cardiac pressure gradients not otherwise available by noninvasive means (Hatle & Angelsen, 1985). The pressure gradient (ΔP) across a cardiac valve is related to the flow velocity (v) as predicted by the simplified Bernoulli equation $\Delta P = 4v^2$. Both aortic outflow and mitral inflow, available through Doppler measurements, are depicted along with other events of the cardiac cycle for the left heart in Figure 1. Doppler measurement of cardiac output (CO) provides an important noninvasive descriptor of heart function. Stroke volume (SV) times heart rate (HR) equals CO, and SV is the product of the integrated Doppler velocity (SV_{int}) signal in the aorta times the cross-sectional aortic root area (Ao) determined from M-mode echocardiography. Therefore, $CO = HR \times Ao \times SV_{int}$.

For the assessment of ventricular function, both at rest and during exercise, the development of new Doppler ultrasound devices has brought this modality into the forefront of clinical research as an attractive application of noninvasive measurement techniques (Teague, 1986). In addition to the measurement of CO, ejection-phase indices of aortic flow velocity and acceleration, and systolic ejection time intervals are readily obtainable. Of these parameters, it appears that aortic acceleration may be the best index to identify contractility changes in left ventricular systolic function. Measurement of inflow through the mitral valve has the promise of assessing diastolic properties of the left ventricle. In summary, the Doppler technology has many attractive features to recommend it for use as a noninvasive technique in cardiovascular behavioral research. Other features include: accuracy of measurement, relatively inexpensive, safety without electrical or radioisotope intrusion, and that the assessments are also valid with moderate activity, e.g., treadmill exercise.

Measurement Considerations

Validity. The validity of the M-mode and 2-D echocardiographic method depends greatly on the skill of the observer and the operator who obtained the data. Accurate measurements of cardiac structures and their movements (function) depend on correct identification of the reflective surfaces producing the echo signals. Since there are many acoustical boundaries that reflect the ultrasonic beam, there is a learning curve to acquire the skills in placement of the transducer and in adjusting the signals for optimum observer interpretation. Doppler devices applied to measurement of aortic outflow for assessment of ventricular systolic function (Rushmer, Baker, Johnson, & Strandness, 1967) are more easily used.

Reliability. Echocardiography has the capability for assessment of many aspects of cardiac structure and function in health and disease states. Probably the most reliable measurement in terms of sensitivity and reproducibility is the assessment of valvular disease and of the presence and magnitude of pericardial effusion. Quantitative measures of wall motion and chamber size are important for clinical assessment, are of intermediate reliability in that setting, and can be made highly reproducible with the subject at rest under research laboratory standards.

Sources of Artifact. Since the ultrasound beam will reflect from discontinuities of acoustic impedance, there is a high probability of receiving echo signals that are not of interest or that are even spurious. This is especially true, for example, in searching for intracardiac thrombi; thus, although echocardiographic examination is highly sensitive with regard to detection of thrombi, it may be less specific. Another source of error may occur in the quantitative assessment of chamber size and function (wall motion). Accurate measurement depends on correct placement and alignment of the transducer (sensor) so that the ultrasound beam intersects cardiac structures through the desired axis. Misalignment will result in over- or underestimation of the measurement.

Conditions for Data Collection

Conditions for Optimal Recording. With correct placement and alignment of the ultrasound transducer for M-mode, 2-D, or Doppler recording, accurate measurements of chamber dimensions, wall motion, or blood flow are expected. Echocardiography is the most precise method for determination of ventricular wall thickness, and therefore for diagnosis of ventricular hypertrophy.

Limitations on Use. There are two main limitations. (1) Not all subjects have an adequate thoracic acoustic window for an interpretable echocardiogram. Patients with chronic obstructive pulmonary disease commonly have a restricted acoustic window due to hyperinflation of the thoracic cage. (2) However, the key limitation for cardiovascular behavioral medicine is the current need to hand-hold the sensor, thereby introducing an obtrusive element. Current technology is readily capable of removing this limitation.

Future Prospects

Three developments for increased future use of echocardiographic methods should be mentioned:

(1) increased use in cardiac measurements with exercise stress testing, (2) simpler and less obtrusive Doppler transducers, and (3) placement of echocardiographic sensors which do not need to be hand-held, thereby removing the observer from contact with the subject, and significantly improving prospects for use in cardiovascular behavioral studies. There is a substantial body of evidence that myocardial contractile performance can be sensed directly by noninvasive Doppler techniques recording aortic flow velocity and peak acceleration in the ascending aorta from a transducer positioned at the sternal notch.

Nuclear Cardiac Imaging

Nuclear cardiac imaging is a valuable and sensitive method to assess: (1) heart function by blood pool imaging, (2) coronary blood supply by quantitative thallium tomography, (3) extent of heart attacks by acute infarct imaging, and (4) abnormal blood flows by shunt detection programs. Since nuclear imaging can examine functional and pathological events of the heart without use of catheters or significant risk to the patient, it has come to be recognized as a first-line test for evaluation of heart function and performance in nearly all diseases that impinge on the human heart (Cohn & Wynne, 1982; Strauss, Pitt, & James, 1974).

Description of Technique

History. Nuclear cardiology emerged from general nuclear medicine which in turn is a composite of nuclear physics, chemistry, physiology, and scientific medicine. The use of a radioactive tracer to study chemical (1913) and biological (1923) events was first described by Hevesy. In 1972, Blumgart and Weiss used this method to measure circulation time, which thus marks the beginning of the field of nuclear cardiology.

The first imaging or visualization of cardiovascular blood pools was in 1958. The technology of blood pool imaging was greatly enhanced by the development of improved scintillation cameras with associated computer analysis and radionuclide tracers, particularly technetium-99m, used as the free [^{99m}Tc]pertechnetate, [^{99m}Tc]albumin, or ^{99m}Tc-labeled red blood cells.

Efforts to effectively assess the distribution of coronary blood flow to the myocardium have evolved over the past two decades into a highly sensitive and specific technique using quantitative thallium (^{201}Tl) tomography (SPECT: single photon emission computerized tomography). Areas of transient ischemia following exercise or pharmacologic induced stress can be determined and sized using this radionuclide. Also, unperfused or poorly perfused regions indicating the presence of infarct and scar tissue can be identified. However, the myocardial distribution of ^{201}Tl, which tracks coronary blood flow (myocardial perfusion), does not indicate the age of the infarct. The search for agents which localize in fresh infarcts or recently irreversibly damaged myocardium resulted in the radiopharmaceutical [^{99m}Tc]stannous pyrophosphate. The infarct avid imaging [^{99m}Tc]phosphate compounds label damaged myocardial areas from recent infarct, blunt trauma, unstable angina, diffuse necrotizing processes, ventricular aneurysm, and damage incidental to open heart surgery (Willerson, 1981).

Two techniques (and camera systems) for determining heart function at rest and during exercise by blood pool imaging have been developed (Konstam & Wynne, 1982). They are: (1) first pass and (2) multiple gated acquisition (MUGA). Each technique has its preferred scintillation camera detector system for data acquisition but similar methods for computer storage and data processing. The multicrystal camera is best for the first pass and the Anger camera, consisting of a large single crystal and a photomultiplier tube array, for MUGA. Both camera systems are also capable of performing: shunt detection programs, infarct imaging, and myocardial perfusion imaging. Other instruments are capable of positron emission tomography (PET); this is an attractive, but currently expensive method, which has much promise for continued development and future widespread use in nuclear cardiology.

An alternative nonimaging method for the assessment of ventricular function on a beat-to-beat basis is the use of the ''nuclear stethoscope.'' This is a specially designed instrument with a micro-pressor and a detector probe which is collimated, but nonimaging. It accepts counts from the region of interest (e.g., left ventricle) and processes them on-line to inscribe a continuous beat-to-beat curve of counts versus time. Thus, end-diastolic, end-systolic, and stroke change in counts over the left ventricle are recorded for each cardiac cycle. Since ejection fraction does not require absolute volumes, but only differences in maximum and minimum counts over the region of interest minus background counts, accurate measures of ejection fraction are possible. The nuclear stethoscope (Wagner *et al.*, 1979) is capable of following dynamic fluctuations in ejection fraction, SV, and CO with high precision over the course of an acute experiment. The SV and CO measures are readily calibrated by MUGA volume determinations.

Physical Parameter Measured

Heart Function. Assessments of heart function, at rest and under conditions of exercise stress, are the most frequently employed nuclear cardiac imaging tests (Iskandrian, 1987). To perform these tests a tracer isotope is injected intravenously to mark the pool of blood flowing through the heart. By imaging with the nuclear camera the internal aspects of cardiac pumping action are visualized; the image data are rapidly sorted and processed by digital computers to present a video motion picture of the beating heart and to give quantitative, direct information for assessment of heart function by hard-copy digital display of: (1) heart chamber volumes, (2) regional wall motion, (3) CO, and (4) estimates of contractility by measurement of ejection fraction and end-systolic volume. Contractility is also estimated by the end-systolic pressure/volume ratio (contractitlity = systolic blood pressure/end-systolic volume). Assessment of heart function by cardiac imaging has vastly improved our ability to accurately detect the presence of coronary disease, to evaluate prognosis for decisions such as cardiac surgery and catheterization, to follow therapeutic benefits or adverse cardiac effects of therapy, e.g., Doxorubicin treatment. The combined exercise stress test with cardiac

imaging developed over the past decade was a major advance for diagnosis and prognosis of patients with ischemic heart disease and those with cardiomyopathy (Wilson, *et al.*, 1984).

Radionuclide Tracers. High-energy gamma rays are emitted upon radioactive decay of an isotope (radionuclide). The resultant radiations, called photons, have characteristic energy levels of thousands of electron volts (keV). Two common nuclear cardiology tracers are: (1) ^{99m}Tc, which has a 6 h half-life and 140 keV energy, and (2) ^{201}Tl, with a 73 h half-life and an energy level of approximately 80 keV. Technetium has single photon emission by isomeric transition from a metastable state (''m'') and thallium decays by k-electron capture with the emission of characteristic X rays.

Positron emission isotopes (carbon-11, oxygen-15, nitrogen-13, potassium-38, and others) create photons with an energy of 511 keV when a positron is ejected from the nucleus, combines with an electron, and annihilates into energy ($E = mc^2$). Two annihilation photons, each with 511 keV, escape at a 180° angle from one another; thus, a time coincidence detector system for cardiac imaging is especially applicable to positron computed tomography (Sorenson, 1980).

Labeling. For gated blood pool studies, the tracer should remain within the vasculature for the entire study to maintain a uniformity of isotope count activity. *In vitro* red blood cell labeling is the best method when both rest and exercise studies are to be performed. We have found that the BNL (Brookhaven National Laboratories) kit produces a consistently high ^{99m}Tc labeling efficiency of $\geq$ 95%. This provides high-quality images and a uniform blood label for 4 to 6 h for serial imaging. *In vivo* red cell labeling with [^{99m}Tc]pertechnetate injected intravenously after stannous pyrophosphate also provides a satisfactory blood pool label for both first pass and gated studies. The reader is referred to key references for detailed methods and for techniques relating myocardial perfusion and metabolism studies using ^{201}Tl and positron imaging.

Theory

Anger Camera. The Anger scintillation camera consists of a large flat NaI(Tl) crystal, fronted by a collimator, and backed by an array of closely packed photomultiplier tubes (PMTs) connected with computing circuitry to determine the $X–Y$ location of scintillations (Anger, 1959). When gamma radiation (photons) strikes the crystal, the resultant scintillations are absorbed by the light-sensitive PMT system, which releases electrons for current flow. The computing circuitry plots the $X–Y$ coordinates, and also sums the total output from all tubes for each event to determine the Z pulse. This output is proportional to the total energy absorbed by the NaI(Tl) crystal for that event. The camera electronics has a pulse-height analyzer which can reject pulses from undesirable sources, such as energy levels different from that being imaged.

Multicrystal Camera. The multicrystal scintillation camera devised by Bender and Blau has a collimator and then 294 small NaI crystals in a rectangular array which are optically coupled to 35 PMTs. The light (scintillations) from each crystal is divided into two equal parts, one for the X coordinate and the other for the Y. The total outputs are passed to a channel analyzer for pulse-height processing. This multicrystal camera system has a higher intrinsic count rate but a lower spatial resolution compared to the Anger single-crystal camera.

Single Photon Emission Computerized Tomography. Imaging facilities to measure coronary blood supply to the heart muscle (myocardial perfusion) under conditions of stress (exercise, drug infusion) and rest are commonly called SPECT or thallium tomography. The purpose of quantitative thallium tomography is to present images of the heart muscle in slices or sections to determine the distribution of coronary blood supply to the heart muscle. In the healthy heart, there is a uniform blood supply, both at rest and under conditions of stress. With coronary heart disease, this homogeneity breaks down first under conditions of stress; this can be visualized by thallium tomography with a very high sensitivity. The region and amount of heart muscle involved can be determined by quantitative thallium thomography. This is of major importance in the evaluation of thrombolytic agents (streptokinase, tissue plasminogen activator) to salvage heart muscle in acute myocardial infarction and to assess the need for coronary angioplasty or bypass graft surgery (Cohn & Wynne, 1982).

PET. Positron imaging has several advantages that are attractive for cardiac evaluations: (1) lead collimation is not required; instead, electronic coincidence circuitry is used to sort out radionuclide location; (2) this system has both high detection efficiency and good spatial resolution; and (3) over half the radionuclides are positron emitters so theoretically we should be able to identify an isotope with desirable characteristics for each imaging use. The tomographic principle is that positron annihilation events originating within a given plane will be in focus and those outside the plane will appear blurred. The major inhibition to widespread use is the lack of conveniently located cyclotron sources and the short half-life of current positrons of interest.

Specific Applications

First-Pass Angiography. Scintigraphy of the cardiac blood pool is performed immediately after intravenous bolus injection of the tracer isotope. Serial cardiac images follow the course of the radioactive tracer through the right heart, lungs, and left heart chambers. Ejection fraction (EF) of the right and left ventricles can be determined from ventricular time–activity curves. (EF = diastolic counts − systolic counts/diastolic counts − background.) Several computer-assisted methods are available to measure background counts. CO and SV can be calculated from classical indicator dilution principles or by first obtaining ventricular volumes using nongeometric techniques of total counts over the ventricular region of interest. Noninvasive evaluation of cardiac shunts is also particularly useful. However, first-pass angiography has limitations in its use for behavioral studies due to: (1) relative obtrusiveness relating to intravenous bolus injections immediately prior to data acquisition, (2) necessity for repeated injections for each additional study, and therefore (3) concern for radiation load (risk) and modification of data by the procedure.

Gated Blood Pool Ventriculography

Equilibrium cardiac blood pool studies have provided a noninvasive clinical method to assess cardiac function. Accurate calculations of left ventricular ejection fraction at rest and during exercise have been accomplished using ECG-synchronized blood-pool images (Borer *et al.*, 1977; Pitt & Strauss, 1977). Quantitation of left ventricular wall motion by computer algorithms has also been developed. Accurate computation of CO and left ventricular volumes using radionuclide imaging techniques has been more difficult. The calculation of volumes from the left ventricular silhouette using geometric assumptions (e.g., prolate-ellipsoid model) is probably not valid during systole and especially cannot be considered correct when there is asynchronous wall motion which is present in many patients who have had a myocardial infarct due to coronary disease. Nuclear cardiac imaging can measure ventricular volumes accurately because geometric assumptions are not necessary and can be avoided (Wilson *et al.*, 1982).

Data Acquisition. Synchronization by electrocardiographic R-wave gating is necessary to align each acquired image because several minutes of data acquisition is necessary to accumulate sufficient counts for high-quality images. MUGA algorithms are used to divide each cardiac cycle into imaging intervals of 20–30 ms; the counts for each interval over the cardiac cycle are summed separately by the computer to arrive at a composite set of images from end-diastole when chamber volume is greatest through systolic ejection to end-systole when chamber volume is least and on to end-diastole of the next cycle (Figures 6 and 7).

Ejection Fraction. This is a clinically important measurement in the evaluation of cardiac function whether determined by noninvasive or invasive methods. In the past, contrast angiography (invasive method) was considered the best method; how-

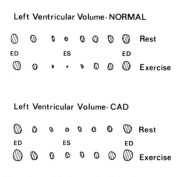

Figure 6. Drawings of left ventricular volumes over the cardiac cycle from a left anterior oblique nuclear ventriculogram which are typical of (top) a normal subject and (bottom) a patient with coronary artery disease (CAD) at rest and during symptom-limited exercise. ED, end-diastole; ES, end-systole. The volume changes are similar at rest, but are divergent with exercise.

ever, gated blood pool ventriculography is now considered to be the most accurate and reproducible method for calculating left ventricular ejection fraction (LVEF). The first pass technique is more accurate for the calculation of right ventricular ejection fraction (RVEF). Since ejection fraction is a ratio, it does not require actual volume determination but only counts over the region of interest (ROI) such as the left or right ventricle. See Definitions below for additional information.

Ventricular Volumes. The method for calculating left ventricular volumes from gated blood pool

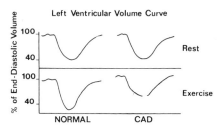

Figure 7. Left ventricular volume curve over the cardiac cycle expressed as a percent of end-diastolic volume for normal subjects and patients with coronary artery disease (CAD) at rest and during symptom-limited exercise. Data obtained by nuclear cardiac imaging. The maximum volume is end-diastolic, the minimum is end-systolic, and the difference is stroke volume. Ejection fraction (the ratio of stroke volume/end-diastolic volume) generally increases in normals with exercise but decreases in CAD patients with exercise-induced myocardial ischemia.

images by on-line attenuation correction to determine absolute left ventricular volumes produces a high correlation ($r = 0.96$) between simultaneously determined thermodilution and radionuclide stroke volumes. The relationship between thermodilution and scintigraphic SV is: thermal SV = 0.999 × radionuclide SV + 1.2 ml. This radionuclide imaging technique for the quantitative determination of absolute left ventricular volumes provides a reliable, noninvasive means to obtain SV and CO in humans, at rest and during exercise, without using geometric assumptions or regression equations (Burow *et al.*, 1982).

Left Ventricular Function. From the radionuclide ventriculographic images, the following data are obtained of left ventricular function at rest and during the last 2 min of each 3-min stage of a graded bicycle exercise stress test: end-diastolic and end-systolic volumes, EF, SV, HR, CO, blood pressures, and a measure of contractility which is independent of changes in both preload (EDV) and afterload (SBP) and is more fully described in the following section on "measurements and equations."

Measurements and Equations. Important applications of nuclear cardiac imaging include the quantitative assessment of global and regional ventricular function at rest and the evaluation of ventricular reserve and the measurement of reversible myocardial ischemia by exercise stress testing.

Definitions:

- *Ejection fraction* (EF) is the fractional amount or percent of blood ejected from the left or right ventricle during the heartbeat. It is expressed as a ratio: EF = stroke volume/end-diastolic volume. It is the current standard for the clinical assessment of ventricular function.
- *Stroke volume* (SV) is the volume of blood ejected from the left or right ventricle with each heartbeat. It is usually expressed in milliliters and is the difference between the maximum and minimum volumes during the cardiac cycle.
- *End-diastolic volume* (EDV) is the maximum

and *end-systolic volume* (ESV) the minimum ventricular volume during the cardiac cycle. SV = EDV − ESV.
- *Cardiac output* (CO) is the volume of blood ejected by either ventricle over time, usually 1 min. Cardiac output in liters per minute is forward blood flow expressed by the equation: CO = SV × heart rate (HR).
- *Index* means a parameter, such as volume or flow, divided by body surface area in meters squared.
- *Left ventricular contractility* (E_{max}) is the maximum value of the ratio between ventricular pressure and volume during cardiac systole (Nivatpumin, Katz, & Scheuer, 1979). The E_{max} occurs very close to end-systole and may be estimated by the ratio: systolic blood pressure/end-systolic volume (SBP/ESV).

Normal Values. The normal range of EF is listed as the mean plus or minus two standard deviations from the mean, and therefore represents the 95% confidence limits. Right ventricular volumes are larger than the left and since both ventricles normally have the same SV, the larger EDV of the right ventricle translates into a smaller EF (EF = SV/EDV). In our nuclear cardiology laboratory, EF and the following cardiac volume and flow values recorded at rest in the supine position have been established as our standards of normal:

- Ejection fraction
  Left ventricle: 65 ± 12%
  Right ventricle: 55 ± 12%
- Left ventricular volume and index
  End-diastolic: < 180 ml and < 100 ml/m²
  End-systolic: < 80 ml and < 45 ml/m²
- Cardiac output index: 3.0 ± 0.5 liters/min m²
- Stroke volume and index: < 100 ml and < 50 ml/m²
  (Both ventricles have the same values.)
- Left ventricular contractility (SBP/ESV): 1.5 to 4.0 mm Hg/ml

Measurement Considerations

Validity. Nuclear cardiac images for evaluation of EF and regional wall motion are the result of common and relatively straightforward procedures in the clinical nuclear cardiology laboratory (Qureshi *et al.*, 1978). They are considered to be important measurements in the management of patients with heart disease. A valid LVEF and regional wall motion study can be obtained on nearly every patient with a regular rhythm regardless of bodily habitus or severity of illness. These tests are also obtained in the exercise laboratory and in the intensive care unit. The accurary of routine clinical ventricular volume determinations may be somewhat lower because there is greater probability of error and interpretation requires more skill or expertise. However, absolute left ventricular volume measurements in our nuclear imaging laboratories during clinical research studies have been highly reproducible (Burow *et al.*, 1982).

Reliability. Measurement of LVEF by gated blood pool techniques is considered to be the most accurate means of obtaining this parameter provided that a standard computer algorithm is used in the determination (Marshall, Berger, Reduto, Gottschalk, & Zaret, 1978). Reproducibility of resting baseline values obtained several days to weeks apart is within 4–5%. This technique is well adapted for cardiac measurement during vigorous exercise (Rergch, Scholz, Sabiston, & Jones, 1980). Variations of volume measures may be greater in the routine clinical laboratory; but the determination of both end-diastolic and end-systolic left ventricular volumes by radionuclide imaging is probably the most reliable and accurate method available.

Sources of Artifact. When there is a highly irregular heartbeat from atrial fibrillation or frequent ectopic atrial or ventricular beats, the quantitative interpretation of cardiac blood pool images is not to be trusted. With controlled atrial fibrillation at heart rates below 80 bpm, left ventricular ejection fraction, volumes, and wall motion are generally considered valid in the clinical arena. These rhythm irregularities do not interfere with interpretation of thallium or positron images. Since the nuclear camera detects tracer radioactivity from the subject, any radioopaque object (e.g., pacemaker) in the path between heart and scintilla-

tion camera will create an artifact of reduced count intensity. Excessive background radioactivity will skew quantitative results. In applications with lower-energy isotope tracers (e.g., thallium, 80 keV), concentrations of activity in overlying bone or muscle may create artifacts in planar images; tomography reduces this as a problem, but may occasionally create artifacts due to low counts in the reconstruction algorithms.

Considerations for Data Collection

Conditions for Optimal Recording. Only persons who have been trained and certified for proper use of radioactive materials, especially with regard to safety, may perform these tests. The scintillation camera should be checked daily for uniformity of field. For blood pool studies it is important to ascertain that the labeling has a high efficiency, the ECG gating is correct, the computer algorithms which control data acquisition are set as desired, and the scintillation camera is viewing the heart. Three views for ventriculography are optimal.

Limitations on Use. The main clinical limitation of gated blood pool ventriculography relates to severe arrhythmias which produce great variations in cardiac cycle durations, thus interfering with accurate summation of gated data to form a valid composite cycle. However, using advanced computer processing, accurate and medically useful information can now be obtained in patients with significant and even life-threatening arrhythmias. The methodological details are beyond the scope of this chapter.

In cardiovascular behavioral research, the principal concern is with radiation dose and thus with subject risk. The dose administered for a nuclear ventriculogram or a thallium study is approximately that received during a routine upper gastrointestinal X-ray exam.

Future Prospects

Increased utilization of clinical nuclear cardiology procedures for diagnosis and management of patients is expected in association with: (1) development of new and improved radiopharmaceutical agents, (2) improvements in computerized tomography techniques, and (3) increased availability of positron imaging facilities.

For cardiovascular behavioral research, the current nuclear cardiac procedures are highly quantitative but moderately obtrusive; reproducible results in a patient population can be attained (Sung, Robinson, Thadani, Lee, & Wilson, 1986; Wilson, Sung, Robinson, Thadani, & Brackett, 1986). Favorable features associated with new clinical developments include: reduced radiation dose, greater accuracy and reproducibility of cardiac function and flow measurements, and the capability to assess cellular metabolic processes noninvasively.

Impedance Cardiography

Measurement of thoracic electrical impedance provides a noninvasive method of assessing cardiac activity, particularly the estimation of SV and myocardial contractility. Impedance techniques have had a mixed history of acceptance, probably due to: a general neglect of noninvasive methods in favor of highly precise invasive techniques in cardiology; poor quality of early studies to validate measurement of SV; and a lack of an adequate model relating the impedance (Z) waveform to specific physical parameters and physiological processes.

The advantages of impedance cardiography are that, properly applied, the technique provides a

completely safe, relatively unobtrusive, inexpensive method for SV and contractility measurements. These characteristics make the technique ideally suited to behavioral studies, and they allow repeated determinations to be made on a long-term basis with good reliability.

Description of Technique

History. Impedance cardiography as presently used dates directly from the work of Kubicek and colleagues (Kubicek *et al.,* 1974). A variety of early techniques in effect measured intrathoracic electrical impedance variations thought to reflect cardiac activity and were based on the principle that changes in the volume of a conductor within a current field produce proportional changes in electrical resistance across that field. The evolution of increasingly sophisticated techniques, through the efforts of such workers as Geddes and Baker (1975), Patterson (1965), and Lamberts, Visser, and Zijlstra (1984), has resulted in theory and practice as described below.

Overview of Principles. The most commonly used application of impedance technology is based on the method of Kubicek *et al.* (1974). Because of the electrical characteristics of both the recording system and the thorax itself, the best impedance recordings are obtained by a system of four electrodes in which the two outer electrodes im-

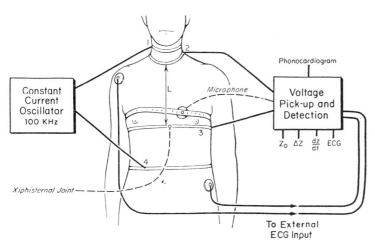

Figure 8. Arrangement of electrodes and phonocardiogram microphone used in impedance cardiography. Electrodes 1 and 4 impose a 100-kHz, 4-mA current along the thorax and electrodes 3 and 4 record the impedance change (ΔZ) on each heartbeat. Electrocardiographic electrodes are shown on the right shoulder and left lower abdomen. The phonocardiogram microphone is shown adjacent to the sternum. From *Instruction manual: Minnesota impedance cardiograph,* Minneapolis: Surcom, Inc.; reprinted by permission.

pose a 100-kHz, 4-mA, sinusoidal current along the thorax (see Figure 8). Two inner recording electrodes detect the potential difference which is then divided by the current to yield the electrical thoracic impedance (Z). The Z tracing can then be seen to vary with each heartbeat (ΔZ).

The ΔZ signal indexes the displacement of a volume of blood on each heartbeat proportional to the change in thoracic resistivity and is thought to reflect two sources of displacement: inflow, due primarily to ejection from the left ventricle, and outflow, due to runoff via the aorta. In order to obtain an estimate of forward flow due to left ventricular ejection, it is necessary to correct the ΔZ signal for either inflow or outflow by extrapolating to zero along the slope of either the descending or ascending limb of the ΔZ curve. In order to avoid certain potential errors in this technique, modern recording systems usually provide a signal which is the first derivative of ΔZ, the dZ/dt. The dZ/dt is thus proportional to flow, making the estimation of SV possible, as shown below.

In practice, the dZ/dt tracing is acquired along with the ECG used to denote the onset of electromechanical systole from the Q wave. The phonocardiogram may also be obtained in order to denote the opening and closing of the aortic valve to assist in determining left ventricular ejection time (LVET). Figure 9 shows a set of simultaneous tracings. In addition, the resistivity of the blood (rho) is a determinant of Z, and therefore rho is estimated using one of a variety of formulas. The one suggested by Kubicek is:

$$rho = 53.2 \ e \ (0.022) \ HEM$$

where HEM is the hematocrit of the blood in percent. Finally, the distance between recording electrodes (L) is obtained in centimeters in order to estimate the volume of tissue being sampled by the system. The Kubicek approach assumes that the thorax is approximated by a cylinder.

After obtaining LVET (in seconds), peak dZ/dt (in ohms per second) by measuring the height of the dZ/dt tracing on a given beat, SV may be estimated using the Kubicek et al. (1974) formula:

$$SV = rho(L/Z_0)^2(LVET) \ (dZ/dt)_{min}$$

where SV is the stroke volume in milliliters; rho is the resistivity of blood derived from the hematocrit (HEM) in percent, given as shown above; L is the

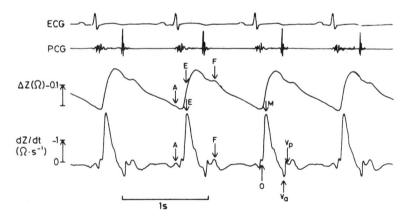

Figure 9. Proposal for the designation of the peaks and troughs in the impedance cardiogram. Twenty-four-year-old male subject, erect position at rest. From top to bottom: ECG, electrocardiogram; PCG, phonocardiogram; ΔZ, heart-synchronous impedance variation; dZ/dt = rate of change of the heart-synchronous impedance variation. Z_0 = 20.2 Ω. A wave (atrial wave) for the small wave which is due to atrial contraction; E wave (ejection wave) for the large wave associated with left ventricular ejection. This E wave has a clear O point (onset point), an M point (minimum point), and is followed by two valve closure points, V_a and V_P associated with aortic and pulmonic valve closure, respectively. During the rapid filling phase of the ventricles, an F wave (filling wave) occurs in the impedance cardiogram. From Lamberts et al. (1984); reprinted by permission.

minimum distance between recording electrodes in centimeters; LVET is the left ventricular ejection time in seconds; $(dZ/dt)_{min}$ is the minimum value of the dZ/dt waveform (point E) measured from the onset of the upsweep (point 0) of the dZ/dt tracing as shown in Figure 9; and Z_0 is the basal thoracic impedance in ohms.

An alternative method for calculation of SV was developed by Sramek (1981). This formula assumes that the volume of tissue sampled by impedance cardiographic units is approximated by a truncated cone rather than a cylinder and that the resistivity of blood can be assumed to be constant at 135 ohm-cm. Thus, under these assumptions,

$$SV = (L^3/4.124)(LVET)[(dZ/dt\ min)/Z_0]$$

By noting the heart rate (HR) over the interval in which SV is being determined, the cardiac output (CO) in liters may be calculated by:

$$CO = HR(SV/1000)$$

A valuable estimate of myocardial contractility (the Heather index, HI) has been proposed by Heather (1969; see also Siegel et al., 1970) based on impedance information. Using the formula

$$HI = (dZ/dt\ min)/Q–M$$

where Q–M is time in seconds from the Q wave of the ECG to the minimum peak of the dZ/dt tracing (M). The HI is thus given in ohms per second per second, which is a measure of acceleration. Various investigations have shown the HI to be superior to the commonly used ratio of preejection period to LVET (PEP/LVET) (Baller, Hurwitz, and Nassirian, 1983) and to compare well with time to maximum left ventricular pressure development (Matsuda et al., 1978; Siegel et al., 1970).

Key References. A classic presentation of most of the early work on impedance was provided by Nijboer (1970). A recent, thorough discussion of impedance cardiography, including an excellent review of the physiological basis of the dZ/dt wave as well as a presentation of the interpretation of some of the qualitative aspects of this waveform, is given in a well-written book by Lamberts et al. (1984). A good short review is that of Miller and Horvath (1978). A comparison of impedance-derived stroke volume in men versus women is provided by McKinney, Buell, and Eliot (1984).

Specific Application

Placement of Sensors. The ΔZ tracing is derived from a system of four adhesive strip electrodes as shown in Figure 8. Placement of the inner recording electrodes is critical because Z_0 is dependent on electrode distance (L) and because the base of the heart must be between these electrodes. The standard calls for placing electrode 2 at the base of the neck and electrode 3 at the xiphisternal joint. This leads to L values of 19 to 27 cm. Lamberts et al. (1984) recommend consistently placing electrode 3 about 22 cm from electrode 2. Since Z_0 in most men is 21 to 24, the value for L/Z_0 in the SV equation then has a value close to unity, which is desirable. In most cases an L of 22 cm should provide optimal recordings. Each recording electrode must be placed at least 3 cm from the outer electrodes. A practical way to accomplish this is to use a short electrode strip on the forehead as electrode 1. Some investigators have achieved valid results using a disk electrode on the forehead (Ebert, Eckberg, Vetrovic, & Cowley, 1984). Either of these approaches avoids electrode-proximity problems likely to occur when both are placed on the neck.

The ECG is best recorded with a lead II configuration (upper right to lower left). This yields a large QRS complex providing a clear demarcation for the onset of electromechanical systole.

The phonocardiogram microphone, if used, is typically placed to one side of the sternum at the second or third intercostal space in order to obtain the clearest aortic valve sounds.

Interpretation and Scoring. Figure 9 shows a set of tracings with a system of designations for landmarks on the dZ/dt signal proposed by Lamberts et al. (1984). Recommended paper speed for recording is at least 25 mm/s. Scoring of single beats is best accomplished by deriving: (1) preejection period as the interval from the Q wave of the

ECG to 0 on the dZ/dt signal; (2) LVET as the interval from 0 to point V_a; and (3) total electromechanical systole as the interval Q to Va. When hand-scoring single beats, the phonocardiogram can provide a useful second reference to confirm that appropriate points associated with the opening and closure of the aortic valve have been detected on dZ/dt. The second peak of the first heart sound usually agrees well with 0, and the peak of the second heart sound corresponds well with V_a. This holds true for normal hearts.

The value for (dZ/dt min) is derived by measuring the vertical distance in ohms per second from 0 to M. SV is then obtained by the above formula. It is usual practice for 5 to 10 single beats to be calculated and averaged to derive a single estimate of SV. Even with the use of dZ/dt to calculate SV, hand-scoring is tedious and places a limit on how much data may be obtained. Recent efforts have been made to automatically score single waveforms and average the results (see McKinney et al., 1985). Another approach has been to acquire an ensemble-averaged waveform by digitizing and averaging a large number of cardiac cycles and calculating SV from the averaged waveform (see Muzi et al., 1985; Muzi, Jeutter, & Smith, 1986).

Ensemble averaging methods employ the same scoring scheme. Instead of digitizing values from a single cardiac cycle, the dZ/dt, ECG, and phonocardiogram signals represent averages of a large number of cardiac cycles (e.g., 50–100) which can then be scored from a single set of the above measurements.

The Heather Index of contractility is derived by obtaining the interval Q–M and applying the formula given above.

Measurement Considerations

Validity. The validity of the impedance method depends on how closely the dZ/dt waveform reflects the volume of blood ejected by the left ventricle. Earlier investigations ruled out the heart muscle itself as a significant contributor to the ΔZ signal. Similarly, the ejection from the right ventricle was ruled out as a significant source of input by determining that the ΔZ signal arises primarily from displacement of volumes in *parallel* with the

equipotential lines of the electromagnetic field between the outer electrodes. The pulmonary artery branches lead laterally from the heart directly to the lungs, and their orientation is primarily at right angles to these lines. The ascending and descending aorta provide sufficient parallel flow for the volume to be detected by the recording system. The other primary signal source is the thoracic inflow along the superior and inferior venae cavae which are also oriented parallel to the field lines. Therefore, the upsweep of the dZ/dt wave is due primarily to aortic outflow.

A primary source of error in the impedance estimate of SV, however, has to do with the resistivity of blood during pulsatile flow. The resistivity of red cells in solution is partly a function of their collective orientation. Red cells are randomly oriented when still, but they become aligned when flowing. Furthermore, the flow rate and pulse rate are important factors determining the degree of alignment. For these reasons, the rho is not constant across the cardiac cycle. Lamberts et al. (1984) conducted an ingenious series of experiments to determine the contribution of erythrocyte orientation to the ΔZ and dZ/dt signals. Their conclusion was that if thoracic impedance drops 37% during a cardiac cycle, 21% would be due to aortic flow and 16% to erythrocyte orientation changes. Thus, if this conclusion is correct, 56% of the change in dZ/dt is due to volume and 44% to changing red cell alignment. These studies point to the fact that ΔZ is a complex signal lacking a simple relationship to volume of flow. However, carefully conducted validity studies do report good agreement between impedance and other techniques.

A second validity issue has to do with the adequacy of the model relating dZ/dt to actual SV. The equation of Kubicek is based on principles of electrical resistance; however, tests of its validity rest on comparing estimates of SV or CO with those obtained by other methods. A review of 23 studies of humans without valve defects or shunts comparing impedance with other methods for measuring SV or CO at rest and during exercise revealed r values ranging from 0.49 to 0.98 with an average of 0.84. In a recent study in our lab conducted on 31 healthy men ages 21–36, we compared resting impedance estimates of SV index with those obtained from nuclear ventriculography. The obtained r value was 0.82, and SV indices were 49 (8.6) and 47 (6.8) ml/m^2 for the two techniques, respectively (Wilson, Sung, Pincomb, & Lovallo, 1988).

Recent attempts at ensemble averaging to obtain impedance estimates of SV allowing a large number of cardiac cycles to be sampled have yielded promising results. Muzi *et al.* (1985) obtained a correlation of 0.87 between ensemble-averaged impedance estimates and thermodilution estimates on 14 patients, some of whom were in cardiac failure. Other studies on normals at rest and during exercise have shown correlations of $r = 0.90$ in SV between averaged impedance signals and the indirect Fick method (Ebert, DeMeersman, Seip, Snead, & Schelhorn, 1988). Advantages of this technique are that random errors are averaged out of the final signal and that averaged dZ/dt waveforms show a clear inflection point on the upsweep denoting the onset of left ventricular ejection. This allows a determination of ejection time without relying on the phonocardiogram, allowing use during exercise. Ebert *et al.* also found that measuring (dZ/dt min) from this point rather than from Z_0 yielded better agreement with the Fick method. Averaged signals would appear to have application in research settings and to permit accurate recordings even during the degree of movement and respiration which occur due to bicycle exercise.

Reliability. Reliability is an estimate of the extent to which a technique obtains the same value on repeated measurements. In prior work in our lab, impedance-derived values were obtained at rest on 15 healthy men aged 20–35 years on two separate occasions. Coefficients of reliability over the two sessions using the Spearman–Brown prophecy formula (Winer, 1971) were as follows: SV (0.96), CO (0.92), HI (0.90) (Pincomb *et al.*, 1985). Ensemble-averaged impedance signals have shown excellent stepwise increases in SV and CO during graded exercise as well as having standard deviations comparable at each stage to SV and CO values derived from indirect Fick determinations (Ebert *et al.*, 1988). Most authors who have con-

ducted such studies have concluded that the reliability of impedance measurements is superior to their overall accuracy.

Sources of Artifact. A review of a large number of studies comparing impedance to other techniques for measuring SV and CO indicates that on the average, impedance can approximate these parameters as measured by other techniques, but that potential sources of error exist making data in the case of any single subject potentially unreliable. There is general agreement that impedance follows very closely the magnitude and direction of change in SV and CO, making it an excellent technique for following trends. The irregularities of blood flow, occurring in cases having heart valve defects or shunts, make impedance much less valid in determining SV and CO when these defects are present.

Two important sources of artifact causing inaccuracy are improper determination of L and rho. Many early and current studies assume a constant value for rho based on assumptions of "average" hematocrit values. Those studies which determined rho for each case revealed better agreement between impedance and other techniques. The other source of uncontrolled variation is the choice of L. The length between recording electrodes is known to influence the value of Z_0. The critical factor for accurate recording is to ensure that the base of the heart including the aortic arch is between these electrodes. Lamberts *et al.* (1984) recommend using 22 cm as the value of L since this produced the most physiologically reasonable SV estimates in their studies. Finally, since the ΔZ signal depends on the alignment of the aortic arch with the equipotential lines along the thorax, a normal position of the heart is critical.

Conclusion. Impedance cardiography can be a valuable technique for measuring SV and CO in the research setting given its advantages outlined above: When the investigation calls for averaging grouped data; when a prime consideration is to note trends in SV or CO; when the observations are being made on structurally normal hearts; and when a reasonable number of determinations can be made, impedance measurements may be worth considering.

In the context of behavioral studies, the value of impedance lies in the fact that by permitting an estimate of CO, the simultaneous measurement of mean blood pressure (MBP) permits calculation of peripheral resistance (PR) by the formula PR = (MBP/CO) 80. This permits blood pressure to be interpreted in terms of the relative contributions of both cardiac and vascular factors.

Studies in our laboratory have demonstrated the value of using impedance cardiography in such a manner. For example, in an initial investigation of the effects of caffeine on cardiovascular function in persons at rest (Pincomb *et al.*, 1985), we measured CO simultaneous with blood pressure. In so doing we found that caffeine elevated resting blood pressure by increasing peripheral resistance with no change in inotropic stimulation of the heart. In other studies we were able to do detailed analyses of hemodynamic patterns associated with exposure to aversive (Lovallo *et al.*, 1985) and apetitive (Lovallo, Pincomb, & Wilson, 1986) behavioral tasks. In each case we were able to unobtrusively measure cardiac function in order to evaluate the integrated cardiovascular response pattern to the challenge of interest.

Conditions for Data Collection

In practice, four sources of error in measurement must be considered. These are: failure to estimate rho by hematocrit, careless placement of recording electrodes leading to unreasonable values for *L,* attempting measurements from persons with valve defects or shunts, and allowing excessive respiration or movement during recording.

Most practitioners have made measurements during end-expiratory apnea, glottis open, to avoid respiratory artifact. In our experience, modest respiration as during quiet rest or work on purely cognitive or behavioral tasks is not a problem. Ebert *et al.* (1988) have reported good validity of ensemble-averaged *dZ/dt* tracings during bicycle exercise during which breathing is heavy but movement is somewhat more restricted than during running.

Qualitative Use of dZ/dt. The fact that *dZ/dt* provides a signal denoting major events in the car-

diac cycle, and due to its sensitivity to valve defects, this signal provides an excellent noninvasive tool for monitoring *qualitative* cardiac function in clinical states. These include comparisons pre- and postsurgery for valve repair, monitoring in cardiac failure, and other states. A full discussion of these uses is beyond the scope of this chapter (see Lamberts *et al.*, 1984).

Future Prospects

Future developments are likely to include improvements in qualitative interpretation of the ΔZ and *dZ/dt* waveforms as clinical experience is gained using impedance measurements. More important for research investigations will be improved reliability and accuracy of measurements via the use of ensemble averaging of waveforms to reduce common sources of artifact. Finally, advances in high-density data storage and rapid analogue-to-digital conversion of incoming signals combined with ensemble averaging will allow ambulatory impedance monitoring to become a reality. This will permit extensive cardiovascular studies to be conducted outside the laboratory in real-life situations.

Summary

This chapter has provided a summary of four techniques for measurement of cardiac function: electrocardiography, echocardiography, nuclear cardiac imaging, and impedance cardiography. These were chosen because they represent the state-of-the-art in noninvasive or minimally invasive methods of cardiac measurement. The choice of techniques for a given research project then becomes a matter of choosing the best method for the purpose. In any event, the researcher now has a good set of tools for use in studies of behavioral–cardiovascular interactions.

ACKNOWLEDGMENTS. Preparation of this chapter was supported in part by funds from the Medical Research Service of the Veterans Administration and by a National Heart, Lung and Blood Institute grant (HL 32050). We gratefully acknowledge the editorial assistance of Carolyn Thorsen and Megan Lerner.

Suggested Readings

Cardiac Function

Berne, R. M., & Levy, M. N. (1972). *Cardiovascular physiology* (pp. 178–182). St. Louis: Mosby.

Jones, N. L. (1982). Mixed venous PCO$_2$ and the measurement of cardiac output. In *Clinical exercise testing*. Philadelphia: Saunders.

Lewis, R. P., Rittgers, S., Forester, W. F., & Boudoulas, H. (1977). A critical review of the systolic time intervals. *Circulation, 56,* 146.

Rushmer, R. F., Watson, N., Harding, D., & Baker, D. (1963). Effects of acute coronary occlusion upon the performance of right and left ventricles in intact unanesthetized dogs. *American Heart Journal, 66,* 522.

Sagawa, K., Sanagawa, K., & Naughan, W. L. (1985). Ventricular end-systolic pressure–volume relations. In H. J. Levine & W. H. Gaasch (Eds.), *The ventricle: Basic and clinical aspects*. The Hague: Nijhoff.

Wilson, M. F., Sung, B. H., Thadani, U., Brackett, D. J., & Burow, R. D. (1985). Efficacy of myocardial contractility index to discriminate coronary disease. *Circulation, 72,* III-103.

Electrocardiography

Goldberger, A. L., & Goldberger, E. (1981). *Clinical electrocardiography: A simplified approach* (2nd ed., pp. 3–34). St. Louis: Mosby.

Goldberger, E. (1953). *Unipolar lead electrocardiography*. Philadelphia: Lea & Febiger.

Manion, C. V., Whitsett, T. L., & Wilson, M. F. (1980). Applicability of correcting the QT interval for heart rate. *American Heart Journal, 99,* 678.

Rushmer, R. F. & Guntheroth, W. G. (1976). Electrical activity of the heart. In R. F. Rushmer (Ed.), *Cardiovascular dynamics* (4th ed., pp. 281–350). Philadelphia: Saunders.

Wilson, F. N., Johnston, F. D., Rosenbaum, F. F., Erlanger, H., Kossmann, C. E., Hecht, H., Cotrim, N., De Oliveira, R. M., Scarsi, R., & Barker, P. S. (1944). The precordial electrocardiogram. *American Heart Journal, 27,* 19.

Echocardiography

Baker, D. W., Rubenstein, S. A., & Lorch, G. S. (1977). Pulsed Doppler echocardiography: Principles and applications. *American Journal of Medicine, 63,* 69.

Cohn, P. F., & Wynne, J. (1982). *Diagnostic methods in clinical cardiology*. Boston: Little, Brown.

Feigenbaum, H. (1976). *Echocardiography* (2nd ed.). Philadelphia: Lea & Febiger.

Hatle, L., & Angelsen, B. (1985). *Doppler ultrasound in cardiology* (2nd ed.). Philadelphia: Lea & Febiger.

Kisslo, J., Adams, D., & Mark, D. B. (1986). *Basic Doppler echocardiography*. Edinburgh: Churchill Livingstone.

Rushmer, R. F., Baker, D. W., Johnson, W. L., & Strandness, D. E. (1967). Clinical applications of a transcutaneous ultrasonic flow detector. *Journal of the American Medical Association, 199,* 104.

Teague, S. M. (1986). Measurement of ventricular function using Doppler ultrasound. In J. Kisslo, D. Adams, & D. B. Mark (Eds.), *Basic Doppler echocardiography* (pp. 147–157). Edinburgh: Churchill Livingstone.

White, D. N. (1982). Johann Christian Doppler and his effect: A brief history. *Ultrasound in Medicine and Biology, 8,* 583.

Nuclear Cardiac Imaging

Borer, J. S., Bacharach, S. L., Green, M. V., Kent, K. M., Epstein, S. E., Johnston, G. S., & Mack, B. (1977). Real-time radionuclide cineangiography in the noninvasive evaluation of global and regional left ventricular function at rest and during exercise in patients with coronary artery disease. *New England Journal of Medicine, 296,* 840.

Iskandrian, A. S. (1987). *Nuclear cardiac imaging: Principles and applications*. Philadelphia: Davis.

Pitt, B., & Strauss, H. W. (1977). Evaluation of ventricular function by radioisotopic techniques. *New England Journal of Medicine, 296,* 1097.

Sung, B. H., Wilson, M. F., Robinson, C., Thadani, U., Lovallo, W. R. (1988). Mechanisms of myocardial ischemia induced by epinephine: Comparison with exercise-induced ischemia. *Psychosomatic Medicine, 50,* 381–393.

Wilson, M. F., Burow, R. d., Brackett, D. J., Sung, B. H., Thadani, U., & Schechter, E. (1982). Quantitative cardiac blood pool scintigraphic evaluation of responses to epinephrine infusion and exercise in normals and coronary disease. *American Journal of Cardiology, 49,* 992.

Impedance Cardiography

Lamberts, R., Visser, K. R., & Zijlstra, W. G. (1984). *Impedance cardiography*. Assen. The Netherlands: Van Gorcum.

McKinney, M. E., Buell, J. C., & Eliot, R. S. (1984). Sex differences in transthoracic impedance: Evaluation of effects on calculated stroke volume index. *Aviation, space, and Environmental Medicine, 55,* 893–895.

Miller, J. C., & Horvath, S. M. (1978). Impedance cardiography. *Psychophysiology, 15,* 80.

Nijboer, J. (1970). *Electrical impedance plethysmography* (2nd ed.). Springfield, IL: Thomas.

References

Anger, H. O. (1959). Scintillation camera. *Review of Scientific Instruments, 29,* 23.

Baker, D. W., Rubenstein, S. A., & Lorch, G. S. (1977). Pulsed Doppler echocardiography: Principles and applications. *American Journal of Medicine, 63,* 69.

Berne, R. M., & Levy, M. N. (1972). *Cardiovascular physiology* (pp. 178–182). St. Louis: Mosby.

Borer, J. S., Bacharach, S. L., Green, M. V., Kent, K. M., Epstein, S. E., Johnston, G. S., & Mack, B. (1977). Real-time radionuclide cineangiography in the noninvasive evaluation of global and regional left ventricular function at rest and during exercise in patients with coronary artery disease. *New England Journal of Medicine, 296,* 840.

Burow, R. D., Wilson, M. F., Heath, P. W., Corn, C. R., Amil, A., & Thadani, U. (1982). Influence of attenuation on radionuclide stroke volume determinations. *Journal of Nuclear Medicine, 23*(9), 781.

Cohn, P. F., & Wynne, J. (1982). *Diagnostic methods in clinical cardiology.* Boston: Little, Brown.

Ebert, T. J., Eckberg, D. L., Vetrovic, G. M., & Cowley, M. J. (1984). Impedance cardiograms reliably estimate beat-by-beat changes in left ventricular stroke volume in humans. *Cardiovascular Research, 18,* 354.

Ebert, T. J., DeMeersman, R. E., Seip, R. L., Snead, D. B., & Schelhorn, J. J. (1988). Signal-averaged impedance cardiograms during continuous exercise in man. Unpublished manuscript, VA Medical Center, Milwaukee, WI.

Feigenbaum, H. (1972). Clinical applications of echocardiography. *Progress in Cardiovascular Diseases, 14,* 531.

Feigenbaum, H. (1976). *Echocardiography* (2nd ed.). Philadelphia: Lea & Febiger.

Geddes, L. E., & Baker, L. E. (1972). Thoracic impedance changes following saline injection into right and left ventricles. *Journal of Applied Psychology, 33,* 278–281.

Goldberger, A. L., & Goldberger, E. (1981). *Clinical electrocardiography: A simplified approach* (2nd ed., pp. 3–34). St. Louis: Mosby.

Goldberger, E. (1953). *Unipolar lead electrocardiography.* Philadelphia: Lea & Febiger.

Hatle, L., & Angelsen, B. (1985). *Doppler ultrasound in cardiology* (2nd ed.). Philadelphia: Lea & Febiger.

Heather, L. W. (1969). A comparison of cardiac output values by the impedance cardiograph and dye dilution techniques in cardiac patients. In W. G. Kubicek, D. A. Witsoe, R. P. Patterson, & A. H. L. From (Eds.), *Development and evaluation of an impedance cardiographic system to measure cardiac output and other cardiac parameters (NASA-CR 101956)* (pp. 247–258). Houston: National Aeronautics and Space Administration.

Iskandrian, A. S. (1987). *Nuclear cardiac imaging: Principles and applications.* Philadelphia: Davis.

Jones, N. L. (1982). Mixed venous PCO_2 and the measurement of cardiac output. In *Clinical exercise testing.* Philadelphia: Saunders.

Kisslo, J., Adams, D., & Mark, D. B. (Eds.). (1986). *Basic Doppler echocardiography.* Edinburgh: Churchill Livingstone.

Konstam, M. A., Wynne, J. (1982). Radionuclide ventriculography. In P. F. Cohn & J. Wynne (Eds.), *Diagnostic methods in clinical cardiology* (pp. 165–198). Boston: Little, Brown.

Kubicek, W. G., Kottke, F. J., Ramos, M. V., Patterson, R. P., Witsoe, D. A., Labree, J. W., Remole, W. Layman, T. E., Schwening, H., & Garamella, J. T. (1974). The Minnesota impedance cardiograph—theory and applications. *Biomedical Engineering, 9,* 410–416.

Lamberts, R., Visser, K. R., & Zijlstra, W. G. (1984). *Impedance cardiography.* Assen, The Netherlands: Van Gorcum.

Lewis, R. P., Rittgers, S., Forester, W. F., & Boudoulas, H. (1977). A critical review of the systolic time intervals. *Circulation, 56,* 146.

Lovallo, W. R., Wilson, M. F., Pincomb, G. A., Edwards, G. L., Tompkins, P., & Brackett, D. J. (1985). Activation patterns to aversive stimulation in man: Passive exposure versus effort to control. *Psychophysiology, 22,* 283.

Lovallo, W. R., Pincomb, G. A., & Wilson, M. F. (1986). Predicting response to a reaction time task: Heart rate reactivity compared with type A behavior. *Psychophysiology, 23,* 648.

Manion, C. V., Whitsett, T. L., & Wilson, M. F. (1980). Applicability of correcting the QT interval for heart rate. *American Heart Journal, 99*(5), 678.

Marshall, R. C., Berger, H. J., Reduto, L. A., Gottschalk, A., & Zaret, B. L. (1978). Variability in sequential measures of left ventricular performance assessed with radionuclide angiography. *American Journal of Cardiology, 41,* 531.

Matsuda, Y., Yamada, S., Kurogani, H., Sato, H., Maeda, K., & Fukuzaki, H. (1978). Assessment of left ventricular performance in man with impedance cardiography. *Japanese Circulation Journal, 42,* 945.

McKinney, M. E., Buell, J. C., & Eliot, R. S. (1984). Sex differences in transthoracic impedance: Evaluation of effects on calculated stroke volume index. *Aviation, Space, and Environmental Medicine, 55,* 893–895.

McKinney, M. E., Miner, M. H., Ruddel, H., McIlvain, H. E., Witte, H., Buell, J. C., Eliot, R. S., & Grant, L. B. (1985). The standardized mental stress test protocol: Test–retest reliability and comparison with ambulatory blood pressure monitoring. *Psychophysiology, 22,* 453.

Miller, J. C., & Horvath, S. M. (1978). Impedance cardiography. *Psychophysiology, 15,* 80.

Muzi, M., Ebert, T. J., Tristani, F. E., Jeutter, D. C., Barney, J. A., & Smith, J. J. (1985). Determination of cardiac output using ensemble-averaged impedance cardiograms. *Journal of Applied Physiology, 58,* 200.

Muzi, M., Jeutter, D. C., & Smith, J. J. (1986). Computer-automated impedance-derived cardiac indexes. *IEEE Transactions on Biomedical Engineering, BME-31,* 42.

Nijboer, J. (1970). *Electrical impedance plethysmography* (2nd ed.). Springfield, IL: Thomas.

Nivatpumin, T., Katz, S., & Scheuer, J. (1979). Peak left ventricular systolic pressure/end-systolic volume ratio: A sensitive detector of left ventricular disease. *American Journal of Cardiology, 43,* 969.

Patterson, R. P. (1965). *Cardiac output determinations using impedance plethysmography.* Unpublished doctoral dissertation, University of Minnesota, Minneapolis.

Pincomb, G. A., Lovallo, W. R., Passey, R. L., Whitsett, T. L., Silverstein, S. M., & Wilson, M. F. (1985). Effects of caffeine on vascular resistance, cardiac output, and myocardial contractility in young men. *American Journal of Cardiology, 56,* 119.

Pitt, B., & Strauss, H. W. (1977). Evaluation of ventricular function by radioisotopic techniques. *New England Journal of Medicine, 296,* 1097.

Qureshi, S., Wagner, H. N., Alderson, P. O., Housholder, D. F., Douglas, K. H., Lotter, M. G., Nickoloff, E. L., Tanobe, M., & Knowles, L. G. (1978). Evaluation of left-ventricular function in normal persons and patients with heart disease. *Journal of Nuclear Medicine, 19,* 135.

Rergch, S. K., Scholz, P. M., Sabiston, D. C., & Jones, R. H. (1980). Effects of exercise training on left ventricular function in normal subjects: A longitudinal study by radionuclide angiography. *American Journal of Cardiology, 45,* 244.

Rushmer, R. F., & Guntheroth, W. G. (1976). Electrical activity of the heart. In R. F. Rushmer (Ed.), *Cardiovascular dynamics* (4th ed. pp. 281–350). Philadelphia: Saunders.

Rushmer, R. F., Watson, N., Harding, D., & Baker, D. (1963). Effects of acute coronary occlusion upon the performance of right and left ventricles in intact unanesthetized dogs. *American Heart Journal, 66,* 522.

Rushmer, R. F., Baker, D. W., Johnson, W. L., & Strandness, D. E. (1967). Clinical applications of a transcutaneous ultrasonic flow detector. *Journal of the American Medical Association, 199,* 104.

Sagawa, K., Sanagawa, K., & Naughan, W. L. (1985). Ventricular end-systolic pressure–volume relations. In H. J. Levine & W. H. Gaasch (Eds.), *The ventricle: Basic and clinical aspects* (pp. 79–103). The Hague: Nijhoff.

Siegel, J. H., Fabian, M., Lankov, C., Levine, M., Cole, A., & Nahmad, M. (1970). Clinical and experimental use of thoracic impedance plethysmography in quantifying myocardial contractility. *Surgery, 67,* 907.

Sorenson, J. A. (1980). Single photon emission computed tomography, and other selected computer topics. *Proceedings, 10th Annual Symposium Society of Nuclear Medicine.* New York: Society of Nuclear Medicine.

Sramek, B. B. (1981). Noninvasive technique for measurement of cardiac output by means of electrical impedance. *Proceedings of the 5th International Conference on Electrical Bioimpedance* (pp. 39–42). Tokyo.

Strauss, H. W., Pitt, B., & James, Jr., A. E. (1974). *Cardiovascular nuclear medicine.* St. Louis: Mosby.

Sung, B. H., Robinson, C., Thadani, U., Lee, R., & Wilson, M. F. (1986). Plasma catecholamine concentrations at onset of myocardial ischemia during supine bicycle exercise. *Federation Proceedings, 45*(3), 281.

Sung, B. H., Wilson, M. F., Robinson, C., Thadani, U., & Lovallo, W. R. (1988). Mechanisms of myocardial ischemia induced by epinephrine: Comparison with exercise-induced ischemia. *Psychosomatic Medicine, 50,* 381–393.

Teague, S. M. (1986). Measurement of ventricular function using Doppler ultrasound. In J. Kisslo, D. Adams, & D. B. Mark (Eds. *Basic Doppler echocardiography* (pp. 147–157). Edinburgh: Churchill Livingston.

Wagner, H. N., Jr., Rigo, P., Baxter, R. H., Alderson, P. O., Douglas, K. H., & Housholder, D. F. (1979). Monitoring ventricular function at rest and during exercise with a nonimaging nuclear detector. *American Journal of Cardiology, 43*(5), 975.

White, D. N. (1982). Johann Christian Doppler and his effect: A brief history. *Ultrasound in Medicine and Biology, 8,* 583.

Willerson, J. T. (1981). *Nuclear cardiology: Cardiovascular clinics.* A. N. Brest (Ed.). Philadelphia: Davis.

Wilson, F. N., Johnston, F. D., Rosenbaum, F. F., Erlanger, H., Kossmann, C. E., Hecht, H., Cotrim, N., De Oliveira, R. M., Scarsi, R., & Barker, P. S. (1944). The precordial electrocardiogram. *American Heart Journal, 27,* 19.

Wilson, M. F., Burow, R. D., Brackett, D. J., Sung, B. H., Thadani, U., & Schechter, E. (1982). Quantitative cardiac blood pool scintigraphic evaluation of responses to epinephrine infusion and exercise in normals and coronary disease. *American Journal of Cardiology, 49,* 992.

Wilson, M. F., Brackett, D. J., Thorsen, C. K., McDaniel, K., Schaefer, C. F., Wilson, M. L., & Folkers, K. (1984). Treatment of dilated cardiomyopathy by coenzyme Q_{10}: Evaluation of benefits by nuclear cardiography. In K. Folkers & Y. Yamamura (Eds.), *Biomedical and clinical aspects of coenzyme Q* (Vol. 4, pp. 403–416). Amsterdam: Elsevier.

Wilson, M. F., Sung, B. H., Thadani, U., Brackett, D. J., & Burow, R. D. (1985). Efficacy of myocardial contractility index to discriminate coronary disease. *Circulation, 72*(4), III–103.

Wilson, M. F., Sung, B. H., Robinson, C., Thadani, U., & Brackett, D. J. (1986). Dose–response effects of epinephrine on hemodynamics and left ventricular function in man with coronary artery disease (CAD). *Federation Proceedings, 45*(3), 196.

Wilson, M. F., Sung, B. H., Pincomb, G. A., & Lovallo, W. R. (in press). Simultaneous measurement of stroke volume by impedance and nuclear ventriculography: Comparison at rest and during exercise. *Annals of Biomedical Engineering.*

Winer, B. J. (1971). *Statistical principles in experimental design* (2nd ed.). New York: McGraw–Hill.

CHAPTER 3

The Experimental Study of Behaviorally Induced Arrhythmias

Vikas Saini and Richard L. Verrier

Introduction

The belief that psychological stress can precipitate major illness has long been accepted in both folk wisdom and medical thinking, but its scientific basis is fragmentary and incomplete.

The experimental study of behavioral factors in the induction of life-threatening arrhythmias constitutes one area in which notable advances have been made. This has been largely due to the development of well-defined behavioral models and the evolution of quantitative methods for assessing myocardial electrical stability. The availability of improved pharmacologic probes to factor out the effects of various components of the nervous system and the refinement of selective denervation procedures have contributed further to elucidation of mechanisms. The successful study of this area requires a continuous cross-fertilization of advanced techniques and concepts between the disciplines of neuroscience and cardiovascular physiology, two areas which are advancing at rapid rates.

This chapter will be guided by four major objectives: (1) to review basic concepts of electrophysiology and arrhythmogenesis and to specify the pathophysiologic features which should guide the development of experimental models; (2) to discuss the proper use and limitations of methods available to assess the influence of behavioral state on susceptibility to arrhythmias; (3) to summarize the current understanding of the mechanisms involved in behaviorally induced arrhythmias; and (4) to discuss how application of the latest developments in the neurosciences and in cardiac electrophysiology could further accelerate our progress in this field.

Basic Electrophysiology

As outlined in Chapters 1 and 2 of this handbook, the maintenance of a coordinated heartbeat in normal rhythm requires the adequate function of the specialized pacemaker and conducting tissue of the heart. A variety of disturbances of rhythm can occur at any point in the sequence of spontaneous depolarization, propagation of the impulse, and myocardial contraction. Many of these pathologic

Vikas Saini • Cardiovascular Laboratories, Harvard University School of Public Health, Boston, Massachusetts 02115.   *Richard L. Verrier* • Department of Cardiology, Tufts University Medical School, Boston, Massachusetts 02115, and Department of Pharmacology, Georgetown University Medical Center, Washington, D.C. 20007. V. S. is a postdoctoral fellow of the American Heart Association, Massachusetts Affiliate.

processes are influenced by neural factors and are thus suitable for behavioral study. Electrocardiography is the central technique for the measurement of normal cardiac electrical function and for the analysis of abnormalities of rhythm. In the following section, we will review those more specific measurement techniques which have been applied most successfully to the study of behavioral factors in arrhythmogenesis.

Classification of Arrhythmias

Examination of the body surface ECG allows, in most cases, the diagnosis of cardiac arrhythmias. These may be classified as follows:

- Supraventricular
    Atrial premature beats (APBs)
    Supraventricular tachycardia (SVT)
    Nonparoxysmal junctional tachycardia (NPJT)
    Multifocal atrial tachycardia (MAT)
    Atrial flutter
    Atrial fibrillation (AF)
- Ventricular
    Ventricular premature beats (VPBs)
    Ventricular tachycardia (VT)
    Ventricular fibrillation (VF)

Electrophysiologic Mechanisms

The study of underlying electrophysiologic mechanisms requires the use of many complex techniques for recording, from the cellular level to the three-dimensional mapping of cardiac electrical activity (Wit, 1985).

As suggested by Hoffman and Cranefield (1964), the primary mechanisms of arrhythmias may be classified into three categories: abnormal impulse initiation, abnormal conduction, or a combination of the two (Table 1).

Abnormal Impulse Initiation

Our current understanding of abnormalities of impulse initiation has resulted primarily from the recording of transmembrane potentials in vitro. Two types of abnormalities are distinguished, those of automaticity and those of triggered activity.

Automaticity, the capacity to initiate the action potential spike spontaneously, is normally limited to the specialized conducting tissue of the heart and is based on the slow phase 4 diastolic depolarization which occurs in these cells. Normally the electrical activity of the sinus node entrains the depolarization

Table 1. Mechanisms for Arrhythmias[a]

I	II	III
		Simultaneous abnormalities of impulse generation and conduction
Abnormal impulse generation	Abnormal impulse conduction	
A. Normal automatic mechanism	A. Slowing and block (e.g., S-A block, A-V block)	A. Parasystole
B. Abnormal automatic mechanism	B. Unidirectional block and reentry 1. Random reentry 2. Ordered reentry 3. Summation and inhibition	B. Slow conduction because of phase 4 depolarization
C. Triggered activity 1. Early afterdepolarization 2. Delayed afterdepolarization	C. Conduction block, electrotonic transmission, and reflection	

[a]From Wit (1985), as modified from Hoffman and Rosen (1981); reprinted by permission.

of the rest of the heart. However, if the resting membrane potential is reduced in lower portions of the conduction system or in portions of the myocardium itself, ectopic foci of spontaneous depolarization may emerge and capture the heart for one or more beats. Triggered activity is impulse initiation resulting from an afterdepolarization, a second depolarization of the membrane following soon after the initial one. Both mechanisms have been invoked to explain a wide variety of arrhythmias, including APBs, VPBs, NPJT, MAT, paroxysmal atrial tachycardia (PAT), and VT. Autonomic factors have been shown to influence both mechanisms. Thus, sympathetic activity is known to enhance automaticity and to cause the occurrence of triggered afterdepolarizations. Parasympathetic activation is known to decrease automaticity.

Abnormalities of Conduction

Fundamental to an understanding of this mechanism of arrhythmia is the concept of reentry. Reentry is said to occur when a propagating impulse returns to reexcite previously depolarized cardiac tissue which has completed its repolarization (Figure 1). The mechanism requires the existence of at least two functionally distinct pathways with some degree of slowing of conduction in one of those pathways and unidirectional block in the other. Thus, an impulse which is critically timed may block in the antegrade direction along one path while conducting slowly down the parallel one. If the recovery of excitability of the first path is then completed, it may be reexcited by the same impulse from the distal end. Clearly, these requirements can be met only for certain critical relationships between conduction velocity, path length, and refractory period. Under some circumstances, these relationships may result in an "endless loop" of excitation which repetitively captures the heart ("ordered reentry"), as in SVT, in which the reentrant loop travels through two pathways within the AV node, and in atrial flutter, in which the reentrant circuit involves a large portion of the atrium. In other settings, if the degree of electrophysiologic inhomogeneity is greater, impulse propagation may fractionate further and further along constantly changing pathways at changing

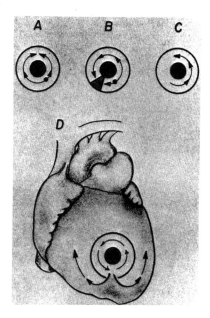

Figure 1. Schematic representation of reentry in a ring of cardiac tissue as described by Mines in 1914. In A, the ring was stimulated in the area indicated by the small black dot; impulses propagated away from the point of stimulation in both directions and collided; no reentry occurred. In B, the cross-hatched area was compressed while the ring was stimulated again at the black dot. The impulse propagated around the ring in only one direction, having been blocked in the other direction by the area of compression. Then immediately after stimulation, the compression was relieved, and in C, the unidirectionally circulating impulse is shown returning to its point of origin and then continuing around the loop. Identical reentry would occur if the cross-hatched area was a region of unidirectional conduction block, with the conduction block in the right-to-left direction. D shows how reentry in a loop of the kind described in A–C might cause arrhythmias if located in the heart. In this example, the loop is composed of ventricular muscle which is separated functionally from the rest of the ventricle along most of its border represented by the heavy black line (perhaps caused by fibrosis), but in functional continuity with the ventricles in one place, at its lower end. The arrows show how excitation waves could propagate into the ventricles from the continuously circulating impulse to cause ventricular tachycardia. From Wit (1985); reprinted by permission.

rates ("random reentry"). This is the essential feature of both AF and VF.

Methods of Investigation

The study of behavioral factors in arrhythmogenesis requires the creation of an adequate model for investigation. Such a model has four essential components: (1) a substrate in which the electrophysiologic mechanisms discussed above are present and sufficient to generate arrhythmia; (2) reliable measurement techniques for assessing arrhythmogenesis; (3) suitable behavioral models which reproduce commonly encountered life situations; (4) techniques for the elucidation of underlying mechanisms of behavioral effects.

Substrates

The model which holds the most interest on clinical grounds and which has been studied thoroughly to date is that of sudden cardiac death (SCD). Epidemiologic studies have confirmed that psychologic factors may provide protection or confer risk in its occurrence. Certain pathophysiologic features of SCD guide the creation of a model, and these need to be reviewed briefly.

Sudden Cardiac Death

There are over 300,000 such deaths in the United States annually, accounting for 15–20% of all natural fatalities and for over half of all fatalities due to coronary artery disease (CAD) (Lown, 1984). The development of resuscitative techniques, intensive care and ambulatory monitoring has unequivocally established VF as the terminal mechanism of death. The association with CAD is also well documented. Fully 75% of cases of SCD have significant multivessel terminal stenosis and myocardial scarring from prior infarctions.

The role of acute ischemia in the precipitation of VF remains to be quantified. Although a majority of those dying suddenly are known to have symptomatic CAD, fully one fourth will have VF as their first and only event. Evidence for acute myocardial infarction (MI) is present in only a minority of cases (Cobb, Werner, & Trobaugh, 1980). However, the occurrence of transient, often asymptomatic episodes of ischemia has been increasingly recognized and is currently the focus of intense investigation. Known mechanisms include (1) coronary vasospasm; (2) platelet aggregation, plugging, and release; and (3) thrombosis with or without reperfusion. The proportion of VF arrests

which are preceded by such episodes of transient ischemia remains to be established. The markedly increased rate of SCD in patients recently hospitalized for unstable angina suggests that the proportion will be high.

The development of the coronary care unit and routine in-hospital monitoring of patients after MI have also established that so-called "late-phase" arrhythmias, including VF, may occur without associated acute ischemia. In this setting, VF is often preceded by some period of sustained tachyarrhythmia of varying hemodynamic stability. Post-MI patients thus constitute a distinct population of SCD patients.

Electrophysiologic Features of Ischemia

The features of SCD discussed above highlight the importance of studying well-specified phases of the natural history of this disease. There is increasing evidence that different phases engender different electrophysiologic mechanisms of arrhythmia (Elharrar & Zipes, 1982).

Within minutes of an acute coronary artery occlusion, bipolar electrogram recordings demonstrate a transient increase in conduction velocity followed by a loss of amplitude and duration and by the delaying of activation, resulting in slowing of conduction. This delay in conduction in the ischemic zone would be an important component in the creation of conditions favoring reentry if it were substantial enough to outlast repolarization of adjacent zones and then reactivate them. The extent of conduction delay has been so correlated with the incidence of spontaneous tachyarrhythmias. Other investigations have demonstrated significant changes in refractory period duration and excitability threshold in the ischemic zone, and these factors undoubtedly influence the generation of arrhythmias, although the exact mechanisms remain to be determined.

If an occlusion is maintained beyond the initial phase, a second phase of spontaneous ventricular arrhythmia ensues. The electrophysiology of this period is not completely elucidated, but these arrhythmias are probably related in part to the increased automaticity of surviving Purkinje fibers in areas of recent infarction.

In humans the propensity to develop so-called "late phase" ventricular tachyarrhythmia, including VF, persists long after an acute MI has healed. Dogs in which only a single coronary artery is permanently occluded are not prone to this type of chronic arrhythmia. However, in recent years, Michelson, Spear, and Moore (1980) have developed methods for the production of infarctions which are more chronically arrhythmogenic. Hypothesizing that the richly developed collateral channels in dogs facilitate well-demarcated healing when single stage occlusions are carried out, these workers have resorted to occlusions with variable periods of release, or to the occlusion of a major vessel and multiple smaller epicardial vessels. The infarcts so produced are typically "mottled," with closely interpenetrated areas of viable and nonviable myocardium. Such infarcts have been found to be extremely susceptible to sustained tachyarrhythmias which are inducible days to months later. The electrophysiologic characteristics of these infarcts have been studied in some detail by El-Sherif and co-workers (El-Sherif, Scherlag, Lazzara, & Hope, 1977a; El-Sherif, Hope, Scherlag, & Lazzara, 1977b). Of note are the findings of delayed, slowly conducting, fractionated electrical activity, and a marked heterogeneity of excitability and refractory period at different sites in close proximity. On theoretical grounds, these findings would all favor the occurrence of reentry. The unique anatomy of these infarcts provides multiple potential conduction pathways which also favor reentrant mechanisms. The finding that the site of stimulation is important for the induction of a tachyarrhythmia underscores the fact that arrhythmogenesis is a complex interaction of geometry and electrophysiology.

Electrophysiology of VF

The sequence of events leading from the normally organized advancing wavefront of electrical activity to the chaotic activity of VF involves several electrophysiologic mechanisms operating at once in a complex, multilayered process. All of these can be present in ischemic heart disease (Surawicz, 1985).

As indicated above, VF, the final common path-

Table 2. Factors That May Enhance Vulnerability to Ventricular Fibrillation[a]

Large mass of myocardium
Local depolarization
Increased automaticity of Purkinje fibers
Transformation of nonpacemaker into pacemaker fibers
Slow conduction
  Localized focal block or preexcitation
  Generalized (including changes in membrane responsiveness)
Uniformly prolonged refractoriness (duration of action potential)
Increased nonuniformity of refractoriness
  Altered differences between Purkinje and ventricular fibers
  Increased dispersion of refractoriness in the ventricular myocardium

[a]From Surawicz (1985); reprinted by permission.

way of SCD, can be seen as an extreme, fractionated form of the phenomenon of reentry. Necessary for its initiation is an appropriately timed excitable stimulus delivered into an electrophysiologic matrix in which certain conditions of geometry, conduction velocity, and refractoriness are present. The subsequent propagation and maintenance of VF throughout the entire heart requires that a critical mass of myocardium be involved in the initial matrix. The premature stimulus may be due to automaticity, triggered activity, reentrant activation, or an artificially delivered electrical pulse. It follows that physiologic influences, including changes in behavioral state, which generate premature impulse formation or which slow conduction velocity or increase inhomogeneity of refractoriness will all increase vulnerability to fibrillation (Table 2) (Han, Garcia de Jalon, & Moe, 1964; Kolman, Verrier, & Lown, 1975; Verrier, 1987).

Techniques for the Measurement of Cardiac Electrical Vulnerability

Two general measurement strategies are available for assessing cardiac electrical instability: (1) passive recording techniques and (2) provocative electrical testing. In practice, there is considerable overlap between the two, and in the more sophisticated techniques the two approaches are complementary. In either case, the object measured may be VF itself, or some component of the electrophysiologic matrix out of which fibrillation emerges.

Recording Techniques/Spontaneous Arrhythmias

The first approach is to vary the substrate in ways known to re-create the conditions of arrhythmia formation, observing its spontaneous development and recording the process with greater or lesser degrees of sophistication. In this approach, the measurement technique generally utilized in behavioral studies to date has been the monitoring and recording of the surface ECG. This technique measures the final electrophysiologic "output" of the system, the ventricular arrhythmia itself. End points for this "noninvasive" measurement approach have included the generation of VPBs, the latency of VT or VF, or the incidence of either arrhythmia.

VPBs. VPBs are a heterogeneous population. They can occur due to the ectopic discharge of a focus of increased automaticity, due to the development of an area in which micro-reentry takes place, or due to macro-reentry. In the development of VF, VPBs could therefore play the role of the triggering premature impulse or merely be a sign of the onset of conditions of reentry. Given the multiple constraints for the development of VF, the experimental induction of VPBs, although clearly indicating alterations in cardiac electrical properties, cannot be considered a surrogate for VF.

A number of classification schemes for VPBs have been developed. In general, these incorporate considerations of frequency, multifocality, or repetitive features. The Lown grading system (Lown and Graboys, 1977) is one such approach (Table 3).

Latency of VT or VF. This is the time required from some experimental intervention which is arrhythmogenic, such as acute coronary artery occlusion or rapid infusion of a toxic dose of ouabain, to the point at which VT or VF emerges. Although this end point has been shown to be influenced by behavioral factors, the elucidation of underlying mechanisms is made more difficult by its physiologically ambiguous nature. It is unclear, for ex-

Table 3. A Grading System for Ventricular Premature Beats[a,b]

Grade	Characteristics of beat
0	No ventricular beats
1A	Occasional, isolated ventricular premature beats (less than 30/h): Less than 1/min
1B	Occasional, isolated ventricular premature beats (less than 30/h): More than 1/min
2	Frequent ventricular premature beats (more than 30/h)
3	Multiform ventricular premature beats
4A	Repetitive ventricular premature beats: Couplets
4B	Repetitive ventricular premature beats: Salvos
5	Early ventricular premature beats (i.e., abutting or interrupting the T wave)

[a]From Lown and Graboys (1977); reprinted by permission.
[b]This grading system is applied to a 24-h monitoring period and indicates the number of hours within that period that a patient has ventricular premature beats of a particular grade.

ample, whether behaviorally induced changes in latency of VF are a result of direct neural effects on electrophysiology or whether they reflect secondary changes in hemodynamic function expressed in the time domain.

Incidence of VF. The incidence of VF in an experimental protocol is the most reliable parameter available in the assessment of spontaneous electrical instability. However, as a relatively global assessment of myocardial electrical stability, its limitations must be acknowledged. Although behavioral states and pharmacological interventions may alter this measure, little information is derived regarding the mediating electrophysiologic mechanism. Furthermore, the need for repeated defibrillations reduces the utility of the method for tracking electrical stability in changing behavioral states.

Recent work in basic electrophysiology has developed more elaborate recording techniques to measure separately the various electrophysiologic components which create the conditions for arrhythmogenesis. Thus, multiple lead systems at the body surface, or, more invasively, at endocardial or epicardial sites, have been used to create maps of ventricular activation sequences, of the fractionation of impulse conduction, and of the dispersion of repolarization. Burgess (1982) and

Abildskov, Burgess, Lux, Wyatt, and Vincent (1976) in particular have developed "vulnerability maps" which graphically display increased dispersion of repolarization after a variety of physiologic interventions known to enhance ventricular vulnerability. This technique requires recording electrograms from 192 body surface sites. The QRS and ST-T, and QRST isoarea maps are created. By subtracting a normal T map from the map to be analyzed, those areas of increased dispersion of ventricular repolarization, the so-called vulnerability map, may be identified.

To date, none of these techniques have been applied to the study of behavioral states.

Cardiac Electrical Testing

The second major approach to the measurement of electrical stability involves the deliberate introduction of an impulse to perturb the system while recording the electrophysiologic consequences. It thus incorporates most features of the first approach while adding an element of control.

VF Threshold. Wiggers and Wegria (1940a,b) first showed the ability of a single electrical pulse to induce VF when delivered during a critical period of diastole. Han *et al.* (1964), utilizing a train of pulses, showed a similar effect. In both methods, the timing and the strength of the pulse were found to be critical factors.

In either case, the method is based on the notion that during the intrinsic inhomogeneity of repolarization, manifest as the T wave on a surface ECG (Figure 2), a vulnerable period exists in which a critically timed stimulus may further increase the dispersion of recovery, facilitate reentry, and so induce VF. Moore and Spear (1975) demonstrated that increasing current intensity induces greater dispersion of refractoriness. If one assumes that a fixed amount of dispersion is necessary to precipitate VF, then the enhanced intrinsic dispersion lowers the current necessary to induce VF. The amount of current required (VF threshold) thus varies inversely with the intrinsic degree of electrical stability and provides a quantitative measure of it.
sure of it.

The technique for measuring the VF threshold

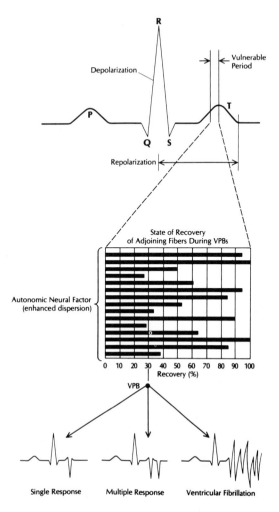

Figure 2. Fibrillation and sudden cardiac death may be presaged by ventricular premature beats (VPBs) that depolarize the ventricles during the vulnerable period of the cardiac cycle. They are particularly dangerous in an electrically unstable myocardium or when acute inputs to the heart, as by neural stimuli, have momentarily altered cardiac excitability to favor repetitive electric discharge. The vulnerable period corresponds to the time during the repolarization phase when there is marked dispersion in refractoriness and conduction velocity among adjacent myofibrils, so that these are at varying stages of recovery. Such conditions would be conducive to fractionation of recirculating wave fronts, resulting in rapid, disorganized activity, i.e., fibrillation (Lown, 1982).

requires attention to several methodologic details. First, appropriate scanning of the vulnerable period is necessary. By using a systematic approach it is possible to search the vulnerable period expeditiously and reliably. The measurements are carried out through a quadripolar electrode catheter which is placed in the right ventricular apex via a jugular vein under fluoroscopic control (Figure 3). The intracavitary ECG is recorded from the proximal pair of electrodes. The single-stimulus technique for VF threshold determination involves ventricular pacing at a constant rate of at least 10 beats above the intrinsic heart rate. Test impulses are generated by a constant-current square wave pulse generator current source (Mansfield, 1967). Timing is synchronized from the pacemaker stimulus. The test stimuli are delivered after every 10–12 paced beats, followed by inhibition of the pacemaker output for 3 s. The initial current strength of the test stimulus is set at 2 mA. Scanning of the vulnerable period begins at the end of the T wave and ends at the effective refractory period. Scanning intervals are of 5 or 10 ms duration, being equal to the width of the test stimulus. Current strength is then increased by 2 mA and scanning is repeated in the opposite direction. The lowest current strength at which VF is elicited defines the VF threshold (Figure 4A,B).

Numerous studies have shown a close corre-

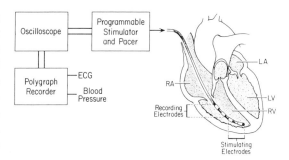

Figure 3. Experimental preparation for determination of the VF threshold. The measurements are made using a quadripolar electrode catheter which is placed in the apex of the right ventricle via a jugular vein. Pacing and test stimuli are delivered through the distal pair of electrodes. The intracavitary ECG is recorded from the proximal set of electrodes.

spondence between changes in the VF threshold and the spontaneous incidence of VF (Figures 5 and 6). Moreover, many interventions which alter dispersion of excitability and refractoriness alter VF threshold in the expected manner (Surawicz, 1985; Moore & Spear, 1975).

Several studies have shown apparent discrepan-

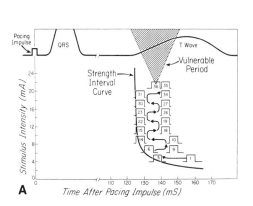

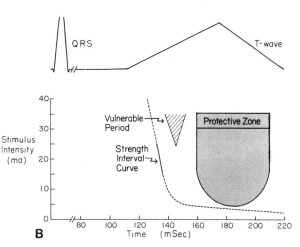

Figure 4. (A) Scanning of the vulnerable period using the single-stimulus technique. This figure is a schematic of the temporal relationships between the T wave of the ECG, strength interval curve, and the vulnerable period. During testing, heart rate is held constant by ventricular pacing. A 5-ms impulse with an initial current strength of 4 mA is delivered to coincide with the apex of the T wave (impulse #1). While the output is held at 4 mA, the vulnerable period is scanned in 5-ms decrements until the refractory period is encountered (impulse #5). The output is then increased to 6 mA (impulse #6) and scanning proceeds in 5-ms increments (impulse #9). In this

way, single pulses of increasing energy are delivered until the vulnerable zone is intercepted (impulse #36) to give a repetitive extrasystole threshold of 20 mA. (B) Location of the protective zone. Temporal relationships between T wave, vulnerable period, strength interval curve, and protective zone. The vulnerable-period curve has a characteristic V shape, the nadir of which coincides temporally with that for provoking ventricular fibrillation. The protective zone is a relatively broad zone which occurs 10 to 20 ms after the VP nadir and is approximately 50 ms in duration (Verrier & Lown, 1982).

Figure 5. Time course of changes in ventricular electrical stability following left anterior descending coronary artery occlusion in the dog. Cardiac response to electrical testing is designated above the bar, while the spontaneous rhythm is denoted inside the bar. VF, ventricular fibrillation; RVR, repetitive ventricular response; VT, ventricular tachycardia (Verrier & Lown, 1978).

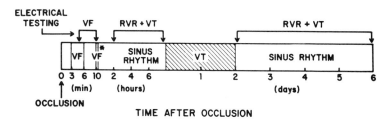

cies in the VF threshold when compared to spontaneous fibrillation (Jaillon, Schnittger, Griffin, & Winkle, 1980; Gaum, Elharrar, Walker, & Zipes, 1977). The method of testing requires careful attention, however (Table 4). The site of stimulation has been shown to be an important variable, especially if it includes ischemic tissue. In addition, the train of stimuli method has several limitations. The existence of a protective zone adjacent to the vulnerable period has been demonstrated (Verrier, Brooks, & Lown, 1978; Verrier & Lown, 1982). When it is activated by a second pulse, fibrillation can be prevented (Figure 4B). Furthermore, trains of pulses can liberate local catecholamines which can themselves distort the VF threshold (Euler, 1980). Thus, the single-stimulus method is preferred. However, it must be recognized that the usefulness of the VF threshold lies in the relative simplicity of the technique and the global assessment of myocardial electrical stability which it

provides. As with spontaneous fibrillation, it has limited usefulness for the elucidation of the complex three-dimensional changes within the electrophysiological substrate which occur in different pathologic conditions. Moreover, the necessity for defibrillation in this method imposes the same limitations on the study of behavioral factors as does the occurrence of spontaneous VF.

Electrical Testing in the Conscious Animal: RE Threshold. The search for a measure of cardiac electrical stability in the freely moving conscious animal led to the development of the repetitive extrasystole (RE) threshold as an index of vulnerability to VF (Matta, Verrier, & Lown, 1976a). As noted above, during VF threshold determination, a gradual increase in the stimulus intensity leads to a progressive increase in the number of spontaneous ventricular depolarizations following the premature stimulus until VF occurs (Figure

Figure 6. Changes in VF threshold induced by a 10-min period of left anterior descending coronary artery occlusion and by release. Note relation between the occurrence of ventricular arrhythmia and the reduction in threshold (solid line). VPB, ventricular premature beats; VTvp, ventricular tachycardia of the vulnerable period (Lown & Verrier, 1976).

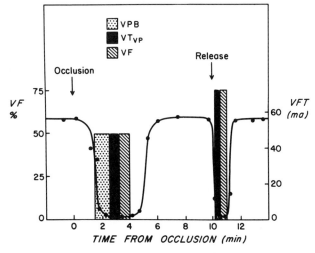

Table 4. Common Pitfalls in the Measurement of VF Threshold

Problems	Underlying causes	Solutions
Improper positioning of electrode catheter within the heart	Lack of suitable activation of myocardial tissue	Placement of catheter in apical region Electrodes should not be in infarcted region
Inadequate spatial separation of bipolar electrodes	Coagulative necrosis of myocardial tissue	Use of interelectrode distance of 1–1.5 cm
Inappropriate scanning technique (train of pulses)	Norepinephrine release within the myocardium Activation of the protective zone	Use of the single-stimulus technique
Inadequate pacing duration between test stimuli	Variable changes in location of the vulnerable period	Sequence of 10 to 12 paced beats before delivering test stimulus

4A). By increasing the current in a step-by-step fashion, we have found that a repetitive extrasystole, i.e., a *single* spontaneous ventricular depolarization after the test stimulus, occurs at approximately two-thirds of the energy required to provoke VF. This relationship holds under diverse experimental interventions which alter cardiac vulnerability (Verrier *et al.*, 1978; Matta *et al.*, 1976a; Lown & Verrier, 1976). As the animals do not perceive the test stimuli, the RE threshold method permits the detailed study of the effects of behavioral state on the vulnerable period threshold (Lown, Verrier, & Corbalan, 1973).

There are, of course, some limitations to the RE threshold method. First, about 8–10% of dogs do not show REs before the attainment of VF. This demonstrates that REs are not a necessary precursor to VF but represent instead a related phenomenon sharing a common electrophysiologic substrate. The use of the RE method therefore requires larger samples. A second limitation of the RE threshold method is seen upon assessing dogs in the postinfarct state when that infarction has been created by the occlusion/reperfusion method. Gang, Bigger, and Livelli (1982) found that in this form of experimental infarction, useful for its ability to create inducible sustained VT, the RE threshold/VF threshold ratio was lowered and the variability was increased. Thus, in experimental infarcts designed to study the electrophysiology of inducible sustained VT, the RE threshold may

have a limited role. On the other hand, sustained VT, especially if hemodynamically stable, would be the more appropriate end point for study in this model.

Electrical Testing for Sustained Tachyarrhythmias. As previously discussed, the electrophysiology of late-phase arrhythmia is different from that of acute ischemia. Electrical testing for the induction of sustained VT proceeds according to a different protocol. As during measurement of VF threshold, the heart is paced at a fixed rate. Unipolar cathodal stimulation at a single site is used for both pacing and premature stimulation. Diastole is similarly scanned in 10-ms decrements until the refractory period is reached. However, in this method of testing, the output of the premature stimulus is fixed at two or three times the middiastolic threshold. If no sustained tachyarrhythmia is induced, the first premature pulse is placed at a fixed coupling interval 10 ms beyond the refractory period, and a second premature impulse of the same intensity is utilized to scan diastole once more. If necessary, a third extra stimulus can be added, but beyond this number there is little increase in yield (Wellens, Brugada, & Stevenson, 1985).

Inducibility of a sustained arrhythmia is influenced by several stimulus parameters as well as by the number of premature extra stimuli.

Rate. Increased pacing rates increase the yield

of sustained VT but also increase the incidence of more nonspecific arrhythmias such as polymorphic VT or VF.

Site. Generally, right ventricular (RV) apical sites of stimulation are used. In theory, small changes in site may be adequate to render the geometry favorable for arrhythmia induction, but such a maneuver creates a problem of methodologic consistency. Use of the RV outflow tract, or even of sites within the LV, increases the yield of VT induction, but again increases the incidence of undesired arrhythmias such as VF.

Current output. By convention, this is generally measured as a multiple of the middiastolic threshold rather than an absolute value. In contrast to the measurement of VF threshold, there is at present little information on the effects of smaller increments of output on the inducibility of sustained VT.

Behavioral Models

Once the substrate for arrhythmia has been established as described above, the investigation of a possible role for psychological factors requires the addition of behavioral variables. Several models have been employed to define the effects of behavioral state on cardiac arrhythmogenesis.

Passive Restraint

Passive restraint models utilize some form of physical restraining device to effect immobilization, and all therefore share the problem of differentiating physical from psychological components of the stress experience. Despite this drawback, useful information can be obtained, as Natelson has shown in his studies of psychosomatic digitalis toxicity (Natelson, Cagin, Donner, & Hamilton, 1978).

Stress Adapation

Because the ability to adapt to recurrent stress appears to be an important determinant of disease outcome, models which incorporate features of repetition of stress or which allow the learning of coping mechanisms would be of interest. Although such approaches have not yet been fully developed in the study of arrhythmias, some work has been carried out. Natelson (1983) has shown that the arrhythmogenic effects of acute passive restraint can be nearly extinguished when repeated daily for 5 days. Another physically less taxing approach has been to examine the effects of an abrupt change in environment alone without any associated physical stress (Skinner, Lie, & Entman, 1975). In some cases, this relatively simple behavioral paradigm has been shown to exert significant effects which are discussed below.

Aversive Conditioning

In an attempt to separate physical from psychological components of stress, several versions of classical aversive conditioning have been employed. Signal–shock pairing utilizes a repetitively delivered signal (a flash of light, a loud tone) which is delivered alone in the control group, but is delivered in association with an aversive stimulus (e.g., cutaneous shock) in the experimental group. After the completion of a conditioning period, the presentation of the signal alone without the associated aversive stimulus is sufficient to elicit the aversive behavioral effects. Another approach is to use two different environments during the conditioning period. In this way, one setting (e.g., a sling) becomes the "stress" environment associated with aversive conditions whereas the other setting (e.g., undisturbed or free-roaming conditions in a cage) becomes the "relaxed" environment. Such paradigms may be refined further to study more specific behavioral components. In shock avoidance protocols, for example, the aspect of control of the environment may be added by including a lever or button which allows the subject to "escape" the stress.

The search for a model of a human emotion thought to confer risk for SCD led to the development of a model of anger in dogs (Verrier, Hagestad, & Lown, 1987). The protocol involves placing a dog in the nonaversive environment for 30 to 40 min. Thereafter, the dog is leashed and allowed to stand. A plate of food is presented and the animal is permitted to take a few bites. Then the plate is placed just out of reach. At this point, a second, provoker dog is brought into the room and allowed to approach the food. Upon observing

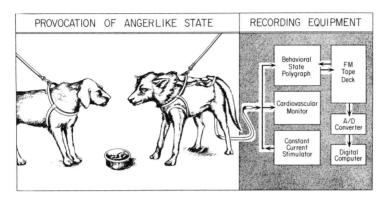

Figure 7. Experimental model of an angerlike state induced by food-access-denial (Verrier & Hohnloser, 1987).

this, the first dog may exhibit an angerlike state as indicated by growling and exposing its teeth. At no time is contact allowed between the animals (Figure 7). The anger response persists as long as the animals remain in sight of each other. These behavioral changes are associated with relatively consistent changes in heart rate and elevation of plasma catecholamine levels.

Techniques for the Elucidation of Underlying Mechanisms

Irrespective of the behavioral model used, when one finds significant effects on arrhythmia, attention naturally focuses on two possible mechanisms: (1) direct neural traffic to the heart and (2) neurohumoral influences. The investigation of neural pathways for the transmission of higher CNS activity to the heart requires study at many levels of the neuraxis. Investigational methods directed at higher levels are fewer, though growing. To date the most successful has been the use of intracranial electrodes to stimulate specific areas or nuclei in the brain, allowing observation of the effects on arrhythmia. The results of these studies and possible techniques for future use are discussed below. Most work has focused on direct autonomic effects on the heart. This is due both to the ready availability of appropriate pharmacologic probes and surgical interventions and to the sometimes forbidding complexity of the higher CNS.

Pharmacologic agents which have been used are diverse and increasing rapidly. They include β-adrenoreceptor agonists and antagonists, mus-

carinic agonists and antagonists, and centrally acting agents which alter autonomic outflow (morphine, diazepam). Surgical techniques include partial cardiac sympathectomy in which the stellate ganglia, ansa subclavia, and rami communicantes from T_2 to T_4 are excised, or complete sympathectomy in which the excision is extended to include the middle cervical ganglia and the upper thoracic trunks to the T_6 level (Schwartz & Stone, 1977). Complete vagotomy in dogs is achieved by bilateral sectioning of the vagosympathetic trunks in the neck. Selective vagotomy can also be accomplished surgically by a single-stage thoracotomy and intrapericardial dissection (Randall, Kaye, Thomas, & Barber, 1980; Randall, Thomas, Barber, & Rinkema, 1983).

Behavioral Factors in Ventricular Vulnerability

Current Knowledge

In the normal heart, passive restraint can reversibly induce unifocal VPBs in guinea pigs. In the conscious pig, severe physical stress can produce VF (Johansson, Jonsson, Lannek, Blomgren, Lindberg, & Poupa, 1974). Aversive conditioning and induction of an angerlike state have both been shown to reduce the RE threshold significantly (Figure 8). The magnitude of the effect is approximately 40–50% and is independent of heart rate *per se,* as this is fixed by pacing.

When the heart is sensitized by experimental

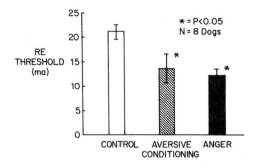

Figure 8. Effects of behavioral stress on the repetitive extrasystole (RE) threshold in normal dogs. Both passive aversive conditioning using a mild electric shock and induction of an angerlike state by food-access-denial produced significant reductions in the vulnerable period threshold. Heart rate was maintained constant during cardiac electrical testing by ventricular pacing (Verrier & Lown, 1984).

digitalis toxicity, passive restraint significantly increases the incidence of death at the lower end of the toxic dose range of the drug; however, adaptation to repeated stresses confers protection. Conditioning with a paired signal–shock during ouabain infusion causes an earlier emergence of VT than would occur in controls (Natelson, 1983).

The effects of stress during acute myocardial ischemia have been examined in more detail. Dogs which are exposed alternately to a nonaversive cage and an aversive sling environment during the occlusion–release sequence show a threefold increase in the incidence of VF during acute coronary artery occlusion in the aversive setting compared to the nonaversive environment (Verrier & Lown, 1979). The episodes of VF occur within 3–5 min of coronary artery occlusion or within 20–30 s following release and reperfusion, corresponding closely to the periods of maximum myocardial electrical instability as exposed by electrical testing. Skinner *et al.* (1975) observed a comparable profibrillatory effect of stress in pigs. Their model involved producing myocardial ischemia in animals prior to and after adaptation to the laboratory environment. In unadapted animals, coronary artery occlusion resulted in fibrillation within a few minutes. However, following 2–3 days of adaptation, the onset of fibrillation was substantially delayed or even entirely prevented.

The effect of stress during permanent coronary artery occlusion has also been explored (Corbalan, Verrier, & Lown, 1974). Exposure of dogs to a stressful environment during the quiescent phase prior to onset of spontaneous arrhythmia or after its termination consistently provoked diverse ventricular arrhythmias including VT and R-on-T extrasystoles. These effects disappeared when the animals were returned to the nonstressful cage setting. The arrhythmic response to psychologic stress waned over a 4- to 5-day period despite persistence of behavioral patterns indicative of stress. This time course corresponds to the recovery of ventricular electrical stability as exposed by cardiac testing with electrical or mechanical stimuli.

Thus, when psychologic stress is imposed during the periods of electrical instability associated with acute myocardial ischemia, VF is likely to be precipitated. When stress is induced during the later phases of one-stage MI, ventricular ectopic activity or VT are the main arrhythmias elicited.

The occlusion/reperfusion model of infarct, known to produce electrically inducible sustained VT, has not been evaluated in behavioral studies.

Mechanisms of Stress-Induced Arrhythmias

Autonomic Factors

The fully denervated heart has an extremely low propensity for ventricular arrhythmia. Autonomic neural pathways have been shown to play an important role in arrhythmogenesis through reflexly induced alterations in cardiac electrical properties even before behavioral factors are considered.

The sympathetic limb of the autonomic nervous system (ANS), acting primarily through direct neural traffic and to a lesser degree through circulating catecholamines, causes enhanced vulnerability to ventricular arrhythmia. The vagus nerve exerts a protective effect which is most pronounced in conditions in which adrenergic tone is increased, consistent with the finding that muscarinic activation results in both pre- and postsynaptic inhibition of noradrenergic transmission (Kolman *et al.*, 1975; Gilmour & Zipes, 1984). When behavioral stressors are superimposed on the system, these capabilities of the ANS are activated and constitute a crucial mediating link between higher nervous activity and the heart.

Normal Heart. Several studies indicate that pharmacologic or surgical sympathectomy in the absence of ischemia is effective in reducing the profibrillatory influence of diverse types of stress. Thus, it has been shown that β-adrenergic blockade completely prevents the effects of aversive conditioning or induction of anger on the vulnerable period threshold. It is noteworthy that unilateral or bilateral stellectomy is only partially effective, suggesting that adrenergic stimuli in addition to those derived from the stellate ganglia affect ventricular vulnerability during behavioral stress. Most probably these additional stimuli derive from other thoracic ganglia and from adrenal medullary catecholamines (Verrier & Lown, 1977; Matta, Lawler, & Lown, 1976b).

Several studies indicate that during biobehavioral stress, vagal activity exerts a protective effect on the normal heart which is not evident in nonstressful environments. This is the case whether vagal tone is due to spontaneous activity or results from administration of a vagomimetic agent such as morphine sulfate (DeSilva, Verrier, & Lown, 1978).

Ischemic Heart. The mechanisms of behaviorally induced arrhythmias during myocardial ischemia and infarction are only partially understood. In dogs, β-adrenergic blockade protects against arrhythmias associated with acute coronary artery occlusion during several forms of behavioral stress (Verrier & Lown, 1984; Rosenfeld, Rosen, & Hoffman, 1978). However, Skinner *et al.* (1975) showed in farm pigs that adaptation to a laboratory environment reduces and delays onset of VF during coronary artery obstruction, but β-adrenergic blockade with propranolol does not afford any protection in unadapted animals. It remains to be determined whether this is due to a failure of propranolol to block adequately adrenergic inputs to the heart, or to the involvement of extraadrenergic factors in the antifibrillatory effect of behavioral adaptation, or to species differences (Benfey, Elfellah, Ogilvie, & Varma, 1984).

The involvement of α-adrenergic receptors in stress-induced arrhythmias is as yet uncertain. This relates to the complexity of their influences, including both direct actions on myocardial excitable properties and indirect effects on insulin secretion, coronary hemodynamic function, and platelet aggregability.

Higher Neural Pathways

Electrical stimulation of various sites in the CNS can profoundly alter cardiac electrical stability and elicit a diversity of arrhythmias.

Excitation of the posterior hypothalamus, for example, substantially lowers the VF threshold in the normal canine heart and results in a tenfold increase in the incidence of spontaneous VF during acute coronary artery occlusion. This effect can be prevented by sympathectomy or β-adrenergic blockade but is not altered by vagotomy (Verrier, Calvert, & Lown, 1975; Manning & Cotten, 1962).

Skinner and Reed (1981) hypothesized that stressful environmental sensory information is integrated in the frontal cortex and impinges on the posterior hypothalamus. They have shown that cryogenic blockade of the cortical–brainstem pathway involved in this putative mechanism completely prevents the occurrence of VF in pigs with acute coronary artery occlusion.

Central Neurochemical Factors

There is a paucity of data on the role of specific neurotransmitter systems in fluctuations of autonomic outflow. Diazepam has been shown to exert an antiarrhythmic effect during behavioral stress, but the mechanism has not been established (Rosenfeld *et al.,* 1978). Blatt, Rabinowitz, and Lown (1979) showed that the intravenous administration of serotonin precursors to anesthetized dogs diminishes sympathetic neural traffic to the heart and increases the RE threshold. These results have not been extended to experiments in which agents are given orally, but this methodology holds promise for new, CNS-directed approaches to the pharmacotherapy of ventricular arrhythmia (Verrier, 1986; Saini, Carr, Hagestad, Lown, & Verrier, 1988).

Future Directions

It is evident that our understanding of behaviorally induced arrhythmias is far from complete. Further progress will depend on continuing advances in techniques in basic cardiac electrophysiology and the neurosciences and on the application of these to behavioral models. Some possible strategies are already evident, while others remain futuristic.

The development of sophisticated mapping techniques for the electrophysiologic study of tachyarrhythmias may provide insights into neural mechanisms at the level of the myocardium (Burgess, 1982; Kramer, Saffitz, Witkowski, & Corr, 1985; Janse, Wilms-Schopman, Wilensky, & Tranum-Jensen, 1985; Wit & Josephson, 1985). The relationship of anatomically inhomogeneous sympathetic and parasympathetic innervation to electrophysiologic inhomogeneity has yet to be elucidated and will undoubtedly require three-dimensional techniques. We can expect such studies to shed new light on the electrophysiologic consequences of sympathetic–parasympathetic interactions. Such information will be crucial to an understanding of behavioral effects.

The development of the occlusion–reperfusion model resulting in "mottled" infarcts with distinct electrophysiologic characteristics can also be used fruitfully in behavioral work. This model of postinfarct arrhythmias represents a large and fairly common management problem for clinicians, and yet no behavioral studies have been undertaken. Underlying neural mechanisms would be expected to be different since the effects of infarcted innervation would have to be considered (Barber, Mueller, Davies, Gill, & Zipes, 1985).

Higher in the neuraxis, the role of various brainstem nuclei in integrating the cardiovascular adaptation to behavioral stress needs to be studied. For example, experiments using the selective ablation of the nucleus tractus solitarius have yielded valuable insights into the role of baroreflex integration in the development of behaviorally induced hypertension (Nathan & Reis, 1977; Nathan, Tucker, Severini, & Reis, 1978). Application of such techniques to the study of behaviorally induced arrhythmias is warranted. Well-localized neuroinjection techniques need to be adapted to the freely moving conscious animal. This would allow the experimental study of specific neurotransmitter systems at specific brain sites and might open new avenues for the pharmacotherapy of arrhythmias.

Behavioral models appropriate to the wide range of human emotions are scarce. Our model of an angerlike state has been applied to the study of arrhythmias. Other models in contemporary use are discussed elsewhere in this handbook.

The neurohumoral component of brain–heart interactions remains largely unexplored. Pituitary secretion of β-endorphin as well as the other hormones may play a role in longer-term fluctuations in cardiac electrophysiologic properties. The recent discoveries of circulating peptides with significant cardiovascular effects (atrial natriuretic factor, γ-MSH, enkephalins) (Holtz, Sommer, & Bassenge, 1986; Sander, Giles, Kastin, Quiroz, Kaneish, & Coy, 1981) add another promising dimension to the study of brain–heart relationships.

ACKNOWLEDGMENT. Supported by Grants HL-32905, HL-33567, and HL-35138 from the National Heart, Lung and Blood Institute, National Institutes of Health.

References

Abildskov, J. A., Burgess, M. J., Lux, R. L., Wyatt, R., & Vincent, G. M. (1976). The expression of normal ventricular repolarization in the body surface distribution of T potentials. *Circulation, 54,* 901–906.

Barber, M. J., Mueller, T. M., Davies, B. G., Gill, R. M., & Zipes, D. P. (1985). Interruption of sympathetic and vagal-mediated afferent responses by transmural myocardial infarction. *Circulation, 72,* 623–631.

Benfey, B. G., Elfellah, M. S., Ogilvie, R. I., & Varma, D. R. (1984). Anti-arrhythmic effects of prazosin and propranolol during coronary artery occlusion and reperfusion in dogs and pigs. *British Journal of Pharmacology, 82,* 717–725.

Blatt, C. M., Rabinowitz, S. H., & Lown, B. (1979). Central serotonergic agents raise the repetitive extrasystole threshold of the vulnerable period of the canine ventricular myocardium. *Circulation Research, 44,* 723–730.

Burgess, M. J. (1982). Ventricular repolarization and electrocardiographic T wave form and arrhythmia vulnerability. In M. N. Levy & M. Vassalle (Eds.), *Excitation and neural control of the heart.* Bethesda: American Physiological Society.

Cobb, L. A., Werner, J. A., & Trobaugh, G. B. (1980). Sudden cardiac death. 2. Outcome of resuscitation; management, and future directions. *Modern Concepts in Cardiovascular Disease, 49,* 37–42.

Corbalan, R., Verrier, R. L., & Lown, B. (1974). Psychological stress and ventricular arrhythmias during myocardial infarction in the conscious dog. *American Journal of Cardiology, 34,* 692–696.

DeSilva, R. A., Verrier, R. L., & Lown, B. (1978). The effects of psychological stress and vagal stimulation with morphine on vulnerability to ventricular fibrillation (VF) in the conscious dog. *American Heart Journal, 95,* 197–203.

Elharrar, V., & Zipes, D. P. (1982). Cardiac electrophysiological alterations during myocardial ischemia. In M. N. Levy & M. Vassalle (Eds.), *Excitation and neural control of the heart.* Bethesda: American Physiological Society.

El-Sherif, N., Scherlag, B. J., Lazzara, R., & Hope, R. R. (1977a). Re-entrant ventricular arrhythmias in the late myocardial infarction period. 1. Conduction characteristics in the infarction zone. *Circulation, 55,* 686–701.

El-Sherif, N., Hope, R. R., Scherlag, B. J., & Lazzara, R. (1977b). Re-entrant ventricular arrhythmias in the late myocardial infarction period. 2. Patterns of initiation and termination of re-entry. *Circulation, 55,* 702–719.

Euler, D. E. (1980). Norepinephrine release by ventricular stimulation: Effect on fibrillation thresholds. *American Journal of Physiology, 238,* H406–H413.

Gang, E. S., Bigger, J. T., Jr., & Livelli, F. D., Jr. (1982). A model of chronic ischemic arrhythmias: The relation between electrically inducible ventricular tachycardia, ventricular fibrillation threshold and myocardial infarct size. *American Journal of Cardiology, 50,* 469–477.

Gaum, W. E., Elharrar, V., Walker, P. D., & Zipes, D. P. (1977). Influence of excitability on the ventricular fibrillation threshold in dogs. *American Journal of Cardiology, 40,* 929–935.

Gilmour, R. F., Jr., & Zipes, D. P. (1984). Evidence for prejunctional and postjunctional antagonism of the sympathetic neuroeffector junction by acetylcholine in canine cardiac Purkinje fibers. *Journal of the American College of Cardiology, 3,* 760–765.

Han, J., Garcia de Jalon, P., & Moe, G. K. (1964). Adrenergic effects on ventricular vulnerability. *Circulation Research, 14,* 516–524.

Hoffman, B. F., & Cranefield, P. F. (1964). The physiological basis of cardiac arrhythmias. *American Journal of Medicine, 37,* 670–684.

Hoffman, B. F., & Rosen, M. R. (1981). Cellular mechanisms for cardiac arrhythmias. *Circulation Research, 49,* 1–15.

Holtz, J., Sommer, O., & Bassenge, E. (1987). Inhibition of sympathoadrenal activity by atrial natriuretic factor in dogs. *Hypertension, 9,* 350–354.

Jaillon, P., Schnittger, I., Griffin, J. C., & Winkle, R. A. (1980). The relationship between the repetitive extrasystole threshold and the ventricular fibrillation threshold in the dog. Non-parallel changes following pharmacological intervention. *Circulation Research, 46,* 599–605.

Janse, M. J., Wilms-Schopman, F., Wilensky, R. J., & Tranum-Jensen, J. (1985). Role of the subendocardium in arrhythmogenesis during acute ischemia. In D. P. Zipes & J. Jalife (Eds.), *Cardiac electrophysiology and arrhythmias.* New York: Grune & Stratton.

Johansson, G., Jonsson, L., Lannek, N., Blomgren, L., Lindberg, P., & Poupa, O. (1974). Severe stress-cardiopathy in pigs. *American Heart Journal, 87,* 451–457.

Kolman, B. S., Verrier, R. L., & Lown, B. (1975). The effect of vagus nerve stimulation upon vulnerability of the canine ventricle: Role of sympathetic–parasympathetic interactions. *Circulation, 52,* 578–585.

Kramer, J. B., Saffitz, J. E., Witkowski, F. X., & Corr, P. B. (1985). Intramural reentry as a mechanism of ventricular tachycardia during evolving canine myocardial infarction. *Circulation Research, 56,* 736–754.

Lown, B. (1982). Clinical management of ventricular arrhythmias. *Hospital Practice, 17*(4), 73–86.

Lown, B. (1984). Cardiovascular collapse and sudden death. In E. Braunwald (Ed.), *Heart disease: A textbook of cardiovascular medicine.* Philadelphia: Saunders.

Lown, B., & Graboys, T. B. (1977). Sudden death: An ancient problem newly perceived. *Cardiovascular Medicine, 2,* 219–233.

Lown, B., & Verrier, R. L. (1976). Neural activity and ventricular fibrillation. *New England Journal of Medicine, 294,* 1165–1170.

Lown, B., Verrier, R. L., & Corbalan, R. (1973). Psychologic stress and threshold for repetitive ventricular response. *Science, 182,* 834–836.

Manning, J. W., & Cotten, M. D. (1962). Mechanism of cardiac arrhythmias induced by diencephalic stimulation. *American Journal of Physiology, 203,* 1120–1124.

Mansfield, P. B. (1967). Myocardial stimulation: The electrochemistry of electrode–tissue coupling. *American Journal of Physiology, 212,* 1475–1488.

Matta, R. J., Verrier, R. L., & Lown, B. (1976a). Repetitive extrasystole as an index of vulnerability to ventricular fibrillation. *American Journal of Physiology, 230,* 1469–1473.

Matta, R. J., Lawler, J. E., & Lown, B. (1976b). Ventricular electrical instability in the conscious dog: Effects of psychologic stress and beta adrenergic blockade. *American Journal of Cardiology, 38,* 594–598.

Michelson, E. L., Spear, J. F., & Moore, E. N. (1980). Electrophysiologic and anatomic correlates of sustained ventricular tachyarrhythmias in a model of chronic myocardial infarction. *American Journal of Cardiology, 45,* 583–590.

Moore, E. N., & Spear, J. F. (1975). Ventricular fibrillation threshold: Its physiological and pharmacological importance. *Archives of Internal Medicine, 135,* 446–453.

Natelson, B. H. (1983). Stress, predisposition and the onset of serious disease: Implications about psychosomatic etiology. *Neuroscience and Biobehavioral Reviews, 7,* 511–527.

Natelson, B. H., Cagin, N. A., Donner, K., & Hamilton, B. E. (1978). Psychomatic digitalis-toxic arrhythmias in guinea pigs. *Life Sciences, 22,* 2245–2250.

Nathan, M. A., & Reis, D. J. (1977). Chronic labile hypertension produced by lesions of the nucleus tractus solitarii in the cat. *Circulation Research, 40,* 72–81.

Nathan, M. A., Tucker, L. W., Severini, W. H., & Reis, D. J. (1978). Enhancement of conditioned arterial pressure responses in cats after brainstem lesions. *Science, 201,* 71–73.

Randall, W. C., Kaye, M. P., Thomas, J. X., & Barber, M. J. (1980). Intrapericardial denervation of the heart. *Journal of Surgical Research, 29,* 101–109.

Randall, W. C., Thomas, J. X., Jr., Barber, M. J., & Rinkema, L. E. (1983). Selective denervation of the heart. *American Journal of Physiology, 244,* H607–H613.

Rosenfeld, J., Rosen, M. R., & Hoffman, B. F. (1978). Pharmacologic and behavioral effects on arrhythmias that immediately follow abrupt coronary occlusion: A canine model of sudden coronary death. *American Journal of Cardiology, 41,* 1075–1082.

Saini, V., Carr, D. B., Hagestad, E. L., Lown, B., & Verrier, R. L. (1988). Antifibrillatory action of the narcotic agonist fentanyl. *American Heart Journal, 115,* 598–605.

Sander, G. E., Giles, T. D., Kastin, A. J., Quiroz, A. C., Kaneish, A., & Coy, D. H. (1981). Cardiopulmonary pharmacology of enkephalins in the conscious dog. *Peptides, 2,* 403–407.

Schwartz, P. J., & Stone, H. L. (1977). Tonic influence of the sympathetic nervous system on myocardial reactive hyperemia and on coronary blood flow distribution in dogs. *Circulation Research, 41,* 51–58.

Skinner, J. E., & Reed, J. C. (1981). Blockade of frontocortical–brain stem pathway prevents ventricular fibrillation of ischemic heart. *American Journal of Physiology, 240,* H156–H163.

Skinner, J. E., Lie, J. T., & Entman, M. L. (1975). Modification of ventricular fibrillation latency following coronary artery occlusion in the conscious pig. The effects of psychological stress and beta-adrenergic blockade. *Circulation, 51,* 656–667.

Surawicz, B. (1985). Ventricular fibrillation. *Journal of the American College of Cardiology, 5,* 43B–54B.

Verrier, R. L. (1986). Neurochemical approaches to the prevention of ventricular fibrillation. *Federation Proceedings, 45,* 2191–2196.

Verrier, R. L. (1987). Mechanisms of behaviorally induced arrhythmias. *Circulation, 76,* I48–I56.

Verrier, R. L., & Hohnloser, S. H. (1987). How is the nervous system implicated in the genesis of cardiac arrhythmias? In D. J. Hearse, A. S. Manning, & M. J. Janse (Eds.), *Life-threatening arrhythmias during ischemia and infarction.* New York: Raven Press.

Verrier, R. L., & Lown, B. (1977). Effects of left stellectomy

on enhanced cardiac vulnerability induced by psychologic stress [abstract]. *Circulation, 55/56,* III80.

Verrier, R. L., & Lown, B. (1978). Influence of neural activity on ventricular electrical stability during acute myocardial ischemia and infarction. In E. Sandøe, D. G. Julian, & J. W. Bell (Eds.), *Management of ventricular tachycardia: Role of mexiletine.* Amsterdam: Excerpta Medica.

Verrier, R. L., & Lown, B. (1979). Influence of psychologic stress on susceptibility to spontaneous ventricular fibrillation during acute myocardial ischemia and reperfusion [abstract]. *Clinical Research, 27,* 570A.

Verrier, R. L., & Lown, B. (1982). Prevention of ventricular fibrillation by use of low-intensity electrical stimuli. *Annals of the New York Academy of Sciences, 382,* 355–370.

Verrier, R. L., & Lown, B. (1984). Behavioral stress and cardiac arrhythmias. *Annual Review of Physiology, 46,* 155–176.

Verrier, R. L., Calvert, A., & Lown, B. (1975). Effect of posterior hypothalamic stimulation on ventricular fibrillation threshold. *American Journal of Physiology, 228,* 923–927.

Verrier, R. L., Brooks, W. W., & Lown, B. (1978). Protective zone and the determination of vulnerability to ventricular fibrillation. *American Journal of Physiology, 234,* H592–H596.

Verrier, R. L., Hagestad, E. L., & Lown, B. (1987). Delayed myocardial ischemia induced by anger. *Circulation, 75,* 249–254.

Wellens, H. J. J., Brugada, P., & Stevenson, W. G. (1985). Programmed electrical stimulation of the heart in patients with life-threatening ventricular arrhythmias: What is the significance of induced arrhythmias and what is the correct stimulation protocol? *Circulation, 72,* 1–7.

Wiggers, C. J., & Wegria, R. (1940a). Ventricular fibrillation due to single, localized induction and condenser shocks applied during the vulnerable phase of ventricular systole. *American Journal of Physiology, 128,* 500–505.

Wiggers, C. J., & Wegria, R. (1940b). Quantitative measurement of the fibrillation thresholds of the mammalian ventricles with observations on the effect of procaine. *American Journal of Physiology, 131,* 296–308.

Wit, A. L. (1985). Cardiac arrhythmias: Electrophysiologic mechanisms. In H. J. Reiser & L. N. Horowitz (Eds.), *Mechanisms and treatment of cardiac arrhythmias: Relevance of basic studies to clinical management.* Munich: Urban & Schwarzenberg.

Wit, A. L., & Josephson, M. E. (1985). Fractionated electrograms and continuous electrical activity: Fact or artifact? In D. P. Zipes & J. Jalife (Eds.), *Cardiac electrophysiology and arrhythmias.* New York: Grune & Stratton.

CHAPTER 4

The Measurement of Blood Pressure

Thomas G. Pickering and Seymour G. Blank

Arterial pressure is one of the most widely measured cardiovascular variables, but the ideal technique has yet to be developed. A number of methods have been described, all of which have their own advantages and disadvantages. Central to any consideration of these is an appreciation of the enormous variability of blood pressure: a single measurement of pressure made at a discrete point in time may have very little meaning. This is particularly relevant to behaviorally oriented studies, where the emphasis is commonly on the transient changes of pressure occurring in response to a behavioral challenge. Therefore, methods capable of taking multiple measurements over a relatively short space of time are desirable. Currently available methods are reviewed below.

The Arterial Pressure Wave

The arterial pressure wave has an initial rapidly rising phase followed by an early systolic peak known as the percussion wave, followed by a second late systolic peak or bulge (the tidal wave). Following this second peak, there is a notch or incisura corresponding to aortic valve closure. During diastole, there is a gradual decrease of

pressure as runoff proceeds to the peripheral circulation. There may be a third wave known as the diastolic or dicrotic wave.

The maximum (systolic) pressure may occur either during the early (percussion) wave or late (tidal) wave; diastolic pressure is taken as the minimum pressure at the end of the runoff period. Pulse pressure is the difference between systolic and diastolic pressure. Mean arterial pressure is the area under the pulse wave divided by the cardiac cycle duration, and is often taken to be diastolic pressure plus one third of the pulse pressure, but this will depend on the shape of the pulse wave (Geddes, 1984). These are shown in Figure 1.

The shape of the arterial pressure wave varies according to a number of factors. The arterial pressure wave can be considered as being the summation of an incident and a reflected wave, and it is generally agreed that wave reflection and the physical properties of the arterial wall are significant factors responsible for propagating arterial pressure pulse changes (O'Rourke, 1984). Progressive changes occur as the wave proceeds to the peripheral circulation, with an increase of pulse pressure and the maximal rate of rise (dp/dt). Thus, because mean pressure decreases slightly at more peripheral sites, there is an increase of systolic pressure and a decrease of diastolic pressure (Kroeker & Wood, 1956). For a person with an aortic pressure of 122/81 mm Hg, the corresponding pressures might be 131/79 in the brachial artery and 136/77 in the radial.

Thomas G. Pickering and Seymour G. Blank • Department of Medicine, Cardiovascular Center, New York Hospital–Cornell Medical Center, New York, New York 10021.

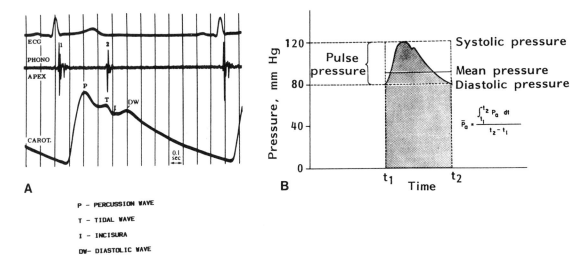

A

P - PERCUSSION WAVE

T - TIDAL WAVE

I - INCISURA

DW- DIASTOLIC WAVE

Figure 1. (A) Contour of the arterial pressure wave and its various components, together with the corresponding timing of the ECG and heart sounds (Phono). (B) Relationship between systolic, diastolic and mean pressure.

Spontaneous Variations of Arterial Pressure

The arterial pressure is subject to a number of types of cyclical variability. The shortest periodicity of these is the sinusoidal variations of pressure that accompany respiration, which were first observed by Stephen Hales in 1733. The relationship between blood pressure and respiratory phase depends on the respiratory rate: at moderate rates of breathing the pressure falls during most of inspiration, but at slower rates pressure rises during inspiration (Dornhorst, Howard, & Leathart, 1952); the amplitude of variation is around 5 mm Hg. The respiratory fluctuations are more pronounced in the upright than the supine position; pulse pressure also fluctuates more widely when upright. This variability may be partly due to vagally mediated effects on heart rate (sinus arrhythmia) because it can be diminished by atropine (Clement, Jordaens, & Heyndrickx, 1984).

During periods of breath-holding (apnea) regular pressure waves may still occur, with a periodicity of 6 per min. These have been variously termed Traube–Hering, or Mayer waves (Heymans & Neil, 1958).

Slower fluctuations, with a periodicity of 90 min, have been described in animals, but their significance in humans is unproven.

Direct Intraarterial Recording

This is generally accepted as the "gold standard" of arterial pressure measurement against which other methods are compared. It has the great advantage of being the only method that can assess beat-to-beat changes of pressure for more than a very short time, but is invasive and not free of risk.

The sites most commonly used for intraarterial pressure recording are the brachial and radial arteries. Although intraarterial recording is potentially the most accurate method, its accuracy may be limited by the frequency response of the recording system. Such recordings are commonly made with a long thin fluid-filled line connecting the artery and the transducer. This low-compliance coupling may adversely affect the fidelity of the intraarterial pressure being recorded, often taking the form of an overshoot of systolic pressure. In addition, such lines may contain small air bubbles, and these factors may interact to cause substantial damping and distortion of the signal (Geddes, 1984). It is now possible to obtain catheter-tip transducers of sufficiently small size to be inserted in the brachial artery, which avoid these problems, and which also give recordings that are free of artifact.

Noninvasive Techniques for Measuring Blood Pressure

Korotkoff Sound Technique

Despite continued efforts to find a superior method, the technique first described by Korotkoff in 1905 is still the most widely used, both for clinical measurement of blood pressure and for automatic recorders. The mechanism of the origin of the Korotkoff sounds has been a subject of debate for many years. The two most popular theories are that they are caused by pressure-induced movement of the arterial wall, or by turbulent flow through the compressed arterial lumen. Most of the evidence favors the former; thus, McCutcheon and Rushmer (1967) showed that the sounds occur before there is any real increase of flow, and Dock (1980), using a model with isolated segments of artery, concluded that they are due to a sudden tautening of the arterial wall.

Several studies have compared measurements taken by the auscultatory Korotkoff sound method and intraarterial recordings, and have generally reported correlations better than 0.9. Systolic pressure is more reliably detected than diastolic pressure, since, as conventionally recorded, there is a gradual diminution in the intensity of the sounds at around diastolic pressure.

There is still no universal agreement as to which phase of the Korotkoff sounds should be used for recording diastolic pressure. Phase four (muffling) is about 8 mm Hg higher than the intraarterial di-

astolic pressure, and is more subject to interobserver error; phase five (disappearance) is about 2 mm Hg higher than the true diastolic pressure (Short, 1976).

The official recommendation of the American Heart Association was formerly to report both the fourth and fifth phases (Kirkendall, Burton, Epstein, & Fries, 1967), but more recently to use the fifth phase, except in children (Kirkendall, Feinlieb, Fries, & Mark, 1981). Most of the large-scale clinical trials which have evaluated the benefits of treating hypertension have used the fifth phase, although the Framingham study, which has given us much of our knowledge about the risks associated with hypertension, used the fourth phase. Most people today use the fifth phase.

A number of factors may lead to inaccuracies with the Korotkoff sound technique. The size of the cuff relative to the diameter of the arm is critical. (See Table 1 and discussion of problems related to age and obesity below.) Blood pressure measurements are also influenced by the position of the arm. Both systolic and diastolic readings may change by as much as 20 mm Hg by moving the arm through 90° (Webster, Newnham, Petrie, & Lovell, 1984).

Observer error and observer bias are important sources of error when conventional sphygmomanometers are used. Differences of auditory acuity between observers may lead to consistent errors, and digit preference is very common, with most observers recording a disproportionate number of readings ending in 5 or 0 (Pickering, 1968). The level of pressure that is recorded may also be profoundly influenced by behavioral factors related to the effects of the observer on the subject; the best known of these is the presence of a physician. It has been known for more than 40 years that blood pressures recorded by a physician can be as much as 30 mm Hg higher than pressures taken by the patient at home, using the same technique and in the same posture (Ayman & Goldshine, 1940). Physicians also record higher pressures than do nurses or technicians (Mancia *et al.*, 1983). In our own population of patients with mild hypertension (diastolic pressures between 90 and 104 mm Hg), we have estimated that approximately 20% have

Table 1. Recommended Cuff Sizes for Auscultatory Measurement of Blood Pressure

Arm circumference (cm)	Cuff type	Cuff size (cm) Kirkendall et al. (1981)	Maxwell et al. (1982)
<7.5	Newborn	3 × 5	
7.5–13	Infant	5 × 8	
13–20	Child	8 × 13	
17–26	Small adult	11 × 17	
24–32	Adult	13 × 24	12 × 23
32–42	Large adult	17 × 32	15 × 33
>42	Thigh	20 × 42	18 × 36

"white coat" hypertension, i.e., pressures that are persistently high in the presence of a physician, but normal at other times. Other factors that influence the pressure that is recorded may include both the race and sex of the observer; Comstock (1957) found that men tended to have higher pressures when measurement was taken by a woman than by a man, whereas the opposite was true for women.

There are also technical sources of error with the auscultatory method, although these are usually much lower when a mercury column is used than with many of the semiautomatic methods (see below). These include the position of the column, which should be at approximately the level of the heart; the mercury should read zero when no pressure is applied; and it should fall freely when the pressure is reduced (this may not occur if the mercury is not clear or if the pinhole connecting the mercury column to the atmosphere is blocked). With aneroid meters, it is essential that they be checked against a mercury column both at zero pressure and when pressure is applied to the cuff. Surveys of such devices used in clinical practice have shown them to be frequently inaccurate (Burke, Towers, O'Malley, Fitzgerald, & O'Brien, 1982).

Random Zero Sphygmomanometer

Some of the sources of observer error, e.g., digit preference, may be reduced by the use of a random zero (Hawksley) sphygmomanometer. This device was developed by Wright and Dore (1970),

and is a mercury sphygmomanometer whose zero point may be varied randomly; after a reading is taken, the zero value is subtracted from it to give the true reading. The elimination of digit preference is more apparent than real, however, because although it may not appear in the final value, it may still occur when the pressures are read off the mercury column. It does not, of course, eliminate the more subtle psychosocial effects due to the interaction of the observer and the subject.

Korotkoff Sound Monitors

A number of investigators have constructed blood pressure tracking devices which can track changes in blood pressure using a servoloop which operates to maintain the Korotkoff sound at a constant intensity (Shapiro, Schwartz, & Tursky, 1972). Because it causes less discomfort and congestion of the arm, diastolic pressure is usually preferred for this purpose. The Korotkoff sounds are detected by a microphone under a sphygmomanometer cuff; if the intensity of the sounds decreases as a result of an increase of arterial pressure, air is pumped into the cuff until the sounds return to the equilibrium level. These devices can measure changes of pressure for periods of about 2 min at a time with reasonable accuracy.

Oscillometric Technique

This was first demonstrated by Marey in 1876, and it was subsequently shown that when the oscillations of pressure in a sphygmomanometer cuff are recorded during gradual deflation, the point of maximal oscillation corresponds to the mean intra-arterial pressure (Mauck, Smith, Geddes, & Bourland, 1980). The oscillations begin above systolic pressure and continue below diastolic, so that systolic and diastolic pressure can only be estimated indirectly according to some empirically derived algorithm. One advantage of the method is that no transducer need be placed over the brachial artery, so that placement of the cuff is not critical. The method works reasonably well in general, but may be seriously in error in some patients (Ramsey, 1979; Yelderman & Ream, 1979).

Ultrasound Techniques

Devices employing this technique use an ultrasound transmitter and receiver placed over the brachial artery under a sphygmomanometer cuff. As the cuff is deflated the movement of the arterial wall at systolic pressure causes a Doppler phase shift in the reflected ultrasound, and diastolic pressure is recorded as the point at which diminution of arterial motion occurs (Ware & Laenger, 1967). Another variation of this method detects the onset of blood flow at systolic pressure, and has been found to be of particular value for measuring pressure in infants and children (Elseed, Shinebourne, & Joseph, 1973; Steinfeld, Dimich, Reder, Cohen, & Alexander, 1978). Such devices compare favorably with other techniques (Hochberg & Solomon, 1971); however, their accuracy in measuring diastolic pressure in infants and children has been questioned (Reder, Dimich, Cohen, & Steinfeld, 1978).

Pulse Transit Time Technique

The velocity of the pulse wave along an artery is proportional to the arterial pressure, and this technique has been used to evaluate changes of blood pressure by measuring changes of pulse wave velocity, by recording either the interval between the R wave of the ECG and the radial pulse, or the interval between brachial and radial pulses. Although the method has the advantages of not requiring a cuff and being theoretically suitable for

beat-to-beat measurement of blood pressure, its accuracy is unacceptably low (Pollack & Obrist, 1983; Steptoe, Smulyan, & Gribbin, 1976). In addition, the correlations between values for pulse wave velocity measured over different parts of the arterial system, e.g., R wave to brachial artery, and brachial to radial artery, are low (Lane, Greenstadt, & Shapiro, 1983).

Finger Cuff Method of Penaz

This interesting method was first developed by Penaz (1973), and works on the principle of the "unloaded arterial wall." Arterial pulsation in a finger is detected by a photoplethysmograph under a pressure cuff. The output of the plethysmograph is used to drive a servoloop which rapidly changes the cuff pressure to keep the output constant, so that the artery is held in a partially opened state. The oscillations of pressure in the cuff are measured, and have been found to resemble the intraarterial pressure wave in most subjects (Molhoek et al., 1983). This method gives an accurate estimate of systolic and diastolic pressure, although both may be underestimated when compared to brachial artery pressures (Wesseling, deWit, Settels, & Klawer, 1982); the cuff can be kept inflated for up to 2 h. It is now available in a commercial form, but is unlikely to be suitable for ambulatory recordings because of movement artifact. A variant of this method has been described by Aaslid and Brubakk (1981), who measured flow with an ultrasound transducer placed over the brachial artery distal to a cuff. A servoloop system operated to keep the artery partly compressed with a constant flow. This method also correlated well with intraarterial pressures.

Korotkoff Signal (K₂) Technique

We have recently described a technique of indirect blood pressure measurement which is based on waveform analysis of the Korotkoff signal (Blank et al., 1988), and uses a specially designed transducer called a foil electret sensor, which gives an accurate rendition of both the low-frequency and high-frequency components of the signal (West, Bush-Vishniac, Harshfield, & Pickering, 1983).

With this technique, we have identified three components, which we have termed K_1, K_2, and K_3 (Figure 2). K_1 is a low-frequency low-amplitude signal that can be detected at cuff pressures above systolic. As cuff pressure is reduced, a high-frequency component (K_2) develops, and we have found that its appearance corresponds precisely to systolic pressure. With further reduction of cuff pressure, a third component (K_3) appears, which resembles the arterial pressure waveform. K_2 disappears at diastolic pressure, and therefore corresponds roughly to the audible Korotkoff sound. The potential advantage of blood pressure measurement by the "K_2 algorithm" is that it can be done on the basis of pattern recognition rather than by an absolute level of sound, which varies greatly from one individual to another. We suspect that K_2 originates from sudden movement of the arterial wall. We have shown that the K_2 method gives readings that are closer to true intraarterial pressure than the auscultatory method. Although this technique is not yet generally available, it can be repli-

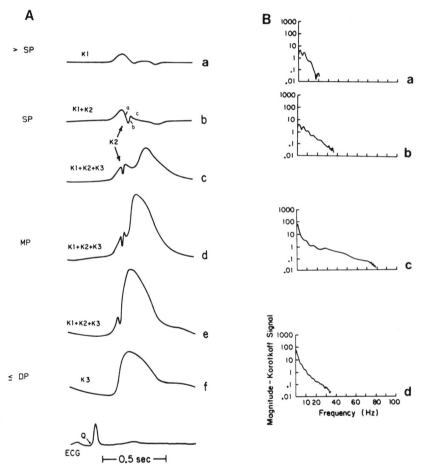

Figure 2. (A) Time domain changes in the Korotkoff signal at various levels of cuff pressure. The timing of each trace is linked to the ECG. (a) Cuff pressure above systolic; (b) cuff pressure at systolic; (c) cuff pressure slightly below systolic; (d) cuff pressure approximately equal to mean arterial pressure; (e) cuff pressure slightly above diastolic; (f) cuff pressure at diastolic and below. (B) Frequency spectral analysis (using 2048-point fast Fourier transform) of corresponding signal in left panel. The ordinate represents the magnitude of the Fourier coefficients. The relative energy contained in the signal is the area under the curve of the square of the magnitude of the Fourier coefficients versus frequency. (a) Above systolic; (b) at systolic; (d) mean arterial pressure; (f) diastolic and below.

cated using any sensor-amplifier system that has an appropriately wide frequency response (including low frequencies).

Automatic and Semiautomatic Blood Pressure Monitors

A large number of devices which monitor blood pressure automatically are now available. Virtually all use a sphygmomanometer cuff, and operate by either Korotkoff sound detection, oscillometry, or ultrasound. Some are suitable for home monitoring of blood pressure, whereas others are better for laboratory studies. They have several obvious advantages: one is that they eliminate observer error and observer bias, and may print out the readings as well as displaying them. We have evaluated a number of such devices, and have come to the following conclusions (Pickering, Cvetkovski, & James, 1986): First, many of the recorders are inaccurate, giving readings that are consistently more than 5 mm Hg in error when compared with simultaneously determined auscultatory values; second, no single method of recording, e.g., oscillometric or Korotkoff sound, is consistently superior; and third, there is no correlation between the price and the accuracy of the recorders. It is essential that any automatic recorder be calibrated against auscultatory readings in each subject.

Measurement of Blood Pressure in Special Populations and Circumstances

Infants and Children

Conventional techniques such as the auscultatory method may give systematic errors in infants, where the true systolic pressure may be underestimated (Elseed *et al.*, 1973). For indirect measurements the best technique is using an ultrasonic flow detector (e.g., a Parks Doppler unit) coupled with an appropriately designed (e.g., Pedisphyg) cuff (Elseed *et al.*, 1973; Steinfeld *et al.*, 1978; Reder *et al.*, 1978). In children over the age of 12

the auscultatory method may be used, provided that the appropriate sized cuff is used (Table 1).

Elderly Subjects

In older people there is often an increase of systolic pressure without a corresponding increase of diastolic. This has been attributed to a diminished distensibility of the arteries with increasing age. In extreme cases this may result in a diminished compressibility of the artery by the sphygmomanometer cuff, so that falsely high readings may be recorded, often referred to as pseudohypertension of the elderly (Spence, Sibbald, & Cape, 1978). In such individuals the only accurate method of measuring the arterial pressure is with direct intraarterial recordings, which may reveal pressures 30 mm Hg lower than noninvasive techniques.

Obese Subjects

It is well known that the accurate estimation of blood pressure using the auscultatory method requires an appropriate match between cuff size and arm diameter. In obese subjects the regular adult cuff (12 × 23 cm) may seriously overestimate blood pressure (Nielsen & Janniche, 1974). Maxwell, Waks, Schroth, Karam, and Dornfeld (1982) compared readings in obese subjects taken with the three available cuff sizes for adults, and recommended that the appropriate cuff size be selected according to the arm diameter, as shown in Table 1. These recommendations are somewhat different than the earlier recommendations of the American Heart Association, also shown in Table 1.

Posture

When a normal subject goes from the lying to the standing position, there is usually no change or a slight fall in systolic pressure, but diastolic pressure increases by a few millimeters. This occurs because blood is shifted from the thorax to the legs, so that stroke volume and cardiac output decrease, but the effects of this on mean arterial pressure are offset by a reflex vasoconstriction. These changes are usually similar in patients with hypertension, but a subgroup has recently been identified with what has been termed orthostatic hypertension (Frohlich, Tarazi, Ulrych, Dustan, & Page, 1967; Streeten *et al.*, 1985), which is defined by a diastolic pressure that is below 90 mm Hg while recumbent, but above it while standing; systolic pressure is typically the same in both positions. The mechanism appears to be an excessive gravitational pooling of blood, with an enhanced reflex vasoconstriction.

Exercise

During dynamic exercise the auscultatory method may underestimate systolic pressure by up to 15 mm Hg, and during recovery it may be overestimated by 30 mm Hg (Henschel, DeLaVega, & Taylor, 1954; Gould, Hornung, Altman, Cashman, & Raftery, 1985). Errors in diastolic pressure are unlikely to be as large, except during the recovery period, when falsely low readings may be recorded (Henschel *et al.*, 1954). This is the reason why the American Heart Association recommends taking the fourth phase of the Korotkoff sound after exercise.

Recommendations for Evaluation of Noninvasive Blood Pressure Monitors and of Observers

Any automatic or semiautomatic blood pressure device that is used in behavioral studies needs to be calibrated against standard methods. Ideally, intraarterial pressures should be used as a reference, but this is often not feasible in practice. Most of the noninvasive methods cannot be expected to give readings that are any more accurate than the auscultatory method, which remains the usual method for comparison. At the present time, there is no automatic or semiautomatic recorder that is universally reliable, so we would strongly recommend that every time such a device is used, it is calibrated against a standard method, which for practical reasons means a mercury sphygmomanometer rather than intraarterial measurement. It is possible that, in the future, the K_2 method may be used rather than the auscultatory method.

Calibration against a mercury column is best performed using readings taken simultaneously from the same arm by the device being tested, and by an observer with a stethoscope placed just distal to the cuff, reading a mercury column connected to the cuff. With this technique, a satisfactory device should give readings that are within 5 mm Hg of the observer's. If this technique is not practical, the observer can take auscultatory readings from the opposite arm. This is less satisfactory for two reasons: there may be differences between the two arms, and it may be difficult to obtain the two sets of readings simultaneously. We have found that with the latter technique two observers with mercury sphygmomanometers can get correlation coefficients between the two arms of 0.98 for systolic and 0.94 for diastolic pressure; 70% of readings should be within 5 mm Hg of each other (Pickering *et al.*, 1986).

Validation of each observer's technique is also necessary; for this purpose, training videotapes are available, and a double-headed stethoscope is advisable, so that two observers may listen to the same Korotkoff sounds. With this technique, differences in auditory acuity can be evaluated; under ideal circumstances more than 90% of readings taken by the two observers should be within 5 mm Hg of each other.

Selection of Method of Measurement and Timing of Readings

One of the implications of the variability of blood pressure is that a single reading is of very little value, so that any measure of pressure should ideally consist of an average of several readings. Given this point, however, the number and timing of readings that are required will depend on the purpose for which they are being taken. In behavioral studies, there are four main reasons for measuring blood pressure. These are: screening; measuring the response to treatment; measuring changes during laboratory (reactivity) testing; and ambulatory monitoring. The optimal methods of measurement, and the timing of readings are different in these different cases.

Screening

The purpose of screening is to characterize individual subjects according to their prevailing level of blood pressure. This requires not only taking several readings (usually two or three) at each session, but also several sessions (also usually two or three) separated by intervals of days or weeks. In the Charlottesville blood pressure survey, 20% of individuals were classified as hypertensive after a single visit, whereas only 9% were after multiple visits (Carey et al., 1976). There are at least two reasons for this trend: regression to the mean, and habituation to the measurement procedure.

The best method for screening is still a mercury sphygmomanometer. Other devices have been tested but found wanting (Labarthe, Hawkins, & Remington, 1973). A recent refinement of categorizing individual subjects' blood pressure is to use home readings as well as clinic readings.

Measuring the Response to Treatment

When nonpharmacological forms of treatment of hypertension are being evaluated, conventional clinic measurements can no longer be relied on for three reasons: observer bias, the placebo effect, and lack of generalization. Observer bias may be minimized by using a semiautomatic or automatic device, provided that it has been validated against a mercury sphygmomanometer in each subject. The placebo effect and the question of generalization of the treatment effect to everyday life are interrelated. The former probably occurs as a result of a diminution of the pressor response associated with a clinic visit (Pickering, Harshfield, Devereux, & Laragh, 1985), rather than a sustained reduction (which, by definition, would be a therapeutic rather than a placebo effect). The latter is important to establish for any behavioral technique learned in a laboratory setting. These questions are best answered by supplementing objectively taken clinic readings by ambulatory monitoring of blood pressure, and perhaps by home readings as well.

Laboratory Testing

In general, blood pressure measurement during laboratory testing requires multiple measurements made at frequent intervals (e.g., every 2 min). Automatic or semiautomatic devices are preferred, using any of the currently available methods, e.g., Korotkoff sound, oscillometry, or ultrasound. For dynamic exercise testing or studies where movement artifact may be a problem, a device such as the Paramed monitor, which has a double transducer (one for subtraction of noise artifact), is preferable.

Ambulatory Monitoring

This topic was reviewed in an earlier section.

References

Aaslid, R., & Brubakk, A. O. (1981). Accuracy of an ultrasound Doppler servo method for noninvasive determination of instantaneous and mean arterial blood pressure. *Circulation, 64,* 753–759.

Ayman, P., & Goldshine, A. D. (1940). Blood pressure determinations by patients with essential hypertension. I. The difference between clinic and home readings before treatment. *American Journal of Medical Science, 200,* 465–474.

Blank, S. G., West, J. E., Mueller, F. B., Cody, R. J., Harshfield, G. A., Pecker, M. S., Laragh, J. H., & Pickering, T. G. (1988). Wideband external pulse recording during cuff deflation: A new technique for evaluation of the arterial pressure pulse and measurement of blood pressure. *Circulation, 77,* 1297–1305.

Burke, M. J., Towers, H. M., O'Malley, K., Fitzgerald, D. J., & O'Brien, E. T. (1982). Sphygmomanometers in hospital and family practice: Problems and recommendations. *British Medical Journal, 285,* 469–471.

Carey, R. M., Reid, R. A., Ayers, C. R., Lynch, S. S., McLain, W. L., & Vaughan, E. D. (1976). The Charlottesville Blood Pressure Survey: Value of repeated blood pressure measurements. *Journal of the American Medical Association, 236,* 847–851.

Clement, D. L., Jordaens, L. J., & Heyndrickx, G. R. (1984). Influence of vagal nervous activity on blood pressure variability. *Journal of Hypertension, 2*(Suppl. 3), 391–393.

Comstock, G. W. (1957). An epidemiologic study of blood pressure levels in a biracial community in the southern United States. *American Journal of Hygiene, 65,* 271–315.

Dock, W. (1980). Occasional notes—Korotkoff sounds. *New England Journal of Medicine, 302,* 1264–1267.

Dornhorst, A. C., Howard, P., & Leathart, G. L. (1952).

Respiratory variations in blood pressure. *Circulation, 6,* 553–558.

Elseed, A. M., Shinebourne, E. A., & Joseph, M. C. (1973). Assessment of techniques for measurement of blood pressure in infants and children. *Archives of Disease in Childhood, 48,* 932–936.

Frohlich, E. D., Tarazi, R. C., Ulrych, M., Dustan, H. P., & Page, I. H. (1967). Tilt test for investigating a neural component in hypertension: Its correlation with clinical characteristics. *Circulation, 36,* 387–393.

Geddes, L. A. (1984). *Cardiovascular devices and their applications.* New York: Wiley.

Gould, B. A., Hornung, R. S., Altman, D. G., Cashman, P. M. M., & Raftery, E. B. (1985). Indirect measurement of blood pressure during exercise testing can be misleading. *British Heart Journal, 53,* 611–615.

Henschel, A., DeLaVega, F., & Taylor, H. L. (1954). Simultaneous direct and indirect blood pressure measurements in man at rest and work. *Journal of Applied Physiology, 5,* 506–508.

Heymans, C., & Neil, E. (1958). *Reflexogenic areas of the cardiovascular system* (pp. 180–181). London: Churchill.

Hochberg, H. M., & Solomon, H. (1971). Accuracy of an automated ultrasound blood pressure monitor. *Current Therapeutic Research, 13,* 129–138.

Kirkendall, W. M., Burton, A. C., Epstein, F. H., & Fries, E. D. (1967). American Heart Association Recommendations for human blood pressure determinations by sphygmomanometers. *Circulation, 36,* 980.

Kirkendall, W. M., Feinlieb, M., Fries, E. D., & Mark, A. L. (1981). American Heart Association Recommendations for human blood pressure determination by sphygmomanometer. *Hypertension, 3,* 510a–519a.

Kroeker, E. J., & Wood, E. H. (1956). Beat-to-beat alterations in relationship to simultaneously recorded central and peripheral arterial pressure pulses during Valsalva maneuver and prolonged expiration in man. *Journal of Applied Physiology, 8,* 483–494.

Labarthe, D. R., Hawkins, C. M., & Remington, R. D. (1973). Evaluation of performance of selected devices for measuring blood pressure. *American Journal of Cardiology, 32,* 546–553.

Lane, J. E., Greenstadt, L., & Shapiro, D. (1983). Pulse transit time and blood pressure: An intensive analysis. *Psychophysiology, 20,* 45–49.

Mancia, G., Bertini, G., Grassi, G., Pomidossi, G., Gregorini, L., Bertinieri, G., Parati, G., Ferrari, A., & Zanchetti, A. (1983). Effects of blood pressure measurement by the doctor on patients' blood pressure and heart rate. *Lancet, 2,* 695–697.

Marey, E. J. (1876). Pression et vitesse du sang. Physiologie Experimentale, Paris. Pratique des hautes etudes lab de M. Marey.

Mauck, G. B., Smith, C. R., Geddes, L. R., & Bourland, J. D. (1980). The meaning of the point of maximum oscillations in cuff pressure in the indirect measurement of blood pressure II. *Journal of Biomechanical Engineering, 102,* 28–33.

Maxwell, M. H., Waks, A. V., Schroth, P. C., Karam, M., &

Dornfeld, L. (1982). Error in blood pressure measurement due to incorrect cuff size in obese patients. *Lancet, 2,* 33–35.

McCutcheon, E. P., & Rushmer, R. F. (1967). Korotkoff sounds: An experimental critique. *Circulation Research, 20,* 149–161.

Molhoek, P. G., Wesseling, K. H., Arntzenius, C., Settels, J. J. M., VanVollenhoven, E., & Weeda, H. W. H. (1983). Initial results of non-invasive measurement of finger blood pressure according to Penaz. *Automedica, 4,* 241–246.

Nielsen, P. E., & Janniche, H. (1974). The accuracy of auscultatory measurement of arm blood pressure in very obese subjects. *Acta Medica Scandinavica, 195,* 403–409.

O'Rourke, M. (1984). Wave reflection and the arterial pulse. *Archives of Internal Medicine, 144,* 366.

Penaz, J. (1973). Photo-electric measurement of blood pressure, volume and flow in the finger. *Digest Tenth International Conference on Medical and Biological Engineering, Dresden,* p. 104.

Pickering, G. W. (1968). *High blood pressure.* London: Churchill.

Pickering, T. G., Harshfield, G. A., Devereux, R. B., & Laragh, J. H. (1985). What is the role of ambulatory blood pressure monitoring in the management of hypertensive patients? *Hypertension, 7,* 171–177.

Pickering, T. G., Cvetkovski, B., & James, G. D. (1986). An evaluation of electronic recorders for self monitoring of blood pressure. *Journal of Hypertension, 4*(Suppl.), S329–S330.

Pollack, M. H., & Obrist, P. A. (1983). Aortic–radial pulse transit time and ECG Q-wave to radial pulse wave interval as indices of beat-to-beat blood pressure change. *Psychophysiology, 20,* 21–28.

Ramsey, M. (1979). Noninvasive automatic determination of mean arterial pressure. *Medical and Biological Engineering and Computing, 17,* 11–18.

Reder, R. F., Dimich, I., Cohen, M. L., & Steinfeld, L. (1978). Evaluating indirect blood pressure measurement techniques: A comparison of three systems in infants and children. *Pediatrics, 62,* 326–330.

Shapiro, D., Schwartz, G. E., & Tursky, B. (1972). Control of diastolic blood pressure in man by feedback and reinforcement. *Psychophysiology, 9,* 296–304.

Short, D. (1976). The diastolic dilemma. *British Medical Journal, 2,* 685–686.

Spence, J. D., Sibbald, W. J., & Cape, R. D. (1978). Pseudohypertension in the elderly. *Clinical Science and Molecular Medicine, 55,* 399s–402s.

Steinfeld, L., Dimich, I., Reder, R., Cohen, M., & Alexander, H. (1978). Sphygmomanometry in the pediatric patients. *Journal of Pediatrics, 92,* 934–938.

Steptoe, A., Smulyan, H., & Gribbin, B. (1976). Pulse wave velocity and blood pressure change: Calibration and applications. *Psychophysiology, 13,* 488–493.

Streeten, D. H. P., Auchincloss, J. H., Anderson, G. H., Richardson, R. L., Thomas, F. D., & Miller, J. W. (1985). Orthostatic hypertension: Pathogenetic studies. *Hypertension, 7,* 196–203.

Ware, R. W., & Laenger, C. J. (1967). Indirect blood pressure measurement by Doppler ultrasonic kinetoarteriography. *Proceedings of the 20th Annual Conference on Engineering in Medicine and Biology, 9,* 27–30.

Webster, J., Newnham, D., Petrie, J. C., & Lovell, H. G. (1984). Influence of arm position on measurement of blood pressure. *British Medical Journal, 228,* 1574–1575.

Wesseling, K. H., deWit, B., Settels, J. J., & Klawer, W. H. (1982). On the indirect registration of finger blood pressure after Penaz. *Funktionale Biologie und Medizin, 245,* 245–250.

West, J. E., Busch-Vishniac, I. J., Harshfield, G. A., & Pickering, T. G. (1983). Foil electret transducer for blood pressure monitoring. *Journal of the Acoustical Society of America, 74,* 680–686.

Wright, B. M., & Dore, C. F. (1970). A random-zero sphygmomanometer. *Lancet, 1,* 337–338.

Yelderman, M., & Ream, A. K. (1979). Indirect measurement of mean blood pressure in the anesthetized patient. *Anesthesiology, 50,* 253–256.

CHAPTER 5

Measurement of Blood Flow and Venous Distensibility

Erling A. Anderson

Measurement of arterial and venous function can provide important insights regarding hemodynamic responses to behavioral stimuli that cannot be obtained from measurement of systemic arterial pressure alone. This chapter describes the use of Doppler flow probes for measuring flow within single arteries or veins, laser Doppler probes for measuring skin blood flow, and venous occlusion plethysmography for measuring limb blood flow. Finally, the use of venous occlusion plethysmography to assess venous distensibility is described. The goal is to provide an overview of the techniques and their relative advantages and disadvantages. References are provided for those wishing to examine techniques in further detail.

Doppler Measurement of Blood Flow

Theory of Doppler Flow Probes

Doppler measurement of blood flow velocity is based on the principle that the frequency shift of sound reflected from moving objects varies with the speed of the objects. Doppler probes emit an ultrasonic beam into tissue. Although reflected by different tissues, only moving blood cells change the frequency of the reflected ultrasound waves. The frequency shift is proportional to the velocity of the blood cells and is expressed by the formula

$$\Delta f = \frac{2 f_t V \cos \Theta}{c}$$

where Δf is the Doppler frequency shift, f_t is the transmitter frequency, V is the velocity of blood cells, Θ is the angle between transmitted beam and blood flow, and c is the sound velocity in tissue (Sumner, 1982).

All Doppler probes use piezoelectric transducer crystals to transmit and receive ultrasonic waves. The crystals vibrate in response to an energizing voltage when emitting a pulse and produce a measurable voltage when vibrated by reflected signals. Intensity of the emitted signal is attenuated as the beam is scattered or absorbed by tissue. Attenuation is greater at higher frequencies (5–10 MHz), and lower frequencies (1–2 MHz) are required to penetrate deeper tissue.

Types of Doppler Probes

The three types of flow velocity probes available are (1) continuous-wave Doppler probes, (2) sin-

Erling A. Anderson • Departments of Anesthesia and Internal Medicine, Cardiovascular and Clinical Research Centers, University of Iowa College of Medicine, Iowa City, Iowa 52242.

gle-crystal pulsed Doppler probes, and (3) dual-crystal pulsed Doppler probes. Continuous-wave and single-crystal pulsed Doppler probes have many clinical applications, e.g., detecting major vessel stenosis. There are numerous excellent books describing their theory and application (Bernstein, 1985; Zwiebel, 1982). Dual-crystal pulsed Doppler probes are relatively new and used primarily in research. The three types of Doppler probes will be described and then compared.

Continuous-Wave Doppler Probes

These employ two crystals and are the simplest and least expensive available. One crystal emits a continuous ultrasonic wave while the second continuously records reflected signals. Since reflected signals originate from all points along the signal path, continuous-wave Doppler probes are good for rapidly locating vessels. Unfortunately, they have a major limitation. The emitted pulse is reflected from many depths and cannot be directed with certainty at a single vessel. This problem is known as "range ambiguity." Further, they cannot be used to measure vessel diameter. Thus, continuous-wave Doppler probes cannot be used transcutaneously to quantify blood flow.*

Single-Crystal Pulsed Doppler Probes

These Doppler probes employ a single crystal which both emits and receives signals. They represent a significant advance over continuous-wave Doppler probes since they can measure blood flow velocity in precisely defined *volume areas* at *differing depths*. The volume area, or "sample size," is determined by the duration of the emitted pulse. The shorter the pulse duration, the smaller is the volume (i.e., length) of the pulse. Thus, at any

---

*Continuous-wave Doppler probes surgically placed around an artery can quantitate blood flow. However, this invasive technique is of limited use in humans. Continuous-wave Doppler probes can be coupled with simultaneous ultrasonic imaging devices used in clinical cardiology to quantitate flow. However, ultrasonic imaging equipment is very expensive and beyond the resources of most laboratories.

given moment, signals are reflected from only the small area of tissue through which the pulse is passing. The depth of measurement is determined by adjusting the time between burst transmission and reception of the reflected signal. The longer the delay, the greater is the depth from which the reflected signal originates.

Adjusting sample volume and measurement depth makes it possible to record flow velocity within a single vessel. Emitted signals may pass through several vessels. However, flow velocity in a single vessel can be measured by activating the receiving crystal only when signals return from the depth of the vessel (Figure 1).

Vessel diameter can be measured with pulsed Doppler probes (Levenson, Peronneau, Simon, & Safar, 1981; Fitzgerald, O'Shaughnessy, & Keaveny, 1983). First, a small sample volume is selected by emitting a short pulse (e.g., 0.5 μs or ≃ 0.4 mm). This small-width signal is stepwise advanced from the depth at which flow is first registered (at the proximal wall) to the point of zero flow (at the distal wall). Diameter is then calculated as the number of steps across the vessel multiplied by the width of each step.

Mean blood flow velocity is measured by increasing sample volume (i.e., pulse duration) to encompass the entire vessel and recording only signals returning from the vessel depth. Knowing

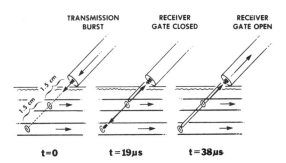

Figure 1. A single-crystal pulsed Doppler probe permits measurement of flow velocity in a single vessel. Increasing the time delay at which the crystal receives returning signals increases the depth of recording. As shown, only signals originating from the deeper vessels are detected since the crystal is opened only during the time of their arrival. From Sumner (1982, p. 37).

vessel diameter and mean flow velocity* permits calculation of absolute flow rate (see below).

However, the accuracy of absolute blood flow measurement obtained with single-crystal probes is questionable because the angle between the vessel and the emitted pulse must be known *and* constant. This angle is critical since the frequency shift of the reflected beam depends on the angle between the beam and moving cells. Small changes in vessel/beam angle can significantly alter flow readings (Shoor, Fronek, & Bernstein, 1979). Accurately determining vessel/beam angle with a single-crystal pulsed probe requires a stereotaxic device and considerable skill. The vessel is first located. Since objects moving perpendicularly to the pulse cause no frequency shift, the probe is moved in the stereotaxic device until there is no Doppler shift. Shifting the probe by 20° results in a 70° Doppler angle. Flow velocity can be quantified if this angle does not change. However, minor movements of the probe or subject are quite difficult to avoid.

Dual-Crystal Pulsed Doppler Probes

The echovar (Alvar Electronics, Chicago) is a dual-crystal pulsed Doppler probe developed in France by Peronneau and Safar. Both sample volume and measurement depth can be adjusted. The Echovar's unique feature is the configuration of the two crystals (both of which transmit and receive). The crystals are mounted in the probe to form a 120° angle (Figure 2). This configuration allows precise and consistent probe positioning so that the angle between transmitted beams and vessel is always 60°. Errors resulting from unknown or changing probe/vessel angle are minimized.

Obtaining a 60° probe/vessel angle is relatively easy. After positioning the probe over the vessel and emitting a long-duration pulse to locate the

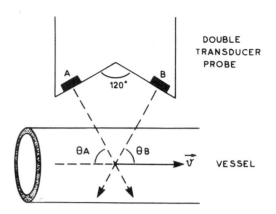

Figure 2. Positioning of the two crystals with the Echovar probe. When equal frequency shifts are detected by both probes, the angles ΘA and ΘB are both 60°. Knowing these angles permits absolute flow to be quantified accurately. From Chauveau *et al.* (1985, p. 701).

vessel, the probe is first moved laterally with a stereotaxic instrument while listening to an audio output from the Doppler. Maximum Doppler shift is obtained when the ultrasound beam crosses the center of the vessel. The longitudinal tilt of the probe is then adjusted to obtain equal Doppler shifts on both transducers. Equal Doppler shifts indicate the angle between the ultrasonic beam and vessel axis is 60° for both probes. This angle can be kept at precisely 60° by periodically comparing the frequency shifts obtained with each probe.

Knowing the exact probe/vessel angle allows accurate measurement of both vessel diameter and mean blood flow velocity. As with a single-crystal pulsed Doppler, diameter is determined by stepwise advancing a short-duration pulse (0.5 μs or 0.4 mm) from the proximal to distal walls of the vessel. Diameter is calculated as with a single-crystal pulsed Doppler. Mean flow velocity is then measured by increasing pulse width (i.e., duration) to that of the vessel diameter. The Doppler shift then reflects mean flow velocity. Absolute blood flow is calculated by the formula: flow = $(\pi D^2/4)$ × mean flow velocity.

The Echovar has been used extensively by Safar and his colleagues (Levenson *et al.*, 1981; Levenson, Simon, Safar, Bouthier, & London, 1985). Both *in vitro* and *in vivo* studies indicate the Echo-

---

*For technical reasons, the ability to quantitate velocity *and* location limits the maximum velocity that can be recorded with pulsed Doppler probes. The maximum frequency shift (Δf) which can be measured is one-half the pulse repetition frequency (e.g., 32 pulses/s). However, velocity in most peripheral arteries is within the limits that can be measured.

var can measure vessel diameter to within ±3.7% and mean flow velocity to within ±5.4% (Chauveau *et al.*, 1985). Flow measurements obtained with the Echovar compare favorably with those obtained by water and strain gauge plethysmographs.

Application and Limitations of Doppler Probes

Doppler systems can be used to measure changes in blood flow velocity within arteries. They can provide a continuous measure of blood flow which cannot be obtained by venous occlusion plethysmography. Doppler probes can therefore assess rapid flow changes in response to acute interventions. They can also be used to measure changes in vessel diameter. Further, they can measure both arterial and venous flow. Arterial and venous flows are easily distinguished by their Doppler frequency shifts. Arterial signals have prominent systolic and diastolic components. Venous signals are not pulsatile, vary with respiration, and have a lower pitch. Finally, compressing the distal extremity increases venous return and greatly augments the Doppler shift.

Continuous-wave Doppler probes cannot be focused on a single vessel ("range ambiguity"). As a result, they may measure arterial and venous flow in both deep and superficial vessels. Thus, despite simplicity and low cost, inherent technological limitations make them of limited use for measuring changes in blood flow in peripheral circulation.

Single-crystal pulsed Doppler probes can measure flow velocity within a single vessel and indicate relative changes in flow velocity. However, precisely determining vessel/probe angle is difficult. Since this angle influences measurement of both vessel diameter and mean velocity, single-crystal pulsed Doppler probes must be used with caution when quantitating blood flow.

The dual-crystal configuration of the Echovar makes it possible to accurately determine probe/vessel angle. This permits accurate and reproducible measurement of flow velocity and vessel diameter. Absolute blood flow can be quantified quite accurately. Thus, of the three types of Doppler probes, the Echovar system would appear best for quantifying blood flow.

Laser Dopplers for Cutaneous Blood Flow

The laser Doppler technique for noninvasive measurement of cutaneous blood flow is relatively recent. Although conceptually similar to ultrasound Doppler probes, laser Dopplers measure only cutaneous blood flow. The technique is based on the fact that laser light (which penetrates only superficial tissue) is backscattered from moving blood cells. The reflected light enters a photo detector, the Doppler shifted frequencies are analyzed, and the output converted to velocity signals in volts.

This technique has advantages over conventional plethysmography. First, the laser Doppler is specific to skin and subcutaneous tissue, whereas plethysmographic recording reflects both muscle and skin blood flow. Second, laser Dopplers can be applied to skin anywhere on the body, whereas plethysmography is limited to extremities. Third, laser Dopplers provide a continuous measurement of cutaneous blood flow, which is not possible with plethysmography.

Laser Dopplers do have disadvantages. First, the light cannot be focused on individual vessels. Skin microvasculature is complex and blood flows in many directions at different velocities. The reflected light is therefore a broad spectrum of frequency shifts and may indicate arterial and venous circulation. Comparison with xenon washout techniques indicates that laser Dopplers probably measure blood flow in arteriovenous anastomoses as well as capillaries and that they overestimate flow in areas with anastomoses (Englehart & Kristensen, 1983).

Further, laser Doppler flow values can vary considerably at different skin sites within the same subject (Johnson, Taylor, Shepherd, & Park, 1984). This presumably reflects differences in the number of capillaries at different sites (Johnson *et al.*, 1984; Englehart & Kristensen, 1983). Thus, laser Doppler probes cannot be used for comparison between subjects or between sites within the same subject. Finally, laser Doppler output (measured in volts) is not convertible to traditional flow units such as milliliters per units of tissue per minute. These disadvantages would indicate that laser Dopplers are best suited to measuring relative blood flow changes within a subject during a single experiment.

Plethysmography

Blood flow in limbs can be quantified by venous occlusion plethysmography. The term *plethysmography* is derived from the Greek words *plethysmos* ("increase") and *graphein* ("to write"). Plethysmography records volume increases after occlusion of venous return and was originally used to measure internal organ blood flow. An excellent history of the technique is presented by Hyman and Winsor (1961).

Plethysmography is noninvasive, involves few assumptions, and had been proved valid (Formel & Doyle, 1957). The technique can be used to measure blood flow to segments of limbs (e.g., forearm, hand, calf, foot). Blood flow to these regions includes skin and muscle flow, and the relative contribution of muscle and skin flow varies (Siggaard-Anderson, 1970; Kontos, Richardson, & Patterson, 1966). Forearm and calf flows reflect flow to both skeletal muscle and skin whereas hand and finger flow reflects primarily skin flow.

Venous occlusion plethysmography involves placing a pneumatic cuff proximal to a plethysmographic recording device and inflating it to a pressure (e.g., 50 mm Hg) sufficient to interrupt venous return but not arterial inflow (i.e., less than diastolic pressure). Increasing limb volume during the first 5–8 s of venous occlusion reflects arterial inflow as blood accumulates in the venous system. The cuff is then deflated for 8–10 s to allow venous drainage. The limb being measured must be elevated above the heart to assure adequate venous drainage. The cycle of cuff inflation, measurement, and cuff deflation allows four to five measurements each minute.

Measuring blood flow to a limb segment (such as forearm or calf) requires placement of a second cuff distal to the plethysmograph. Inflating this distal cuff to suprasystolic levels (200 mm Hg) interrupts blood flow to the distal extremity. In the case of forearm blood flow, placing this cuff at the wrist temporarily excludes the hand circulation which is primarily skin flow.

There are at least three major assumptions underlying the use of venous occlusion plethysmography to measure blood flow. First, the initial venous occlusion must not impede arterial inflow. Second, there must be complete arrest of venous return. Third, the increase in venous pressure during occlusion must not alter arterial inflow. These assumptions have been widely tested and found valid (see Hyman & Winsor, 1961, or Formel & Doyle, 1957).

There are several types of plethysmographic recording devices for measuring limb expansion during venous occlusion. These include displacement (volumetric) plethysmographs, and the more frequently used strain gauge plethysmograph introduced by Whitney (1953).*

Volumetric Plethysmographs

Volumetric plethysmographs use water- or air-filled chambers to directly measure volume changes. With water-filled plethysmographs, the limb being measured is placed in a rubber sleeve inside a rigid container filled with water (Figure 3). Limb expansion during venous occlusion displaces an equal amount of water. A transducer connected to a polygraph records the volume changes as water rises in a column. Water plethysmographs are calibrated by injecting known volumes of water into the chamber (e.g., 10 ml). Blood flow can be expressed as milliliters per minute per 100 ml of tissue by measuring limb volume. Limb volume is determined by withdrawing the limb from the plethysmograph and measuring the water volume needed to refill the plethysmograph.

Water plethysmographs are extremely sensitive and directly measure volume displacement. Unfortunately, they are cumbersome, can leak, and require immobilization of the limb throughout the study.

*Water-filled plethysmographs, Whitney strain gauges, and the automated cuff inflation device used with both can be obtained from Medical Instruments, 8 Medical Laboratories, University of Iowa, Iowa City, Iowa 52242.

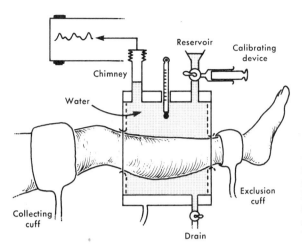

Figure 3. Schematic of a water-filled plethysmograph for recording volume expansion of the calf during venous occlusion. Inflating the distal ("exclusion") cuff to 200 mm Hg eliminates circulation to the foot during recording. Calf expansion during venous occlusion displaces an equal amount of water in the chimney. From Sumner (1985, p. 70).

Air-filled plethysmographs are conceptually similar to water plethysmographs. Limb expansion is indicated by the volume of air displaced or the increase in air pressure within a closed chamber. The plethysmograph is calibrated by injecting a known volume of air and recording pressure or volume changes. However, the high thermal expansion coefficient of air makes this method quite sensitive to temperature changes. Enclosing the limb can increase air temperature. Thus, frequent recalibration is needed unless temperature is kept constant by cooling the chamber. This disadvantage is serious and air plethysmographs are used infrequently. However, a modified air plethysmograph (which uses pressure-sensitive cuffs similar to blood pressure cuffs) has been developed. This system may overcome some limitations of air chamber devices. A thorough discussion of air-cuff plethysmographs is presented by Siggaard-Anderson (1970).

Strain Gauge Plethysmography

Strain gauge plethysmography is the most commonly used method for measuring limb blood flow. The method yields flow measurements comparable to those obtained with water plethysmographs (Lind & Schmid, 1972). Strain gauge plethysmographs measure changes in limb circumference and do not measure volume directly. Changes in circumference are measured by placing a mercury-filled Silastic tube around the limb (e.g., forearm).

A DC current is passed through the mercury. Changes in tube length (i.e., limb circumference) produce proportional changes in electrical resistance. Strain gauges are calibrated by shortening the Silastic tubing by known amounts (e.g., 1 mm) and noting the change in electrical resistance. Shortening is usually done by means of a calibration screw mounted on a Wheatstone bridge to which the Silastic tube is attached (Figure 4).

Circumference changes during venous occlusion are indicated by changes in resistance across the mercury-filled tube. Since the percent change in volume is twice the percent change in circumference, the increase in circumference can be converted to volume increase in milliliters per minute per 100 ml limb volume (see Whitney, 1953, or Williams, 1984, for discussion of conversion formulas).

Measurement for Venous Distensibility

The systemic veins are a reservoir from which blood is pumped by the heart. The venous system, which holds as much as 70% of blood volume, is not a passive reservoir but a dynamic one which is actively controlled by both neural and hormonal mechanisms (see Mark & Eckstein, 1968; Abboud, Schmid, Heistad, & Mark, 1976; Rowell, 1986, for reviews). The characteristics and re-

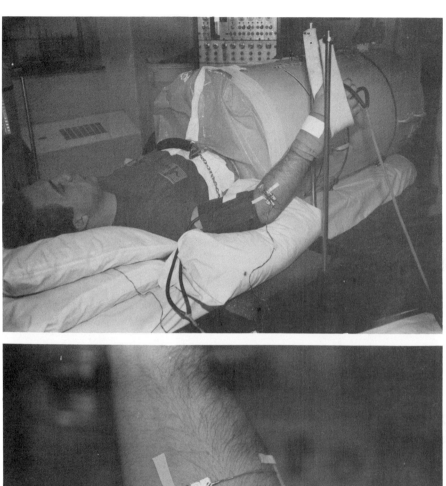

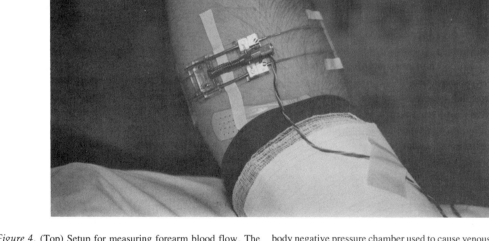

Figure 4. (Top) Setup for measuring forearm blood flow. The cuff placed around the biceps is inflated to 500 mm Hg to occlude venous return. The wrist cuff is inflated to a suprasystolic level to arrest hand circulation. Whitney strain gauge is placed around the widest section of the forearm. Subject is shown in a lower body negative pressure chamber used to cause venous pooling in the legs. (Bottom) Close-up of strain gauge. Mercury-filled Silastic tube connected to gauge is passed around the arm. Calibration screw (surrounded by a spring) is in the center of the gauge.

sponses of the venous system are best studied by defining pressure–volume relationships. This contrasts with the pressure–flow relationships used to characterize the behavior of resistance vessels.

The venous system may play an important role in hemodynamic responses to behavioral stimuli. For example, increased venomotor tone can increase right atrial pressure which, in part, controls cardiac output (Mark & Eckstein, 1968). The venous system has, to date, been largely ignored in the field of behavioral medicine.

Venous occlusion plethysmography can be used to measure distensibility of venous capacitance vessels. The relationship between transmural venous pressure and venous volume (pressure–volume relationship) reflects venous distensibility. Changes in pressure–volume relationship reflect altered venomotor tone. Two techniques for determining venous distensibility are the *equilibration* and *occluded limb* techniques (Abboud *et al.*, 1976; Rowell, 1986).

Equilibration Technique

The equilibration technique can be performed with water or strain gauge plethysmographs. When using a water-filled plethysmograph, the limb is placed in a plethysmograph filled with a sufficient volume of water to collapse the veins. It is critical to have a low, reproducible baseline transmural venous pressure since veins are quite distensible at low pressures. Thus, even small differences in baseline transmural venous pressure can have significant effects on measurements of venous distensibility. Arterial inflow drives up venous pressure (measured by venous catheter) to a level slightly higher than the external water pressure. The difference between the pressure within the vessel and the external water pressure is the distending, or transmural, pressure.

Changes in forearm venous volume are then recorded during stepwise increases (of 5 or 10 mm Hg) in transmural venous pressure to 30 mm Hg. Transmural venous pressure is increased by inflating a cuff on the limb proximal to the plethysmograph. Venous volume at each pressure is reflected by increasing forearm volume. Venous pressure–volume curves are calculated by plotting changes

in forearm volume (in ml/100 ml of tissue) against corresponding levels of transmural venous pressure (Figure 5).

Venous pressure–volume relationships can also be determined with strain gauge plethysmography. The limb is first positioned above the heart to collapse veins and obtain a low, reproducible baseline transmural venous pressure. A congesting cuff is placed proximal to the plethysmograph and inflated slowly until a slight increase in limb volume is registered by the plethysmograph. The cuff pressure producing this initial increase is considered to represent zero cuff pressure ("cuff zero"). The cuff is then inflated by increments of 5 to 10 mm Hg allowing time at each pressure for forearm circumference to plateau ("equilibrate"). Increased forearm circumference at different pressures reflects increased venous volume. Venous volume–pressure slopes can be plotted or the results expressed as change in forearm volume per 100 ml of tissue at a given transmural venous pressure (e.g., 30 mm Hg).

Although noninvasive and easier to use than water plethysmographs, strain gauge plethysmographs measure only circumference changes at a single point and not total volume increases. Further, use of a congesting cuff makes it difficult to precisely increase transmural venous pressure by known amounts since cuff pressure, which may not be transmitted entirely to the veins, may not reflect venous pressure. Thus, this method is probably less accurate than water plethysmographs for measuring venous distensibility.

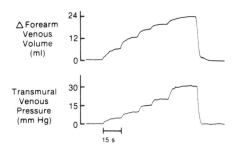

Figure 5. Illustration of the equilibration technique for measuring venous distensibility. Changes in forearm venous volume are recorded by a water plethysmograph during stepwise increases in transmural venous pressure. From Takeshita and Mark (1979, p. 203).

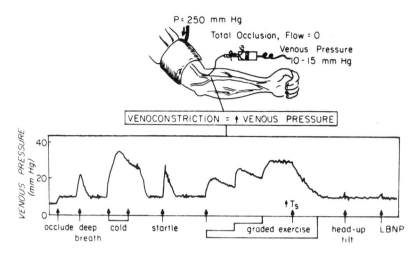

Figure 6. Schematic showing the occluded limb technique for measuring venomotor responses to stimuli. Note the marked venoconstriction with a startle response. This technique can be used to study reflex neural responses but not humoral influences. From Rowell (1986, p. 67).

Occluded Limb Technique

Venous tone can be measured by the "occluded limb" technique (Samueloff, Bevegard, & Shepherd, 1966). In this technique a cuff placed proximal to the plethysmograph is inflated to suprasystolic levels, which completely arrests limb circulation. Veins in the occluded limb therefore contain a constant blood volume. Subsequent changes in venous pressure (measured by venous catheter) reflect changes in venomotor tone. Venomotor responses to stimuli such as stress can be determined (Figure 6).

The occluded limb technique is simple to perform and is a sensitive measure of reflex changes in venous tone. A disadvantage of the technique is that only reflex neural responses can be assessed. It cannot be used to evaluate effects of humoral factors, structural changes in venous distensibility, or basal venous tone.

Future

Doppler flow probes and venous occlusion plethysmography can yield considerable information on acute circulatory responses to behavioral interventions. Future areas of research employing these techniques might include the effects of salt loading on arterial and venous responses to stress. Of particular importance is how responses to stress may be different in those at risk for heart disease or hypertension. Further, pharmacological manipulations can be used to assess specific neural and humoral control of regional blood flow during stress.

ACKNOWLEDGMENTS. The writing of this chapter was supported by National Research Service Award HL-07385; by Grants HL-24962 and HL-36224 from the National Heart, Lung and Blood Institute; by Grant RR59 from the General Clinical Research Center's Program, Division of Research Resources, National Institutes of Health; by a grant-in-aid from the Iowa Affiliate of the American Heart Association; and by research funds from the Veterans Administration.

References

Abboud, F. M., Schmid, P. G., Heistad, D. D., & Mark, A. L. (1976). Regulation of peripheral and coronary circulations. In H. J. Levine (Ed.), *Clinical cardiovascular physiology* (pp. 143–205). New York: Grune & Stratton.

Chauveau, M., Levy, B., Dessanges, J. F., Savin, E., Bailliart, O., & Martineaud, J. P. (1985). Quantitative Doppler blood flow measurement method and *in vivo* calibration. *Cardiovascular Research, 19,* 700–706.

Englehart, M., & Kristensen, J. K. (1983). Evaluation of cutaneous blood flow responses by [133]Xenon washout and a laser-Doppler flowmeter. *Journal of Investigative Dermatology, 80,* 12–15.

Fitzgerald, D. E., O'Shaughnessy, A. M., & Keaveny, V. T. (1983). Pulsed Doppler: A classification of results of diameter, velocity and volume flow measurement in diseased common carotid arteries. *Cardiovascular Research, 17,* 122–126.

Formel, P. F., & Doyle, J. T. (1957). Rationale of venous occlusion plethysmography. *Circulation Research, 5,* 351–356.

Hyman, C., & Winsor, T. (1961). History of plethysmography. *Journal of Cardiovascular Surgery, 35,* 506–518.

Johnson, J. M., Taylor, W. F., Shepherd, A. P., & Park, M. K. (1984). Laser-Doppler measurement of skin blood flow: Comparison with plethysmography. *Journal of Applied Physiology, 56,* 798–803.

Kontos, H. A., Richardson, D. W., & Patterson, J. L. (1966). Blood flow and metabolism of forearm muscle in man at rest and during sustained concentration. *American Journal of Physiology, 211,* 869.

Levenson, J. A., Peronneau, P. A., Simon, A., & Safar, M. E. (1981). Pulsed Doppler: Determination of diameter, blood flow velocity, and volumic flow of brachial artery in man. *Cardiovascular Research, 15,* 164–170.

Levenson, J., Simon, A. C., Safar, M. E., Bouthier, J. D., & London, G. M. (1985). Elevation of brachial arterial blood velocity and volumic flow mediated by peripheral β-adrenoreceptors in patients with borderline hypertension. *Circulation, 71,* 663–668.

Lind, A. R., & Schmid, P. G. (1972). Comparison of volume and strain-gauge plethysmography during static effort. *Journal of Applied Physiology, 32,* 552–554.

Mark, A. L., & Eckstein, J. W. (1968). Venomotor tone and central venous pressure. *Medical Clinics of North America, 52,* 1077–1090.

Rowell, L. B. (1986). *Human circulation regulation during physical stress.* London: Oxford University Press.

Samueloff, S. L., Bevegard, B. S., & Shepherd, J. T. (1966). Temporary arrest of circulation to a limb for the study of venomotor reactions in man. *Journal of Applied Physiology, 21,* 341.

Shepherd, J. T., & Vanhoutte, P. M. (1979). *The human cardiovascular system.* New York: Raven Press.

Shoor, P. M., Fronek, A., & Bernstein, E. F. (1979). Quantitative transcutaneous arterial velocity measurements with Doppler flowmeters. *Archives of Surgery, 114,* 922–928.

Siggaard-Anderson, J. (1970). Venous occlusion plethysmography on the calf. *Danish Medical Bulletin, 17*(Suppl. I), 1–68.

Sumner, D. S. (1982). Ultrasound. In R. F. Kempczinski & J. S. T. Yao (Eds.), *Practical noninvasive vascular diagnosis* (pp. 21–47). Chicago: Year Book Medical.

Sumner, D. S. (1985). Volume plethysmography in vascular disease: An overview. In E. F. Bernstein (Ed.), *Noninvasive diagnostic techniques in vascular disease* (pp. 97–118). St. Louis: Mosby.

Takeshita, A., & Mark, A. L. (1979). Decreased venous distensibility in borderline hypertension. *Hypertension, 1,* 202–206.

Whitney, R. J. (1953). The measurement of volume changes in human limbs. *Journal of Physiology, 121,* 1–27.

Williams, R. B. (1984). Measurement of local blood flow during behavioral experiments: Principles and practice. In A. J. Herd, A. M. Gotto, P. G. Kaufmann, & S. M. Weiss (Eds.), *Cardiovascular instrumentation.* National Institutes of Health Publication No. 84-1654, pp. 207–217.

Zwiebel, W. J. (Ed.). (1982). *Introduction to vascular ultrasonography.* New York: Grune & Stratton.

CHAPTER **6**

Autonomic Function Testing

E. D. Dunlap and M. A. Pfeifer

Many lines of evidence suggest that behavioral and neuroendocrine factors are related to cardiovascular disease and hypertension. Methods of testing cardiovascular autonomic function can provide an explanation to the relationship between behavioral factors and cardiovascular disease. Successful treatments can then be developed based on that knowledge.

The objective of this chapter is to provide information on the methods available to assess cardiovascular autonomic function. The description of each method contains a discussion of the theory behind each test, how each test is administered, the portion of the autonomic nervous system (ANS) assessed by the particular test, and advantages and drawbacks to each method.

To be practical, diagnostic tests should fulfill certain criteria. They need to be simple, noninvasive, easy for both operator and subject, reproducible, and must clearly distinguish between normal and abnormal results. The conclusions of autonomic reactivity and integrity should be based on the results of several tests. Results based on one test are limited by the sensitivity and accuracy of that test. Almost all autonomic tests assess reflex arc function. A typical reflex arc involves one or

more sensors, an afferent branch, central processing, an efferent branch, neuroeffector junctions, and an end organ (see Figure 1). Most tests of autonomic function measure a change in end organ function in response to a stimulus. The assumption that a change in end organ function is correlated to changes in efferent nerves is a common but perhaps incorrect assumption. Nevertheless, assessing reflex arcs still provides a simple noninvasive method of testing the cardiovascular system.

There are a large number of reflexes which involve the cardiovascular system. The baroreceptor reflex is one which is very relevant to autonomic testing. Baroreceptors are arterial stretch receptors (sensors) located in carotid sinuses and the aortic arch. Afferent impulses from the carotid sinus receptors travel to the brain via the carotid sinus nerves, which are branches of the glossopharyngeal nerves (Thomas & Eliasson, 1984). Impulses from the aortic baroreceptors ascend to the brain via the aortic nerves, which are branches of the vagus nerves (Thomas & Eliasson, 1984). Sympathetic and vagal parasympathetic fibers constitute the efferent limbs of the baroreceptor reflex.

Baroreceptors discharge impulses at a frequency directly related to the mean arterial pressure in the carotid sinuses and aortic arch (Koizumi & Brooks, 1980). An increased frequency of impulses during increased blood pressure causes a reflex reduction in activity of efferent sympathetic fibers and increased activity in efferent vagal

E. D. Dunlap and M. A. Pfeifer • Division of Endocrinology and Metabolism, Veterans Administration Medical Center, Louisville, Kentucky 40202.

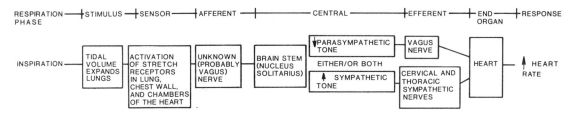

Figure 1. Components of the reflex arc involved in the RR-variation reflex.

fibers. This results in decreased heart rate, diminished vasomotor tone, and diminished atrial and ventricular contractility.

The presence of autonomic neuropathy disrupts the flow of impulse transmission to the end organ. This results in abnormal end organ responses to a sensor stimulus. Abnormal cardiovascular responses can result from problems anywhere in the reflex arc. A strict definition of autonomic neuropathy should include only abnormalities which result from an autonomic efferent nerve abnormality. However, it is difficult to determine where the abnormality exists within a reflex arc. Therefore, a more practical definition of autonomic neuropathy would be an abnormal reflex arc response to a standardized stimulus.

Importance of Assessment of Cardiovascular ANS

The assessment of the cardiovascular ANS has many implications in both clinical research and therapeutic behavioral medicine. Recently, studies have tested the hypothesis that behavior influences the cardiovascular system and that altered cardiovascular responses have consequences in the pathogenesis of arteriosclerosis, arterial hypertension, and sudden cardiac death. Specifically, behavioral stress has been related to an increased vulnerability to ventricular fibrillation and arrhythmia (Verrier & Lown, 1984). Schwartz and Stone demonstrated a correlation between weak vagal reflexes and increased susceptibility to ventricular fibrillation in postinfarction dogs (Schwartz & Stone, 1985). Exercise was able to

increase vagal reflexes and dramatically reduce mortality in these dogs. Findings such as these help clarify the relationship between behavior and cardiovascular disease and suggest possible modes of therapy to reduce the occurrence of ventricular fibrillation and sudden death.

In clinical practice, assessment of the cardiac ANS can help direct the proper management of a patient. For example, individuals with a "Type A" behavior pattern have enhanced physiologic cardiovascular responses (increased reactivity) compared to individuals with a non-coronary-prone "Type B" behavior pattern (Manuck, Kaplan, & Clarkson, 1983). Cardiovascular ANS tests may be used to detect increased cardiovascular reactivity in individuals with a Type A behavior pattern. This information can then help indicate which patients would benefit from behavior modification.

Assessment of Cardiovascular ANS

Difficulties

Tests which use reflex arc responses to evaluate ANS function have several inherent difficulties. A change in end organ function after an applied stimulus can result from an alteration at any point in the reflex arc, not necessarily the efferent autonomic pathway. For example, there is decreased baroreceptor sensitivity in patients with hypertension (Eckberg, 1980). Studies in the Dahl salt-sensitive (DS) rat (an animal model of hypertension) have confirmed that afferent discharge from aortic baroreceptors is also impaired in prehypertensive DS rats (Ferrari, Gordon, & Mark, 1984). When the baroreceptor is impaired, the reflex decrease in heart rate and blood pressure in response to elevated blood pressure is diminished. This decrease is not due to an abnormality in the efferent autonomic nerves but rather in the sensor (baroreceptor). Subjects should be screened for ANS abnormalities before behavioral ANS testing is performed. Test results will not be valid if obtained from a person with an abnormal ANS.

Also, many organ systems innervated by autonomic nerves have dual parasympathetic and sympathetic innervation with opposing effects. This can confound the interpretation of results. For example, an increase in heart rate after an applied stimulus may reflect an increase in sympathetic nervous system (SNS) tone, a decrease in parasympathetic nervous system (PNS) tone, or both. Fortunately, pharmacologic agents are available which specifically block either PNS or SNS activity and allow differentiation.

Other difficulties involved in cardiovascular autonomic testing include the presence of diseases which cause autonomic dysfunction. For example, autonomic neuropathy is a common complication of diabetes mellitus. It is estimated that from 17 to 40% of randomly selected diabetics exhibit abnormal ANS responses (Ewing, 1984). Syndromes of autonomic dysfunction include: postural hypotension, cardiac denervation, and exercise intolerance.

Orthostatic hypotension, cardiac denervation syndrome, and exercise intolerance are three examples of disturbed cardiovascular autonomic function. The presence of any of these three can suggest an abnormal ANS. If abnormal ANS function is present, results of reactivity testing will not be valid. It is important to eliminate sources of abnormal results before initiating reactivity testing.

Postural Hypotension

A generally accepted definition of postural hypotension is a decrease, upon standing, of 10 mm Hg diastolic blood pressure or 30 mm Hg systolic blood pressure. Postural hypotension is characterized by posture-related weaknesses, dizziness, visual impairment, and may include syncope. A detailed discussion of the causes of postural hypotension is provided in an excellent review by Thomas, Schirger, Fealey, and Sheps (1981). Normally, after a sudden change in body position, the blood pressure, heart rate, and volume of cardiac output are maintained by the "postural reflex" in which baroreceptors initiate increased cardiac peripheral vascular sympathetic efferent activity. The increase in SNS activity to the peripheral vasculature results in increased plasma concentration of norepinephrine (Burke, Sundlof, & Wallin, 1977; Cryer, 1980; Ziegler, Lake, & Kopin, 1977). Orthostatic hypotension associated with autonomic neuropathy is believed to reflect vascular sympathetic dysfunction of the ANS. Its presence indicates a defect within the ANS and will interfere with interpretation of test results.

Cardiac Denervation Syndrome

Cardiac denervation syndrome is another complication of cardiovascular autonomic neuropathy. A fixed pulse rate of 80–90 beats/min which is unresponsive to mild exercise, stress, or sleep indicates nearly complete cardiac denervation (Clarke, Ewing, & Campbell, 1979; Hosking, Bennett, & Hampton, 1978; Lloyd-Mostyn & Watkins, 1976). The presence of cardiac denervation syndrome generally indicates the presence of severe autonomic damage. Cardiac denervation has been proposed as an explanation of the increased incidence of painless myocardial ischemia and infarction in diabetic patients (Bradley & Schonfield, 1962; Clarke et al., 1979; Ewing, Campbell, & Clarke, 1980a).

Sudden death in patients with cardiac denervation syndrome may result from adrenergic supersensitivity secondary to cardiac denervation (Clarke et al., 1979; Ewing, 1984; Ewing, Campbell, & Clarke, 1980b). According to this theory, as a result of fewer nerve impulses from neurons innervating the heart, the sensitivity and/or numbers of postsynaptic receptors are increased. Too much stimulation to an end organ primed for activity may increase occult cardiac arrhythmias. Preliminary studies support the theory of denervation supersensitivity (Burke et al., 1977; Hilsted et al., 1981).

Exercise Intolerance

The presence of exercise intolerance may also be an indicator of cardiovascular autonomic neuropathy.

Changes in the ANS are important in the circulatory, hormonal, and metabolic responses to exercise. In subjects with cardiac autonomic neuropathy, evaluated using graded exercise, it was found that the worse the neuropathy, the more abnormal were the cardiovascular performance, systemic peripheral resistance, and change in heart rate in response to exercise (Dysberg, Benn, Sandahl-Christiansen, Hilsted, & Nerup, 1981; Freyschuss, 1970; Kent & Cooper, 1974).

Specific Methods

RR Variation

It has long been known that heart rate is more rapid during inspiration and slows during expiration. This sinus arrhythmia is measured as the beat-to-beat variation in R–R interval and is referred to as RR variation.

RR variation is primarily under cardiac parasympathetic control (Wheeler & Watkins, 1973). Blocking parasympathetic tone with atropine will greatly attenuate RR variation (Wheeler & Watkins, 1973). However, there is also a small sympathetic component to RR variation, since administration of propranolol to remove sympathetic stimulation causes a slight decrease in RR variation (Weinberg & Pfeifer, 1986). β-Adrenergic stimulation with isoproterenol will also greatly decrease RR variation (Pfeifer et al., 1982).

How the PNS and SNS influence RR variation is illustrated in Figure 2. Work by Kollai and Koizumi (1979, 1981) has shown in dogs that during normal respiration there are bursts of sympathetic nerve activity from the stellate ganglion during inspiration which alternate with bursts of parasympathetic vagal nerve activity during exhalation. The combination of alternating parasympathetic and sympathetic nerve activity results in RR variation. In the normal resting state, parasympathetic nerve activity contributes more to the amount of RR variation than does sympathetic nerve activity. Therefore, when vagal nerve activity is blocked with atropine, there is a large decrease in RR variation (Figure 3). When sympathetic nerve action is blocked using propranolol, there is only a small decrease in RR variation (Weinberg & Pfeifer, 1986) (Figure 4). β-Adrenergic stimulation using isoproterenol causes an increased heart rate which overwhelms the effects of the SNS and PNS nerves that regulate resting RR variation. The result of the overwhelming SNS stimuli is a suppression of RR variation (Figure 5).

In summary, resting RR variation reflects activity of both sympathetic and parasympathetic nerves. Use of propranolol can eliminate any sympathetic influence; thus, results would reflect only

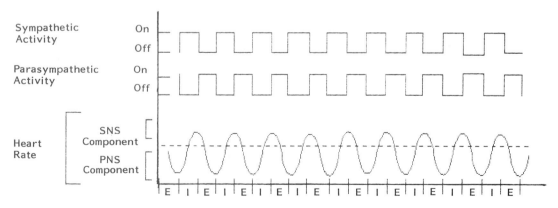

Figure 2. Nervous system regulation of RR variation in the normal resting state. E, exhalation; I, inhalation; dashed line is the intrinsic heart rate in the absence of nervous system influence.

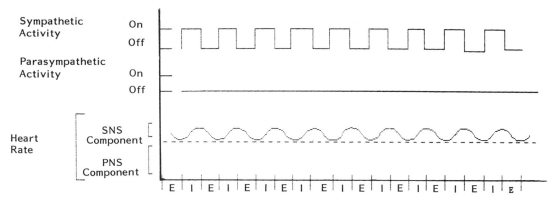

Figure 3. Effect of parasympathetic blockade on RR variation. E, exhalation; I, inhalation; dashed line is the intrinsic heart rate in the absence of nervous system influence.

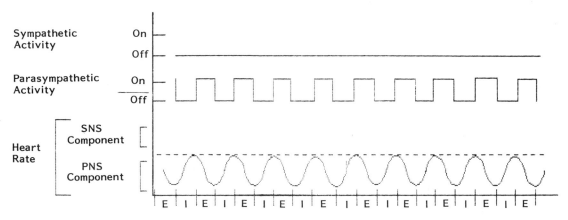

Figure 4. Effect of sympathetic blockade on RR variation. E, exhalation; I, inhalation; dashed line is the intrinsic heart rate in the absence of nervous system influence.

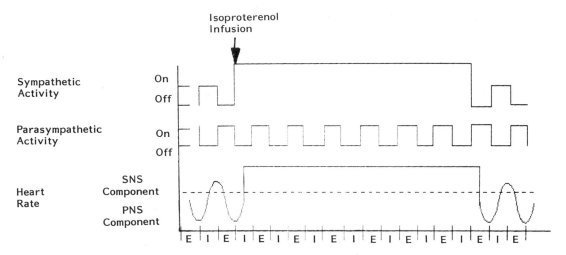

Figure 5. Effect of sympathetic stimulation on RR variation. E, exhalation; I, inhalation; dashed line is the intrinsic heart rate in the absence of nervous system influence.

parasympathetic activity. However, use of atropine to remove parasympathetic influences removes such a large portion of RR variation that accurate measurements can no longer be made. Also, the presence of too much sympathetic stimuli (i.e., stress, hypoglycemia, MI, or anxiety) can overwhelm the modulating effects of alternating PNS and SNS stimuli and suppress RR variation.

Several techniques have been proposed to analyze RR variation. Ewing et al. (Ewing, Borsey, Bellavere, & Clarke, 1981) published a review which compared five ways of describing RR variation. They concluded that the two most accurate procedures were: (1) calculating the standard deviation of the mean R–R interval during a period of quiet breathing and (2) finding the difference between the maximum and minimum heart rate recorded during deep breathing at a rate of six breaths per minute.

A new method is the circular mean resultant method (Weinberg & Pfeifer, 1984). It is based on vector analysis of RR variation during each breathing cycle. It eliminates the effects of trends of heart rate over time and removes the effect of ectopic beats on RR variation. It also has the advantage of determining how well the subject is following the prescribed breathing rate of five breaths per minute. The RR variation technique has also been defined for use in the rat (Dunlap, Samols, Waite, & Pfeifer, 1987). The presence of an animal model for measuring RR variation makes possible many experiments not possible in human subjects.

Several specific protocols for measurement of RR variation are available (Bennett, Farquhar, Hosking, & Hampton, 1978; Ewing, 1984; Hosking et al., 1978; Weinberg & Pfeifer, 1984). These protocols generally involve continuous electrocardiographic measurements of heart rate over a defined period of time. A standard breathing rate of five or six breaths per minute has been shown to produce maximal RR variation (Pfeifer et al., 1982).

Patient position affects RR variation (Bennett et al., 1977). Therefore, protocols require a standardized patient position. The authors prefer the supine position since volume changes during upright posture may result in increased SNS tone

which may in turn alter RR variation (Pfeifer & Peterson, 1987).

Other factors may potentially alter RR variation. Since vascular SNS activity is affected by eating (Eckberg, 1979), coffee (Pincomb et al., 1985; Robertson et al., 1979; Robertson, Wade, Workman, Woosley, & Oates, 1981), and smoking (Gash, Karliner, Janowsky, & Lake, 1978), these factors should be avoided before RR-variation testing. Medications should also be examined for their possible autonomic effects. In particular, sodium salicylate has an affect on RR variation (Figure 6). Therefore, patients should not use aspirin while taking part in RR-variation studies. It has also been shown that RR variation decreases with age (Pfeifer, Halter, et al., 1983). Thus, an abnormal result for a 20-year-old may not be abnormal for a 60-year-old.

In order to avoid as many interfering factors as possible, the following protocol is recommended (Pfeifer & Peterson, 1987).

Studies should be performed:

- In the morning.
- After an overnight (7 h) fast.
- In a quiet, relaxed atmosphere.

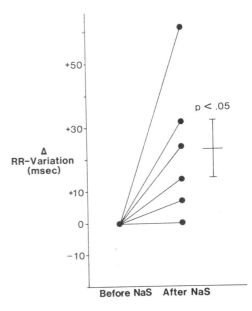

Figure 6. Effect of sodium salicylate (NaS) on RR variation.

- With assistance of a timed breathing indicator.
- After the patient has practiced the procedure.
- After 30 min of supine rest.
- After the patient has avoided tobacco products for 8 h, ethanol for 24 h, and over-the-counter medicines for 8 h.
- In patients who have avoided prescription medicines for at least 8 h.
- In patients who have not experienced vigorous exercise or severe emotional upset in the last 24 h.
- In patients who have not experienced acute illness in the last 48 h.
- In patients breathing at a rate of five breaths per minute.

Diabetic patients require additional precautions:

- They should not have taken insulin for at least 8 h (unless they are on an insulin pump in which case they should maintain basal infusion rate).
- They should not have had a hypoglycemic episode in the last 8 h.

Use of β blockade (propranolol) is recommended because it removes possible confounding effects of the SNS on the RR-variation response (Pfeifer *et al.*, 1982; Pfeifer, Halter, *et al.*, 1983; Pfeifer, Weinberg, Cook, Halter, & Porte, 1983).

Normal values and reproducibility of RR variation vary according to the protocol and method of analysis.

The RR-variation technique is straightforward and easy to perform. It is a sensitive and accurate method of assessing parasympathetic innervation to the heart.

Valsalva Maneuver

The Valsalva maneuver consists of forced expiration against a standardized resistance for a specific period of time. A continuous recording is made of either blood pressure or heart rate before, during, and after the maneuver. The response of blood pressure to the Valsalva maneuver has both SNS and PNS components, whereas changes in heart rate reflect only PNS activity (Bennett, Hosking, & Hampton, 1976; Lloyd-Mostyn & Watkins, 1975). A normal Valsalva heart rate response is shown in Figure 7.

There are four phases to the Valsalva maneuver, and they were well described by Pfeifer and Peterson (1987). In phase I, at onset of exhalation, there

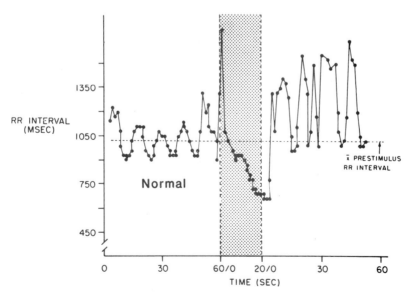

Figure 7. Normal heart rate response to Valsalva maneuver.

is a transient rise in blood pressure due to increased intrathoracic and intraabdominal pressure and an increase in stroke volume. Phase II occurs during the continued strained expiration. Venous return is reduced and cardiac output falls, producing a decreased blood pressure which in turn causes reflex tachycardia.

At release of the strain (phase III) there is further fall in blood pressure and cardiac output for a few beats due to release of the increased intrathoracic pressure and consequent rise in venous capacity. Phase IV is marked by rebound hypertension which causes a reflex bradycardia due to increased PNS tone. This post-Valsalva bradycardia can be eliminated by atropine (Leon, Shaver, & Leonard, 1970), and the post-Valsalva hypertension can be eliminated by SNS blockade (Ewing, 1978).

The Valsalva maneuver is standardized by asking the subject to blow into a mouthpiece attached to a manometer at a pressure of 40 mm Hg for 20 s while a continuous heart recording or intraarterial blood pressure recording is made. The subject should be given two or three practice trials before a recording is made.

Initially, measurement of the response to the Valsalva maneuver was assessed by relating the increase in diastolic blood pressure after the maneuver to the decrease in pulse pressure during the maneuver (Ewing, 1984). A more recent method has been to relate the decrease in heart rate after the maneuver to the resting heart rate (Akselrod *et al.*, 1981). A third commonly used method is to calculate the Valsalva ratio (Ewing *et al.*, 1980b). The Valsalva ratio is the maximum heart rate during the maneuver divided by the slowest heart rate after the maneuver. Classically, a Valsalva ratio greater than 1.5 is normal (Levin, 1966). However, 1.2 has been suggested to be the lower limit of normal by one group of investigators (Ewing, 1984; Ewing *et al.*, 1980b).

Calculation of the Valsalva ratio has several advantages over the other two methods. The Valsalva ratio is simple to measure and provides reproducible results. It is noninvasive, whereas continuous measurement of blood pressure during the Valsalva maneuver is invasive. The Valsalva ratio is well standardized, and results clearly separate normal from abnormal responses. Finally, evaluation of heart rate changes in response to the Valsalva maneuver reflect only cardiac parasympathetic activity whereas the blood pressure changes reflect an undefined combination of PNS and SNS tone.

The Valsalva ratio is less sensitive than RR variation (Pfeifer, Weinberg, *et al.*, 1983). Pfeifer *et al.* determined both RR variation and the Valsalva ratio for normal subjects before and after graded doses of atropine (PNS blockade). RR variation was significantly reduced after only 0.7 mg of atropine whereas the Valsalva ratio was not significantly reduced until 2.0 mg was given.

Finally, there may be difficulty in interpreting Valsalva responses of patients with autonomic damage or cardiovascular disease. Patients with cardiovascular disease may have difficulty maintaining straining during expiration for the time necessary to initiate reflex responses. Also, patients with congestive heart failure do not experience the same arterial pressure and volume changes as do normal subjects in response to the Valsalva maneuver. This alters the reflex changes in blood pressure and heart rate which normally occur. Eckberg (1980) provides a thorough explanation of problems involved in interpretation of responses from patients with cardiovascular disease.

Plasma Catecholamines

Plasma norepinephrine arises primarily from spillover from postganglionic sympathetic neuromuscular junctions. Although norepinephrine is also present in the adrenal gland, adrenalectomy does not influence plasma norepinephrine levels (Cryer, 1976). In humans, plasma levels of norepinephrine increase with mild or severe stress and upon standing after being in a recumbent position (Pfeifer & Peterson, 1987). Thus, plasma norepinephrine appears to be an index of vascular SNS activity.

In contrast to norepinephrine, epinephrine is believed to come solely from the adrenal medulla. Epinephrine is not detectable in plasma after adrenalectomy (Pfeifer & Peterson, 1987). It is not used as an index of vascular SNS activity because, although levels increase during severe stress [i.e., hypoglycemia or maximal exercise (Cryer, 1980; Lloyd-Mostyn & Watkins, 1976)], mild stress does not affect plasma epinephrine levels (Cryer, 1980; Metz, Halter, & Robertson, 1980). There is a larger increase in norepinephrine levels than epinephrine levels in response to physiologic stimuli (Dimsdale, 1984; Hilsted, 1982). Despite the greater response of norepinephrine, results from many experiments include levels of both epinephrine and norepinephrine.

Elevated resting levels of plasma catecholamines have been found in some, but not all, patients with essential hypertension (DeQuattro *et al.*, 1984). The elevation of catecholamines implies that increased SNS activity or decreased catecholamine degradation may be involved in the development of essential hypertension. When measuring plasma catecholamines, factors which may alter SNS tone need to be controlled. These include obesity, eating, coffee, and cigarettes. Because of peripheral uptake of norepinephrine, arterial values of catecholamines may be more reflective of vascular SNS activity than are venous blood samples (Hilsted, Christensen, & Madsbad, 1983).

Plasma epinephrine and norepinephrine may be measured using a laboratory radioenzymatic assay (Cryer, 1976; Evans, Halter, & Porte, 1978; Passon & Peuler, 1973). The enzyme promotes formation of radiolabeled metanephrine and normetanephrine from epinephrine and norepinephrine, respectively. The compounds are then separated and quantified by liquid scintillation counting.

Although plasma catecholamines can be measured in a resting subject and analyzed by comparison to ''normals,'' a more accurate method of assessing vascular SNS tone is by measuring the change in catecholamine levels in response to a stimulus. Examples of this include measuring catecholamine levels before and after exercise, stress, or postural changes. These are discussed in greater detail in their respective sections (see Exercise, Mental Stress, Postural Testing, and Cold Pressor Test).

Postural Testing

Several methods are available to assess the cardiovascular ANS during changes in posture

(Ewing, 1978; Ewing, Campbell, Murray, Neilson, & Clarke, 1978; Sundkvist, Lilja, & Almer, 1980). These are based on the observation that changes in posture result in compensatory alterations in autonomic tone to maintain adequate tissue perfusion. Both heart rate and blood pressure responses to standing can be used to assess cardiac autonomic tone.

When a subject assumes an erect posture, brachial systolic pressure is unaffected while diastolic pressure is raised about 7 mm Hg (Pfeifer, Halter, *et al.*, 1983). There is a fall in cardiac vagal activity (Scher, Ohm, Bumgarner, Boynton, & Young, 1971) and a rise in SNS activity to muscle (Burke *et al.*, 1977) resulting in elevation of plasma norepinephrine (Vendsalu, 1960).

This test can be easily performed by measuring blood pressure with a sphygmomanometer, first with the subject supine, and then after standing. Conventionally, a fall of diastolic blood pressure of more than 10 mm Hg or a systolic fall of more than 30 mm Hg is regarded as abnormal.

The immediate heart rate response to standing is another method of ANS assessment (Ewing *et al.*, 1978). In normal subjects there is an immediate and rapid increase in heart rate after standing followed by a relative slowing to a level slightly faster than the recumbent heart rate. Maximum heart rate is reached around the 15th beat after standing, and a relative bradycardia is reached around the 30th beat. The reflex tachycardia is thought to be mediated by a decrease in the PNS since the response can be abolished with atropine but not with propranolol (Ewing *et al.*, 1978).

This test is easily performed by asking the subject to lie quietly while the heart rate is recorded on an ECG. The subject is then asked to stand up as quickly as possible (within 2–3 s) and remain standing. Measurement of the shortest R–R interval after starting to stand (usually around beat 15) and the longest R–R interval (around beat 30) enables the 30 : 15 ratio to be calculated. A ratio less than 1.0 is considered abnormal.

Several precautions must be observed. Do not derive conclusions from reduced values still in the normal range. Borderline results should be confirmed by other methods of testing. This will improve the accuracy of results. Also, a misleading ratio will be produced either if the trace is counted from where the subject completes standing or if beats 15 and 30 are too rigidly adhered to. This test should not be performed using a tilt table since the characteristic heart rate changes occur only upon standing.

A final method of postural testing involves measuring the change in catecholamine levels which occurs upon standing. As discussed earlier, in normal subjects there is reflex SNS activation upon standing. This results in an elevation of plasma catecholamine levels upon standing. Figure 8 gives values which are considered normal and abnormal for this response. Once again, to get a clear value of SNS function, factors which influence SNS activity must be avoided, i.e., coffee, eating, smoking, and medications.

To assess changes in plasma catecholamine levels, the subject should be in a relaxed supine posi-

tion for 30 min before testing. Blood samples are taken 5 min before standing, at the moment of standing, and 2, 5, and 10 min after standing. Plasma catecholamines are assayed as discussed in the Plasma Catecholamines section.

Neck Suction

This technique assesses parasympathetic innervation by stimulating carotid baroreceptors with neck suction (Eckberg, 1979). The neck suction technique requires the use of a neck chamber which applies vacuum pressure to the carotid area in order to stimulate increased blood pressure and thus stimulate baroreceptors. Stimulation of baroreceptors will result in a reflex increase in parasympathetic tone. The neck chamber is able to monitor changes in arterial pressure and heart rate. Neck suction has been commonly used to study baroreflex responses in hypertension (Eckberg, 1979; Leon et al., 1970). Normal subjects should experience a decrease in heart rate and blood pressure in response to increased baroreceptor activity. Most (Bristow, Honour, Pickering, Sleight, & Smyth, 1969; Eckberg, 1979), but not all (Mancia, Ludbrook, Ferrari, Gregorini, & Zanchetti, 1978) studies indicate that baroreflex-mediated sinus node inhibition is reduced in patients with hypertension.

There are several difficulties with this system. The magnitude of arterial baroreflex responses is determined in part by the rate and duration of onset of stimuli (Eckberg, 1980). Therefore, it is important that the rate and duration be strictly standardized in the study protocol. It is inappropriate to compare results from studies in which rate and duration of pressure change are not the same.

Lower Body Negative Pressure (LBNP)

Reflex changes in circulation and heart rate in response to accumulation of blood in the lower body have been examined using this technique (Brown, Goei, Greenfield, & Plassaras, 1966). LBNP involves the use of a large box enclosing the lower body of a supine subject. The box is connected to a vacuum pump which removes air to a pressure of −70 mm Hg. The negative pressure is

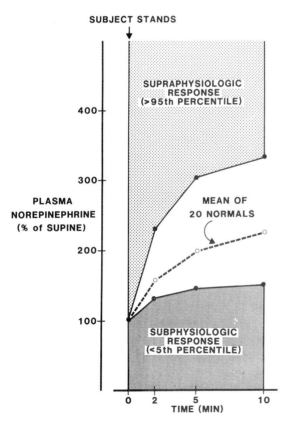

Figure 8. Normal plasma catecholamine response to standing..

usually maintained for several minutes and causes displacement into the lower body of approximately 10 g of blood per kg total body weight (Brown *et al.*, 1966).

The cardiovascular response to LBNP is similar to that due to postural changes (Brown *et al.*, 1966). As blood is sequestered, heart rate increases and blood pressure decreases and then slightly recovers. Proposed advantages to LBNP include: pressures can be changed quicker than postures, and transmural pressure is altered uniformly in all exposed areas of the supine subject. In postural changes, there is a gradient of transmural pressure in erect subjects caused by gravity. This does not occur with LBNP.

The release of blood at the end of suction has the effect of a large, rapid autotransfusion. Arterial pressure increases to greater than resting values, reaching a maximum within 4 s, and then declines to resting levels (Brown *et al.*, 1966). As a result, there is bradycardia and then a return to resting heart rate. Heart rate effects are mediated through baroreceptor reflexes whereas blood pressure changes are mediated by sympathetic vasoconstrictor nerves (Brown *et al.*, 1966).

Handgrip

Fatiguing muscle exercise such as sustained handgrip results in a reflex rise in heart rate and blood pressure. This response is mediated afferently by fibers activated by metabolic products of anaerobic metabolism (Hague, Scarpello, Sladen, & Cullen, 1978; Mark, Victor, Nerhed, & Wallin, 1985). The response consists of a temporarily increased heart rate and blood pressure due to increased SNS activity. This results in increased blood flow to the ischemic muscle. The response to the handgrip test is expressed as the change in blood pressure rather than change in heart rate since the heart rate response during early exercise results primarily from PNS withdrawal rather than SNS activation (Hollander & Bouman, 1975; Mark *et al.*, 1985).

The handgrip technique requires only a handgrip dynamometer and sphygmomanometer. The subject is first asked to grip a dynamometer as hard as possible for a few seconds, to register the maximum grip. The dynamometer is set at a standard value, usually 30% of maximum, and the subject is asked to grip at this level as long as possible (usually between 2 and 4 min) while blood pressure is periodically recorded.

The response to the test is taken as the difference in diastolic pressure just before releasing the grip and the resting value. Most normal subjects show an increase of diastolic blood pressure by at least 15 mm Hg. Apart from subjects with mechanical obstructions in the heart (such as mitral valve stenosis), the only subjects known to have abnormally low blood pressure responses are those with damaged autonomic pathways (Eckberg, 1980). Subjects can cheat by not gripping maximally but if the grip is at least 15% of their maximum it will still become fatiguing and provide accurate results. This test is quick, simple to perform, and provides good reproducibility. It gives reliable information about peripheral sympathetic vasoconstrictor nerves.

Mental Stress

Mental stress such as arithmetic, loud noise, and pain cause an increase in sympathetic activity. This results in an increase in blood pressure and heart rate in normal subjects (Pfeifer & Peterson, 1987).

One example of this technique requires the subject to do a sequential subtraction as fast as possible (Falkner, Kushner, Gaddo, & Angelakos, 1981). Measurements of blood pressure and heart rate are made before and during a 10-min timed behavioral task. Sympathetic response to this technique has also been assessed by measuring plasma norepinephrine and epinephrine levels (Falkner *et al.*, 1981; Hilsted *et al.*, 1983). It has been proposed that the neuroendocrine response to physiologic stimuli include greater plasma levels of norepinephrine whereas responses to psychologic stimuli include greater plasma levels of epinephrine (Hilsted, 1982; LeBlanc, Cote, Tobin, & Labrie, 1979).

Problems with this method include easy adaptation and variability of responses so that an absent response may be seen even in a control subject (Bennett, Hosking, & Hampton, 1975). Dimsdale

(1984) reported that field experience can provide a much greater source of mental stress than routine laboratory tests. As compared to routine office determinations, field studies of behaviorally elicited blood pressure increases are a better predictor of complications from hypertension (Dimsdale, 1984). However, field studies also include greater variability of response. Repeat testing using mental stress is hampered by a learning effect. The amount of time allowed between tests will also influence results.

Exercise

In normal subjects, low levels of exercise cause an increase in heart rate due to withdrawal of vagal tone (Dysberg et al., 1981). At higher work loads, an increase in heart rate and blood pressure occurs due to activation of the SNS (Dysberg et al., 1981; Freyschuss, 1970; Kent & Cooper, 1974). The increase in SNS activity can be assessed by measuring either heart rate, blood pressure, or catecholamine response to exercise. When examining the response to exercise, baseline samples need to be taken from each subject and another sample at the time of exhaustion. This allows each subject to serve as his or her own control. Results can then be expressed as the percent change or absolute change from the baseline value. Different responses can be expected depending on the type of exercise (e.g., isometric versus dynamic exercise) employed (Stein et al., 1984).

An example of isometric exercise is the handgrip test mentioned earlier. A treadmill test or pedaling an ergometer cycle are examples of dynamic exercise.

Drug Testing

Pharmacologic methods of testing are most often used to specifically block or stimulate the ANS. The drug is administered as a bolus or infusion and the change in a measured physiologic response is related to the portion of the nervous system affected. For example, induction of pharmacologic hypertension by phenylephrine stimulates arterial baroreceptors and is occasionally used in assessing baroreceptor function (Eckberg et al., 1980).

A major difficulty with provocative testing is the presence of drug-induced side effects. Ideally, each subject should receive the same concentration of drug at the desired site of action if results are to be accurate. The large number of factors which influence drug distribution make this nearly impossible to achieve. It must be decided whether to administer the drug as a bolus or infusion and it is crucial that the drug effect be measured at a constant time period after administration. Each of these factors needs to be accurately reproduced for each subject. Thus, a standard stimulus is not easily achieved in provocative testings.

Drugs are more commonly used as a means of clarifying the source of a response; e.g., propranolol is routinely given during RR-variation testing to eliminate possible interference from the SNS. Also, if a response is abolished by propranolol, it can be assumed the response was mediated through the SNS. In the same way, administration of atropine can indicate if the response is mediated by the PNS. More information on pharmacologic testing is provided by Julius (this volume).

Cold Pressor Test

Several variations of the cold pressor test have been developed (Hosking et al., 1978; Lloyd-Mostyn & Watkins, 1975; 1976). These include feet immersion, arm immersion, or face immersion into cold water. The normal response consists of a reflex increase in sympathetic tone resulting in increased blood pressure, heart rate, and catecholamine levels. A drawback to this test is that the cold stimulus is often considered very painful.

Power Spectrum Analysis

Power spectrum analysis of heart rate fluctuation has recently been proposed as a method which provides a sensitive, quantitative, and noninvasive measure of the cardiovascular control systems: sympathetic, parasympathetic, and renin–angiotensin systems (Akselrod et al., 1981). Use of power spectrum analysis requires instruments to measure heart rate fluctuation and the ability to perform the necessary power spectrum analysis on data.

This method involves analyzing the frequency content of heart rate fluctuations by measuring their power spectrum. In addition to the well-known fluctuation in heart rate associated with respiration (which predominantly reflects PNS activity), there are also fluctuations in heart rate which cluster at other frequencies. Akselrod et al. (1981) proposed that these other frequency clusters are associated with SNS activity and renin–angiotensin activity. Power spectrum analysis is a recent development which has not yet received wide use as an investigative tool.

Summary and Conclusions

Studies of cardiovascular behavioral medicine should not base conclusions on the results of one autonomic test. A thorough battery of autonomic tests should be administered before a conclusion is reached. The tests to be administered should be determined by several factors. (1) They should be simply and rapidly performed. (2) They should clearly distinguish between normal and abnormal results. (3) Results must be reproducible. The tests to be used will also be determined by the section of the ANS which the investigator wishes to examine (PNS or SNS). Table 1 outlines the techniques discussed in this chapter, the portion of the nervous system assessed, and references for further information.

Several of the tests presented here have been widely studied and well characterized. The range of normal and abnormal results in the standard protocol is well known. However, other tests require standardization by each investigator for the individual protocol. An abnormal result from these tests is determined by comparison to a group of normal subjects. Results are more accurate if the study is designed so that the subjects can serve as their own control, e.g., by comparing responses in the same person before and after a stimulus.

Tests which have well-defined protocols and responses include the Valsalva ratio, heart rate response to standing (30:15 ratio), blood pressure response to submaximal handgrip, blood pressure

Table 1. Methods for Assessment of Cardiovascular Autonomic Function

Test	Predominant branch of ANS assessed	References[a]
RR variation	PNS	1–3
Valsalva maneuver	Both	2, 4, 5
Plasma catecholamines	SNS	6–8
Postural testing		
30:15 ratio	Both	9
Catecholamine response to standing	SNS	7, 10
Blood pressure response to standing	SNS	11
Neck suction	PNS	12–16
Maximal handgrip	SNS	1, 9, 17–19
Mental stress	SNS	20–24
Cold pressor test	SNS	20, 22, 25–27
Exercise	SNS	19, 28
Drug testing	Both	14, 29
Lower body negative pressure	Both	14, 30
Power spectrum analysis	Both	31

[a]References: 1, Ewing et al. (1980b); 2, Robertson et al. (1979); 3, Wheeler and Watkins (1973); 4, Bennett et al. (1976); 5, Lloyd-Mostyn and Watkins (1975); 6, Christensen (1979); 7, Clarke et al. (1979); 8, Passon and Peuler (1973); 9, Ewing et al. (1974); 10, Herd (1984); 11, Thomas et al. (1981); 12, Bristow et al. (1969); 13, Eckberg et al. (1975); 14, Eckberg (1980); 15, Ernsting and Parry (1957); 16, Evans et al. (1978); 17, Ewing (1984); 18, Falkner et al. (1981); 19, Sharpey-Schafer (1965); 20, Bennett et al. (1975); 21, Freyschuss (1970); 22, Leon et al. (1970); 23, Lloyd-Mostyn and Watkins (1976); 24, Mancia et al. (1978); 25, Bennett et al. (1978); 26, Friedman et al. (1984); 27, Hasegawa and Rodbard (1979); 28, Dysberg et al. (1981); 29, Smyth et al. (1969); 30, Brown et al. (1966); 31, Akselrod et al. (1981).

response to standing, catecholamine response to standing, and some of the RR-variation techniques. These tests have the advantage of not requiring individual standardization and determination of what constitutes an abnormal result.

Tests which will require individual standardization include neck suction, response to exercise, mental stress, cold pressor test, and some RR-variation methods.

The relationship between behavioral medicine and cardiovascular changes is a rapidly expanding field. An important component of this research lies in the identification of pathophysiologic mechanisms that may translate behaviorally related risk factors into cardiovascular disease. Work in this field has already defined a relationship between the Type A personality and heart disease. Type A persons show greater increases in heart rate, blood pressure, and catecholamine secretion in response to behavioral tasks (Herd, 1984). Similar work is now being done on persons with essential hypertension and atherosclerosis.

Both sympathetic and parasympathetic mechanisms are thought to be involved in cardiovascular diseases (Verrier & Lown, 1984). Cardiovascular reactivity testing can help define the influence of the ANS on arteriosclerosis, essential hypertension, and vulnerability to sudden death. It is not until these factors have been defined that effective treatments and preventive measures can be developed.

ACKNOWLEDGMENTS. Special thanks to Ms. Pat Hagan and Ms. Janice Blair for their assistance in the preparation of the manuscript. The work discussed herein was supported in part by the Veterans Administration, The Cecil E. and Mamie M. Bales Medical Research Fund, and The Adolph O. Pfingst Fund for Medical Research.

References

Akselrod, S., Gordon, D., Ubel, F. A., Shannon, D. C., Barger, A. C., & Cohen, R. J. (1981). Power spectrum analysis of heart rate fluctuation: A quantitative probe of beat-to-beat cardiovascular control. *Science, 213,* 220–222.

Bennett, T., Hosking, D. J., & Hampton, J. R. (1975). Cardiovascular control in diabetes mellitus. *British Medical Journal, 2,* 585.

Bennett, T., Hosking, D. J., & Hampton, J. R. (1976). Baroreflex sensitivity and responses to the Valsalva maneuver in subjects with diabetes mellitus. *Journal of Neurology, Neurosurgery, and Psychiatry, 39,* 178–183.

Bennett, T., Fentem, P. H., Fitton, D., Hampton, J. R., Hosking, D. J., & Riggott, P. A. (1977). Assessment of vagal control of the heart in diabetes: Measures of RR-interval variation under different conditions. *British Heart Journal, 39,* 25.

Bennett, T., Farquhar, I. K., Hosking, D. J., & Hampton, J. R. (1978). Assessment of methods for estimating autonomic nervous control of the heart in patients with diabetes mellitus. *Diabetes, 27,* 1167.

Bradley, R. F., & Schonfield, A. (1962). Diminished pain in diabetic patients with acute myocardial infarction. *Geriatrics, 17,* 322–326.

Bristow, J. D., Honour, A. J., Pickering, B. W., Sleight, P., & Smyth, H. S. (1969). Diminished baroreflex sensitivity in high blood pressure. *Circulation, 39,* 48–54.

Brown, E., Goei, J., Greenfield, A. D. M., & Plassaras, G. (1966). Circulatory responses to simulated gravitational shifts of blood in man induced by exposure of the body below the iliac crests to sub-atmospheric pressure. *Journal of Physiology (London), 183,* 607–627.

Burke, D., Sundlof, G., & Wallin, B. G. (1977). Postural effects on muscle nerve sympathetic activity in man. *Journal of Physiology (London), 272,* 399.

Christensen, N. J. (1979). Catecholamines and diabetes mellitus. *Diabetologia, 16,* 211.

Clarke, B. F., Ewing, D. J., & Campbell, I. W. (1979). Diabetic autonomic neuropathy. *Diabetologia, 17,* 195.

Cryer, P. E. (1976). Isotope derivative measurement of plasma norepinephrine and epinephrine in man. *Diabetes, 25,* 1074.

Cryer, P. E. (1980). Physiology and pathophysiology of the human sympathoadrenal neuroendocrine system. *New England Journal of Medicine, 303,* 436.

DeQuattro, V., Sullivan, P., Minagawa, R., Kopin, I., Bornheimer, J., Foti, A., & Barndt, R. (1984). Central and peripheral noradrenergic tone in primary hypertension. *Federation Proceedings, 43,* 47–51.

Dimsdale, J. E. (1984). Generalizing from laboratory studies to field studies of human stress physiology. *Psychosomatic Medicine, 46*(5), 463–469.

Dunlap, E. D., Samols, E., Waite, L. C., & Pfeifer, M. A. (1987). Development of a method to determine autonomic nervous system function in the rat. *Metabolism, 36*(2), 193–197.

Dysberg, T., Benn, J., Sandahl-Christiansen, J., Hilsted, J., & Nerup, J. (1981). Prevalence of diabetic autonomic neuropathy measured by simple bedside tests. *Diabetologia, 20,* 190.

Eckberg, D. L. (1979). Carotid baroreflex function in young men with borderline blood pressure elevation. *Circulation, 59,* 632–636.

Eckberg, D. (1980). Parasympathetic cardiovascular control in human disease: A critical review of methods and results. *American Journal of Physiology, 239,* H581–H593.

Eckberg, D. L., Cavanaugh, M. S., Mark, A. L., & Abboud, F. M. (1975). A simplified neck suction device for activation of carotid baroreceptors. *Journal of Laboratory and Clinical Medicine, 85,* 167.

Ernsting, J., & Parry, D. J. (1957). Some observations on the effects of stimulating the stretch receptors in the carotid artery of man. *Journal of Physiology (London), 137,* 45P–46P.

Evans, M. I., Halter, J. B., & Porte, D., Jr. (1978). Comparison of double and single isotope enzymatic derivative methods for measuring catecholamines in human plasma. *Clinical Chemistry (New York), 24,* 567.

Ewing, D. J. (1978). Cardiovascular reflexes and autonomic neuropathy. *Clinical Science and Molecular Medicine, 55,* 321.

Ewing, D. J. (1984). Cardiac autonomic neuropathy. In R. J. Jarrett (Ed.), *Diabetes and heart disease* (p. 122). Amsterdam: Elsevier.

Ewing, D. J., Irving, J. B., Ken, F., Wildsmith, J. A. W., & Clarke, B. F. (1974). Cardiovascular responses to sustained handgrip in normal subjects and subjects with diabetes mellitus. A test of autonomic function. *Clinical Science and Molecular Medicine, 46,* 295.

Ewing, D. J., Campbell, I. W., Murray, A., Neilson, J. M. M., & Clarke, B. F. (1978). Immediate heart rate response to standing: Simple test for autonomic neuropathy in diabetes. *British Medical Journal, 1,* 145.

Ewing, D. J., Campbell, I. W., & Clarke, B. F. (1980a). Assessment of cardiovascular effects in diabetic autonomic neuropathy and prognostic implications. *Annals of Internal Medicine, 92*(Pt. 22), 308.

Ewing, D. J., Campbell, I. W., & Clarke, B. F. (1980b). The natural history of diabetic autonomic neuropathy. *Quarterly Journal of Medicine, 49,* 95–108.

Ewing, D. J., Borsey, D. Q., Bellavere, F., & Clarke, B. F. (1981). Cardiac autonomic neuropathy in diabetes: comparison of measure of RR-interval variation. *Diabetologia, 21,* 18.

Falkner, B., Kushner, H., Gaddo, O., & Angelakos, S. (1981). Cardiovascular characteristics in adolescents who develop essential hypertension. *Hypertension, 3,* 521–527.

Ferrari, A., Gordon, F., & Mark, A. (1984). Impairment of cardiopulmonary baroreflexes in Dahl salt-sensitive rats fed low salt. *American Journal of Physiology, 247,* H119–H123.

Freyschuss, U. (1970). Cardiovascular adjustment to somatomotor activation. *Acta Physiologica Scandinavica, Supplementum, 342,* 1–63.

Friedman, H. S., Sacerdote, A., Bandu, I., Jubay, F., Herrera, A. G., Vasavada, B. C., & Bleicher, S. J. (1984). Abnormalities of the cardiovascular response to cold pressor test in Type I diabetes. Correlation with blood glucose control. *Archives of Internal Medicine, 144,* 43.

Gash, A., Karliner, J. S., Janowsky, D., & Lake, C. R. (1978). Effects of smoking marijuana on left ventricular performance and plasma norepinephrine. Studies in normal men. *Annals of Internal Medicine, 89,* 448.

Hague, R., Scarpello, J., Sladen, G., & Cullen, D. (1978). Autonomic function tests in diabetes mellitus. *Diabetes and Metabolism, 4,* 227.

Hasegawa, M., & Rodbard, S. (1979). Effect of posture on

arterial pressures, timing of the arterial sounds and pulse wave velocities in the extremities. *Cardiology, 64,* 122.

Herd, J. (1984). Cardiovascular disease and hypertension. In W. D. Gentry (Ed.), *Handbook of behavioral medicine* (pp. 222–279). New York: Guilford Press.

Hilsted, J. (1982). Pathophysiology in diabetic autonomic neuropathy: Cardiovascular, hormonal, and metabolic studies. *Diabetes, 31,* 730.

Hilsted, J., Madsbad, S., Krarup, T., Sestoft, L., Christensen, N. J., Tronier, B., & Galbo, H. (1981). Hormonal, metabolic, and cardiovascular responses to hypoglycemia in diabetic autonomic neuropathy. *Diabetes, 30,* 626.

Hilsted, J., Christensen, N. J., & Madsbad, S. (1983). Whole body clearance of norepinephrine. *Journal of Clinical Investigation, 71,* 500–505.

Hollander, A. P., & Bouman, L. N. (1975). Cardiac acceleration in man elicited by a muscle–heart reflex. *Journal of Applied Physiology, 38,* 272–278.

Hosking, D. J., Bennett, T., & Hampton, J. R. (1978). Diabetic autonomic neuropathy. *Diabetes, 27,* 1043.

Kent, K. M., & Cooper, T. (1974). The denervated heart. *New England Journal of Medicine, 290,* 1017–1021.

Koizumi, K., & Brooks, C. (1980). The autonomic nervous system and its role in controlling body functions. In V. Mountcastle (Ed.), *Medical physiology* (Vol. I). St. Louis: Mosby.

Kollai, M., & Koizumi, K. (1979). Reciprocal and non-reciprocal action of the vagal and sympathetic nerves innervating the heart. *Journal of Autonomic Nervous System Function, 1,* 33–52.

Kollai, N. M., & Koizumi, K. (1981). Cardiovascular reflexes and interrelationships between sympathetic and parasympathetic activity. *Journal of Autonomic Nervous System Function, 4,* 135–148.

LeBlanc, J., Cote, J., Tobin, M., & Labrie, A. (1979). Plasma catecholamines and cardiovascular responses to cold and mental activity. *Journal of Applied Physiology, 47,* 1207–1211.

Leon, D. F., Shaver, J. A., & Leonard, J. J. (1970). Reflex heart rate control in man. *American Heart Journal, 80,* 729.

Levin, A. B. (1966). A simple test of cardiac function based upon the heart rate changes induced by the Valsalva manoeuvre. *American Journal of Cardiology, 18,* 90.

Lloyd-Mostyn, R. H., & Watkins, P. J. (1975). Defective innervation of heart in diabetic autonomic neuropathy. *British Medical Journal, 3,* 15–17.

Lloyd-Mostyn, R. H., & Watkins, P. J. (1976). Total cardiac denervation in diabetic autonomic neuropathy. *Diabetes, 25,* 748.

Mancia, G., Ludbrook, J., Ferrari, A., Gregorini, L., & Zanchetti, A. (1978). Baroreceptor reflexes in human hypertension. *Circulation Research, 43,* 170–177.

Manuck, S. B., Kaplan, J. R., & Clarkson, T. B. (1983). Behaviorally induced heart rate reactivity and atherosclerosis in cynomolgus monkeys. *Psychosomatic Medicine, 45*(2), 95–106.

Mark, A., Victor, R. G., Nerhed, C., & Wallin, B. G. (1985). Microneurographic studies of the mechanisms of sympathetic nerve responses to static exercise in humans. *Circulation Research, 57,* 461–469.

Metz, S., Halter, J., & Robertson, R. P. (1980). Sodium salicylate potentiates neurohumoral responses to insulin-induced hypoglycemia. *Journal of Clinical Endocrinology and Metabolism, 51,* 93.

Passon, P. G., & Peuler, J. D. (1973). A simplified radiometric assay for plasma norepinephrine and epinephrine. *Analytical Biochemistry, 51,* 618.

Pfeifer, M. A., & Peterson, H. (1987). Cardiovascular autonomic neuropathy. In P. J. Dyck, P. K. Thomas, A. K. Asbury, A. I. Winegrad, & D. Porte (Eds.), *Diabetic neuropathy.* Philadelphia: Saunders.

Pfeifer, M. A., Cook, D., Brodsky, J., Tice, D., Reenan, A., Swedine, S., Halter, J. B., & Porte, D., Jr. (1982). Quantitative evaluation of cardiac parasympathetic activity in normal and diabetic man. *Diabetes, 31,* 339.

Pfeifer, M. A., Halter, J. B., Weinberg, C. R., Cook, D., Best, J., Reenan, A., & Porte, D., Jr. (1983). Differential changes of autonomic nervous system function with age in man. *American Journal of Medicine, 75,* 249.

Pfeifer, M. A., Weinberg, C. R., Cook, D., Halter, J., & Porte, D., Jr. (1983). Sensitivity of RR-variation and the Valsalva ratio in the assessment of diabetic autonomic neuropathy. *Clinical Research, 31,* 394.

Pincomb, G. A., Lovallo, W. R., Passey, R. B., Whitsett, T. L., Silverstein, S. M., & Wilson, M. (1985). Effects of caffeine on vascular resistance, cardiac output, and myocardial contractility in young men. *American Journal of Cardiology, 56,* 119–122.

Robertson, D., Johnson, F. A., Robertson, R. M., Nies, A. S., Shand, D. G., & Oates, J. A. (1979). Comparative assessment of stimuli that release neuronal and adrenomedullary catecholamines in man. *Circulation, 59,* 637.

Robertson, D., Wade, D., Workman, R., Woosley, R. L., & Oates, J. A. (1981). Tolerance to the humoral and hemodynamic effects of caffeine in man. *Journal of Clinical Investigation, 67,* 1111.

Scher, A. M., Ohm, W. W., Bumgarner, K., Boynton, R., & Young, A. C. (1971). Sympathetic and parasympathetic control of heart rate in the dog, baboon, and man. *Federation Proceedings, 31,* 1219.

Schwartz, P. J., & Stone, H. L. (1985). The analysis and modulation of autonomic reflexes in the prediction and prevention of sudden death. In K. Zipes & D. Jalife (Eds.), *Cardiac electrophysiology and arrhythmias.* New York: Grune & Stratton.

Smyth, H. S., Sleight, P., & Pickering, G. W. (1969). Reflex regulation of arterial pressure during sleep in man. *Circulation Research, 24,* 109–121.

Stein, D. T., Lowenthal, D. T., Porter, R. S., Falkner, B., Bravo, E., & Hare, T. (1984). Effects of nifedipine and verapamil on isometric and dynamic exercise on normal subjects. *American Journal of Cardiology, 54,* 386–389.

Sundkvist, G., Lilja, B., & Almer, L. O. (1980). Abnormal diastolic blood pressure and heart rate reactions to tilting in diabetes mellitus. *Diabetologia, 19,* 433.

Thomas, J. E., Schirger, A., Fealey, R. D., & Sheps, S. G. (1981). Orthostatic hypotension. *Mayo Clinic Proceedings, 56,* 117.

Thomas, P. K., & Eliasson, S. G. (1984). Diabetic neuropathy. In P. Dyck, P. K. Thomas, E. Lamber, & R. Bunge (Eds.), *Peripheral neuropathy.* Saunders.

Vendsalu, A. (1960). Studies on adrenaline and noradrenaline in human plasma. *Acta Physiologica Scandinavica, Supplementum, 173,* 49–70.

Verrier, R., & Lown, B. (1984). Behavioral stress and cardiac arrhythmias. *Annual Review of Physiology, 46,* 155–176.

Weinberg, C. R., & Pfeifer, M. A. (1984). An improved method for measuring heart rate variability: Assessment of cardiac autonomic function. *Biometrics, 40,* 855.

Weinberg, C. R., & Pfeifer, M. A. (1986). Development of a predictive model for symptomatic neuropathy in diabetes. *Diabetes, 35,* 873–880.

Wheeler, T., & Watkins, P. J. (1973). Cardiac denervation in diabetes. *British Medical Journal, 4,* 584.

Ziegler, M. G., Lake, C. R., & Kopin, I. J. (1977). The sympathetic nervous system defect in primary orthostatic hypotension. *New England Journal of Medicine, 296,* 293.

CHAPTER **7**

Microneurographic Measurement of Sympathetic Nerve Activity in Humans

Erling A. Anderson and Allyn L. Mark

Introduction

Microneurography is a technique in which electrodes are inserted percutaneously into peripheral nerves in humans for recording of single or multiunit action potentials. The technique has been used to study (1) sensory innervation of skin, (2) proprioceptive innervation of skeletal muscle, and (3) sympathetic innervation of autonomic effector organs in muscle and skin (Hagbarth, 1979).

Microneurography was developed by Hagbarth and Vallbo in Sweden during the 1960s (Hagbarth & Vallbo, 1968) and has been employed extensively by Wallin and his colleagues during the past 15 years to characterize the regulation of sympathetic nerve activity (SNA) to muscle and skin in humans (Wallin, 1979). The technique is primarily a research tool with few clinical applications and requires considerable training. It is relatively safe and well tolerated when performed properly (Hagbarth, 1979). However, some subjects report mild and transient paresthesias or muscle weakness in the distal extremity or an ache at the recording site following the procedure. In over 500 studies in our

laboratory, symptoms have occurred in 7% of subjects. Symptoms following microneurography usually persist less than 1 week. In over 1000 studies, Hagbarth (1979) reported only three subjects in whom paresthesias persisted for 30 days. We have observed one subject in whom mild paresthesias persisted for 35 days but we have not encountered permanent symptoms or complications after microneurography.

The microneurography technique can be used to record from any nerve which is accessible percutaneously. These include the radial, median, tibial, and sural nerves, but for practical reasons, most recordings of SNA have been made from a peroneal nerve adjacent to the fibular head below the knee. In this region the peroneal nerve has identifiable landmarks (the fibular head) and is often palpable. In addition, the peroneal nerve often provides a stable recording site with minimal electromyographic artifacts. Finally, the peroneal nerve below the knee has a high frequency of relatively pure nerve fascicles to muscle or skin.

Although different types of afferent and efferent nerve activity can be recorded using microneurography, this chapter will focus on measurement of postganglionic activity along unmyelinated, type C sympathetic fibers innervating muscle and skin. This activity represents efferent vasoconstrictor activity which is of interest to in-

Erling A. Anderson and Allyn L. Mark • Departments of Anesthesia and Internal Medicine, Cardiovascular and Clinical Research Centers, University of Iowa College of Medicine, Iowa City, Iowa 52242.

vestigators studying the influence of psychosocial factors on the sympathetic nervous system.

Description of Equipment

Equipment required for microneurography includes a nerve stimulator and stimulus isolation unit, a preamplifier, a nerve traffic analyzer, a storage oscilloscope, and an audio amplifier. The preamplifier has a gain of 1000. The nerve traffic analyzer allows further amplification (1–100), high- and low-pass filters (bandwidth 700–2000 Hz), and integration (time constant 0.1 s). Tungsten wire electrodes (30–40 mm long, 0.2 mm wide tapering to a tip of 1 to 5 μm) are used for recording. Use of such small electrodes allows percutaneous insertion without local anesthetic and with minimal discomfort to subjects.

Procedure

The general procedure for locating and recording from a nerve is similar for all nerves and will be described for the peroneal nerve. The procedure involves three basic steps: (1) percutaneous electrical stimulation to map the position of the nerve, (2) insertion of the electrode into the nerve using weak electrical stimulation through the electrode, and (3) fine adjustments of electrode position to obtain a satisfactory recording site.

The leg is positioned as shown in Figure 1 for recording from the peroneal nerve. The preamplifier is positioned at the knee. A ground for the percutaneous external stimulation is attached to the ankle. The path of the peroneal nerve adjacent to the fibular head is determined by percutaneous stimulation at 40 to 120 V, 0.2 ms, and 1 Hz. Percutaneous stimulation over the nerve elicits in-

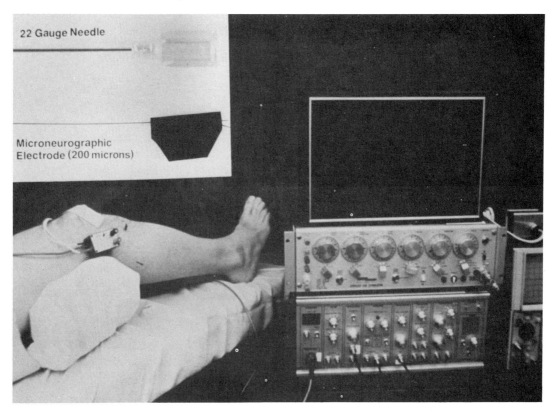

Figure 1. Experimental setup for microneurographic recording from the peroneal nerve at the fibular head. The knee is slightly elevated and stabilized to minimize movement. A preamplifier is attached at the knee immediately proximal to the recording site. Insert shows the tungsten microelectrode.

voluntary contractions and/or paresthesias in the distribution of the nerve. After marking the course of the nerve, the investigator inserts two electrodes. No special skin preparation is required. An uninsulated reference electrode is placed subcutaneously approximately 1–2 cm from the recording electrode. An insulated electrode, which will be used as the recording electrode, is inserted percutaneously over the path of the nerve (Fig. 2).

The recording electrode is advanced toward the nerve while stimulating through one electrode at 4–5 V, 0.2 ms, and 1 Hz. Upon entering the nerve, stimulation produces an involuntary muscle twitch and/or paresthesias in the distal extremity. An involuntary muscle twitch without paresthesias elicited by low-voltage stimulation (< 3 V) indicates that the electrode is in a nerve fascicle to muscle. Paresthesias without a muscle twitch indicate that the electrode is in a nerve fascicle to skin.

The electrode is then switched from a stimulating to a recording mode. The investigator confirms the position of the electrode in a nerve fascicle by determining that it is possible to detect evoked afferent activity. Specifically, if the electrode is in a nerve fascicle to muscle, tapping or stretching the muscle or tendon will elicit detectable afferent activity. If the electrode is in a nerve fascicle to skin, afferent activity is detected during stroking of the innervated skin. When the electrode is in a nerve fascicle, minor adjustments are made to obtain a site with spontaneous action potentials characteristic of SNA to skin or muscle and with a favorable signal-to-noise ratio.

There is considerable evidence that activity regarded as sympathetic action potentials is indeed postganglionic, efferent SNA and not motor or sensory activity. First, the activity is eliminated by nerve block proximal, but not distal, to the record-

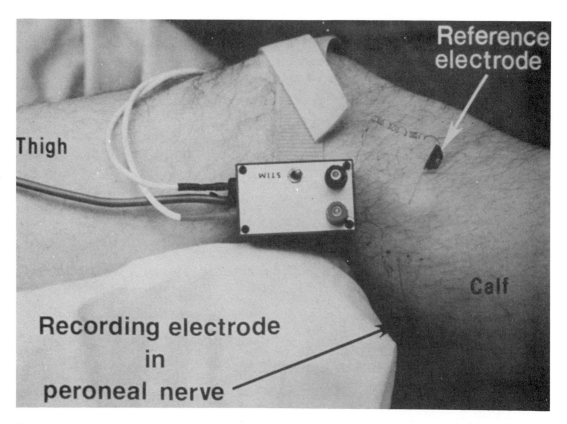

Figure 2. Close-up of microelectrode placement in the leg (peroneal nerve). Black dots indicate the path of the nerve as determined by percutaneous stimulation. Preamplifier at the knee can be switched from stimulation to recording mode.

ing site (Hagbarth & Vallbo, 1968; Delius, Hagbarth, Hongell, & Wallin, 1972a). Second, the activity is reversibly eliminated by ganglionic blockade (Delius et al., 1972a; Hagbarth, Hallin, Hongell, Torebjörk, & Wallin, 1972). Third, the conduction velocity (~ 1 m/s) is similar to that of sympathetic unmyelinated C fibers (Hagbarth & Vallbo, 1968; Delius et al., 1972a). Fourth, changes in activity are accompanied by directional changes in vascular resistance and in skin by changes in sudomotor activity (Delius, Hagbarth, Hongell, & Wallin, 1972b).

Since there are profound differences in the characteristics and control of SNA to muscle versus skin, the sympathetic activity to those two vascular beds will be discussed separately.

Muscle SNA

Characteristics

There are three steps in obtaining a satisfactory recording of SNA to muscle. Low-voltage stimulation through the microelectrode elicits a twitch without paresthesias. Further, afferent activity is elicited by stretching or tapping the innervated muscle or tendon but not by stroking the overlying skin. Finally, muscle SNA has a characteristic pattern (Figure 3). The activity occurs in intermittent, pulse synchronous bursts (Delius et al., 1972b). Muscle SNA frequently occurs in short sequences separated by periods of neural silence. The burst sequences tend to occur during the periodic spontaneous reductions in arterial pressure, whereas the SNA is suppressed during increases in arterial pressure. As discussed below, these characteristics indicate strong baroreceptor modulation of muscle SNA.

Simultaneous recordings from two muscle nerves (e.g., radial and peroneal nerves) reveal remarkable similarity in the pattern and number of sympathetic bursts at rest (Sundlöf & Wallin, 1977). This indicates that a recording of resting muscle SNA from one nerve is representative of resting muscle SNA from another nerve. In a broader context, these observations suggest that postganglionic muscle SNA to various regions is under a relatively uniform preganglionic influence. It should be emphasized, however, that these observations apply only to muscle SNA under resting conditions. As discussed later, there is increasing evidence for a regional difference in muscle SNA during autonomic stimuli including mental stress.

The frequency of resting muscle SNA is quite reproducible in a given individual during an experimental session and in repeated recordings spanning weeks to months (Sundlöf & Wallin, 1977). However, between individuals, resting levels of muscle SNA vary considerably (from less than 5 up to 50–60 bursts/min).

The control of SNA to muscle has been studied extensively. These studies have revealed a strong influence of baroreceptors. Both cardiopulmonary (low pressure) and carotid (high pressure) baroreceptors exert pronounced effects on muscle SNA. Inhibition of cardiopulmonary baroreceptors by lower body negative pressure produces a marked and sustained increase in muscle SNA (Sundlöf & Wallin, 1978).

Stimulation of carotid arterial baroreceptors by application of neck suction produces a profound, though transient, reduction in SNA (Wallin & Eckberg, 1982). The transient nature of this response may stem from the fact that blood pressure decreases during neck suction. A decrease in blood pressure induced by carotid baroreceptor stimulation would be expected to decrease aortic baroreceptor activity. The opposing influence of aortic baroreceptors could counter and abbreviate the sympathoinhibitory influence of carotid baroreceptors. In this regard, we have recently observed that

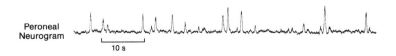

Peroneal Neurogram

10 s

Figure 3. Neurogram showing characteristic pattern of resting muscle SNA recorded from the peroneal nerve. Bursts of muscle SNA occur in short sequences separated by periods of neural silence.

concerted stimulation of aortic and carotid bar-oreceptors (from increases in arterial pressure produced by phenylephrine) causes sustained inhibition of muscle SNA (Aylward, Anderson, Kempf, & Mark, 1986). Thus, it appears that both arterial and cardiopulmonary baroreceptors can trigger sustained reflex changes in muscle SNA.

Muscle SNA in humans is also responsive to exercise and stimulation of chemically sensitive muscle afferents. Mark, Victor, Nerhed, and Wallin (1985) reported that static handgrip of 30% of maximal voluntary contraction (MVC) increased muscle SNA. Further, posthandgrip muscle ischemia (stimulation of chemically sensitive muscle afferents) maintained striking increases in SNA. These studies indicate that stimulation of chemically sensitive muscle afferents is a potent stimulus to muscle SNA in humans and suggest that these chemically sensitive muscle afferents are a trigger to increases in muscle SNA during static handgrip. Interestingly, Victor, Seals, and Mark (1987) demonstrated that rhythmic handgrip at 10 to 50% MVC failed to increase muscle SNA presumably because rhythmic handgrip is associated with less muscle ischemia than sustained handgrip and therefore fails to reach the threshold for activation of chemosensitive muscle afferents.

Rhythmic contraction of larger muscle groups (arm cycling) is associated with increases in muscle SNA, but the increases in muscle SNA do not occur at low work loads (Victor et al., 1987). Moreover, increases in muscle SNA during higher work loads of arm cycling lag behind increases in heart rate. These observations emphasize the differential control of heart rate and muscle SNA during exercise.

Svendenhag, Wallin, Sundlöf, and Henriksson (1984) found no difference in resting muscle SNA between trained racing cyclists and age-matched, untrained cyclists. Further, an 8-week training program did not change resting muscle SNA in previously untrained subjects. These studies suggest that endurance exercise training does not reduce resting muscle SNA and cannot account for the large variation in resting muscle SNA in different individuals. However, it is not known if endurance exercise training attenuates the sympathetic response to exercise.

Muscle SNA is increased by stimulation of cutaneous as well as muscle afferents. Victor, Leimbach, Wallin, and Mark (1985) demonstrated that immersion of the hand in ice water (a cold pressor test) increases muscle SNA as well as heart rate.

These studies have provided considerable information on the reflex mechanisms controlling muscle sympathetic nerve activity. However, of perhaps even greater interest to researchers in the field of behavioral medicine is the influence of psychological stress on sympathetic nerve traffic.

Stress and Muscle SNA

It is well known that psychologic stress influences the sympathetic nervous system as evidenced by elevation in circulating catecholamine levels (Ward et al., 1983). However, until recently there have been only sporadic reports of the effects of stress on muscle SNA (Delius et al., 1972b; Wallin, Delius, & Hagbarth, 1974; Wallin, 1981b).

Mental stress has long been assumed to increase blood flow to skeletal muscle, although Rusch, Shepherd, Webb, and Vanhoutte (1981) reported that mental stress increases blood flow to the forearm but not to the calf. The importance of tonic sympathetic vasoconstrictor activity in regulating blood flow to skeletal muscle suggests that altered sympathetic outflow may be involved in these blood flow changes. We recently tested the hypothesis that mental stress alters sympathetic outflow to the arm and the leg (Anderson, Wallin, & Mark, 1987). We found that stress (mental math) increases muscle SNA in the leg (peroneal nerve; see Fig. 4) but not in the arm (radial nerve).

These findings are interesting for several reasons. First, they illustrate the complex and unique sympathetic response to mental stress and indicate that mental stress can differentially alter sympathetic outflow to different regions of the skeletal muscle circulation. Second, the results suggest that the sympathoexcitatory influence of mental stress may override baroreceptor control of SNA. Finally, and perhaps most importantly, these findings demonstrate the value of microneurographic recording techniques to the fields of psychophysiology and behavioral medicine.

Although the term "sympathetic reactivity" is

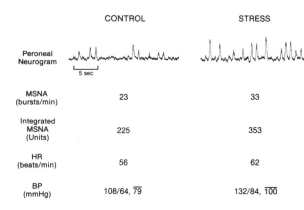

Figure 4. Neurogram of muscle SNA (MSNA) from the leg (peroneal nerve) in one subject during rest and mental stress. Mental stress (mental math performed under pressure) was associated with increased MSNA. Heart rate and blood pressure also increased during mental stress.

often used when studying psychosocial influences on blood pressure in different groups such as Type A and B persons, the term is loosely defined and nearly meaningless. One reason is the profound difference in sympathetic outflow to various vascular beds, e.g., muscle and skin. Another reason is that "sympathetic reactivity" can reflect different facets of sympathetic function. These include the frequency of sympathetic nerve discharge, amount of neurotransmitter released, efficiency of reuptake and metabolism of neurotransmitter, adrenergic receptor density and affinity, and the characteristics of vascular muscle.

Microneurography allows direct measurement of sympathetic nerve discharge in humans, and thus permits study of central sympathetic outflow to skeletal muscle or skin. Microneurographic studies of SNA in individuals assumed to be "sympathetically hyperreactive" could help determine if these individuals have augmented sympathetic outflow.

Skin SNA

There are three steps in obtaining a recording of skin SNA. Low-voltage stimulation through the electrode must elicit paresthesias but not a muscle twitch. Further, afferent activity is elicited by lightly stroking the skin but not by stretching muscle. Finally, the site must have spontaneous action potentials characteristic of skin SNA.

The characteristics of skin SNA are markedly different from those of muscle SNA. Skin and muscle SNA differ both in the resting state and in response to different interventions. Whereas muscle SNA is primarily vasoconstrictor, skin includes vasoconstrictor, sudomotor, and piloerector activity (Hagbarth, 1979). Further, skin SNA is not pulse-synchronous and does not vary with spontaneous fluctuations in blood pressure (Delius *et al.,* 1972c; Hagbarth *et al.,* 1972). These observations indicate little baroreceptor influence on skin SNA.

Blood flow to skin is important in regulating body temperature and it is not surprising that skin SNA changes with alterations in body temperature. Body cooling tends to increase skin SNA, presumably vasoconstrictor activity. Subsequent body warming initially reduces skin SNA and then causes a progressive increase as subjects begin to perspire (Wallin, 1981b). This increase in skin SNA at high temperatures reflects augmented sudomotor activity.

Mental stimuli also have a major influence on skin SNA. In general, skin SNA increases during mental stress and declines during periods of relaxation. Novel stimuli, both pleasant and unpleasant, cause a sudden increase in skin SNA when first presented (Hagbarth *et al.,* 1972). As with electrodermal responses, skin SNA responses to novel stimuli decline after several repetitions. Changes in skin SNA during stress have been found to correlate with blood flow to the innervated cutaneous tissue (Wallin *et al.,* 1974). By correlating changes in skin resistance responses and skin SNA recorded from the median nerve, Lidberg and Wallin (1981) concluded that changes in skin resistance may provide a reasonable index of sympathetic outflow of skin.

However, since there is little relationship between muscle and skin SNA at rest or in response to different interventions, skin SNA does not provide an index of muscle SNA. These findings have significant implications for investigators who study electrodermal responses as a measure of sympathetic activation.

Consideration for Design, Analysis, and Interpretation

A variety of factors must be considered during data collection. First, when recording SNA, considerable care must be taken to ensure that a pure muscle or skin site has been obtained because of the profound differences in characteristics and control of muscle and skin SNA. Second, muscle SNA has been shown to increase upon going from a supine to sitting position (Burke, Sundlöf, & Wallin, 1977). Therefore, posture must be standardized within a study. Third, when recording from skin nerves, changes in ambient temperature and extraneous noise must be minimized and time allowed for the subject to adjust to the laboratory setting.

For purposes of analysis, SNA can be quantified in three ways: (1) bursts per minute, (2) integrated SNA which is calculated as burst frequency times mean burst amplitude, and (3) bursts per 100 heartbeats. In these integrated mean voltage neurograms from multifiber recordings, burst frequency should theoretically not be the most accurate measure of sympathetic outflow since bursts of small amplitude are weighted equally with large-amplitude bursts. Integrated activity should be a more accurate indication of SNA. However, burst amplitude is determined by amplifier gain and the proximity of the electrode to a nerve fascicle. Therefore, one cannot compare burst amplitude or integrated activity across different recording sessions or between subjects. Instead, analysis of integrated SNA is valuable in examining changes in

SNA during interventions performed during an experimental session with a stable recording site.

For comparison between subjects or across sessions, burst frequency provides the best index of SNA. As mentioned previously, there are theoretical limitations to the analysis of SNA as burst frequency. However, in a given study analysis of changes in SNA as bursts per minute and as integrated activity usually yields similar conclusions. In addition, muscle SNA expressed as bursts per minute correlates with forearm venous norepinephrine (Morlin, Wallin, & Eriksson, 1983). Moreover, resting muscle SNA expressed as bursts per minute is quite reproducible in a given individual from one experimental session to another. Thus, despite some theoretical limitations, measurement of muscle SNA expressed as bursts per minute can be used to compare muscle SNA between sessions and subjects. However, caution should be exercised in interpreting the significance of small or no differences.

Finally, it should be noted that microneurographic studies of SNA may be slightly biased toward individuals with moderate to high levels of sympathetic activity. This stems from the fact that obtaining a satisfactory recording site depends to some degree on the frequency of resting SNA. Locating a site in a subject with very low levels of resting SNA is more difficult.

Future

We consider the microneurographic technique for direct, *in vivo* recording of SNA in humans to be an important and underutilized tool for studying the impact of psychosocial factors on the sympathetic nervous system and its role in blood pressure regulation. When performed properly, microneurography is a safe procedure which allows measurement of central sympathetic neural outflow to muscle or skin. This information cannot be gained by other methods such as measurement of catecholamine levels, regional blood flow, galvanic skin responses, heart rate, or blood pressure which are influenced by numerous factors.

Recent studies of the effects of mental stress on SNA are promising and suggest that mental stress may have a unique impact on the sympathetic nervous system. Future areas of research in this field might include systematic study of (1) SNA in Type A and B individuals, (2) sympathetic nerve responses to stress in individuals hypothesized to be sympathetically hyperreactive, (3) sympathetic nerve responses to stress in normotensive and hypertensive subjects, and (4) the effects of pharmacologic agents on sympathetic responses to mental stress.

ACKNOWLEDGMENTS. Studies by the authors and their colleagues reviewed in this chapter were supported by a National Research Service Award Grant (HL-07385) and by research grants HL-24962 and HL-36224 from the National Heart, Lung and Blood Institute and by grant RR59 from the General Clinical Research Center's Program, Division of Research Resources, National Institutes of Health; by a Grant-In-Aid from the Iowa Affiliate of the American Heart Association; and by research funds from the Veterans Administration.

References

Anderson, E. A., Wallin, B. G., & Mark, A. L. (1987). Dissociation of sympathetic nerve activity to arm and leg during mental stress. *Hypertension, 9,* III-114–III-119.

Aylward, P. E., Anderson, E. A., Kempf, J. S., & Mark. A. L. (1986). Arterial baroreceptors can produce sustained inhibition of sympathetic nerve activity in humans. *Circulation, 74,* II69.

Burke, D., Sundlöf, G., & Wallin, B. G. (1977). Postural effects on muscle nerve sympathetic activity in man. *Journal of Physiology (London), 272,* 399–414.

Delius, W., Hagbarth, K. E., Hongell, A., & Wallin, B. G. (1972a). General characteristics of sympathetic activity in human muscle nerves. *Acta Physiologica Scandinavica, 84,* 65–81.

Delius, W., Hagbarth, K. E., Hongell, A., & Wallin, B. G. (1972b). Manoeuvres affecting sympathetic outflow in human muscle nerves. *Acta Physiologica Scandinavica, 84,* 82–94.

Delius, W., Hagbarth, K. E., Hongell, A., & Wallin, B. G. (1972c). Manoeuvres affecting sympathetic outflow in human skin nerves. *Acta Physiologica Scandinavica, 84,* 177–186.

Hagbarth, K. E. (1979). Exteroceptive, proprioceptive, and sympathetic activity recorded with microelectrodes from human peripheral nerves. *Mayo Clinic Proceedings, 54,* 353–365.

Hagbarth, K. E., & Vallbo, A. B. (1968). Pulse and respiratory grouping of sympathetic impulses in human muscle nerves. *Acta Physiologica Scandinavica, 74,* 96–108.

Hagbarth, K. E., Hallin, R. G., Hongell, A., Torebjörk, H. E., & Wallin, B. G. (1972). General characteristics of sympathetic activity in human skin nerves. *Acta Physiologica Scandinavica, 84,* 164–176.

Lidberg, L., & Wallin, B. G. (1981). Sympathetic skin nerve discharges in relation to amplitude of skin resistance responses. *Psychophysiology, 18,* 268–270.

Mark, A. L., Victor, R. G., Nerhed, C., & Wallin, B. G. (1985). Microneurographic studies of the mechanisms of sympathetic nerve responses to static exercise in humans. *Circulation Research, 57,* 461–469.

Morlin, C., Wallin, B. G., & Eriksson, B. M. (1983). Muscle sympathetic activity and plasma noradrenaline in normotensive and hypertensive man. *Acta Physiologica Scandinavica, 119,* 117–121.

Rusch, N. J., Shepherd, J. T., Webb, R. C., & Vanhoutte, P. M. (1981). Different behavior of the resistance vessels of the human calf and forearm during contralateral isometric exercise, mental stress, and abnormal respiratory movements. *Circulation Research, 48,* I118–I130.

Sundlöf, G., & Wallin, B. G. (1977). The variability of muscle nerve sympathetic activity in resting recumbent man. *Journal of Physiology (London), 272,* 399–414.

Sundlöf, G., & Wallin, B. G. (1978). Effect of lower body negative pressure on human muscle nerve sympathetic activity. *Journal of Physiology (London), 278,* 525–532.

Svendenhag, J., Wallin, B. G., Sundlöf, G., & Henriksson, J. (1984). Skeletal muscle sympathetic activity at rest in trained and untrained subjects. *Acta Physiologica Scandinavica, 120,* 499–504.

Victor, R., Leimbach, W., Wallin, G., & Mark, A. (1985). Microneurographic evidence for increased central sympathetic neural drive during the cold pressor test. *Journal of the American College of Cardiology, 5,* II415.

Victor, R. G., Seals, D. R., & Mark, A. L. (1987). Differential control of heart rate and sympathetic nerve activity during dynamic exercise: Insight from direct intraneural recordings in humans. *Journal of Clinical Investigation, 79,* 508–516.

Wallin, B. G. (1979). Intraneural recording and autonomic function in man. In R. Bannister (Ed.), *Autonomic failure* (pp. 36–51). London: Oxford University Press.

Wallin, B. G. (1981a). New aspects of sympathetic function in man. In E. Stalberg & R. R. Young (Eds.), *Neurology I. Clinical neurophysiology* (pp. 145–167). London: Butterworths.

Wallin, B. G. (1981b). Sympathetic nerve activity underlying electrodermal and cardiovascular reactions in man. *Psychophysiology, 18,* 470–476.

Wallin, B. G., & Eckberg, D. L. (1982). Sympathetic transients caused by abrupt alterations of carotid baroreceptor activity in humans. *American Journal of Physiology, 242,* H185–H190.

Wallin, B. G., Delius, W., & Hagbarth, K. E. (1974). Regional control of sympathetic outflow in human skin and muscle nerves. In W. Umbach & H. P. Koepchen (Eds.), *Central rhythmic and regulation* (pp. 190–195). Stuttgart: Hippokrates Verlag.

Ward, M. M., Mefford, I. N., Parker, S. D., Chesney, M. A., Taylor, C. B., Keegan, D. L., & Barchas, J. D. (1983). Epinephrine and norepinephrine responses in continuously collected human plasma to a series of stressors. *Psychosomatic Medicine, 45,* 471–486.

CHAPTER 8

Measurement of Volume Regulation
Renal Function

Bonita Falkner

Introduction

Investigation of the involvement of the renal function in behavioral medicine is an area in which little study has been done to date. An overall concept of renal physiology is that the kidneys respond to excesses or deficits in nutrient and fluid supply by excretion or conservation. The kidneys adjust numerous specific functional parameters to maintain total body fluid and electrolyte homeostasis. The kidneys also respond to stimuli mediated through the autonomic nervous system and extrarenal hormonal factors. Unlike the cardiovascular response to similar stimuli which is quite rapid, the renal response to stimuli is slower. Renal adjustments to neurogenic stressor or altered electrolyte loads will occur over hours to days. Therefore, methodologic issues addressing renal participation in behavior-related disorders will require a design which addresses means of investigating a system which functions under slower stimulus–response rate. This chapter will discuss the basic elements of renal function, and those which may be altered by behavioral factors. The standard methods of

evaluating renal function and factors which effect functional variations will also be presented.

The two kidneys in man are composed of two million nephrons or specialized functional units. The function of each nephron varies somewhat depending on its regional location. However, it is generally convenient to consider all nephrons collectively in determinations of renal function. Despite this known heterogeneity among nephrons, parameters of renal function in humans will provide composite values which reflect the total glomerular function, the total proximal tubular function, the total distal tubular function, and so forth.

The kidney is considered an excretory organ. However, excretion *per se* is but one portion of the kidney's primary role in fluid volume and chemical homeostasis. Figure 6 of Chapter 1 is a very simplified depiction of the body's fluid compartments. In a normally hydrated 70-kg male, the total body water is approximately 60% of the total body mass, or in this case 42 liters of water. This body water is contained in two fluid compartments: the intracellular fluid space (ICF) consisting of about 40% of the total body mass, and the extracellular fluid space (ECF) consisting of about 20% of the total body mass. The ECF can be further divided into interstitial fluid space (IF) and plasma volume (PV). Total blood volume is approximately 7% of body weight. When the volume

Bonita Falkner • Department of Pediatrics, Hahnemann University, Philadelphia, Pennsylvania 19102.

of blood due to red blood cells is subtracted, the remainder is the PV. Assuming the average hematocrit of 45%, the circulating plasma will be 3.8–4% of body mass. Therefore, a 70-kg man will have 2.8 liters of plasma fluid. It is this 2.8 liters that is delivered to the two million glomeruli for filtration. The normal glomerular filtration rate is 125 ml/min per 1.73 m^2. At the normal rate of filtration in a 70-kg male, 180 liters of filtrate will be produced in 24 h. This daily glomerular filtrate will contain over 1 kg of sodium chloride and other plasma constituents in similar large amounts. The total volume of fluid excreted as urine will be less than 2 liters. Also, equally small fractions of the other substances from the filtrate will be excreted daily. Hence, the renal tubules function to reabsorb the filtrate. The filtered water must be restored to the ECF to replace the PV. In addition to reabsorbing sodium and chloride, other filtered substances including glucose, bicarbonate, and amino acids must also be reabsorbed. At certain tubular sites, some substances, in particular potassium and hydrogen ion, will be secreted and added to the filtrate. Fluid and volume homeostasis is accomplished by reabsorption of the bulk of the filtrate and excretion of a small fraction. The process of tubular reabsorption and tubular secretion modifies the composition of the filtrate. The composition and volume of the urine excreted is the final product of this process.

The overall concept of renal function is that of a steady filtering of total body water through rapid recycling of plasma fluid. This is accomplished by three major components of nephron activity: (1) glomerular filtration, (2) tubular reabsorption, and (3) tubular secretion. These functional components respond to a variety of other factors including renal blood flow, neuroendocrine effects, and the fluid and nutrient supply to the body. A detailed discussion of each aspect of renal physiology is beyond the scope of this chapter. The reader is referred to other sources for more expanded detail (Brenner, Zatz, & Ichikawa, 1986; Pitts, 1974; Fawcett, 1986; Hepinstall, 1983). This chapter will discuss the major components of renal function, the response to extrarenal factors, and the current methods of investigation of renal function.

Renal Blood Flow

The two kidneys of an adult man weigh about 300 g (about 0.5% of body weight). Relative to other vascular beds, the vascular resistance in the kidneys is low. Under resting conditions, the kidneys are perfused with 1.2 liters of blood per min which represents about 25% of the cardiac output.

The organizational pattern of the vascular supply to the kidney is related to varying components of renal function (Bargen & Herd, 1971). The basic pattern of flow is through a main renal artery branching from the descending aorta. The renal artery branches at the hilus of the kidney into the interlobar arteries which enter the renal parenchyma and ascend to the corticomedullary junction. They then form the arcuate arteries which give off the interlobular arteries. The afferent arterioles emerge from the interlobular arteries. The afferent arteriole subdivides into a capillary network which forms the glomerular tuft and the reemergence of this glomerular capillary network forms the efferent arteriole (Figure 7 of Chapter 1). These vessels proceed into a capillary network in the cortex and in the medulla and then into venous channels. The vasa recta also emerge from the efferent arteriole. The vasa recta are vascular bundles which extend deep into the medulla.

The renal vessels have characteristic histologic structures which are very relevant to certain aspects of nephron function. The afferent and efferent arterioles have smooth muscle cells and nerve endings. Electron microscopic studies have identified adrenergic and cholinergic fibers in these vessels. The afferent arteriole has epithelioid cells at the site where the arteriole is adjacent to the mascula densa of the ascending tubule. Together these structures form the juxtaglomerular apparatus which is the site of renin formation (Figure 1). The vasa recta vessels in the deep medulla have a large number of endothelial cells. This feature is related to the function of the countercurrent exchange mechanism for concentration (Fawcett, 1963).

Blood flow into the kidney from the main renal artery does not have a uniform distribution throughout the kidney. Approximately 93% of the

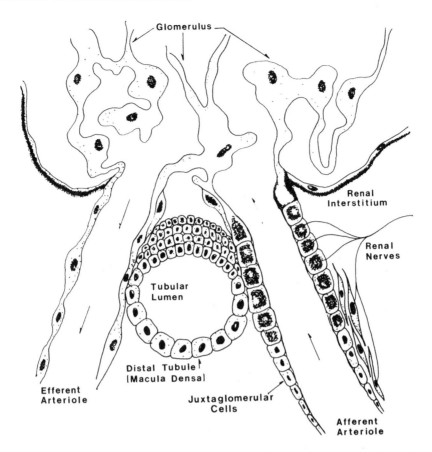

Figure 1. The microscopic anatomy of the juxtaglomerular apparatus. Blood flows through the afferent arteriole, enters the glomerular capillary network, and following filtration exits the glomerulus through the efferent arteriole. Afferent and efferent arterioles are positioned adjacent to the macula densa, which is a segment of the distal renal tubule. The juxtaglomerular cells are the renin-producing cells and are located in the wall of the afferent arteriole and adjacent to the macula densa. Renin released from the juxtaglomerular cells is regulated by volume signals transmitted from the afferent arteriole or/and from the macula densa, reflecting the volume of tubular filtrate entering the distal tubules.

total renal blood flow (RBF) goes to the renal cortex which comprises 75% of the renal mass. The rate of cortical flow is about 500 ml/min per 100 g of kidney. The rate of medullary flow is about 100 ml/min per 100 g of kidney in the outer zone and 25 ml/min per 100 g in the inner zone (Thurau & Levine, 1971). Accordingly, with this distribution, detectable changes in RBF will largely reflect changes in flow in the cortex (Spitzer, 1978).

Factors which control RBF are the systemic arterial pressure, circulating volume, and renal vascular resistance. The vascular resistance in the kidneys resides at the level of the arterioles. These vessels respond to extrinsic nervous and hormonal mechanisms which can modify resistance. Also, there is an internal autonomous mechanism which regulates resistance.

Under basal conditions, the tonic vasoconstrictor activity of the kidney is minimal or absent (Pomeranz, Birtch, & Bargen, 1968). Direct neural stimulation will induce mild vasoconstriction of the afferent arterioles reflected by a decrease in RBF (DiBona, 1983). This effect can be abolished by α blockers such as reserpine and guanethidine which would indicate that the vasoconstrictive effect is mediated by sympathetic α receptors (Di-Salvo & Fell, 1971; Gomer & Zimmerman, 1972).

Renal denervation increases RBF but only in the anesthetized animal where sympathetic tone has been elevated by the prior use of barbiturate anesthesia (Berne, 1952). Overall, neurogenic mechanisms do not regulate RBF under basal physiologic conditions. However, they may be invoked in circumstances which threaten homeostasis.

Several hormonal factors may affect RBF. Both epinephrine and norepinephrine have a constrictive effect on renal vessels. Small doses will reduce RBF significantly. A larger dose will produce a large decrease in RBF and also affect glomerular filtration. A similar dose-related effect occurs with renin and angiotensin. Stimulation of the renal nerves or the administration of norepinephrine or angiotensin II has been shown to raise the level of prostaglandins in renal venous blood. Conversely, prostaglandin inhibitors enhance the vasoconstrictive effect of norepinephrine and angiotensin II (Burton-Opitz & Lucas, 1981).

Autoregulation of RBF was first described in 1981 (Burton-Optiz & Lucas, 1981) and has been repeatedly confirmed in experimental models. In the kidneys, autoregulation consists of a constancy of RBF as the arterial pressure varies between 80 and 180 mm Hg. The changes in vascular resistance, which explain this constancy of RBF, occur in the denervated and isolated kidney, thereby demonstrating the intrarenal origin of the control (Spitzer, 1978; Berne, 1952). Several hypotheses have been developed to explain autoregulation, but precise confirmation of the mechanism has not been established.

RBF is reduced by exercise, intense mental stress, norepinephrine, stimulation of certain areas in the CNS, and also by anything which reduces systemic blood pressure. A lowering of systemic blood pressure generally results in a much greater reduction in RBF than that which can be explained by the reduction in pressure alone. This is due to increases in renal vascular resistance, a counter-response to maintain central volume (Bargen & Herd, 1971; Thurau & Levine, 1971). RBF is also reduced by most of the drugs that reduce blood pressure. However, the reduction of RBF is lessened when systemic blood pressure is reduced with antihypertensive drugs because the vasoconstrictive response to systemic pressure reduction is usually inhibited by the drug.

It is apparent that measurement of RBF must be performed under basal conditions to avoid activation of potentially confounding factors such as fluctuation in blood pressure or sympathetic nervous system excitation. Methods for measurement of RBF can be technically difficult. A standard method is that of measuring clearance of a substance which is completely extracted from the plasma on a single passage through the kidney. Para-aminohippuran (PAH) is a substance which has been used for determination of RBF. Techniques developed in nuclear medicine using radioisotope labeling of substances which are completely extracted from the renal vasculature have simplified the procedural involvement. Methods have been developed to determine effective renal plasma flow using [^{131}I]hippuran. An intravenous injection of [^{131}I]hippuran results in a biexponential plasma disappearance curve. Timed postinjection samples of plasma are then counted for concentration of the isotope. From these data and the hematocrit, the RBF can be calculated by formulas using slopes and intercept (Blaufox, 1972; Brenner et al., 1986). Another method of determining RBF is by scintillation counting of activity over the kidneys following an intravenous injection of a known quantity of ^{99}Tc. The current instrumentation of most nuclear medicine laboratories includes computerized systems to generate blood flow curves based on the measured isotope activity.

Although current methods for measuring RBF in well human subjects are technically difficult and expensive, there are reports indicating that variations in RBF are detectable at early phases of essential hypertension and may reflect an interrelationship with CNS activity. Changes in RBF have been identified in early mild essential hypertension and also in normotensive offspring of parents with essential hypertension (Hollenberg & Adams, 1974; Bianchi et al., 1978). Hollenberg, Williams, and Adams demonstrated that during psychologic stimuli, RBF decreases and plasma renin activity increases in patients with essential hypertension as well as in normotensive adult off-spring of parents with essential hypertension.

Very extensive investigations of systemic and renal hemodynamics were performed by London, Safar, Sassard, Levenson, and Simon (1984) on patients with mild essential hypertension and normotensive subjects. These investigators demonstrated a reduced RBF and a decreased RBF/cardiac output (CO) ratio in the hypertensives. Administration of the centrally acting drugs clonidine and α-methyldopa reversed these changes. The β blocker propranolol did not normalize the reduced RBF/CO as the centrally acting agent did. These studies provide data indicating that changes in renal perfusion are present in individuals with essential hypertension as well as those at risk for hypertension. Furthermore, these variations in RBF may be related to a variation in central adrenergic control. This relationship is one that warrants further investigation.

Glomerular Filtration Rate

The filtering function of the kidney resides in the glomerulus, which is a specialized capillary network interposed between the afferent and efferent arterioles. Filtration occurs from the intracapillary space across the capillary wall into the urinary space of the glomerular capsule (Figure 7 of Chapter 1). The permeability of the glomerular capillary wall is far greater than that of other capillaries of the body. This enhanced permeability, for the purpose of filtration, is related to the microstructure of the capillaries, including increased number and size of pores in the endothelial cells on the inner lumen and also the specialized structure of the capillary basement membrane (i.e., glomerular basement membrane).

The factors which regulate glomerular filtration include glomerular membrane permeability, capillary blood pressure, the intracapsular hydrostatic pressure and colloid osmotic pressure (Baylis & Brenner, 1978; Brenner & Humes, 1977).

Glomerular permeability generally remains constant in the absence of pathologic conditions. The total area available for filtration depends on the number of glomeruli and the glomerular size. The available area then is affected by growth and body size.

The major variable in regulation of the rate of glomerular filtration is the intracapillary hydrostatic pressure. The intracapillary hydrostatic pressure is dependent on systemic arterial pressure and the resistance of the glomerular arterioles. Constriction of the afferent arteriole will lower the capillary pressure; dilation of the afferent arteriole will raise the capillary pressure to the level of systemic pressure. On the other hand, constriction of the efferent arteriole will raise intracapillary pressure and dilation of the efferent arteriole will lower the intracapillary pressure. As noted earlier, arteriolar constriction is under neural control and also responds to hormonal factors.

Intracapsular hydrostatic pressure is the pressure created by the volume of filtrate in the capsule of the glomerulus. This represents a force opposing filtration. Under normal physiologic conditions, this pressure is slight and of little significance. However, in conditions of a massive solute diuresis, the volume of fluid in the capsule increases, raising the hydrostatic pressure and opposing filtration. Pathologic conditions which obstruct tubular flow also increase the intracapsular pressure.

The colloid osmotic pressure is a force opposing filtration and is created by the osmotic effect of the plasma proteins. This force is roughly equivalent to a hydrostatic pressure of 25–30 mm Hg. The plasma protein concentration is relatively stable under usual physiologic conditions so that colloid osmotic pressure is probably not a significant variable in regulating the glomerular filtration rate. However, due to the presence of this force opposing filtration, when the intracapillary hydrostatic pressure falls to 25–30 mm Hg, glomerular filtration will cease (Brenner & Humes, 1977).

The measurement of glomerular filtration is central to the evaluation of renal function. The difference between the rate at which a substance is filtered at the glomerulus and excreted in the urine reflects the rate of tubular activity by reabsorption or secretion.

The measurement of glomerular filtration rate

(GFR) is based on the excretion of a given substance which can be neither reabsorbed nor secreted by the tubules. Thus, the rate of excretion of this substance will be equal to the rate of filtration at the glomeruli. The basic formula is as follows:

$$U_x V = \text{GFR} \times P_x$$

or

$$\text{GFR} = U_x V / P_x$$

U_x is the urine concentration of the X, P_x the plasma concentration of X, and V the urine flow expressed in milliliters per minute.

Inulin is generally accepted as the reference substance by which GFR is measured since it is freely filtered at the glomerulus and neither reabsorbed nor secreted in the tubules. The expression $U_x V / P_x$ denotes clearance (C_x), which refers to the volume of plasma required to supply substance X at a rate at which it is excreted in the urine. The term "clearance" denotes that volume of plasma which yields its entire content for renal excretion and is thus cleared of the substance in question. The clearance of inulin (or similar inert substances such as creatinine) can then be compared with some other substance to assess tubular reabsorption or secretion. The amount of a given substance (X) filtered will be the product of the plasma concentration of X times the GFR, expressed as the clearance of inulin (C_{in}). The difference in the amount filtered and the amount excreted will be the amount transported by the tubules in reabsorption or secretion. The basic formulas are as follows:

$$\text{Filtered X} = C_{in} P_x$$
$$\text{Excreted X} = U_x V$$
$$\text{Transported X} = \text{Filtered X} - \text{Excreted X}$$

or

$$T_x = C_{in} P_x - U_x V$$

A positive value for T_x indicates reabsorption. A negative value indicates tubular secretion.

Measurement of GFR by inulin clearance in humans is often technically difficult. The most commonly used substance for approximating glomerular filtration is creatinine. The clearance of endogenously produced creatinine from muscle cell metabolism is quite constant on a daily basis. Although there is some tubular secretion of creatinine in humans which would result in somewhat higher determinations of GFR, the clearance of creatinine is fairly close to that of inulin.

Determination of creatinine clearance can then be used as a stable reflection of GFR and as such can be used as a reference in the calculation of quantities of other substances filtered and delivered to the tubules for reabsorption. The normal value for GFR based on creatinine clearance is 100–125 ml/min per 1.73 m². Women tend to have values in the lower range of normal, whereas men produce values in the upper portion of the normal range. The formula is:

$$C_{cr} = U_{cr} V / P_{cr}$$

where U_{cr} is the concentration of creatinine in the collected urine (mg/ml), V the urine flow or the volume of urine produced during the collection period (ml/min), and P_{cr} the plasma concentration of creatinine (mg/100 ml).

The value obtained will be the creatinine clearance or GFR of a given subject. In clinical evaluations this value will then be corrected to a body surface of 1.73 m² so that the GFR can be compared to the normal range.

Example: Creatinine clearance is to be determined on a 28-year-old female who weighs 50 kg and is 160 cm tall. Directions given to the subject for the urine collection are as follows: At 7:00 a.m., completely empty the bladder and discard. Save all subsequent urine in a container. At 7:00 a.m. the next day, empty bladder and add this volume to the total collection. The 24-h urine collection is brought to a laboratory, at which time a blood sample is obtained for serum creatinine. The laboratory results are as follows:

Serum creatinine:	0.6 mg/dl
Total volume:	1680 ml
Urine creatinine:	886 mg/total volume or
	527 mg/liter

Creatinine clearance $= U_{cr}V/P_{cr}$

where

$$U_{cr} = 886 \text{ mg}/1680 \text{ ml}$$
$$V = 1680 \text{ ml}/1440 \text{ min}$$
$$P_{cr} = 0.6 \text{ mg}/100 \text{ ml}$$

$$C_{cr} = \frac{886 \text{ mg}/1680 \text{ ml} \times 1680 \text{ ml}/1440 \text{ min}}{0.6 \text{ mg}/100 \text{ ml}}$$

$$= \frac{886 \text{ mg}/1440 \text{ min}}{0.6 \text{ mg}/100 \text{ ml}}$$

$$= 102.5 \text{ ml/min}$$

The subject's creatinine clearance is 102.5 ml/min. Next, make the correction for surface area: Subject's weight is 50 kg, height 160 cm, surface area 1.50 m².

$$102.5 \text{ ml/min}/1.50 \text{ m}^2 = x \text{ ml/min per } 1.73 \text{ m}^2$$
$$\text{Corrected } C_{cr} = 118 \text{ ml/min per } 1.73 \text{ m}^2$$

There is some developmental variation in normal GFR relevant to age. Newborn infants have a low GFR even when corrected for body surface area. This low GFR presumably reflects continued functional development of the nephrons. By 12 months of life, the corrected GFR is in the adult range. In the elderly, there will be a decline in GFR due to loss of functioning nephrons.

Many clinical diseases, particularly intrinsic renal disease, alter GFR through pathologic processes which directly affect the structure and functioning number of glomeruli. Prolonged uncontrolled hypertension can result in target organ damage to the kidney, manifested by arteriolar nephrosclerosis. The structural changes of this process will reduce the intracapillary flow through the glomeruli and reduce GFR. Diabetes mellitus is another condition which frequently produces alterations in GFR. In the early phases of diabetes, the elevated plasma glucose will raise the plasma osmotic pressure. This will result in a raised intracapillary hydrostatic pressure and result in a force enhancing filtration. Thus, the GFR will be higher than normal in the earlier phases of diabetes. As the disease progresses and the diabetic glomerulopathy occurs, these structural

changes will result in reduced available glomerular filtering surface and hence a reduction in GFR. Therefore, human subjects having GFR values outside of the normal range should be excluded from investigations of behavioral–renal interaction.

Renal Tubular Function

The composition of the glomerular filtrate, as it enters the renal tubular system, is identical to plasma devoid of protein. One of the most striking aspects of the mammalian kidney is the capacity to produce urine which differs greatly in solute composition from the plasma from which it is derived. Under normal conditions, the composition of the body fluid is maintained within very narrow limits despite wide fluctuations in intake and extrarenal fluid losses. When the body fluids are diluted by excessive water intake, the urine becomes dilute and the excess water is rapidly excreted. Conversely, when the concentration of the body fluid increases due to excessive solute intake or excessive water loss, the urine becomes greatly concentrated so that solute excretion is enhanced and water is conserved. This process will reestablish normal solute concentrations. Electrolyte concentrations of the extracellular system are similarly maintained within a narrow range despite broad ranges of intake. Excesses are excreted, and during conditions of deficient intake, maximum conservation of these constituents will occur through adjustments in tubular reabsorption and secretion.

The anatomy of the renal tubules is given in Figure 7 of Chapter 1. Briefly, two populations of nephrons exist. The cortical nephrons reside more peripherally in the outer cortex and have relatively short loops of Henle. The juxtamedullary nephrons reside in the inner cortex. These nephrons have very long loops of Henle which extend deep into the renal medulla. Due to their extension into the medullary regions of high tonicity, the tubules of the juxtamedullary nephrons have more powerful concentrating capacity.

The tubules may be divided anatomically and functionally into four basic segments: (1) proximal convoluted tubule, (2) loop of Henle, (3) distal convoluted tubule, and (4) collecting tubule. Each of these segments can be subdivided further relative to type and function of the tubular epithelial cells. Transport mechanisms, which cause the movement of water and solutes from the tubular lumen to the ECF compartment, vary at the different tubular sites. The transport of solutes and water may follow one of two pathways. Active transport consists of a transcellular pathway in which the ion moves into the epithelial cell. Movement across the luminal epithelial surface is governed by an established concentration, or electrochemical gradient. The substance then is pumped into the interstitium by an active transport mechanism. The other course of movement is the paracellular pathway. Solutes and water may move across the intercellular spaces in a passive manner. The passive movement occurs down gradients created by active transport. The rate of passive movement is also contingent on the relative permeability of the intercellular junctions (Herbert, Schafer, & Andreoli, 1981; Aronson, 1981).

Proximal Tubular Segments

At least 60% of the glomerular filtrate is reabsorbed in the proximal tubular segments. The transport process is isosmotic, with movement across the tubular lumen directed by electrical potential gradients. The first phase of proximal reabsorption affects the preferential reabsorption of the essential nutrients including sugars, amino acids, bicarbonate, and organic metabolites. These are sodium-coupled transport processes. Water transport follows solute transport in this first phase of proximal tubule reabsorption and is driven passively by a small osmotic gradient.

The second phase of proximal tubule reabsorption affects sodium and chloride reabsorption. In this phase, new gradients are created by the preceding removal of bicarbonate, sodium, and organic solutes. Chloride and sodium move from the tubular lumen into the tubular cell and then are actively pumped into the interstitium in this phase with some further passive water transport. Movement of reabsorbed water and solute from the renal interstitum into the peritubular capillaries is then determined by Starling forces which govern fluid movement across all capillaries.

Organic ions and many drugs are removed from the plasma by secretion in the proximal tubules. This process occurs at the second phase level. The organic ion secretions occur by an active transport step from plasma across the base of the epithelial cell. The raised intracellular concentration and increased permeability at the luminal side of the epithelial cell then permits passive movement into the tubular lumen. Endogenous compounds secreted at this level include prostaglandins, dopamine, epinephrine, histamine, and serotonin. Some of the drugs secreted at this level include chlorothiazide, furosemide, salicylates, atropine, and morphine (Grantham, 1982).

Loop of Henle

The loop of Henle consists of the thin descending limb and the thin ascending limb. These segments have unique permeability characteristics which govern their role in urinary concentration and dilution. Tubular fluid entering the thin descending limb from the proximal nephron is isosmotic relative to plasma with a concentration of about 300 mosm. This segment is very permeable to water and relatively impermeable to solutes. Thus, as the tubular fluid is exposed to the progressively hypertonic medullary interstitium, water moves from tubular lumen to interstitium.

At the bend of Henle's loop, the thin ascending limb begins. This portion of the loop is water impermeable and highly permeable to NaCl. The tubular fluid then flows along a course of gradually decreasing interstitial osmolarity. Sodium and chloride then move out of the tubular lumen, rendering the tubular fluid progressively less concentrated. The absence of any significant water permeability permits the tubular epithelium to maintain the osmotic gradients (Kokko, 1982).

Distal Tubular Segments

The distal tubular segments consist of the thick ascending limb and the distal convoluted tubule. The transition point between the two segments is the area of the macula densa.

The thick ascending limb, which functions to dilute the tubular fluid, actively transports sodium and chloride. The sodium transport processes at this level are similar to the sodium transport mechanisms occurring in the proximal tubule. However, a major difference is that the transepithelial electrical potential difference is the reverse in the thick ascending limb (lumen positive) of that in the proximal tubule (lumen negative). This results in the transport of potassium from cell to tubular lumen. Several diuretics act in the thick ascending limb. Furosemide is one of the diuretics which acts at this site, but only from the lumen, and inhibits NaCl reabsorption (Burg & Good, 1983).

The macula densa separates the thick ascending limbs from the distal convoluted tubule (Figure 1). This portion of the distal nephron is in contact with the afferent arteriole entering the glomerulus and the efferent arteriole exiting the glomerulus. Together these tubular and vascular structures make up the juxtaglomerular apparatus. Granular cells in the afferent arteriole secrete renin, the enzyme essential for generation of angiotensin II. These cells, which are tubular and vascular cells, act as a syncytium. When sodium concentration is low or tubular volume is low, renin release is activated, ultimately resulting in stimulation of aldosterone secretion and enhanced sodium conservation.

Tubular fluid emerging from the thick ascending limb and entering the distal convoluted tubule is hypotonic relative to plasma. The distal tubule is very impermeable to water. Further dilution of tubular fluid occurs by active transport of sodium with further NaCl reabsorption in the absence of water movement. Calcium reabsorption also occurs in this segment (Imai & Nakamura, 1982).

Collecting Tubules

The first portions of the collecting tubules are designated connecting tubule and initial cortical collecting tubule. Following these segments, the tubules of nephrons begin to join. The progressive confluence of nephrons results in an increasing collecting tubule diameter.

The collecting tubule segments are the sites for final regulation of sodium, potassium, hydrogen ion, water, and urine excretion. Different cell types are present in the collecting tubule which regulates these various transport functions. Active transport mechanisms are efficient enough to produce urine with a sodium concentration of 1 meq/liter during conditions of sodium deprivation. The rate of sodium reabsorption in the cortical collecting tubules is regulated by mineralocorticoid hormones such as aldosterone.

Most of the filtered potassium is reabsorbed before the tubular fluid reaches the collecting tubule. Cells of the collecting tubule are capable of both potassium reabsorption and potassium secretion, depending on dietary intake. However, the actual function of reabsorption or secretion is performed by different cell types (Stokes, 1982).

The collecting tubules are the sites of hormonal regulation. Parathormone and calcitonin affect calcium secretion and act at the initial portion of the collecting tubules. Aldosterone produced by the zona glomerulosa of the adrenal cortex stimulates sodium reabsorption, potassium secretion, and hydrogen ion secretion. The water permeability of the collecting tubules is controlled by vasopressin (ADH) secreted by the brain. This is the mechanism by which the final concentration of the tubular fluid (i.e., urine) is achieved (Jamison & Kriz, 1982).

Under usual conditions, urine flow is relatively low and has an osmotic concentration well in excess of plasma. If a large volume of water is ingested (1000 ml), there will be no change in the urine concentration for 15–20 min. Urine flow then increases and reaches a maximum approximately 40–60 min after water ingestion. Urine flow will remain high until most of the ingested water has been excreted. It will then drop rapidly to the control level. If positive water balance is maintained by continued water intake, the high rate of urine flow will be sustained. The changes in urine flow rates are due to changes in the rate of water excretion. The rate of glomerular filtration will be unchanged.

Regulation of water and osmotic balance by the renal tubular system is maintained through a hypothalamic–pituitary–renal axis. The major parts of this system include (1) thirst and drinking, (2) ADH secretion, and (3) a renal tubular mechanism for concentration or dilution by water transport.

The cerebral cortex may influence drinking behavior. Specific areas within the hypothalamus are critical to regulating water balance and tonicity by stimulating thirst. Also, osmoreceptors transmit stimuli for ADH secretion from the posterior pituitary gland. Thirst is stimulated by increasing osmolarity in the extracellular fluid and also by changing extracellular fluid volume by stimuli believed to be relayed by arterial and thoracic baroreceptors. Also of note is the direct stimulation of thirst by circulating angiotensin II in the hypothalamus. Angiotensin II is considered the most powerful known dipsogen.

Hypothalamic synthesis and posterior pituitary release of ADH are effected by changes in extracellular tonicity. Slight increases of plasma osmolarity, in the range of 10 mosm, will provoke a substantial increase in ADH secretion. Slight decreases in plasma osmolarity can reduce ADH secretion to minimal levels as measured by radioimmunoassay. ADH secretion is stimulated by pain, emotional stress, and is also altered by several drugs (Table 1). Therefore, nonosmotic factors may lead to alterations of water excretion independent of shifts in body fluid osmolarity.

The tubular site for ADH activity is the collecting tubule. ADH binds to the receptor on the peritubular surface. In the presence of ATP, adenyl cyclase generates cyclic AMP. This process results in an alteration of the tubular membrane permeability to water. Water then moves from the tubular lumen, resulting in an increase in concentration of the filtrate (Handler & Orloff, 1981).

Table 1. Drugs That Alter ADH Secretion

Increase ADH Secretion
   Narcotics
   Tricyclic antidepressants
   Cyclophosphamide
   Clofibrate
   Vincristine
   Nicotine
Decrease ADH secretion
   Ethanol
   Narcotic antagonists
   Phenytoin
   Caffeine

Investigative Maneuvers

The kidneys function primarily to maintain fluid and electrolyte homeostasis. This is accomplished through reabsorption for conservation, and excretion of excesses and toxic products. Renal function is altered by deficits or excesses or exogenous load and also by changes in endogenous hormonal factors. Thus, any factors which alter endogenous hormonal activity such as catecholamines, renin–angiotensin, or aldosterone may also alter renal function. It is also likely that levels of function may be controlled by genetic factors which direct cellular function, either by means of hormonal regulation or by means of transport mechanisms.

Investigative techniques to challenge renal function generally involve loading and depletion maneuvers. The investigative subject is shifted from its current fluid and/or electrolyte steady state by depletion or loading. Renal response and function during the altered steady state can then be determined. Very elegant models for loading and depletion have been developed by Weinberger and associates (see Weinberger, this volume). In these studies, sodium and volume loading was accomplished by intravenous saline infusions or by oral sodium intake. Sodium depletion was accomplished by administration of furosemide or by reduction of dietary sodium intake. Factors which were monitored were blood pressure change, body weight change, excretion rates for sodium and potassium, and renin–aldosterone response. Through these experimental investigations, Weinberger *et al.* have demonstrated racial and age differences in the renal–endocrine response to shifts in sodium balance. They also demonstrated heterogenicity of ''sodium sensitivity'' within populations.

When studies of renal function and response are designed, certain characteristics of renal function should be considered. First, relative to the cardiovascular system, the renal excretory system is slower in its adaptive response to external stimuli. The response to loading or depletion will take from hours to days to reach a new steady state. When loading is performed by intravenous infusion, the volume expansion is accomplished by completion of the infusion and the renal response will begin within hours. However, oral loading with NaCl will occur more slowly and the renal response to this perturbation of sodium balance may require several days.

Another important issue in experimental design is the effect of loading or depletion on regulatory hormones. For example, volume loading will suppress plasma levels of renin, aldosterone, and catecholamines and stimulate atrial natriuretic factor. Volume depletion will have the reverse effect. Similarly, loading and depletion may affect other parameters of renal solute regulation. For example, in the sodium loading studies of Weinberger *et al.*, when sodium excretion was greatly increased by high sodium intake, enhanced potassium excretion also occurred.

Therefore, the imposed shift in renal function requires a longer time for stabilization. Hormonal and electrolyte factors must be monitored. Finally, another factor to be considered is that kidneys function at a level relative to body size. Therefore, a given dose (e.g., 10 g NaCl) will not necessarily represent the same stimulus to all subjects due to variation in body size. It is advisable to adjust dose to body size (e.g., mg/kg per day).

Investigation of the interaction of the central nervous system and renal function is a very challenging area in behavioral medicine research. Careful investigations which have incorporated loading and central stressors have produced very provocative results in experimental animals and in humans.

In a series of experiments by Anderson, Kearns, and Worden (1983a), dogs became hypertensive following a combination of avoidance conditioning and saline infusions. In a subsequent study, these investigators demonstrated that this pressor effect could be attenuated by administration of potassium (Anderson, Kearns, & Wordern, 1983b).

A few investigations have been performed in human subjects, which have provided some initial reports on the relationships of renal electrolyte regulation and sympathetic nervous system activity. Falkner, Onesti, and Angelakos (1981) investigated the interaction of stress and sodium intake on blood pressure in adolescents who varied in their genetic risk for essential hypertension. Normotensive offspring of hypertensive parents (FH$^+$) were compared to normotensive offspring of normoten-

sive parents (FH$^-$). The cardiovascular response to the stress of mental arithmetic was compared before and after 14 days of sodium loading with 10 g/day NaCl in addition to their usual diets. The sodium loading resulted in no significant blood pressure change in the FH$^-$ subjects, whereas in the FH$^+$ subjects the baseline blood pressure values were greater in addition to higher levels of blood pressure during the stress. This study indicated that normotensive children with a low genetic risk for hypertension were resistant to the effect of sodium loading, whereas the FH$^+$ subjects were sensitive to the sodium.

In a subsequent study, these investigators demonstrated that 53% of normotensive young black adults exhibited a sodium-sensitive response to chronic oral sodium loading. The stress response was augmented in the sodium-loaded condition and the greatest stress-induced response occurred in those who were both sodium-sensitive and had a positive family history of hypertension (Falkner, Katz, Canessa, & Kushner, 1986).

Further work has demonstrated that the apparent pressor effect of sodium loading in some can be altered by other cations. The observation by Sullivan *et al.* (1980) of higher serum and urinary potassium levels in young borderline hypertensives, who were resistant to dietary sodium load, suggested that potassium blunted the effect of the high sodium intake. Hypertensive patients given potassium chloride supplementation along with a high salt intake gained less weight and had less increase in plasma volume and cardiac output than those without added potassium. Plasma norepinephrine levels were lower in those supplemented with potassium, suggesting a reduction in adrenergic activity (Fujita & Ando, 1984). Skrabal *et al.* (1984) studied the effect of a low-sodium high-potassium diet on 20 young normotensive adults, 10 of whom had a family history of hypertension. The high-potassium diet reduced the diastolic blood pressure (5 mm Hg) of 10 of the 20 subjects; of the 10, 7 had a family history of essential hypertension. In all subjects, the low-sodium/high-potassium diet reduced the blood pressure rise from norepinephrine infusion, or from mental stress. These studies have provided data which indicate that the renal adjustment to changes in sodium and potassium intake indirectly alters the hemodynamic response to sympathetic stimulation. However, this response occurs in some but not all individuals.

In another study, Light, Koepke, Obrist, and Willis (1983) compared the renal response to competitive stress in young adults with high risk versus low risk for essential hypertension. Those designated as high risk had slight blood pressure elevation, high heart rate reactivity, and most had a strong family history of hypertension. By means of water drinking, a high urine flow was established. During the prolonged stress of competitive tasks, the high-risk group demonstrated a drop in urine flow and a decrease in sodium excretion. These observations indicated that the potential hypertensives had a renal response of increased sodium reabsorption to the central stress. These investigations have demonstrated not only the existence of important relationships, but they have also demonstrated the need for continued well-designed studies on the effects of the CNS on renal physiology.

References

Anderson, D. E., Kearns, W. D., & Worden, T. J. (1983a). Progressive hypertension in dogs by avoidance conditioning and saline infusions. *Hypertension, 5,* 286–291.

Anderson, D. E., Kearns, W. D., & Worden, T. J. (1983b). Potassium infusion attenuates avoidance saline hypertension in dogs. *Hypertension, 5,* 415–420.

Aronson, P. S. (1981). Identifying secondary active transport in epithelia. *American Journal of Physiology, 45,* F1–F11.

Bargen, A. C., & Herd, J. A. (1971). The renal circulation. *New England Journal of Medicine, 284,* 482.

Baylis, C., & Brenner, B. M. (1978). The physiologic determinants of glomerular ultrafiltration. *Reviews of Physiology, Biochemistry, and Pharmacology, 80,* 1–46.

Berne, R. M. (1952). Hemodynamics and sodium excretion of the denervated kidney in anesthesized and unanesthesized dog. *American Journal of Physiology, 171,* 148.

Bianchi, G., Picotti, G. B., Bratchi, G., Cusi, D., Datti, M., Lupi, D. P., Ferrari, P., Barlassina, G., Colambo, G., & Cori, B. (1978). Familial hypertension and hormonal profile, renal hemodynamics, and body fluids of young normotensive subjects. *Clinical Science and Molecular Medicine, 55,* 367.

Blaufox, M. D. (1972). Compartmental analysis of radiorenogram on kinetics of I-131 hippuran. *Progress in Nuclear Medicine, 2,* 107–124.

Brenner, B. M., & Humes, H. D. (1977). Mechanics of glomerular ultrafiltration. *New England Journal of Medicine, 297,* 148–154.

Brenner, B. M., Zatz, R., & Ichikawa, I. (1986). The renal circulation. In B. M. Brenner & F. C. Rector, Jr. (Eds.), *The kidney* (3rd ed.). Philadelphia: Saunders.

Burg, M. B. & Good, D. (1983). Sodium chloride coupled transport in mammalian nephrons. *Annual Review of Physiology, 45,* 533–547.

Burton-Opitz, R., & Lucas, D. R. (1981). The blood supply of the kidney: Vs the influence of the vagus nerve upon the vascularity of the left organ. *Journal of Experimental Medicine, 13,* 308.

DiBona, G. F. (1983). The function of the renal nerves. *Reviews of Physiology, Biochemistry, and Pharmacology, 94,* 75–181.

DiSalvo, J., & Fell, C. (1971). Changes in renal blood flow during renal nerve stimulation. *Proceedings of the Society for Experimental Biology and Medicine, 136,* 150.

Falkner, B., Onesti, G., & Angelakos, E. T. (1981). The effect of salt loading on the cardiovascular response to stress in adolescents. *Hypertension, 3*(Suppl. II), 195–199.

Falkner, B., Katz, S., Canessa, M., & Kushner, H. (1986). The response to long-term oral sodium loading in young blacks. *Hypertension, 8*(Suppl. I), I-165–I-168.

Fawcett, D. W. (1963). Comparative observations of the fine structure of blood capillaries. In J. L. Orbison & D. W. Smith (Eds.), *The peripheral blood vessels.* Baltimore: Williams & Wilkins.

Fawcett, D. W. (1986). *Textbook of histology* (11th ed.). Philadelphia: Saunders.

Fujita, T., & Ando, K. (1984). Hemodynamic and endocrine changes associated with potassium supplementation in sodium-loaded hypertensives. *Hypertension, 6,* 184–192.

Gomer, S. K., & Zimmerman, B. G. (1972). Determination of sympathetic vasodilator responses during renal stimulation. *Journal of Pharmacology and Experimental Therapeutics, 181,* 75.

Grantham, J. J. (1982). Studies of organic anion and cation transport in isolated segments of proximal tubules. *Kidney International, 22,* 519–525.

Handler, J. S., & Orloff, J. (1981). Antidiuretic hormone. *Annual Review of Physiology, 42,* 611–624.

Hepinstall, R. H. (1983). *Pathology of the kidney* (3rd ed.). Boston: Little, Brown.

Herbert, S. C., Schafer, J. A., & Andreoli, T. E. (1981). Principles of membrane transport. In B. M. Brenner & F. C. Rector, Jr. (Eds.). *The kidney* (2nd ed.). Philadelphia: Saunders.

Hollenberg, N. K., & Adams, D. F. (1974). Renal circulation in hypertensive disease. *American Journal of Medicine, 60,* 773.

Hollenberg, N. K., Williams, G. H., & Adams, D. F. (1981). Essential hypertension: Abnormal renal vascular and endocrine response to mild psychogenic stimulus. *Hypertension, 3,* 11.

Imai, M., & Nakamura, R. (1982). Function of distal convoluted and connecting tubules studied by isolated nephron fragments. *Kidney International, 22,* 465–472.

Jamison, R. L., & Kriz, W. (1982). *Urinary concentrating mechanism: Structure and function.* London: Oxford University Press.

Kokko, J. P. (1982). Transport characteristics of the thin limbs of Henle. *Kidney International, 22,* 449–453.

Light, K. C., Koepke, J. P., Obrist, P. A., & Willis, P. W. (1983). Psychological stress induces sodium and fluid retention in men at risk for hypertension. *Science, 220,* 429.

London, G. M., Safar, M. E., Sassard, J. D., Levenson, J. A., & Simon, A. C. (1984). Renal and systemic hemodynamics in sustained hypertension. *Hypertension, 6,* 743–754.

Pitts, R. F. (1974). *Physiology of the kidney and body fluids* (3rd ed.). Chicago: Year Book Medical.

Pomeranz, B. H., Birtch, A. G., & Bargen, A. C. (1968). Neural control of intrarenal blood flow. *American Journal of Physiology, 215,* 1067.

Skrabal, F., Herholz, H., Newyman, M., Hamberger, L., Ledochowski, M., Sporer, H., Hortnagl, H., Schwartz, X., & Schonitzer, D. (1984). Salt sensitivity in humans is linked to enhanced sympathetic responsivity to enhanced proximal tubular reabsorption. *Hypertension, 6,* 152–158.

Spitzer, A. (1978). Renal physiology and functional development. In C. M. Edelman, Jr. (Ed.), *Pediatric kidney diseases* (Vol. 1). Boston: Little, Brown.

Stokes, J. B. (1982). Ion transport by the cortical and outer medullary collecting tubule. *Kidney International, 22,* 473–484.

Sullivan, J. M., Ratts, T. E., Taylor, J. C., Kraus, D. H., Barton, B. R., Patrick, D. R., & Reed, S. W. (1980). Hemodynamic effects of dietary sodium in man. *Hypertension, 2,* 506.

Thurau, K., & Levine, D. Z. (1971). The renal circulation. In C. Roullier & A. F. Huller (Eds.), *The kidney* (Vol. 3). New York: Academic Press.

Chemistries and Hormonal Measurement

Section Editor: Joel E. Dimsdale

Cardiovascular reactivity studies explore the communication between organ systems. Section I of this book discusses the analysis of bioelectrical and mechanical communication; this section considers chemical communication. Our bodies swim in a bouillon of exquisite complexity, filled with spices (compounds) whose composition varies and affects organ systems at a distance.

This section considers techniques of measurement of electrolytes, glucose regulation, and hormonal/neuroendocrine activity. Throughout this section, the contributors have discussed certain common questions: (1) What is the physiological meaning of an elevated level of the compound? (2) How rapidly will the compound have its onset and offset in response to stimulation? (3) What are the implications of measuring the compound at various sites? (4) What are the assay techniques for measuring the compound? (5) What are known confounders to measurement of the compound?

Weinberger in Chapter 9 discusses electrolytes—sodium, potassium, calcium, and magnesium. He points to dietary effects, as well as the interaction between sodium, for instance, and hormonal systems such as the sympathetic nervous system or renin–angiotensin system. Although sodium and potassium are easy to measure, he cautions about certain ways of handling samples that can introduce substantial artifact to such measurement. Relatively little behavioral medicine research has examined calcium or magnesium, although both have prominent cardiovascular effects.

Skyler in Chapter 10 considers the vitally important complex area of carbohydrate metabolism, with special reference to its assessment in diabetic patients. There have been dramatic developments in techniques for assessing carbohydrate metabolism. For instance, glycosylated hemoglobin levels can give one an impression of the habitual state of glycemic control of an individual. Similarly, loop and clamp techniques allow one to examine insulin action *in vivo*.

The sympathetic nervous system and adrenomedullary system are of central relevance to cardiovascular regulation. In Chapter 11 Ziegler discusses the difficulty of drawing inferences regarding such activity from plasma levels, as well as the confusion regarding the precise meaning of a urinary catecholamine measurement. For decades, we have been improving our measurement strategies for assessing catecholamines. However, we are still far from an acceptable biochemical measure of such activity, as well as from an understanding of the true physiological significance of a level.

Adrenocortical and gonadal steroids are also of considerable interest in behavioral medicine. Kuhn notes in Chapter 12 that secretory patterns are not constant for these systems. Cortisol, for instance,

Joel E. Dimsdale • Department of Psychiatry, University of California, San Diego Medical Center, San Diego, California 92103.

has a pulsatile release and, of course, gonadal steroids are profoundly influenced by menstrual cycle. She notes that there are surprisingly easy opportunities for evaluating these systems noninvasively by sampling from saliva. Although there are some complexities concerning salivary pH, rate of flow, and preservation strategies (Reid, 1984), sampling from this compartment is likely to provide a wealth of future data in behavioral medicine research.

Koob and Bissette in Chapter 13 consider the measurement and function of neuropeptides in a chapter which focuses primarily on corticotropin-releasing factor. The chapter provides an excellent overview of radioimmunoassays which underlie so much of today's hormonal studies.

It is not sufficient to assume that an elevated hormonal level will account for the end organ response; rather, the hormone's receptors themselves are under dynamic control. In Chapter 14 Robertson, Parfyonova, Menshikov, and Hollister, review this important area with particular reference to adrenoreceptors. They provide an excellent background discussion of receptor physiology. This is an understudied area in behavioral medicine.

Discussing hormonal systems in isolation is appealingly simple but misleading given the tremendous overlap across systems. In Chapter 15 Atlas reviews measurement strategies and implications for four interacting compounds—renin, angiotensin, aldosterone, and atrial natriuretic factor (ANF). The latter has kindled considerable interest because of its recent discovery in the wall of the heart, as well as its apparent opposition to certain activities of the sympathetic nervous system. Relatively few studies in humans have examined the role of behavioral factors in regulating ANF. Similarly, although there are clear linkages between sympathetic nervous system functioning and the renin–angiotensin system, this area deserves further study.

This section thus spans an enormous range of physiology—brain, kidney, adrenal, heart, sympathetic nervous tissue, reproductive glands, pancreas. Furthermore, at various points the chapters discuss the unique opportunities and problems of measuring hormonal activity in saliva, urine, blood, or tissue. We must acknowledge the arbitrariness of our choice of chapters. These particular topics seem to be today's most promising targets for hormonal research in cardiovascular behavioral medicine. The field, however, is growing with such rapidity that one could well imagine a future edition of this book focusing on entirely different hormonal systems. Although such systems will have their own unique problems of measurement, we believe the general methodological issues discussed in this edition will prove useful.

Reference

Reid, G. F. (Ed.). (1984). *Immunoassays of steroids in saliva: Proceedings of the 98th Tenovus Workshop*. Cardiff, Wales: Alpha Omega Publishing.

CHAPTER 9

Electrolytes

Myron H. Weinberger

Electrolytes are minerals present in variable concentrations in all biological fluids. They are essential for maintenance of body fluid balance and in the function of all cells, tissues, and organs. The concentration of specific electrolyte ions and the gradients that they establish control the flow of nutrients and fluids between cells and body compartments. This chapter will deal with the major electrolytes influencing hemodynamic behavior and about which the most is known. These include sodium, potassium, calcium, and magnesium. Each electrolyte will be examined in terms of its relative concentrations in various compartments, its effects on biological function, factors influencing its effects on biological function and metabolism, and its role in disease states.

Sodium

Distribution

Sodium is the most abundant electrolyte in the extracellular fluid space, its concentration being 135–145 mM (meq/liter). As such, it is the major determinant of the osmotic concentration and volume of body fluids. The intracellular sodium concentration (range 3–30 mM) is much lower than

that of extracellular fluid and, thus, the large gradient in concentration between cells and extracellular fluid requires a sophisticated system for preventing excessive sodium entry into cells, which would also bring with it fluid because of the powerful osmotic effect of the sodium ion. Such an unrestricted osmotic influx of sodium and water would swell and rupture cells. Thus, to prevent this passive diffusion of sodium and water, all cells contain active and passive "pumps" to extrude sodium. Some of these systems are energy-dependent ($Na^+,K^+-ATPase$), whereas others involve exchange of sodium for ions of like ionic charge normally required in higher concentrations inside the cell than outside (hydrogen, potassium). The maintenance of the manifold concentration gradient of sodium between extracellular fluid and cells (Table 1) represents the single metabolic activity requiring the greatest amount of energy for mammals. Alterations in sodium balance also are the primary determinants of changes in extracellular fluid volume.

Sources

The primary source of sodium is dietary. Sodium is abundant in most foods. Its content in the soil varies: Foods grown near the sea are richer in sodium than those from inland areas. Carnivorous diets are many times higher in sodium than are herbivorous ones due to the abundance of sodium in animal tissues. The sodium content of the con-

Myron H. Weinberger • Department of Medicine, Indiana University School of Medicine, Indianapolis, Indiana 46223.

Table 1. Range of Normal Electrolyte Constituents

	Intracellular	Extracellular	Diet
Na	3–30 mM	135–145 mM	25–800 meq/day
K	100–160 mM	4.0–5.5 mM	25–200 meq/day
Ca	100 nM?	2.5 mM	200–2000 mg/day
Mg	1–2 mM?	1.5–2.0 mM	150–350 mg/day

temporary diet is artificially high because of the addition of sodium in the preparation, preservation, and flavoring of food. The average daily American diet contains about 175 ± 50 (S.D.) meq of sodium, although the range of intake among Americans (and humans in general) is very great (25–600 meq/day).

Gross Metabolism

The human physiologic machinery has evolved several remarkably efficient mechanisms for conserving sodium. Under normal physiologic circumstances, virtually all of the ingested sodium is absorbed across the gastrointestinal mucosa, primarily in the small intestine, and enters the circulation. Sodium is freely filtered with water by the glomerulus and reabsorbed at different sites in the nephron. In situations of balance (where intake and losses are not being altered), the amount of sodium excreted in the urine is equal to intake minus insensible losses (via sweat and respiration) which are normally minimal and constant. Thus, careful collection of timed urine samples, under conditions of balance, provides an estimate of dietary sodium intake. There is a diurnal rhythm in sodium excretion, being highest in proximity to meals, and, thus, 24-h urine collections are most accurate.

Measurement

Sodium can be measured in body fluids and tissues by flame photometry, usually utilizing automated procedures. The precision and accuracy of such measurements are great and rarely vary by more than 1–2%. In normal individuals, plasma (or serum) sodium concentration ranges from 135 to 145 mM (meq)/liter. Artifactual increases in plasma sodium concentration may result from the use of sodium heparin as an anticoagulant. Alterations in this normal range are rarely due to alterations in sodium intake unless there are abnormalities of gastrointestinal absorption or excessive losses of sodium. Most of the aberrations in plasma or serum sodium concentration observed are due to abnormalities of water metabolism leading to hemodilution or hemoconcentration, or replacement of sodium by other osmotically active particles not usually present in plasma in high concentrations (e.g., glucose, urea, lipoproteins).

Estimates of sodium intake are made as previously stated, in conditions of balance, and in the absence of gastrointestinal or renal disease, congestive heart failure, or hepatic cirrhosis with ascites. In such conditions, the urinary excretion of sodium is equal to its intake, over a 24-h period. It is possible to utilize shorter urine collection periods but the utility of such must consider such factors as the diurnal variation in sodium excretion, the influence of the proximity of dietary intake, alterations in posture, and the accuracy of bladder emptying. Completeness of urine collection can be estimated by measuring the creatinine content of the urine. Creatinine excretion is relatively constant for a given individual although the amount excreted is a reflection of muscle mass and body weight. Thus, creatinine excretion varies markedly between individuals. It is possible to express the urinary excretion of sodium on the basis of creatinine, but this has the limitation of segregating individuals on the basis of sex and body weight. Within the same individual, however, urinary creatinine excretion should vary by less than 15% in 24-h urine collections, if obtained carefully and completely. The bulk of sodium consumed is excreted within hours of ingestion; thus, nocturnal excretion of sodium is much less than excretion during the day. However, carefully timed urine collections obtained during the nocturnal or sleep period can be used to characterize sodium intake as high or low, if accurately obtained and verified by creatinine content (Luft, Weinberger, Grim, Henry, & Fineberg, 1980). Short-term urine collections require complete bladder emptying before and at the end of the collection period. This generally requires a reasonably high rate of urine flow before the collection is begun and assumption of the upright posture in men to enable maximum bladder drainage. Although a liberal water load will help increase urine flow, it may also alter the sodium excretion rate or promote changes in extracellular fluid volume which can lead to alterations in sodium excretion apart from the experimental measures.

Need

There are no data clearly defining the minimum amount of sodium required for survival. Experimental studies demonstrate that with sodium-free intake, humans can reduce their urinary sodium excretion to 1 meq/day (23 mg) or less (MacGregor, 1983). Epidemiologic studies have identified primitive societies, living in jungle or highland areas, where sodium is scarce, who have a daily urinary sodium excretion of much less than 10 meq/day (MacGregor, 1983). A small amount of sodium is excreted in sweat fluid and even less with respiration. Sodium losses by such mechanisms may be increased in hot environments, during exercise involving profuse perspiration, or during febrile illnesses. In addition, acute or chronic gastrointestinal disease or surgical removal of large surfaces of the small bowel can reduce sodium absorption. Notwithstanding these abnormal conditions, it would appear that the minimal daily requirement for sodium does not exceed 10 meq/day (230 mg/day). The evolution of very highly efficient sodium-conserving mechanisms doubtless permitted human survival in prehistoric times in areas where sodium was scarce and the climate very hot. However, these same mechanisms, which permitted survival during evolutionary times, may have created a biologic disadvantage in the current era of sodium surfeit. A review of these mechanisms provides insight into the effect of sodium on hemodynamic function.

Renal Handling

All of the sodium transported to the glomerulus is freely filtered with water and, with the other filtered solutes and fluid, constitutes renal tubular fluid. Approximately 90–95% of the filtered sodium is reabsorbed by the proximal tubule as an active, energy-requiring process as well as by passive diffusion. However, a significant portion escapes obligatory reabsorption and enters more distal parts of the nephron where variable reabsorption occurs or else sodium is excreted in the urine. The latter component of sodium reabsorption is also energy-dependent and is largely, but not wholly, influenced by aldosterone. This adrenal cortical hormone initiates a sequence of events at the renal tubular membrane which causes the absorption of sodium from tubular fluid into the interstitial and intracellular space in exchange for hydrogen and potassium ions, which are secreted into the urine. Aldosterone production is regulated by at least three factors, the chief of which is angiotensin II. This peptide is generated by the action of a proteolytic enzyme, renin, which is released by specialized kidney cells (the juxtaglomerular apparatus) in response to small changes in renal perfusion pressure or renal tubular sodium content which this structure is uniquely positioned to monitor. Other factors modulating aldosterone production are ACTH from the pituitary and the potassium ion concentration of adrenal cortical cells (see Atlas, this volume).

Renin–Angiotensin–Aldosterone System

Manipulation of dietary sodium intake has a marked effect on the renin–aldosterone system. The system is stimulated maximally when sodium intake is low and is suppressed during high sodium intake. The threshold for stimulation and/or suppression of the renin–aldosterone system is variable among humans and appears to be genetically determined. Certainly the ability to excrete a fixed sodium load has been shown to be highly variable (Luft & Weinberger, 1982).

Demographic Aberrations in Sodium Handling

Among normotensive individuals, those at highest likelihood to develop hypertension (blacks, individuals over age 40, first-degree relatives of hypertensive subjects) have been demonstrated to have an abnormality in their ability to excrete a sodium load (Luft & Weinberger, 1982). The mechanism for these abnormalities is not clear. Since renal handling of sodium is determined, in large part, by an active pumping mechanism, interest in the behavior of cellular pumps for sodium handling has been stimulated. From the study of red blood cells in these pumps, a variety of abnormalities as well as racial differences have been described in hypertensive subjects.

Stress and Sodium Excretion

Recent studies suggest that enhanced sympathetic nervous system (SNS) activity can increase proximal tubular sodium reabsorption (Skrabal et al., 1984). These authors further suggested that this can be responsible for salt-sensitive blood pressure. Light, Koepke, Obrist, and Willis (1983) demonstrated a relationship between stress and sodium and fluid retention, presumably mediated by the SNS in men. Thus, stress and SNS activity must be considered in evaluating sodium handling.

Pathophysiology of Sodium Handling

Given the magnitude of filtered sodium [24,191 mM (meq)/24 h], a subtle abnormality of reabsorption, leading to retention of an extra 1 mM (meq) of sodium per day over a period of years, could markedly increase total body sodium content and extracellular fluid volume. Such small aberrations in sodium balance cannot be detected by current balance techniques. Therefore, it is necessary to manipulate the physiologic mechanisms in a more vigorous manner in order to demonstrate abnormalities in metabolism and the hemodynamic effects of sodium.

Sodium Loading Studies

We conducted such a study in 16 normotensive young men (age 18–40) without a known parental history of hypertension (Luft et al., 1979). After an initial baseline evaluation, these subjects began a 7-day period of dietary sodium restriction (10 meq/day) during which sodium and potassium balance, blood pressure, cardiac output determined by an echocardiographic technique, creatinine clear-

ance, plasma renin activity, aldosterone and plasma and urinary catecholamines were carefully measured. At the end of this period, incremental changes in sodium intake to 300; 600; 800 or 1000; 1200 or 1500 meq/day for 3 days each were made. All other nutrients were continued at the same level as during the 10 meq period. Careful measurements were again obtained at the end of each incremental change in sodium intake. With increasing levels of sodium intake, significant suppression of plasma renin activity and aldosterone were observed beginning with the 300 meq/day level and with values reaching the lower limits of assay detectability (i.e., being virtually completely suppressed) at the 1000–1200 meq/day level. Plasma and urinary catecholamines similarly decreased with sodium loading, but never reached levels of nondetectability. Creatinine clearance increased and reached maximal values at 600–800 meq/day. At the end of each period, urinary sodium excretion approximated intake, indicative of steady-state (balance) conditions. Urinary potassium excretion exceeded intake at levels of sodium intake above 300 meq/day and, thus, progressive net potassium depletion (negative balance) occurred. Cardiac output increased at the higher levels of sodium intake, and blood pressure, at the end of the study, was significantly higher than at the beginning. This study clearly demonstrated that sodium could raise blood pressure in healthy, normotensive men. Large increases in sodium intake, beyond normal daily consumption, were required to mimic the more subtle and insidious impact of the cumulative effect of a miniscule abnormality in sodium handling over decades of a normal sodium intake.

Racial Differences

This study also revealed several important aspects. Not every subject participating in the study demonstrated a rise in blood pressure, although the mean value for the entire group did increase significantly. There was marked heterogeneity of blood pressure responsiveness to sodium. When the blood pressure responses of the eight black subjects were compared to those of the white subjects, the blacks were found to have a lower threshold and a greater magnitude of blood pressure increase (Luft *et al.*, 1979).

Influence of Sodium on Blood Pressure

The rise in blood pressure in these studies was apparently not due to angiotensin II since renin was virtually completely suppressed above 300 meq of sodium per day (Luft *et al.*, 1979). Norepinephrine, although reduced by sodium loading, was not so completely suppressed (Luft *et al.*, 1979). We conducted another study to determine whether the pressor effect of norepinephrine could be influenced by the state of sodium balance (Rankin, Henry, Weinberger, Gibbs, & Luft, 1981). We compared the blood pressure response to incremental arterial infusion of norepinephrine in normotensive subjects after achieving balance on 10 and 800 meq sodium diets. Norepinephrine caused a significantly greater rise in blood pressure for the high-sodium diet when compared to the low-sodium diet.

Sodium Sensitivity and Resistance

A variety of recent studies have confirmed the heterogeneity of human blood pressure responsiveness to sodium. Falkner, Katz, Canessa, and Kushner (1986) separated sodium-sensitive from sodium-insensitive black adults on the basis of a rise of mean arterial pressure of 5 mm Hg after 14 days of dietary sodium supplementation (10 g/day). Other investigators have utilized the blood pressure changes occurring from the end of a 7- to 10-day period of low dietary sodium intake (9 meq) compared to that following 3–5 days of 259 meq/day intake (Kawasaki, Delea, Bartter, & Smith, 1978). However, the amount of sodium retained with the high sodium intake during the latter maneuver may be, in part, dependent on the magnitude of aldosterone stimulation at the end of the low-sodium period which is highly variable among individuals. Several studies have attempted to examine sodium sensitivity of blood pressure by comparing the blood pressure change with rapid changes in dietary sodium intake, going from low to high or vice versa (Dustan, Tarazi, & Bravo, 1972).

We developed a protocol for rapid sodium and volume expansion followed by contraction in order to study neurohumoral mechanisms in blood pressure control (Grim, Weinberger, Higgins, & Kramer, 1977). The protocol induced sodium and volume expansion by the intravenous infusion of 2 liters of normal (0.9%) saline over a 4-h period. This was followed, the next day, by a 10 meq sodium intake and three 40-mg doses of furosemide, each given orally to induce sodium and volume contraction. We compared the blood pressure change from the end of the saline infusion to that at the end of sodium and volume contraction in 378 normotensive and 198 hypertensive subjects (Weinberger, Miller, Luft, Grim, & Fineberg, 1986). We observed sodium-sensitive (fall in mean arterial pressure $\geq$ 10 mm Hg) as well as sodium-resistant individuals (fall in pressure < 5 mm Hg and including those with a *rise* in blood pressure after the low-sodium diet and diuretic) in both populations. The hypertensive subjects were significantly more likely to be sodium-sensitive (51%) than were the normotensives (26%) who were more frequently sodium-resistant. These studies were the first to show heterogeneity of sodium responsiveness of blood pressure in normotensives as well as hypertensives. In addition, the sodium-sensitive subjects were significantly older than resistant subjects and had lower levels of plasma renin activity. Decreased plasma renin activity suggests that these subjects had retained more sodium than those who were sodium-resistant and that they had a relatively expanded extracellular fluid space. The relationship of sodium sensitivity to age suggests that the age-related increase in blood pressure, observed only in societies where sodium intake is abundant, may be a result of sodium sensitivity. We have previously reported that normotensives over age 40 years, as a group, do not excrete the sodium load given intravenously as quickly or completely when compared to younger normotensives (Luft & Weinberger, 1982). A genetic basis for sodium sensitivity has also been suggested by our recent observations of a disproportionately higher incidence of sodium sensitivity among subjects with haptoglobin (Hpl-1 phenotype than those with 2-1 or 2-2 (Weinberger *et al.*, 1987).

Potassium Influences Sodium Response

The dietary sodium-loading study described previously was confounded by net potassium loss which was observed at levels of sodium intake greater than 300 meq/day (Luft *et al.*, 1979). Deficiencies in potassium intake have been associated with blood pressure elevation in some studies. It has been suggested that the ratio of sodium to potassium intake or that of sodium and calcium may be the determinants of the blood pressure response rather than the amount of sodium alone (Langford, 1983). In order to determine whether there was an interaction between potassium loss and sodium excess in the sodium-induced blood pressure rise, we repeated the study in several subjects, replacing potassium losses daily (as potassium supplementation) as they occurred during incremental sodium loading (Weinberger *et al.*, 1982). During the potassium supplement study, the blood pressure increase with sodium loading was significantly blunted.

Potassium

Concentration and Distribution

Potassium is the major electrolyte in the intracellular space, existing in concentrations of 100–160 mM in mammalian cells, and has a major role in maintaining the integrity as well as the electrical activity of many cells. The critical importance of potassium is most evident in cardiac muscle cells where it is the major determinant of the electrogenic membrane action potential. In its distribution in body fluids, potassium generally opposes sodium (see Table 1). The intracellular concentration of potassium is 20-fold or more greater than that of extracellular fluid (4.0–5.5 mM) and an active, energy-dependent mechanism is required to keep potassium inside the cell and sodium out.

Sources

Potassium is provided primarily in the diet, being highest in green or yellow vegetables, in fruit, milk, and fresh meat. The primitive diet of our hunter-gatherer forebears probably contained more than 200 meq/day potassium and very little sodium. The current average American diet contains about 55 meq/day potassium, but like sodium, there is considerable variability in intake. Since potassium-rich foods may be more costly, potassium intake is generally lower among underprivileged socioeconomic groups than in more affluent groups. Specifically, potassium intake is lower in blacks than in whites (Langford, 1983).

Metabolism

Potassium is absorbed almost entirely in the small bowel and enters the circulation where it is freely filtered by the glomerulus. In the proximal renal tubule and the loop of Henle, 90% of the tubular fluid potassium is reabsorbed. Potassium is also secreted into the urine at the distal portion of the nephron in exchange for aldosterone-mediated sodium reabsorption. The magnitude of this route of urinary potassium loss is dependent on the degree of stimulation of the renal–angiotensin–aldosterone system and the amount of sodium presented to the mineralocorticoid receptors at the distal tubular site. In steady-state conditions, the urinary excretion of potassium is equivalent to intake. Net potassium conservation generally occurs during a reduced sodium intake, although the level of sodium restriction required for such conservation in man is not clearly defined and probably is dependent on the magnitude of increase in aldosterone associated with the reduced sodium intake. Net loss of potassium occurs at levels of sodium intake above 300 meq/day, even in the face of marked suppression of aldosterone (Luft *et al.*, 1979).

Measurement

Potassium, like sodium, is easily and accurately measured by flame photometry. Variability in potassium measurement is approximately 2%. Since the intracellular concentration of potassium is approximately 20-fold higher than that in extracellular fluid, factors influencing efflux of potassium from the cellular to the extracellular compartment can have a profound effect on the concentration of the latter. A diurnal variation for potassium has been described with a peak at noon and a nadir at midnight.

Variation in Potassium Measurements

Serum has a potassium concentration 0.4 meq/liter higher than those of plasma, owing to release of potassium from erythrocytes during clot formation and retraction in the preparation of serum. This is increased if the serum remains in contact with the clot for longer than 15–20 min or if it is shaken vigorously. If the blood is collected and handled in the cold, potassium enters serum or plasma. The prolonged use of a tourniquet for venipuncture or repeated exercise during venipuncture can raise potassium concentration in plasma or serum by contributing potassium-rich tissue juice. A factor which can artificially raise the apparent concentration of potassium in serum is hemolysis of red blood cells, which contain high amounts of potassium. The use of potassium-based anticoagulants can also artifactually raise plasma potassium concentration. Potassium flux in or out of cells is influenced by the pH of extracellular fluid. When acidosis occurs, potassium leaves the intracellular compartment and enters the extracellular fluid space. With alkalosis, the reverse occurs. Insulin increases cellular influx of potassium and β_2-adrenergic stimulation increases the shift of potassium from extracellular fluid into skeletal muscle cells.

Aberrations in Potassium Concentration

Diuretics acting on the proximal tubule of the kidney, and to a lesser extent, on the loop of Henle, inhibit potassium reabsorption in the tubule and promote potassium loss (hypokalemia). In addition, diuretics stimulate renin release by decreasing intravascular volume. This increases aldosterone production which stimulates sodium–potassium exchange at the distal nephron site (see sodium section) and further increases potassium loss. Hypokalemia can also be caused by impairment of gastrointestinal absorption (bowel resection, gastroenteritis, diarrhea, laxative abuse) or by vomiting. When renal function is compromised, thereby reducing the filtration of blood, hy-

perkalemia results. Another cause of hyperkalemia can be an abnormality of low aldosterone production (Schambelan, Stockigt, & Biglieri, 1973), decreasing distal tubular sodium–potassium exchange. This is most commonly encountered in older individuals and in diabetics in whom the renin response is subnormal as well as some patients with parenchymal renal disease. Several drugs can also promote hyperkalemia. These include potassium-sparing diuretics, potassium supplements, angiotensin-converting enzyme inhibitors, and nonsteroidal antiinflammatory agents of the prostaglandin synthetase inhibitor group. Pseudohyperkalemia can be the result of cell lysis during venipuncture in individuals with thrombocytosis or marked leukocytosis.

Vascular Effects of Potassium

The effects of potassium on vascular smooth muscle are dual. Acute intravascular administration of potassium can induce vasoconstriction and increase vascular resistance (Chen, Brace, Scott, Anderson, & Haddy, 1972). Chronic dietary potassium supplementation appears to dilate the vasculature, and, in the case of the spontaneously hypertensive rat, decreases the incidence of cerebral vascular hemorrhage commonly associated with untreated hypertension in this animal model (Tobian, Lange, Ulm, Wold, & Iwai, 1985).

Cardiac Effects

Potassium dynamics appear to be critical factors in the genesis of cardiac arrhythmias ranging from premature ventricular contractions and atrial tachyarrhythmias to ventricular fibrillation and sudden cardiac death (Curry, Fitchett, & Stubbs, 1976). Decreases in myocardial cell potassium concentration alter the contractile threshold and increase ventricular arrhythmias (Stewart, Ikram, Espiner, & Nicholls, 1985).

Catecholamine (β_2) Effects

A potentially lethal interaction between catecholamines and potassium has recently been elucidated (Brown, Brown, & Murphy, 1983).

Stimulation of the β_2-adrenergic receptors by catecholamines drives potassium into skeletal muscle cells and out of plasma and cardiac muscle. This flux can occur rapidly in the presence of bursts of catecholamine release, such as with exercise, stress, or acute myocardial infarction. In addition, catecholamine-induced stimulation of cardiac β_1 receptors increases both heart rate and cardiac contractility. When this occurs in association with rapid changes in membrane action potential threshold due to sudden potassium efflux in a heart with ischemic tissue or an irritable focus, ventricular fibrillation may occur and progress to sudden death if not corrected.

Calcium

Calcium is a critical electrolyte in most intracellular functions. It is a key component of the action and release of hormones and peptides, nerve function, and the contraction and relaxation of muscle cells. Calcium is maintained in an inactive form in the cell by specific binding proteins and is activated rapidly by a complex process.

Concentration

There is a large concentration gradient (roughly 1000-fold) for calcium between extracellular and intracellular compartments (see Table 1). Much of the calcium in both compartments is protein-bound. In blood, 45% of calcium is ionized and readily available, 40% is protein-bound, and 15% is nonionized. Protein binding of calcium can be altered by pH. Rapid induction of alkalosis can cause manifestations of hypocalcemia (tetany, seizures) in the presence of normal levels of total serum calcium by increasing bound calcium and decreasing the ionized fraction. The ionized fraction in blood is the most meaningful physiologically since it is the accessible form and its amount is not dependent on dissociation from protein-bound stores.

Measurement

The measurement of calcium concentrations in blood requires sensitive techniques because of the relatively low concentration of calcium (~ 2.5 mM). Intracellular concentrations require greater sensitivity. Ion-specific electrodes and atomic absorption spectrophotometry provide reasonable sensitivity and precision but special techniques are required to quantify ionized and bound calcium fractions.

Metabolism

Calcium is absorbed by the gut, primarily the jejunum, under the influence of vitamin D and its metabolites. Absorption is variable, influenced by intake, and incomplete (30–35%). Fecal excretion of calcium accounts for substantial loss of consumed calcium. There is a dynamic flux of calcium into and out of bone. Generally, the rates of bone absorption and formation in adults are equal and, thus, no net change in calcium balance is induced by this pool. Calcium is filtered by the glomerulus and 1–1.5% of this load is excreted in the urine. About 90% of calcium is reabsorbed in the proximal tubule and Henle's loop. Distal calcium secretion is influenced by parathyroid hormone. Unlike sodium and potassium, however, urinary calcium excretion, even under steady-state conditions, does not equal intake because of variable absorption of this ion and its sizable fecal excretion. The urinary excretion of calcium is influenced by a variety of factors including: volume expansion or contraction, diuretic administration, parathyroid hormone, acid–base status, phosphate intake, magnesium balance, and other hormones such as thyroid hormone, adrenal corticoids, and perhaps calcitonin.

Sources

Major dietary sources of calcium include dairy products, eggs, and baked goods. The average daily American diet contains 500–1000 mg varying by age and sex. A role for calcium-deficient diets in the pathogenesis of essential hypertension has been proposed based on epidemiologic surveys (McCarron, 1985). The accuracy of estimates of calcium intake, based on dietary recall, is questionable. Studies have shown both direct and indirect correlations between calcium and blood pressure (MacGregor, 1985; Kaplan, 1986). Curiously, demographic groups known to have an increased prevalence of hypertension (blacks and the elderly) frequently have an acquired lactase deficiency and a reduced calcium intake.

Effect of Intervention

Some studies have suggested that calcium supplementation may lower blood pressure in some hypertensive subjects (McCarron & Morris, 1985; Belizan, Villar, & Pineda, 1983; Resnick, Muller, & Laragh, 1986). It is clear that this is not a consistent observation in all hypertensives and appears to be most effective in patients with low renin levels (Resnick et al., 1986). These individuals are most often black and/or elderly. The effects of calcium on blood pressure are confounded by its ability to promote natriuresis. Thus, calcium supplementation may be most effective in sodium-sensitive individuals or in the presence of increased dietary sodium intake. A recent report suggests similar heterogeneity in the blood pressure response of normotensive subjects to calcium supplementation (Lyle, Melby, Hyner, Edmondson, & Weinberger, 1987).

Magnesium

Magnesium is the second most abundant intracellular electrolyte and has important neurohumoral, renal, and adrenal effects. Magnesium deficiency also appears to play a role in cardiac arrhythmias and may induce vasoconstriction and increase peripheral resistance.

Concentration

Magnesium exists in plasma in ionized, complexed, and protein-bound forms. The normal plasma concentration ranges from 1.5 to 2.0 meq/liter (see Table 1). Magnesium is absorbed from the gastrointestinal mucosa passively, but incompletely.

Sources

The dietary intake of magnesium usually ranges from 200 to 325 mg/day, primarily in the form of vegetables and cereals. Phosphate can bind magne-sium and impair its absorption, and calcium can also limit magnesium transport.

Metabolism

An inverse relationship appears to exist between magnesium balance and its gastrointestinal absorption. The majority of plasma magnesium is filtered by the glomerulus. Although some magnesium reabsorption occurs in the proximal tubule, most of the reabsorption occurs in the ascending limb of Henle's loop. The determinants of magnesium metabolism by the kidney are not clearly understood but do not appear to be linked to a specific hormone or receptor system. Because of variable fecal losses of magnesium, urinary excretion does not consistently reflect intake. Magnesium deficiency has been observed in a wide range of gastrointestinal, hepatic, renal, and nutritional disorders as well as in alcoholism. Thus, measuring plasma magnesium concentration to identify and help correct deficiencies is particularly appropriate in such disorders. Considerable parallelism has been noted between potassium and magnesium deficiency with diuretic therapy and in physiologic states characterized by hyperaldosteronism. It has been suggested that renal magnesium loss is mediated by aldosterone but convincing evidence is lacking. Spironolactone and amiloride both reduce renal losses of magnesium as well as potassium.

Measurement

Because of the low magnesium concentrations in plasma, sensitive and precise techniques such as atomic absorption spectrophotometry are required for quantification. In view of the high intracellular concentration, care must be taken in withdrawing and preparing blood samples for measurement to avoid the artifactual influence of intracellular magnesium stores on plasma or serum. Future studies should clarify the poorly understood control of magnesium absorption and excretion and identify the role of this electrolyte in human disease.

Summary

Sodium, potassium, calcium, and magnesium are important in cellular function and have been implicated in various cardiovascular disorders. Information concerning the effects of these electrolytes is important in conducting and analyzing biobehavioral studies. Sodium metabolism is the easiest of these ions to follow since, in steady-state conditions, urinary excretion is a good reflection of intake. Potassium balance can be less precisely estimated by its urinary excretion because of other factors influencing its handling. Calcium and magnesium metabolism are quite complex and no single approach can be relied on to quantify its handling. In short-term studies, administration of measured quantities of all four of these electrolytes is the best way of determining intake.

References

Belizan, J. M., Villar, J., & Pineda, O. (1983). Reduction of blood pressure with calcium supplementation in young adults. *Journal of the American Medical Association, 249,* 1161–1165.

Brown, M. S., Brown, D. C., & Murphy, M. D. (1983). Hypokalemia from beta 2 receptor stimulation by circulating epinephrine. *New England Journal of Medicine, 23,* 1414–1419.

Chen, W. T., Brace, R. A., Scott, J. B., Anderson, D. K., & Haddy, F. J. (1972). The mechanism of the vasodilator action of potassium. *Proceedings of the Society for Experimental Biology and Medicine, 140,* 820–824.

Curry, P., Fitchett, D., & Stubbs, W. (1976). Ventricular arrhythmias and hypokalemia. *Lancet, 2,* 231–233.

Dustan, H. P., Tarazi, R. C., & Bravo, E. L. (1972). Physiologic characteristics of hypertension. *American Journal of Medicine, 52,* 610–622.

Falkner, B., Katz, S., Canessa, M., & Kushner, H. (1986). The response to long-term oral sodium loading in young blacks. *Hypertension, 8,* I-165–I-168.

Grim, C. E., Weinberger, M. H., Higgins, J. T., Jr., & Kramer, N. J. (1977). Diagnosis of secondary forms of hypertension: A comprehensive protocol. *Journal of the American Medical Association, 237,* 1331–1335.

Kaplan, N. M. (1986). The calcium deficiency hypothesis of hypertension: A critique. *Annals of Internal Medicine, 105,* 947–955.

Kawasaki, T., Delea, C. S., Bartter, F. C., & Smith, H. (1978). The effect of high sodium intakes on blood pressure and other related variables in human subjects with idiopathic hypertension. *American Journal of Medicine, 64,* 193–198.

Langford, H. G. (1983). Dietary potassium and hypertension: Epidemiologic data. *Annals of Internal Medicine, 98,* 770–772.

Light, K. C., Koepke, J. P., Obrist, P. A., & Willis, P. W.

(1983). Psychological stress induces sodium and fluid retention in men at risk for hypertension. *Science, 220,* 429–431.

Luft, F. C., & Weinberger, M. H. (1982). Sodium intake and essential hypertension. *Hypertension, 4*(Suppl. III), III-14–III-19.

Luft, F. C., Rankin, L. I., Bloch, R., Weyman, A. E., Willis, L. R., Murray, R. H., Grim, C. E., & Weinberger, M. H. (1979). Cardiovascular and humoral responses to extremes of sodium intake in normal white and black men. *Circulation, 60,* 697–703.

Luft, F. C., Weinberger, M. H., Grim, C. E., Henry, D. P., & Fineberg, N. S. (1980). Nocturnal urinary electrolyte excretion and its relationship to the renin system and sympathetic activity in normal and hypertensive man. *Journal of Laboratory and Clinical Medicine, 95,* 395–406.

Lyle, E. M., Melby, C. L., Hyner, G. C., Edmondson, J. W., & Weinberger, M. H. (1987). Blood pressure and metabolic effects of calcium supplementation in normotensive white and black males. *Journal of the American Medical Association, 257,* 1772–1776.

MacGregor, G. A. (1983). Sodium and potassium intake and blood pressure. *Hypertension, 5,* III-79–III-84.

MacGregor, G. A. (1985). Sodium is more important than calcium in essential hypertension. *Hypertension, 7,* 628–637.

McCarron, D. A. (1985). Is calcium more important than sodium in the pathogenesis of essential hypertension? *Hypertension, 7,* 607–627.

McCarron, D. A., & Morris, C. D. (1985). Blood pressure response to oral calcium in persons with mild to moderate hypertension. *Annals of Internal Medicine 103*(Suppl. 1), 825–831.

Rankin, L. I., Henry, D. P., Weinberger, M. H., Gibbs, P. S., & Luft, F. C. (1981). Sodium intake alters the effects of norepinephrine on blood pressure. *Hypertension, 3,* 650–656.

Resnick, L. M., Muller, F. B., & Laragh, J. H. (1986). Calcium-regulating hormones in essential hypertension: Relation to plasma renin activity and sodium metabolism. *Annals of Internal Medicine, 105,* 649–654.

Schambelan, M., Stockigt, J. R., & Bigheri, E. G. (1973). Isolated hypoaldosteronism in adults. *New England Journal of Medicine, 287,* 573–576.

Skrabal, F., Herholz, H., Neumayr, M., Hamberger, L., Ledochowski, M., Sporer, H., Hortnagl, N., Schwarz, S., & Schonitzer, D. (1984). Salt sensitivity in humans is linked to enhanced sympathetic responsiveness and to enhanced proximal tubular reabsorption. *Hypertension, 6,* 152–158.

Stewart, D. E., Ikram, H., Espiner, E. A., & Nicholls, M. G. (1985). Arrhythmiogenic potential of diuretic-induced hypokalemia in patients with mild hypertension and ischemic heart disease. *British Heart Journal, 54,* 290–297.

Tobian, L., Lange, J., Ulm, K., Wold, K., & Iwai, J. (1985). Potassium reduces cerebral hemorrhage and death rate in hypertensive rats, even when blood pressure is not lowered. *Hypertension, 7,* I-110–I-114.

Weinberger, M. H., Luft, F. C., Bloch, R., Henry, D. P.,

Pratt, J. H., Weyman, A. E., Rankin, L. I., Murray, R. H., Willis, L. R., & Grim, C. E. (1982). The blood pressure-raising effects of high dietary sodium intake: Racial differences and the role of potassium. *Journal of the American College of Nutrition, 1,* 139–148.

Weinberger, M. H., Miller, J. Z., Luft, F. C., Grim, C. E., & Fineberg, N. S. (1986). Definitions and characteristics of sodium sensitivity and blood pressure resistance. *Hypertension, 8,* II-127–II-134.

Weinberger, M. H., Miller, J. Z., Grim, C. E., Luft, F. C., Fineberg, N. S., & Christian, J. C. (1987). Sodium sensitivity and resistance of blood pressure are associated with different haptoglobin phenotypes. *Hypertension, 10,* 443–446.

CHAPTER **10**

Methods for Study of Carbohydrate Metabolism

Jay S. Skyler

Introduction

This chapter will consider issues involved in the study of carbohydrate metabolism and of diabetes mellitus and its complications. As will become apparent from this introductory section, the study of carbohydrate metabolism and of diabetes mellitus are important considerations for investigators interested in cardiovascular behavioral medicine.

One in every 20 Americans has diabetes, an estimated 10.8 million people, many of whom are undiagnosed (National Diabetes Data Group, 1985). Diabetes, with its complications, is the number three cause of death by disease in the United States. People with diabetes are twice as prone to coronary and cerebral vascular disease. Peripheral vascular disease is markedly increased in the presence of diabetes. Diabetes accounts for more than half of all amputations performed annually in the United States. Diabetes is the leading cause of new blindness in adults aged 20 to 74. Diabetic patients are 17 times more prone to kidney disease, and diabetes is now the leading known cause of end stage renal disease in the United States. Diabetic neuropathies may impair

function of nerves throughout the body and involve any organ system.

Diabetes mellitus is recognized by elevated levels of plasma glucose (hyperglycemia), and is monitored by measuring the variation in glycemia. Current classification divides primary diabetes into two major categories, known as Type I and Type II (WHO Expert Committee on Diabetes Mellitus, 1980; National Diabetes Data Group, 1979, 1985). Type I, or insulin-dependent diabetes mellitus (IDDM), is characterized by absolute insulin deficiency and thus a dependence on insulin therapy for the preservation of life. In contrast, in Type II, or non-insulin-dependent diabetes mellitus (NIDDM), insulin therapy is not generally required for the maintenance of life, but may be necessary for the control of symptoms or for the correction of disordered metabolism.

Chronic diabetes management involves careful attention to food intake, energy expenditure (activity), and medication (insulin injections or sulfonylurea tablets). In both types of diabetes, the patient must be involved in the treatment program on a daily basis, including attention to the various components of treatment and the monitoring of therapy. Thus, motivation and patient behavior are critical factors in the therapeutic plan.

Glycemic control may become decompensated as a consequence of intercurrent stress, either

Jay S. Skyler • Departments of Medicine, Pediatrics, and Psychology, University of Miami, Miami, Florida 33101.

physiological or psychological (Woods, Smith, & Porte, 1981). This is a result of the secretion of neurohumoral stress hormones, including: catecholamines, cortisol, growth hormone, and glucagon. The biological consequences of these hormones include stimulation of glucose production, lipolysis and ketogenesis, and proteolysis. In nondiabetic individuals, the secretion of these stress hormones is counteracted by incremental insulin secretion, which serves to maintain constancy of glycemia. In individuals with diabetes, especially Type I diabetes, such modulation by insulin is not possible. Thus, stress serves to disrupt glycemic control and leads to metabolic decompensation.

As a function of time, many diabetic patients suffer the ravages of the chronic complications of the disease—vascular, neurological, and organ-specific (particularly retinal and renal) (Keen & Jarrett, 1982; Watkins, 1986). The frequency, severity, and progression of many of the chronic complications appear to be related to the degree of hyperglycemia and associated metabolic derangements, as well as the duration of the disease (Skyler, 1979, 1987). In addition, other factors influence the emergence of diabetic complications, as well as morbidity and mortality. One such factor is blood pressure. For example, the appearance and severity of diabetic retinopathy and diabetic nephropathy is related to blood pressure elevation and hemodynamic considerations (Zatz & Brenner, 1986). Moreover, the rate of progression of diabetic renal disease is profoundly influenced by the effectiveness and method of control of coexisting hypertension (Parving *et al.*, 1983, 1987). Conversely, diabetic renal disease and other cardiovascular changes secondary to diabetes may result in blood pressure elevation.

The cardiovascular complications of diabetes fall into three categories: (1) micoangiopathy—a characteristic small blood vessel (capillary) disease, associated more or less specifically with diabetes mellitus, and clinically manifested principally in the retina (diabetic retinopathy) (Klein, 1985) and kidney (diabetic nephropathy) (DeFronzo, 1985); (2) macroangiopathy—accelerated atherosclerotic disease of large blood vessels (arteries) (Colwell, Lopes-Virella, Winocour, &

Halushka, 1988), clinically manifested principally in coronary arteries, cerebral vasculature, and peripheral vessels in the lower extremities (National Diabetes Data Group, 1985); and (3) cardiovascular autonomic neuropathy—with increased heart rate, altered heart rate control, and the possibility of exercise intolerance, postural hypotension, and/or cardiac denervation syndrome (including painless myocardial infarctions), and increased mortality from sudden death (Ewing, Campbell, & Clarke, 1980; Ewing & Clarke, 1986). Mild cardiovascular autonomic neuropathy primarily afflicts the parasympathetic nervous system, whereas the sympathetic system also becomes impaired in severe autonomic neuropathy.

Classification

As noted, there are two major categories of primary diabetes mellitus: IDDM and NIDDM. These two major clinical patterns of the diabetic syndrome appear to be distinct entities in terms of etiology, pathogenesis, clinical presentation, and requisite treatment strategies. In addition, other subtypes have been recognized, including: "tropical malnutrition diabetes" (called "Type III" by some) (McMillan & Geevarghese, 1979), maturity-onset diabetes of the young (MODY) (Tattersall & Fajans, 1975), and a relatively newly defined subtype that occurs in young blacks that has some features of IDDM and some of NIDDM (Winter *et al.*, 1987). Moreover, secondary diabetes mellitus refers to hyperglycemia caused by some other primary pancreatic disease, e.g., pancreatic surgery or chronic pancreatitis; or secondary to medication use of some other disease (such as Cushing's syndrome, acromegaly, or chronic steroid therapy). Diabetes mellitus is also associated with a number of relatively uncommon genetic conditions.

Characteristics of Type I Diabetes

IDDM (previously labeled juvenile-onset diabetes or ketosis-prone diabetes) is characterized by greatly decreased numbers of insulin-producing beta cells in the pancreatic islets, resulting in an absolute deficiency of endogenous pancreatic insulin secretion, insulinopenia, hypoinsulinemia, proneness to ketosis, with dependency on daily insulin administration for the maintenance of life (Skyler, 1986). This is the rarer, although more severe form of the disease. IDDM usually has its onset in childhood, with a peak incidence between ages 10 and 13, although it may occur at any age. Patients are usually thin. Chronic management involves two or more daily insulin injections; careful attention to food intake, energy expenditure (activity), and insulin dosage; and routine daily patient self-monitoring of blood pressure.

Current formulation (Skyler & Rabinovitch, 1987) of the pathogenesis of IDDM includes: (1) a genetic predisposition, conferred by diabetogenic genes on the short arm of chromosome 6 in close proximity to the HLA region, including a clear association with HLA antigens DR3 and DR4; (2) environmental triggers (? viral infections, noxious chemicals, and/or other as yet unidentified environmental factors) which in genetically susceptible individuals appear to initiate damage to pancreatic islet beta cells; and (3) an immune mechanism gone awry, leading to slow, progressive, further damage to pancreatic islet beta cells and eventual beta cell destruction, such islet beta cell destruction often reflected by circulating islet cell antibodies (ICA), particularly at the onset of IDDM.

Characteristics of Type II Diabetes

NIDDM (previously labeled maturity-onset diabetes or ketosis-resistant diabetes) is characterized by retention of endogenous pancreatic insulin secretion, although with altered insulin secretory dynamics; the absence of ketosis; and insulin resistance due to diminished target cell response to insulin (Lebovitz & Feinglos, 1986; Skyler, 1984). Patients with NIDDM are usually not dependent on insulin for prevention of ketosis or maintenance of life, although they may require insulin for correction of symptomatic or persistent, fasting hyperglycemia if this cannot be achieved with the use of diet or oral agents. This is the

milder, although more common form of the disease. It generally has its onset after age 40, although the disease rarely may make its appearance as early as adolescence. The majority (80–90% in the United States) are obese, and the nonobese may represent a separate subtype. Indeed, there likely is a spectrum of subtypes of NIDDM. Chronic management involves weight reduction, increased physical activity, balanced nutrition, and medication (insulin injections or sulfonylurea tablets). Effective weight reduction may lead to complete normalization of glycemia.

Both genetic and environmental factors appear to be involved in the etiopathogenesis of NIDDM (Zimmet, 1982). The specific nature of genetic predisposition to NIDDM remains to be established. That environmental factors play a role in the pathogenesis of NIDDM has become evident from studies of ''primitive'' societies undergoing ''Westernization'' (Zimmet, 1979). The development of a sedentary life-style, particularly when coupled with the emergence of obesity, leads to marked increase in prevalence of NIDDM. Other diabetogenetic factors are aging and multiparity.

The major pathogenetic mechanisms in NIDDM are impaired islet beta-cell function and impaired insulin action (Porte & Halter, 1982; Lebovitz & Feinglos, 1986). Impaired islet beta-cell function (impaired insulin secretion) is manifested in at least three ways (Porte *et al.*, 1982): (1) blunted or absent first phase insulin response to glucose; (2) decreased sensitivity of insulin response to glucose, such that insulin response to glucose is attenuated, and that the islet beta cell shows a relative ''blindness'' to hyperglycemia; (3) decreased overall insulin secretory capacity, particularly in more severe NIDDM. The impairment in insulin secretory response is not static, but dynamic. Chronic hyperglycemia may, of itself, aggravate the impairment in insulin secretion. Thus, with deterioration of NIDDM, there is concomitant deterioration in insulin secretory response. Moreover, when there is correction of hyperglycemia, there is some reversal of the impairment in endogenous insulin response to a meal challenge, i.e., demonstrable improvement in insulin secretion.

Impaired insulin action (insulin resistance) is due to an impairment of insulin action at target cells (Olefsky, 1981). The target cell defects include: (1) receptor binding defects—decreased insulin binding to cellular receptors as a consequence of reduced numbers of receptors; and (2) postbinding ("postreceptor") defects—defective insulin action as a consequence of defects in the effector system beyond the level of insulin binding to cellular receptors, including a decrease in glucose transport capacity, although other additional defects cannot be excluded. The defects in insulin action are not static, but dynamic. Thus, it is possible to alter insulin binding. Indeed, insulin receptors are highly regulated and influenced by a variety of factors, including diet, activity, hormones, pharmacological agents, and circulating concentrations of insulin itself. This can be taken advantage of therapeutically. Moreover, the apparent postreceptor defects also can be substantially reversed by vigorous insulin therapy, and these too probably are also subject to a complex regulatory scheme.

State of Carbohydrate Tolerance

Diabetes mellitus, in the untreated state, is recognized on the basis of chronic elevation of plasma glucose (hyperglycemia) (Table 1) (National Diabetes Data Group, 1979, 1985). Specifically, diabetes mellitus is reflected by fasting plasma glucose greater than 140 mg/dl (on two occasions) or by plasma glucose levels greater than 200 mg/dl at two time points after a 75-g glucose challenge, including the 2-h value. This is an oral glucose tolerance test (OGTT). Normal glucose tolerance is defined as a fasting plasma glucose of 115 mg/dl or less, and a 2-h value on OGTT of 139 mg/dl or less. Impaired glucose tolerance (IGT) is defined as a glycemic response to a standard glucose challenge intermediate between normal and diabetic, and can therefore only be determined by an OGTT. The criteria for IGT are a fasting plasma glucose between 116 and 139 mg/dl and a 2-h OGTT between 140 and 200 mg/dl. The above definitions apply to nonpregnant adults. During childhood and during pregnancy, slightly different criteria are used (Table 1).

The OGTT should be performed under carefully defined conditions (National Diabetes Data Group, 1979). The subject should be free of intercurrent illness, should be following his/her usual activity program, and should be on an unrestricted diet (containing at least 150 g of carbohydrate daily) for 3 days prior to testing (in order to avoid "starvation" diabetes). The OGTT should commence in the morning, preceded by an overnight fast of 10–16 h. Glucose is usually administered as a solution consisting of 200–300 ml, consumed over a 5-min period. Samples are taken at baseline, and half-hourly for 2 h.

Assessment of Metabolic Control

Metabolic control fluctuates and may influence whatever outcome variable is being measured in a research study. Thus, it is important that research subjects be carefully characterized. This should include assessment not only of metabolic control, but also specification of the treatment program being used at the time of assessment of metabolic control. For insulin doses, for comparative purposes, this should be expressed in units per kilogram per day. A number of control parameters may be measured. They are reviewed below.

Glycated Hemoglobin

The formation of glycated (or glycosylated) hemoglobin occurs by the process of nonenzymatic glycosylation (glycation) (Figure 1) (Bunn, 1981). Glycation of proteins occurs both at N-terminal amino groups and at epsilon amino groups of intrachain amino acids (e.g., lysine). It involves the addition of glucose to protein by a slow continuous reaction that is a function of the duration of contact between the reactants and the integrated glucose concentration during the time of contact. Glycated hemoglobin thus is a direct indicator of the average plasma glucose. The most abundant glycated hemoglobin is HbA1c.

Over the past decade, the measurement of glycated hemoglobin has emerged as the most important clinical tool in the assessment of chronic

Table 1. Criteria for Diagnosis of Diabetes

I. *Diabetes mellitus in nonpregnant adults*
   Any one of the following is diagnostic of diabetes:
   A. Classic symptoms (e.g., polyuria, polydipsia, ketonuria, rapid weight loss) together with gross and unequivocal elevation of random plasma glucose (> 200 mg/dl)
   B. Elevated fasting glucose (on more than one occasion):
      1. Venous plasma ≥ 140 mg/dl
      2. Whole blood ≥ 120 mg/dl
   C. Sustained elevated glucose during OGTT on more than one occasion. *Both* the 2-h sample and some other sample ($\frac{1}{2}$, 1, or $1\frac{1}{2}$ h) must meet the following criteria:
      1. Venous plasma ≥ 200 mg/dl
      2. Venous whole blood ≥ 180 mg/dl
      3. Capillary whole blood ≥ 200 mg/dl
II. *Diabetes mellitus in children*
    Same as I above, except both B and C must be met
III. *Impaired glucose tolerance (IGT) in nonpregnant adults*
     Three criteria must be met:
     A. Fasting glucose below that in I.B
     B. Two-hour sample on OGTT must be between normal and diabetic values
     C. One other sample ($\frac{1}{2}$, 1, or $1\frac{1}{2}$ h) must be unequivocally elevated (by criteria in I.C)
IV. *Impaired glucose tolerance (IGT) in children*
    Two criteria must be met:
    A. Fasting glucose below that in I.B
    B. Two-hour sample on OGTT must exceed values usually used for fasting, i.e., those in I.B
V. *Normal glucose levels in nonpregnant adults*

	Venous plamsa	Venous whole blood	Capillary whole blood
Fasting	<115	<100	<100
$\frac{1}{2}$, 1, $1\frac{1}{2}$ h OGTT	<200	<180	<200
2-h OGTT	<140	<120	<140

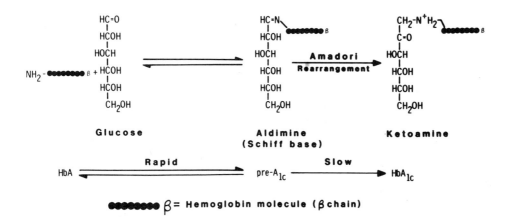

Figure 1. Schematic representation of the process of nonenzymatic glycation of hemoglobin at the terminal amino group of the hemoglobin β chain. Adapted from Bunn (1981).

glycemic control (Nathan, Singer, Hurxthal, & Goodson, 1984). It has become the "gold standard" in assessment, by virtue of the fact that it reflects integrated glycemia over several weeks, specifically over the life span of the hemoglobin molecule. The correlations are strongest for glycemic control 4–8 weeks before glycated hemoglobin determination, and determinations are thus made every 2–3 months. Values appear to be more sensitive to deterioration in control than improvement in control.

A number of different assays have been developed to measure glycated hemoglobin (Goldstein, Little, Wiedmeyer, England, & McKenzie, 1986). Each has advantages and disadvantages, and each measures different glycated hemoglobin components. The most common assays have been chromatographic, based on cation-exchange chromatography. The chromatographic methods are influenced by a number of circumstances, including uremia, alcoholism, pregnancy, thalassemia, and certain hemoglobinopathies. Chemically based methods include colorimetric techniques, a fluorometric technique, and affinity chromatography. Electrophoretic methods include isoelectric focusing on polyacrylamide slab gels, and agar gel electrophoresis. A radioimmunoassay, specific for measurement of HbA1c, has also been developed, but has only had limited use. Each method should be carefully standardized with appropriate quality control. All of the methods show excellent correlation with each other. The absolute numbers obtained by one or another method, or between laboratories, cannot be directly compared, however.

Glycated Albumin and/or Serum Fructosamine

These are also products of nonenzymatic glycation, but involve components that turn over at a more rapid rate than hemoglobin (Lloyd, Nott, & Marples, 1985). Thus, their measurement reflects shorter-term glycemic control. These are used in conjunction with glycated hemoglobin to ascertain the relative degree of glycemic control over the short term in comparison with the longer term, thus indicating whether control is improving or deteriorating.

Glucose

Plasma or whole blood glucose may be measured by several procedures. Plasma values are generally 15% higher than whole blood values. Most laboratories perform plasma determinations. The most commonly used methods are enzymatic using glucose oxidase, which is specific for glucose (Clark & Lyons, 1962; Guilbault, 1982). The reaction is:

$$O_2 + glucose \xrightarrow{\text{Glucose oxidase}} H_2O_2 + gluconic\ acid$$

There are a number of ways to measure the reaction, including uptake of oxygen with a gas membrane electrode, recording the peroxide or oxygen polarographically, measuring the signal electrochemically with a platinum electrode, or using one of the products in a second enzymatic reaction which can be detected colorimetrically (Guilbault, 1982). Other methods involve the enzyme hexokinase rather than glucose oxidase.

Periodic plasma glucose determinations have long been used as a means of monitoring diabetic control. Unfortunately, the lability of plasma glucose in many diabetic patients is such that intermittent random glucose determinations give little insight into chronic glucose regulation (Service, O'Brien, & Rizza, 1987). On the other hand, in stable patients with Type II diabetes, the *fasting* plasma glucose is often an excellent index of overall glycemic control (Holman & Turner, 1979), and is highly correlated with glycosylated hemoglobin determinations.

Plasma *glucose profiles* are commonly used to assess glucose fluctuations during the course of the day. The pattern of glycemia can thus be assessed (Figure 2). In addition, the *mean glucose level* (mean plasma glucose, MPG) may be calculated. Periodic samples may be measured on a portable glucose meter, used either by the patient or by a member of the investigative team. Although a general assessment of pattern of glycemia and mean glucose level can be made on patient-determined samples using a portable meter, ideally research profiles should be based on laboratory determinations, performed in a research unit or hospital, or

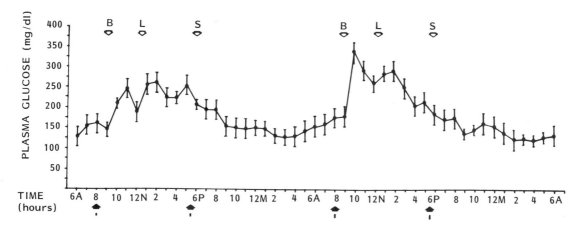

Figure 2. Plasma glucose profile on an hourly basis over a 48-h period. Each point is the mean value for ten subjects with Type I diabetes mellitus. The major meals are indicated by the open arrows labeled B (breakfast), L (lunch), and S (supper). Each subject was treated with a twice-daily insulin program, given at the times indicated by the black arrows. From Reeves, Seigler, Ryan, and Skyler (1982).

on samples collected by the patient and brought to the laboratory in special capillary tubes (Clark, Bilous, Keen, & Keen, 1982). The greater the number of samples obtained during the profile day, the more valuable is the profile. As a minimum, preprandial and bedtime determinations should be made. This may be supplemented by postprandial and some overnight values, or for some studies, hourly (or even half-hourly) determinations may be made. Continuous glucose monitors also are available, but are cumbersome and require that the subject be tethered to the machine throughout the study period.

Glycemic Lability and Stability

If one wishes to approach the glycemic pattern in a more sophisticated manner, a number of in-dices have been used to assess the degree of *lability/stability* of glycemia (Service & Nelson, 1980; Service *et al.*, 1987). Two that have been used for characterizing lability of glycemia in diabetic patients are: (1) the *mean amplitude of glycemic excursion* (MAGE), as a quantitative measure of within-day glucose fluctuations that quantifies the extent of glucose swings over a defined period (Figure 3); and (2) the *mean of daily differences* (MODD), as a numerical expression for between-day glucose fluctuations, thus quantifying the variability of glucose from day to day (Figure 4). Coupled with the *mean plasma glucose,* the MAGE and MODD values provide useful information for quantifying the lability of glycemia in any given individual. Another useful parameter is the *"M" value* of Schlictkrull, a weighted average of glucose values obtained at de-

Figure 3. Derivation of mean amplitude of glycemic excursions (MAGE), calculated from 24-h glucose profile. Each amplitude of glycemic excursion (AGE) that exceeds 1 standard deviation (SD) of the mean plasma glucose (MPG) (in this example, MPG = 84, SD = 16) is used in the calculations. In this case, there are four such excursions, calculated from peak to nadir. From Service and Nelson (1980).

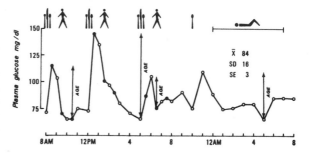

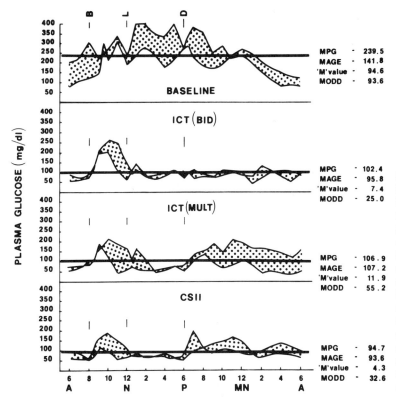

Figure 4. Curves representing various indices of glycemic lability and stability in a subject with Type I diabetes treated with four different insulin programs. The glucose profiles in each curve are depicted as solid lines showing the 24-h glucose profiles obtained on two consecutive days. The dotted area in between the curves depicts the between-day differences used to calculate the mean of daily differences (MODD). The solid horizontal line designates the mean plasma glucose (MPG). Also listed for each set of curves are the MAGE and "M" values. From Skyler, Reeves, Seigler, and Ryan (1983).

fined time points. Thus, it is possible to define the degree of lability or stability of diabetic individuals with quantitative parameters useful for research evaluations.

Urine Glucose

Until the advent of patient self-monitoring of blood glucose during the past decade, urine glucose determinations were commonly used as an index of diabetic control (Kohler, 1978). Glucose in the glomerular filtrate is quantitatively reabsorbed by the proximal tubule. As the concentration of glucose in the plasma increases, the amount of glucose presented to the tubules eventually exceeds their capacity to reabsorb glucose. The maximum tubular reabsorptive capacity for glucose (T_m for glucose) is usually about 300 mg glucose/min, although this is not the same for all tubules. Urinary glucose excretion is thus related to plasma glucose concentration, glomerular filtration rate, and T_m for glucose, and in normal human

beings does not occur until plasma glucose concentration is approximately 160–200 mg/dl, known as the *renal threshold for glucose*. The renal threshold varies between individuals, with age, and is altered by changes in kidney function. Thus, in order to understand the significance of urine glucose determinations as an index of control, it is necessary to have some approximation of the renal threshold. It should also be noted that the maintenance of physiologic blood glucose does not allow the usual renal threshold to be exceeded. In addition, urine glucose concentration will be influenced by degree of hydration. For these reasons, and because many factors may cause fluctuations in renal threshold, most experts have abandoned urine glucose determination as an index of glucose control.

"Quantitative" (or "fractional" or "block") urine specimens permit quantification of glycosuria over a defined time interval and are correlated with the mean simultaneously recorded and continuously analyzed blood glucose (Service, Molnar,

& Taylor, 1972; Forman, Goldstein, & Genel, 1974). They involve collection of all urine produced during that interval, with the measurement of both concentration and volume of the pooled specimen so that the quantity of glucose (in grams) lost during the interval can be defined.

Two general classes of methods are used for urine glucose determination (Skyler, 1982a). Methods based on copper reduction detect all reducing substances. Enzymatic tests involve the use of glucose oxidase to specifically detect glucose.

Urine Ketones

Urinary ketone determinations can be used as an important parameter for monitoring diabetic status (James & Chase, 1974). Ketosis and ketonuria are a consequence of one of four conditions: (1) *insulin deficiency* and uncontrolled diabetes; (2) *starvation* (insufficient calorie intake); (3) *posthypoglycemia* in response to secretion of counterregulatory hormones (catecholamines, glucagon, growth hormone, and cortisol) which are lipolytic; and (4) in response to *stress* with attendant hormonal secretion (again, of catecholamines, glucagon, growth hormone, and cortisol), be that stress physical (e.g., illness, infection, vomiting) or emotional. Ketone production rate also increases during exercise but ketosis and ketonuria generally occur only if there is concomitant insulin deficiency.

All of the commercial methods for urinary ketone determination are based on the nitroprusside reaction in which acetoacetate and acetone (but not β-hydroxybutyrate) produce a purple color, the intensity of which provides a qualitative estimate of the degree of ketosis. Humidity adversely affects the reagent such that false-negative readings may occur (Rosenbloom & Malone, 1978).

Lipid Profiles

Abnormalities in plasma lipids and lipoproteins have been correlated with inadequacy of diabetic control (Goldberg, 1981). Thus, increased concentrations of cholesterol and triglyceride, and decreased levels of HDL-cholesterol may be indicative of inadequate diabetic control, particularly in the presence of fasting hyperglycemia. These val-

ues often can be corrected, albeit slowly over weeks, with the attainment of improved diabetic control. Extent of lipid abnormality has been shown to correlate with glycosylated hemoglobin level, and may be an additional indicator of long-term diabetic control.

Frequency of Hypoglycemia

It is desirable to quantify the frequency of hypoglycemia, particularly in insulin-treated diabetic patients. At times, attainment of good metabolic control is at the price of an excessive frequency of hypoglycemic episodes (DCCT Research Group, 1987). Distinction should be made between asymptomatic chemical hypoglycemia (determined by patient self-monitoring of blood glucose) and symptomatic hypoglycemia. Suspected hypoglycemic symptoms should be documented by concomitant blood glucose determination.

Serum Ketones, Bicarbonate, Anion Gap

Obviously, in markedly uncontrolled diabetes, there will be elevations of serum ketones, bicarbonate, and a widening of the calculated anion gap (Brenner, 1985). Such individuals are not candidates for most research studies, until their acute metabolic decompensation is corrected.

Assessment of Insulin Secretion

Insulin is synthesized in pancreatic islet beta cells. It is a peptide hormone consisting of two chains, called A and B chains, linked by disulfide bridges. Insulin is produced from a higher-molecular-weight, single precursor molecule, proinsulin (Figure 5) (Steiner, 1977; Chan, Kwok, & Steiner, 1981). The A and B chains are linked by an additional polypeptide sequence known as the "connecting peptide," or C-peptide. The precursor molecule proinsulin is cleaved to insulin and C-peptide within the beta cells. Insulin and C-peptide are then released into the circulation concurrently, on an equimolar basis, when the secretory granules liberate their contents, although there is no known function of C-peptide. As a consequence, mea-

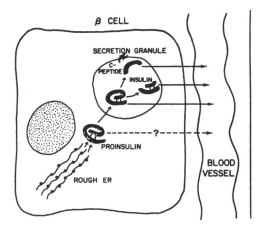

Figure 5. Schematic depiction of a pancreatic islet beta cell, demonstrating initial biosynthesis of proinsulin, which is then packaged in an insulin secretion granule, in which proinsulin is cleaved to insulin and C-peptide. When the granule liberates its contents, insulin and C-peptide are liberated on an equimolar basis. From Rubenstein, Horwitz, and Steiner (1975).

surement of C-peptide serves as an index of islet beta-cell function.

Glucose is the primary physiological stimulus for insulin secretion (Lacy, 1977). The kinetics of insulin secretion after a glycemic challenge involves an asynchronous biphasic discharge (Figure 6) (Porte & Pupo, 1969). The initial first phase of insulin secretion is from a rapidly mobilizable

pool. Second-phase insulin release is from a larger compartment which is replenished by newly synthesized insulin if the stimulus is prolonged. Other factors influencing insulin secretion include gastrointestinal hormones, protein ingestion, and neural control mechanisms (Porte *et al.,* 1982).

The important physiological event is that in response to nutrient ingestion there is *substrate-mediated* (particularly glucose-mediated) *insulin secretion.* Insulin secretion is timely and occurs in concert with the glycemic challenge and abates abruptly as glycemia diminishes and the signal abates. Nevertheless, in the absence of substrate stimulation, insulin secretion is not absent but continues at a low basal rate (*basal insulin secretion*) that is crucial in modulating intermediary metabolism, particularly in maintaining hepatic glucose production equivalent to non-insulin-mediated basal glucose utilization.

Circulating insulin concentration is the primary regulator of fuel metabolism, coordinating the mobilization of fuel into and out of the various fuel storage depots in order to meet the needs of the organism depending on the availability or lack thereof of fuel in the environment (Cahill, 1971). In response to nutrient input, i.e., the "fed" state, insulin secretion is stimulated, and insulin stimulates the utilization of substrates and the assimilation of substrates into their storage forms.

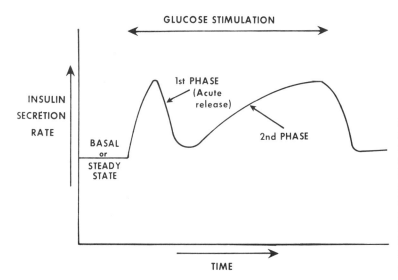

Figure 6. The biphasic insulin response to a constant glucose stimulus. A theoretical response to a constant square-wave infusion of glucose is shown. The peak of the first phase in man is between 3 and 5 min and lasts 10 min. The second phase begins at 2 min but is not evident until 10 min has passed. It continues to increase slowly for at least 60 min or until the stimulus stops. From Porte and Halter (1982).

Thus, relatively high levels of insulin herald the "fed" state. In contrast, in the interval between feeding (the "fasted" state), fuel is efficiently mobilized from storage depots to meet energy demands. Low circulating basal levels of insulin characterize the "fasted" state and facilitate fuel mobilization.

In Type I diabetes, initially there may be some preservation of endogenous insulin secretion, but this progressively declines over the first year or two of diabetes, and eventuates in essentially absent endogenous insulin production (Ludvigsson & Heding, 1976; Ludvigsson, Heding, Larsson, & Leander, 1977).

In Type II diabetes, there is impaired islet beta-cell function (Pfeifer, Halter, & Porte, 1981; Porte et al., 1982; Pfeifer et al., 1984), which as noted is manifested in at least three ways: (1) blunted or absent first-phase insulin response to glucose. It is the first phase of the normally biphasic response (Figure 6) which is the critical determinant of the magnitude of hyperglycemia following carbohydrate intake. The decrease in first-phase insulin secretion results in an overall delayed insulin secretory response to glucose. Although variable, in most circumstances, however, second-phase insulin response is sufficient to restore postprandial plasma glucose excursions to basal (preprandial) levels before the next meal, albeit after a prolonged interval. (2) Decreased sensitivity of insulin response to glucose, such that insulin response to glucose is attenuated, and that the islet beta cell shows a relative "blindness" to hyperglycemia (Porte et al., 1982). In spite of significant hyperglycemia, the islet fails to generate an adequate insulin response. The blindness is selective for glucose, in that the islet responds to nonglucose stimuli, e.g., isoproterenol, arginine, glucagon, secretin, theophylline. (3) Decreased overall insulin secretory capacity, particularly in more severe NIDDM (Reaven, Bernstein, Davids, & Olefsky, 1976). The declining insulin response in more severe NIDDM is illustrated by "Starling's law of the pancreas" (Figure 7), in which there is compensatory insulin release in response to increasing hyperglycemia in nondiabetic individuals, and in patients with IGT (impaired glucose tolerance), but decreased insulin response

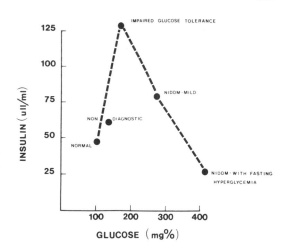

Figure 7. Plot of the mean plasma insulin (vertical axis) versus the mean plasma glucose (horizontal axis) in five groups of subjects: nondiabetic individuals, individuals with nondiagnostic (borderline) glucose tolerance tests, individuals with impaired glucose tolerance, individuals with mild NIDDM with normal fasting plasma glucose, and individuals with moderate and severe NIDDM with significant fasting hyperglycemia. From Skyler (1982b), redrawn using data of Reaven et al. (1976).

to increasing hyperglycemia once NIDDM is present.

Measurements: Insulin versus C-peptide

Insulin and C-peptide each may be measured by specific and sensitive radioimmunoassays (Heding, 1972, 1975). In nondiabetic individuals and in many of those with Type II diabetes, it is possible to measure plasma insulin response directly. On the other hand, in insulin-treated individuals with Type I or Type II diabetes, it is necessary to distinguish endogenous insulin production from exogenously administered insulin. In such circumstances, and for the reasons cited above, it is possible to use plasma C-peptide levels as an index of endogenous insulin secretion (Polansky et al., 1986), since this molecule is secreted along with insulin by islet beta cells and is not contained in commercial insulin preparations. Moreover, the measurement of C-peptide obviates the technical problems of insulin antibodies interfering with the radioimmunoassay of insulin. Since insulin antibodies are formed in the vast majority of insulin-treated patients, this has the potential of being a serious problem. The presence of insulin anti-bodies also may prolong insulin availability in the circulation, and thus alter insulin action. Thus, it may be desirable in some studies to determine both antibody-"bound" and "free" insulin levels (Kuzuya, Blix, Horwitz, Steiner, & Rubenstein, 1977). This is accomplished by measuring "total" insulin, and by determining "free" insulin after polyethylene glycol precipitation of antibody-bound insulin. It is also possible to quantify the levels of insulin antibodies (Reeves, 1983), which may be desirable in some studies.

Insulin/Glucose Ratios

Because glucose stimulates insulin secretion, one would expect a greater insulin response in the presence of higher ambient levels of plasma glucose. In view of this, some workers believe that it is best to express the insulin response as an "insulin/glucose ratio," to facilitate comparison of data among subjects studied at different levels of glycemia.

Basal versus Challenged Values

Since insulin secretion is profoundly influenced by substrate, it is important that the conditions of measurement be carefully defined. Basal or fasting insulin levels are influenced by basal glycemia, adiposity, degree of physical training, and other factors. Thus, their utility is limited in many studies. When used, it is important to define the period of time in which the subject has been maintained in the basal state prior to sampling. Many investigators obtain two or three basal samples 5–15 min apart, and report the mean value.

In most studies, it is best to assess insulin (or C-peptide) response to a provocative challenge under standardized conditions. The subject is generally studied in the basal state, either fasting or after a specific overnight preparation to assure either stability of glycemia within the subject and/or uniformity of glycemia among subjects. The challenge usually is conducted in the morning to avoid the confounding influence of diurnal rhythms. A number of challenges have been used, and include

the following: (1) *oral glucose*. This is performed in a manner similar to the diagnostic OGTT (see above), with plasma insulin (or C-peptide) response being measured in addition to plasma glucose (National Diabetes Data Group, 1979; Small, Cohen, Beastall, & MacCulsh, 1985). (2) *Standardized meal*. A standardized mixed meal (e.g., 400 kcal with fixed proportions of carbohydrate, fat, and protein) is often used in lieu of oral glucose, in order to provide a more physiological challenge. This is often a formula meal, e.g., Sustacal, but may be a defined portion of food, e.g., a "standard" breakfast (Schade, Eaton, Mitchell, & Ortega, 1980). Although many investigators focus only on the peak response (e.g., the 60- or 90-min C-peptide value), others make serial determinations over several hours, in order to obtain sufficient data points to calculate secretion rates. (3) *Intravenous glucose*. An intravenous glucose challenge, e.g., 1.75 g/kg body weight, provides a rapid stimulus to insulin secretion in a reproducible fashion that bypasses the vagaries of variation in gastrointestinal motility. On the other hand, it also bypasses the cephalic and gastrointestinal stimuli to insulin secretion and is unphysiologic. Recent investigations, however, have demonstrated that the early insulin secretory response (in the first 5 min after giving an intravenous bolus of glucose) is diminished early in the course of evolving Type I diabetes, prior to either clinical disease and even prior to abnormalities in oral glucose tolerance (Srikanta, Ganda, Eisenbarth, *et al.*, 1983; Srikanta, Ganda, Jackson, *et al.*, 1983; Vardi *et al.*, 1987). More prolonged intravenous glucose challenges have been used by some investigators seeking to define the kinetics of insulin secretion, and to distinguish "first-phase" insulin secretion from "second-phase" insulin secretion (Cerasi & Luft, 1977). (4) *Nonglucose secretagogues*. A variety of nonglucose secretagogues have also been used to assess beta-cell response. A popular challenge for assessing the intactness (or lack thereof) of insulin secretory response in Type I diabetes is the C-peptide response to an intravenous dose of 1 mg of glucagon (Ludvigsson & Heding, 1977; Faber & Binder, 1977; Small *et al.*, 1985). Samples are obtained at baseline and 6 min after the administration of the glucagon, for measurement of C-peptide. The measurement of an acute insulin response to an intravenous dose of either arginine, isoproterenol, or tolbutamide has been used to demonstrate the specific "blindness" to glucose seen in Type II diabetes (Figure 8) (Pfeifer, Halter, Graf, & Porte, 1980; Pfeifer, Halter, & Porte, 1981; Porte & Halter, 1982; Porte et al., 1982). In these individuals, there is no acute response to glucose, whereas the responses to these other agents remain intact.

Assessment of Insulin Action

The first step in the action of insulin at target cells is the binding of insulin to a specific receptor on the surface membrane of the cell (Figure 9) (Roth, 1981; Olefsky, 1981). The measurement of insulin binding to insulin receptors has become a useful tool in the study of insulin action. Indeed, decreased insulin binding to cellular receptors, as a consequence of apparent reduced numbers of re-

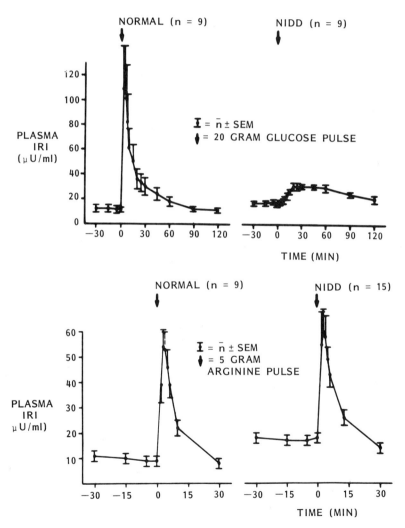

Figure 8. (Top) Insulin levels during 20-g intravenous glucose tolerance tests in normal and NIDDM subjects. The first phase is completely lacking in all NIDDMs, while the second phase is variably preserved. (Bottom) Insulin levels before and after a 5-g rapid injection of arginine in normal and NIDDM subjects. The insulin responses are not different in the two groups. From Pfeifer et al. (1980).

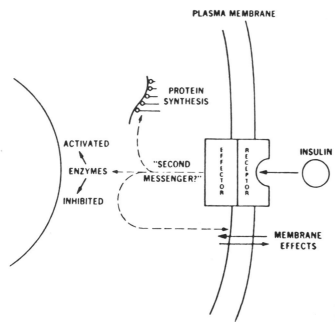

Figure 9. Schematic depictions of insulin action at target cells. The first step in the action of insulin is its binding to a specific receptor on the surface membrane of the cell. This initiates the sequence of events that effect insulin's biological actions. From Kahn *et al.* (1975).

ceptors, has been found to be a characteristic feature of most patients with Type II diabetes as well as most obese individuals (Kolterman, Insel, Saekow, & Olefsky, 1980; Kolterman *et al.*, 1981; Olefsky, Clarall, & Kolterman, 1985).

The receptor not only recognizes the insulin molecule, but also triggers a series of biochemical events within the target cell, leading to the biological effects of insulin. This effector mechanism appears to involve the receptor acting as a protein kinase, possibly activating a kinase cascade (Kahn *et al.*, 1985). The effector mechanisms may also involve the generation of intracellular mediator(s) (Jarett, Klechle, Parker, & Macauley, 1983; Larner, 1983). As a consequence of these intracellular signaling systems, there is modification of the various enzymes and transport systems responsible for the biological effects of insulin, e.g., glucose transport and glucose metabolism. Collectively, all of these effector steps have been referred to as ''postreceptor'' events in the insulin action sequence (although ''postbinding'' would be a more accurate term since the initial events in the effector mechanism do include the activated receptor as a protein kinase). In contrast to the widespread measurement of insulin binding to insulin

receptors, direct measurement of postbinding events is in its infancy.

Insulin resistance may be defined as being present whenever normal concentrations of insulin elicit a less than normal biological response (Kahn, 1978). In nondiabetic individuals (e.g., obesity), insulin resistance may be recognized by the presence of hyperinsulinemia in the absence of hypoglycemia. In any subject, insulin resistance can be demonstrated by a subnormal response to exogenous insulin under controlled conditions. Although there may be circulating factors responsible for insulin resistance (such as high titers of antiinsulin antibodies in rare patients with immunological insulin resistance, or antibodies directed against the insulin receptor), most insulin resistance is a consequence of impaired insulin action at the level of target cells. This is the case for the most common causes of insulin resistance, obesity and Type II diabetes.

Insulin Action in Vivo (Whole Man)

Insulin action may be quantified by measuring the biological response to exogenous insulin under controlled conditions. A number of protocols have been devised to standardize the conditions for insulin administration (the challenges) and to provide uniformity of measurement of the response variables (Reaven, 1983). Several of the more commonly used protocols are discussed below.

Insulin Tolerance Tests

Insulin tolerance tests involve the administration of a fixed dose of insulin (e.g., 0.1 U/kg) either subcutaneously or as an intravenous bolus, with the response variable generally being the decline of plasma glucose (Figure 10). These tests are felt by many workers to have relatively limited utility due to non-steady-state plasma insulin levels, variable counterregulatory hormone response, and the notion that the rate of change of plasma glucose may be influenced by the basal plasma glucose level. Nevertheless, some investigators find that the rate of decline of plasma glucose (the K_1 value) is a simple determination (obtained from serial samples over a short period, i.e., 30–60 min) that correlates well with other measures of insulin action (Figure 10) (Lebovitz, Feinglos, Bucholtz, & Lebovitz, 1977; Lebovitz & Feinglos, 1980). Its value may be enhanced by its calculation following several different dose levels of insulin (on separate days) (Lebovitz & Feinglos, 1980). Another role of the subcutaneous test is the identification of in-

dividuals who have disproportionate impaired insulin action to subcutaneous insulin, in comparison to intravenous insulin (Pickup, Home, Bilous, Keen, & Alberti, 1981).

Insulin/Glucose Infusion Test with Insulin Suppression

Several protocols have been devised which are based on the premise that infusion of fixed amounts of glucose and insulin will result in steady-state glucose concentrations that reflect overall responsiveness to insulin, assuming that endogenous insulin is suppressed (Shen, Reaven, & Farquhar, 1970; Reaven & Miller, 1979; Harano *et al.*, 1977; Ratzmann, Besch, Witt, & Schulz, 1981). These protocols have achieved such suppression with infusions either of epinephrine plus propranolol (Figure 11) or of somatostatin. In such protocols, high steady-state plasma glucose concentrations (Figure 12) signify insulin resistance.

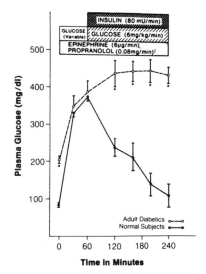

Figure 11. Protocol for insulin suppression test, involving quadruple infusion of glucose, insulin, epinephrine, and propranolol. Endogenous insulin is suppressed by epinephrine and propranolol, so that equivalent steady-state plasma insulin is achieved in all subjects. Under these circumstances, steady-state plasma glucose (SSPG) reflects insulin action at target cells. Insulin resistance is evidenced by high levels of SSPG. From Ginsberg, Kimmerling, Olefsky, and Reaven (1975).

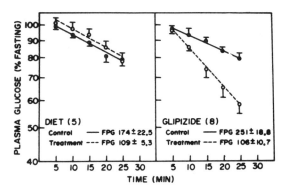

Figure 10. Decrement in plasma glucose following intravenous insulin (0.1 U/kg) in patients treated with diet or the sulfonylurea glipizide. Data are shown as mean ± S.E. for each group. FPG is fasting plasma glucose. From Lebovitz *et al.* (1977).

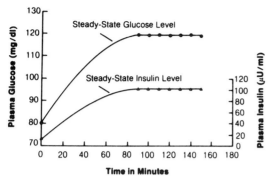

Figure 12. Schematic curves demonstrating steady-state levels of plasma glucose and plasma insulin achieved during an insulin suppression test. From Reaven (1983).

Insulin Clamp

In the insulin clamp technique (DeFronzo, Tobin, & Andres, 1979), insulin is infused at a fixed rate designed to achieve a steady-state plasma insulin concentration (Figure 13). Plasma glucose level is maintained constant (clamped) at a predetermined level (usually either euglycemia or the basal plasma glucose level, depending on the protocol) by virtue of continuous infusion of a variable amount of glucose, the amount determined by sampling every 1–5 min of plasma glucose, with computer-guided adjustment of the glucose infusion. Once steady-state glucose infusion rates are achieved, these are considered a parameter of insulin action, since the glucose infusion rate would equal the rate of glucose metabolism (less any urinary glucose losses) (Figure 14). If the clamp is performed at basal glucose concentration, glucose clearance (glucose infusion rate divided by plasma glucose) may serve as a parameter of insulin action.

Greater precision of measurement can be achieved by simultaneously determining glucose fluxes using isotopic glucose. This permits calculation of hepatic glucose production and peripheral glucose utilization (Kolterman *et al.,* 1980, 1981; DeFronzo, Simonson, & Ferrannini, 1982; Finegood, Bergman, & Vranic, 1987). Even greater understanding of the components of insulin action can be achieved by coupling the insulin clamp technique to simultaneous indirect calorime-

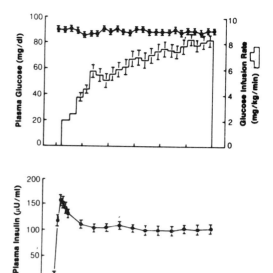

Figure 13. Protocol for euglycemic insulin clamp study. A primed-continuous insulin infusion is given to achieve a constant level of insulinemia (lower panel). Euglycemia is maintained by giving a variable dextrose (glucose) infusion, the rate of infusion being determined by a feedback control algorithm based on frequent (every 1 to 5 min) measurement of plasma glucose. At steady state, the rate of glucose infusion reflects the rate of glucose utilization and is thus a parameter of insulin action. From DeFronzo *et al.* (1979).

try, thus identifying how the glucose is being metabolized (DeFronzo *et al.,* 1981). It is also possible to measure responses of nonglucose parameters (e.g., free fatty acids, lactate, ketones, amino acids) during the clamp procedure.

Several laboratories have performed euglycemic insulin clamp measurements at multiple different plasma insulin levels (Kolterman *et al.,* 1980, 1981; Rizza, Mandarino, & Gerich, 1981a,b). This permits determination of the dose–response characteristics of insulin action (Figure 15). Two features of the functional form of the dose–response curve are important in characterizing insulin action: the maximal response that can be achieved no matter how high the insulin concentration; and the sensitivity of the insulin response, generally represented by the insulin concentration that produces half-maximal stimulation of re-

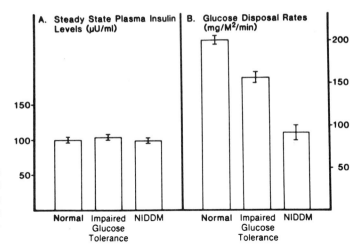

Figure 14. Data from insulin clamp studies in normal subjects, subjects with impaired glucose tolerance (IGT), and subjects with NIDDM. The reduced glucose disposal rates in IGT and NIDDM signify insulin resistance. From Olefsky (1981).

sponse (Kahn, 1978; Olefsky, 1981). Using these constructs, insulin resistance may be characterized by: decreased sensitivity to insulin, decreased maximal responsiveness to insulin, or a combination of both (Figure 16).

Closed Loop Systems

Closed loop systems may be programmed to achieve a constant level of glycemia, either by infusing a constant amount of dextrose and ascertaining the amount of insulin infusion required to maintain constancy of glycemia, or by infusing a constant amount of insulin and ascertaining the amount of dextrose infusion required to maintain constancy of glycemia. In either case, the infusion rate may be taken as a parameter which is a reflection of insulin action (Massi-Benedetti, Burrin, Capaldo, & Alberti, 1981; Raptis *et al.,* 1981). This has been used by some investigators effectively, provided the target glucose levels are achieved.

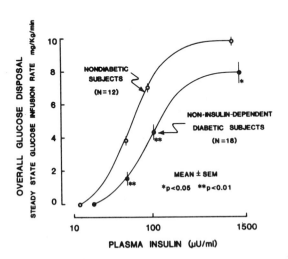

Figure 15. Dose–response curves in nondiabetic and NIDDM subjects, based on insulin clamp studies at several different levels of plasma insulin. From Mandarino and Gerich (1984).

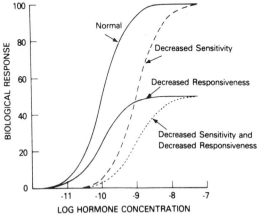

Figure 16. Types of insulin resistance as defined by theoretical insulin dose–response curves. This demonstrates the constructs used to define decreases in insulin sensitivity, insulin responsiveness, or both. From Kahn (1978).

Insulin Action in Vitro (Isolated Cells)

In order to better define mechanisms of insulin action and insulin resistance, *in vivo* studies are correlated with *in vitro* observations on isolated cells obtained from the experimental subjects. Such cells might include circulating cells (e.g., erythrocytes, monocytes) (Olefsky, 1976a; Kahn *et al.*, 1981), adipocytes (obtained by biopsy of adipose tissue) (Kolterman *et al.*, 1981), or cultured fibroblasts (obtained by skin biopsy) (Prince, Tsai, & Olefsky, 1981). The latter are useful for determining whether abnormalities are genetic or environmental, since fibroblasts maintained in culture will faithfully reflect the genetic composition of the organism, and can be compared with other cells freshly obtained from the experimental subject, which reflect the metabolic milleu at that point in time (Prince *et al.*, 1981).

Parameters of insulin action that have been measured in human subjects include: insulin receptor binding (receptor concentration and affinity), glucose uptake and/or oxidation (Olefsky, 1976b), glucose transport (Ciraldi, Kolterman, Scarlett, & Olefsky, 1982) and/or number of glucose transporters (Karnieli, Hissin, Simpson, Salans, & Cushman, 1981), and receptor kinase activity (Kahn *et al.*, 1985). With the exception of receptor binding, which is a widely available assay, only a few laboratories have established the other techniques.

Glucose Counterregulation

Insulin is the preeminent hormone regulating glucose metabolism. Glucose is counterregulated by an array of hormones working in concert. These include glucagon, the catecholamines (epinephrine and norepinephrine), growth hormone, and cortisol. Often it is desirable to test the intactness of the counterregulatory response and/or to assess relative levels of counterregulatory hormones and insulin. The latter might be performed by intermittent sampling around the clock (MacGillivray *et al.*, 1982). The testing of counterregulatory responsiveness is generally in response either to an intravenous (Cryer, 1981) or subcutaneous (Bolli,

Dimitriadis, *et al.*, 1984) insulin bolus or an intravenous insulin infusion (White *et al.*, 1983; Bolli, DeFeo, *et al.*, 1984). In addition to measurements of the counterregulatory hormones, an important component of the assessment of counterregulatory response is the recovery of plasma glucose from hypoglycemic levels (White *et al.*, 1983).

Conclusions

There has been growing interest in the relationship between cardiovascular reactivity, behavior, and diabetes mellitus (Kemmer *et al.*, 1986; Surwit & Feinglos, 1988; Ryan, 1988). In addition, issues related to carbohydrate metabolism may be of importance in the study of subjects involved in protocols evaluating other aspects of cardiovascular behavioral medicine. This chapter has attempted to provide a background and serve as a primer for investigators wishing to study carbohydrate metabolism and/or diabetes in the context of behavioral medicine. A recent volume may provide insights into other useful methods (Clarke, Larner, & Pohl, 1986).

ACKNOWLEDGMENTS. Supported by Grants P01-HL36588 and R01-DK34901 from the National Institutes of Health.

References

Bolli, G. M., Dimitriadis, G. D., Pehling, G. B., Baker, B. A., Haymond, M. W., Cryer, P. E., & Gerich, J. E. (1984). Abnormal glucose counterregulation after subcutaneous insulin on insulin-dependent diabetes mellitus. *New England Journal of Medicine, 310,* 1706–1711.

Bolli, G. E., DeFeo, P., DeCosmo, S., Perriello, G., Ventura, M. M., Massi-Benedetti, M., Santeusanio, F., Gerich, J. E., & Brunetti, P. (1984). A reliable and reproducible test for adequate glucose counterregulation on type I diabetes mellitus. *Diabetes, 33,* 732–737.

Brenner, B. E. (1985). Clinical significance of the elevated anion gap. *American Journal of Medicine, 79,* 289–296.

Bunn, H. F. (1981). Nonenzymatic glycosylation of protein: Relevance to diabetes. *American Journal of Medicine, 70,* 325–330.

Cahill, G. F. (1971). Physiology of insulin in man. *Diabetes, 20,* 785–799.

Cerasi, E., & Luft, R. (1977). Insulin secretion and the development of diabetes in the adult. *Acta Medica Scandinavica Supplementum, 601,* 111–148.

Chan, S. J., Kwok, S. C. M., & Steiner, D. F. (1981). The biosynthesis of insulin: Some genetic and evolutionary aspects. *Diabetes Care, 4,* 4–10.

Claraldi, T. P., Kolterman, O. G., Scarlett, J. A., & Olefsky, J. M. (1982). Role of glucose transport in the post-receptor defect of non-insulin-dependent diabetes mellitus. *Diabetes, 31,* 1016–1024.

Clark, A. J. L., Bilous, R. W., Keen, W. L., & Keen, H. (1982). Capillary tubes for blood glucose sampling. *Diabetologia, 23,* 539–540.

Clark, L. C., & Lyons, C. (1962). Electrode systems for continuous monitoring in cardiovascular surgery. *Annals of the New York Academy of Sciences, 102,* 29–45.

Clarke, W. L., Larner, J., & Pohl, S. L. (Eds.). (1986). *Methods in diabetes research: Vol. II. Clinical methods.* New York: Wiley.

Colwell, J. A., Lopes-Virella, M. F., Winocour, P. D., & Halushka, P. V. (1988). New concepts about the pathogenesis of atherosclerosis in diabetes mellitus. In M. E. Levin & L. W. O'Neal (Eds.), *The diabetic foot* (4th ed., pp. 51–70). St. Louis: Mosby.

Cryer, P. E. (1981). Glucose counterregulation in man. *Diabetes, 30,* 261–264.

DCCT Research Group. (1987). Diabetes control and complications trial (DCCT): Results of feasibility study. *Diabetes Care, 10,* 1–19.

DeFronzo, R. A. (1985). Diabetes and the kidney: An update. In J. M. Olefsky & R. S. Sherwin (Eds.), *Diabetes mellitus: Management and complications* (pp. 159–222). Edinburgh: Churchill Livingstone.

DeFronzo, R. A., Robin, J. D., & Andres, R. (1979). Glucose clamp technique: A method for quantifying insulin secretion and resistance. *American Journal of Physiology, 6,* E214–E223.

DeFronzo, R. A., Jacot, E., Jequier, E., Maeder, E., Wahren, J., & Felber, J. P. (1981). The effect of insulin on the disposal of intravenous glucose: Results from indirect calorimetry and hepatic and femoral venous catheterization. *Diabetes, 30,* 1000–1007.

DeFronzo, R. A., Simonson, D., & Ferrannini, E. (1982). Hepatic and peripheral insulin resistance: A common feature of type II (non-insulin-dependent) and type I (insulin-dependent) diabetes mellitus. *Diabetologia, 23,* 313–319.

Ewing, D. J., & Clarke, B. F. (1986). Diabetic autonomic neuropathy: Present insights and future prospects. *Diabetes Care, 9,* 648–665.

Ewing, D. J., Campbell, I. W., & Clarke, B. F. (1980). The natural history of diabetic autonomic neuropathy. *Quarterly Journal of Medicine, 49,* 95–108.

Faber, O. K., & Binder, C. (1977). C-peptide response to glucagon: A test for the residual beta-cell function in diabetes mellitus. *Diabetes, 26,* 605–610.

Finegood, D. T., Bergman, R. N., & Vranic, M. (1987). Estimation of endogenous glucose production during hyperin-sulinemic–euglycemic glucose clamps. *Diabetes, 36,* 914–924.

Forman, B. H., Goldstein, P. S., & Genel, M. (1974). Management of juvenile diabetes mellitus: Usefulness of 24-hour fractional quantitative urine glucose. *Pediatrics, 53,* 257–263.

Ginsberg, H., Kimmerling, G., Olefsky, J. M., & Reaven, G. M. (1975). Demonstration of insulin resistance in untreated adult onset diabetic subjects with fasting hyperglycemia. *Journal of Clinical Investigation, 55,* 451–461.

Goldberg, R. B. (1981). Lipid disorders in diabetes. *Diabetes Care, 4,* 561–572.

Goldstein, D. E., Little, R. R., Wiedmeyer, H. M., England, J. D., & McKenzie, E. M. (1986). Glycated hemoglobin: Methodologies and clinical applications. *Clinical Chemistry (Winston-Salem, North Carolina), 32,* B64–B70.

Guilbault, G. (1982). Enzymatic glucose electrodes. *Diabetes Care, 5,* 181–183.

Harano, Y., Ohgaku, S., Hidake, H., Haneda, K., Kikkawa, R., Shigeta, Y., & Abe, H. (1977). Glucose, insulin and somatostatin infusion for the determination of insulin sensitivity. *Journal of Clinical Endocrinology and Metabolism, 45,* 1124–1127.

Heding, L. G. (1972). Determination of total serum insulin (IRI) in insulin-treated diabetic patients. *Diabetologia, 8,* 260–266.

Heding, L. G. (1975). Radioimmunological determination of human C-peptide in serum. *Diabetologia, 11,* 541–548.

Holman, R. R., & Turner, R. C. (1979). Maintenance of basal plasma glucose and insulin concentration in maturity-onset diabetes. *Diabetes, 28,* 1039–1057.

James, R. C., & Chase, G. R. (1974). Evaluation of some commonly used semiquantitative methods for urinary glucose and ketone determinations. *Diabetes, 23,* 474–479.

Jarett, L., Kiechle, F. L., Parker, J. C., & Macauley, S. L. (1983). The chemical mediators of insulin action: Possible targets for post-receptor defects. *American Journal of Medicine, 74*(1A), 31–38.

Kahn, C. R. (1978). Insulin resistance, insulin insensitivity, and insulin unresponsiveness: A necessary distinction. *Metabolism, 27,* 1893–1902.

Kahn, C. R., Soll, A. H., Neville, D. M., Goldfine, I. D., Archer, J. A., Gorden, P., & Roth, J. (1975). The insulin receptor in obesity and other states of altered insulin sensitivity. In G. A. Bray (Ed.), *Obesity in perspective* (DHEW Publication No. NIH 75-708, pp. 301–311). Washington, DC: U.S. Government Printing Office.

Kahn, C. R., Baird, K. L., Flier, J. S., Grunfeld, C., Harmon, J. T., Harrison, L. C., Karlsson, F. A., Kasuga, M., King, G. L., Lang, U. C., Podskainy, J. M., & Van Obberghen, E. (1981). Insulin receptors, receptor antibodies, and the mechanisms of insulin action. *Recent Progress in Hormone Research, 37,* 477–538.

Kahn, C. R., White, M. F., Grigorescu, F., Takayama, S., Haring, H. U., & Crettaz, M. (1985). The insulin receptor protein kinase. In M. P. Czech (Ed.), *Molecular basis of insulin action* (pp. 67–94). New York: Plenum Press.

Karnieli, E., Hissin, P. J., Simpson, I. A., Salans, L. B., & Cushman, S. W. (1981). A possible mechanism of insulin resistance in the rat adipose cell in streptozotocin-induced diabetes mellitus. *Journal of Clinical Investigation, 68,* 811–814.

Keen, H., & Jarrett, J. (Eds.). (1982). *Complications of diabetes* (2nd ed.). London: Arnold.

Kemmer, F. W., Bisping, R., Steingruber, H. J., Baar, H., Hardtmann, F., Schlaghecke, R., & Berger, M. (1986). Psychological stress and metabolic control in patients with type I diabetes mellitus. *New England Journal of Medicine, 314,* 1078–1084.

Klein, R. (1985). Retinopathy and other ocular complications in diabetes. In J. M. Olefsky & R. S. Sherwin (Eds.), *Diabetes mellitus: Management and complications* (pp. 101–158). Edinburgh: Churchill Livingstone.

Kohler, E. (1978). On materials for testing glucose in urine. *Diabetes Care, 1,* 64–67.

Kolterman, O. G., Insel, J., Saekow, M., & Olefsky, J. M. (1980). Mechanisms of insulin resistance in human obesity—Evidence for receptor and postreceptor defects. *Journal of Clinical Investigation, 65,* 1273–1284.

Kolterman, O. G., Gray, R. S., Griffin, J., Burstein, P., Insel, J., Scarlett, J. A., & Olefsky, J. M. (1981). Receptor and post-receptor defects contribute to insulin resistance in non-insulin dependent diabetes mellitus. *Journal of Clinical Investigation, 68,* 957–969.

Kuzuya, H., Blix, P. M., Horwitz, D. L., Steiner, D. F., & Rubenstein, A. H. (1977). Determination of free and total insulin and C-peptide in insulin treated diabetes. *Diabetes, 26,* 22–29.

Lacy, P. E. (1977). The physiology of insulin release. In B. W. Volk & K. F. Wellman (Eds.), *The diabetic pancreas* (pp. 211–230). New York: Plenum Press.

Larner, J. (1983). Mediators of postreceptor action of insulin. *American Journal of Medicine 74*(1A), 38–51.

Lebovitz, H. E., & Feinglos, M. N. (1980). Therapy of insulin independent diabetes mellitus: General considerations. *Metabolism, 29,* 474–481.

Lebovitz, H. E., & Feinglos, M. N. (1986). Noninsulin-dependent diabetes mellitus. In P. O. Kohler (Ed.), *Clinical endocrinology* (pp. 574–602). New York: Wiley.

Lebovitz, H. E., Feinglos, M. N., Bucholtz, H. K., & Lebovitz, F. L. (1977). Potentiation of insulin action: A probable mechanism for the anti-diabetic action of sulfonylurea drugs. *Journal of Clinical Endocrinology and Metabolism, 45,* 601–604.

Lloyd, D. R., Nott, M., & Marples, J. (1985). Comparison of serum fructosamine with glycosylated serum protein (determined by affinity chromatography) for the assessment of diabetic control. *Diabetic Medicine, 2,* 474–478.

Ludvigsson, J., & Heding, L. G. (1976). C-peptide in children with diabetes mellitus. *Diabetologia, 12,* 627–630.

Ludvigsson, J., & Heding, L. G. (1977). C-peptide in diabetic children after stimulation of glucagon compared with fasting C-peptide levels in non-diabetic children. *Acta Endocrinologica, 85,* 364–371.

Ludvigsson, J., Heding, L. G., Larsson, Y., & Leander, E. (1977). C-peptide in juvenile diabetics beyond the postinitial remission period. *Acta Paediatrica Scandinavica, 66,* 177–184.

MacGillivray, M. H., Voorhees, M. L., Putnam, T. I., Li, P. K., Schaefer, P. A., & Bruck, E. (1982). Hormone and metabolic profiles in children and adolescents with type I diabetes mellitus. *Diabetes Care, 5*(Suppl. 1), 38–47.

Mandarino, L. J., & Gerich, J. E. (1984). Prolonged sulfonylurea administration decreases insulin resistance and increases insulin secretion in non-insulin-dependent diabetes mellitus: Evidence for improved insulin action at a postreceptor site in hepatic as well as extrahepatic sites. *Diabetes Care, 7*(Suppl. 1), 89–99.

Massi-Benedetti, M., Burrin, J. M., Capaldo, B., & Alberti, K. G. M. M. (1981). A comparative study of the activity of biosynthetic human insulin and pork insulin using the glucose clamp technique in normal subjects. *Diabetes Care, 4,* 163–167.

McMillan, D. E., & Geevarghese, P. J. (1979). Dietary cyanide and tropical malnutrition diabetes. *Diabetes Care, 2,* 202–208.

Nathan, D. M., Singer, D. E., Hurxthal, K., & Goodson, J. D. (1984). The clinical information value of the glycosylated hemoglobin assay. *New England Journal of Medicine, 310,* 341–346.

National Diabetes Data Group. (1979). Classification of diabetes mellitus and other categories of glucose intolerance. *Diabetes, 28,* 1039–1057.

National Diabetes Data Group. (1985). *Diabetes in America* (U.S. Public Health Service Publication No. 85-1468). Washington, DC: NIADDKD, NIH.

Olefsky, J. M. (1976a). The insulin receptor: Its role in insulin resistance of obesity and diabetes. *Diabetes, 25,* 1154–1164.

Olefsky, J. M. (1976b). Effects of fasting on insulin binding, glucose transport, and glucose oxidation in isolated rat adipocytes: Relationships between insulin receptors and insulin action. *Journal of Clinical Investigation, 58,* 1450–1460.

Olefsky, J. M. (1981). Insulin resistance and insulin action: An in vitro and in vivo perspective. *Diabetes, 30,* 148–162.

Olefsky, J. M., Ciarali, T. P., & Kolterman, O. G. (1985). Mechanisms of insulin resistance in non-insulin-dependent (type II) diabetes. *American Journal of Medicine, 79*(3), 12–22.

Parving, H. H., Andersen, A. R., Smidt, U. M., Christiansen, J. S., Oxenboli, B., & Svendsen, P. A. (1983). Diabetic nephropathy and arterial hypertension. *Diabetes, 32*(Suppl. 2), 83–87.

Parving, H. H., Andersen, A. R., Smidt, U. M., Hommel, E., Mathiesen, E. R., & Svendsen, P. A. (1987). Effect of antihypertensive treatment on kidney function in diabetic nephropathy. *British Medical Journal, 294,* 1443–1447.

Pfeifer, M. A., Halter, J. B., Graf, R., & Porte, D. (1980). Potentiation of insulin secretion to nonglucose stimuli in normal man by tolbutamide. *Diabetes, 29,* 335–340.

Pfeifer, M. A., Halter, J. B., & Porte, D. (1981). Insulin

secretion in diabetes mellitus. *American Journal of Medicine, 70,* 579–588.

Pfeifer, M. A., Halter, J. B., Judzewitsch, R. G., Beard, J. C., Best, J. D., Ward, W. K., & Porte, D. (1984). Acute and chronic effects of sulfonylurea drugs on pancreatic islet function in man. *Diabetes Care, 7*(Suppl. 1), 25–34.

Pickup, J. C., Home, P. D., Bilous, R. W., Keen, H., & Alberti, K. G. M. M. (1981). Management of severely brittle diabetes by continuous subcutaneous and intramuscular insulin infusions: Evidence for a defect in subcutaneous insulin absorption. *British Medical Journal, 282,* 347–350.

Polansky, K., Frank, B., Pugh, W., Addis, A., Karrison, T., Meler, P., Tager, H., & Rubenstein, A. (1986). The limitations to and valid use of C-peptide as a marker of the secretion of insulin. *Diabetes, 35,* 379–386.

Porte, D., & Halter, J. B. (1982). The endocrine pancreas and diabetes mellitus. In R. H. Williams (Ed.), *Textbook of endocrinology* (6th ed., pp. 716–843). Philadelphia: Saunders.

Porte, D., & Pupo, A. A. (1969). Insulin responses to glucose: Evidence for a two pool system in man. *Journal of Clinical Investigation, 48,* 2309–2319.

Porte, D., Pfeifer, M. A., Halter, J. B., Beard, J. C., Best, J. D., & Ward, W. K. (1982). Impaired B-cell function in noninsulin-dependent diabetes mellitus: The essential lesion? In J. S. Skyler (Ed.), *Insulin update 1982* (pp. 1–23). Princeton: Excerpta Medica.

Prince, M. J., Tsai, P., & Olefsky, J. M. (1981). Insulin binding, internalization, and insulin-receptor regulation in fibroblasts from type II noninsulin dependent diabetic subjects. *Diabetes, 30,* 596–600.

Raptis, S., Karalskos, C., Enzmann, F., Hatzidakis, D., Zoupas, C., Souvatzoglou, A., Diamantopoulos, E., & Moulopoulos, S. (1981). Biological activities of biosynthetic human insulin in healthy volunteers and insulin dependent diabetic patients monitored by the artificial endocrine pancreas. *Diabetes Care, 4,* 140–143.

Ratzmann, K. P., Besch, W., Witt, S., & Schulz, B. (1981). Evaluation of insulin resistance during inhibition of endogenous insulin and glucagon secretion by somatostatin in nonobese subjects with impaired glucose tolerance. *Diabetologia, 21,* 192–197.

Reaven, G. M. (1983). Insulin resistance in non-insulin dependent diabetes mellitus. Does it exist and can it be measured? *American Journal of Medicine, 74*(1A), 3–17.

Reaven, G. M., & Miller, R. G. (1979). An attempt to define the nature of chemical diabetes using a multidimensional analysis. *Diabetologia, 16,* 17–24.

Reaven, G. M., Bernstein, R., Davids, B., Olefsky, J. M. (1976). Nonketotic diabetes mellitus: Insulin deficiency or insulin resistance? *American Journal of Medicine, 60,* 80–88.

Reeves, M. L., Seigler, D. E., Ryan, E. A., & Skyler, J. S. (1982). Glycemic control in insulin-dependent diabetes mellitus: Comparison of outpatient intensified conventional therapy with continuous subcutaneous insulin infusion. *American Journal of Medicine, 72,* 673–680.

Reeves, W. B. (1983). Insulin antibody determination: The-

oretical and practical consideration. *Diabetologia, 24,* 399–403.

Rizza, R. A., Mandarino, L. J., & Gerich, J. E. (1981a). Mechanism and significance of insulin resistance in noninsulin-dependent diabetes mellitus. *Diabetes, 30,* 990–995.

Rizza, R. A., Mandarino, L. J., & Gerich, J. E. (1981b). Mechanisms of insulin resistance in man. Assessment using the insulin dose–response curve in conjunction with insulin receptor binding. *American Journal of Medicine, 70,* 169–176.

Rosenbloom, A. L., & Malone, J. I. (1978). Recognition of impending ketoacidosis delayed by ketone reagent strip failure. *Journal of the American Medical Association, 240,* 2462–2464.

Roth, J. (1981). Insulin binding to its receptor: Is the receptor more important than the hormone? *Diabetes Care, 4,* 27–32.

Rubenstein, A. H., Horwitz, D. L., & Steiner, D. F. (1975). Clinical significance of circulating proinsulin and C-peptide. In K. E. Sussman & R. J. S. Metz (Eds.), *Diabetes mellitus* (4th ed., pp. 9–14). New York: American Diabetes Association.

Ryan, C. (1988). Neurobehavioral complications of type I diabetes. Examination of possible risk factors. *Diabetes Care, 11,* 86–93.

Schade, D. S., Eaton, R. P., Mitchell, W., & Ortega, T. (1980). Glucose and insulin response to high carbohydrate meals in normal and maturity onset diabetic subjects. *Diabetes Care, 3,* 242–244.

Service, F. J., & Nelson, R. L. (1980). Characteristics of glycemic instability. *Diabetes Care, 3,* 58–62.

Service, F. J., Molnar, G. D., & Taylor, W. F. (1972). Urine glucose analyses during continuous blood glucose monitoring. *Journal of the American Medical Association, 222,* 294–298.

Service, F. J., O'Brien, P. C., & Rizza, R. A. (1987). Measurements of glucose control. *Diabetes Care, 10,* 225–237.

Shen, S. W., Reaven, G. M., & Farquhar, J. (1970). Comparison of impedance to insulin-mediated glucose uptake in normal subjects and in subjects with latent diabetes. *Journal of Clinical Investigation, 49,* 2151–2160.

Skyler, J. S. (1979). Complications of diabetes mellitus: Relationship to metabolic dysfunction. *Diabetes Care, 2,* 499–509.

Skyler, J. S. (1982a). Nondiabetic melliturias. In B. N. Brodoff & S. J. Bleicher (Eds.), *Diabetes mellitus and obesity* (pp. 407–413). Baltimore: Williams & Wilkins.

Skyler, J. S. (1982b). On the pathogenesis and treatment of non-insulin-dependent diabetes mellitus. In J. S. Skyler (Ed.), *Insulin update 1982* (pp. 247–259). Princeton: Excerpta Medica.

Skyler, J. S. (1984). Non-insulin dependent diabetes mellitus—A clinical strategy. *Diabetes Care, 7*(Suppl. 1), 118–129.

Skyler, J. S. (1986). Insulin-dependent diabetes mellitus. In P. O. Kohler (Ed.), *Clinical endocrinology* (pp. 491–573). New York: Wiley.

Skyler, J. S. (1987). Why control blood glucose? *Pediatric Annals, 16,* 713–724.

Skyler, J. S., & Rabinovitch, A. (1987). Etiology and pathogenesis of insulin-dependent diabetes mellitus. *Pediatric Annals, 16,* 682–692.

Skyler, J. S., Reeves, M. L., Seigler, D. E., & Ryan, E. A. (1983). Self-monitoring of blood glucose and intensive conventional therapy: Comparison with continuous subcutaneous insulin infusion in insulin-dependent diabetes mellitus. In P. Brunetti, K. G. M. M. Alberti, A. M. Albisser, K. D. Hepp, & M. Massi-Benedetti (Eds.), *Artificial systems for insulin delivery* (pp. 329–338). New York: Raven Press.

Small, M., Cohen, H. N., Beastall, G. H., & MacCuish, A. C. (1985). Comparison of oral glucose loading and intravenous glucagon injection as stimuli to C-peptide secretion in normal man. *Diabetic Medicine, 2,* 181–183.

Srikanta, S., Ganda, O. P., Eisenbarth, G. S., & Soeldner, J. S. (1983). Islet-cell antibodies and beta-cell function in monozygotic triplets and twins initially discordant for type I diabetes mellitus. *New England Journal of Medicine, 308,* 322–325.

Srikanta, S., Ganda, O. P., Jackson, R. A., Gleason, R. E., Kaldany, A., Garovoy, M. R., Milford, E. L., Carpenter, C. B., Soeldner, J. S., & Eisenbarth, G. S. (1983). Type I diabetes mellitus in monozygotic twins: Chronic progressive beta cell dysfunction. *Annals of Internal Medicine, 99,* 320–326.

Steiner, D. F. (1977). Insulin today. Banting Memorial Lecture. *Diabetes, 26,* 322–340.

Surwit, R. S., & Feinglos, M. N. (1988). Stress and autonomic nervous system in type II diabetes. A hypothesis. *Diabetes Care, 11,* 83–85.

Tattersal, R. B., & Fajans, S. S. (1975). A difference between the inheritance of classical juvenile-onset and maturity-onset type diabetes of young people. *Diabetes, 24,* 44–53.

Vardi, P., Dib, S. A., Tuttleman, M., Connelly, J. E., Grinbergs, M., Radizabeh, A., Riley, W. J., MacLaren, N. K., Eisenbarth, G. S., & Soeldner, J. S. (1987). Competitive insulin autoantibody assay. Prospective evaluation of subjects at high risk for development of type I diabetes mellitus. *Diabetes, 36,* 1286–1291.

Watkins, P. J. (Ed.). (1986). Long-term complications of diabetes. *Clinics in Endocrinology and Metabolism, 15*(4). London: Saunders.

White, N. H., Skor, D. A., Cryer, P. E., Levandoski, L., Bier, D. M., & Santiago, J. V. (1983). Identification of type I diabetic patients at increased risk for hypoglycemia during intensive therapy. *New England Journal of Medicine, 308,* 485–491.

WHO Expert Committee on Diabetes Mellitus. (1980). Second Report. Technical Report Series 646. Geneva: WHO.

Winter, W. E., MacLaren, N. K., Riley, W. J., Clarke, D. W., Kappy, M. S., & Spillar, R. P. (1987). Maturity-onset diabetes of youth in black americans. *New England Journal of Medicine, 316,* 285–282.

Woods, S. C., Smith, P. H., & Porte, D. (1981). The role of the nervous system in metabolic regulation and its effect on diabetes and obesity. In M. Brownlee (Ed.), *Handbook of diabetes mellitus* (Vol. 3, pp. 208–271). New York: Garland.

Zatz, R., & Brenner, B. M. (1986). Pathogenesis of diabetic microanglopathy. The hemodynamic view. *American Journal of Medicine, 80,* 443–453.

Zimmet, P. (1979). Epidemiology of diabetes and its macrovascular manifestations in pacific populations: The medical effects of social progress. *Diabetes Care, 2,* 144–153.

Zimmet, P. (1982). Type 2 (non-insulin-dependent) diabetes— An epidemiological overview. *Diabetologia, 22,* 399–411.

CHAPTER 11

Catecholamine Measurement in Behavioral Research

Michael G. Ziegler

Introduction

The catecholamines norepinephrine (NE), epinephrine (E), and dopamine (DA) are released from nerves and the adrenal into blood, cerebrospinal fluid (CSF), and urine. E is released from the adrenal medulla into the bloodstream where it acts as a hormone by stimulating α- and β-adrenergic receptors. Blood levels of E provide a good guide to adrenomedullary stimulation. A small increase in a resting subject's blood E levels from a low normal of 20 pg/ml to a high normal of 80 pg/ml is sufficient to alter glucose metabolism. NE is also present in the adrenal, but most blood NE comes from sympathetic nerves. Blood levels of NE in the normal range for a resting, recumbent subject (150–500 pg/ml) have little physiologic effect, but blood levels of 1000 pg/ml cause subtle hemodynamic changes. NE has its major effect following release from sympathetic nerves across a synapse onto adjacent adrenergic receptors. A small fraction of this NE finds its way into the bloodstream. Blood levels of NE correlate with sympathetic nerve activity and double 5 min after one stands from a recumbent posture. Blood levels of the catecholamines are a potentially valuable guide to sympathetic nervous activity. Unfortunately, the use of catecholamine levels as a research tool has sometimes preceded adequate understanding of their chemistry or biology.

Catecholamines in aqueous solution without preservatives decay in hours and catecholamines in the circulation have a half-life of minutes. There is a long history of erroneous plasma catecholamine measurements in the scientific literature. The first fluorometric assays were plagued by interfering compounds and gave plasma NE levels 10 to 100 times too high. As assay techniques improved, basal catecholamine levels in laboratory animals were reported 10 to 100 times too high because the effects of the stress of routine handling on an animal's catecholamine release were not appreciated.

Serious problems in catecholamine measurements persist in 1987. Basal levels reported for NE in CSF vary over a fourfold range. Assay techniques provide poor reproducibility. The origin of urinary catecholamines is unknown. This chapter will provide the information necessary to evade the common pitfalls in catecholamine measurements. There is so much we do not know about catecholamine biochemistry that the wise investigator will remain wary of unforeseen pitfalls.

Michael G. Ziegler • Department of Medicine, University of California, San Diego Medical Center, San Diego, California 92103.

Catecholamine Assay Techniques

Catecholamines are present in human plasma in a concentration of less than one part per billion. Because it is difficult to assay these tiny amounts, current assay systems have problems with reliability and reproducibility. All of the currently available assay techniques have idiosyncratic situations in which they perform poorly so that it is necessary to know something about the assay techniques just to read the catecholamine literature adequately.

Fluorometric Assay

Many chemicals absorb light of one wavelength and then fluoresce by emitting light of another wavelength. Fluorometric assays quantitate these chemicals by measuring the intensity of the emitted light.

Catecholamines fluoresce with an excitation maximum of 285 nm and emission maximum at 325 nm. Reaction of the catecholamines with trihydroxyindole or ethylenediamine enhances native fluorescence. There are many materials in human plasma and urine that fluoresce at similar wavelengths and provide falsely high estimates of catecholamines. Most of the catecholamine assays in the literature published before 1970 were based on fluorescence techniques and provide values that are clearly higher than those seen with current assay methods. Hjemdahl (1984) reported that two of three laboratories using current fluorometric techniques estimated catecholamine levels about five times as high as those found by radioenzymatic assays. Other fluorometric techniques (Miura, Campese, DeQuattro, & Meyer, 1977) reported very low catecholamine levels.

Radioenzymatic Assays

In a radioenzymatic assay the compound to be measured is incubated with a radioactive substrate and an enzyme that catalyzes a reaction between them (Figure 1). The amount of radioactive metabolite formed can be measured and is proportional to the level of the compound initially present.

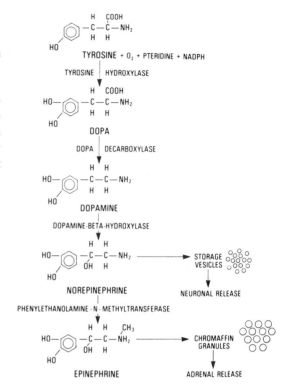

Figure 1. Enzymes in the synthesis of the catecholamines. NE is stored in small vesicles in nerve endings. E is stored in large vesicles in the adrenal medulla.

Catechol-O-methyltransferase (COMT)

COMT is a nonspecific enzyme which will *O*-methylate almost any molecule with a catechol group by transferring a methyl group from *S*-adenosylmethionine (SAM). In its simplest form, the catecholamines in unextracted plasma are incubated in a buffer solution with magnesium and radiolabeled SAM. The derived radiolabeled E and NE metabolites can then be oxidized to radiolabeled vanillin, which is extracted into toluene and counted by liquid scintillation spectroscopy.

COMT converts E to metanephrine, NE to normetanephrine, and DA to 3-methoxytyramine. A more specific form of the assay separates these metabolites by thin-layer chromatography to measure individual catecholamines. Since COMT is nonspecific, it will methylate compounds as small as catechol and as large as the drug dobutamine.

Many drugs such as isoproterenol, dobutamine, and methyldopa can interfere with the assay, but when the assay is combined with appropriate separation techniques, these other catechol drugs can also be measured (Durrett & Ziegler, 1980). COMT is strongly inhibited by calcium which must be chelated out of solution by EGTA to bind inhibiting calcium and with magnesium to stimulate enzymatic activity. Plasma proteins, some compounds in urine, aluminum, and ascorbic acid also interfere with the enzymatic activity of COMT and can provide spurious assay values (Durrett & Ziegler, 1980). After chromatographic separation, E and NE can be measured more reliably than DA, because of high blank values in the DA measurement. Since samples are separated by thin-layer chromatography, very high levels of one compound may contaminate an adjacent chromatographic band, thus artifactually elevating levels of the adjacent compound. Besides all these individual technical difficulties, the COMT assay for catecholamines is quite complex and subject to error from pipetting and standardization.

The COMT assay for catecholamines has advantages in several situations. The assay can be performed on 50 μl of plasma 0.5 μl of urine and can measure several catechol drugs and drug metabolites (Durrett & Ziegler, 1980). The assay is sensitive enough to measure basal levels of plasma E and is applicable to measuring large numbers of samples at one time.

PNMT Radioenzymatic Assay for Catecholamines

Phenylethanolamine - *N* - methyltransferase (PNMT) converts NE to E in the adrenal medulla. PNMT can be purified from cow adrenal glands and [³H]-SAM can be used as a methyl donor to convert NE to [³H]-E. Unlike COMT, the enzyme PNMT is relatively specific for β-hydroxylated phenylethanolamines so that it does not appreciably label DA or further label E. It can be adapted to measure large numbers of samples (Lake, Ziegler, & Kopin, 1976) and is applicable in a number of circumstances where other assay techniques are not effective.

Since PNMT is not inhibited by aluminum, catecholamines can be concentrated on alumina prior to assay so that the assay can be made very sensitive when large volumes of plasma are concentrated onto alumina and then eluted into 0.1 ml of acid solution. This preconcentration step eliminates inhibiting substances that might interfere with the assay, so that standardization of the PNMT assay is easier than that of the COMT assay. However, the very specificity of the PNMT assay limits the number of compounds it can measure.

HPLC Assay Techniques

Assays using HPLC separate catecholamines or their metabolites and an internal standard into sharp peaks. After separation, the catecholamines can be detected by native fluorescence, by the fluorescence of their chemical derivatives, or by electrochemical detection. Recent 5- to 10-μm reverse-phase and cation exchange materials have increased the efficiency of HPLC to 25,000 plates/m and allow short columns which decrease the time needed to perform analysis. Reverse-phase HPLC columns have been used directly to separate catecholamines but most frequently they have been modified using "soap" chromatography with the addition of sodium heptylsulfonate or sodium octylsulfate to the mobile phase. These hydrophobic, anionic detergents are strongly absorbed to the stationary phase and transform it into a cation exchange column. This column will separate neutral and anionic substances as well as catecholamines. Microparticulate cation exchange HPLC columns have recently become more popular in separation of catecholamines.

Because the catecholamines easily oxidize, they can be detected electrochemically when they are passed by a carbon electrode with an electrical potential in the range of +600 mV. The resulting electric current passing across the electrode is proportional to the amount of catecholamine present. Unfortunately, the electrical potential of the catecholamine group is similar to that of uric acid, which is present in plasma at 10,000-fold higher concentrations than the catecholamines. For this reason, catecholamine-containing solutions usually need to be purified on ion exchange columns and on alumina prior to injection into the HPLC. Even with these precautions, there is often a peak that elutes near the NE peak, which may be a caffeic acid metabolite. This process provides detection limits in the range of 25 pg/ml (Yui & Kawai, 1981) so that when the system is performing optimally it can detect human plasma catecholamine levels. Slight degradation in characteristics of the electrochemical detector or small amounts of electrical noise can interfere with the assay technique and make it insufficiently sensitive for measuring basal levels of plasma E.

Catecholamines can also be detected by fluorescence. Natural fluorescence of the catecholamines requires several nanograms for detection but derivatized fluorescence techniques can greatly enhance sensitivity. Catecholamines may be derivatized by the trihydroxyindole, ethylenediamine, ninhydrin, fluorescamine, or *O*-phthalaldehyde methods to enhance their fluorescence. One study (Yui & Kawai, 1981) compared the sensitivity of these techniques and concluded that postcolumn derivatization with trihydroxyindole was the most sensitive and specific detection system. However, this technique has not been very widely applied and to date is used in only a few laboratories.

Gas Chromatography

Volatile compounds can be separated by gas chromatography. The catecholamines are unsuitable for direct use in gas chromatographic separation but are small enough to allow volatile derivatives to be made. These derivatives can be separated by gas chromatography and then can be detected by flame ionization, electron capture, or mass spectroscopy. Electron capture is sensitive enough but lacks specificity; however, mass spectroscopy has both sensitivity and specificity sufficient for reliable detection of catecholamine levels. Gas chromatography with mass spectroscopy (GCMS) is very accurate because it can be standardized by the addition of deuterated catecholamines which differ slightly in molecular weight but in no other characteristics. GCMS provides a reference standard against other less

rigorous procedures and has been used to verify the accuracy of the PNMT radioenzymatic assay (Ziegler, Lake, Foppen, Shoulson, & Kopin, 1976). However, the technique is so time-consuming and expensive that it is not suitable for routine catecholamine analysis.

In a comparison of 34 laboratories performing 41 plasma catecholamine assays (Hjemdahl, 1984), the COMT, PNMT, HPLC, and fluorometric techniques all had problems with accuracy and reproducibility. Fluorometric techniques gave by far the largest variation. The other techniques gave roughly comparable results which can only be described as disappointing. The coefficient of variance between laboratories not using fluorometric techniques was about 40% when measuring very low catecholamine concentrations and about 20% when measuring high concentrations of the catecholamines. Several of the laboratories reported fivefold differences between catecholamine levels of samples that were actually duplicates. The mean catecholamine concentrations determined by nonfluorometric techniques were roughly similar except for plasma DA levels which were considerably higher when measured by radioenzymatic techniques than by HPLC methods. One can conclude that plasma DA determinations are probably not reliable, that low-level plasma catecholamine determinations such as measurements of E in resting subjects show wide variances, that high levels of plasma catecholamines can be determined with about a 20% coefficient of variance, and that some samples will show an extremely high error in measurement on the order of 500%.

For several years a radioimmunoassay of catecholamines was commercially available. This assay measured both catecholamines and sulfate-conjugated catecholamines so that reported "catecholamine" levels had very high baseline levels and showed minimal physiologic variation. This assay technique has now been replaced by an HPLC method.

The choice of an assay system to measure catecholamines depends on individual needs. If only NE is to be measured, the PNMT radioenzymatic technique is relatively rapid and sensitive. HPLC provides the greatest flexibility in measuring catecholamines and metabolites. The COMT radioenzymatic assay's sensitivity permits use of smaller blood volumes than does HPLC. All of these assays are difficult, so it is best to obtain the advice of a laboratory with experience in a particular technique before using it. A recent book describes catecholamine assay techniques in detail (Krstulovic, 1986).

Catecholamine Stability

If one places catecholamines in distilled water, the clear solution will pass through color changes, first becoming pink and then brown as the catecholamines oxidize and cyclize to adrenochromes. Catecholamines are conjugated to sulfates in humans and to catecholamine sulfates and glucuronides in rodents. They can be metabolized to active catecholamines and may have minor biological effects. These conjugated catecholamines are normally present in biological fluids and can be broken down by heat and acid to catecholamines. The catecholamines themselves are very labile under oxidizing conditions or at basic pH or high temperature. Storage in acid decreases catecholamine breakdown, but may artifactually raise catecholamine levels by cleavage of catecholamine conjugates. Fortunately, catecholamines are quite stable in blood or plasma (Weir, Smitt, Round, & Betteridge, 1986). Heparinized blood or plasma can safely be held at room temperature for ½ h, in wet ice for 2 h, or at −20°C for 2 weeks or at −70°C for 1 year without apparent degradation. Catecholamines in urine are usually preserved by addition of acid, an antioxidant, or cold. Catecholamine conjugates are excreted into urine and

so are present there in relatively high levels. Preservation of urine with acid, particularly if the sample is not kept cold, can lead to cleavage of these conjugates and erroneously high catecholamine measurements. Antioxidants such as sodium metabisulfite are probably adequate to prevent destruction of catecholamines in urine if samples are kept refrigerated. Unfortunately, there have been no good studies of preservation methods for catecholamines in urine that consider potential for cleavage of catecholamine conjugates by acid or by bacteria.

In contrast to blood where NE is stable at room temperature for at least 30 min, NE is extremely labile in CSF as can be seen in Table 1. Ascorbic acid, which is both an antioxidant and an acidifying agent, helps preserve NE in CSF, as does freezing. Samples collected on ice without preservative can lose three-fourths of their NE content in 1 h. The best technique we have found for collecting CSF is to have it drip directly from the lumbar puncture needle into a tube containing an antioxidant with the collection tube placed in a container of dry ice. These exacting conditions have only rarely been followed in studies of CSF catecholamines so that degradation of the catecholamines is an important factor to consider in evaluating most of the literature on CSF catecholamine levels.

Circadian Rhythms

Plasma NE

As shown in Figure 2, plasma NE has a striking circadian rhythm with lowest levels at 03:00 and

Table 1. Norepinephrine in Cerebrospinal Fluid Preserved by Different Means[a]

N	29	9	18	9
Age	29 ± 2	42 ± 5	34 ± 3	42 ± 5
Preservative	Ascorbic acid in 60 min	Ascorbic acid in 30 min	Ascorbic acid immediately	Ascorbic acid immediately
Temperature	2°C immediately −70°C by 60 min	2°C immediately −70°C by 30 min	−70°C immediately	−70°C immediately
NE (pg/ml)	91 ± 6	242 ± 72	373 ± 38	408 ± 61

[a]All subjects were normal volunteers with lumbar puncture performed in left lateral decubitus position. The CSF sample was taken after 12 ml of CSF was removed. Samples stored at −70°C immediately were collected on dry ice.

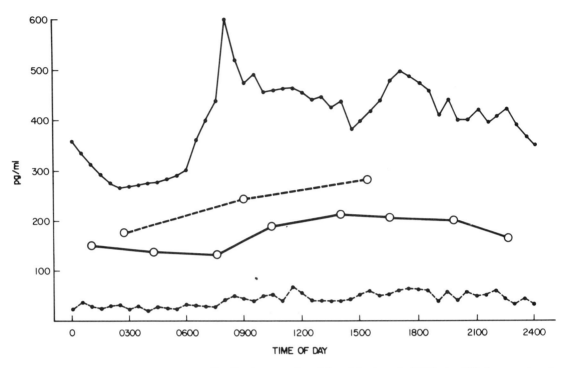

Figure 2. Circadian rhythm of catecholamines. ●—●, plasma NE in humans; ○- -○, CSF NE in humans; ○—○ CSF NE in monkeys; ●- -●, plasma E in humans. The plasma data are adapted from Linsel *et al.* (1985); the CSF data are adapted from Ziegler, Lake, and Kopin (1976b).

peak levels occurring shortly after awakening. This circadian rhythm is the result of the effects of sleep which lower NE (Lake *et al.*, 1976; Linsel, Lightman, Mullen, Brown, & Causon, 1985). Even in recumbent subjects there is a circadian rhythm for plasma NE (Kato *et al.*, 1980) which may be partly the result of sleep and feeding (Young, Rowe, Pallotta, Sparrow, & Landsberg, 1980). This sharp rise in NE just prior to 09:00 has been implicated in the peak of cardiovascular mortality that occurs at 09:00; it is only partly the result of an increase in NE with upright posture (Figure 3).

Plasma E

Basal plasma E levels are quite low so that it has been more difficult to demonstrate the circadian rhythm for E (Barnes, Fitzgerald, Brown, & Dollery, 1980; Linsel *et al.*, 1985). The E rhythm does not appear to be affected by posture and no dif-ference between sleeping and waking states has been demonstrated. Studies of urinary secretion of catecholamines suggest that the E rhythm is present even in the absence of sleep (Akerstedt, 1979). Although there is a significant correlation between the diurnal changes in E and NE, there may be separate factors controlling circulating levels of each compound.

CSF NE Circadian Rhythm

NE in CSF is not contaminated by plasma NE to any significant extent. Intravenous infusions of radiolabeled NE in monkeys cause peak CSF levels of the label amounting to only 2% of peak plasma concentrations. Chronic increases in peripheral NE from a pheochromocytoma are not reflected in CSF NE levels (Ziegler, Lake, Wood, Brooks, & Ebert, 1977). There is a prominent circadian rhythm for CSF NE which roughly parallels that of plasma NE and E. This rhythm has been demon-

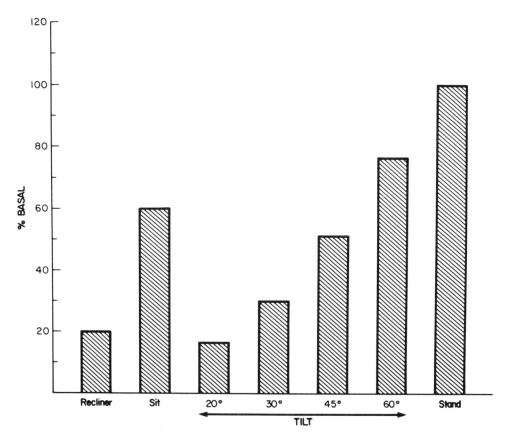

Figure 3. The percent of baseline recumbent NE levels in subjects who were nearly horizontal in a recliner chair, sat, were tilted from 20° to 60° above horizontal, or who stood. Data from Lake *et al.* (1976), Rosenthal, Cbircy, Osikowska, and Sever (1978), Hesse, Ring-Larson, Neilsen, and Christiansen (1978), and Lake and Ziegler (1985).

strated in both humans and monkeys and was not affected when a monkey's light cycle was reversed (Ziegler, Lake, Wood, & Ebert, 1976).

Ultradian Rhythm of Plasma Catecholamines

Levin, Goldstein, and Natelson (1978) reported an ultradian rhythm of plasma NE in monkeys. Subsequent studies have shown an ultradian rhythm for both plasma NE and E in monkeys (Hansen *et al.*, 1982), for NE in rats (Tapp, Levin, & Natelson, 1981), and for NE and E in humans (Levin & Natelson, 1980). This ultradian fluctuation of plasma NE in humans is very large with the highest values typically twice as great as the lowest values obtained over a several hour period. The

rhythm cycles over about 90 min and the plasma NE and E levels generally correlate with one another. They have generally not been shown to correlate with blood pressure or even with heart rate. This may be explained by the observation that levels of plasma NE and E alternate from one side of the body to the other and that NE levels drawn from one arm may frequently be twice as high as NE levels from the contralateral arm (Kennedy, Ziegler, & Shannahoff-Khalsa, 1986).

The local variations in NE levels could be the result of variations in blood flow, catecholamine clearance, or catecholamine release. This phenomenon deserves further study since it may be an important contribution to the "noise" level of plasma catecholamines when samples are taken at a single time point. It may account for the observation that plasma NE levels are poorly reproducible over time in an individual although the mean NE level of a group remains constant.

Catecholamine Kinetics

Plasma catecholamine levels are a function of the rate of release of catecholamines into the circulation and the rate of clearance out of the circulation. If the rate at which NE is cleared from the plasma is known and the plasma level of NE is known, then the rate at which NE appears in the plasma can be calculated. This is known as the "spillover rate," "NE appearance rate," or "NE release rate." Clearance of NE has been measured by two infusion techniques. In one technique, NE is infused at a rate which increases plasma levels but has no marked effect on hemodynamics. Blood is sampled to measure plateau levels of NE and NE decay rates to determine the rate of NE clearance (Grimm, Weidmann, Keusch, Meier, & Gluck, 1980). A technically simpler method for evaluating NE clearance rates is to infuse radiolabeled NE and then measure the disappearance rate of radioactivity by alumina absorption of the $[^3H]$-NE in sequential blood samples (Esler, Jackman, Leonard, et al., 1980; Esler, Jackman, et al., 1981). Results of these two techniques have not been entirely identical since $[^3H]$-NE infusions take longer to reach plateau level than do unlabeled NE. Both techniques indicate that the initial half-life of NE after infusion has stopped is in the range of 2–3 min in humans.

Catecholamine Kinetics in Regional Vascular Beds

During radiolabeled NE infusion, it is possible to sample arterial $[^3H]$-NE blood levels and the venous drainage of $[^3H]$-NE from individual organs. When these data are combined with measurements of endogenous plasma NE, the contribution of individual vascular beds to release and clearance of NE can be calculated. Arterial and venous catecholamine sampling do not represent the same things. Arterial blood catecholamines are representative of the mixed venous drainage from the lungs, an organ that is very active in cate-

cholamine uptake and release. Venous catecholamines represent arterial catecholamine levels further modified by the venous organ drained; usually the forearm and hand. Most published values are for venous blood obtained from the forearm. The lung, kidney, and skeletal muscle contribute the largest fractions both to NE clearance and to NE release (Esler et al., 1984; Christensen et al., 1984). NE is both cleared and released in capillary beds with the net effect that venous plasma NE levels are higher than arterial levels (Lake et al., 1976) and NE clearance based on venous levels appears larger than NE clearance based on arterial levels (Christensen et al., 1984). When the forearm and hand are kept warm, blood is shunted from the arterial circulation into the venous circulation so that venous forearm blood NE should be higher when the hand is kept cold than when it is warm. Such variables may explain why Christensen et al. (1984) found no correlation between NE clearance values based on venous and arterial sampling since local factors such as hand temperature will alter venous NE levels without affecting arterial NE levels. E is cleared and metabolized in the forearm but is not synthesized there so that the fractional excretion of E across vascular beds can be calculated. E extraction by the forearm ranged from 33 to 51% (Best & Halter, 1982).

Catecholamines are known to be cleared by reuptake into nerves (referred to as uptake 1) and by uptake into nonneuronal tissue (referred to as uptake 2). NE is cleared more by uptake 1 than the other catecholamines; E and isoproterenol are cleared predominately by uptake 2. Catecholamines can stimulate their own clearance, so subjects with a high NE level have a shorter half-life for NE (Ziegler, Chernow, et al., 1986). E is even more potent than NE in stimulating metabolic clearance of catecholamines (Clutter, Bier, Shah, & Cryer, 1980). β blocking drugs diminish uptake 2 clearance of the catecholamines into nonneuronal tissues (Ziegler, Chernow, et al., 1986). Antidepressant agents such as desipramine block uptake 1 by interfering with the neuronal "pump" for catecholamine reuptake, prolonging the half-life of NE (Esler, Jackman, et al., 1981). NE levels increase with age, primarily due to increased NE release from sympathetic nerves, but partly due to decreased NE clearance (Esler, Skews, *et al.*, 1981). Infusion of unlabeled NE to measure half-life may also affect subsequent plasma NE measurements by loading the nerves and other tissues with high levels of NE. Infusion of 9 μg/min of NE for 60 min led to increased plasma NE levels for 10 days subsequent to the infusion (Pequignot, Claustre, & Peyrin, 1979).

Drugs such as the β blockers can increase NE levels by decreasing NE clearance. In this case, plasma NE levels do not accurately reflect NE release but behavioral scientists are more interested in NE release rate since it reflects sympathetic nervous system activity (SNS). At steady state: plasma NE level × clearance of NE = apparent release rate or spillover into plasma. This rate is one step closer to a real measure of SNS activity than plasma NE levels alone. It does not measure the amount of NE released into the synapse, but no techniques currently available do that. If the rate of NE clearance is normal, then NE levels may be adequate for determination of SNS activity. NE clearance varies widely between normal individuals, however (Fitzgerald *et al.*, 1979), and there are many diseases wherein NE clearance is grossly abnormal. For example, in autonomic neuropathy plasma NE levels seriously underestimate the deficit in SNS activity (Esler, Jackman, Kelleher, *et al.*, 1980). NE clearance has been reported to be abnormal in depression, hypertension, in patients receiving tricyclic antidepressants, monoamine oxidase inhibitors, β blockers, and several other drugs. It is not safe to simply assume that a drug or disease does not affect catecholamine clearance or that an isolated plasma catecholamine level actually represents systemic SNS activity.

Catecholamines in Urine

Catecholamines are much more concentrated in urine than plasma, so that older fluorometric assays could detect urine but not plasma catecholamines. As a result, a large clinical literature on urinary catecholamines evolved before it was possible to evaluate plasma catecholamines. With the advent of more accurate assays for measuring plasma catecholamines, it has become apparent

that most urinary catecholamines are not derived from plasma. Levels of urinary DA are quite high while plasma DA levels are so low as to be nearly undetectable. There is so much NE and E in urine that they cannot possibly be derived from glomerular filtration of plasma catecholamines. In fact, removal of both adrenals in humans did not change the urinary excretion of E (Von Euler, Ikkos, & Luft, 1961) and urinary E concentration increased when adrenalectomized rats were subjected to a cold stress (Leduc, 1961). Some urinary catecholamines are derived from intrarenal sympathetic nerves. Other potential sources for urinary catecholamines are circulating catecholamine sulfates which might be deconjugated by a renal sulfatase and circulating L-dopa which might be converted to dopamine by renal dopa decarboxylase. The exact origin of urinary catecholamines is unknown but it is apparent that urinary catecholamines do not simply reflect filtered plasma catecholamines. It is impossible to provide a reasonable physiologic interpretation of the meaning of urinary catecholamines at the present time but there are a large number of empiric observations about changes in urinary catecholamines. (See Table 2 for the effect of various factors on catecholamine levels.)

Forsman (1981) has shown that urine samples obtained at 75-min intervals following successive periods of stress and inactivity have measurably different catecholamine levels. Urinary levels of NE and E are low during nighttime at rest and increase gradually during morning hours and reach a peak between 12:00 and 14:00 (Akerstedt & Levi, 1978). Urine E has a somewhat more pronounced diurnal pattern than does NE and is relatively independent of sleep–wakefulness patterns. Urine NE levels reflect variations in both posture and activity. Following reversal of sleep–wakefulness patterns, urine catecholamine levels did not reverse their pattern until approximately 1 week later (Dahlgren, 1981). The total amount of urinary catecholamines tends to increase with age but when urinary catecholamines are expressed per unit body surface area, their levels are roughly constant from age 13 to 38 (De Schaepdryver, Hooft, Delbeke, & Van den Noortgaete, 1978). Urinary NE levels of old men are higher than those

Table 2. The Effect of Various Factors on Catecholamine Levels[a]

	Reference	Effect[b]
Diet		
Carbohydrate	Welle, Lilavivanthana, and Campbell (1981)	↑
Obesity	Tuck, Sowers, Dornfeld, Kledzik, and Maxwell (1981)	↑
Sodium	Henry, Luft, Weinberger, Fineberg, and Grim (1980)	↓
Fasting	Leiter, Grose, Yale, and Marliss (1984)	↓
Diseases that alter hemodynamics		
Renal failure	Lake, Ziegler, Coleman, and Kopin (1979a)	↑ ↓
Burns	Becker *et al.* (1980)	↑
Cirrhosis	Nicholls *et al.* (1985)	↑
Heart failure	Cohn *et al.* (1984)	↑
Sodium depletion	Brosnihan, Szilagyi, and Ferrario (1981), Lake and Ziegler (1978)	↑
Essential hypertension	Goldstein (1981), Lake *et al.* (1981)	↑ −
Secondary hypertension	Lake *et al.* (1984)	↑ −
Chronic obstructive pulmonary disease	Henriksen, Christensen, Kok-Jensen, and Christiansen (1980)	↑
Thyroid disease	Christensen (1979)	↑ ↓
Diseases that alter autonomic nerves		
Shy–Drager syndrome	Ziegler, Lake, and Kopin (1977)	↓ −
Orthostatic hypotension	Ziegler, Lake, and Kopin (1977), Ziegler (1980), Ziegler and Lake (1984, 1985), Bravo and Tarazi (1982)	↑ ↓
Familial dysautonomia	Ziegler, Lake, and Kopin (1976a)	↓
Depression	Esler *et al.* (1982), Lake *et al.* (1982)	↑
Parkinsonism	Teychenne, Lake, and Ziegler (1980)	↓
Other diseases		
Dystonia	Ziegler, Lake, Eldridge, and Kopin (1976)	↑
Lesch–Nyhan syndrome	Lake and Ziegler (1977)	↓
Autism	Lake, Ziegler, and Murphy (1977)	↑ −
Hyperactivity	Mikkelsen, Lake, Brown, Ziegler, and Ebert (1980)	↑
Duodenal ulcer	Christensen (1979)	↑
Migraine	Gotoh, Komatsumoto, Araki, and Gomi (1984)	↓ ↑
Iron deficiency	Voorhess, Stuart, Stockman, and Oski (1975)	↑ −
Schizophrenia	Castellani *et al.* (1982), Lake *et al.* (1980)	
Huntington's chorea	Shoulson, Ziegler, and Lake (1976)	↓
Amyotrophic lateral sclerosis	Ziegler, Brooks, Lake, Wood, and Enna (1980)	↑ ↓
Hypoglycemia	Chalew *et al.* (1984)	
Drugs that alter hemodynamics		
Antihypertensives	Ziegler (1983), Chernow, Zaloga, Lake, Coleman, and Ziegler (1984)	↑ ↓
Theophylline	Biberstein, Ziegler, and Ward (1984)	↑
Chlorpromazine	Castellani *et al.* (1982)	↑
Diuretics	Lake, Ziegler, Coleman, and Kopin (1979b)	↑
Nitroglycerine	Ogasaware, Ogawa, and Sassa (1981)	↑

Table 2. (Continued)

	Reference	Effect[b]
Other drugs		
Disulfiram	Lake, Major, Ziegler, and Kopin (1977)	↑
Lead	Goldman, Hejmancik, Williams, and Ziegler (1980)	↑
Oxygen	Hesse *et al.* (1981)	↓
Probenecid	Lake, Wood, Ziegler, Ebert, and Kopin (1978)	↑
Lithium	Rosenblatt, Lake, van Kammen, Ziegler, and Bunney (1979)	↑ ↓
Stress, physical		
Head injury	Clifton, Ziegler, and Grossman (1981)	↑
Aerobic fitness	Hull, Young, and Ziegler (1984)	↓ −
Venipuncture	Ziegler, Milano, and Hull (1985)	↑
Posture	Ziegler, Milano, and Hull (1985), Burke, Sundlof, and Walli (1977)	↑
Exercise	Ziegler, Milano, and Hull (1985), Robertson *et al.* (1979)	↑
Cold	Palmer, Ziegler, and Lake (1978), Robertson *et al.* (1979)	↑
Age	Palmer *et al.* (1978), Ziegler, Lake, and Kopin (1976b)	↑
Alcohol withdrawal	Hawley, Major, Schulman, and Lake (1981)	↑
Exercise training	Peronnet *et al.* (1981)	↑
Caffeine	Robertson *et al.* (1978, 1979)	↑ −
Digitalis	Nechay, Jackson, Ziegler, and Neldon (1981)	↑
Propranolol	Ziegler, Chernow, *et al.* (1986)	↑
Drugs that alter autonomic function		
Bromocriptine	Ziegler, Lake, Williams, *et al.* (1979)	↓
Physostigmine	Kennedy, Janowsky, Risch, and Ziegler (1984)	↑
Clonidine	Chernow *et al.* (1984), Chernow, Lake, Ziegler, Zaloga, and Coleman (1983)	↓
Fenfluramine	Chernow, Lake, Cook, *et al.* (1983)	↓
Amphetamine	Ziegler, Lake, and Ebert (1979)	↑
Tobacco	Cryer, Haymond, Santiago, and Shah (1976)	↑
Antidepressants	Esler, Jackman, *et al.* (1981), Veith *et al.* (1983)	↑
L-Dopa	Ziegler, Kennedy, Holland, Murphy, and Lake (1985)	↑
Dopamine	Ziegler, Kennedy, *et al.* (1985)	↑
Stress, psychological		
Sexual activity	Wiedeking, Lake, Ziegler, Muske, and Jorgensen (1977)	↑
Vasovagal fainting	Ziegler, Echon, *et al.* 1986)	↓
Psychological testing	Dimsdale and Moss (1980a)	↑
Anxiety	Dimsdale and Moss (1980a,b)	↑

[a]Usually norepinephrine.

[b]Minus indicates no change under some circumstances. Many of these conditions and drugs cause complex responses, or an elevation under some circumstances and a decrease under others (↑ ↓). The reader is referred to the original report by reference listed.

of young men and NE responses following stress seem to be higher in old men (Aslan, Nelson, Carruthers, & Lader, 1981). In general, the diurnal, age- and stress-related changes in urine catecholamines parallel those reported for plasma catecholamines.

Low levels of exercise do not have much effect on urinary catecholamine levels but at high work loads catecholamine levels increase substantially. Mental work such as monotonous vigilance tasks or rapid complex cognitive efforts induce an increase in E excretion in urine (Lundberg & Forsman, 1979). Both pleasant and unpleasant emotional stimuli increase urine E (Patkai, 1971). A lack of control over the pace of one's work and extremely high or extremely low work loads are associated with high levels of urinary catecholamines (Frakenhaeuser & Johasson, 1976; Rassler, 1977). Research at Three Mile Island near the sight of the 1979 nuclear power plant accident suggested that continuing uncertainty and perceived threat are associated with chronic elevations in both urinary E and NE. General levels of catecholamines were higher in subjects living near the damaged plant than in control subjects living in other areas (Baum, Lundberg, Grunberg, Singer, & Gatchel, 1985).

During rest and relaxation, there are generally no differences between urine catecholamines of men and women after adjusting for body weight. However, sex differences have been found during intelligence testing and stress testing (Baum *et al.*, 1985). Data suggest that performance efficiency in men is more closely associated with E excretion than it is in women since men tend to excrete higher levels of urinary E in response to testing. More recently, pronounced E responses have been recorded for women in nontraditional occupational roles such as female engineering students (Collins & Frankenhauser, 1978). Rural villagers have been found to have lower urinary catecholamine levels and lower blood pressure than workers, students, or laborers (Baum *et al.*, 1985). This may be due to a large variety of factors since increased catecholamine excretion has been related to job stress, caffeine consumption, cigarette use, life frustration, and disturbing life events.

In summary, a great deal of research has linked urinary catecholamine levels with physical and psychological stress. Urinary E appears especially responsive to these stresses. It is not at all clear where urinary catecholamines originate.

Other Indices of Catecholamine Release

NE is synthesized by the enzyme dopamine-β-hydroxylase (DBH) and E is synthesized from NE by PNMT. NE and E are stored in granules with DBH and chromogranins and are released along with DBH, chromogranins, enkephalins, and neuropeptide Y. NE is inactivated by *O*-methylation to normetanephrine. These compounds are acted on by monoamine oxidase to form vanillylmandelic acid (VMA) or the corresponding reduced compound 3-methoxy-4-hydroxyphenylglycol (MHPG). Catecholamines that escape these enzymes may be sulfated by phenylsulfotransferase. All of these metabolites are excreted into urine.

DBH is a large glycoprotein that is released with NE and E into the bloodstream and is broken down by the reticuloendothelial system. Blood levels of DBH are a function of the rate of release and rate of destruction. In laboratory rodents, destruction of DBH is quite rapid, blood levels are low, and many stresses increase DBH levels. Animals higher up the phylogenetic tree have higher blood DBH levels. In humans, genetic factors are the major determinant of DBH levels as people can inherit DBH that breaks down rapidly or slowly. As a result, DBH levels in human plasma are slightly altered by activity and greatly dependent on the rate of DBH degradation. One exception is Robertson's syndrome where DBH is apparently absent from sympathetic nerves and not measurable in plasma (Robertson *et al.*, 1986). DBH is present in very low levels in human CSF. CSF DBH is technically difficult to measure, but appears to reflect brain noradrenergic activity (Major, Lerner, & Ziegler, 1984).

Catecholamines are metabolized to metanephrines and further metabolized to VMA and MHPG. These compounds are excreted in the urine and their levels change in response to gross changes in catecholamine synthesis such as occur with pheochromocytoma. MHPG is the major metabolite of brain NE, but most MHPG in urine originates outside the brain. The ratio of MHPG to VMA excreted depends on the redox potential of mitochondria so that some foods such as ethanol enhance production of the reduced metabolite MHPG at the expense of the oxidized metabolite VMA.

Catecholamines can be sulfated and glucuronidated in rodents, but glucuronidation is not an important pathway in humans. The enzyme phenylsulfotransferase is present in platelets and the gut, so that dietary ingestion of catecholamines increases plasma catecholamine sulfates (Davidson, Vandongen, & Beilen, 1981; Dunne et al., 1984). Exercise increases catecholamine levels, but decreases plasma levels of catecholamine sulfates (Davidson, Vandongen, Beilin, & Arkwright, 1984). Catecholamine sulfate levels in CSF are not affected by blood levels (Kuchel, Hausser, Buu, & Tenneson, 1985). Some studies suggest that low levels of catecholamine sulfates may be associated with impaired catecholamine inactivation (Kuchel et al., 1981).

Chromogranin A is the major soluble protein in catecholamine storage vesicles. It is released along with NE and E and has a half-life of about 18 min in humans, intermediate between that of catecholamines and DBH. It has a much narrower normal range than DBH and levels respond to stimuli of the SNS, such as upright posture and hypoglycemia (O'Connor & Bernstein, 1984). It can be measured by radioimmunoassay whereas catecholamine measurements require more difficult assays. It is useful in detecting endocrine tumors, and may prove useful in evaluating stress.

In summary, levels of catecholamines and related compounds can provide a useful guide to SNS activity, but many factors can artifactually alter levels. Catecholamine assays have recently improved, but remain quite variable. The catecholamines are unstable compounds that degrade under improper storage and are rapidly cleared from blood and CSF. Catecholamine levels in blood change rapidly in response to minor stresses and may show 100-fold variations in response to major stress. Even at rest, there are circadian and ultradian rhythms for catecholamines.

Catecholamine levels in plasma depend on rate of release and rate of clearance. Clearance is rapid and varies in response to drugs, disease, and catecholamine levels. Since clearance is rapid, sampling site is important and catecholamine levels vary between venous and arterial blood and even between right and left arms. Blood sampling sites need to be uniform, but there is no one best site for all circumstances.

Urinary catecholamines may come from plasma, renal nerves, or blood metabolic substrates such as L-dopa. Although the origin of urinary catecholamines is not resolved, their levels parallel changes in plasma catecholamine levels.

References

Akerstedt, T. (1979). Altered sleep wake patterns and circadian rhythms. Laboratory and field studies of sympatho-adrenal medullary, and related variables. *Acta Physiologica Scandinavica, 1,* 469.

Akerstedt, T., & Levi, L. (1978). Circadian rhythms from the secretion of cortisone, adrenaline, and noradrenaline. *European Journal of Clinical Investigation, 8,* 57–58.

Aslan, S., Nelson, L., Carruthers, N., & Lader, M. (1981). Stress and age effects on catecholamines in normal subjects. *Journal of Psychosomatic Research, 25,* 33–41.

Barnes, P., Fitzgerald, G., Brown, M., & Dollery, C. (1980). Nocturnal asthma and changes in circulating epinephrine, histamine, and cortisol. *New England Journal of Medicine, 303,* 263–267.

Baum, A. S., Lundberg, U., Grunberg, N. E., Singer, J. E., & Gatchel, R. J. (1985). Urinary catecholamines in behavioral research stress. In C. R. Lake & M. G. Ziegler (Eds.), *The catecholamines in psychiatric and neurologic disorders* (pp. 55–72). Woburn: Butterworths.

Becker, R. A., Vaughn, G. M., Goodwin, C. W., Ziegler, M. G., Harrison, T. S., Mason, A. D., Jr., & Pruitt, B. A., Jr. (1980). Plasma norepinephrine, epinephrine, and thyroid hormone interactions in severely burned patients. *Archives of Surgery, 115,* 439–443.

Best, J. D., & Halter, J. B. (1982). Release and clearance rates of epinephrine in man: Importance of arterial measurements. *Journal of Clinical Endocrinology and Metabolism, 55,* 263–268.

Biberstein, M. G., Ziegler, M. G., & Ward, D. M. (1984). Use of beta-blockade and hemoperfusion for acute theophylline poisoning. *Western Journal of Medicine, 141,* 485–490.

Bravo, E. L., & Tarazi, R. C. (1982). Plasma catecholamines in clinical investigation: A useful index or a meaningless number? *Journal of Laboratory and Clinical Medicine, 100,* 155–160.

Brosnihan, K. B., Szilagyi, J. E., & Ferrario, C. M. (1981). Effect of chronic sodium depletion on cerebrospinal fluid and plasma catecholamines. *Hypertension, 3,* 233–239.

Burke, D., Sundlof, G., & Wallin, B. G. (1977). Postural effects on muscle nerve sympathetic activity in man. *Journal of Physiology* (London), *272,* 399–440.

Castellani, S., Ziegler, M. G., van Kammen, D. P., Alexander, P. E., Siris, S. G., & Lake, C. R. (1982). Plasma norepinephrine and dopamine-beta-hydroxylase activity in schizophrenia. *Archives of General Psychiatry, 39,* 1145–1149.

Chalew, S. A., McLaughlin, J. V., Mersey, J. H., Adams, A. J., Cornblath, M., & Kowarski, A. (1984). The use of the plasma epinephrine response in the diagnosis of idiopathic postprandial syndrome. *Journal of the American Medical Association, 251,* 612–615.

Chernow, B., Lake, C. R., Cook, D., Coyle, J., Hughes, P., Coleman, M., & Ziegler, M. G. (1983). Fenfluramine lowers plasma norepinephrine in overweight subjects. *International Journal of Clinical Pharmacological Research, 3,* 233–237.

Chernow, B., Lake, C. R., Ziegler, M. G., Zaloga, G. P., & Coleman, M. D. (1983). The effect of clonidine on sympathetic nervous system activity in essential hypertension. *International Journal of Clinical Pharmacological Research, 3,* 9–15.

Chernow, B., Zaloga, G. P., Lake, C. R., Coleman, M. D., & Ziegler, M. G. (1984). Effect of antihypertensive therapy on sympathetic nervous system activity in patients with essential hypertension. *Federation Proceedings, 43,* 72–77.

Christensen, N. J. (1979). The role of catecholamines in clinical medicine. *Acta Medica Scandinavica, Supplementum, 624,* 9–18.

Christensen, N. J., Galbe, H., Gjerris, A., Henriksen, J. H., Hilsted, J., Kjaer, M., & Ring-Larsen, H. (1984). Whole body and regional clearances of noradrenaline and adrenaline in man. *Acta Physiologica Scandinavica, Supplementum, 527,* 17–20.

Clifton, G. L., Ziegler, M. G., & Grossman, R. G. (1981). Circulating catecholamines and sympathetic activity after head injury. *Neurosurgery, 8,* 10–14.

Clutter, W. E., Bier, D. M., Shah, S. D., & Cryer, P. E. (1980). Epinephrine plasma metabolic clearance rates and physiologic thresholds for metabolic and hemodynamic actions in man. *Journal of Clinical Investigation, 66,* 94–101.

Cohn, J. N., Levine, T. B., Olivari, M. T., Gerberg, V., Lura, D., Francis, G. S., Simon, A.B., & Rector, T. (1984). Plasma norepinephrine as a guide to prognosis in patients with chronic congestive heart failure. *New England Journal of Medicine, 311,* 819–823, 850–851.

Collins, A., & Frankenhauser, M. (1978). Stress responses in male and female engineering students. *Journal of Human Stress, 4,* 43–48.

Cryer, P. E., Haymond, M. W., Santiago, J. V., & Shah, S. D. (1976). Norepinephrine and epinephrine release and adrenergic mediation of smoking-associated hemodynamic and metabolic events. *New England Journal of Medicine, 295,* 573–577.

Dahlgren, K. (1981). Shift work, circadian rhythms and sleep. Field studies of different shift systems. *Reports from the Department of Psychology, University of Stockholm. Supplement 53.*

Davidson, L., Vandongen, R., & Beilin, L. J. (1981). Effect of eating bananas on plasma free and sulfate-conjugated catecholamines. *Life Sciences, 29,* 1773–1778.

Davidson, L., Vandongen, R., Beilin, L. J., & Arkwright, P. D. (1984). Free and sulfate-conjugated catecholamines during exercise in man. *Journal of Clinical Endocrinology and Metabolism, 58,* 415–418.

De Schaepdryver, A. F., Hooft, D., Delbeke, M. J., & Van den Noortgaete, M. (1978). Urinary catecholamines and metabolites in children. *Journal of Pediatrics, 93,* 266–268.

Dimsdale, J. E., & Moss, J. (1980a). Short-term catecholamine response to psychological stress. *Psychosomatic Medicine, 42,* 493–497.

Dimsdale, J. E., & Moss, J. (1980b). Plasma catecholamines in stress and exercise. *Journal of the American Medical Association, 243,* 340–342.

Dunne, J. W., Davidson, L., Vandongen, R., Beilin, L. J., Tunney, A. M., & Rogers, P. B. (1984). The effect of ascorbic acid on the sulphate conjugation of ingested noradrenaline and dopamine. *British Journal of Clinical Pharmacology, 17,* 356–360.

Durrett, L. R., & Ziegler, M. G. (1980). A sensitive radioenzymatic assay for catechol drugs. *Journal of Neuroscience Research, 5,* 587–598.

Esler, M., Jackman, G., Leonard, P., Bobik, A., Skews, H., Jennings, G., Kelleher, D., & Korner, P. (1980). Determination of noradrenaline uptake, spillover to plasma, and plasma concentration in patients with essential hypertension. *Clinical Science, 59,* 311s–313s.

Esler, M., Jackman, G., Kelleher, D., Skews, H., Jennings, G., Bobik, A., & Korner, P. (1980). Norepinephrine kinetics in patients with idiopathic autonomic insufficiency. *Circulation Research, Suppl.* 46(6), 147–148.

Esler, M., Jackman, G., Leonard, P., Skews, H., Bobik, A., & Korner, P. (1981). Effect of norepinephrine uptake blockers on norepinephrine kinetics. *Clinical Pharmacology and Therapeutics, 29,* 12–20.

Esler, M., Skews, H., Leonard, P., Jackman, G., Bobik, A., & Korner, P. (1981). Age-dependence of noradrenaline kinetics in normal subjects. *Clinical Science, 60,* 217–219.

Esler, M., Turbott, J., Schwartz, R., Leonard, P., Bobik, A., Skews, H., & Jackman, G. (1982). The peripheral kinetics of norepinephrine in depressive illness. *Archives of General Psychiatry, 39,* 295–300.

Esler, M., Jennings, G., Leonard, P., Sacharias, N., Burke, F., Johns, J., & Blombery, P. (1984). Contribution of individual organs to total noradrenaline release in humans. *Acta Physiologica Scandinavica, Supplementum, 527,* 11–16.

Fitzgerald, G. A., Hossmann, V., Hamilton, C. A., Reid, J. L., Davies, D. S., & Dollery, C. T. (1979). Interindividual variation in kinetics of infused norepinephrine. *Clinical Pharmacology and Therapeutics, 26,* 669–675.

Forsman, L. (1981). Note on estimating catecholamines in urine sampled after 75 minutes of mental work and inactivity. *Journal of Psychosomatic Research, 25,* 223–225.

Frakenhaeuser, N., & Johasson, G. (1976). Task demand as reflected in catecholamine excretion and heart rate. *Journal of Human Stress, 2*, 15–23.

Goldman, D., Hejmancik, M. G., Williams, B. J., & Ziegler, M. G. (1980). Altered noradrenergic systems in the lead-exposed neonatal rat. *Neurobehavioral Toxicology and Teratology, 2*, 337–343.

Goldstein, D. S. (1981). Plasma norepinephrine in essential hypertension: A study of the studies. *Hypertension, 3*, 48–52.

Gotoh, F., Komatsumoto, S., Araki, N., & Gomi, S. (1984). Noradrenergic nervous activity in migraine. *Archives of Neurology, 41*, 951–955.

Grimm, M., Weidmann, P., Keusch, G., Meier, A., & Gluck, Z. (1980). Norepinephrine clearance and pressor effect in normal and hypertensive man. *Klinische Wochenschrift, 58*, 1175–1181.

Hansen, B. C., Schielke, G. P., Jen, K. L. C., Wolfe, R. A., Movahed, H., & Pek, S. B. (1982). Rapid fluctuations in plasma catecholamines in monkeys under undisturbed conditions. *American Journal of Physiology, 242*, E40–E46.

Hawley, R. J., Major, L. F., Schulman, E., & Lake, C. R. (1981). CSF levels of norepinephrine during alcohol withdrawal. *Archives of Neurology, 38*, 289–292.

Henriksen, J. H., Christensen, N. J., Kok-Jensen, A., & Cnristiansen, I. B. (1980). Increased plasma noradrenaline concentration in patients with chronic obstructive lung disease: Relation to haemodynamics and blood gases. *Scandinavian Journal of Clinical Laboratory Investigation, 40*, 419–427.

Henry, D. P., Luft, F. C., Weinberger, M. H., Fineberg, N. S., & Grim, C. E. (1980). Norepinephrine in urine and plasma following provocative maneuvers in normal and hypertensive subjects. *Hypertension, 2*, 20–28.

Hesse, B., Ring-Larson, H., Nielsen, I., & Christiansen, N. H. (1978). Renin stimulation by passive tilting: The influence of anti-gravity suit on postural changes in plasma renin activity, plasma noradrenaline concentration, and kidney function in normal man. *Scandinavian Journal of Clinical Laboratory Investigation, 38*, 163–169.

Hesse, B., Kanstrup, I. L., Christensen, N. J., Ingemann-Hansen, T., Hansen, J. F., Halkjaer-Kristensen, J., & Petersen, F. B. (1981). Reduced norepinephrine response to dynamic exercise in human subjects during O_2 breathing. *The American Physiological Society, 81*, 176–178.

Hjemdahl, P. (1984). Inter-laboratory comparison of plasma catecholamine determinations using several different assays. *Acta Physiologica Scandinavica, 527*, 43–54.

Hull, E. M., Young, S. H., & Ziegler, M. G. (1984). Aerobic fitness affects cardiovascular and catecholamine responses to stressors. *Psychophysiology, 2*, 353–360.

Kato, K., Hashitmot, Y., Nagatsu, T., Shinoda, T., Okada, T., Takeuchi, T., & Umezawa, H. (1980). Twenty-four hour rhythm of human plasma noradrenaline and the effect of fusaric acid, a dopamine-beta-hydroxylase inhibitor. *Neuropsychobiology, 6*, 61–65.

Kennedy, B., Janowsky, D. S., Risch, D. S., & Ziegler, M. G. (1984). Central cholinergic stimulation causes adrenal epinephrine release. *Journal of Clinical Investigation, 74*, 972–975.

Kennedy, B., Ziegler, M. G., & Shannahoff-Khalsa, D. S. (1986). Alternating lateralization of plasma catecholamines and nasal patency in humans. *Life Sciences, 38*, 1203–1214.

Krstulovic, A. M. (1986). *Quantitative analysis of catecholamines and related compounds.* Wiley, New York.

Kuchel, O., Buu, N. T., Hamet, P., Larochelle, P., Bourque, M., & Genest, J. (1981). Essential hypertension with low conjugated catecholamines imitates pheochromocytoma. *Hypertension, 3*, 347–355.

Kuchel, O., Hausser, C., Buu, N. T., & Tenneson, S. (1985). CSF sulfoconjugated catecholamines in man: Their relationship with plasma catecholamines. *Journal of Neural Transmission, 62*, 91–97.

Lake, C. R., & Ziegler, M. G. (1977). Lesch–Nyhan syndrome: Low dopamine-beta-hydroxylase activity and diminished sympathetic response to stress and posture. *Science, 196*, 905–906.

Lake, C. R., & Ziegler, M. G. (1978). Effect of acute volume alterations on norepinephrine and dopamine-beta-hydroxylase in normotensive and hypertensive subjects. *Circulation, 57*, 774–778.

Lake, C. R., & Ziegler, M. G. (1985). Techniques for assaying the catecholamines in psychiatric patients. In C. R. Lake & M. G. Ziegler (Eds.), *The catecholamines in psychiatric and neurologic disorders* (pp. 1–34). Woburn: Butterworths.

Lake, C. R., Ziegler, M. G., & Kopin, I. J. (1976). Use of plasma norepinephrine for evaluation of sympathetic neuronal function in man. *Life Sciences, 18*, 1315–1326.

Lake, C. R., Major, L. F., Ziegler, M. G., & Kopin, I. J. (1977). Increased sympathetic nervous system activity in alcoholic patients treated with disulfiram. *American Journal of Psychiatry, 134*, 1411–1414.

Lake, C. R., Ziegler, M. G., & Murphy, D. L. (1977). Increased norepinephrine levels and decreased dopamine-beta-hydroxylase activity in primary autism. *Archives of General Psychiatry, 34*, 553–556.

Lake, C. R., Wood, J. D., Ziegler, M. G., Ebert, M. H., & Kopin, I. J. (1978). Probenecid-induced norepinephrine elevations in plasma and CSF. *Archives of General Psychiatry, 35*, 237–240.

Lake, C. R., Ziegler, M. G., Coleman, M. D., & Kopin, I. J. (1979a). Plama levels of norepinephrine and dopamine-beta-hydroxylase in CRF patients treated with dialysis. *Cardiovascular Medicine, 4*, 1099–1111.

Lake, C. R., Ziegler, M. G., Coleman, M. D., & Kopin, I. J. (1979b). Sustained sympathetic hyperactivity in hydrochlorothiazide-treated hypertensives. *Clinical Pharmacology and Therapeutics, 26*, 428–432.

Lake, C. R., Sternberg, D. E., van Kammen, D. P., Ballenger, J. C., Ziegler, M. G., Post, R. M., Kopin, I. J., & Bunney, W. E., Jr. (1980). Schizophrenia: Elevated cerebrospinal fluid norepinephrine. *Science, 207*, 331–333.

Lake, C. R., Gullner, H. G., Polinski, R. J., Ebert, M. H., Ziegler, M. G., & Bartter, F. C. (1981). Essential hypertension: Central and peripheral norepinephrine. *Science, 211,* 955–957.

Lake, C. R., Pickar, D., Ziegler, M. G., Lipper, I. S., Slater, S., & Murphy, D. L. (1982). High plasma norepinephrine levels in patients with major affective disorders. *American Journal of Psychiatry, 139,* 1315–1318.

Lake, C. R., Chernow, B., Goldstein, D., Glass, D. G., Coleman, M., & Ziegler, M. G. (1984). Plasma catecholamine levels in normal subjects and in patients with secondary hypertension. *Federation Proceedings, 43,* 52–56.

Leduc, J. (1961). Excretion of catecholamines in rats exposed to cold. *Acta Physiologica Scandinavica, 51,* 94.

Leiter, L. A., Grose, M., Yale, J. F., & Marliss, E. B. (1984). Catecholamine responses to hypocaloric diets and fasting in obese human subjects. *Journal of The American Physiologic Society, 84,* 190–197.

Levin, B. E., & Natelson, B. H. (1980). The relationship of plasma norepinephrine and epinephrine levels over time in humans. *Journal of the Autonomic Nervous System, 2,* 315–325.

Levin, B. E., Goldstein, A., & Natelson, B. H. (1978). Ultradian rhythm of plasma noradrenaline in rhesus monkeys. *Nature, 272,* 164–166.

Linsel, C. R., Lightman, S. L., Mullen, P. E., Brown, M. J., & Causon, R. C. (1985). Circadian rhythms of epinephrine and norepinephrine in man. *Journal of Clinical Endocrinology and Metabolism, 60,* 1210–1215.

Lundberg, U., & Forsman, L. (1979). Adrenal medullary and adrenal cortical responses to under-stimulation and over-stimulation—Comparison between type A and type B persons. *Biological Psychiatry, 9,* 797–798.

Major, L. F., Lerner, P., & Ziegler, M. G. (1984). Norepinephrine and dopamine-beta-hydroxylase in cerebrospinal fluid: Indicators of central noradenergic activity. In M. G. Ziegler & C. R. Lake (Eds.), *Norepinephrine* (pp. 117–141). Baltimore: Williams & Wilkins.

Mikkelsen, E., Lake, C. R., Brown, G. L., Ziegler, M. G., & Ebert, M. H. (1980). The hyperactive child syndrome: Peripheral sympathetic nervous system function and the effect of d-amphetamine. *Psychological Research, 4,* 157–169.

Miura, Y., Campese, V., DeQuattro, V., & Meyer, D. (1977). Plasma catecholamines via an improved fluorimetric assay: Comparison with an enzymatic method. *Journal of Laboratory and Clinical Medicine, 89,* 421–427.

Nechay, R. B., Jackson, R. E., Ziegler, M. G., & Nelson, S. L. (1981). Effects of chronic digitalization on cardiac and renal Na$^+$ + K$^+$-dependent adenosine triphosphate and circulating catecholamines in the dog. *Circulation Research, 49,* 655–660.

Nicholls, K. M., Shapiro, M. D., Van Putten, V. J., Kluge, R., Chung, H. M., Bichet, D. G., & Schrier, R. W. (1985). Elevated plasma norepinephrine concentrations in decompensated cirrhosis. *Circulation Research, 56,* 459–461.

O'Connor, D., & Bernstein, K. N. (1984). Radioimmunoassay of chromogranin A in plasma as a measure of exocytotic sympathoadrenal activity in normal subjects and patients

with pheochromocytoma. *New England Journal of Medicine, 311,* 764–795.

Ogasaware, B., Ogawa, K., & Sassa, H. (1981). Effects of nitroglycerin ointment on plasma norepinephrine and cyclic nucleotides in congestive heart failure. *Journal of Cardiovascular Pharmacology, 3,* 867–875.

Palmer, G. J., Ziegler, M. G., & Lake, C. R. (1978). Response of norepinephrine and blood pressure to stress increases with age. *Journal of Gerontology, 33,* 482–487.

Patkai, P. (1971). Catecholamine excretion in pleasant and unpleasant situations. *Acta Psychologica, 35,* 352–363.

Pequignot, J. M., Claustre, J., & Peyrin, L. (1979). Evolution de la noradrenalinemie chez l'homme a court et a long terme apres perfusion d'amine exogene. *Archives Internationales de Physiologie et de Biochimie, 87,* 509–524.

Peronnet, F., Cleroux, J., Perrault, H., Cousineau, D., de Champlain, J., & Nadeau, R. (1981). Plasma norepinephrine response to exercise before and after training in humans. *Journal of Applied Physiology, 51,* 812–815.

Rassler, A. (1977). Stress reactions at work and after work during a period of quantitative overload. *Aergonomics, 20,* 13–16.

Robertson, D., Frolich, J. C., Carr, R. K., Watson, J. T., Hollifield, J. W., Shand, D. G., & Oates, J. A. (1978). Effects of caffeine on plasma renin activity, catecholamines, and blood pressure. *New England Journal of Medicine, 298,* 181–186.

Robertson, D., Johnson, G. A., Robertson, R. M., Nies, A. S., Shand, D. G., & Oates, J. A. (1979). Comparative assessment of stimuli that release neuronal and adrenomedullary catecholamines in man. *Circulation, 59,* 637–643.

Robertson, D., Goldberg, M. R., Onrot, J., Hollister, A. S., Wiley, R., Thompson, G., & Robertson, R. M. (1986). Isolated failure of autonomic noradrenergic neurotransmission. *New England Journal of Medicine, 314,* 1494–1497.

Rosenblatt, J. E., Lake, C. R., van Kammen, D. P., Ziegler, M. G., & Bunney, W. E., Jr. (1979). Interactions of amphetamine, pimozide, and lithium on plasma norepinephrine and dopamine-beta-hydroxylase in schizophrenic patients. *Psychiatric Research, 1,* 45–52.

Rosenthal, T., Cbircy, M., Osikowska, B., & Sever, E. S. (1978). Changes in plasma noradrenaline concentration following sympathetic stimulation by gradual tilting. *Cardiovascular Research, 12,* 144–147.

Shoulson, I., Ziegler, M. G., & Lake, C. R. (1976). Huntington's disease (HD): Determination of plasma norepinephrine (NE) and dopamine-beta-hydroxylase (DBH). *Society for Neuroscience Abstracts, 2,* 800.

Tapp, W. N., Levin, B. E., & Natelson, B. H. (1981). Ultradian rhythm of plasma norepinephrine in rats. *Endocrinology, 109,* 1781–1783.

Teychenne, P. F., Lake, C. R., & Ziegler, M. G. (1980). Cerebrospinal fluid studies in Parkinson's disease: Norepinephrine and gamma-aminobutyric acid concentrations. In J. H. Wood (Ed.), *Neurobiology of cerebrospinal fluid* (pp. 197–206). New York: Plenum Press.

Tuck, M. L., Sowers, J., Dornfeld, L., Kledzik, G., & Maxwell, M. (1981). The effect of weight reduction on blood pressure, plasma renin activity, and plasma aldosterone levels in obese patients. *New England Journal of Medicine, 304,* 930–933.

Veith, R. C., Raskind, M. A., Barnes, R. F., Gumbrecht, G., Ritchie, J. L., & Halter, J. B. (1983). Tricyclic antidepressants and supine, standing, and exercise plasma norepinephrine levels. *Clinical Pharmacological Therapy, 33,* 770–775.

Von Euler, U. S., Ikkos, D., & Luft, R. (1961). Adrenaline excretion during resting conditions and after insulin in adrenalectomized human subjects. *Acta Endocrinologica, 38,* 441.

Voorhess, M. L., Stuart, M. J., Stockman, J. A., & Oski, F. A. (1975). Iron deficiency anemia and increased urinary norepinephrine excretion. *Journal of Pediatrics, 86,* 542–547.

Weir, T. B., Smitt, C. C., Round, J. N., & Betteridge, D. J. (1986). Stability of catecholamines in whole blood plasma and platelets. *Clinical Chemistry, 32,* 882–883.

Welle, S., Lilavivanthana, U., & Campbell, R. G. (1981). Thermic effect of feeding in man: Increased plasma norepinephrine levels following glucose but not protein or fat consumption. *Metabolism, 30,* 953–958.

Wiedeking, C., Lake, C. R., Ziegler, M. G., Muske, E., & Jorgensen, G. (1977). Plasma noradrenaline and dopamine-beta-hydroxylase during sexual activity. *Psychological Medicine, 32,* 143–148.

Young, J. B., Rowe, J. W., Pallotta, J. A., Sparrow, D., & Landsberg, L. (1980). Enhanced plasma norepinephrine response to upright posture and oral glucose administration in elderly human subjects. *Metabolism, 29,* 532.

Yui, Y., & Kawai, C. (1981). Comparison of the sensitivity of various post-column methods for catecholamine analysis by high-performance liquid chromatography. *Journal of Chromatography, 206,* 586–588.

Ziegler, M. G. (1980). Postural hypotension. *Annual Review of Medicine, 31,* 239–245.

Ziegler, M. G. (1983). Antihypertensives. In B. Chernow & C. R. Lake (Eds.), *The pharmacological approach to the critically ill patient* (pp. 303–330). Baltimore: Williams Wilkins.

Ziegler, M. G., & Lake, C. R. (1984). Autonomic degeneration and altered blood pressure control in humans. *Federation Proceedings, 43,* 62–66.

Ziegler, M. G., & Lake, C. R. (1985). Noradrenergic responses to postural hypotension: Implications for therapy. In C. R. Lake & M. G. Ziegler (Eds.), *The catecholamines in psychiatric and neurologic disorders* (pp. 121–136). Woburn: Butterworths.

Ziegler, M. G., Lake, C. R., Foppen, F. H., Shoulson, I., & Kopin, I. J. (1976). Norepinephrine in cerebrospinal fluid.

Brain Research, 108, 436–440.

Ziegler, M. G., Lake, C. R., Wood, J. H., & Ebert, M. H. (1976). Circadian rhythm in cerebrospinal fluid noradrenaline of man and monkey. *Nature, 264,* 656–658.

Ziegler, M. G., Lake, C. R., Eldridge, R., & Kopin, I. J. (1976). Plasma norepinephrine and dopamine-beta-hydroxylase in dystonia. *Advances in Neurology, 14,* 307–318.

Ziegler, M. G., Lake, C. R., & Kopin, I. J. (1976a). Deficient sympathetic nervous response in familial dysautonomia. *New England Journal of Medicine, 294,* 630–633.

Ziegler, M. G., Lake, C. R., & Kopin, I. J. (1976b). Plasma noradrenaline increases with age. *Nature, 261,* 333–335.

Ziegler, M. G., Lake, C. R., Wood, J. H., Brooks, B. R., & Ebert, M. H. (1977). Relationship between norepinephrine in blood and cerebrospinal fluid in the presence of a blood–cerebrospinal fluid barrier for norepinephrine. *Journal of Neurochemistry, 28,* 677–679.

Ziegler, M. G., Lake, C. R., & Kopin, I. J. (1977). The sympathetic nervous system defect in primary orthostatic hypotension. *New England Journal of Medicine, 296,* 293–297.

Ziegler, M. G., Lake, C. R., Williams, A. C., Teychenne, P. F., Shoulson, I., & Steinsland, O. (1979). Bromocriptine inhibits norepinephrine release. *Clinical Pharmacology and Therapeutics, 25,* 137–142.

Ziegler, M. G., Lake, C. R., & Ebert, M. H. (1979). Norepinephrine elevations in cerebrospinal fluid after D- and L-amphetamine. *European Journal of Pharmacology, 57,* 127–133.

Ziegler, M. G., Brooks, B. R., Lake, C. R., Wood, J. H., & Enna, S. J. (1980). Norepinephrine and gamma-aminobutyric acid in amyotrophic lateral sclerosis. *Neurology, 30,* 98–101.

Ziegler, M. G., Kennedy, B., Holland, O. B., Murphy, D., & Lake, C. R. (1985). The effects of dopamine agonists on human cardiovascular and sympathetic nervous systems. *International Journal of Clinical Pharmacology Therapy and Toxicology, 23,* 175–179.

Ziegler, M. G., Milano, A. J., & Hull, E. (1985). The catecholaminergic response to stress and exercise. In C. R. Lake & M. G. Ziegler (Eds.), *The catecholamines in psychiatric and neurologic disorders* (pp. 37–53). Woburn: Butterworths.

Ziegler, M. G., Chernow, B., Woodson, L., Coyle, J., Cruess, D., & Lake, C. R. (1986). The effect of propranolol on catecholamine clearance. *Clinical Pharmacology and Therapeutics, 40,* 116–119.

Ziegler, M. G., Echon, C., Wilner, K. D., Specho, P., Lake, C. R., & McCutchen, J. A. (1986). Sympathetic nervous withdrawal in the vasodepressor (vasovagal) reaction. *Journal of the Autonomic Nervous System, 17,* 273–278.

CHAPTER 12

Adrenocortical and Gonadal Steroids in Behavioral Cardiovascular Medicine

Cynthia M. Kuhn

Introduction

The purpose of this chapter is to provide guidelines for the evaluation of steroid hormone secretion as they relate to cardiovascular function. As aldosterone is covered elsewhere in a discussion of renin–angiotensin–aldosterone secretion (see Atlas, this volume), this chapter will focus on glucocorticoid and gonadal steroids. Parameters relevant to cardiovascular function are emphasized rather than classical endocrinologic methods for assessing adequacy of hormone secretion. This involves somewhat different strategies, as changes in hormone secretion rather than absolute hormone levels are of considerable importance, particularly in understanding the role of behavioral variables in cardiovascular disease.

The most important consideration in evaluating the relevance of hormone secretion in cardiovascular disease is the careful experimental determination of the relationship of a given level of secretion to the physiology or pathology of interest. The danger in simply measuring blood hormone levels in certain disease states or experimental regimens is that the measure itself *does not* imply a causal role in pathology. Although it has become methodologically simple to measure levels of glucocorticoid hormones, causal relationships between these hormone levels and cardiovascular physiology have only rarely been established. Therefore, these measures should be approached with a considerable degree of skepticism until their physiologic significance has been established.

Adrenocortical Hormones

Adrenocortical Steroids and Cardiovascular Function

Cortisol secreted by the adrenal cortex plays a major role in maintaining almost every physiologic function, particularly those that are vital during periods of physiologic demand, or ''stress.'' Cortisol helps maintain blood glucose, lipid, protein, and nucleic acid synthesis, regulates immune function, and controls growth and development of many tissues. In addition, it also modulates behavior, through actions on diverse neuronal systems in the brain. Cortisol has most of its actions through interactions with specific intracellular receptors, which are thought to transport cortisol into the nucleus where the steroid–receptor complex binds to DNA, and alters the transcription of mRNA coding

Cynthia M. Kuhn • Department of Pharmacology, Duke University Medical Center, Durham, North Carolina 27710.

for specific proteins. The actions of steroids often complement, or are "permissive" to, the actions of other hormones which serve related functions. Notable among these, for the purposes of the present discussion, are other stress-related hormones like catecholamines.

Maintenance of cardiovascular function is one of the most important physiologic actions of cortisol secretion. A basal level of cortisol secretion is necessary for maintenance of normal cardiac output, with glucocorticoid insufficiency leading to circulatory collapse (Wilson & Foster, 1980). The physiologic mechanism for this action is unclear, although recent studies suggest that cortisol secretion acts synergistically with the sympathetic nervous system at the heart and blood vessel to facilitate necessary cardiovascular adaptations to challenge (Schomig, Luth, Dietz, & Gross, 1976; Surwit et al., 1982). In addition, an association between cortisol and atherosclerosis has been suggested in both epidemiologic and biochemical studies (Rosenfeld, Marmorston, Sobel, & White, 1960; Bjorkerud, 1974). Although the biochemical mechanism mediating the latter effect is unknown, effects of cortisol on lipid metabolism and on the secretion and action of other agents like catecholamines are being investigated.

The profound stimulation of adrenocortical hormone secretion during "stress" represents an area of even greater interest to behavioral cardiovascular medicine. The cortisol response to a multitude of psychologic and physical stimuli is one of the hallmarks of the "stress response," a badly misused term which has been applied to almost any environmental factor viewed as threatening, unpleasant, and/or physiologically arousing. Despite the imprecision of this term, there is tremendous interest in the links between stress and cardiovascular disease, particularly in physiologic mechanisms by which stress contributes to atherosclerosis, myocardial infarction, and hypertension.

The magnitude, predictability, and "chronicity" of stress-induced cortisol secretion make it a likely mediator of pathologies associated with stress. In both human and animal studies, environmental stressors have been shown to stimulate cortisol secretion two- to fivefold, a stimulation which can persist for days to months (Henry, Kross, Ste-

phens, & Watson, 1976; Friedman et al., 1960; Rose, Jenkins, Hurst, Livingston, & Hasell, 1982). Abnormal secretion of this magnitude could possibly mediate pathology associated with stress.

Understanding the neural mechanisms which regulate stress-induced cortisol secretion is vital for understanding both the physiology and psychology of normal stress responses, as well as the possible contribution of these effects to stress-induced cardiovascular disease. For example, individuals who have personality characteristics like "Type A" behavior show exaggerated cortisol responses to behavioral challenge which may be associated with cardiovascular pathology (Williams et al., 1982). It is possible that the neural integration of physiologic responses to stress is abnormal in such individuals, and that the abnormal responses which result when such individuals are stressed lead to cardiovascular pathology.

Characterization of behavioral stimuli which evoke cortisol secretion and induce cardiovascular pathology represents an important aspect of this problem which can have direct clinical implications for behavioral cardiology. One important goal of behavioral cardiology is to identify those situations which provoke inappropriate cortisol secretion in patients at risk for cardiovascular disease. Although cortisol secretion was originally characterized as a "nonspecific" response to any environmental disturbance, more sophisticated psychologic studies suggest that cortisol responds to situations which possess certain common characteristics. These have been described as those which are "threatening," involve "loss of control," or are novel, unpleasant, and arousing. This affective state can be generated by an intense external stimulus, or it might be generated internally, by personality variables which cause a situation to be anxiety-provoking. A good example of the latter is the cortisol secretion elicited by presenting phobics with the object of their fear (Frederikson, Sundin, & Frankenhaeuser, 1985).

Despite the well-known association of cortisol secretion with "stressful" situations, there are few careful laboratory studies of cortisol secretion evoked by precisely defined behavioral/psychologic stimuli. The majority of published studies of stress-induced cortisol secretion in humans involve instead single determinations following very intense manipulations like surgery, parachute jumping, depression, exercise to exhaustion, or similarly unusual events which are difficult to quantitate (Estep *et al.,* 1968; Pinter, Peterfy, & Cleghorn, 1975; Rose & Hurst, 1975). Cardiovascular pathology has been associated more with *chronic* stimulation produced by more subtle but persistent stimuli, or even by personality variables or other neurobehavioral factors which augment cortisol responses to environmental stimuli. Therefore, studies of cortisol secretion during everyday life and laboratory studies of evoked cortisol secretion represent a necessary step in studying the relevance of cortisol secretion to behavioral issues in cardiovascular medicine. Hopefully, the present chapter will provide some guidelines for designing such studies.

Patterns of Basal and Stress-Induced Secretion

Normal Secretion

Cortisol is secreted from the adrenal cortex under the influence of adrenocorticotrophic hormone (ACTH). Cortisol secretion is strongly controlled by feedback inhibition of ACTH secretion at the pituitary and inhibition of corticotropin releasing factor (CRF) secretion in the hypothalamus. ACTH acts through a cell surface receptor to stimulate synthesis of cyclic AMP, which then increases the first step in cortisol synthesis, the cleavage of the side chain of cholesterol to form Δ^5-pregnenolone (for reviews see Wilson & Foster, 1980; Bondy & Rosenberg, 1980; Streeten *et al.,* 1982). ACTH secretion in turn is controlled by the secretion of CRF from the hypothalamus. Cortisol is not secreted at a constant rate, being secreted in bursts (about 7–13 per day) which are superimposed on a circadian rhythm that has its peak in the early morning hours and its nadir at the beginning of sleep (Figure 1). During a burst, cortisol levels can rise severalfold in the space of 10–30 min. After a secretory burst, cortisol levels fall with a half-life of about 60–90 min. Cortisol is removed mainly by metabolism in the liver, where it is converted by at least four different routes:

reduction of the 3-ketone, oxidation of the 11β hydroxyl, side chain cleavage, and formation of glucuronide and sulfate conjugates of these and other minor metabolites (Figure 2). Greater than 90% of circulating cortisol is bound to protein, mainly the specific corticosteroid binding globulin, and to a much lesser extent to albumin. At high levels of secretion, cortisol in the circulation exceeds the capacity of the binding sites, and the amount of free hormone increases. However, at low or normal levels, protein binding is fairly constant.

Stress-Induced Secretion

Careful studies of the dynamics of stress-induced cortisol secretion which take into account the rhythmicity of basal secretion have only recently been conducted. However, it is clear that cortisol secretion rises predictably in response to a number of "stressors." The response is somewhat sluggish in comparison to cardiovascular variables, as a lag of 5–15 min is imposed by the secretion of ACTH, its diffusion to the adrenal, and the stimulation of steroid output (Orth *et al.,* 1983). Therefore, while cardiovascular variables respond in seconds and plasma norepinephrine and epinephrine in minutes, cortisol responses are best seen 20–30 min after a stimulus. A good example is given in Figure 3, which shows cortisol responses to a mental arithmetic challenge. Furthermore, although cortisol secretion generally increases in proportion to the intensity of the stimulus, the intensity of stimulation required to evoke a significant change in cortisol secretion could well exceed that capable of evoking measurable changes in heart rate or blood flow. A good example of this disparity is found in the sequence of response observed during exercise. While heart rate (and plasma norepinephrine, a good correlate of sympathetic stimulation) rises almost immediately, changes in cortisol are much slower, and occur only at higher levels of effort (Hartley *et al.,* 1972). Therefore, experimental protocols which evoke small changes in cardiovascular parameters might not elicit measurable changes in cortisol secretion.

Another major consideration in understanding

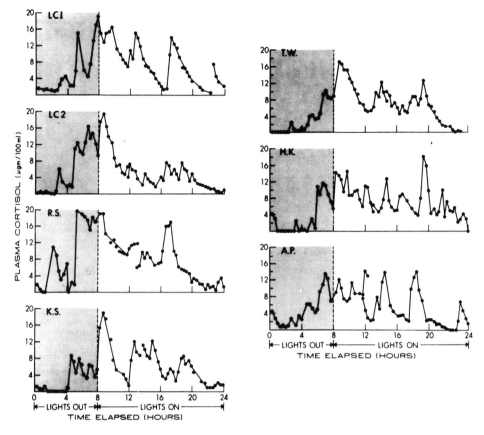

Figure 1. Plasma cortisol values of subjects taken at 20-min intervals for 24 h. From Weitzman *et al.* (1971).

the relationship between cortisol and cardiovascular responses to stress is that these may respond to quite different components of a given experimental environment. As mentioned above, cortisol secretion responds more profoundly to affective state than to physical demand. For example, the delayed rise during exercise might not occur until unpleasant levels of effort are achieved. Similarly, cortisol secretion, like blood pressure, can rise *in anticipation* of a disruption in the environment (Mason *et al.*, 1973), while responses to a psychologically neutral physical task might be minimal.

Finally, it must be emphasized that from the standpoint of cardiovascular function, there may be no "appropriate" hormone level as there is for thyroid hormone, gonadal steroids, or other endocrine measures. Cortisol secretion is so intimately linked to the environment that evaluating the change evoked by a challenge is much more relevant than measuring a basal level, although the magnitude of the evoked response must exceed the variations occurring from normal secretory bursts. This is the one characteristic of secretion that is frequently misunderstood in designing experimental protocols for studying cortisol secretion.

Pathologic Changes in Secretion

The boundary between physiologic and pathologic levels of cortisol secretion in relation to behavioral control of cardiovascular function is unclear. While frank hyper- and hyposecretion of cortisol are well described clinical entities with known cardiovascular pathology, these are fairly rare, and can be resolved by medical intervention.

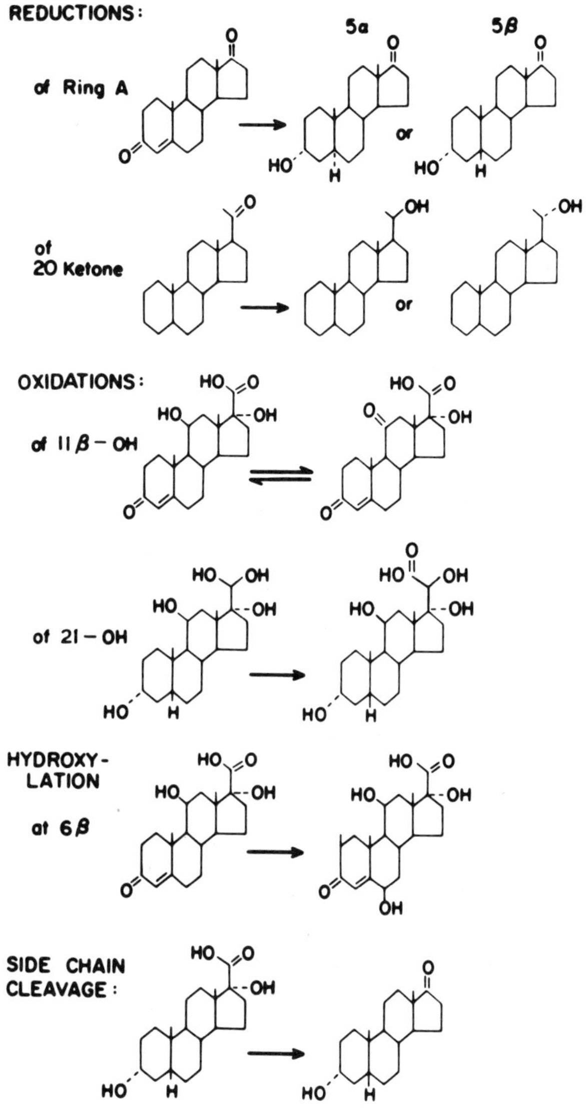

REDUCTIONS:

of Ring A

of 20 Ketone

OXIDATIONS:

of 11β — OH

of 21 — OH

HYDROXY-
LATION

at 6β

SIDE CHAIN
CLEAVAGE:

Figure 2. Reactions occurring in metabolism of corticosteroids. Adapted from Bondy and Rosenberg (1980).

The more important question for the present topic is the association of sustained elevations within the high physiologic range with cardiovascular pathology.

Chronic elevation of cortisol secretion has been described following a number of behavioral manipulations which cause cardiovascular pathology, in both humans and animals. For example, the stress of group living in previously isolated mice produces a chronic sympathoadrenal and adrenocortical activation and concomitant hypertension (Henry, Stephens, & Santisteban, 1975). Similarly, extended periods of work stress in "Type A" humans are associated with chronic adrenocortical activation and concomitant cardiovascular pathology (Troxler, Sprague, Albanese, Fuchs, & Thompson, 1977). The degree of endocrine disruption and possible mechanisms by which altered hormone secretion contributes to cardiovascular pathology represent an important goal of current research. A related but more difficult task would be to demonstrate a relationship between acute

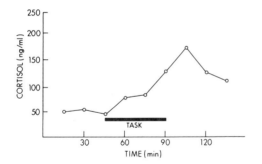

Figure 3. Plasma cortisol values in a single individual before, during, and after a mental arithmetic task (indicated by solid bar).

changes in cortisol secretion evoked in laboratory settings and cardiovascular pathology.

Experimental Evaluation of Cortisol Secretion

Measurement of those characteristics of cortisol secretion that are relevant to cardiovascular function differs considerably from classical assessment of adrenocortical function. Measurement of total daily steroid synthesis and secretion is of considerable importance for diagnosis of Addison's or Cushing's disease. However, it is presently unknown if variations in secretion within the normal range are relevant to cardiovascular pathology. This question can be answered only by future studies of evoked secretion in the laboratory, basal secretion in various environmental circumstances, and naturalistic studies of urinary excretion.

Hormone to Be Measured

In most studies, measurement of cortisol provides the most useful information about the HPA axis with minimal methodologic difficulty. The major theoretical reason for evaluating cortisol rather than CRF or ACTH is that the former represents the most likely source of cardiovascular pathology (excluding the proposed central actions of pituitary and hypothalamic peptides which will be covered elsewhere). However, as mentioned previously, cortisol secretion occurs only after ACTH secretion has stimulated the adrenal cortex, and

concurrent measurement of ACTH theoretically could provide additional useful information. ACTH levels respond more quickly to challenge, and provide a useful index in conjunction with cardiovascular variables. Furthermore, comparison of ACTH and cortisol responses provides information about adrenal responsivity to ACTH, a regulatory mechanism that is of increasing interest. Unfortunately, at this time ACTH determinations are methodologically more challenging, time-consuming, and costly. The few commercially available kits lack the careful standardization of methods utilized by those few research laboratories which have developed their own radioimmunoassay (RIA) methods. Therefore, measurement of ACTH remains a largely unexplored potential.

Another reason why cortisol is the optimal choice for most behavioral studies of adrenocortical secretion is that there is no single metabolite that constitutes the majority of secreted cortisol. Instead, cortisol is metabolized to multiple, structurally related compounds which can be quantitated only with extensive biochemical procedures (Zumoff, Fukushima, & Hellman, 1974). Therefore, although there is a theoretical advantage to measuring total urinary excretion of metabolic products to assess total adrenocortical activity, this is not practical in most laboratory settings. Therefore, most investigators determine the levels of unchanged cortisol in a given biological fluid that has been collected over a specified period of time, understanding that this measure is proportional but not equal to total secretion. For example, although urine cortisol represents less than 5% of the cortisol that has been secreted, it is proportional to that percentage of circulating cortisol that is not bound to plasma protein, and so approximates that amount of secreted hormone that is biologically active.

Sampling Compartment

Cortisol measures that are relevant to studies of cardiovascular function can be made in urine, blood, and saliva. Adrenal steroid content, or the venous drainage of the adrenal (a strategy used by clinicians) are neither practical nor necessary for behavioral studies. The choice of sampling compartment depends on the information which is needed, and the available methodology. The period of time over which secretion is measured, the setting in which the analysis will be conducted (i.e., in the hospital, with nursing personnel, or in a laboratory or naturalistic setting), and the analytic methods available for assay all contribute to this choice. As a first approximation, urinary excretion is most useful for measuring cortisol secretion over a period of hours or days, salivary secretion over hours, while plasma must be sampled to evaluate minute-by-minute changes in secretion.

Urine output has been used historically primarily for methodologic reasons: the original assays for measuring glucocorticoid hormones were not sensitive enough to detect the levels of cortisol found in blood. Methodologic developments now permit quantitation of either unchanged cortisol or total excretory products of the adrenal gland. However, the latter analysis is quite complex because cortisol is so extensively metabolized, as mentioned above. Although measurement of urine cortisol represents only a fraction of total steroid secretion (less than 5%), it is thought to be proportional to free cortisol in blood, and so probably reflects transient secretory events better than the less sensitive fluorometric assays which detect a combination of cortisol and its metabolites. The contribution of metabolites to the latter measure automatically integrates the measure of secretion over a longer period of time.

Quantitation of urinary steroid output still gives the best estimate of total secretion over a long time period (hours rather than minutes), because the total activity of the adrenal gland over the urine collection period is automatically "integrated." This contrasts with measures of plasma cortisol, which reflect only adrenocortical activity of the preceding several minutes. The former approach provides a definite advantage in studies of chronic behavioral influences on cardiovascular pathology. Furthermore, changes in urinary cortisol excretion in response to acute interventions can be detected with appropriate experimental paradigms (Frankenhaeuser, 1982; Zumoff et al., 1974). Therefore, measurement of urinary cortisol excretion represents a viable option where it is difficult to obtain multiple blood samples.

One major difficulty in obtaining accurate urinary measures of adrenocortical hormones in experimental studies is a simple pragmatic issue: obtaining a complete urine sample for the time period under investigation. This is particularly true for long collection times. However, the major limitations of 24-h urinary cortisol measures are not methodologic, but theoretical: it is difficult to evaluate the physiologic significance of changes below the pathologic range. Furthermore, a profound secretory response to one or several environmental events of cardiovascular significance (e.g., exercise, "stressful" events) can be significantly diluted by the secretion occurring during the remainder of the day.

Evaluation of plasma cortisol provides a more sensitive index of transient secretory events. However, it must be reemphasized that measurement of a single plasma sample, or even two samples taken at the diurnal peak and nadir of secretion, are of less value than sequential samples taken at fairly short intervals (5–15 min) preceding, during, and following a specific experimental manipulation that alters secretion. Obviously, such determinations can be made only in fairly sophisticated laboratory settings. However, the strength of this approach is that these measures permit more detailed correlation with cardiovascular assessments. Furthermore, the psychologic aspects of the environment can be controlled to provide information about the neural pathways and personality variables that contribute to cortisol responses. Finally, it should be mentioned that cortisol secretion, like cardiovascular function, is markedly affected by a number of commonly used drugs. Nicotine, caffeine, and β-adrenergic antagonists are all known to alter either basal or stimulated cortisol secretion (Streeten et al., 1982). These variables would provide an unwanted complication of experimental studies.

The measurement of certain hormones in saliva has provided a new opportunity for evaluation of hormone levels in environmental settings in which it was previously impossible (Umeda et al., 1981; Read-Fahmy, Reat, & Walker, 1982; Landon, Smith, Perry, & Al-Ansari, 1984; Walker, Joyce, Dyas, & Read-Fahmy, 1984). For example, steroid secretion can be determined by nonmedical personnel in infants, or in school or work settings where blood collections are impossible. This approach is based on the lipid solubility of the biologically important steroids: cortisol, estradiol, progesterone, and testosterone all diffuse rapidly into the salivary fluid, so that concentration in this compartment rapidly equilibrates with that percentage of circulating cortisol that is not bound to plasma protein. Therefore, salivary concentrations approximate those of unbound plasma steroids under most conditions. Diffusion of steroids is a rapid and passive process, so there is no substantial difference in the concentration of steroids in saliva from different salivary glands, or in salivary concentrations at different rates of salivary secretion. All the normal patterns of steroid secretion that are observed in blood also can be seen in saliva. Diurnal rhythms in secretion, rises with administration of exogenous steroids, suppression with dexamethasone, stimulation by insulin and other conventional evocative tests of secretion all have been verified by simultaneous collection of plasma and saliva samples. An excellent review of this topic is provided in Read-Fahmy et al. (1982).

Saliva collection is simple. The standard method involves stimulating the flow of saliva with a piece of candy, or with a mild acid, and collecting saliva into a Lashley cup or other container. Although fresh saliva is quite viscous and difficult to pipette, freezing alleviates this problem (Read-Fahmy et al., 1982). If small (0.5 ml) sample sizes are taken, multiple samples can be taken over a period of several hours. Even larger samples can be taken with sampling intervals of hours rather than minutes, although most steroid RIAs can detect steroids even in the smaller sample sizes.

There are several special considerations in measuring salivary production of cortisol. First, amounts are equal to the unbound portion of cortisol in blood. These levels are very low (1–15% of total plasma levels), and increase disproportionately in relation to blood levels when secretion exceeds the capacity of plasma binding sites (at very high physiologic levels of secretion). These low levels are most easily measured by RIA, and detection by less sensitive measures requires collections of inconveniently large (several milliliters) samples. Second, changes in saliva levels can differ from plasma somewhat, lagging by minutes during rises, but falling more rapidly (Figure 4). Therefore, the timing of samples must be somewhat different. As salivary cortisol determinations have not been used extensively in behavioral studies, there is not yet a large data base available for comparison, and parallel determinations of plasma and salivary levels would be advisable when starting a new experimental protocol. Finally, some authors report a small amount of metabolism of cortisol to cortisone in saliva, although this does not seem to cause marked changes in salivary concentrations.

Despite the drawbacks, salivary cortisol determinations offer several definite advantages in assessing glucocorticoid output. As salivary cortisol is proportional to the fraction of cortisol in blood that is not bound to plasma protein, it reflects the concentration of the "biologically active" fraction of circulating glucocorticoid. Therefore, the disproportionate increase observed during stress might better reflect the concentration of hormone that is delivered to tissues. For this reason, and the considerable convenience of collection techniques in comparison to obtaining blood samples, salivary cortisol determinations will probably be used increasingly in the future.

Timing of Sample

Obviously, different timing strategies are appropriate with different measures of glucocorticoid output. Urinary cortisol is commonly measured either as a 24-h output or as total excretion over a stated amount of time (generally in hours rather than minutes). As mentioned earlier, the challenge of using urinary measures is that complete collection during the time period is assured, and that results be normalized to body weight (by creatinine clearance or some other method) to control for the known variation of cortisol output with body weight. Salivary collections are most useful if collected as sequential samples over several hours. When validating the use of salivary assessments to detect changes in hormone secretion, parallel determination of plasma cortisol is optimal in establishing the behavioral protocol, as mentioned above. The timing of blood sampling is critical in

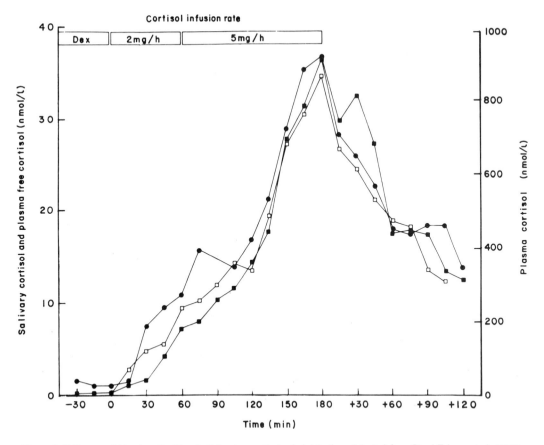

Figure 4. Salivary and blood cortisol levels following cortisol administration. Adapted from Read-Fahmy *et al.* (1982).

assessment of cortisol responses to experimental manipulations. The most sophisticated methodology is the continuous withdrawal of blood with an exfusion pump over 5- to 20-min intervals. This method provides an integrated sample of secretion over the sampling period, and so includes secretory bursts that might be missed by single blood samples. It is critical to implant the withdrawal catheter a significant (at least 1 h) period of time before the experiment, and to make several baseline determinations well before the start of the manipulation. The latter samples are necessary to detect "anticipatory" rises in secretion as well as to assess baseline secretion. As mentioned above, changes in cortisol secretion frequently are slower than changes in cardiovascular parameters, and can be harder to elicit. Therefore, the particular

experimental manipulation must be intense and prolonged enough to elicit a change in ACTH secretion.

Methodology for Assessing Cortisol Secretion

Adrenocortical steroid determinations that are useful for behavioral studies differ considerably from those required by clinicians to identify specific disorders of steroid metabolism. While the latter can involve extensive methodologic verification of many different cortisol precursors and metabolites, behavioral studies require measurement of a single hormone, cortisol itself. However, large numbers of samples must be processed, and multiple sampling often severely limits the size of each individual sample. Furthermore, these studies are often conducted in an environment which lacks extensive technical support. Therefore, the assays must be sensitive, convenient for processing large sample numbers, simple enough for relatively unskilled laboratory personnel, and relatively inexpensive. The current methodologies for evaluating adrenocortical steroids are reviewed below, with these considerations in mind.

Fluorometric Assays

Historical evaluation of adrenocortical secretion was based on the fluorescent product of the 17-hydroxycorticoids and phenylhydrazine (the Porter–Silber reaction; Silber & Porter, 1954). The advantages of this methodology are its simplicity, low cost, and the broad base of historical data on which to evaluate determinations. The disadvantages are that it represents a combined measurement of cortisol and several of its hydroxylated metabolites (e.g., cortisone, tetrahydrocortisol) as well as a number of common drugs including spironolactone and chlordiazepoxide. It has basically been replaced by other methodologies. Furthermore, the large sample sizes needed (0.5–1 ml of plasma) limit the utility of this method for measuring steroids in multiple, small blood samples like those obtained from indwelling catheters.

Corticosteroid Binding Protein Assays

The radioligand binding assay of Murphy (Murphy, Engelberg, & Patter, 1963; Murphy, 1968) is one of the most common methods used in clinical laboratories for assessing cortisol levels in biologic fluids. This assay is based on the binding of a radiolabeled compound (generally cortisol) to a semipurified preparation of the corticosteroid binding globulin (CBG). Cortisol levels in experimental samples are measured as the displacement of radiolabel from the binding protein by unlabeled hormone in the sample. The method involves simply incubating label and binding protein for a short period of time to allow equilibration of hormone with the binding protein. Protein-bound and unbound hormone are separated by adsorption of free

hormone onto any one of a number of substances, including charcoal and florisil. Cortisol is quantitated by measuring the amount of label displaced from the binding site by the cortisol in the sample. The advantages of this technique are its greater sensitivity relative to the fluorometric technique, its simplicity, low cost, and specificity. However, the procedure is fairly time-consuming, and the specificity of the CBG is not absolute: progesterone, 11-deoxycortisol, testosterone, and corticosterone interfere. Although plasma concentrations of these substances are low, this lack of specificity presents a problem in situations where levels of any of these steroids have been elevated for some reason.

RIA

The advent of practical RIA techniques for steroids provided a methodologic improvement which greatly facilitated large-scale studies of cortisol secretion (Abraham, 1974). This advance was made possible by the development of techniques for generating antibodies to small molecules through covalent linkage to antigenic proteins. RIA methods are identical in principle to the CBG method described above, with the simple substitution of an antibody for the CBG as a binding site. The binding of steroid at equilibrium in an RIA is somewhat more stable than in CBG assays, a characteristic which offers some advantage in the separation of bound and free protein, and facilitates the processing of larger numbers of samples.

The commercial availability of sensitive and specific antisera for cortisol has made RIA the method of choice in most laboratories. The specificity of most commercial antisera now available is good enough that assays can be conducted without any sample purification. The availability of radioactive tracers labeled with ^{125}I instead of ^3H has greatly increased assay sensitivity, although slightly more elaborate laboratory safety precautions are required for handling gamma-emitting radiation. The advantages of RIA are the greater sensitivity (although poor antisera will approximate the sensitivity of the CBG method), ease, and speed. Most experimental studies which involve repetitive blood sampling require high sensitivity and easy processing of large numbers of samples, which are most easily adapted to RIA.

Most RIA methods for cortisol simply involve combining a small amount of plasma (5–100 μl), antiserum, and radioactive hormone and allowing them to incubate for a period of hours, followed by separation of bound and free hormone by the charcoal method mentioned above, or by a second antibody technique. Radioactivity in samples is simply counted, as in the CBG method. The recent availability of "solid-phase" assays in which the antiserum is bound to a solid support has facilitated this process even further.

Rigid quality controls must be conducted to control for variability in assay performance. The biggest problems are generally assay-to-assay variability and differences in performance among assays from different suppliers (Ritchie, Varroll, Olton, Shively, & Feinberg, 1985). The best strategy for assuring reproducibility and accuracy of cortisol determinations is to conduct these determinations in a laboratory environment with a historical background of normal values for the particular assay and patient population. Experimental design of longitudinal studies must include control for variability in assay performance over time. The optimal method for comparing such samples is to collect samples over a period of time, and conduct the assays simultaneously.

One final variant of the RIA method which has recently been applied to assay of cortisol is the development of enzyme-linked immunosorbent (ELISA) assays (Lewis & Elder, 1985) incubating a sample on a microtiter plate on which the antibody for cortisol has been immobilized. Following this incubation, the plates are incubated with a second antibody linked to peroxidase followed by a substrate for the enzyme. The color developed on the plate is read by a specialized spectrophotometer that is adapted to use with the 12-well plastic dishes in which the assay is conducted. The color measured is inversely proportional to the amount of cortisol bound to the first antibody. The advantage of this technique is that it does not require the use of any radioactive reagents, and therefore is safer and more economical than standard RIAs. The disadvantage is that a certain amount of specialized equipment that is not yet common to most endocrine laboratories is required, and that the sensitivity does not quite approach that available with standard RIA. Nevertheless, this technique is rapidly gaining popularity.

Other Methods

Cortisol can also be measured by gas chromatography–mass spectrometry (GC-MS), HPLC followed by fluorometric detection and double isotope derivative techniques. While these methods are more specific and accurate, they are also considerably more time-consuming, and require much more complicated instrumentation. Therefore, they are of most benefit in validating more convenient assay techniques.

Sample Preparation

Fortunately, steroid hormones are very stable in urine, plasma, and saliva. Therefore, no extraordinary measures are necessary for preservation. Samples should be kept cold (including 24-h urine samples) to prevent bacterial growth. Blood samples should be centrifuged promptly after collection, although this is not as critical an issue as it is for determination of certain peptides. Fresh saliva is quite viscous and difficult to pipette. However, simply freezing the saliva and centrifuging it briefly or sonicating it usually eliminates this problem. Urine, plasma, or saliva samples can be stored frozen (preferably at −30–80°C) for months without loss of hormone.

For RIA, sample volume is almost never a consideration, because the volume needed for assay is so small (5–100 μl of plasma). However, for other techniques, the size of the sample (0.1–1.0 ml) must be determined by the sensitivity of the assay.

Gonadal Steroids

Gonadal Steroids and Cardiovascular Function

The role of gonadal steroids in cardiovascular function is incompletely understood. However, numerous epidemiologic studies are suggestive of a role for gonadal steroids in some cardiovascular diseases. The greater prevalence of cardiovascular disease in males than in females up until the age of menopause forms the basis of much of the current interest in gonadal steroid hormones (Hazzard, 1984, 1985). However, there has been considerably less investigation of other issues, including the responsivity of gonadal steroids to behavioral stimuli, the adverse cardiovascular consequences of excessive androgen or estrogen administration and the cardiovascular pathology associated with abnormal endocrine states (e.g., the hypertension of pregnancy). Hopefully, a clear description of the appropriate measures will facilitate these important areas of research.

Gonadal steroids have been implicated in several specific biochemical changes associated with cardiovascular pathology. In males, a relationship of gonadal steroids, elevated levels of low-density lipoproteins (LDL) and low levels of high-density lipoproteins (HDL), and atherosclerosis has been suggested (Luria *et al.*, 1982). Whether this pattern is caused by testosterone or its metabolism to active derivatives (estradiol or dihydrotestosterone) is not clear. The reported association between estradiol production in males and increased incidence of atherosclerosis and myocardial infarction supports the latter hypothesis (Knopp, Walden, & Wahl, 1981; Klaibern *et al.*, 1982; Phillips, Castell, Abbott, & McNamara, 1983). However, only a few studies have reported levels of these hormones, and these have been in seriously ill patients (following myocardial infarction) in whom it was impossible to determine if the abnormal hormone levels were a cause or a result of the pathology. The converse question has been studied in females: the purported relationship between gonadal function and a "protective" pattern of high plasma levels of HDL and a reversal of this pattern at menopause.

The responsivity of gonadal steroid secretion to behavioral stimuli is particularly relevant to the present topic. A growing literature demonstrates that certain behavioral states are associated with marked changes in gonadal steroid secretion. Many different "stressors" have been associated with suppression of gonadal function in both males

and females (Mason *et al.*, 1968; Nakashima *et al.*, 1975; Gray, Smith, Damassa, Ehrenkranz, & Davidson, 1978). However, the psychologic "domain" to which testosterone responds is probably considerably different from cortisol. Gonadal steroid secretion seems to be strongly controlled by behavioral cues related to social status, reproductive success, and aggression. For example, gonadal steroid production and status in a dominance hierarchy are highly related in several primate social groups. In both males and females, elevated status is usually associated with increased secretion of gonadal steroids and improved reproductive performance (Rose, Gordon, & Bernstein, 1972; Leshner, 1980; Adams, Kaplan, Clarkson, & Koritnik, 1984; Kaplan, Manuck, Clarkson, Lusso, & Taub, 1982; Kaplan, Adams, Clarkson, & Koritnik, 1984). Furthermore, these changes in hormone secretion are associated with demonstrable changes in cardiovascular function, specifically with the degree of atherosclerosis. Furthermore, the direction of change is opposite in males and females. In one primate study, the incidence of atherosclerosis in dominant females was significantly lower than in submissive females, and directly correlated with gonadal function (Adams *et al.*, 1984; Kaplan *et al.*, 1984). In males, social dominance is also associated with higher levels of gonadal steroids, and in this case, with enhanced rather than reduced atherosclerosis (Kaplan *et al.*, 1982; Rose *et al.*, 1972).

Behaviorally induced changes in gonadal steroid secretion have been demonstrated less frequently under controlled experimental conditions. Again, these changes seem to reflect different aspects of the environment. For example, plasma testosterone increases in response to sexual but not violent content of movies (Hellhammer, Hubert, & Schurmeyer, 1985; Christiansen, Knussmann, & Couwenbergs, 1985). However, acute changes in LH, estradiol, or testosterone secretion to behavioral manipulations are being investigated in laboratory settings, as is cortisol, as a "marker" for neural mechanisms associated with personality/behavioral traits and/or neural pathways that are relevant for cardiovascular pathology. For example, our studies have shown transient increases in testosterone secretion in males during vigilant observation of sensory stimuli (Williams *et al.*, 1982). Recent studies suggest that behavioral stimuli can modulate gonadal steroid production either through regulation of LH secretion from the pituitary, or through the described sympathetic innervation of the ovaries and testes (Kawakami, Kubo, Uemura, Nagase, & Hayashi, 1981).

The relationship between falling estradiol and progesterone production during menopause and increasing levels of atherosclerosis remains a major focus of studies of age-related change in gonadal steroid secretion and cardiovascular pathology. Another possibility which has been investigated is the relationship between falling testosterone, increasing estradiol, and coronary artery disease in males. Long-term changes in gonadal steroid production might play a significant role in cardiovascular pathology to an even greater extent than cortisol.

Patterns of Gonadal Steroid Secretion

Normal Secretion

Testosterone and estradiol, the major gonadal steroids in males and females respectively, are synthesized in the testes and ovaries by side chain cleavage of cholesterol under the influence of luteinizing hormone (LH) secreted by the pituitary (for review see Griffin & Wilson, 1980; Bondy & Rosenberg, 1980; Streeten *et al.*, 1982). LH secretion from the pituitary is regulated by LH-releasing hormone (LHRH) from specific hypothalamic neurons. In the male, secretion of LHRH in small pulses throughout the day maintains a fairly stable level of testosterone in blood, although careful monitoring over a 24-h period can demonstrate the true pulsatility of the secretion, as well as the small diurnal variation in secretion (Figure 5). Testosterone, like cortisol, is removed from the circulation quickly by metabolism in the liver via 3-hydroxylation, 17-oxidation, and the formation of glucuronide and sulfate conjugates of these polar metabolites. However, a small percentage of testosterone (10–15%) is converted in peripheral tissues to active hormones (Figure 5). Dihydrotestosterone is produced in specific target tissues where it is the active hormone. In addition, a small amount is aromatized in peripheral tissues to estradiol, a process which increases with aging.

In females, cyclic release of LHRH establishes the monthly pattern of estradiol and progesterone secretion. The phases of steroid secretion are best understood in relation to the midcycle surge of LH and resultant ovulation. Estradiol secretion rises to a peak during the first half (follicular) of the cycle, reaching maximal levels just before ovulation. Subsequently, secretion falls briefly, then rises to higher plateau levels during the (second) luteal phase of the cycle. Progesterone is secreted mainly during the luteal phase of the cycle by the developing corpus luteum (Figure 5). Estradiol is removed by metabolism in the liver, mainly by 17-oxidation to estrone and further 16-hydroxylation to estriol, which is the major urinary metabolite. While estradiol production is tightly controlled by LH and therefore vulnerable to behaviorally induced changes in LH secretion, progesterone secretion by the corpus luteum appears to be more autonomous.

Cyclic hormone secretion in females necessarily requires careful standardization of experimental studies to a particular point in the cycle. Such standardization requires considerable cooperation from the experimental subject, as evaluation of basal body temperature and/or measurements of luteal-phase progesterone are necessary to verify cycle status. The inconvenience of such assessments has discouraged studies of cardiovascular function in females, and hopefully these can be outlined sufficiently in this chapter to facilitate such studies in the future.

Stress-Induced Changes in Secretion

As mentioned above, basal secretory rates for testosterone and estradiol within the normal range may be of considerable importance in cardiovascular function. In males, for example, the ratio of estradiol to testosterone has been related to the incidence of myocardial infarction. Similarly, in females, the presence or absence of cyclic hormone changes and the absolute level of estrogen and progesterone are probably quite important.

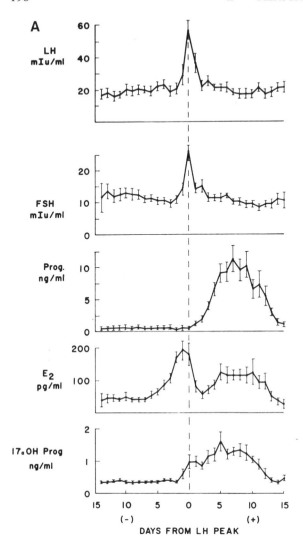

Figure 5. Patterns of daily secretion of reproductive hormones in females (A) and males (B). Daily samples were collected in women through an entire menstrual cycle. Samples in men were collected from an indwelling cannula at 20-min intervals over 24 h, to demonstrate pulsatility of testosterone secretion. A from Thorneycroft *et al.* (1971); B from Griffin and Wilson (1980).

Therefore, evaluation of basal hormone levels has greater utility than baseline determinations. Furthermore, changes over long periods of time, as during the years of menopause, or during the months following a disruption of social environment may be of considerable significance. Therefore, cross-sectional studies across the life span, or longitudinal studies of specific individuals represent important areas of investigation.

Stress-induced changes in gonadal steroid production might also contribute to cardiovascular pathology. Both increases and decreases in LH and estradiol or testosterone production can occur, de-

pending on the behavioral stimulus. These changes can be detected within minutes, but they tend to be small in magnitude. Although stress is conventionally thought to suppress gonadal function, recent studies suggest that some acute interventions might increase LH, through CNS mechanisms stimulatory to LHRH release, or through a recently described sympathetic innervation of the testes and ovaries which is activated by general sympathetic arousal. The latter obviously has greater significance in understanding possible gonadal steroid contributions to behaviorally induced changes in cardiovascular function. Careful studies of the be-

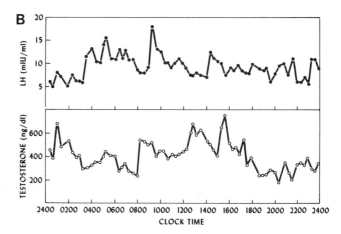

Figure 5. (Continued)

havioral manipulations which increase or decrease gonadal function, analogous to the published studies of cortisol secretion, represent an important future direction for investigation of gonadal steroids and cardiovascular function.

Experimental Evaluation of Steroid Secretion

Three different aspects of gonadal steroid production should be studied experimentally. First is the simple evaluation of basal levels of testosterone, estradiol, progesterone, or more rarely, evaluation of secretion over a 24-h period through analysis of urinary secretion. Second, recent studies strongly suggest that experimental investigation of evoked secretion will be of increasing importance. Finally, evaluation of menstrual status will be discussed, as the perceived difficulty of this measure has probably significantly hampered important research in the area of sex differences in cardiovascular function.

Hormone to Be Measured

Two different strategies can be used to evaluate hormone secretion. Levels of the major active hormone secreted by the gonads (estradiol and progesterone for females, testosterone for males) can be assessed, or some metabolite or combination of metabolites can be determined. For example, extragonadal production of estradiol is thought to be important in cardiovascular pathology in aging males.

Urinary measures of unchanged hormone have been used historically, mainly because available methods were limited to the high concentrations present in this biological fluid. Furthermore, estradiol and testosterone are extensively degraded to metabolites that also are derived from adrenal steroids. Therefore, evaluation of metabolite levels is less appropriate in most cases. Measurement of unchanged steroid provides a more accurate measure for most studies of behaviorally relevant changes in hormone secretion. In this regard, such studies differ considerably from conventional endocrinologic evaluation of gonadal steroid production, in which careful analysis of different metabolite patterns is vital for determining the source of inappropriate or inadequate hormone secretion.

The determination of LH in place of the gonadal steroids is a strategy which has been underutilized in studies of gonadal steroids and cardiovascular pathology. LH is markedly responsive to stress in most mammals, and necessarily responds more promptly than gonadal steroids. As measurement of ACTH secretion has supplanted cortisol in those few laboratories which have an accurate RIA for ACTH, in certain studies, evaluation of LH might be more appropriate than testosterone or estradiol. The benefit of measuring gonadal steroids is that blood levels of the active hormone are measured. However, LH determination provides the advantage of greater sensitivity to acute manipulations.

Sampling CompartmentTiming of Sampling Collection

Such an approach would be particularly appropriate in studies of neural mechanisms mediating changes in gonadal steroid production, where a more sensitive index of hypothalamopituitary gonadal function would be beneficial. Many good RIAs of LH are available, unlike ACTH. Therefore, there is less methodologic limitation to this approach. The major consideration in these studies is the difficulty of determining changes in secretion rate despite the pulsatile nature of normal LH secretion.

Sampling Compartment

Estradiol and testosterone are both extremely lipid soluble, and so measurement in plasma, saliva, and urine provides indices of secretion rates. The differences among these measures are similar to those for sampling of cortisol in these three compartments. Urinary measures provide an integrated value of secretion over a long period (24 h, or the duration of the sampling). Therefore, they provide the best measure for total secretion over an extended time period (Jeffcoate, 1975). However, unchanged steroid represents only a small fraction of secreted estradiol and testosterone, and true evaluation of total hormone production would require either complex pharmacokinetic analysis of injected steroid, or equally difficult determination of total metabolites in urine. This approach should be used only when total secretion over a long period of time must be determined.

Estradiol and testosterone levels in saliva reflect the small percentage of total circulating hormone (1–10%) that is not bound to plasma protein, and is therefore free for diffusion into saliva (Luisi *et al.*, 1980; Chearskul, Rincon-Rodriguez, Sofi, Donaldson, & Jeffcoate, 1982; Ferguson, 1984). As with cortisol, this provides a convenient and accurate measure of the physiologically active pool of circulating hormone, and has been shown in many studies to reflect changes in gonadal steroid production associated with different phases of the menstrual cycle, pregnancy, and disorders of steroid production. The physicochemical factors determining estradiol, progesterone, and testosterone movement into saliva are similar to those for

cortisol. Therefore, the strengths and limitations of this approach are about the same. However, salivary assessment of gonadal steroids has been used more extensively than that of cortisol. Therefore, there is a broader base of information about normal values. Furthermore, salivary assessments might be particularly useful in plotting cyclic changes in progesterone secretion, e.g., because sample collection at daily intervals would be much easier and safer than daily blood withdrawal. However, as for cortisol, laboratory studies of evoked changes in secretion over a period of minutes during behavioral challenge would require validation of this approach first.

Measurement of plasma hormone levels represents the most useful strategy for assessing gonadal steroid production over short time periods. However, they represent only hormone that is being actively secreted, and do not necessarily reflect secretion over an extended period of time. As with cortisol, total gonadal secretion could only be determined through continuous blood withdrawal over a 24-h period. However, normative values are well described, current assay methodologies are sensitive enough for these determinations, and the methodology, unlike some peptide determinations, is readily available in most medical centers.

Timing of Sampling Collection

Basal Secretion. Evaluation of basal hormone levels can be achieved through a single or, optimally, several pooled baseline samples. Testosterone is secreted in small pulses during the day. Therefore, a single determination of pooled blood from several sequential samples taken at 20-min intervals at any time of day provides an accurate assessment (Yen & Jaffe, 1986). As discussed below, single determinations of estradiol or progesterone have little meaning unless taken at a defined point in the menstrual cycle.

Episodic or Evoked Secretion. As described for cortisol, the most accurate assessment of blood levels of hormones that are secreted episodically is obtained through repetitive blood sampling with an indwelling venous catheter. This technique is vital for measurement of LH, but is rarely used for estradiol or testosterone. For experimental determination of correlations between cardiovascular indices and levels of gonadal steroids, sequential collection of several samples provides a more accurate measure than does a single sample. Such studies, as described for cortisol, are absolutely necessary to determine behaviorally induced changes in secretion. They are even more vital for evaluation of testosterone and estradiol, as the changes in evoked secretion are smaller, and therefore closer in size to the magnitude of a spontaneous pulse in secretion.

Like cortisol, testosterone and estradiol production lag behind changes in LH secretion. Therefore, changes are rarely observed sooner than 20–30 min following a manipulation which produces marked changes in LH secretion. Furthermore, changes relevant to cardiovascular function often occur even more slowly, over a period of weeks, months, or years. For example, reported decreases in testosterone production occurred over a period of weeks of basic training in Army recruits (Kreuz, Rose, & Jennings, 1972) and the changes in gonadal steroid production in aging populations are even more gradual (Steger, 1982).

Evaluation of Menstrual Status. Evaluation of menstrual status is obligatory even in studies of basal or stress-evoked secretion of gonadal steroids in females, in order to establish the physiologic significance of levels. It is probably of even greater importance in the growing number of studies of sex differences in physiologic or behavioral rather than endocrine parameters. Recent studies suggest that variations in behavioral measures and cardiovascular physiology occur during the menstrual cycle (Abplanalp, Livingston, Rose, & Sanwisch, 1977; Hastrup & Light, 1984; Collins, Eneroth, & Landgren, 1985). Many studies report sex differences in various cardiovascular parameters without any regard to possible cyclic changes in these measures in the female populations. Although the optimal method for establishing cyclicity involves daily blood samples, several alternative strategies can be used in establishing menstrual status and in choosing an appropriate

time for study. The goal of these evaluations is to establish (1) the time of ovulation, (2) the presence of the follicular (postmenstrual) phase, and (3) the presence of the luteal (postovulatory) phase.

The choice of when to conduct studies is another vital issue. For studies of normal females in comparison to males, many investigators choose an arbitrary point midway through the follicular phase, avoiding the pronounced and rapid endocrine fluctuations at ovulation and those preceding menstruation. The latter strategy provides the most stable endocrine baseline, but prevents detection of effects mediated by the high progesterone levels which occur only during the luteal phase of the cycle. For studies of cyclic changes, obviously, studies must be conducted at each phase of the cycle. These can be quite difficult, as the exact timing of ovulation can be somewhat variable; verification of the cycle requires more extensive endocrine evaluation.

The most inaccurate method of evaluating cycle status is to rely upon self-report of cycle length, with success rates only at about the 50% level. However, this is the method most frequently used. This problem results more from variabilities in cycle length than in failure of the subject to report accurately. Therefore, one situation in which this can be used successfully is in establishing the presence of the follicular phase by counting a specific number of days from the onset of menses, which can be used to approximate midfollicular phase.

The presence of ovulation and significant progesterone secretion during the luteal phase of the cycle results in an increase in basal body temperature that can be determined simply without any invasive procedures. Although this method has been used successfully in fertility control, it has several obvious limitations. First, the amount of rise is variable, and will not be adequate in all individuals. Second, it requires at least several daily measures, and therefore considerable cooperation on the part of the experimental subject. Therefore, it is of limited utility without verification by measurement of progesterone.

The presence of ovulation and a successful luteal phase is best established by progesterone measurement. However, levels of hormones are variable enough from individual to individual that determining the rise in progesterone after ovulation by taking a measure before and after is preferable to a single determination. Therefore, a single determination is only useful if conducted in a setting with a considerable data base on which to evaluate a single measure.

Daily assessment of estradiol, progesterone, and LH represents the only definitive method for establishing the cycle. However, these parameters are rarely known until after the experiment has been conducted, and so these are of most utility if a single subject is being tested repeatedly throughout a cycle. Obviously, these determinations are time-consuming and expensive, and probably are unnecessary if the goal is simply to study a normal female population.

Methodology

Methodology for measurement of gonadal steroids has followed much the same history as cortisol determination. Original studies were based on fluorometric reactions following chromatographic separation of the hormone of interest. These assays originally lacked the sensitivity for detection of plasma hormone levels. Protein binding assays followed which were subject to the same advantages and limitations as the CBG assay. As the methodology for RIA of steroids became widely available, this became the method of choice for estradiol and testosterone determinations (Nieschlag & Wickins, 1978).

There are currently many commercially available RIA kits for estradiol and testosterone. These vary in sensitivity, specificity, and other assay details. The relevant differences, as with cortisol, are specificity and sensitivity. Chromatographic purification of samples is required for kits with antisera that show some cross-reactivity with other circulating steroids. This obviously involves considerably more work, and more opportunity for error. As production of antisera with better specificity progresses, availability of commercial kits that can be used without elaborate sample preparation is improving.

Sensitivity of assays is more of an issue for testosterone, estradiol, and progesterone than for cortisol, because salivary levels are at the limit of sensitivity for some assays. This has been dealt with in two ways. First, radioactive tracers labeled with ^{125}I instead of ^{3}H have been used. Second, more sensitive and specific antisera have been utilized in salivary assays.

Sample preparation involves most of the same considerations as discussed previously for corticosterone. Estradiol, progesterone, and testosterone are all extremely stable in biologic fluids. Samples should be kept refrigerated, and stored frozen as described for cortisol. The major consideration is the amount of purification required by the particular assay. Some assays simply require inactivation of the binding protein. Others require a single solvent extraction (petroleum ether for progesterone, methylene chloride or similar solvent for testosterone or estradiol).

References

Abplanalp, J. M., Livingston, L., Rose, R., & Sanwisch, D. (1977). Cortisol and growth hormone responses to psychological stress during the menstrual cycle. *Psychosomatic Medicine, 39,* 158–177.

Abraham, G. E. (Ed.). (1974). Radioimmunoassay of steroids in biological fluids. *Acta Endocrinologica Supplementum, 183.*

Adams, M. R., Kaplan, J. R., Clarkson, T. B., & Koritnik, D. R. (1984). Ovariectomy, social status and atherosclerosis in cynomolgus monkeys. *Arteriosclerosis, 5,* 192–200.

Bjorkerud, S. (1974). Effect of adrenocortical hormones on the integrity of rat aortic endothelium. In Shettler, G., & Weizler, A. (Eds.), *Atherosclerosis III* (pp. 245–249). Berlin: Springer.

Bondy, P. K., & Rosenberg, L. (1980). *Metabolic control and disease* (8th ed.). Philadelphia: Saunders.

Chearskul, S., Rincon-Rodriguez, I., Sofi, S. B., Donaldson, A., & Jeffcoate, L. (1982). Simple, direct assays for the measurement of estradiol and progesterone in saliva. In *Radioimmunoassay and related procedures in medicine* (pp. 265–274). Vienna: IAEA.

Christiansen, K., Knussmann, R., & Couwenbergs, C. (1985). Sex hormones and stress in the human male. *Hormones and Behavior, 19,* 426–440.

Collins, A., Eneroth, P., & Landgren, B. M. (1985). Psychoneuroendocrine stress responses and mood as related to the menstrual cycle. *Psychosomatic Medicine, 47,* 512–527.

Estep, H. L., Island, D. P., Neu, R. L., & Liddle, G. W. (1968). Pituitary adrenal dynamics during surgical states. *Journal of Clinical Endocrinology and Metabolism, 23,* 419–425.

Ferguson, D. B. (1984). Physiological considerations in the use of salivary steroid estimation for clinical investigations. *Frontiers of Oral Physiology, 5,* 1–20.

Frankenhaeuser, M. (1982). The sympathetic and pituitary–adrenal response to challenge: Comparison between the sexes. In T. Dembroski, T. H. Schmidt, & G. Blumchen (Eds.), *Biobehavioral basis of coronary heart disease* (pp. 91–106). Basel: Karger.

Frederikson, M., Sundin, O., & Frankenhaeuser, M. (1985). Cortisol excretion during the defense reaction in humans. *Psychosomatic Medicine, 47,* 313–319.

Friedman, M., George, S., Byers, S. O., & Rosenman, R. H. (1960). Excretion of catecholamines, 17-ketosteroids, 17-hydroxycorticoids and 5-hydroxyindole in men exhibiting a particular behavior pattern (A) associated with high incidence of clinical coronary artery disease. *Journal of Clinical Investigation, 39,* 758–764.

Gray, G. D., Smith, E. R., Damassa, D. A., Ehrenkranz, J. R. L. & Davidson, J. M. (1978). Neuroendocrine mechanisms mediating the suppression of circulating testosterone levels associated with chronic stress in male rats. *Neuroendocrinology, 25,* 247–256.

Griffin, J. E., & Wilson, J. D. (1980). The testis. In P. K. Bondy & L. E. Rosenberg (Eds.), *Metabolic control and disease* (pp. 1535–1620). Philadelphia: Saunders.

Hartley, H. L., Mason, J. W., Hogan, R. P., Jones, L. G., Kotchen, T. A., Moughey, E. H., Wherry, F. E., Pennington, L. L., & Ricketts, P. T. (1972). Multiple hormonal responses to graded exercise in relation of physical training. *Journal of Applied Physiology, 33,* 602–606.

Hastrup, J. L., & Light, K. C. (1984). Sex differences in cardiovascular stress responses: Modulation as a function of menstrual cycle phases. *Journal of Psychosomatic Research, 28,* 475–483.

Hazzard, W. R. (1984). The sex differential in longevity. In R. A. Andres & E. L. Bierman (Eds.), *Principles of geriatric medicine* (pp. 72–81). New York: McGraw-Hill.

Hazzard, W. R. (1985). Atherogenesis: Why women live longer. *Geriatrics, 40,* 42–54.

Hellhammer, D. H., Hubert, W., & Schurmeyer, H. T. (1985). Changes in saliva testosterone after psychological stimulation in men. *Psychoneuroendocrinology, 10,* 77–81.

Henry, J. P., Stephens, P. M., & Santisteban, G. A. (1975). A model of psychosocial hypertension showing reversibility and progression of cardiovascular complications. *Circulation Research, 36,* 156–164.

Henry, J. P., Kross, M. E., Stephens, P. M., & Watson, F. M. C. (1976). Evidence that differing psychosocial stimuli lead to adrenal cortical stimulation by autonomic or endocrine pathways. In E. Usdin (Ed.), *Catecholamines and stress* (pp. 457–468). New York: Raven Press.

Jeffcoate, S. L. (1975). *Methods of hormone analysis.* New York: Wiley.

Kaplan, J. R., Manuck, S. B., Clarkson, T. B., Lusso, T. B., & Taub, D. M. (1982). Social status environment in atherosclerosis in cynomolgus monkeys. *Arteriosclerosis, 2,* 359–367.

Kaplan, J. R., Adams, M. R., Clarkson, T. B., & Koritnik, D. R. (1984). Psychosocial influences on female protection among cynomolgus macaques. *Atherosclerosis, 53,* 283–295.

Kawakami, M., Kubo, K., Uemura, T., Nagase, M., & Hayashi, R. (1981). Involvement of ovarian innervation in steroid secretion. *Endocrinology, 109,* 136–145.

Klaibern, E. L., Broverman, D. M., Haffajee, C. I., Hochman, J. S., Sacks, G. M., & Dalen, J. E. (1982). Serum estradiol levels in men with acute myocardial infarction. *American Journal of Medicine, 73,* 872–881.

Knopp, R. H., Walden, C. E., & Wahl, P. W. (1981). Oral contraceptive and postmenopausal estrogen effects on lipoprotein triglyceride and cholesterol in an adult female population: Relationships to estrogen and progestin potency. *Journal of Clinical Endocrinology and Metabolism, 53,* 1123–1132.

Kreuz, M. A. J., Rose, R. M., & Jennings, J. R. (1972). Suppression of plasma testosterone levels and pyschological stress, *Archives of General Psychology, 26,* 479–482.

Landon, J., Smith, D. S., Perry, L. A., & Al-Ansari, A. A. K. (1984). The assay of salivary cortisol. In G. F. Read, D. Read-Fahmy, R. F. Walker, & K. Griffiths (Eds.), *Immunoassays of steroids in saliva* (pp. 301–307). London: Alpha Omega Publishing.

Leshner, A. I. (1980). The interaction of experience and neuroendocrine factors in determining behavioral adaptations to aggression. *Progress in Brain Research, 53,* 427–438.

Lewis, J. G., & Elder, P. A. (1985). An enzyme-linked immunosorbent assay (ELISA) for plasma cortisol. *Journal of Steroid Biochemistry, 22,* 673–676.

Luisi, M., Bernini, G. P., Del Genovese, A., Birindelli, R., Barletta, D., Gasperi, M., & Franchi, F. (1980). Radioimmunoassay for free testosterone in human saliva. *Journal of Steroid Biochemistry, 12,* 513–516.

Luria, M. H., Johnson, M. W., Pego, R., Seuc, C. A., Manubens, S. J., Wieland, M. R., & Wieland, R. G. (1982). Relationship between sex hormones, myocardial infarction and occlusive coronary disease. *Archives of Internal Medicine, 142,* 42–44.

Mason, J. W., Kenion, C. C., Collins, D. R., Mougey, E. H., Jones, J. A., Driver, G. C., Brady, J. V., & Beer, B. (1968). Urinary testosterone response to 72-hr avoidance session in the monkey. *Psychosomatic Medicine, 30,* 721–732.

Mason, J. W., Hartley, L. H., Kotchen, T. A., Moughey, E. H., Ricketts, P. T., & Jones, L. G. (1973). Plasma cortisol and norepinephrine responses in anticipation of muscular exercise. *Psychosomatic Medicine, 35,* 406–414.

Murphy, B. E. P. (1968). Clinical evaluation of urinary cortisol determinations by competitive protein binding. *Journal of Endocrinology and Met. 28,* 343–348.

Murphy, B. E. P., Engelberg, W., & Patter, C. J. (1963). Simple method for determination of plasma corticoids. *Journal of Clinical Endocrinology and Metabolism, 23,* 293–300.

Nakashima, A., Koshiyama, K., Uozimi, T., Monden, Y., Hamanaka, Y., Kurachi, K., Aono, T., Mizutani, X., &

Matsumoto, K. (1975). Effects of general anaesthesia and severity of surgical stress on serum LH and testosterone in males. *Acta Endocrinologica, 78,* 258–269.

Nieschlag, E., & Wickins, E. J. (1978). The role of testosterone in the evaluation of testicular function. In G. E. Abraham (Ed.), *Radioassay systems in clinical endocrinology* (pp. 169–196). New York: Dekker.

Orth, D. N., Jackson, R. V., DeCherney, G. S., DeBold, C. R., Alexander, A. N., Island, D. P., Rivier, J., Rivier, C., Speiss, J., & Vale, W. (1983). Effects of ovine synthetic corticotropin releasing factor: Dose response of plasma adrenocorticotropin and cortisol. *Journal of Clinical Investigation, 71,* 587–595.

Phillips, G. B., Castell, W. P., Abbott, R. D., & McNamara, P. M. (1983). Association of hyperestrogenemia and coronary heart disease in men in the Framingham cohort. *American Journal of Medicine, 74,* 863–869.

Pinter, E. J., Peterfy, G., & Cleghorn, J. M. (1975). Studies in endocrine and affective functions in complex flight manoeuvres. *Psychotherapy and Psychosomatics, 26,* 93–100.

Read-Fahmy, D., Read, G. F., & Walker, R. F. (1982). Steroids in saliva for assessing endocrine function. *Endocrine Reviews, 3,* 367–395.

Ritchie, J. C., Varroll, B. J., Olton, P. R., Shively, V., & Feinberg, M. (1985). Plasma cortisol determination for the dexamethasone suppression test. *Archives of General Psychiatry, 42,* 493–497.

Rose, R. M., & Hurst, M. W. (1975). Plasma cortisol and growth hormone responses to intravenous catheterization. *Journal of Human Stress, 1,* 22–36.

Rose, R. M., Gordon, T. P., & Bernstein, I. S. (1972). Plasma testosterone levels in the male rhesus monkey: Influence of sexual and social stimuli. *Science, 178,* 643–645.

Rose, R. M., Jenkins, D., Hurst, M., Livingston, L., & Hasell, R. P. (1982). Endocrine activity in air traffic controllers at work. 1. Characterization of cortisol and growth hormone levels during the day. *Psychoneuroendocrinology, 7,* 101–111.

Rosenfeld, S., Marmorston, J., Sobel, H., & White, A. E. (1960). Enhancement of experimental atherosclerosis by ACTH in the dog. *Proceedings of the Society for Experimental Biology and Medicine, 103,* 83–86.

Schomig, A., Luth, B., Dietz, R., & Gross, F. (1976). Changes in vascular smooth muscle sensitivity to vasoconstrictor agents induced by corticosteroids, adrenalectomy, and differing salt intake in rats. *Clinical Science and Molecular Medicine, 51,* 51–63.

Silber, R. H., & Porter, C. C. (1954). The determination of 17,21-dihydroxy-20-ketosteroids in urine and plasma. *Journal of Biological Chemistry, 210,* 923–932.

Steger, R. W. (1982). Age dependent changes in the responsiveness of the reproductive system to pharmacologic agents. *Pharmacology and Therapeutics, 17,* 1–64.

Streeten, D. H. P., Anderson, G. H., Dalakos, T. G., Seeley, D., Mallov, J. S., Eusebio, R., Sunderlin, F. S., Badawy, S. Z. A., & King, R. B. (1982). Normal and abnormal function of the hypothalamic–pituitary adrenocortical system in man. *Endocrine Reviews, 5,* 371–394.

Surwit, R. S., Allen, L. M., Gilgor, R. S., Schanberg, S., Kuhn, C., & Duvuc, M. (1982). Neuroendocrine response to cold in Raynaud's syndrome. *Life Sciences, 32,* 995–1000.

Thorneycroft, I. H., Mishell, D. R., Stone, S. C., Kharma, K. M., & Nakamura, R. M. (1971). The relation of serum 17-hydroxyprogesterone and estradiol-17-beta levels during the human menstrual cycle. *American Journal of Obstetrics and Gynecology, 111,* 947–951.

Troxler, R. G., Sprague, E. A., Albanese, R. A., Fuchs, R., & Thompson, A. J. (1977). The association of elevated plasma cortisol and early atherosclerosis as demonstrated by coronary angiography. *Atherosclerosis, 26,* 151–162.

Umeda, T., Hiramatsu, R., Iwaoka, T., Shimada, T. R., Miura, R., & Sato, T. (1981). Use of saliva for monitoring unbound free cortisol levels in serum. *Clinica Chimica Acta, 110,* 245–253.

Walker, R. F., Joyce, B. G., Dyas, J., & Read-Fahmy, D. (1984). Cortisol: Monitoring changes in normal adrenal activity. In G. F. Read, D. Read-Fahmy, R. F. Walker, & K. Griffiths (Eds.), *Immunoassay of steroids in saliva* (pp. 309–324). London: Alpha Omega Publishing.

Weitzman, E. D., Fukushima, D., Nogeire, C., Roffwarg, H., Gallagher, T. F., & Hellman, L. (1971). 24 hour pattern of the episodic secretion of cortisol in normal subjects. *Journal of Clinical Endocrinology and Metabolism, 33,* 14–22.

Williams, R. B., Lane, J. D., Kuhn, C. M., Melosh, W., White, A. D., & Schanberg, S. (1982). Type A behavior and elevated physiological and neuroendocrine responses to cognitive tasks. *Science, 218,* 483.

Wilson, J. D., & Foster, D. W. (1980). *Williams textbook of endocrinology.* Philadelphia: Saunders.

Yen, S. S. C., & Jaffe, R. B. (1986). *Reproductive endocrinology.* Philadelphia: Saunders.

Zumoff, B., Fukushima, D. K., & Hellman, L. (1974). Intercomparison of four methods for measuring cortisol production. *Journal of Clinical Endocrinology and Metabolism, 38,* 169–180.

CHAPTER **13**

Measurement and Function of Neuropeptides
Focus on Corticotropin-Releasing Factor and Arginine Vasopressin

George F. Koob and Garth Bissette

Introduction

Peptides are now known to be a class of intercellular messengers that are widely distributed throughout the central nervous system, peripheral nervous system, and various organs of the gastrointestinal tract. An intercellular messenger may be defined as "a substance released from one cell that is capable of modifying the functional activity of another neighboring or distant cell" (Brown & Fisher, 1984). Intercellular messengers may be hormones as in the classical sense or neurotropic substances that interact as neurotransmitters in the CNS. Most of the evidence for the action of neuropeptides as neurotransmitters centers on physiological and pharmacological-like activity of peptides administered exogenously, as well as identification of peptide receptors and to a limited extent the use of peptide antagonists. The actual measure-

ment of release of neuropeptides has been limited, particularly as regards a neurotropic role in the CNS.

The explosion of research on neuropeptides precludes an in-depth examination of the measurement and function of each relevant substance. However, work with a recently discovered hypothalamic releasing factor—corticotropin-releasing factor (CRF)—provides an opportunity to discuss one peptide in depth in terms of measurement and physiology. CRF is a particularly appropriate choice given the wealth of information available and its relevance to stress.

Differences between Neuropeptides and Other Neurotransmitters

There are some major differences between neuropeptides and other neurotransmitters. Intraneuronal catecholamines such as norepinephrine maintain constant levels by replacement of released transmitter by: (1) synthesis in the nerve ending, (2) reuptake from the extraneuronal space through an active mechanism, (3) replenishment of amine in storage vesicles from the cell body via

George F. Koob • Division of Preclinical Neuroscience and Endocrinology, Research Institute of Scripps Clinic, La Jolla, California 92037.   *Garth Bissette* • Laboratory of Psychoneuroendocrinology, Department of Psychiatry, Duke University Medical Center, Durham, North Carolina 27710.

axonal transport. However, peptides are synthesized by direct translational products of genes whereas other neurotransmitters are formed indirectly via enzymes acting on intracellular substrates. Peptides in the CNS are synthesized in the nerve cell body rather than the axon terminal as for the catecholamines. Thus, release is hypothetically much more dependent on axonal transport and large reserves near release sites (Hokfelt, Johansson, Ljungdahl, Lundberg, & Schultzberg, 1980). Peptides are probably produced only by the ribosomes of the cell body in the form of a larger precursor prohormone molecule, without local synthesis in the nerve endings. Peptides are then further processed to a releasable form during axonal transport and packaging in vesicles. As there is no reuptake mechanism known to operate for peptides, every peptide molecule that is released from a nerve ending must be replaced by axonal transport.

These properties may be reflected in significant differences in the dynamics of synaptic events at peptide synapses (Hokfelt *et al.*, 1980). Peptides may be released intermittently and not tonically since there appears to be no mechanism for rapid replenishment in the presynaptic terminal such as synthesis or reuptake. There may be a slower onset of action after release followed by a longer duration of postsynaptic action. The total releasable amounts of peptides may be smaller than those of classical neurotransmitters such as the catecholamines. Indeed, the concentration of neuropeptides is estimated to be 1000 times lower than that of the catecholamines and 100,000 times lower than that of the amino acids (Hokfelt *et al.*, 1980). Finally, peptides may activate receptors at much lower levels than do other neurotransmitters.

Biochemical Indices of Peptide Neuron Activity

Although neuropeptides and several classical chemical neurotransmitters are both made from amino acids and many amino acids themselves are neurotransmitters, most of the classical chemical neurotransmitters are synthesized from a single amino acid precursor whereas neuropeptides represent from 2 to 44 amino acids linked by peptide bonds. The functional state of catecholamines and several other classical chemical neurotransmitters can be quantified using measures of synthesis, release, and degradation. However, at present, one is technologically limited to measurement of static levels of a neuropeptide; measures of neuropeptide synthesis, release, and degradation are not available. Thus, if there is an increase in concentration of a particular peptide in an experimental group compared to controls, one presently cannot directly differentiate between the vastly different functional mechanisms that could cause such an increase: either continued neuropeptide synthesis without concomitant release or increased synthesis and release but decreased degradation.

Attempts to answer such a question indirectly involve measurement of peptide receptors and determining if receptor down-regulation accompanies increased concentrations, which would indicate increased release of the neuropeptide. Alternatively, measurement of the expression of mRNA for the neuropeptide or its precursor molecule will indicate if synthesis is increased. The ''front line'' of neuropeptide research laboratories is now wedding the three approaches of (1) radioimmunoassay of neuropeptide concentrations, (2) measurement of the number and affinity of the neuropeptide's specific receptors, and (3) molecular neurobiological determination of the amount of transcription and translation of neuropeptide prohormones in order to measure peptide turnover.

Except for the opioid neuropeptides and a few other peptides, good specific receptor antagonists are not available for neuropeptides (see Table 1). Thus, pharmacological blockade of the transduction of neuropeptide signals that approximate decreased neuropeptide activity is not usually possible. At present we are therefore limited to examining the biological effects of increased neuropeptide activity by administration of exogenous synthetic neuropeptides. This inability to specifically induce a neuropeptide deficit is most unsatisfactory and severely limits our investigation of the physiological role of these neurotransmitters. Nevertheless, significant progress has been made in elucidating the particular physiological and behavioral effects of more than a few of the 40–50 presently known neuropeptides.

These differences all have implications for un-

Table 1. Peptide Antagonists for Opioids, CRF, and AVP: Approximate in Vivo Antagonist (μg)/Agonist (μg) Ratio

Opioid antagonist	
Naloxone[a]	100:1
CRF antagonist	
α-Helical CRF 9–41[b]	10:1
AVP antagonists	
V-1 receptor	
dPtyr(Me)AVP[c]	5:1
d(Ch2)5[Tyr(Me)]AVP[d]	1:1
V-2 receptor	
d(Ch2)5(D-Ile2, Abu4)AVP[d]	3:1

[a]Loh *et al.* (1976).
[b]Rivier *et al.* (1984).
[c]Bankoski *et al.* (1978).
[d]Manning and Sawyer (1984).

derstanding the functional significance of peptide measurements in bodily fluids. For example, neuropeptide levels in the brain at steady state may more accurately reflect peptide function than do the monoamines which have a high turnover. However, during a homeostatic challenge, neuropeptides may be capable of showing a large initial response but incapable of rapidly replacing depleted stores.

Diversity of Neuropeptides

Another major difference between neuropeptides and other transmitters is the rich diversity of potential neurotropic substances. The list of potential neuropeptide neurotransmitters is growing rapidly; there are more than 30 neuropeptides iden-

tified in the brain by chemical or immunohistochemical means (see Table 2). Some of these neuropeptides act as both hormones and possible neurotropic substances. Arginine vasopressin, oxytocin, opioid peptides, and ACTH are all released from the pituitary but also have putative neurotropic actions.

Even more intriguing has been the new work with the hypothalamic releasing factors where significant functional roles for these substances in the CNS have been identified that are homologous to their classic hormonal action (see Table 3). According to such a homology hypothesis, neuropeptides may via their CNS distribution have functional roles that exaggerate or parallel those functions served by their classical hormonal role. For example, LHRH releases LH which controls sex hormone secretion and LHRH by itself may also have a role in mediating sexual behavior. This provides an excellent framework by which to explore the problems, challenges, and significance of peptide measurement and function. This homology of function hypothesis is perhaps most dramatically elaborated by the recent work with CRF.

CRF

After nearly 30 years of effort, Vale and associates characterized and synthesized a CRF with great potency and intrinsic activity for *in vitro* and *in vivo* stimulation of adrenocorticotropic hormone (ACTH) and β-endorphin (Vale, Spiess, Rivier, & Rivier, 1981). A 41-amino-acid polypeptide, CRF

Table 2. Peptides Found in the Brain by Chemical or Immunologic Identification Methods

Thyrotropin-releasing factor	Oxytocin	Motilin
Luteinizing hormone-releasing factor	Vasopressin	Secretin
Somatostatin-14	β-Endorphin	Gastric inhibitory polypeptide
Somatostatin-28, 1–12	Dynorphins	Vasoactive intestinal peptide
Somatostatin-28	Met-enkephalin and Leu-enkephalin	Cholecystokinin
Corticotropin-releasing factor	Neurotensin	Calcitonin gene-related peptide
Growth hormone-releasing factor	Substance P	Carnosine
Melanotropin-inhibiting factor	Bradykinin	Neuropeptide Y
Adrenocorticotropic hormone	Bombesin	Atrial natriuretic factor
Prolactin	Angiotensin II	Kassinin
Thyrotropin	Insulin	Substance K
Growth hormone	Glucagon	Eledoisin
α-Melanocyte-stimulating hormone	Gastrin	Neuromedin K

Table 3. Pituitary Gland and Brain Actions of the Hypothalamic Hypophysiotropic Regulatory Peptides

Peptide	Pituitary gland action	Brain actions
Thyrotropin-releasing factor	Stimulates thyrotropin secretion	Increases motor activity, heart rate, blood pressure, and sympathetic nervous system activity; produces hyperthermia; antagonizes a variety of hypnotic and sedative drug actions; inhibits growth hormone secretion
Luteinizing hormone-releasing factor	Stimulates luteinizing hormone and follicle-stimulating hormone secretion	Stimulates libido and mating behavior
Somatostatin-14 and somatostatin-28	Inhibits growth hormone and thyrotropin secretion	Somatostatin-28 and related analogues inhibit adrenal epinephrine and pituitary gland adrenocorticotropin secretion; increase pituitary gland thyrotropin secretion; produce hyperthermia
Corticotropin-releasing factor	Stimulates adrenocorticotropin secretion	Increases sympathetic and decreases parasympathetic nervous system activity; increases heart rate and blood pressure; behavioral activation and increased behavioral response to stress
Growth hormone-releasing factor	Stimulates growth hormone secretion	Increases food intake at low doses; decreases food intake and produces sedation at high doses

was presumably the long-sought-after hypothalamic neurohumor with the specific function of releasing ACTH from the anterior pituitary, and thus may be considered the final common pathway for the neurohumoral control of ACTH.

The significance of the chemical identification of CRF is best understood in terms of classical stress theory. A generally accepted definition of stress is that it "is the nonspecific (common) result of any demand upon the body" (Selye, 1980). Probably the most reliable indication that a state of stress exists is variation in the production of ACTH. The latter is derived from a large precursor molecule called pro-opiomelanocortin (POMC) which is synthesized in the anterior pituitary (Akil *et al.*, 1984). Internal or external demands are conveyed in the form of stimuli to the anterior pituitary via neurohumoral means (presumably CRF), and the pituitary responds with a secretion of ACTH. ACTH, in turn, stimulates the adrenal cortex to secrete glucocorticoids, which have widespread effects on metabolism such as gluconeogenesis, hyperinsulinemia, lysis of lymphoid tissue, increased gastric secretion, and reduced inflammatory and antibody responses (see Selye, 1980, and also Kuhn, this volume). These physiological changes in response to increased hypothalamic–pituitary action are paralleled by alterations in

behavior that have been associated with increases in alertness and attention (De Wied, 1977).

There is, however, an alternate means by which behavioral or physiological responses to stress or anxiety might be mediated by the hypothalamic–pituitary system in an organism, i.e., via direct neurotropic action of CRF in the CNS itself. Thus, just as pathways project to the hypothalamus from the limbic areas to activate, via CRF, the pituitary–adrenal axis, so might CRF feedback to these same areas mediate appropriate behavioral responses to stress.

Physiological Effects of CNS CRF

CRF injected intracerebroventricularly (i.c.v.) produces a prolonged elevation of plasma norepinephrine, epinephrine, glucagon, and glucose in rats and dogs (Brown, Fisher, Rivier, *et al.*, 1982; Brown, Fisher, Spiess, *et al.*, 1982). CRF (i.c.v.) also increases heart rate and blood pressure in rats (Brown, Fisher, Rivier, *et al.*, 1982; Fisher *et al.*, 1982) and suppresses gastric acid secretion (Taché *et al.*, 1983; Taché & Gunion, 1985). Both the metabolic and cardiovascular changes are reversed by chlorisondamine, an autonomic ganglionic blocker, but not by angiotensin or vasopressin antagonists. These results suggest that the

CRF effects are mediated by a sympathetic autonomic activation and not by a release of angiotensin or vasopressin. Hypophysectomy or adrenalectomy also does not block these CRF-induced changes (Fisher *et al.*, 1982), suggesting that these effects are not mediated by the hypothalamic–pituitary–adrenal axis. More importantly, a weak CRF antagonist, α-helical CRF (9–41), attenuated the epinephrine increase associated with hemorrhage, suggesting a possible role for endogenous CRF in the CNS sympathetic response to stress (Brown, Gray, & Fisher, 1986). Thus, CRF appears to have a direct neurotropic action in the brain to activate the sympathetic nervous system, eventually through an action on peripheral catecholamine systems, an activation observed with many kinds of stress (Brown, Fisher, Rivier, *et al.*, 1982).

CRF injected i.c.v. also produces a profound dose-dependent activation of the electroencephalogram (EEG) (Ehlers, Henriksen, Bloom, Rivier, & Vale, 1983), and at higher doses this appear to progress to a pathological overactivation not unlike that seen for convulsant stimulants. For example, doses of 1.5–3.75 nmoles produce consistent amygdala interictal spikes and afterdischarges and, after a delay of 4 to 7 h, some motor seizures. At the more cellular level, CRF has been shown to produce a pronounced depolarization and excitation of hippocampal pyramidal cells (Aldenhoff, Gruol, & Siggins, 1983). Intracellular recordings demonstrated that the excitation arose from reduction of the afterhyperpolarizations that followed bursts of spikes (Siggins, Gruol, Aldenhoff, & Pittman, 1985), and it was hypothesized that CRF may alter potassium conductance either directly or via a change in calcium conductances. These results may provide a cellular basis for the EEG changes observed following i.c.v. injection.

Behavioral Effects of CNS CRF

The autonomic and electrophysiological activation produced by i.c.v. injection of CRF is paralleled by a behavioral activation that is dose and situation dependent. CRF injected i.c.v. in rats produces a dose-dependent locomotor activation (Sutton, Koob, Le Moal, Rivier, & Vale, 1982).

This activation, particularly at lower doses (15–150 pmoles), is characterized by increased locomotion, sniffing, grooming, and rearing-behavior consistent with a general behavioral arousal. In these studies, rats are repeatedly exposed individually to a familiar photocell cage environment where without treatment they typically go to sleep within 30 min. CRF has a stimulant-like effect, causing the animals to continue to be awake and active for hours (see Koob & Bloom, 1985). At higher doses (1500 pmoles CRF), more bizarre behavioral effects were observed, e.g., elevated walking and repetitive locomotion such as moving forwards and backwards in a straight line and pawing rapidly against the sides of the cage. Given the marked changes in EEG described at these doses (Ehlers *et al.*, 1983), these behavioral changes at high doses may reflect preconvulsant activity.

This behavioral activation appears to be independent of the pituitary–adrenal system in that hypophysectomized rats chronically treated with rat growth hormone so that they gained 3.5 g/day showed consistent and reliable increases in activity in the photocell cages following i.c.v. administration of CRF, similar to the increases observed in sham-operated animals (Eaves, Thatcher-Britton, Rivier, Vale, & Koob, 1985). This suggests that the CRF effects are mediated directly in the CNS and not via activation of the pituitary–adrenal axis to release ACTH or corticosterone.

Perhaps of more importance for the conceptualization of CRF as a peptide involved in the organism's behavioral response to stress were the experiments showing that CRF can potentiate the effects of exposure to a novel, presumably aversive, environment. Rats tested in a novel open field following i.c.v. injection of CRF (0.0015–0.15 nmoles) showed responses that are consistent with an increased "emotionality" or increased sensitivity to the stressful aspects of the situation. Here rats showed *decreases* in locomotion and rearing. In this open field test, a typical saline-injected rat rapidly circled the outer squares of the open field during the first 3–4 min of the 5-min test. During the last 1–2 min of the test, these saline-injected animals then made some forays into the center of the open field, usually accompanied by rearing on their hind legs. Typically a rat injected with 150 pmoles of CRF and placed 60 min later in the open field moved hesitantly to the outer squares and then either circled the open field remaining close to the floor or remained in one of the corners grooming or hesitantly moving forwards and backwards (Sutton *et al.*, 1982).

In an operant conflict test, CRF produced a significant decrease in punished responding, an effect opposite to that observed with benzodiazepines, and this "anxiogenic" effect was reversed by concurrent treatment with a benzodiazepine (Thatcher-Britton, Morgan, Rivier, Vale, & Koob, 1985). However, this increased sensitivity to aversive events was not paralleled by an increased sensitivity to pain. Similar interactions with benzodiazepines were observed with CRF in the acoustic startle response (Swerdlow, Geyer, Vale, & Koob, 1986). CRF (1 μg i.c.v.) potentiated the acoustic startle response and this effect also was dose-dependently reversed by chlordiazepoxide (Swerdlow *et al.*, 1986). CRF also decreases food intake and muscimol-, norepinephrine-, dynorphin-, and insulin-induced feeding, effects attributed to a stress-related suppression of food intake (Levine, Rogers, Kwerp, Grace, & Morley, 1982; Morley & Levine, 1983). Thus, exogenously administered CRF exaggerates stress effects or produces effects similar to stress and these effects are reversed by antistress (anxiolytic) drugs.

The unusual interaction of CRF with the stress produced by aversive events suggested that an investigation using a stress-induced fighting paradigm might exaggerate this phenomenon. This fighting test was previously shown to be sensitive to environmental parameters such as stress level (Tazi, Dantzer, Mormede, & Le Moal, 1985) and to be modulated by peptides (Tazi, Dantzer, Mormede, & Le Moal, 1983). CRF doses of 0.01 and 0.1 μg injected intraventricularly significantly facilitated fighting at a moderate shock level (0.5 mA). CRF at the highest dose and highest shock level totally disrupted the behavior of the animals. A slightly higher shock level (0.6 mA) produced a higher fighting frequency in control animals that had not received exogenously administered CRF. More importantly, this fighting was reversed by 5

and 25 μg of α-helical CRF (9–41), a CRF antagonist (Tazi, Dantzer, Le Moal, & Koob, 1987). This antagonist has been shown to decrease both *in vitro* and *in vivo* baseline release of ACTH, as well as stress-induced ACTH secretion (Rivier, Rivier, & Vale, 1984). These results suggest that under certain conditions of high arousal and stress, endogenous CNS CRF systems may play a role in mediating behavioral responses.

Summary of Effects of CRF

These results describing neuronal activation, sympathetic activation, EEG arousal, general behavioral activation, and stress-enhancing actions of CRF all suggest a possible role for CRF as a fundamental activating system (see Table 4). The functional significance of this system may have developed as a means for an organism to mobilize not only the pituitary–adrenal system, but also the

Table 4. Summary of CRF Effects

Hypothalamic–pituitary axis
    Potent stimulation of the secretion of ACTH
    Potent stimulation of the secretion of other proopiomelanocortin products such as β-endorphin
Autonomic nervous system
    Elevation of plasma epinephrine and norepinephrine concentrations
    Stimulation of blood pressure and heart rate
    Production of hyperglycemia
    Suppression of gastric acid secretion
Limbic system
    CRF in doses of 0.1–10 μg (15–1500 pmoles) injected intracerebroventricularly increases locomotor activity in a familiar photocell environment
    CRF facilitates the acoustic startle response
    CRF facilitates acquisition of a visual discrimination task
    CRF produces increased responsiveness to "stress" in an open field test
    CRF has an "anxiogenic-like" effect in an operant conflict test
    CRF at low doses (0.01 μg, 1.5 pmoles) facilitates avoidance behavior, but at higher doses (1.0 μg, 150 pmoles) disrupts avoidance behavior
    CRF produces a similar dose-dependent facilitation and disruption of stress-induced fighting
    A weak CRF antagonist, α-helical CRF 9–41, injected intracerebroventricularly blocks stress-induced fighting

CNS in response to environmental challenge. Indeed, results in our laboratory suggest that treatment with CRF can improve performance in learning tasks and this is dose and task related (Koob & Bloom, 1985). Aversive situations appear much more sensitive to exogenous CRF and preliminary results suggest that these aversive states may be sensitive to administration of a weak CRF antagonist. Clearly, a hypothetical CNS activation system definitively linked to the pituitary–adrenal system, that can improve behavioral performance at low levels of output would be of certain survival value. The attenuation of behavioral performance at high levels of output may reflect an overactivity of such a basic CNS activation system (the other side of the U-shaped curve relating arousal to performance). Thus, it is not difficult to imagine a possible role for such a system in clinical disorders such as anxiety, affective disorders, and other psychopathology.

Arginine Vasopressin (AVP)

Physiological Effects

The main physiological role for AVP is the conserving of water for which AVP called antidiuretic hormone. AVP is synthesized in the hypothalamic–hypophysial system and released into the bloodstream from the posterior lobe of the pituitary. Its antidiuretic action is effected by making the distal renal tubules more permeable to water (Sawyer, 1964). Another important nonrenal action of AVP is its pressor effect from which the peptide derives its name (Sawyer, 1964). This vasopressor effect is mediated directly as vasoconstriction on the smooth muscles of the vascular system (Altura, 1967), and may be physiologically significant during hypovolemic or hypotensive crises (Rocha, Silva, & Rosenberg, 1969). This vasopressor effect requires higher doses of AVP than needed for maximal antidiuretic action (Straus, 1957).

AVP is by itself a relatively weak stimulator of ACTH release, but markedly potentiates the activity of CRF *in vivo* and *in vitro* (Yates *et al.,*

1971; Gillies, Linton, & Lowry, 1982). Thus, AVP may play a physiological role in the regulation of ACTH secretion but only in response to severe physical stress.

The usual physiological stimulus for the release of AVP from the posterior pituitary is dehydration or plasma hyperosmolarity. Inhibition in the release of AVP results in a diuresis of dilute urine, a condition known as diabetes insipidus. Lesions placed all along the hypothalamic–neurohypophysial system are associated with permanent diabetes insipidus. AVP secretion into the systemic circulation also is increased during certain types of stress, particularly those involving severe physical stress. Ether (Gibbs, 1984), hypoglycemia (Plotsky, Bruhn, & Vale, 1985), and hypoxia (Stegner, Leake, Palmer, Oakes, & Fisher, 1984) all increase AVP secretion in animals and pain has been shown to increase plasma AVP in humans (Kendler, Weitzman, & Fisher, 1978).

Behavioral Effects

AVP also produces important behavioral effects in addition to its classical endocrine actions. Administered to rats subcutaneously in a dose of 1–5 μg/rat, it prolongs extinction of active avoidance (De Wied, 1971; Koob *et al.,* 1981), and enhances retention of inhibitory (passive) avoidance (Bohus, Kovacs, & De Wied, 1978). These studies led De Wied and colleagues to suggest that AVP has a physiological role in "memory," particularly memory consolidation, and that this action is mediated directly in the CNS (De Wied & Versteeg, 1979).

More recent work with vasopressin antagonist peptides questions this simple interpretation. All the behavioral actions of systemically administered AVP studied to date are reversed by a pressor AVP antagonist analogue [1-deaminopenicillamine, 2-(O-methyl)tyrosine]AVP (Bankoski, Manning, Halder, & Sawyer, 1978) (Le Moal *et al.,* 1981; Koob *et al.,* 1986; Lebrun *et al.,* 1984; Ettenberg, Le Moal, Koob, & Bloom, 1983; Ettenberg, 1985). Based on these data, Koob *et al.* (1985) have hypothesized that the behavioral effects of systemically administered AVP are mediated by the arousal changes secondary to peripheral visceral changes such as increases in blood pressure (see Koob *et al.,* 1985, for details).

Physiological and Behavioral Effects of CNS AVP

AVP administered directly into the CNS in nanogram quantities (0.5–10 ng/rat i.c.v.) also has behavioral actions that have been interpreted as a facilitation of "memory." AVP (i.c.v.) prolongs extinction of active avoidance and inhibitory avoidance (De Wied, 1976; Koob *et al.,* 1986). These doses do not significantly increase systemic blood pressure (Koob *et al.,* 1986). Higher doses of centrally administered AVP can produce analgesia (Berkowitz & Sherman, 1982) and suppress fever (Kasting, Veale, & Cooper, 1982), and also can increase systemic blood pressure (Pittman, Lawrence, & McLean, 1982).

AVP is present in CSF and a prominent daily rhythm has been found in CSF of rats, and monkeys, that is independent of systemic plasma levels (Schwartz, Coleman, & Reppert, 1983; Perlow *et al.,* 1982). Studies of changes in CSF levels of AVP with different physiological challenges have revealed mixed results to date. There is a report of increased AVP release into the ventricular system (Barnard & Morris, 1982) and into push–pull perfusates of the septum (Demotes-Mainard, Chauveau, Rodriguez, Vincent, & Poulain, 1986) with a hypertonic saline challenge. Others have failed to observe increases in CSF AVP of rats under water deprivation or when rats were forced to drink 2% NaCl (Mens, Bouman, Baker, & van Wimersma Greidanus, 1980). However, some CSF changes in AVP have been observed during inhibitory avoidance learning (Laczi, Gaffori, Fekele, de Kloet, & De Wied, 1984). What does appear to be clear is that centrally released AVP is controlled separately from the release of the peptide into blood (Coleman & Reppert, 1985).

Measurement of Neuropeptides— General Considerations

The most generally used method for quantification of neuropeptides in biological tissue or fluids

in the last decade has been the radioimmunoassay (RIA). This technique combines a great simplicity and sensitivity with the well-known specificity of immunological reactions. In an RIA, the concentration of the peptide being studied in a tissue or fluid extract is determined by comparing the inhibitory effect of a known amount of the extract on the binding of a radiolabeled peptide using a limited amount of antibody to the inhibitory effect of given amounts of cold standard peptide. Measurement with the RIA requires three basic steps: (1) preparation of the extracts for RIA, (2) incubation with a specific antiserum and tracer, and (3) separation of bound and free tracer and calculation of the amount of displacement of the bound tracer.

Preparation of Tissue Extracts

The best extraction technique would be one where the desired neuropeptide is exclusively soluble in a solvent and not allowed to be broken down before being extracted. Thus, considerations of solubility, stability, and the presence of other peptides and peptide-degrading enzymes are important. Tissue should be rapidly removed from the animal and extracted as soon as possible. If not extracted immediately, samples should be stored at $-20°C$ or below in aqueous solutions of low salt content.

CRF Extraction

There are a variety of extraction methods in use today for solubilizing neuropeptides and separating them from other subcellular components. Most are empirically derived and require the recovery of the major part of the sample to be measured without significant loss of immunoreactivity. In tissues such as brain, acidic extraction (0.1–1.0 N ice-cold HCl or 0.1–2.0 N acetic acid) is usually adequate and results in greater than 90% recovery of added synthetic CRF. Boiling or heating the sample should be avoided unless rapid degradation is known to be a problem. For CSF samples, unless there is nondilutable, nonspecific interference in the assay, there is no need to extract the neuropeptides as long as artificial CSF of equal volume to the sample is added to the standard curve to control for the presence of CSF salts. Measurement of CRF in serum or plasma requires separation of the peptide from blood proteins and lipids that interfere in the assay. Sep-Pak-18 cartridges (contain C-18 μBondapak silicate) using silicate resins are often employed for these samples. Estimation of recovery of added synthetic CRF is essential in developing any extraction procedure. Immunoreactivity must remain dilutable before and after extraction.

The half-life of neuropeptides varies greatly between tissues and physiological compartments and usually is inversely correlated with available peptidase concentration. With notable exceptions, in human postmortem brain much of the available peptide immunoreactivity is unchanged at up to 72 h without refrigeration. Use of animal tissues with measurement of neuropeptide recovery at various times is still necessary when characterizing the stability of a particular peptide or tissue. Frozen ($-70°C$) tissues have no appreciable peptide degradation for 3 months to 2 years. Because CSF has relatively low concentrations of peptidases, most neuropeptides are not degraded in this fluid. For example, slow degradation is seen with β-endorphin in the CSF of a freely moving rhesus monkey (Rossier, Bayon, et al., 1977). However, brain extracts promoted the rapid disappearance of β-endorphin immunoreactivity, the half-life being 47 min (Rossier, Bayon, et al., 1977). Most neuropeptides are subject to oxidative damage in dilute solutions, including CSF, after prolonged storage (months) and with repeated freeze-thawing. Again, addition of synthetic standard to pooled CSF and calculation of recovery at different times and with different conditions is necessary to establish the stability of a particular peptide in CSF. As CRF is known to be cleared from CSF at six times the rate of passive absorption, a significant gradient probably exists between the brain and spinal CSF (Oldfield et al., 1985).

Most neuropeptides examined to date have relatively short (minutes) half-lives in serum or plasma. For example, Met- and Leu-enkephalin are very susceptible to degradation by peptidases. In serum the half-life of Met-enkephalin is 2 min (Hambrook, Morgan, Rance, & Smith, 1976). However, β-endorphin is quite resistant to serum peptidases. Use of commercial peptidase inhibitors and chelating agents is usually required to successfully preserve peptide immunoreactivity in serum or plasma. Even then, rapid extraction and separation of the peptide from other sample components is usually necessary. There are conflicting reports of the half-life of exogenous synthetic CRF in humans after intravenous injection. One report (Stalla, Hartwimmer, Schopohl, von Werder, & Muller, 1986) showed that ovine CRF had a serum half-life of 18 min whereas rat/human CRF had a half-life of 9 min in humans. Another study (Schulte et al., 1984) reported a fast component ($t_{1/2}$ 11.6 min) and a slow component ($t_{1/2}$ 73 min) for degradation of rat/human CRF in human plasma.

Detection of Neuropeptides—Species Specificity

The amino acid sequence for neuropeptides has changed during the course of evolution and this change has generally been conservative, retaining biological function of the molecule. Using CRF as an example, rat and human CRF are virtually identical whereas ovine CRF has only 83% homology with human CRF. These changes can greatly affect immunochemical recognition depending on what species the antiserum was raised.

Because antisera recognize from three to six amino acids in a peptide chain, the possibility always exists that a similar sequence in another protein could be recognized by the antisera. Because an RIA is based on the relative amounts of radioactive tracer bound in the presence of various concentrations of cold, synthetic peptide in the standard curve, displacement of tracer by any substance will read as though there is more of the endogenous peptide being examined. It is disconcerting how many investigators claim "specificity" for their particular antiserum based on the inability of a wide variety of neuropeptides without any similar sequences of amino acids to displace tracer. Only by using fragments of the original peptide molecule or homologues from other species that contain significant amounts of similar peptide sequences can specificity be determined. Depending on how the peptide is bound to the hapten of choice (most peptides are too small to be

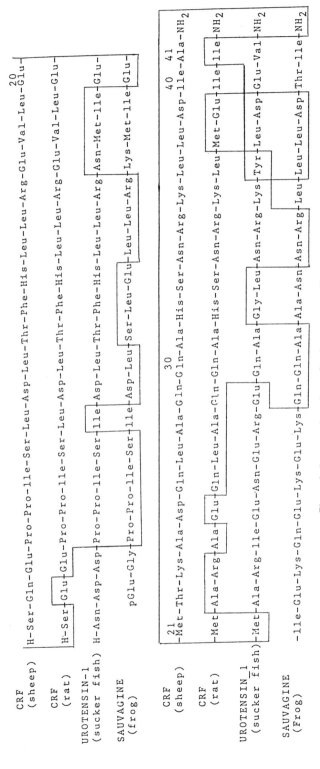

Figure 1. Sequence homology of various neuropeptides.

adequately antigenic alone), one can usually direct the antisera toward the C- or N-terminus by linking the opposite end to the hapten. For CRF, the neuropeptides urotensin I (from suckerfish) and sauvagine (from frogs) have significant sequence homology with CRF and are excellent in testing the specificity of antisera (see Figure 1). If an antiserum has picogram sensitivity for a particular peptide, nanogram amounts of homologues or fragments that are not recognized should not be able to displace the tracer.

RIA for Detection of Neuropeptides— Sources of Artifact

The tissue or fluid extract is placed in a container that can be handled by a gamma counter and predetermined amounts of specific antibody and of a radiolabeled peptide in an effective buffer. The extract may contain chemicals that interfere with the antigen–antibody reaction or degrade the antigen and/or antibody.

An effective control for nonspecific chemical interactions is to add the same amount of tissue fluid extract to the standards after removing the substance being measured. High concentrations of salts, high concentrations of acid, and high concentrations of buffer have all been shown to inhibit peptide antigen-antibody reactions (Straus & Yalow, 1977). The optimum parameters should be empirically derived for each antigen and antiserum used in the assay. In one example of the problems that can arise with nonspecific interference, a dye used to visualize the cerebral ventricles in humans was shown to significantly interfere with the antibody in CSF measurements of β-endorphin, producing false-positive readings (Fessler, Brown, Rachlin, Mullan, & Fang, 1984).

Another possible source of artifact is the degradation of the antigen or antibody during incubation. This problem may be suspected when the binding of tracer to a particular dilution of antisera is significantly different between the binding assay used to characterize the tracer and measurement of actual samples in the RIA. Usually more thorough extraction of the samples is the only way to correct this problem.

Radioactive Tracer

Most RIAs incorporate the γ-emitter ^{125}I in the native molecule to allow measurement of the amount of binding to the antiserum. Native molecules containing amino acids with aromatic side chains can be iodinated directly with the iodine being held in resonance covalent binding to the aromatic ring. Peptides without Tyr, His, or Trp in the native sequence must have these residues substituted at some point in the peptide sequence. When using a substituted molecule, it is important to establish that the substitution does not occur in the recognition sequence or immunoreactivity may be lost. Adding the substituted amino acid at the N-terminus usually avoids this problem. Best results are obtained when the tracer molecule is as structurally identical as possible to the molecule being measured. For example, an antiserum raised in rabbits to ovine CRF does not measure rat/human CRF when Tyr° ovine CRF is used as the tracer, but does quite well when Tyr° rat/human CRF is the tracer.

Physical-Chemical Separation. There are two points in the performance of an RIA where physical-chemical separation techniques are employed. Separation of bound and free tracer is necessary to calculate displacement and a variety of methods are currently employed. Some laboratories use a second, species-specific antiserum to precipitate the primary antiserum–antigen complex, others use staphylococcal membranes, dextran-coated charcoal, talc, or polyethylene glycol to precipitate or bind the antiserum–antigen complex. All of these methods are valid and vary slightly in the sensitivity of the resulting assay.

When purifying radioactive tracer or determining the exact molecular identity of the immunoreactive species being examined, HPLC or liquid column chromatography are currently methods of choice. HPLC is much faster and usually can separate much more closely related molecules than can column chromatography but is also much more expensive. Both methods separate molecules based on charge differences and/or differences in molecular weight. The various fractions resulting from these techniques must be analyzed by RIA to determine where the optimum immunoreactivity is eluted.

Significance of Plasma and CSF Levels of Neuropeptides

Plasma levels of neuropeptides have the advantage that they are the most accessible to the clinical researcher. However, the lack of any functional significance of most of these measures at present gives considerable doubt to their utility at this time. For CRF, plasma levels cannot be reliably measured without the use of an immunoaffinity column and even if measured it is not clear at this time whether these levels would reflect hypothalamic–pituitary activity, CNS CRF, or some other, as yet to be discovered, ectopic sources of CRF. One promising clinical technique has involved intravenous challenge with synthetic ovine CRF (Gold et al., 1984). This procedure shows that patients with unipolar depression have a blunted ACTH response to exogenously administered CRF. Gold et al. interpret this as a receptor subsensitivity resulting from a chronic oversecretion of hypothalamic CRF.

For vasopressin, plasma levels can be reliably determined, because blood is where this hormone is released and plasma levels have been demonstrated to respond to osmotic and emotional stress. Although it has not been directly proven, these AVP changes probably do reflect the release of posterior pituitary AVP and probably not a significant amount of CSF AVP. Indeed, as discussed above, plasma levels probably do not reflect internal CNS activity. Thus, if the hypothesis involves a question of pituitary activation by some independent variable, plasma levels may provide such an indication. However, systematic basic research studies are needed to define the dynamics of these systems. Unknown areas are the capacity for depletion, resynthesis, and turnover of AVP.

Determination of CSF levels of neuropeptides and their correlation with CNS functional measures would seem to be conceptually clearer. Levels of neuropeptides in the CSF are assumed to

reflect the activity of brain neuropeptide systems. However, at present, there are no data directly correlating brain neuropeptide activity with CSF measurements. Nevertheless, much remains to be gained from characterizing and defining the dynamics of this system. Sampling in humans is a problem because of the difficulties associated with permission for spinal taps. Despite these problems, there are now several promising new studies of changes in CSF or brain levels of neuropeptides in psychopathological states such as Alzheimer's disease and depression.

Alterations in CRF Levels in Humans

There are currently two areas of psychiatry where CRF systems are implicated in the resulting neuropathology: depression and Alzheimer's disease. It has been known for some time that patients suffering from endogenous depression (major depression, melancholia) have an altered hypothalamic–pituitary–adrenal (HPA) axis. Sachar et al. (1973) demonstrated that such patients had increased concentrations of serum cortisol and Carroll et al. (1981) and others demonstrated that pituitary regulation of ACTH release was not inhibited by the administration of a synthetic glucocorticoid (dexamethasone) in these patients. Nemeroff et al. (1984) and Banki, Bissette, Arato, O'Connor, and Nemeroff (1987) reported increased CSF concentrations of CRF in depressed patients compared to controls, suggesting that central hypersecretion of CRF may be the stimulus that provokes the HPA axis alterations.

In Alzheimer's disease, specific neuronal pathways containing acetylcholine degenerate and brain concentrations of the neuropeptide somatostatin have been shown to be decreased compared to age-matched controls. Bissette, Reynolds, Kilts, Widerlov, and Nemeroff (1985) and DeSouza, Whitehouse, Kuhar, Price, and Vale (1986) have now reported that CRF concentrations are reduced in several cortical and subcortical areas of postmortem Alzheimer's brain compared to controls and DeSouza et al. have further documented a corresponding up-regulation of CRF receptors.

Concluding Remarks

Any successful RIA must be characterized for sensitivity and specificity. Specificity is established by knowing the amino acid sequence of the molecule that the antiserum recognizes, the ability of immunoreactivity to be diluted, and the absence of cross-reactivity of fragments or homologues without the required amino acid recognition sequence. Nonspecific binding should be less than 5% of the total amount of bound radioactive tracer in the absence of cold ligand and the concentrations of cold ligand needed to displace 50% of the radioactive tracer (IC_{50}) should not change from assay to assay. Calculation of the recovery of added synthetic standard at several concentrations is essential to correct for extraction efficiencies. At the risk of stating the obvious, all assay parameters such as buffer constituents, method of tracer iodination, choice of tracer ligand, method of separation of bound and free tracer, and time intervals between addition for each antiserum tracer and separation must be empirically derived for each antiserum. It is probably safe to say that the sensitivity of any existing RIA can be improved by slight adjustments of the appropriate assay parameters.

Thus, to summarize, neuropeptides are ubiquitous intercellular messengers in the body acting both as hormones and hypothesized to be neurotropic (neurotransmitter-like) substances in the CNS. Studies with CRF provide a model by which to explore the methods available to measure and assess the functional significance of a neuropeptide. Exogenous administration of CRF produces profound cellular, physiological, and behavioral actions. New work with a CRF antagonist points to a possible role of endogenous CRF in physiological and behavioral functions associated with stress. CRF levels can be readily measured using RIA and the principles important for CRF measures apply to most other neuropeptides. Finally, CRF has been measured in brain and CSF of humans and these measures may reflect an important role for brain and pituitary CRF in neuropsychiatric disorders.

References

Akil, H., Watson, S. J., Young, E., Lewis, M. E., Khachaturian, H., & Walker, J. M. (1984). Endogenous opioids: Biology and function. *Annual Reviews of Neuroscience, 7,* 223–255.

Aldenhoff, J. B., Gruol, D. L., & Siggins, G. R. (1983). Corticotropin releasing factor decreases postburst hyperpolarizations and excites hippocampal neurons. *Science, 221,* 875–877.

Altura, B. M. (1967). Evaluation of neurohumoral substances in local regulation of blood flow. *American Journal of Physiology, 212,* 1447–1454.

Banki, C. M., Bissette, G., Arato, M., O'Connor, L., & Nemeroff, C. B. (1987). Cerebrospinal fluid corticotropin-releasing factor-like immunoreactivity in depression and schizophrenia. *American Journal of Psychiatry, 144,* 873–877.

Bankoski, K., Manning, M., Halder, J., & Sawyer, W. H. (1978). Testing of potent antagonists of the vasopressor response to arginine vasopressin. *Journal of Medicinal Chemistry, 21,* 850–853.

Barnard, R. R., & Morris, M. (1982). Cerebrospinal fluid vasopressin and oxytocin: Evidence for an osmotic response. *Neuroscience Letters, 29,* 275–279.

Berkowitz, B. A., & Sherman, S. (1982). Characterization of vasopressin analgesia. *Journal of Pharmacology and Experimental Therapeutics, 220,* 329–334.

Bissette, G., Reynolds, G. P., Kilts, C. D., Widerlov, E., & Nemeroff, C. B. (1985). Corticotropin-releasing factor-like immunoreactivity in senile dementia of the Alzheimer's type. *Journal of the American Medical Association, 254,* 3067–3069.

Bohus, B., Kovacs, G. L., & De Wied, D. (1978). Oxytocin, vasopressin and memory: Opposite effects on consolidation and retrieval processes. *Brain Research, 157,* 414–417.

Brown, M. R., & Fisher, L. A. (1984). Brain peptides as intercellular messengers. *Journal of the American Medical Association, 251,* 1310–1315.

Brown, M. R., Fisher, L. A., Rivier, J., Spiess, J., Rivier, C., & Vale, W. (1982). Corticotropin-releasing factor: Effects on the sympathetic nervous system and oxygen consumption. *Life Sciences, 30,* 207–210.

Brown, M. R., Fisher, L. A., Spiess, J., Rivier, J., Rivier, C., & Vale, W. (1982). Comparison of the biologic actions of corticotropin-releasing factor and sauvagine. *Regulatory Peptides, 4,* 107–114.

Brown, M. R., Gray, T. S., & Fisher, L. A. (1986). Corticotropin releasing factor receptor antagonist: Effects on the autonomic nervous system and cardiovascular function. *Regulatory Peptides, 16,* 321–329.

Carroll, B. J., Feinberg, M., Greden, J. F., Tarika, J., Albata,

A. A., Haskett, R. F., James, N., Kronofol, Z., Lohr, N., Steiner, M., Virne, J. P., & Young, E. (1981). A specific laboratory test for the diagnosis of melancholia. *Archives of General Psychiatry, 38,* 15–22.

Coleman, R. J., & Reppert, S. M. (1985).The cerebrospinal fluid vasopressin rhythm is effectively insulated from osmotic regulation of blood pressure. *American Journal of Physiology, 248,* E346–E352.

Demotes-Mainard, J., Chauveau, J., Rodriguez, F., Vincent, J. D., & Poulain, D. A. (1986). Septal release of vasopressin in response to osmotic, hypovolemic and electrical stimulation in rats. *Brain Research, 381,* 314–321.

DeSouza, E. B., Whitehouse, P. J., Kuhar, M. J., Price, D. L., & Vale, W. W. (1986). Reciprocal changes in corticotropin-releasing factor (CRF)-like immunoreactivity and CRF receptors in cerebral cortex of Alzheimer's disease. *Nature, 319,* 593–595.

De Wied, D. (1971). Long term effect of vasopressin on the maintenance of a conditioned avoidance response in rats. *Nature, 232,* 58–60.

De Wied, D. (1976). Behavioral effects of intraventricularly administered vasopressin and vasopressin fragments. *Life Sciences, 19,* 685–690.

De Wied, D. (1977). Behavioral effects of neuropeptides related to ACTH, MSH and β-LPH. In D. Krieger & W. Ganong (Eds.), *ACTH and related peptides: Structure, regulation and action* (pp. 263–274). New York: *Annals of the New York Academy of Sciences.*

De Wied, D, & Versteeg, D. H. G. (1979). Neurohypophyseal principles and memory. *Federation Proceedings, 38,* 2348–2354.

Eaves, M., Thatcher-Britton, K., Rivier, J., Vale, W., & Koob, G. F. (1985). Effects of corticotropin releasing factor on locomotor activity in hypophysectomized rats. *Peptides, 6,* 923–926.

Ehlers, C. L., Henriksen, S. J., Bloom, F. E., Rivier, J., & Vale, W. W. (1983). Corticotropin releasing factor produces increases in brain excitability and convulsive seizures in rats. *Brain Research, 278,* 332–336.

Ettenberg, A. (1985). Intracerebroventricular application of a pressor antagonist of vasopressin prevents both the "memory" and "aversive" actions of vasopressin. *Behavior and Brain Research, 14,* 201–211.

Ettenberg, A., Le Moal, M., Koob, G. F., & Bloom, F. E. (1983). Vasopressin potentiation in the performance of a learned appetitive task: Reversal by a pressor antagonist analog of vasopressin. *Pharmacology, Biochemistry and Behavior, 18,* 645–647.

Fessler, R. G., Brown, F. D., Rachlin, J. R., Mullan, S., & Fang, V. S. (1984). Elevated β-endorphin in cerebrospinal fluid after electrical brain stimulation: Artifact of contrast infusion? *Science, 224,* 1017–1019.

Fisher, L. A., Rivier, J., Rivier, C., Spiess, J., Vale, W., & Brown, M. (1982). Corticotropin releasing factor (CRF): Central effects on mean arterial pressure and heart rate in rats. *Endocrinology, 110,* 2222–2224.

Gibbs, D. M. (1984). Dissociation of oxytocin, vasopressin and corticotropin secretion during different types of stress. *Life Sciences, 35,* 487–491.

Gillies, G. E., Linton, E. A., & Lowry, P. J. (1982). Corticotropin releasing activity of the new CRF is potentiated several times by vasopressin. *Nature, 299,* 355–357.

Gold, P. W., Chrousos, G., Kellner, C., Post, R., Roy, A., Augerines, P., Schultes, H., Oldfield, E., & Loriaux, D. L. (1984). Psychiatric implications of basic and clinical studies with corticotropin-releasing factor. *American Journal of Psychiatry, 141,* 619–627.

Hambrook, J. M., Morgan, B. A., Rance, M. J., & Smith, C. F. C. (1976). Mode of deactivation of the enkephalins by rat and human plasma and rat brain homogenates. *Nature, 262,* 782–783.

Hokfelt, T., Johansson, O., Ljungdahl, A., Lundberg, J. M., & Schultzberg, M. (1980). Peptidergic neurons. *Nature, 284,* 515–521.

Kasting, N. W., Veale, W. L., & Cooper, K. E. (1982). Vasopressin: A homeostatic effector in the febrile process. *Neuroscience and Biobehavioral Research, 6,* 215–222.

Kendler, K. S., Weitzman, R. E., & Fisher, D. A. (1978). The effect of pain on plasma arginine vasopressin concentration in man. *Clinical Endocrinology, 8,* 89–94.

Koob, G. F., & Bloom, F. E. (1985). Corticotropin-releasing factor and behavior. *Federation Proceedings, 44,* 259–263.

Koob, G. F., Le Moal, M., Gaffori, O., Manning, M., Sawyer, W. H., Rivier, J., & Bloom, F. E. (1981). Arginine vasopressin and a vasopressin antagonist peptide: Opposite effects on extinction of active avoidance in rats. *Regulatory Peptides, 2,* 153–163.

Koob, G. F., Lebrun, C., Martinez, J. L., Jr., Bluthe, R. M., Dantzer, R., Bloom, F. E., & Le Moal, M. (1985). Use of arginine vasopressin antagonists in elucidating the mechanism of action for the behavioral effects of arginine vasopressin. In R. W. Schrier (Ed.), *Vasopressin* (pp. 195–201). New York: Raven Press.

Koob, G. F., Dantzer, R., Bluthe, R. M., Lebrun, C., Bloom, F. E., & Le Moal, M. (1986). Central injections of arginine vasopressin prolong extinction of active avoidance. *Peptides, 7,* 213–218.

Laczi, F., Gaffori, O., Fekele, M., de Kloet, E. R., & De Wied, D. (1984). Levels of arginine vasopressin in cerebrospinal fluid during passive avoidance behavior in rats. *Life Sciences,* 2385–2391.

Lebrun, C. J., Rigter, H., Martinez, J. L., Jr., Koob, G. F., Le Moal, M., & Bloom, F. E. (1984). Antagonism of effects of vasopressin (AVP) on inhibitory avoidance by a vasopressor antagonist peptide (dPtyr(Me)AVP). *Life Sciences, 35,* 1505–1512.

Le Moal, M., Koob, G. F., Koda, L. Y., Bloom, F. E., Manning, M., Sawyer, W. J., & Rivier, J. (1981). Vasopressor receptor antagonist prevents behavioral effects of vasopressin. *Nature, 291,* 491–493.

Levine, A. S., Rogers, B., Kwerp, J., Grace, M., & Morley, J. E. (1982). Effect of centrally administered corticotropin releasing factor (CRF) on multiple feeding paradigms. *Neuropharmacology, 22,* 337–339.

Loh, H. H., Tseng, L. F., Wei, E., & Li, C. H. (1976). β-Endorphin is a potent analgesic agent. *Proceedings of the National Academy of Sciences of the United States of America, 73*, 2895–2898.

Manning, M., & Sawyer, W. H. (1984). Design and uses of selective agonist and antagonistic analogs of the neuropeptides oxytocin and vasopressin. *Trends in Neuroscience, 7*, 6–9.

Mens, W. B. J., Bouman, H. J., Baker, E. A. D., & van Wimersma Greidanus, T. B. (1980). Differential effects of various stimuli on AVP levels in blood and cerebrospinal fluid. *European Journal of Pharmacology, 68*, 89–92.

Morley, J. E., & Levine, A. S. (1983). Corticotropin-releasing factor, grooming and ingestive behavior. *Life Sciences, 31*, 1459–1464.

Nemeroff, C. B., Widerlov, E., Bissette, G., Walleus, H., Karlsson, I., Ecklund, K., Kilts, C. D., Loosen, P. T., & Vale, W. (1984). Elevated concentrations of CSF corticotropin-releasing factor like immunoreactivity in depressed patients. *Science, 226*, 1342–1344.

Oldfield, E. H., Schulte, H. M., Chrousos, G. P., Rock, J. P., Kornblith, P. A., O'Neill, D. L., Poplack, D. G., Gold, P. W., Cutter, G. B., Jr., & Loriaux, L. (1985). Active clearance of corticotropin-releasing factor from the cerebrospinal fluid. *Neuroendocrinology, 40*, 80–87.

Perlow, M. J., Reppert, S. M., Artman, H. A., Fisher, D. A., Seif, S. M., & Robinson, A. G. (1982). Oxytocin, vasopressin, and estrogen-stimulated neurophysin: Daily patterns of concentration in cerebrospinal fluid. *Science, 216*, 1416–1418.

Pittman, G. J., Lawrence, D., & McLean, L. (1982). Central effects of arginine vasopressin on blood pressure in rats. *Endocrinology, 110*, 1058–1061.

Plotsky, P. M., Bruhn, T. O., & Vale, W. (1985). Hypophysiotropic localization of vasopressin, oxytocin and neurophysin in the rat; its relationship with corticotropin function. *Brain Research, 168*, 275–286.

Rivier, J., Rivier, C., & Vale, W. (1984). Synthetic competitive antagonists of corticotropin-releasing factor: Effect on ACTH secretion. *Science, 224*, 889–891.

Rocha E. Silva, M., Jr., & Rosenberg, M. (1969). The release of vasopressin in response to haemorrhage and its role in the mechanism of blood pressure regulations. *Journal of Physiology 202*, (London) 535–557.

Rossier, J., Bayon, A., Vargo, T. M., & Ling, N. (1977). Radioimmunoassay of brain peptides: Evaluation of a methodology for the assay of β-endorphin and enkephalin. *Life Sciences, 21*, 847–852.

Rossier, J., Vargo, T. M., Minick, S., Ling, N., Bloom, F. E., & Guillemin, R. (1977). Regional dissociation of β-endorphin and enkephalin contents in rat brain and pituitary. *Proceedings of the National Academy of Sciences of the United States of America, 74*, 5162–5165.

Sachar, E. J., Hellman, L., Roffwang, H. P., Halpern, F. S., Fukushima, D. K., & Gallagher, T. F. (1973). Disrupted 24-hour patterns of cortisol secretion in psychotic depression. *Archives of General Psychiatry, 28*, 19–24.

Sawyer, W. H. (1964). Vertebrate neurohypophysial principles. *Endocrinology, 75*, 981–990.

Schulte, H. M., Chrousos, G. P., Booth, J. D., Oldfield, E. H., Gold, P. W., Cutter, G. B., Jr., & Loriaux, D. L. (1984). Corticotropin-releasing factor: Pharmacokinetics in man. *Journal of Clinical Endocrinology and Metabolism, 58*, 192–196.

Schwartz, W. J., Coleman, R. J., & Reppert, S. M. (1983). A daily vasopressin rhythm in rat cerebrospinal fluid. *Brain Research, 263*, 105–112.

Selye, H. (1980). *Selye's guide to stress research* (pp. v–xiii). Princeton, NJ: Van Nostrand–Reinhold.

Siggins, G. R., Gruol, D., Aldenhoff, J., & Pittman, Q. (1985). Electrophysiological actions of corticotropin-releasing factor in the central nervous system. *Federation Proceedings, 44*, 237–242.

Stalla, G. K., Hartwimmer, J., Schopohl, J., von Werder, K., & Muller, O. A. (1986). Intravenous application of ovine and human corticotropin-releasing factor (CRF): ACTH, cortisol and CRF levels. *Neuroendocrinology, 42*, 1–5.

Stegner, H., Leake, R. D., Palmer, S. M., Oakes, G., & Fisher, D. A. (1984). The effect of hypoxia on neurohypophyseal hormone release in fetal and maternal sheep. *Pediatric Research, 18*, 188–191.

Straus, M. B. (1956). *Body water in man* (pp. 82–104). Boston: Little, Brown.

Straus, E., & Yalow, R. S. (1977). Specific problems in the identification and quantitation of neuropeptides by radioimmunoassay. In H. Gainer (Ed.), *Peptides in neurobiology* (pp. 39–61). New York: Plenum Press.

Sutton, R., Koob, G., Le Moal, M., Rivier, J., & Vale, W. (1982). Corticotropin releasing factor (CRF) produces behavioral activation in rats. *Nature, 299*, 331–333.

Swerdlow, N., Geyer, M., Vale, W. W., & Koob, G. F. (1986). Corticotropin releasing factor potentiates acoustic startle in the rats: Blockade by chlordiazepoxide. *Psychopharmacology, 88*, 142–152.

Tache, Y., & Gunion, M. (1985). Corticotropin-releasing factor: Central action to influence gastric secretion. *Federation Proceedings, 44*, 255–258.

Tache, Y., Goto, Y., Gunion, M., Vale, W., Rivier, J., & Brown, M. (1983). Inhibition of gastric acid secretion in rats by intracerebral injection of corticotropin-releasing factor. *Science, 222*, 935–937.

Tazi, A., Dantzer, R., Mormede, R., & Le Moal, M. (1983). Effects of post-trial administration of naloxone and β-endorphin on shock-induced fighting in rats. *Behavioral and Neural Biology, 39*, 192–202.

Tazi, A., Dantzer, R., Mormede, R., & Le Moal, M. (1985). Effects of post-trial injection of β-endorphin on shock-induced fighting are dependent on baseline of fighting. *Behavioral and Neural Biology, 43*, 322–326.

Tazi, A., Dantzer, R., Le Moal, M., & Koob, G. F. (1987). Corticotropin-releasing factor antagonist blocks stress-induced fighting in rats. *Regulatory Peptides, 18*, 37–42.

Thatcher-Britton, K., Morgan, J., Rivier, J., Vale, W., & Koob, G. F. (1985). Chlordiazepoxide attenuates CRF-induced response suppression in the conflict test. *Psychophar-macology, 86,* 150–174.

Vale, W., Spiess, J., Rivier, C., & Rivier, J. (1981). Characterization of a 41-residue ovine hypothalamic peptide that stimulates the secretion of corticotropin and β-endorphin. *Science, 213,* 1394–1397.

Yates, F. E., Russell, S. M., Dallman, M. F., Hedge, G. A., McCann, S. M., & Dhariwal, A. P. A. (1971). Potentiation by vasopressin of corticotropin release induced by corticotropin-releasing factor. *Endocrinology, 88,* 3–15.

CHAPTER **14**

Receptors

David Robertson, Yelena Parfyonova, Mikhail Menshikov, and Alan S. Hollister

Introduction

In the past ten years, binding sites for more than two dozen neurotransmitters and hormones have been identified. With the exception of the thyroid and steroid hormone receptors, all neurotransmitter and peptide receptors have thus far been localized to the cell surface of the target organ. It has become clear that the membranes of most cells are endowed with a remarkably heterogeneous population of receptor sites.

Historically, we learned about receptors from observing the biological response of intact isolated organs to the application of agonists or antagonists. Such responses were, of course, indirect, since several steps often separate the initial drug–receptor interaction from the biological response and each intervening step adds greatly to the complexity of data interpretation. These problems are particularly acute in studying the interactions of antagonists (Gaddum, 1957; Kenakin, 1984).

Since the 1970s, a second approach has been

widely employed in studying receptors: the measurement of drug binding to tissue homogenates. The successful exploitation of this technique became possible with the development of drugs with high affinity for the receptor site as well as high specific radioactivity. Both direct and indirect methods have been used. The direct method usually involves the incubation of labeled agonists or antagonists followed by separation of the receptor–ligand complex from the free ligand by filtration, centrifugation, or precipitation. The most commonly employed indirect method of assessment is equilibrium dialysis.

In their enthusiasm to exploit radioligand binding methodology to address research problems, investigators have sometimes neglected the biological response correlates. Of even greater concern, the importance of confirming the authenticity of identified binding sites by the saturability, specificity, and reversibility criteria has sometimes also been neglected. For this reason, premature or erroneous conclusions relating binding to physiology have been made.

There are a number of excellent monographs dealing with the theory and practice of radioligand binding methodology. Perhaps the most complete monograph is that of Limbird (1986). An excellent monograph on human adrenoreceptors has recently appeared (Insel & Motulsky, 1987) with an extremely readable and concise section on how to

David Robertson, Yelena Parfyonova, Mikhail Menshikov, and Alan S. Hollister • Departments of Medicine and Pharmacology, Vanderbilt University Medical Center, Nashville, Tennessee 37232.
Y. P. and M. M. were exchange scholars from the Myasnikov Institute of the All-Union Cardiological Research Center, Moscow, U.S.S.R.

perform receptor ligand binding studies. In this chapter, insofar as possible, we have adopted Limbird's terminology and abbreviations, for the convenience of the reader who may be referring to her text. Other helpful monographs also exist (Levitzki, 1984; Molinoff, Wolfe, & Weiland, 1981; Weiland & Molinoff, 1981). Some authors have also addressed the use of the computer in radioligand binding studies (Munson & Rodbard, 1980; DeLean, Hancock, & Lefkowitz, 1982). The classical pharmacology of drug–receptor interactions is dealt with in pharmacology textbooks (Goldstein, Aronow, & Kalman, 1974) and will not be reiterated here except when it relates directly to radioligand binding methodology.

Theoretical Basis

Much of the theoretical underpinning of receptor ligand binding methodology was developed to explain the effect of agonists on isolated organ systems in the era before agonist–receptor interactions could be more directly assessed (Ariëns, 1954; Nickerson, 1956; Stephenson, 1956; Van Rossum & Ariëns, 1962). The mathematical derivation of these formulas is usually emphasized in introductions to receptor methods, but understanding these derivations, though intellectually satisfying, must not be seen as a substitute for an intuitive grasp of the concepts used in the description of receptors and their coupling.

The binding of a hormone or drug (D) to its receptor (R) can be described in terms of the following equations:

$$D + R \underset{k_2}{\overset{k_1}{\rightleftharpoons}} DR \qquad (1)$$

where D is a hormone, drug, or ligand, R is a receptor, DR is a complex of receptor with hormone, k_1 is the association rate constant, and k_2 is the dissociation rate constant.

k_1 and k_2 can be related to the equilibrium dissociation constant (K_D) in the following manner:

$$K_D = \frac{k_2}{k_1} = \frac{[D][R]}{[DR]} \qquad (2)$$

The K_D is commonly used to describe the affinity of a receptor for a drug. It is the concentration of drug or hormone that half-maximally occupies the receptor at equilibrium. The units of K_D are therefore molar and an increase in K_D reflects a decrease in affinity.

The total number of receptors is the sum of those without attached ligand (R) and those with attached ligand (DR):

$$R_{TOT} = [R] + [DR] \qquad (3)$$

where R_{TOT} is the total number of receptor sites = B_{max}.

It is useful to define the fractional saturation of receptors in order to obtain a more helpful formulation:

$$\bar{Y} = \frac{[DR]}{R_{TOT}} = \frac{B}{B_{max}} \qquad (4)$$

where $\bar{Y}$ is the fractional saturation of R with D, and B is the concentration of D bound to R.

Now substituting from equations (2) and (3), we obtain:

$$\bar{Y} = \frac{[D]}{K_D + [D]} \qquad (5)$$

When incubations are performed with receptor concentration held constant while ligand concentration is varied, a plot of $\bar{Y}$ versus [D] will yield a rectangular hyperbola (Figure 1). Because the form of this plot resembles that derived by Langmuir for absorption of a gas to a surface at a constant temperature, such curves are often called "binding isotherms." If log [D] rather than [D] is plotted on the x axis, a sigmoid curve results (Figure 2). With either curve, K_D can be estimated at half-saturation of $\bar{Y}$.

Equation (5) can be rearranged, substituting [F] for [D], to yield

$$B = \frac{[F] B_{max}}{K_D + [F]} \qquad (6)$$

where [F] is the concentration of free hormone.

Furthermore, equation (6) can be transformed into a linear expression of the form $y = mx + b$:

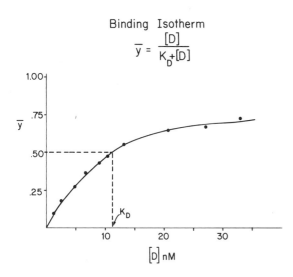

Binding Isotherm

$$\bar{y} = \frac{[D]}{K_D + [D]}$$

Figure 1. Binding isotherm, a plot of fractional saturation of R with D as a function of the concentration of D. See equation (5).

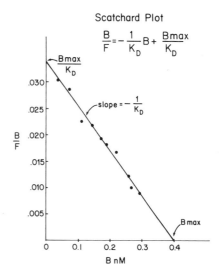

Scatchard Plot

$$\frac{B}{F} = -\frac{1}{K_D} B + \frac{Bmax}{K_D}$$

Figure 3. Scatchard plot of B/F versus B. See equation (7).

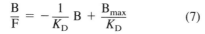

$$\frac{B}{F} = -\frac{1}{K_D} B + \frac{B_{max}}{K_D} \qquad (7)$$

Now if B/F is plotted against B (Figure 3) for a system at equilibrium, a straight line of slope $-1/K_D$ will result (assuming a single type of binding site). Extrapolation to the intercept on the x axis gives B_{max}, the total concentration of receptor sites. Such a representation is usually called a Scatchard plot, although it is sometimes referred to as a Rosenthal plot. The Scatchard plot is the most widely used graphic representation of binding phenomena.

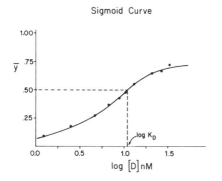

Sigmoid Curve

Figure 2. The plot in Figure 1, but with the logarithm of [D] on the x axis. See equation (5).

Another widely used data representation is the Hill plot. It is used to determine if the ligand and receptor of interest interact via a bimolecular reaction in conformity with the mass action law. When $\log (B/(B_{max}-B))$ is plotted against $\log [D]$ (Figure 4), the slope will be unity if B/B_{max} is proportional to the fraction of sites occupied ($\bar{Y}$).

When the slope of the Hill plot is not unity, this may be due to positive cooperativity (slope > 1.0) or heterogeneous binding or negative cooperativity (slope < 1.0).

The study of competitive inhibitors of receptor ligand binding requires the use of the Cheng and Prusoff equation [equation (8)], which was originally developed to describe the behavior of enzyme inhibitors:

$$K_I = \frac{EC_{50}}{1 + [D^*]/K_{D^*}} \qquad (8)$$

where K_I is the equilibrium dissociation constant for competitor, K_{D^*} is the equilibrium dissociation constant for radioligand, and EC_{50} is the concentration of competitor which effectively competes for 50% of the specific radioligand binding.

A number of criteria must be met for the Cheng and Prusoff equation to be applied to a receptor system:

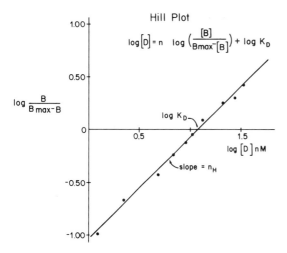

Figure 4. Hill plot of log $(B/(B_{max} - B))$ versus log D. Slope (n) is 1.0 when a single receptor site, which obeys the law of mass action, is present.

1. The tritiated or iodinated ligand must interact with a single population of receptors with a constant affinity for the radioligand; furthermore, the competitor must meet the same restrictions.
2. The receptor concentration must be much less than the K_D of the radioligand or the competitor.
3. Steady state must have been reached.
4. The concentration of unbound receptors should be much lower than the K_D of the radioligand.

The careful use of these formulas and graphic representations can provide an enormous amount of information concerning diverse receptors in a great many tissues.

Methods

At first glance the application of the theoretical principles outlined above may seem strikingly simple. A radioactively labeled drug with selectivity for the relevant receptor is mixed with tissue containing that receptor type. After equilibration, unbound radioactivity is removed, usually by filtration or centrifugation, and the radioactivity still associated with the tissue is taken as an index of receptor binding. In reality, there are many pitfalls

in the conduct of binding studies that make their interpretation problematical.

It is obvious that before determinations of receptor number and affinity can be made, preliminary investigations are required to determine the appropriate amount of tissue to be used in each incubation tube, the appropriate concentration of radioligand in the incubation, the nonspecific binding, the stability of the radioligand in the incubation mixture, the time required for equilibration to occur, the saturability of binding, the agreement of independent methods of deriving the equilibration dissociation constant, and the proportionality of tissue concentration and specific binding of radioligand. Satisfying these criteria to support the biological relevance of the receptor in question is often a difficult and time-consuming exercise. Nevertheless, its importance is very great; almost all the errors in the receptor literature have resulted from a failure to address adequately one or more of these issues.

Nonspecific Binding

Although radioligands are designed to bind only to specific receptor sites, in practice there is almost always a significant amount of nonspecific binding. It can be appreciated that the small number of receptor sites (often only a few hundred per cell) constitute a miniscule portion of a membrane surface. This surface usually has many thousands of other receptor sites in addition to nonreceptor structures to which ligand may become nonspecifically attached.

Fortunately, it is usually possible to study the displacement of the labeled ligand with a series of agonists and antagonists of distinct chemical structures which nevertheless possess the same pharmacological properties as the binding ligand.

In studying nonspecific binding in any given system, it is important to consider the possibility that some binding occurs to nontissue sites. For example, insulin has been shown to bind to talcum powder in the nanomolar range, substance P can bind to glass, and glass fibers can sometimes selectively bind the levorotatory isomer of an opiate.

For adrenoreceptors, 0.1–1.0 mM $(-)$-isoproterenol is usually used to test for specificity of binding to β receptors and 10 μM phentolamine or

100 μM (−)-epinephrine is usually used for α receptors. With these concentrations, it is generally assumed that specific adrenoreceptor sites are blocked and that any bound radioactivity must therefore be attached to nonspecific sites. This amount of radioactivity should therefore be subtracted from the total radioligand binding in the absence of competing ligands in order to obtain an estimate of specific binding.

Binding Saturability

Because there are a limited number of receptor sites per cell, it is clear that the dose–response curve for radioligand binding should reveal saturability of receptor binding. The high-affinity and low-capacity binding which is characteristic of most receptor sites of physiological interest is usually distinguishable from the high-capacity and low-affinity nonspecific binding which is virtually nonsaturable.

Saturability is usually studied in binding experiments with a fixed concentration of tissue and various concentrations of radioligand at equilibrium. Two important variables can be derived from the saturation binding curve as shown in the previous section [equation (7)]. The maximal binding (B_{max}) is a measure of the total number of receptors in the tissue. The equilibrium dissociation constant, K_D, which is the concentration of radioligand required to bind half the receptor sites, is an inverse reflection of receptor affinity. A low K_D reflects high-affinity binding and a high K_D reflects low-affinity binding.

If an attempt is made to measure changes in receptor number on the basis of a single saturating concentration of radioligand, erroneous results will be obtained. In the face of the very high concentration of radioligand that may be required to saturate the receptors, nonspecific binding may be increased as well. Moreover, with a single concentration of radioligand, it is not possible to distinguish alterations in K_D from those in B_{max}.

Binding Reversibility

Since neurotransmitters and hormones act in a reversible manner, the binding of these agents would also be expected to be reversible. More-over, the neurotransmitter or hormone should be able to be recovered in its nonmetabolized form.

In practice, the rate of association (the "on-rate") of radioligand and receptor can be determined by incubating the radioligand with the relevant tissue and measuring the amount of specific binding at appropriate intervals. The binding will reach a plateau at steady state. The time required for this equilibrium to be achieved depends on the concentration of radioligand and receptor in the incubation, with higher concentrations causing more rapid development of equilibrium. Adrenoreceptor radioligands usually have association rate constants of 10^7 to 10^9 M^{-1} min^{-1}. When adrenoreceptor assays are conducted at 25–37°C, equilibrium is usually reached in 30 to 90 min.

There are two potential errors in estimating the rate of association of radioligand and receptor. The first is that an underestimation of equilibration time may be made if the on-rate experiment is not performed with a low concentration of radioligand. Second, competitive binding experiments will require a longer time to reach equilibrium than would be predicted from the simple on-rate experiment. These issues have been elegantly treated by Motulsky and Mahan (1984).

To measure the rate of dissociation, radioligand is initially allowed to bind to receptor sites. The binding reaction is then blocked and the amount of specific radioligand binding at various times thereafter is measured. Blocking the binding reaction is accomplished by addition of excess unlabeled compound or by greatly diluting the reaction mixture (thus reducing radioligand concentration).

Dissociation of radioligand binding usually follows a monoexponential decay curve. If this dissociation occurs too rapidly (e.g., if it occurs during the few seconds required for separation of bound and free ligand), subsequent experiments may be seriously flawed in their interpretation. In such cases, it is necessary to speed up the separation process (e.g., by using centrifugation rather than filtration) or to retard the dissociation (perhaps by using cold buffer when washing filters).

Competition Binding

When the binding of an appropriate radioligand to an adrenoreceptor has been worked out, much additional information can be learned by assessing the capacity of unlabeled drugs to compete for that specific binding. There are an exceptionally large number of compounds which bind to α and β adrenoreceptors and the relative potencies of the binding of these compounds at the receptor site of interest can aid not only in determining the subtype of receptor being examined, but may also confirm the stereoselectivity of binding of some asymmetric molecules.

The IC_{50}, the concentration of competitor that competes for half the radioligand binding, usually approximates the K_I of the competitor. Because this relationship depends on the concentration of radioligand and the K_D of the receptors for the radioligand, the relationship between IC_{50} and K_I is not fixed. The Cheng and Prusoff equation (8) describes this relationship. The Hill slope quantitates the steepness of a competition curve. A finding of a Hill slope at unity supports the hypothesis that both radioligand and competitor bind to a single class of receptors, and confirms the validity of calculating the K_I from the IC_{50}.

Natural History of Receptors

Structure

Neurotransmitter receptors are just now being characterized through the techniques of molecular biology. Some astonishing similarities and differences across receptor types are beginning to emerge. Two families of receptors are now recognized by structural and functional criteria.

The first family includes the β-adrenoreceptor (Lefkowitz & Caron, 1986), the muscarinic receptor (Kubo et al., 1986), and rhodopsin (Benovic, Mayor, Somers, Caron, & Lefkowitz, 1986) which possess a high degree of homology to each other. These receptors interact with G proteins (Bourne, 1986) and adenylate cyclase and have a structure that includes seven traverses of the cell membrane.

The second family includes the nicotinic receptor, the glycine receptor (Grenningloh et al., 1987), and the $GABA_A$ receptor. These receptors share subunit homology and function as ion channels. It has been startling to learn that the mus-

carinic cholinergic receptor resembles the β-adrenoreceptor more closely than it does the nicotinic cholinergic receptor. Recognition that these families have significant stretches of conserved structure should lead to widespread investigations with synthetic nucleotide probes for yet other family members of either group. There may also prove to be new families.

Metabolism

The metabolism of α- and β-adrenoreceptors can now be studied in intact cells using a variety of direct and indirect approaches (Mahan, Motulsky, & Insel, 1985; Motulsky, Cunningham, DeBlasi, & Insel, 1986; Mahan, McKernan, & Insel, 1987). Both α- and β-adrenoreceptors are metabolized slowly in vitro under basal conditions (no agonist exposure). Half lives are usually hours or days, somewhat slower than is observed with other hormones and neurotransmitter classes. Half lives of different adrenoreceptors, even if expressed on the same cell and in the same environment, may differ.

Treatment of cells with agonists shortens the half-life of α_1- and β-adrenoreceptors (Mahan et al., 1987); the shortened half-life results primarily from enhanced receptor loss from the plasma membrane rather than from agonist-induced attenuation of receptor appearance.

In general, adrenoceptors in the CNS appear to have a longer half-life than those in the periphery (Mahan et al., 1987).

Peripheral Adrenoreceptors

The most extensively studied human adrenoreceptors are those occurring on circulating blood cells. The inherent advantages of a readily accessible tissue that can be repeatedly sampled in human subjects are obvious.

Platelet α_2-Adrenoreceptors

Catecholamines act via α_2-adrenoreceptors to initiate platelet aggregation and secretion (Berthelsen & Pettinger, 1977), and to inhibit platelet adenylate cyclase activity. Since α_2-adrenoreceptors exist in the human vascular bed where they mediate an increase in blood pressure (Goldberg & Robertson, 1984; Robertson, Goldberg, Hollister, Wade, & Robertson, 1983; Robertson, Goldberg, Hollister, *et al.*, 1986), the partial agonist [^{3}H]clonidine (Shattil, McDonough, Turnbull, & Insel, 1981) and the selective antagonist radioligand, [^{3}H]yohimbine, have been used to characterize α_2-adrenoreceptors in both intact and membrane preparations of human platelets (Motulsky & Insel, 1982; Motulsky, O'Connor, & Insel, 1983; Goldberg & Robertson, 1983; Goldberg, Hollister, & Robertson, 1983; Hollister, FitzGerald, Nadeau, & Robertson, 1983; Cameron, Smith, Hollingsworth, Nesse, & Curtis, 1984). Although in certain tissues clonidine itself does not appear to elicit the desensitization one would expect of a full agonist (Villeneuve, Carpene, Berlan, & Lafontan, 1985), alterations in platelet α_2-adrenoreceptor character after catecholamine infusion have been demonstrated in humans. These studies have confirmed the α_2-adrenergic classification of these platelet receptors, have identified influences of sodium and magnesium on α_2-adrenoreceptor agonist binding affinity, and have demonstrated high and low agonist affinity states of the receptor, which are modulated by guanine nucleotides.

Exposure of platelets to high concentrations of catecholamines *in vitro* has been reported to alter the number of assayable platelet α_2-adrenoreceptors (Brodde, Daul, O'Hara, & Khalifa, 1985), either through a reduction in receptor number or by retention of agonist in the preparation (Karliner, Motulsky, & Insel, 1982). Exposure to catecholamines at concentrations below 10^{-5} M did not alter the number of platelet α_2-adrenoreceptors. *In vivo* studies in which catecholamine concentrations ranged from 10^{-7} to 10^{-10} M have yielded contradictory results. It has been reported that patients with high levels of plasma catecholamines (Bravo, Tarazi, Gifford, & Stewart, 1979) due to pheochromocytoma have low or normal numbers of receptors (Snavely, Motulsky, O'Connor, Ziegler, & Insel, 1982; Greenacre & Conolly, 1978), and patients with idiopathic orthostatic hypotension have high or normal receptor density (Chobanian, Tifft, Sackel, & Pitruzella, 1982). However, in several physiological circumstances, α_2-adrenoreceptors in platelets have not appeared to change in number (Pfeifer *et al.*, 1984).

In contrast to the results with α_2 receptor number and antagonist affinity described above, agonist affinity of platelet α_2-adrenoreceptors occasionally is found to be altered. In competition studies with yohimbine, mean platelet receptor affinity for *l*-epinephrine was decreased 3.4-fold after 2 h of upright posture and exercise (Hollister *et al.*, 1983). This change in agonist affinity correlated significantly with the increases in plasma epinephrine and norepinephrine that were stimulated by upright posture and exercise. Supine subjects infused with *l*-norepinephrine or *l*-epinephrine for 2 h also averaged a 3.3- and a 2.7-fold decrease in platelet α_2-adrenoreceptor affinity for agonist with no change in receptor number or antagonist affinity. The α_2-adrenoreceptor agonist affinity changes were specific for α agonists since they were blocked by phentolamine and incubation with 10^{-5} M isoproterenol produced no change in α_2-adrenoreceptor affinity for *l*-epinephrine.

In vitro exposure of intact human platelets to 10^{-6} to 10^{-10} M *l*-epinephrine for 2 h produced a concentration-related decrease in α_2-adrenoreceptor affinity for agonist (Hollister *et al.*, 1983; Hollister, Onrot, *et al.*, 1986). Average slope factors approached 1.0 as affinity decreased, which is consistent with a heterogeneous receptor population that becomes more homogeneous after agonist exposure. Incubation of platelet-rich plasma with 10^{-6} to 10^{-8} M *l*-epinephrine resulted in a dose- and time-related loss of aggregatory response to *l*-epinephrine; this demonstrates that agonist affinity changes are correlated with changes in receptor sensitivity.

These observations demonstrate that physiological variations in plasma catecholamines acutely modulate the intact human platelet α_2-adrenoreceptor's affinity for agonist, and can thereby alter the sensitivity of platelets to α_2-adrenergic agonists.

Leukocyte β_2-Adrenoreceptors

Catecholamines interact with β-adrenoreceptors and result in the activation of adenylate cyclase with consequent cAMP accumulation within the cells (Harden, 1983). However, because of rapid desensitization, this response may be transient (DeBlasi, Lipartiti, *et al.*, 1986). In early studies of human β-adrenoreceptors, changes in number and agonist affinity were determined before the process of internalization was fully able to be addressed (Krall, Connelly, & Tuck, 1980; Fraser, Nadeau, Robertson, & Wood, 1981; Feldman *et al.*, 1983; Feldman, Limbird, Nadeau, Robertson, & Wood, 1984a,b). Recent studies have demonstrated that desensitization is accompanied by translocation of the receptor site due to the process of internalization (sometimes called redistribution or sequestration) (Motulsky *et al.*, 1986).

The incubation of whole blood with agonist for periods of 10 to 30 min will decrease isoproterenol-stimulated cAMP accumulation in mononuclear leukocytes by about 50% (DeBlasi, Lipartiti, Motulsky, Insel, & Fratelli, 1985). Concomitantly, 70 to 80% of β-adrenoreceptors are internalized. Although these internalized receptors are inaccessible to hydrophilic compounds such as CGP-12177 and isoproterenol, they are measured by iodocyanopindolol (Engel, Hoyer, Berthold, & Wagner, 1981).

Early studies using membrane preparations showed that the number of β-adrenoreceptors on mononuclear leukocytes and isoproterenol-stimulated cAMP production increased following exercise (Cundell, Danks, Phillips, & Davies, 1984; Butler, Kelly, O'Malley, & Pidgeon, 1983; Brodde, Daul, & O'Hara, 1984). There was some uncertainty as to the appropriate interpretation of this finding since the total number of mononuclear leukocytes is known to increase with exercise (Edwards *et al.*, 1984; Soppi, Varjo, Eskola, & Laitinen, 1982). However, in one recent careful collaborative study, no increase in receptor number on intact mononuclear leukocytes was detected although isoproterenol-stimulated cAMP accumulation did increase after exercise (DeBlasi, Maisel, *et al.*, 1986). This increase was not, however, accompanied by an increase in cAMP accumulation stimulated by either forskolin or prostaglandin E_1. There was also an increase in isoproterenol-stimulated cAMP accumulation after assumption of upright posture. The relation of circulating catecholamine levels to β-adrenoreceptor concentrations remains controversial (Sowers,

Connelly-Fittinghoff, Tuck, & Krall, 1983; Tohmen & Cryer, 1980; Brodde, 1986). Changes can be seen in response to chronic states of catecholamine excess and in the face of sympathomimetic amines (Colucci *et al.*, 1981).

The earlier demonstration that upright posture reduced both receptor affinity for agonist and isoproterenol-stimulated adenylate cyclase activity in mononuclear leukocyte membranes (Feldman *et al.*, 1983) would appear to be in conflict with the above finding. However, the critical determinant may be the importance of added GTP. Whereas the previous data were obtained in an assay without added GTP, this reduction in adenylate cyclase activity did not occur when excess GTP was included in the assay. Agonist-stimulated adenylate cyclase activity in the absence of added GTP must depend on the presence of guanine nucleotides retained in the membrane preparations. Therefore, the differences in postural change might be due to either a differential retention of guanine nucleotides or a differential sensitivity of adenylate cyclase to GTP, rather than to desensitization of maximum β-adrenoreceptor stimulated adenylate cyclase activity.

In summary, the results of recent β-adrenoreceptor radioligand binding studies on mononuclear leukocytes in human subjects underscore the complexity of such analysis and the limited validity of conclusions drawn concerning the character and function of receptors distant from those being analyzed.

Hypertension and Adrenoreceptors

Many early investigations of the role of the sympathetic nervous system in human hypertension concentrated on attempts to detect elevated plasma catecholamines in hypertensive subjects. Although these studies varied greatly in design, the data do not generally support the hypothesis that catecholamine excess is the sole cause of hypertension. However, numerous studies have shown that hypertensive subjects display enhanced pressor responsiveness to catecholamine and sympathomimetic amine infusions. These findings are consistent with the proposal that vasoconstrictor α-adrenoreceptors of hypertensive subjects are more sensitive to catecholamines than are those of normotensives.

Increased responsiveness of adrenergic receptors may be secondary to an increase in the number of receptors and/or an increase in receptor–effector coupling efficiency (Stiles, Caron, & Lefkowitz, 1984; Aarons, Nies, Gal, Hegstrand, & Molinoff, 1980). It seems clear that alterations in β-receptor–effector coupling are present in patients with hypertension (Feldman *et al.*, 1984a). The situation with α_2-adrenoreceptors is much less clear (Boon *et al.*, 1983). However, several reports have described normal numbers of platelet α_2-adrenoreceptors in hypertensive subjects, suggesting that the enhanced sensitivity of hypertensives to catecholamines is not associated with an increase in adrenoreceptor number (for review, see Alexander, 1987).

Both α_2-adrenoreceptor density and affinity for and sensitivity to agonist on intact platelets of normotensive and hypertensive subjects were measured before and after physiological increases in plasma catecholamines (Hollister, Onrot, *et al.*, 1986). In normotensives, posture-induced rises in plasma catecholamines correlated with reduced α_2-adrenoreceptor agonist affinity and fewer high-affinity receptors. Platelet aggregation and inhibition of adenylate cyclase by *l*-epinephrine also were reduced. Hypertensive subjects had similar rises in plasma catecholamines with upright posture, but showed no change in receptor affinity or sensitivity. No change in platelet α_2-adrenoreceptor number occurred in these studies.

In vitro incubation with *l*-epinephrine revealed that platelets from hypertensives had slower desensitization than those from normotensives. Binding studies at different temperatures and with varying sodium concentrations found no thermodynamic or sodium-dependent differences between normotensive and hypertensive groups (Hollister, Onrot, *et al.*, 1986). These studies demonstrate that platelets from hypertensive subjects exhibit a defect in the ability of physiological concentrations of agonist to desensitize the α_2-adrenoreceptor.

Aging

Efforts to use a α- and β-adrenoreceptor binding methodology to study aging are in their infancy but

seem to support a β-adrenoreceptor defect (Docherty & O'Malley, 1985; Guarnieri, Filburn, Zitnik, & Lakatta, 1980; Reinhardt, Zehmisch, Becker, & Nagel-Hiemke, 1984; Hoeldtke & Climi, 1985) perhaps due to reduced β-adrenoreceptor affinity (Feldman *et al.*, 1984b; Pan, Hoffman, Pershe, & Blaschke, 1986).

Hyperthyroidism

Hundreds of reports have dealt with the relation of thyroxine and adrenoreceptor function (for review, see Cryer, 1987). Several things seem clear from these studies: (1) plasma norepinephrine and epinephrine are not raised in hyperthyroidism; (2) adrenoreceptor sensitivity to catecholamines is different in different tissues (Bilezikian & Loeb, 1983); (3) altered adrenoreceptor function can only partly explain tissue effects of thyroxine on catecholamine response (Malbon, Graziano, & Johnson, 1984).

Some have found no differences when mononuclear leukocytes from thyrotoxic individuals were compared with euthyroid controls (Hui, Wolfe, & Conolly, 1982), yet short-term triiodothyronine-induced thyrotoxicosis did produce increased numbers of mononuclear cells in other studies (Ginsberg, Clutter, Shah, & Cryer, 1981; Ratge, Hansel-Bessey, & Wisser, 1985; Andersson, Nilsson, & Kuo, 1983). Decreased β-adrenoreceptor number in hypothyroidism has also been seen (Cognini *et al.*, 1983).

Adrenoreceptors in the CNS

Several laboratories have recently begun to employ radioligand binding methodology to the problems of neurological and psychiatric disorders in human subjects and animal models of human disease, but our knowledge in this area is unfortunately still extremely limited. Our understanding of adrenoreceptors in neurological disease is therefore best illustrated in the set of disorders most readily investigated by this technique. These are the disorders of the autonomic nervous system. Obviously, the receptors studied in such disorders are actually peripheral adrenoreceptors.

Human autonomic dysfunction includes many disease processes, having as their final common pathway the interruption of the efficient functioning of the autonomic nervous system. Severe autonomic dysfunction occurs in one in approximately 5000 people. Usually, such patients have an acquired disorder affecting both parasympathetic and sympathetic nervous systems, but occasional patients have enzymatic defects such as dopamine-β-hydroxylase deficiency (Robertson, Goldberg, Onrot, *et al.*, 1986).

One of the most striking features of autonomic dysfunction is the marked hypersensitivity that develops to various pressor and depressor stimuli (Mohring *et al.*, 1980; Robertson *et al.*, 1984). The loss of the buffering capacity of the baroreceptors and cardiopulmonary receptors undoubtedly contributes to the hypersensitivity, but there is evidence that changes in the function of adrenergic receptors are also involved.

In 12 well-characterized patients with autonomic dysfunction of the Bradbury–Eggleston type (peripheral autonomic failure), we assessed adrenergic receptor sensitivity using standard tests of autonomic responsiveness. All these patients had plasma norepinephrine levels under 50 pg/ml (patients: 28 ± 3 pg/ml; controls: 368 ± 24 pg/ml. On assumption of upright posture, all the patients had a fall in systolic blood pressure greater than 60 mm Hg. None of the patients was able to remain standing longer than 60 s without therapy. Using boluses of phenylephrine and isoproterenol, we documented a 6-fold hypersensitivity of α_1-adrenoreceptors and a 6- to 17-fold hypersensitivity of β_1- and β_2-adrenoreceptors (Robertson *et al.*, 1984).

In 1981, Bannister and co-workers used tritiated dihydroalprenolol (DHA) to study β-adrenergic receptors on lymphocyte membranes of patients with multiple system atrophy in whom supersensitivity to isoproterenol had been observed. There was a sixfold increase in the number of [^{3}H]-DHA sites with no change in [^{3}H]-DHA affinity when incubation was carried out at 37°C, but this increase was smaller at lower incubation temperatures.

Similar observations have been made in other patients. One was a 48-year-old woman who probably had a paracarcinomatous autonomic neuropathy (Hui & Conolly, 1981). She had an approximately threefold hypersensitivity to the chronotropic effect of isoproterenol and a doubling in the number of her lymphocyte β-adrenergic receptor sites as detected using [^{125}I]iodohydroxybenzylpindolol. In addition, Chobanian *et al.* (1982) found a 60% increase in [^{3}H]-DHA binding site number in the polymorphonuclear leukocytes of patients with mild to moderate autonomic failure whose plasma norepinephrine levels were approximately half normal. Thus, there is marked β-adrenergic hypersensitivity in autonomic failure that is accompanied by an increase in the number of β-adrenergic receptors on circulating lymphocytes.

These observations have been extended by examining the increase of cAMP in response to isoproterenol during the incubation of lymphocytes from three patients with multiple system atrophy, three patients with the Bradbury–Eggleston syndrome, and seven normal subjects. Surprisingly, this was not the case in the lymphocytes of the Bradbury–Eggleston patients. It is unclear why these individuals should not manifest the same evidence of supersensitivity as the patients with multiple system atrophy, although it might be noted that the patients discussed by Jennings, Bobik, and Esler (1981) had mean circulating norepinephrine levels of 160 ± 4 pg/ml, suggesting that they were in the mildly affected subgroup of Bradbury–Eggleston patients.

Comparing eight subjects with multiple system atrophy to five normal male volunteers, Davies *et al.* (1982) used [^{3}H]dihydroergocryptine (DHE) and found a sevenfold greater number of [^{3}H]-DHE sites per platelet in the patients as in the normal subjects, with no difference in [^{3}H]-DHE affinity between the two groups. Using the same radioligand, Chobanian *et al.* (1982) found significant increases in platelet receptor number in six patients with orthostatic hypotension as compared to 22 control subjects. It is noteworthy that the absolute differences in numbers of [^{3}H]-DHE sites found by Chobanian *et al.* were much more modest than those observed by Davies *et al.*: there was slightly less than a doubling of receptor number in the patient group. At least one of the patients studied by Chobanian *et al.* had hypotension associated with the anephric state rather than autonomic failure and this may have contributed to the differences in results obtained. Chobanian *et al.* reported similar values for platelet α-adrenergic receptors in four patients in whom ergotamine was studied as a therapeutic agent; there may be overlap in the patients in this and in the previous study.

More recently, Kafka *et al.* (1984), also using [^{3}H]-DHE, reported that there was a mean 50% increase in platelet α-adrenergic receptor number in patients with idiopathic orthostatic hypotension and multiple system atrophy. However, the interindividual variation was quite large and 80% of patients had [^{3}H]-DHE binding density below 350 fmoles/mg protein, a level found in some normal subjects.

However, radioligand binding studies utilizing [^{3}H]-DHE have been demonstrated to be less reliable for estimation of platelet α_2-adrenergic receptor number, as compared to [^{3}H]yohimbine. Brodde *et al.* (1985) reported an approximate doubling in platelet α_2-adrenergic receptor number determined using [^{3}H]yohimbine binding in a patient with diabetic polyneuropathy. In view of this observation and because the patient had manifested a tenfold hypersensitivity to phenylephrine, Brodde *et al.* reasoned that yohimbine might be helpful in the treatment of their patient. In fact, the patient reportedly did well for 6 months on a regimen of 12.5 mg oral yohimbine daily. We have also had favorable results using yohimbine in some autonomic dysfunction patients (Onrot *et al.*, 1987).

Assessing the number and function of adrenoreceptors in response to behavioral stimuli and in psychiatric disease is of great interest. Studies in humans present special difficulties because of the inaccessibility of the relevant tissue, unlike the situation in autonomic dysfunction. However, some significant inroads are being made and brief mention will be made of them below. Some of the most stimulating observations, although they were not developed in human subjects, are the observations that administration of caffeine (Goldberg, Curatolo, Tung, & Robertson, 1982), chronic tricyclic antidepressants (Banerjee, Kung, Riggi, & Chanda, 1977), monoamine oxidase inhibitors, and electroconvulsant therapy (Pandey, Heinze, Brown, & Davis, 1979) reduce β-adrenoreceptor binding in the rodent brain and also reduce norepinephrine-stimulated cAMP production (Vetulani & Sulser, 1975). Decreases in α_2-adrenoreceptor binding and functional activity have also been observed in rat brain following tricyclic antidepressants or monoamine oxidase inhibitors. Because these therapeutic interventions are chronically but not acutely effective in treating depression in human subjects, the time course of the development of these changes in rat brain has encouraged investigators to believe the animal observations may have important human implications. The recent observation of elevated dopamine D_2 receptors in the brains of schizophrenic subjects has increased excitement among investigators about the applicability of the newer methodology (Wong *et al.*, 1986).

Attention has focused on both the cholinergic (Snyder, 1984; Nadi, Nurnberger, & Gershon, 1984) and the adrenergic systems, but our focus in this chapter is on the latter. Because platelets with their amine uptake sites bear a certain resemblance to neurons, one can imagine that a supersensitivity of α_2-adrenoreceptors in the brain might also be manifest in the platelet (Metz *et al.*, 1983). A number of investigators have sought to utilize the assessment of platelet α_2-adrenoreceptor number and affinity in an effort to discover abnormalities in patients with psychiatric disorders. Garcia-Sevilla, Zia, Hollingsworth, Greden, and Smith (1981) found a 29% higher number of sites for clonidine binding in the platelets of depressed but drug-free subjects. Kafka and Paul (1983) found 41% more binding in affective disorder patients as compared to normal controls. In subsequent studies, patients with unipolar depression had significantly reduced cAMP production following prostaglandin E_1 stimulation. However, others (Daiguji, Meltzer, Tang, & U'Prichard, 1981) were not able to find differences in the two groups.

The recent data of Wolfe, Cohen, and Gelenberg (1987) and the accompanying discussion provide a useful overview of the current data with respect to platelet α_2-adrenoreceptors in depression. These investigators found that affinity of α_2-adrenoreceptors was increased in depressed patients but that there was no significant difference in receptor number.

Fewer studies of β-adrenoreceptor function in psychiatric illness have been carried out. Reduced sensitivity of β-adrenoreceptors on lymphocytes has been seen in patients with depression and psychomotor agitation (Mann *et al.*, 1985). The relationship of these findings to circulating catecholamine levels has not been clearly identified. The clearly demonstrable reduction in sympathetic activation during the relaxation response (Hoffman *et al.*, 1982) may also prove to be reflected in β-receptor affinity for agonist.

In an attempt to focus on α_2-adrenoreceptor responsiveness, studies have been done to assess the growth hormone, MHPG, and blood pressure response to clonidine administration in depressed subjects. One study has shown a blunted decrease in plasma MHPG in the first hour following intravenous clonidine (2 μg/kg) in depressed patients, but similar studies using slightly different protocols did not yield precisely the same result. At least three studies have failed to find a difference between patients and controls in the hypotensive response to clonidine.

Special Applications

Autoradiography

With the advent of suitable radioligands, it has been possible to apply radioligand binding methodology to morphological detection of receptor sites in the CNS. Beginning in the late 1970s, Kuhar and Unnerstall (1985) made great inroads in the tissue analysis of receptor sites by application of photographic materials to the radioligand-exposed tissue slice. Concentrations of receptor sites in different locations were clearly demonstrated. When labeled α_2-adrenoreceptor ligand localized to tissues containing substantial quantities of epinephrine and phenylethanolamine-*N*-methyltransferase, the physiological relevance of this technique was particularly appreciated. This technique of autoradiography has also been applied to various peptides or hormones and neurotransmitters. The ability to localize neurotransmitter (by other techniques) and to compare this with the location of receptor sites for that transmitter (by auto-radiography) constitutes an extremely powerful set of investigative strategies.

Hormone Assay

The presence of receptors with high affinity can sometimes be exploited to assay hormones, drugs, and neurotransmitters. Atrial natriuretic peptide (ANF) inhibits aldosterone production in the adrenal zona glomerulosa (DeLean *et al.*, 1984). It is a 28-amino-acid peptide released from the human atrium which seems to counterbalance many of the effects of the renin–angiotensin system (Hollister, Tanaka *et al.*, 1986). Adrenal cortex membranes possess high-affinity binding sites for ANF (K_D in the picomolar range), and through use of a synthetic 24-amino-acid radioligand, a remarkable assay sensitivity for ANF in human plasma has been achieved (2 fmoles per assay tube) (Bürgisser, Raine, Erne, Kamber, & Bühler, 1986).

Positron Emission Tomography (PET)

One of the most exciting new avenues for investigation of adrenoreceptors in human subjects is PET scanning (Wagner *et al.*, 1983; Garnett, Firnau, & Nahmias, 1983). As positron-emitting ligands suitably selective for adrenoreceptors are identified, it should be possible to measure directly the functional status of target receptors in the brain and to monitor their changes in response to various stimuli or over the course of the waxing and waning of, for example, depression. This technique has already been applied with great success to the identification of dopamine receptors in the brain. In MPTP-treated nonhuman primates, progressive dopamine receptor damage has been inferred via PET scanning (Hantraye *et al.*, 1986). Moreover, schizophrenic patients have been shown to have elevated numbers of D_2 receptors by this technique (Wong *et al.*, 1986). Information about both number and kinetics of receptors in brain has been obtained (Farde, Hall, Ehrin, & Sedvall, 1986). It is likely that in the coming decade, PET scanning will provide the most fundamental information about the relation of psychological stresses and psychiatric conditions to adrenoreceptor number and function.

ACKNOWLEDGMENTS. Supported in part by NIH Grants HL-14192 and HL-31419, General Clinical Research Center Grant RR-00095, and the U.S.–U.S.S.R. Health Cooperative Agreement.

References

Aarons, R. D., Nies, A. S., Gal, J., Hegstrand, L. R., & Molinoff, P. B. (1980). Elevation of beta-adrenergic receptor density in human lymphocytes after propranolol administration. *Journal of Clinical Investigation, 65*, 949–957.

Alexander, R. W. (1987). Adrenergic receptors in cardiovascular disease. In P. A. Insel (Ed.), *Adrenergic receptors in man*. New York: Dekker.

Andersson, R. G. G., Nilsson, O. R., & Kuo, J. F. (1983). Beta-adrenoceptor–adenosine 3′-5′ monophosphate system in human leukocytes before and after treatment for hyperthyroidism. *Journal of Clinical Endocrinology and Metabolism, 56*, 42–45.

Ariëns, E. J. (1954). Affinity and intrinsic activity in the theory of competitive inhibition. Part I. Problems and theory. *Archives Internationales de Pharmacodynamie, 99*, 32–49.

Banerjee, S. P., Kung, L. S., Riggi, S. J., & Chanda, S. K. (1977). Development of beta adrenergic receptor subsensitivity by antidepressants. *Nature, 268*, 455–456.

Bannister, R., Boylston, A. W., Davies, I. B., Mathias, C. J., Sever, P. S., & Sudera, D. (1981). Beta-receptor numbers and thermodynamics in denervation supersensitivity. *Journal of Physiology (London) 319*, 369–377.

Benovic, J. L., Mayor, F., Jr., Somers, R. L., Caron, M. G., & Lefkowitz, R. J. (1986). Light-dependent phosphorylation of rhodopsin by β-adrenergic receptor kinase. *Nature, 321*, 869–872.

Berthelsen, S., & Pettinger, W. A. (1977). A functional basis for classification of α-adrenergic receptors. *Life Sciences, 21*, 595–606.

Bilezikian, J. P., & Loeb, J. N. (1983). The influence of hyperthyroidism and hypothyroidism on alpha- and beta-adrenergic receptor systems and adrenergic responsiveness. *Endocrine Reviews, 4*, 378–388.

Boon, N. A., Elliott, J. M., Davies, C. L., Conway, F. J., Jones, J. V., Grahame-Smith, D. G., & Sleight, P. (1983). Platelet α₂-adrenoreceptors in borderline and established essential hypertension. *Clinical Science, 65*, 207–208.

Bourne, H. R. (1986). One molecular machine can transduce diverse signals. *Nature, 321*, 814–816.

Bravo, E. L., Tarazi, R. C., Gifford, R. W., & Stewart, B. H. (1979). Circulating and urinary catecholamines in pheochromocytoma. Diagnostic and pathophysiologic implications. *New England Journal of Medicine, 301*, 682.

Brodde, O.-E. (1986). Molecular pharmacology of β-adrenoceptors. *Journal of Cardiovascular Pharmacology, 8* (Suppl. 4), S16–S20.

Brodde, O.-E., Daul, A., & O'Hara, N. (1984). Beta-adrenoceptor changes in human lymphocytes induced by dynamic exercise. *Naunyn-Schmiedebergs Archives of Pharmacology, 325*, 190.

Brodde, O.-E., Daul, A. E., O'Hara, N., & Khalifa, A. M. (1985). Properties of α- and β-adrenoceptors in circulating blood cells of patients with essential hypertension. *Journal of Cardiovascular Pharmacology, 7*(Suppl. 6), S162–S167.

Bürgisser, E., Raine, A. E. G., Erne, P., Kamber, B., & Bühler, F. R. (1986). Human cardiac plasma concentrations of atrial natriuretic peptide quantified by radioreceptor assay. *Biochemical and Biophysical Research Communications, 133*, 1201–1209.

Butler, J., Kelly, J. G., O'Malley, K., & Pidgeon, F. (1983). Beta-adrenergic adaptation to acute exercise. *Journal of Physiology (London), 344*, 1131.

Cameron, O. G., Smith, C. B., Hollingsworth, P. J., Nesse, R. M., & Curtis, G. C. (1984). Platelet α₂ adrenergic receptor binding and plasma catecholamines. *Archives of General Psychiatry, 41*, 1144–1148.

Chobanian, A. V., Tifft, C. P., Sackel, H., & Pitruzella, A. (1982). Alpha and beta adrenergic receptor activity in circulating blood cells of patients with idiopathic orthostatic hypotension and pheochromocytoma. *Clinical and Experimental Hypertension, A4*, 793–806.

Cognini, G., Piantanelli, L., Paolinelli, E., Orlandoni, P., Pelligrini, A., & Masera, N. (1983). Decreased beta-adrenergic receptor density in mononuclear leukocytes from thyroidectomized patients. *Acta Endocrinologica, 103*, 1–5.

Colucci, W. S., Alexander, R. W., Williams, G. H., Rude, R. E., Holman, B. L., Konstam, M. A., Wynne, J., Mudge, G. H., Jr., & Braunwald, E. (1981). Decreased lymphocyte beta-adrenergic receptor density in patients with heart failure and tolerance to the beta-adrenergic agonist pirbuterol. *New England Journal of Medicine, 305*, 185–189.

Cryer, P. E. (1987). Adrenergic receptors in endocrine and metabolic diseases. In P. A. Insel (Ed.), *Adrenergic receptors in man* (pp. 285–301). New York: Dekker.

Cundell, D., Danks, J., Phillips, M. J., & Davies, R. J. (1984). Effect of exercise on isoprenaline-induced lymphocyte cAMP production in atopic asthmatics and atopic and non-atopic, non-asthmatic subjects. *Clinical Allergy, 24*, 433.

Daiguji, M., Meltzer, H. Y., Tang, C., & U'Prichard, D. C. (1981). Alpha-2-adrenergic receptors in platelet membranes of depressed patients: No change in number of ³H-yohimbine affinity. *Life Sciences, 29*, 2059–2064.

Davies, I. B., Sudera, D., Sagnella, G., Marchesi-Saviotti, E., Mathias, C., Bannister, R., & Sever, P. (1982). Increased numbers of alpha receptors in sympathetic denervation supersensitivity in man. *Journal of Clinical Investigation, 69*, 779–784.

DeBlasi, A., Lipartiti, M., Motulsky, H. J., Insel, P. A., & Fratelli, M. (1985). Agonist-induced redistribution of beta-adrenergic receptors on intact human mononuclear leukocytes: Redistributed receptors are nonfunctional. *Journal of Clinical Endocrinology and Metabolism, 61*, 1081.

DeBlasi, A., Cotecchia, S., Fratelli, M., & Lipartiti, M. (1986). Agonist-induced beta-adrenoceptor internalization of intact human mononuclear leukocytes: Effects of temperature of mononuclear separation. *Journal of Laboratory and Clinical Medicine, 107,* 86.

DeBlasi, A., Maisel, A. S., Feldman, R. D., Ziegler, M. G., Fratelli, M., Dilallo, M., Smith, D. A., Lai, C. Y. C., & Motulsky, H. J. (1986). In vivo regulation of β-adrenergic receptors on human mononuclear leukocytes: Assessment of receptor number, location, and function after posture change, exercise, and isoproterenol infusion. *Journal of Clinical Endocrinology and Metabolism, 63,* 847–853.

DeLean, A., Hancock, A. A., & Lefkowitz, R. J. (1982). Validation and statistical analysis of a computer modeling method for quantitative analysis of radioligand-binding data for mixtures of pharmacological receptor subtypes. *Molecular Pharmacology, 21,* 5–16.

DeLean, A., Racz, K., Gutkowska, J., Nguyen, T. -T., Cantin, M., & Genest, J. (1984). Specific receptor-mediated inhibition by synthetic atrial natriuretic factor of hormone-stimulated steroidogenesis in cultured bovine adrenal cells. *Endocrinology, 115,* 1636–1638.

Docherty, J. R., & O'Malley, K. (1985). Aging and alpha-adrenoceptors. *Clinical Science, 68*(Suppl. 10), 133S–136S.

Edwards, A. J., Bacon, T. H., Elms, C. A., Verardi, R., Felder, M., & Knight, S. C. (1984). Changes in the populations of lymphoid cells in human peripheral blood following physical exercise. *Clinical and Experimental Immunology, 58,* 420.

Engel, G., Hoyer, D., Berthold, R., & Wagner, H. (1981). (±)-^{125}Iodocyanopindolol, a new ligand for β-adrenoceptors: Identification and quantitation of subclasses of β-adrenoceptors in guinea-pig. *Naunyn-Schmiedeberg's Archives of Pharmacology, 317,* 277–285.

Farde, L., Hall, H., Ehrin, E., & Sedvall, G. (1986). Quantitative analysis of D2 dopamine receptor binding in the living human brain by PET. *Science, 231,* 258–261.

Feldman, R. D., Limbird, L. E., Nadeau, J. H., FitzGerald, G. A., Robertson, D., & Wood, A. J. J. (1983). Dynamic regulation of leukocyte beta adrenergic receptor–agonist interactions by physiological changes in circulating catecholamines. *Journal of Clinical Investigation, 72,* 164.

Feldman, R. D., Limbird, L. E., Nadeau, J. H. J., Robertson, D., & Wood, A. J. J. (1984a). Alterations in leukocyte β-receptor affinity with aging: A potential explanation for altered β-adrenergic sensitivity in the elderly. *New England Journal of Medicine, 310,* 815–819.

Feldman, R. D., Limbird, L. E., Nadeau, J. H., Robertson, D., & Wood, A. J. J. (1984b). Leukocyte beta-receptor alterations in hypertensive subjects. *Journal of Clinical Investigation, 73,* 648.

Fraser, J. A., Nadeau, J. H. J., Robertson, D., & Wood, A. J. J. (1981). Regulation of human leukocyte beta receptors by endogenous catecholamines: Relationship of leukocyte beta receptor density to the cardiac sensitivity to isoproterenol. *Journal of Clinical Investigation, 67,* 1777–1784.

Gaddum, J. H. (1957). Theories of drug antagonism. *Pharmacological Reviews, 9,* 211–217.

Garcia-Sevilla, J. A., Zia, A. P., Hollingsworth, P. J., Greden,

J. F., & Smith, C. B. (1981). Platelet alpha$_2$-adrenergic receptors in major depressive disorder: Binding of tritiated clonidine before and after tricyclic antidepressant drug treatment. *Archives of General Psychiatry, 38,* 1327–1333.

Garnett, E. S., Firnau, G., & Nahmias, C. (1983). Dopamine visualized in the basal ganglia of living man. *Nature, 305,* 137–138.

Ginsberg, A. M., Clutter, W. E., Shah, S. D., & Cryer, P. E. (1981). Triiodothyronine-induced thyrotoxicosis increases mononuclear leukocyte beta-adrenergic receptor density in man. *Journal of Clinical Investigation, 67,* 1785–1791.

Goldberg, M. R., & Robertson, D. (1983). Yohimbine: A pharmacological probe for study of the α$_2$-adrenergic receptor. *Pharmacological Reviews, 35,* 143–180.

Goldberg, M. R., & Robertson, D. (1984). Evidence for the existence of vascular α$_2$-adrenoreceptors in man. *Hypertension, 6,* 551–556.

Goldberg, M. R., Curatolo, P. W., Tung, C. S., & Robertson, D. (1982). Caffeine down-regulates β-adrenoreceptor density in rat forebrain. *Neuroscience Letters, 31,* 47–52.

Goldberg, M. R., Hollister, A. S., & Robertson, D. (1983). Influence of yohimbine on blood pressure, autonomic reflexes and plasma catecholamines. *Hypertension, 5,* 772–778.

Goldstein, A., Aronow, L., & Kalman, S. M. (1974). *Principles of drug action: The basis of pharmacology* (2nd ed., pp. 82–111). New York: Wiley.

Greenacre, J. K., & Conolly, M. E. (1978). Desensitization of the beta-adrenoceptor of lymphocytes from normal subjects and patients with phaeochromocytoma: Studies in vivo. *British Journal of Pharmacology, 5,* 191–197.

Grenningloh, G., Rienitz, A., Schmitt, B., Methfessel, C., Zensen, M., Beyreuther, K., Gundelfinger, E. D., & Betz, H. (1987). The strychnine-binding subunit of the glycine receptor shows homology with nicotinic acetylcholine receptors. *Nature, 328,* 215–220.

Guarnieri, T., Filburn, C. R., Zitnik, G. S., & Lakatta, E. G. (1980). Contractile and biochemical correlates of beta-adrenergic stimulation of the aged heart. *American Journal of Physiology, 239,* H501–H508.

Hantraye, P., Loc'h, C., Tacke, U., Riche, D., Stulzaft, O., Doudet, D., Guibert, B., Naquet, R., Maziere, B., & Maziere, M. (1986). "In vivo" visualization by positron emission tomography of the progressive striatal dopamine receptor damage occurring in MPTP-intoxicated non-human primates. *Life Sciences, 39,* 1376–1378.

Harden, T. K. (1983). Agonist-induced desensitization of the beta-adrenergic receptor-linked adenylate cyclase. *Pharmacological Reviews, 35,* 5.

Hoeldtke, R. D., & Climi, K. M. (1985). Effects of aging on catecholamine metabolism. *Journal of Clinical Endocrinology and Metabolism, 60,* 479–484.

Hoffman, J. W., Benson, H., Arns, P. A., Stainbrook, G. L., Landsberg L., Young, J. B., & Gill, A. (1982). Reduced sympathetic nervous system responsivity associated with the relaxation response. *Science, 215,* 190–192.

Hollister, A. S., FitzGerald, G. A., Nadeau, J. H. J., & Robertson, D. (1983). Acute reduction in human platelet α$_2$-

adrenoreceptor affinity for agonist by endogenous and exogenous catecholamines. *Journal of Clinical Investigation, 72,* 1498–1505.

Hollister, A. S., Onrot, J., Lonce, S., Nadeau, J. H. J., & Robertson, D. (1986). Plasma catecholamine modulation of α_2-adrenoreceptor agonist affinity and sensitivity in normotensive and hypertensive human platelets. *Journal of Clinical Investigation, 77,* 1416–1421.

Hollister, A. S., Tanaka, I., Imada, T., Onrot, J., Biaggioni, I., Kincaid, D., Robertson, D., & Inagami, T. (1986). Sodium loading and posture modulate human atrial natriuretic factor plasma levels. *Hypertension, 8,* II-106–II-111.

Hui, K. K. P., & Conolly, M. E. (1981). Increased numbers of beta receptors in orthostatic hypotension due to autonomic dysfunction. *New England Journal of Medicine, 304,* 1473–1476.

Hui, K. K. P., Wolfe, R. N., & Conolly, M. E. (1982). Lymphocyte beta-adrenergic receptors are not altered in hyperthyroidism. *Clinical Pharmacology and Therapeutics, 32,* 161–165.

Insel, P. A., & Motulsky, H. J. (1987). *Adrenergic receptors in man.* New York: Raven Press.

Jennings, G., Bobik, A., & Esler, M. (1981). Beta receptors in orthostatic hypotension. *New England Journal of Medicine, 305,* 1019.

Kafka, M. S., Polinsky, R. J., Williams, A., Kopin, I. J., Lake, C. R., Ebert, M. H., & Tokola, N. A. (1984). Alpha-adrenergic receptors in orthostatic hypotension syndromes. *Neurology, 34,* 1121–1125.

Karliner, J. S., Motulsky, H. J., & Insel, P. A. (1982). Apparent "down-regulation" of human platelet alpha$_2$-adrenergic receptors is due to retained agonist. *Molecular Pharmacology, 21,* 36–43.

Kenakin, T. P. (1984). The classification of drugs and drug receptors in isolated tissues. *Pharmacological Reviews, 36,* 165–222.

Krall, J. F., Connelly, M., & Tuck, M. L. (1980). Acute regulation of beta adrenergic catecholamine sensitivity in human lymphocytes. *Journal of Pharmacology and Experimental Therapeutics, 214,* 554.

Kubo, T., Fukuda, K., Mikami, A., Maeda, A., Takahashi, H., Mishina, M., Haga, T., Haga, K., Ichiyama, A., Kangawa, K., Kojima, M., Matsuo, H., Hirose, T., & Numa, S. (1986). Cloning, sequencing, and expression of complementary DNA encoding the muscarinic acetylcholine receptor. *Nature, 323,* 411–416.

Kuhar, M., & Unnerstall, J. R. (1985, February). Quantitative receptor mapping by autoradiography: Some current technical problems. *Trends in Neurological Science,* 49–53.

Lefkowitz, R. J., & Caron, M. G. (1986). Regulation of adrenergic receptor function by phosphorylation. *Journal of Molecular and Cellular Cardiology, 18,* 885–895.

Levitzki, A. (1984). *Receptors: A quantitative approach.* Menlo Park: Benjamin/Cummings.

Limbird, L. E. (1986). *Cell surface receptors: A short course on theory and methods.* The Hague: Nijhoff.

Mahan, L. C., Motulsky, H. J., & Insel, P. A. (1985). Do agonists promote rapid internalization of β-adrenergic receptors? *Proceedings of the National Academy of Sciences of the United States of America, 82,* 6566–6570.

Mahan, L. C., McKernan, R. M., & Insel, P. A. (1987). Metabolism of alpha- and beta-adrenergic receptors in vitro and in vivo. *Annual Reviews of Pharmacology and Toxicology, 27,* 215–235.

Malbon, C. C., Graziano, M. P., & Johnson, G. L. (1984). Fat cell beta-adrenergic receptor in the hypothyroid rat: Impaired interaction with the stimulatory regulatory component of adenylate cyclase. *Journal of Biological Chemistry, 259,* 3254–3260,

Mann, J. J., Brown, R. P., Halper, J. P., Sweeney, J. A., Kocsis, J. H., Stokes, P. E., & Bilezikian, J. P. (1985). Reduced sensitivity of lymphocyte beta-adrenergic receptors in patients with endogenous depression and psychomotor agitation. *New England Journal of Medicine, 313,* 715–720.

Metz, A., Cowen, P. J., Gelder, M. G., Stump, K., Elliott, J. M., & Grahame-Smith, D. G. (1983). Changes in platelet alpha$_2$-adrenoceptor binding post-partum: Possible relation to maternity blues. *Lancet, 1,* 495.

Mohring, J., Glanzer, K., Marciel, J. A., Jr., Dusing, R., Kramer, H. J., Arogast, R., & Koch-Weser, J. (1980). Greatly enhanced pressor response to antidiuretic hormone in patients with impaired cardiovascular reflexes due to idiopathic orthostatic hypotension. *Journal of Cardiovascular Pharmacology, 2,* 367–376.

Molinoff, P. B., Wolfe, B. B., & Weiland, G. A. (1981). Quantitative analysis of drug–receptor interactions. II. Determination of the properties of receptor subtypes. *Life Sciences, 29,* 427–443.

Motulsky, H. J., & Insel, P. A. (1982). Adrenergic receptors in man: Direct identification, physiologic regulation, and clinical alterations. *New England Journal of Medicine, 307,* 18–28.

Motulsky, H. J., & Mahan, L. C. (1984). The kinetics of competitive radioligand binding predicted by the law of mass action. *Molecular Pharmacology, 25,* 1–9.

Motulsky, H. J., O'Connor, D. J., & Insel, P. A. (1983). Platelet α_2-adrenergic receptors in treated and untreated essential hypertension. *Clinical Science, 64,* 265–272.

Motulsky, H. J., Cunningham, E. M. S., DeBlasi, A., & Insel, P. A. (1986). Agonists promote rapid desensitization and redistribution of beta adrenergic receptors on intact human mononuclear leukocytes. *American Journal of Physiology, 250,* E583.

Munson, P. J., & Rodbard, D. (1980). LIGAND: A versatile computerized approach for characterization of ligand-binding systems. *Analytical Biochemistry, 107,* 220.

Nadi, N. S., Nurnberger, J. I., & Gershon, E. S. (1984). Muscarinic cholinergic receptors on skin fibroblasts in familial affective disorder. *New England Journal of Medicine, 311,* 225–230.

Nickerson, M. (1956). Receptor occupancy and tissue response. *Nature, 78,* 697–698.

Onrot, J., Goldberg, M. R., Biaggioni, I., Wiley, R., Hollister, A. S., & Robertson, D. (1987). Oral yohimbine in human autonomic failure. *Neurology, 37*, 215–220.

Pan, H. Y. -M., Hoffman, B. B., Pershe, R. A., & Blaschke, T. F. (1986). Decline in beta adrenergic receptor-mediated vascular relaxation with aging in man. *Journal of Pharmacology and Experimental Therapeutics, 239*, 802–807.

Pandey, G. N., Heinze, W. J., Brown, B. D., & Davis, J. M. (1979). Electroconvulsive shock treatment decreases beta-adrenergic receptor sensitivity in rat brain. *Nature, 280*, 234–235.

Pfeifer, M. A., Ward, K., Malpass, T., Stratton, J., Halter, J., Evans, M., Beiter, H., Harker, L. A., & Porte, D., Jr. (1984). Variations in circulating catecholamines fail to alter human platelet alpha$_2$-adrenergic receptor number or affinity for [^{3}H]yohimbine or [^{3}H]dihydroergocryptine. *Journal of Clinical Investigation, 74*, 1063–1072.

Ratge, D., Hansel-Bessey, S., & Wisser, H. (1985). Altered plasma catecholamines and numbers of α- and β-adrenergic receptors in platelets and leucocytes in hyperthroid patients normalized under antithyroid treatment. *Acta Endocrinologica, 110*, 75–82.

Reinhardt, D., Zehmisch, T., Becker, B., & Nagel-Hiemke, M. (1984). Age-dependency of alpha- and beta-adrenoceptors on thrombocytes and lymphocytes of asthmatic and non-asthmatic children. *European Journal of Pediatrics, 142*, 111–116.

Robertson, D., Goldberg, M. R., Hollister, A. S., Wade, D., & Robertson, R. M. (1983). Clonidine raises blood pressure in idiopathic orthostatic hypotension. *American Journal of Medicine, 74*, 193–199.

Robertson, D., Hollister, A. S., Carey, E. L., Tung, C. S., Goldberg, M. R., & Robertson, R. M. (1984). Increased vascular β$_2$-adrenergic hypersensitivity in autonomic dysfunction. *Journal of the American College of Cardiology, 3*, 850–856.

Robertson, D., Goldberg, M. R., Hollister, A. S., Tung, C. S., & Robertson, R. M. (1986). Use of α$_2$ adrenoreceptor agonists and antagonists in the functional assessment of the sympathetic nervous system. *Journal of Clinical Investigation, 78*, 576–581.

Robertson, D., Goldberg, M. R., Onrot, J., Hollister, A. S., Wiley, R., Thompson, J. G., & Robertson, R. M. (1986). Isolated failure of autonomic noradrenergic neurotransmission: Evidence for impaired β-hydroxylation of dopamine. *New England Journal of Medicine, 314*, 1494–1497.

Shattil, S. J., McDonough, M., Turnbull, J., & Insel, P. A. (1981). Characterization of alpha-adrenergic receptors in human platelets using [^{3}H]clonidine. *Molecular Pharmacology, 19*, 179–183.

Snavely, M. D., Motulsky, H. J., O'Connor, D. T., Ziegler, M. G., & Insel, P. A. (1982). Adrenergic receptors in human and experimental pheochromocytoma. *Clinical and Experimental Hypertension, 4*, 829–848.

Snyder, S. H. (1984). Cholinergic mechanisms in affective disorders. *New England Journal of Medicine, 311*, 254–255.

Soppi, E., Varjo, P., Eskola, J., & Laitinen, L. A. (1982). Effect of strenuous physical stress on circulating lymphocyte number and function before and after training. *Clinical and Laboratory Immunology, 8*, 43.

Sowers, J. R., Connelly-Fittinghoff, M., Tuck, M. L., & Krall, J. F. (1983). Acute changes in noradrenaline levels do not alter lymphocyte beta-adrenergic receptor concentrations in man. *Cardiovascular Research, 17*, 184.

Stephenson, R. P. (1956). A modification of receptor theory. *British Journal of Pharmacology, 11*, 379–393.

Stiles, G. L., Caron, M. G., & Lefkowitz, R. J. (1984). Beta-adrenergic receptors: Biochemical mechanisms of physiological regulation. *Physiological Reviews, 64*, 661–743.

Tohmen, J. F., Cryer, P. E. (1980). Biphasic adrenergic modulation of beta-adrenergic receptors in man: Agonist-induced early increment and late decrement in beta-adrenergic receptor number. *Journal of Clinical Investigation, 65*, 836.

Van Rossum, J. M., & Ariëns, E. J. (1962). Receptor reserve and threshold phenomena. II. Theories on drug-action and a quantitative approach to spare receptors and threshold values. *Archives Internationales de Pharmacodynamie, 136*, 385–413.

Vetulani, J., & Sulser, F. (1975). Action of various antidepressant treatments reduces reactivity of noradrenergic cyclic AMP generating system in the limbic forebrain of the rat. *Nature, 257*, 495–496.

Villeneuve, A., Carpene, C., Berlan, M. D., & Lafontan, M. (1985). Lack of desensitization of alpha$_2$-mediated inhibition of lipolysis in fat cells after acute and chronic treatment with clonidine. *Journal of Pharmacology and Experimental Therapeutics, 233*, 433–440.

Wagner, H. N., Burns, H. D., Dannals, R. F., Wong, D. F., Langstrom, B., Duelfer, T., Frost, J. J., Ravert, H. T., Links, J. M., Rosenbloom, J. B., Luckas, S. E., Kramer, A. V., & Kuhar, M. J. (1983). Imaging dopamine receptors in the human brain by positron tomography. *Science, 221*, 1264–1266.

Weiland, G. A., & Molinoff, P. B. (1981). Quantitative analysis of drug–receptor interactions. I. Determination of kinetic and equilibrium properties. *Life Sciences, 29*, 313–330.

Wolfe, N., Cohen, B. M., & Gelenberg, A. J. (1987). Alpha-2-adrenergic receptors in platelet membranes of depressed patients: Increased affinity for ^{3}H-yohimbine. *Psychiatric Research, 20*, 107–116.

Wong, D. F., Wagner, H. N., Jr., Tune, L. E., Dannals, R. F., Pearlson, G. D., Links, J. M., Tamminga, C. A., Broussolle, E. P., Ravert, H. T., Wilson, A. A., Toung, J. K. T., Malat, J., Williams, J. A., O'Tuama, L. A., Snyder, S. H., Kuhar, M. J., & Gjedde, A. (1986). Positron emission tomography reveals elevated D$_2$ dopamine receptors in drug-naive schizophrenics. *Science, 234*, 1558–1562.

CHAPTER **15**

The Renin–Angiotensin–Aldosterone System and Atrial Natriuretic Factor

Steven A. Atlas, Jean E. Sealey, and John H. Laragh

Introduction

The purpose of this chapter is to provide an overview of physiological, biochemical, and methodological considerations concerning two hormonal systems that appear to play opposing roles in the physiological regulation of the circulation. Emphasis is placed on those issues pertinent to the needs of investigators involved in cardiovascular and behavioral research, in terms of selection of methods, adequacy of experimental design, and interpretation of data. The bulk of the information presented is directed toward assessment of hormone levels in blood or urine, but brief consideration is also given to measurements in other tissues which might be entertained in certain experimental studies. In addition, a description is given of available pharmacological probes which can be used to assess the functional significance of these hormones.

The renin–angiotensin system plays an integral role in the homeostatic control of blood pressure and fluid balance through the actions of angiotensin II, a peptide whose best characterized proper-

ties are arteriolar vasoconstriction and stimulation of aldosterone biosynthesis. Since the discovery of renin by Tigerstedt and Bergman (1898), there has accumulated a wealth of information regarding the biochemical and physiological characteristics of this hormonal system, thus permitting establishment of well-validated methodologies and experimental approaches to study its functions. These developments, combined with the availability of specific antagonists of the system, have led to a considerable understanding of its importance in several physiological and pathological processes.

More recently it has been learned that the cardiac atria secrete a polypeptide hormone which may also be involved in circulatory homeostasis. Discovered by deBold, Borenstein, Veress, and Sonnenberg (1981) as a potent natriuretic principle in atrial extracts, this atrial natriuretic factor (ANF) has been shown to have, in addition, major hemodynamic effects and interactions with other hormonal systems, notably the renin–angiotensin–aldosterone system. The availability of advanced technologies and the intense interest among the scientific community have together resulted in rapid accumulation of knowledge concerning its fundamental properties, and specific assays have been developed which at least clearly establish its hormonal nature. Although unequivocal statements about its exact physiological role or relative

Steven A. Atlas, Jean E. Sealey, and John H. Laragh • Cardiovascular Center and Department of Medicine, Cornell University Medical College, New York, New York 10021.

importance are not yet possible, available data suggest that it is a counterregulatory hormone involved in volume and cardiovascular homeostasis.

The Renin–Angiotensin–Aldosterone System

Components of the Renin–Angiotensin System

Renin is a proteolytic enzyme of the aspartyl (acid) protease family which is found most abundantly in the kidney (Inagami, 1981). Renin also appears to be synthesized in other organs, including brain, pituitary, blood vessels, gonads, and adrenal (Deschepper, Mellon, Cumin, Baxter, & Ganong, 1986), where it may have significant local actions. The kidney is, however, the major, if not sole, source of active renin secreted into the circulation of higher mammals (Sealey, White, Laragh, & Rubin, 1977), and it is this renal enzyme whose functional significance has been best characterized.

The catalytically inactive precursor of renin (prorenin) is also released by the kidney and is, in fact, the major circulating form in humans, accounting for 70–95% of the total plasma renin in normal subjects (Sealey, Atlas, & Laragh, 1980). Plasma prorenin is also partly derived from extrarenal tissues, where prorenin may be the major product of renin biosynthesis. It has been hypoth-

esized that locally released prorenin may serve as a "reservoir" for local, and possibly reversible, formation of active renin without affecting systemic functions (Itskovitz & Sealey, 1987). Although there is no evidence that circulating prorenin is converted to renin in the blood, its presence in plasma has major implications with regard to the measurement of renin (see below).

Renin has several properties that distinguish it from the other acid proteases: it has a pH optimum (ca. pH 6 in humans) closer to the physiological range of extracellular fluid; it is not appreciably inhibited by the known major classes of plasma protease inhibitors; and it has an extremely narrow substrate specificity. As illustrated in Figure 1, its only known catalytic function is to cleave a decapeptide (angiotensin I) from the N-terminus of angiotensinogen, a plasma glycoprotein of hepatic origin. There is evidence that angiotensinogen may also be synthesized *in situ* in brain and other tissues where renin may act locally (Campbell & Habener, 1986).

The concentration of renin is the major rate-limiting factor in angiotensin formation. Plasma angiotensinogen concentration is normally in the range of its Michaelis constant (K_m) for renin, so that variations in angiotensinogen levels may also influence the rate of angiotensin I formation to some degree. Plasma angiotensinogen levels are relatively constant within an individual and vary over a rather narrow range (0.7–2 μM) in normal subjects (Sealey, Gerten-Banes, & Laragh, 1972),

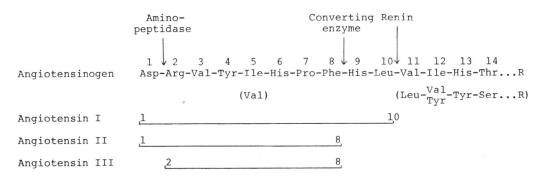

Figure 1. N-terminal sequence of human angiotensinogen, indicating hydrolytic cleavages mediated by renin and other peptidases to produce the angiotensin peptides. Amino acid substitutions found in pig, horse, and rat angiotensinogen are shown in parentheses.

but hepatic synthesis of this protein is markedly induced by estrogens, glucocorticoids, and possibly thyroxine (Krakoff & Eisenfeld, 1977; Campbell & Habener, 1986); consequently, in several conditions, plasma levels may be elevated (pregnancy, Cushing's syndrome) or depressed (adrenal insufficiency, hepatic disease).

Angiotensin I, which is itself probably devoid of important physiological actions, is converted to the active octapeptide hormone angiotensin II by the action of angiotensin converting enzyme (Soffer, 1981), a dipeptidyl hydrolase which cleaves the C-terminal dipeptide of angiotensin I (and, at least *in vitro,* other peptides). Although converting enzyme is found in blood, angiotensin II is mainly formed by the enzyme bound to the plasma membrane of vascular endothelial cells. This reaction probably always occurs as a first-order process (i.e., one which is dependent upon the ambient concentration of angiotensin I), and there is at present no evidence that alterations in the density of converting enzyme have significant impact on plasma angiotensin II levels under most circumstances. Angiotensin II may be formed locally in several vascular beds (by either circulating or locally synthesized renin or angiotensin I); however, a major site of conversion appears to be in the

pulmonary microcirculation, so that newly formed angiotensin II is quantitatively delivered into the arterial tree (Ng & Vane, 1968). This, together with the fact that the peptide is extensively metabolized in peripheral tissues, leads to lower venous (compared to arterial) plasma levels. Although most of the shorter breakdown products (some of which are present in blood) have little or no biological activity, a heptapeptide metabolite (angiotensin III), formed by the action of an aminopeptidase, may have comparable activity in some target tissues (e.g., adrenal) in some species, but apparently not in humans (Carey, Vaughan, Peach, & Ayers, 1978); the functional importance of this metabolite is uncertain.

Physiological Operation of the System

The principal regulatory step in the renin–angiotensin cascade (Figure 2) is the control of renin secretion by the kidney, where renin is synthesized and stored in modified myoepithelial cells [juxtaglomerular (JG) cells] that predominantly line the afferent arteriole of the glomerulus. Renin release is regulated by two intrarenal mechanisms that are stimulated by a decrease in renal perfusion: 1) activation of a renal baroreceptor, which probably

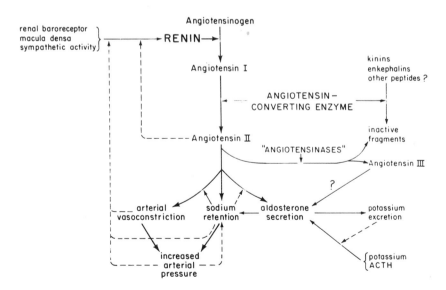

Figure 2. Schematic representation of the renin–angiotensin-aldosterone system. Solid arrows indicate direct pathways or facilitating effects and dashed arrows indicate inhibitory or antagonistic effects. Reproduced from Atlas and Case (1981).

comprises direct sensitivity of the JG cells to stretch; and (2) a decrease in NaCl load to the distal tubule, which is sensed by a cluster of specialized epithelial cells (the macula densa) that lie in close apposition to the JG cells (see Laragh & Sealey, 1973, and Keeton & Campbell, 1981, for review). The latter mechanism is also largely responsible for the stimulation of renin by chronic sodium depletion. In addition to these mechanisms, renin release is also under sympathetic nervous system control (β_1-adrenergic stimulation and possible α-adrenergic inhibition); an increase in renal sympathetic outflow is provoked by deactivation of cardiopulmonary (low-pressure) stretch receptors, which likely contributes to stimulation of renin release with upright posture or systemic hypotension. Additional implications of sympathetic control of renin release will be considered subsequently.

Upon release into the blood, renin accelerates the generation of angiotensin II, which in turn causes a prompt, direct increase in systemic vascular resistance. By its action on the outer (glomerulosa) zone of the adrenal cortex, angiotensin also stimulates the biosynthesis and release of aldosterone, which leads to expansion of extracellular volume by promoting sodium reabsorption at the distal nephron. Angiotensin also has direct renal actions (renal vasoconstriction and effects on proximal tubular epithelium) which further promote sodium conservation and sustain glomerular perfusion. In addition, systemically or locally formed angiotensin may also influence central nervous system function (stimulating drinking, release of vasopressin, ACTH, and other pituitary hormones, and raising blood pressure) and adrenergic transmission (by stimulating local catecholamine release) to further promote fluid conservation and increase arteriolar tone (Laragh & Sealey, 1973; Re, 1984).

In concert, these actions serve to defend the circulation when hypersecretion of renin is appropriately provoked by systemic signals such as volume contraction, upright posture, or hypotension. Normally, restoration of volume and of renal perfusion serves to turn off the signals that increase renin secretion; in addition, direct feedback inhibition of renin release by angiotensin II probably contributes to regulation of plasma renin levels, although this mechanism appears to be overwhelmed when stimuli to renin release persist (Laragh & Sealey, 1973).

These homeostatic responses, which are illustrated schematically in Figure 2, are impaired in several pathological states. In conditions where the arterial circulation is selectively compromised (e.g., heart failure, cirrhosis with ascites), stimulation of renin release leads to elevations in angiotensin II levels which contribute to pathological fluid accumulation while attempting to maintain arterial pressure. On the other hand, when hypersecretion of renin is autonomous (i.e., renin-secreting tumors) or is provoked by selective underperfusion of the kidneys (e.g., renal artery stenosis or renal vasculitis), the inappropriate elevations in plasma renin and angiotensin II will induce systemic hypertension.

Measurements of Plasma Renin, Angiotensinogen, and Angiotensins

The ideal measurement for evaluating activity of the circulating renin system would be direct assay of plasma angiotensin II, the effector hormone of the system. Moreover, the angiotensin II feedback mechanism suggests that factors which influence renin secretion may serve ultimately to regulate plasma concentrations of angiotensin II, rather than of renin *per se*. The issue of sensitivity and other practical considerations have led, however, to more widespread use of plasma renin assays.

Enzymatic Assays of Renin

The most widely used assay, and one that continues to have the greatest practical application for physiological studies, is measurement of *plasma renin activity* (PRA). This assay measures the rate of angiotensin I formation by the action of plasma active renin on endogenous angiotensinogen, during incubation of plasma at 37°C under conditions that favor linear accumulation of product (Helmer & Judson, 1963; Sealey, Gerten-Banes, & Laragh, 1972). Under proper conditions, prolonged incubation of plasma can be used to provide a method with extremely good sensitivity.

Blood is generally collected using EDTA as the anticoagulant, since this will provide effective inhibition of plasma converting enzyme, which is critical during subsequent incubation *in vitro*. Although other anticoagulants (e.g., heparin or citrate) can be used, EDTA will then have to be added prior to incubation. Very high concentrations of heparin can inhibit the renin reaction *in vitro*, but this is not a problem at the usual concentrations in anticoagulated blood. It should be noted, however, that if a single blood sample is to be collected for simultaneous analysis of other peptide hormones, EDTA is probably the best universal anticoagulant (see below). Human blood can be safely collected and processed at room temperature, since there is no appreciable accumulation of an angiotensin I "blank" (see below) under these conditions and since renin itself is quite stable in plasma at temperatures under 40°C. Collection of blood on ice may be necessary to prevent angiotensin I accumulation in other species, but prolonged exposure of blood or plasma to low temperatures must be avoided since this will cause inadvertent activation of plasma prorenin, particularly in human plasma (Sealey, Moon, Laragh, & Alderman, 1976; Sealey, Moon, Laragh, & Atlas, 1977). This phenomenon can lead to significant overestimation of active renin levels, particularly when renin secretion is either suppressed (e.g., in patients with primary aldosteronism or other low-renin forms of hypertension) or absent (e.g., in anephric patients). If the same blood sample is to be used for measurement of other peptides, where collection on ice is frequently necessary, it is recommended that the sample be centrifuged and processed within an hour. The plasma obtained should be stored in a non-self-defrosting freezer, preferably at −40°C or below.

In addition to EDTA, other peptidase inhibitors must be added prior to incubation for maximum protection of the formed angiotensin I; phenylmethylsulfonyl fluoride (PMSF) is the inhibitor currently preferred by most authorities, although other combinations have been advocated. Addition of a bacteriostatic agent (e.g., neomycin) is also necessary when prolonged incubation times are used (see below). Most investigators incubate plasma at the pH optimum of renin (pH 5.5–6.0 for human and dog, somewhat higher in other species), since buffering of plasma at this pH provides greater stability of the reaction, improved sensitivity, and (in the case of the lower pH for human and dog plasma) more effective inhibition of angiotensin degradation. These considerations, and a detailed description of the method used in our laboratories, have recently been reviewed in greater depth (Sealey, 1981; Preibisz, Sealey, Aceto, & Laragh, 1982).

The formed angiotensin I is now generally measured by direct radioimmunoassay (RIA), although perfectly valid bioassay procedures have been used as well. These assays are of sufficient sensitivity that small aliquots of incubated plasma can be assayed directly without prior extraction. Since measurement of PRA is, properly speaking, a rate determination, it is theoretically necessary to measure angiotensin I prior to incubation as well, so that one can calculate the net angiotensin I formed per unit time (generally expressed as ng/ml per h). However, nonspecific plasma interference and/or cross-reacting substances contribute substantially to the low levels of angiotensin I-like immunoreactivity in unincubated, unextracted plasmas, so that subtraction of such "blank" values may be invalid and is generally not advocated (Preibisz *et al.*, 1982). In practice, what is done is to incubate plasma for a sufficient period of time so that the "blank" immunoreactivity becomes negligible. A 2- to 3-h incubation at 37°C is satisfactory for normal renin levels, but many advocate a longer incubation (up to 18 h) for greater precision in discriminating subnormal levels.

Extreme elevations of plasma renin may lead to false underestimation of PRA values if there is significant consumption of plasma angiotensinogen during incubation *in vitro*, and shorter incubation times (e.g., 0.5–1 h) and/or verification of linearity of product formation may be required. Such situations are quite infrequent, and, moreover, are unlikely to lead to gross misperceptions since estimated PRA will still be very high even if this is not taken into account. Nonetheless, for very precise comparisons of PRA, measurement of plasma angiotensinogen (see below) may be useful; generally speaking, the reaction rate can be considered relatively constant as long as angiotensinogen levels fall by less than 10% during the course of the incubation.

Some investigators, particularly in Europe and Australia, have advocated measuring renin activity in the presence of excess angiotensinogen (usually using semipurified heterologous sources), in order to approximate zero-order kinetics of the reaction. Such *plasma renin concentration* (PRC) assays (Stockigt, Collins, & Biglieri, 1971) provide a more stringent measure of enzyme concentration *per se,* since they lessen the impact of angiotensinogen consumption on reaction rate *in vitro* and also minimize interindividual differences in endogenous angiotensinogen levels. These assays do not necessarily provide a superior physiological assessment, however, since PRA measurements are more likely to reflect circulating angiotensin II levels. In other words, higher endogenous angiotensinogen levels are normally likely to induce compensatory suppression of renin secretion (via indirect and direct feedback effects of angiotensin II) in order to maintain normal plasma angiotensin levels. Indeed, early studies suggested that when plasma angiotensinogen levels are increased by estrogen treatment, there is a close direct correlation between PRA and angiotensin II levels, whereas the latter are actually inversely correlated with PRC (Catt, Cain, & Menard, 1972). In addition, it is important to note that early published methods for PRC employed an acidification step in order to destroy endogenous angiotensinogen (Brown, Davies, Lever, Robertson, & Tree, 1964; Skinner, 1967); it is now known that prorenin can be activated by acidification (Sealey, Atlas, & Laragh, 1980), so that results obtained with such methods, used in many older reports in the literature, may have limited physiological significance.

Direct Immunoassays of Renin

RIAs of human renin, which provide direct estimates of its concentration in plasma and other biological fluids, were first developed in 1980 following successful purification of the enzyme and development of monospecific antibodies (Galen *et al.,* 1979; Guyenne, Galen, Devaux, Corvol, & Menard, 1980). The classical displacement RIAs used initially were of limited sensitivity and

required a continuing supply of pure renin to be used as a tracer; moreover, the antisera used recognized prorenin as well as active renin, making such assays of limited value for physiological studies. More recently, several monoclonal antibodies to renin have become available and solid-phase "sandwich" or immunometric assays have been devised, in which the second of a pair of antibodies is labeled either radioactively or enzymatically (Galen *et al.,* 1984; Menard *et al.,* 1985). In at least one commercial assay currently being tested, the second antibody has little or no affinity for prorenin and available results suggest that this assay may be specific for active renin. Its sensitivity is sufficient to distinguish elevated from normal plasma renin levels, indicating that such assays may prove to have utility for certain diagnostic purposes; however, greater sensitivity will be required to discriminate suppressed renin levels or to evaluate changes in renin secretion within the physiological range. Aside from the latter issue, there are as yet no indications that direct immunoassays will prove superior to PRA methods for the purpose of physiological assessments, since it may be preferable to measure activity rather than active renin concentration, as discussed above.

Measurement of Angiotensinogen

Traditionally, angiotensinogen concentrations in plasma and other tissues have been measured enzymatically as the amount of angiotensin I formed by incubation to exhaustion with excess semipurified renin (Sealey, Gerten-Banes, & Laragh, 1972). In theory, 1 mol of angiotensin I is formed per mol of angiotensinogen. More recently, with the advent of complete purification of angiotensinogen, direct RIAs have been developed which have been useful in physiological studies (Genain, Bouhnik, Tewksbury, Corvol, & Menard, 1984), although these are not widely available at present.

RIA of Angiotensins I and II

As mentioned above, direct RIA of angiotensin I has been used extensively to measure product formation in enzymatic assays for renin and angiotensinogen. Such assays can also be used to measure basal, endogenous levels of plasma angiotensin I if precautions are taken to avoid *in vitro* generation of the peptide by renin (Morton *et al.,* 1976). Although continued accumulation of angiotensin I does not occur in human plasma, even at room temperature, it is probable that supraphysiological amounts are formed within a few minutes of ordinary blood collection. Inclusion of one of the new, potent renin inhibitors in the collection tube may obviate this problem (see below). In addition, extraction of plasma may be necessary to remove nonspecific interference with the assay. There is little evidence, however, that direct measurement of endogenous angiotensin I concentration adds significantly to the information provided by measurement of renin activity.

Direct RIAs for angiotensin II have been available for many years, but most methods in use have problems with both sensitivity and specificity. Extraction of plasma (e.g., by precipitation of protein with polar organic solvents or, more recently, by application to prepacked reversed-phase cartridges) is used to reduce interference by nonspecific cross-reacting substances and to concentrate the sample (Morton *et al.,* 1976). Nonetheless, most procedures that have been developed still have poor discrimination of subnormal versus normal values. All available antisera show considerable cross-reactivity with angiotensin III and other metabolites and, more importantly, cross-react to some extent with angiotensin I. The latter is especially problematic in evaluating the effects of converting enzyme inhibitors *in vivo,* since administration of these drugs results in angiotensin I accumulation which is further compounded by the sometimes marked stimulation of renin secretion. Recently, high-resolution chromatographic procedures (e.g., reversed-phase HPLC) have been used to separate angiotensin peptides in plasma extracts prior to RIA (Kubo *et al.,* 1985; Nussberger, Brunner, Waeber, & Brunner, 1985). Such approaches offer a high degree of specificity and have indeed demonstrated, contrary to earlier reports, that converting enzyme inhibition leads to profound suppression of plasma angiotensin II levels. However, these assays are cumbersome and are, at present, impractical for studies involving a large number of samples. It is

possible, however, that inclusion of a renin inhibitor in the collection tube may sufficiently suppress angiotensin I formation so that chromatographic separation becomes unnecessary (Nussberger, Brunner, Waeber, & Brunner, 1988).

Measurements in Other Tissues

The aforementioned assay procedures have all been employed to measure components of the renin–angiotensin system in tissues such as kidney, brain, adrenal, vessel wall, and gonads. There are three general methodological issues of which investigators in this area should be aware. First, proteases other than renin are capable of generating angiotensinlike immunoreactivity *in vitro*. These include other acid proteases, notably cathepsin D, which cleave angiotensin I from angiotensinogen (Dorer, Lentz, Kahn, Levine, & Skeggs, 1978), trypsinlike enzymes, which can generate larger N-terminal fragments (Skeggs, Dorer, Kahn, Lentz, & Levine, 1981) which may cross-react in some immunoassays, and a cathepsin G-like protease (tonin) which has been shown to cleave angiotensin II directly from angiotensinogen in certain tissues (Schiffrin & Genest, 1983). Second, additional inhibitors may be required to prevent angiotensin I or II degradation by tissue peptidases. And third, direct immunoassays may show interference from nonspecific cross-reacting substances when low levels of antigen are being measured; for instance, chromatographic procedures appear to be required for added specificity in measurements of brain angiotensin II (Phillips & Stentstrom, 1985).

In interpreting very low levels of tissue components, it should also be borne in mind that contamination from blood may be a significant problem. Therefore, in recent years many investigators have turned to measurement of tissue mRNA levels for renin or angiotensinogen (Deschepper *et al.,* 1986; Campbell & Habener, 1986) in order to more critically address the question of *in situ* biosynthesis.

Measurements of Aldosterone

Assays of both urine and plasma aldosterone are widely available. Although accurate collection of a

24-h urine sample is required, the urinary assays may be preferable for screening or diagnostic purposes since plasma aldosterone levels may fluctuate markedly with posture or time of day (see below). Steroid excretion rates generally parallel secretion rates, and measurements of urinary steroids or their metabolites have largely replaced the older double isotope dilution methods for directly estimating secretion rate (Ulick, Laragh, & Lieberman, 1958). On the other hand, plasma aldosterone measurements are useful for assessing short-term effects of interventions and may, in some circumstances, have greater physiological relevance since they are not, over the long term, affected by changes in clearance rate.

Urinary Aldosterone Excretion

The most widely used assay takes advantage of a steroid metabolite unique to aldosterone, i.e., the C_{18}-glucuronide which is formed in kidney and liver and is readily excreted in the urine (Tait, Tait, Little, & Laumas, 1961; Bledsoe et al., 1966). Unlike other polar steroid conjugates, the C_{18}-glucuronide is quantitatively hydrolyzed at low pH; therefore, following extraction of free steroids in urine with nonpolar organic solvents, acidification and reextraction of the urine results in selective isolation of aldosterone (Sealey, Buhler, Laragh, Manning, & Brunner, 1972). Subsequent quantitation by RIA thus provides a highly specific assay even if the antibody used has significant cross-reactivity with other steroids. Although aldosterone-18-glucuronide is a relatively minor metabolite, accounting for roughly 10% of the total aldosterone produced by the adrenal, measurement of the excretion rate of this metabolite correlates quite well with more direct estimates of aldosterone secretory rate in most instances (Sealey, Buhler, et al., 1972). There is also quite a good correlation with the excretion of the major metabolite, tetrahydroaldosterone-3-glucuronide, which accounts for about 35% of the daily output (Gomez-Sanchez & Holland, 1981). Measurement of this metabolite has been advocated by some investigators, but such methods are more difficult because they require more tedious chromatographic procedures to isolate it from cross-reacting steroids.

Because steroid excretion rates generally parallel secretory rates, they may be influenced by alterations in metabolic clearance. That is, since feedback control of secretion is determined by the level of hormone reaching its particular target cell(s), factors which alter clearance ultimately will alter secretion rate in a parallel direction in order that plasma level is maintained in the normal range. In the case of steroids, thyroid hormone is known to significantly stimulate hepatic reduction of the A ring (leading to formation of tetrahydro metabolites), so that secretion and excretion rates may be either increased (hyperthyroidism) or depressed (hypothyroidism) while plasma levels are relatively normal (Luetscher et al., 1963). In addition, formation and/or excretion of steroid metabolites may be considerably impaired in patients with advanced renal or liver disease. In such instances, measurement of plasma aldosterone may provide better assessment of homeostatic control mechanisms, provided that samples are obtained under carefully controlled circumstances.

Plasma Aldosterone

Extraction of free aldosterone from plasma (e.g., with immiscible organic solvents) is required for adequate sensitivity in most available RIAs (Bühler, Sealey, & Laragh, 1974). Since most commercially available antisera show appreciable cross-reactivity with other steroids, which are coextracted with aldosterone, additional purification procedures are required, making such assays more difficult than measurement of the acid-labile metabolite in urine. Highly specific antialdosterone antibodies do exist (McKenzie & Clements, 1974) but these are not widely available.

Factors Influencing Measurements

Sampling Sites

Both renin and aldosterone are mainly cleared by the liver, so that peripheral venous and arterial levels of these substances are quite similar. Measurements of arteriovenous differences of renin (across the kidney) or of aldosterone (across the adrenal) are common diagnostic procedures, and in each case inferior vena cava samples (obtained below the renal or adrenal veins, respectively) can be substituted for arterial samples. In the case of renin, secretion rate can be calculated if renal plasma flow is measured simultaneously.

Because angiotensin II is in large part formed in the pulmonary microcirculation and is degraded in the periphery (see above), levels of this peptide are generally higher in arterial, compared to venous, blood. For comparative purposes, venous sampling is probably perfectly valid, but it must be borne in mind that arterial levels are more likely to reflect angiotensin concentration at its target tissues.

Age, Sex, and Race

Plasma renin levels tend to decline with increasing age (Kaplan *et al.*, 1976), although the differences in the white adult population are subtle if subjects with hypertension (who frequently have low PRA) are excluded (Sealey, 1981). PRA is, on average, lower in normotensive black subjects (Kaplan *et al.*, 1976), and the effect of increasing age is more apparent in this population. Plasma angiotensinogen concentration tends to be higher in females, blacks, and older subjects (Sealey, 1981). Although the latter may in part be a compensation for the tendency toward reduced renin

secretion, the mechanisms responsible for these differences have not been definitely established. Cyclical changes in renin in menstruating females are discussed below.

Physiological Factors

The principal factors influencing plasma renin and aldosterone levels are summarized in Tables 1 and 2, respectively. The major short-term variable influencing plasma renin, angiotensin, and aldosterone levels is posture (Laragh & Sealey, 1973). The principal mechanism responsible for this effect is the increase in renin secretion with upright posture; there is conflicting evidence whether a decrease in aldosterone clearance, due to a decrease in hepatic blood flow, may contribute to the postural rise in plasma aldosterone (Williams, Cain, Dluhy, & Underwood, 1972), but in any event this is likely to be a transient effect and not sustained under steady-state conditions. An extreme postural stimulus (e.g., head-up tilt) may also induce a stress-related ACTH surge which can contribute to the rise in aldosterone (Morganti, Sealey, Lopez-Ovejero, Pickering, & Laragh, 1979). Renin and aldosterone have biological half lives of approximately 15 and 20–30 min, respectively, so that 60–90 min is required to approximate steady-state conditions when posture is changed. Although angiotensin II itself has a far shorter half-life, the functional half-time of changes in its plasma level is dictated by that of

Table 1. Physiological Factors Affecting Renin Secretion

Factor	Effect on plasma renin	Major mechanism
Posture	Increase with upright posture	Sympathetic reflex
Circadian rhythm	Variable peak between midnight and 6 a.m.	Sympathetic discharge?
Sodium balance	Increase with sodium depletion	NaCl load to macula densa
Menstrual cycle[a]	Variable increase during luteal phase	Natriuretic effect of progesterone?
Age	Slight decrease with age	?
Race	Lower in blacks versus whites	?

[a]In addition, plasma prorenin (but not renin) increases transiently at the time of ovulation, presumably reflecting ovarian secretion of prorenin.

Table 2. Factors Affecting Plasma Aldosterone Concentration

Stimulus	Major mechanisms
Upright posture	Increased secretion due to: Increased angiotensin II; Increased ACTH (head-up tilt)?; Decreased metabolic clearance rate (short-term)?
Circadian rhythm	Variation in secretion due to rhythm in ACTH release (normally evident only during maintained recumbency)
Sodium depletion	Increased secretion due to: Increased angiotensin II; Increased adrenal sensitivity to angiotensin II (and other agonists)
Dietary potassium	Increased secretion due to direct effect of K^+

renin. It is critical that baseline measurements be obtained under close to steady-state conditions when assessing the responses of hormone levels to acute interventions. For diagnostic purposes, ambulatory PRA measurements are generally recommended since the postural stimulus provides greater discrimination between suppressed and elevated levels (Laragh & Sealey, 1973).

Diurnal changes also occur in renin and aldosterone levels. Plasma renin generally increases between midnight and 6 a.m. (Gordon, Wolfe, Island, & Liddle, 1966), possibly due to a surge in sympathetic outflow during sleep. A circadian rhythm in aldosterone is generally not apparent in ambulatory humans due to the postural variations in renin and angiotensin. In supine subjects, however, aldosterone varies in parallel with plasma cortisol due to the rhythm in ACTH (Katz, Romfh, & Smith, 1972). This may also be apparent during marked suppression of the renin–angiotensin system, as can occur with ingestion of a high-salt diet or as frequently occurs in primary aldosteronism due to an aldosterone-secreting adenoma (Ganguly, Dowdy, Luetscher, & Melada, 1973), a finding which may be useful diagnostically.

Dietary sodium intake has an important effect on renin secretion and PRA levels increase sharply over a period of several days during marked sodium deprivation. Nomograms relating PRA to concurrent urinary sodium excretion rates (which reflect sodium intake in the steady state and which provide an important index of the state of sodium balance) are very useful in assessing the normalcy or appropriateness of renin levels (Brunner, Sealey, & Laragh, 1972; Laragh & Sealey, 1973). Plasma and urinary aldosterone levels exhibit a similar close relationship to sodium excretion rate, mainly due to the parallel variation in PRA (Bühler, Laragh, Sealey, & Brunner, 1974); in addition, these relationships may be amplified by an increased adrenal sensitivity to angiotensin II induced by sodium depletion.

Dietary potassium has an important influence on aldosterone levels, since even subtle increases in extracellular potassium concentration can markedly increase aldosterone secretion (Laragh & Sealey, 1973). Marked hypokalemia may also mask angiotensin-induced increases in aldosterone and may even lead to apparent ''normalization'' of aldosterone in patients with primary aldosteronism. Consideration of urinary potassium excretion (reflecting dietary intake) is therefore useful for precise interpretation of aldosterone levels. Marked potassium loading has also been shown to depress (and potassium depletion to stimulate) plasma renin levels (Laragh & Sealey, 1973); the effect appears to be more subtle than that on aldosterone and may not have significant impact in the usual ranges of potassium intake, although further study is needed in this regard.

Plasma renin and aldosterone levels increase to a variable extent during the luteal phase of the menstrual cycle (Katz & Romfh, 1972; Glorioso, Atlas, Laragh, Jewelewicz, & Sealey, 1986). This effect is probably related to the natriuretic effect of progesterone, which antagonizes the action of aldosterone in the distal nephron. Recently it has been shown that there is an abrupt and transitory rise in plasma prorenin coincident with the LH surge at the time of ovulation (Glorioso et al., 1986; Itskovitz & Sealey, 1987). Active renin levels do not rise concurrently, and it appears that this increase is due to ovarian secretion of prorenin.

Pharmacological Agents

A variety of pharmacological agents, including virtually all drugs used to treat hypertension or edematous disorders, have marked effects on renin secretion (Keeton & Campbell, 1981). In general, all drugs which cause volume depletion, reflex sympathetic stimulation, decreased renal perfusion pressure, or interruption of angiotensin II formation will stimulate renin secretion, whereas those which cause volume retention or inhibition of sympathetic activity will depress it. Direct actions of, or withdrawal responses to, nicotine, caffeine, alcohol, or other agents affecting the sympathetic nervous system may also influence plasma renin levels. With the possible exception of chloralose, virtually all anesthetic and hypnotic agents stimulate renin secretion and should be avoided in studies in experimental animals.

Physiological Relevance of Measurements

Studies employing a variety of pharmacological probes have suggested that the renin–angiotensin system is involved in the regulation of systemic vascular resistance, aldosterone secretion, and renal function under physiological conditions and in several pathological states. As reviewed by Ondetti and Cushman (1982), the agents frequently used include angiotensin analogues which are receptor antagonists but which also have partial agonist properties; peptidic and orally active inhibitors of angiotensin converting enzyme; and the more recently developed peptidic renin inhibitors. Although each class has its own problems in specificity, the strikingly similar results obtained with all of these agents provide solid evidence for the role of the renin–angiotensin system.

Regarding its role in blood pressure regulation, much has been made of the fact that when one considers the broad spectrum of normal and pathological states, levels of PRA or angiotensin II bear if anything an *inverse* relationship to concurrently measured blood pressure or calculated peripheral resistance. But this is not at all surprising when one takes into account that the renin–angiotensin system is homeostatically involved in car-

diovascular regulation, serving to maintain arterial pressure in the face of circulatory collapse but able to induce hypertension when renin secretion is inappropriate. Thus, it has been shown that the decreases in blood pressure or vascular resistance induced by blockade of the system are directly related to the baseline level of PRA or angiotensin II (Cody, Laragh, Case, & Atlas, 1983). Such findings do not rule out the contribution of extrarenal renin or of locally formed angiotensin II to such responses, but they clearly indicate that valid measurements of these components in plasma provide an important index of the functional status of the renin–angiotensin system.

Atrial Natriuretic Factor

Structure and Tissue Sources

ANF is a small polypeptide derived from the C-terminus of a 126-amino-acid residue precursor (proANF) which is stored in secretory granules present in atrial myocytes (deBold, 1985; Cantin & Genest, 1985; Laragh, 1985; Maack, Camargo, Kleinert, Laragh, & Atlas, 1985; Needleman et al., 1985; Atlas, 1986). Lesser quantities of immunoreactive ANF and/or ANF-specific mRNA have been localized in other tissues, including ventricular muscle, pituitary, hypothalamus, and other brain structures, but the atrium is the major, if not sole, source of circulating ANF in mammals.

Several structurally related peptides derived from the C-terminus of proANF, ranging between 21 and 35 amino acids, were originally isolated from rat atrial muscle (Figure 3), but these probably resulted in large part from nonspecific proteolysis of proANF during extraction and purification procedures. Recent evidence suggests that the 28-residue peptide (ANF 99–126) isolated by Flynn, deBold, and deBold (1983) and by Kangawa and Matsuo (1984) is the major circulating form in rat, and probably human, blood (Schwartz et al., 1985; Thibault et al., 1985). On the other hand, N-terminally deleted 24- and 25-residue peptides (ANF 103–126 and ANF 102–126), originally isolated from rat atrium by Currie et al. (1984) and Atlas et

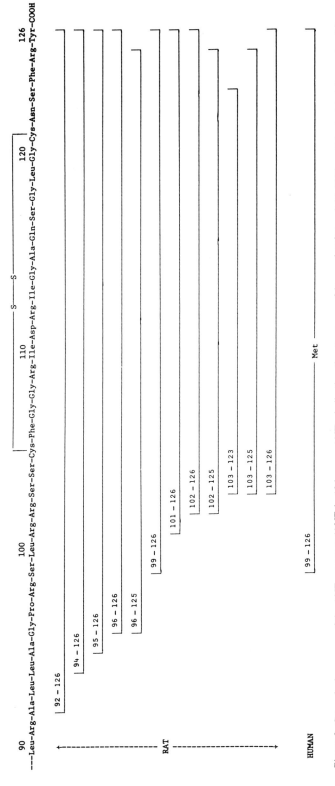

Figure 3. C-terminal sequence of the ANF precursor (ANF 1–126 or proANF), indicating the structures of low-molecular-weight ANF peptides isolated from rat and human atria. Reproduced from Atlas (1986).

al. (1984), respectively, appear to be the major forms present in brain and spinal cord (Shiono *et al.*, 1986), where ANF is presumed to exert a neurotransmitter or neuromodulatory action (Skofitsch, Jacobowitz, Eskay, & Zamir, 1985; Quirion *et al.*, 1984). This finding suggests an alternate mode of precursor processing in neural tissue.

Although proANF appears to be the major storage form in the atrial granules (deBold, 1985), little or no intact proANF is found in blood under normal circumstances (see below). At present, the exact mechanism and site of biosynthetic processing of the precursor to yield the mature hormone have not been elucidated. Recent studies suggest that the precursor is cleaved within the heart, since ANF appears to be cosecreted on an equimolar basis with the N-terminal fragment (i.e., probably ANF 1–98) in both the rat (Michener, Gierse, Seetharam, Fok, & Needleman, 1986) and human (Sala, Camargo, *et al.*, 1987). This fragment, which is not detected by routine ANF immunoassays, appears to accumulate in blood owing to its slower, renal clearance; its biological function, if any, is unknown.

Regulation of Secretion

ANF appears to be released mainly via the coronary sinus, so that the hormone produced by the right and left atria exit the heart together (Espiner *et al.*, 1985); however, direct secretion from the atria (e.g., via the thebesian veins) has not been ruled out. Whatever the case, indirect lines of evidence suggest that secretion by the right and left atria may be regulated independently under certain circumstances (Imada, Takayanagi, & Inagami, 1985).

Atrial Distension

The major factor that has been shown to increase ANF secretion is an increase in right or left atrial stretch or wall tension. This has been demonstrated experimentally with maneuvers such as acute volume expansion (Lang *et al.*, 1985), mechanical distension of the atria (Ledsome, Wilson, Courney, & Rankin, 1985), infusion of pressor agents

(Manning, Schwartz, Katsube, Holmberg, & Needleman, 1985), and increases in central blood volume induced by water immersion to the neck (Epstein *et al.*, 1986). The cellular mechanism of stretch secretion coupling has not been determined.

Increased atrial wall tension is likely to account for the transient increases in plasma ANF observed during induction of atrial tachyarrhythmias (Yamaji, Ishibashi, Nakaoka, *et al.*, 1985) and for the chronically elevated levels found in patients with poorly compensated congestive heart failure (Shenker, Sider, Ostafin, & Grekin, 1985; Cody *et al.*, 1986) or in conditions associated with marked generalized expansion of extracellular volume, such as chronic renal parenchymal disease or mineralocorticoid excess (Rascher, Tulassay, & Lang, 1985; Yamaji, Ishibashi, Sekihara, *et al.*, 1986). Dietary sodium loading has also been reported to increase plasma ANF levels modestly, again possibly related to increases in atrial stretch (Sagnella, Markandu, Shore, & MacGregor, 1985).

Other Factors

Glucocorticoids, and possibly thyroid hormone, have been shown to stimulate ANF gene transcription rate *in vitro* (Matsuo & Nakazato, 1987). Thus, these hormones may have long-term effects on plasma ANF levels by increasing hormone biosynthesis.

A variety of hormonal and other factors (including osmolality and sodium concentration) have been postulated to influence ANF secretion *per se,* but the physiological significance of these has yet to be established. The large increases in plasma ANF induced by supraphysiological doses of vasopressin, angiotensin II, α-adrenergic agonists, and other pressor substances can probably be explained by their effects on atrial stretch (Manning *et al.*, 1985), and there is considerable controversy concerning effects of such agents in *in vitro* systems (Sonnenberg & Veress, 1984; LaChance, Garcia, Gutkowska, Cantin, & Thibault, 1986). Thus, although it is probable that significant modulators of ANF secretion will be identified by further work, their existence remains somewhat speculative at present.

Finally, it should be mentioned that levels of ANF mRNA have been shown to increase in cardiac ventricular muscle in experimental models of ventricular hypertrophy (Day et al., 1987). This may be related to dedifferentiation, since it is known that secretory granules appear in ventricle, as well as atrium, in lower vertebrates and during mammalian embryogenesis (deBold, 1985). Although secretion from ventricular muscle has not been demonstrated, it remains possible that the ventricle may contribute to increased plasma ANF levels in certain pathological conditions.

Physiological Actions

A comprehensive discussion of the myriad actions of ANF described to date is beyond the scope of this chapter, and the reader is referred to several recent reviews for additional details and primary reference sources (Cantin & Genest, 1985; Laragh, 1985; Maack et al., 1985; Atlas & Laragh, 1986; Atlas & Maack, 1987). It should be noted at the outset that the relative physiological importance of each of these actions has not been determined.

ANF is a potent natriuretic and diuretic substance that also inhibits renin secretion. These renal actions appear to be in large part dependent upon complex renal hemodynamic effects, including an increase in glomerular filtration rate, although direct actions on the JG cell and on collecting duct sodium reabsorption appear to contribute to renin suppression and natriuresis, respectively. ANF also inhibits adrenal steroidogenesis. Its most prominent action in this regard is inhibition of agonist-induced aldosterone biosynthesis and release; inhibition of glucocorticoid production has been described in some species, and both inhibitory and stimulatory effects on gonadal steroidogenesis have been reported in vitro.

Inhibition of vasopressin secretion has also been documented, and several studies suggest possible inhibition of the release of ACTH, LH, and other anterior pituitary hormones, probably via actions on the hypothalamus. Other central effects, such as inhibition of thirst and salt appetite and lowering of systemic blood pressure, have been described following intracerebroventricular administration of the peptide. ANF exerts a marked smooth muscle relaxant effect on isolated arteries contracted with angiotensin II and other hormonal agonists or neurotransmitters. This action may contribute to the lowering of blood pressure induced by ANF infusion, but reductions in cardiac output, possibly due to intravascular volume contraction and/or to interactions with neural reflex mechanisms, have also been observed. In addition to its natriuretic action, ANF appears to reduce intravascular volume by inducing fluid shifts to the extravascular space, possibly by increasing capillary hydraulic permeability.

As is apparent from the foregoing summary, ANF opposes the renin–angiotensin system at several levels, by inhibiting renin release and by antagonizing the actions of angiotensin II on aldosterone production and on vascular tone. In addition, the central inhibitory effects of ANF on hormone secretion, thirst, and blood pressure are antagonistic to known central effects of angiotensin II. Thus has arisen the concept that a major aspect of ANF action is as a functional antagonist to the renin–angiotensin–aldosterone system (Laragh, 1985; Atlas & Maack, 1987).

Although the unavailability of specific antagonists of ANF makes it difficult to study the physiological significance of each of these actions, it has long been known that distension of the atria induces many of the phenomena that are mimicked by ANF infusion, particularly diuresis and natriuresis, and inhibition of renin, aldosterone, and vasopressin release (Goetz, Bond, & Bloxham, 1975). In all probability, increased ANF release participates in these short-term events; however, as indicated in Figure 4, neural reflex mechanisms, evoked by activation of cardiopulmonary stretch receptors, clearly contribute to these responses, and the precise contribution of ANF is currently uncertain (see below).

Measurements of ANF and Related Substances

Assays for ANF have only recently been developed (Lang et al., 1985; Shenker et al., 1985; Cody et al., 1986; Gutkowska et al., 1986) and the precise requirements for proper sample collection and assay performance have not been studied ex-

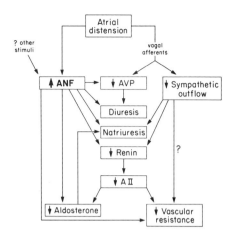

Figure 4. Schematic representation of the interactive effects of ANF and neurally mediated reflexes on renal function and the renin–angiotensin system during distension of the atria. Reproduced from Atlas (1986).

tensively. As with most peptide assays, blood samples should probably be collected on ice and processed relatively quickly. EDTA has been widely used as the anticoagulant since it effectively inhibits many peptidases; some investigators also add aprotinin to the blood, but the need for such additional protease inhibitors has not been clearly established. Most investigators currently extract plasma samples using octadecylsilane (C_{18}) cartridges or other methods, and assays using unextracted plasma generally give higher results; this is probably due to interference with nonspecific cross-reacting substances or other immunoassay artifacts, although this point has not been proven. Extraction also serves to concentrate the plasma sample and thereby improve sensitivity.

In most published reports, detection of ANF has been accomplished by direct RIA. The significance of reported assay results thus depends heavily on the specificity of the antibodies used, and the existing characterization data are incomplete. One of the most widely used antibodies, supplied from a commercial source (Peninsula Laboratories), is directed at the C-terminal sequence of ANF, and its sensitivity is markedly reduced by deletion of the C-terminal tyrosine residue (which is not essential for biological activity). This antibody exhibits 40% cross-reactivity with intact proANF (Sala, Camargo, *et al.*, 1987). Studies from

several laboratories have shown, however, that intact proANF is a very minor component in rat or human plasma (Lang *et al.*, 1985; Yamaji, Ishibashi, & Takaku, 1985; Epstein *et al.*, 1986). In our experience, proANF levels are appreciable mainly in plasma samples from patients with marked chronic hypersecretion of ANF (e.g., congestive heart failure) and proANF levels do not change during acute stimulation of ANF secretion. The major form of immunoreactive ANF recognized by most ANF antisera in human plasma extracts has a retention from time on reversed-phase HPLC identical to that of synthetic ANF 99–126 (Yamaji, Ishibashi, & Takaku, 1985; Epstein *et al.*, 1986). Significant amounts of at least one earlier eluting peak have also been detected, however; this probably represents a metabolite or oxidized form of the peptide. Since the biological activity of this additional peak is unknown, further work is needed to determine whether its contribution to total immunoreactivity varies in different experimental or clinical conditions.

Direct RIA has also been used to measure levels of ANF immunoreactivity in extracts of atrium, ventricle, and other tissues. In these cases, the cross-reactivity of most available antisera with proANF becomes an issue of critical importance. For instance, proANF has been shown to be the major storage form in atrial tissue using highly stringent extraction conditions designed to minimize proteolysis (deBold, 1985), and variations in such conditions can lead to appreciable nonspecific cleavage of the precursor to smaller peptides with increased antibody crossreactivity. Consequently, differences in tissue levels of immunoreactivity may reflect variability in nonspecific proteolysis as well as in molar peptide concentrations, and chromatographic analysis may be necessary for proper interpretation of such assay results.

Several investigators have also employed adrenal membrane preparations to develop radioreceptor assays for ANF (Raine *et al.*, 1986). In theory, such an approach may provide results with more certain biological significance. To date, qualitatively similar findings have been reported with these assays, but a rigorous comparison of this method with direct RIA has not been published as yet.

As mentioned earlier, one or more fragments derived from the N-terminal portion of proANF coexist with ANF in the blood. These fragments are not detected in ANF assays employing antisera which recognize only the mature hormone (i.e., ANF 99–126), but can be measured in plasma extracts by routine RIA procedures using antisera prepared against specific peptide sequences in the N-terminal region (Michener *et al.,* 1986; Sala, Camargo, *et al.,* 1987). The major peptide detected in blood by these assays has chromatographic properties that are consistent with the intact propeptide (i.e., ANF 1–98), although smaller degradation products are also present in patients with end-stage renal disease and extremely high levels (Sala, Camargo, *et al.,* 1987). Total N-terminal fragment levels are more than 20-fold higher than ANF levels, suggesting accumulation due to slower metabolic clearance. Following acute stimuli to ANF release, comparable absolute increments in propeptide levels occur (suggesting co-release by the heart on an equimolar basis), but the percentage increase is far smaller—for instance, a two-fold acute increase in plasma ANF may be accompanied by only a 5–10% increase in propeptide levels. Consequently, such assays may prove useful in reflecting long-term changes in ANF biosynthesis and release.

Another parameter which may prove useful in studies of ANF release and action is measurement of cyclic guanosine monophosphate (cGMP) in urine or blood. Early studies demonstrated that ANF raises cGMP levels in many tissues (Hamet *et al.,* 1984), an effect which is due to ANF receptor-mediated stimulation of particulate guanylate cyclase (Waldman, Rapoport, & Murad, 1984). Although this latter action is unique to ANF among all known mammalian substances, other factors may potentially influence cGMP levels (e.g., through stimulation of the cytosolic form of cyclase). Nonetheless, available data suggest a striking correlation between plasma ANF and cGMP levels across the spectrum of health and disease. Moreover, acute stimulation of ANF secretion is associated with parallel changes in plasma levels and urinary excretion rates of cGMP (Sala, Pecker, *et al.,* 1987). Consequently, such measurements may offer additional insights regarding the biological relevance of ANF assay results. There are several commercially available kits providing reagents for direct RIA of cGMP, using either [3]H- or ^{125}I-labeled nucleotide as tracer. These assays can be applied directly to dilutions of urine or to ethanol extracts of plasma. Blood collected on ice in EDTA is appropriate, since the latter provides for effective inhibition of phosphodiesterase.

Factors Influencing Measurements

In view of the limited time that ANF assays have been available, understanding of this issue is necessarily limited. It should be noted that the range of normal values reported in most series to date is extremely broad (Shenker *et al.,* 1985; Cody *et al.,* 1986), and this is not explained by any of the factors influencing ANF levels thus far identified.

Sampling Sites

Because ANF is secreted by the heart and metabolized or cleared peripherally, levels of the peptide are consistently higher in arterial compared to peripheral venous plasma (Cody *et al.,* 1986; Raine *et al.,* 1986). Levels in mixed venous blood (i.e., obtained from the right ventricle or pulmonary artery) are on average similar to arterial levels, as expected with secretion from the coronary sinus; one report suggests a slight decrement in ANF concentration across the pulmonary bed, consistent with slight metabolism in the lung, but this has not been confirmed. There is a considerable decrease in ANF concentration in renal venous plasma, suggesting that the kidney is a major site of metabolism.

It should be noted that the gradient in ANF concentration across the heart should be increased when cardiac output is decreased, and available data in patients with heart failure confirm this (Cody *et al.,* 1986). Acute decreases in cardiac output could thus conceivably increase arterial ANF concentration even without a change in secretion rate; this might contribute to the marked increase in plasma ANF reported following infusion of pharmacological doses of pressor agents in rats, where blood was sampled by decapitation (Manning *et al.*, 1985). Thus, in assessing changes in ANF secretion in intact animals, analyses of both venous and arterial blood are probably necessary for proper interpretation of responses to acute interventions that simultaneously alter cardiac output.

Age, Sex, and Race

Limited data are available on the influence of these parameters. There are several reports which demonstrate a weak direct relationship between plasma ANF levels and age, suggesting that age must be controlled for in defining normal ranges. Our unpublished data in normal volunteers suggest that plasma ANF levels tend to be slightly higher in females versus males and in blacks versus whites; however, these trends are not statistically significant.

Physiological Factors

The biological half-life of ANF is quite short, being on the order of 3 min in humans (Yandle *et al.*, 1986). Consequently, steady-state responses to acute interventions occur relatively rapidly (Epstein *et al.*, 1986). As might be predicted with an atrial stretch mechanism, plasma ANF levels tend to be higher in the supine versus the upright position. Available data suggest that the effect of posture is relatively subtle and variable on low or normal salt intakes, but may become quite pronounced following sodium loading (Sagnella *et al.*, 1985). Marked increases in dietary sodium intake clearly increase plasma ANF levels, but the effect appears to be relatively modest (about twofold); there is a weak positive relationship between ANF and urinary sodium excretion over the initial few days of increased dietary salt intake (Shenker *et al.*, 1985), but the precise relationship between plasma ANF and sodium balance requires additional study. Finally, although there is a report suggesting that there may be a nocturnal peak in ANF similar to that observed for plasma renin (Donckier, Anderson, Yeo, & Bloom, 1986), recent work from our laboratories suggests that this is merely a consequence of recumbent posture (Bell *et al.*, 1988).

Pharmacological Agents

Drugs which alter plasma volume, cardiac contractility or heart rate, and arterial or venous tone are all likely to alter atrial wall tension and, thus, ANF secretion. Concerning specific agents, very little rigorously obtained data have thus far been reported in the literature. With the exception of pentobarbital, most anesthetic agents have a marked stimulatory effect on plasma ANF in rats (Gutkowska *et al.*, 1986).

Physiological Significance of Measurements

In contrast to the renin–angiotensin system, the current state of knowledge regarding the physiological significance of ANF is rudimentary, in part due to the lack of specific antagonists. As outlined above, there are certain inferences that can be drawn from the documented responses to ANF infusion and from current understanding of the regulation of ANF secretion. In addition, there are some more direct lines of evidence suggesting that ANF may generally be involved in the regulation of intravascular volume, at least over the short term. Resection of the atrial appendages has been shown in some (but not all) studies to blunt the natriuretic response to acute volume expansion (Veress & Sonnenberg, 1984; Kobrin, Kardon, Trippodo, Pegram, & Frolich, 1985), and administration of monoclonal antibodies to ANF to intact rats has been shown to nearly abolish the natriuresis induced by autologous blood transfusion (Hirth *et al.*, 1986). Certain technical aspects of most studies reported to data do not permit such findings to be extrapolated to more physiological conditions of volume expansion, and more specific antagonists of ANF will probably be required to definitively assess its relative importance.

Based on the chromatographic characteristics of immunoassayable ANF, one can make the tentative conclusion that at least some of the RIA data reported in the literature reflect biologically active hormone. Furthermore, as already noted, the broad range of endogenous ANF levels encountered in a variety of physiological and pathological states shows extremely good correlation with plasma levels of cGMP. Since stimulation of membrane-bound guanylate cyclase is a documented action of ANF in many target cells *in vitro* (Waldman, Rapoport, & Murad, 1984), this finding at least suggests that variations in measured levels reflect alterations in cellular metabolism at one or more target organs.

For the moment, therefore, it appears that current approaches to measurement of ANF provide meaningful assessments of its biological action. Clearly, further work is needed to validate the current concept that this hormone is involved in the short-term regulation of intravascular volume and to define its importance in long-term volume control in normal and pathological states.

References

Atlas, S. A. (1986). Atrial natriuretic factor: A new hormone of cardiac origin. *Recent Progress in Hormone Research, 42,* 207–249.

Atlas, S. A., & Case, D. B. (1981). Renin in essential hypertension. *Clinical Endocrinology and Metabolism, 10,* 537–575.

Atlas, S. A., Kleinert, H. D., Camargo, M. J. F., Januszewicz, A., Sealey, J. E., Laragh, J. H., Schilling, J. W., Lewicki, J. A., Johnson, L. K., & Maack, T. (1984). Purification, sequencing and synthesis of natriuretic and vasoactive rat atrial peptide. *Nature, 309,* 717–720.

Atlas, S. A., & Laragh, J. H. (1986). Physiological actions of atrial natriuretic factor. In P. J. Mulrow & R. Schrier (Eds.), *Atrial hormones and other natriuretic factors* (pp. 53–76). Bethesda: American Physiological Society.

Atlas, S. A., & Maack, T. (1987). Effects of atrial natriuretic factor on the kidney and the renin–angiotensin–aldosterone system. *Endocrinology and Metabolism Clinics of North America, 16,* 107–143.

Bell, G. M., Pecker, M., Atlas, S. A., James, G., Sealey, J. E., & Laragh, J. H. (1988). Diurnal and postural variations in plasma ANF, cGMP and sodium excretion. *American Journal of Hypertension, 1,* 108A.

Bledsoe, T., Liddle, G. W., Riondel, A., Island, D. P., Bloomfield, D., & Sinclair-Smith, B. (1966). Comparative fates of intravenously and orally administered aldosterone: Evidence for extrahepatic formation of acidlabile conjugate in man. *Journal of Clinical Investigation, 45,* 264–269.

Brown, J. J., Davies, D. L., Lever, A. F., Robertson, J. I. S., & Tree, M. (1964). Estimation of renin in human plasma. *Biochemical Journal, 93,* 594–600.

Brunner, H. R., Sealey, J. E., & Laragh, J. H. (1972). Renin subgroups in essential hypertension. Further analysis of their pathophysiological and epidemiological characteristics. *Circulation Research, 32–33*(Suppl. 1), 99–109.

Bühler, F. R., Laragh, J. H., Sealey, J. E., & Brunner, H. R. (1974). Plasma aldosterone–renin interrelationships in various forms of essential hypertension. In J. H. Laragh (Ed.), *Hypertension manual* (pp. 353–369). New York: Dun–Donnelley.

Bühler, F. R., Sealey, J. E., & Laragh, J. H. (1974). Radioimmunoassay of plasma aldosterone. In J. H. Laragh (Ed.), *Hypertension manual* (pp. 655–669). New York: Dun–Donnelley.

Campbell, D. J., & Habener, J. F. (1986). Angiotensin gene is expressed and differentially regulated in multiple tissues of the rat. Journal of Clinical Investigation, 78, 31.

Cantin, M., & Genest, J. (1985). The heart and the atrial natriuretic factor. *Endocrine Reviews, 6,* 107–127.

Carey, R. M., Vaughan, E. D., Jr., Peach, M. J. & Ayers, C. (1978). Activity of [des-aspartyll]-angiotensin II and angiotensin II in man—Differences in blood pressure and adrenocortical responses during normal and low sodium intake. *Journal of Clinical Investigation, 40,* 2026–2042.

Catt, K. J., Cain, M. D., & Menard, J. (1972). Radioimmunoassay studies of the renin–angiotensin system in human hypertension and during estrogen treatment. In J. Genest & E. Koiw (Eds.), *Hypertension '72* (pp. 591–604). Berlin: Springer-Verlag.

Cody, R. J., Atlas, S. A., Laragh, J. H., Kubo, S. H., Covit, A. B., Ryman, K. S., Shaknovich, A., Pondolfino, K., Clark, M., Camargo, M. J. F., Scarborough, R. M., & Lewicki, J. A. (1986). Atrial natriuretic factor in normal subjects and heart failure patients: Plasma levels and renal, hormonal and hemodynamic responses to peptide infusion. *Journal of Clinical Investigation, 78,* 1362–1372.

Cody, R. J., Laragh, J. H., Case, D. B., & Atlas, S. A. (1983). Renin system activity as a determinant of response to treatment in hypertension and heart failure. *Hypertension, 5*(Suppl. 3), 36–42.

Currie, M. G., Geller, D. M., Cole, B. R., Siegel, N. R., Fok, K. F., Adams, S. P., Eubanks, S. R., Galluppi, G. R., & Needleman, P. (1984). Purification and sequence analysis of bioactive atrial peptides (atriopeptins). *Science, 223,* 67–69.

Day, M. L., Schwartz, D., Weigand, R. C., Stockman, P. T., Brunnert, S. R., Tolunay, H. E., Currie, M. G., Standaert, D. F., & Needleman, P. (1987). Ventricular atriopeptin: Unmasking of messenger RNA and peptide synthesis by hypertrophy or dexamethasone. *Hypertension, 9,* 485–491.

deBold, A. J. (1985). Atrial natriuretic factor: A hormone produced by the heart. *Science, 230,* 767–770.

deBold, A. J., Borenstein, H. B., Veress, A. T., & Sonnenberg, H. (1981). A rapid and potent natriuretic response to intravenous injection of atrial myocardial extract in rats. *Life Sciences, 28,* 89–94.

Deschepper, C. F., Mellon, S. H., Cumin, F., Baxter, J. D., & Ganong, W. F. (1986). Analysis by immunocytochemistry and in situ hybridization of renin and its mRNA in kidney, testis, adrenal, and pituitary of the rat. *Proceedings of the National Academy of Sciences of the United States of America, 83,* 7552–7556.

Donckier, J., Anderson, J. V., Yeo, T., & Bloom, S. R.

(1986). Diurnal rhythm in the plasma concentration of atrial natriuretic peptide [Letter]. *New England Journal of Medicine, 315,* 710.

Dorer, F. E., Lentz, K. E., Kahn, J. R., Levine, M., & Skeggs, L. T. (1978). A comparison of the substrate specificities of cathepsin D and pseudorenin. *Journal of Biological Chemistry, 253,* 3140–3142.

Epstein, M., Loutzenhiser, R., Friedland, E., Aceto, R. M., Camargo, M. J. F., & Atlas, S. A. (1986). Increases in circulating atrial natriuretic factor during immersion-induced central hypervolemia in normal humans. *Journal of Hypertension, 4*(Suppl. 2), S93–S99.

Espiner, E. A., Crozier, I. G., Nicholls, M. G., Cuneo, R., Yandle, T. G., & Ikram, H. (1985). Cardiac secretion of atrial natriuretic peptide. *Lancet, 2,* 398–399.

Flynn, T. G., deBold, M. L., & deBold, A. J. (1983). The amino acid sequence of an atrial peptide with potent diuretic and natriuretic properties. *Biochemical and Biophysical Research Communications, 117,* 859–865.

Galen, F. X., Devaux, C., Atlas, S. A., Guyenne, T., Menard, J., Corvol, P., Simon, D., Cazaubon, C., Richer, P., Badouaille, G., Richaud, J. P., Gros, P., & Pau, B. (1984). New monoclonal antibodies directed against human renin. Powerful tools for the investigation of the renin system. *Journal of Clinical Investigation, 74,* 723–735.

Galen, F. X., Guyenne, T. T., Devaux, C., Auzan, C., Corvol, P., & Menard, J. (1979). Direct radioimmunoassay of human renin. *Journal of Clinical Endocrinology and Metabolism, 48,* 1041–1043.

Ganguly, A., Dowdy, A. J., Luetscher, J. A., & Melada, G. A. (1973). Anomalous postural response of plasma aldosterone concentration in patients with aldosterone-producing adrenal adenoma. *Journal of Clinical Endocrinology and Metabolism, 36,* 401–402.

Genain, C., Bouhnik, J., Tewksbury, D., Corvol, P., & Menard, J. (1984). Characterization of plasma and CSF human angiotensinogen and des-angiotensin I angiotensinogen by direct radio-immunoassay. *Journal of Clinical Endocrinology and Metabolism, 59,* 478–484.

Glorioso, N., Atlas, S. A., Laragh, J. H., Jewelewicz, R., & Sealey, J. E. (1986). Prorenin in high concentrations in human ovarian follicular fluid. *Science, 233,* 1422–1424.

Goetz, K. L., Bond, G. C., & Bloxham, D. D. (1975). Atrial receptors and renal function. *Physiological Reviews, 55,* 157–205.

Gomez-Sanchez, C. E., & Holland, O. B. (1981). Urinary tetrahydroaldosterone and aldosterone-18-glucuronide excretion in white and black normal subjects and hypertensive patients. *Journal of Clinical Endocrinology and Metabolism, 52,* 214–219.

Gordon, R. D., Wolfe, L. K., Island, D. P., & Liddle, G. W. (1966). A diurnal rhythm in plasma renin activity in man. *Journal of Clinical Investigation, 45,* 1587–1592.

Gutkowska, J., Horky, K., Schiffrin, E. L., Thibault, G., Garcia, R., De Lean, A., Hamet, P., Tremblay, J., Anand-Srivasta, M. B., Januszewicz, P., Genest, J., & Cantin, M. (1986). Atrial natriuretic factor: Radioimmunoassay and ef-

fects on adrenal and pituitary glands. *Federation Proceedings, 45,* 2101–2105.

Guyenne, T. T., Galen, F. X., Devaux, C., Corvol, P., & Menard, J. (1980). Direct radioimmunoassay of human renin. Comparison with renin activity in plasma and amniotic fluid. *Hypertension, 2,* 465–470.

Hamet, P., Tremblay, J., Pang, S. C., Garcia, R., Thibault, G., Gutkowska, J., Cantin, M., & Genest, J. (1984). Effect of native and synthetic atrial natriuretic factor on cyclic GMP. *Biochemical and Biophysical Research Communications, 123,* 515–527.

Helmer, O. M., & Judson, W. E. (1963). The quantitative determination of renin in the plasma of patients with arterial hypertension. *Circulation, 27,* 1050–1060.

Hirth, C., Stasch, J. -P., John, A., Kazda, S., Morich, F., Neuser, D., & Wohlfeil, S. (1986). The renal response to acute hypervolemia is caused by atrial natriuretic peptides. *Journal of Cardiovascular Pharmacology, 8,* 268–275.

Imada, T., Takayanagi, R., & Inagami, T. (1985). Changes in the content of atrial natriuretic factor with the progression of hypertension in spontaneously hypertensive rats. *Biochemical and Biophysical Research Communications, 133,* 759–765.

Inagami, T. (1981). Renin. In R. L. Soffer (Ed.), *Biochemical regulation of blood pressure* (pp. 39–71). New York: Wiley.

Itskovitz, J., & Sealey, J. E. (1987). Ovarian prorenin–renin–angiotensin system. *Obstetrical & Gynecological Survey, 42,* 545–551.

Kangawa, K., & Matsuo, H. (1984). Purification and complete amino acid sequence of alpha-human atrial natriuretic polypeptide (alpha-hANP). *Biochemical and Biophysical Research Communications, 118,* 131–139.

Kaplan, N. M., Kem, D. C., Holland, O. B., Kramer, N. J., Higgins, J., & Gomez-Sanchez, C. (1976). The intravenous furosemide test. A simple way to evaluate renin responsiveness. *Annals of Internal Medicine, 84,* 639–645.

Katz, F. H., & Romfh, P. (1972). Plasma aldosterone and renin activity during the menstrual cycle. *Journal of Clinical Endocrinology and Metabolism, 34,* 819–821.

Katz, F. H., Romfh, P., & Smith, J. A. (1972). Episodic secretion of aldosterone in supine man. Relationship to cortisol. *Journal of Clinical Endocrinology and Metabolism, 35,* 178.

Keeton, T. K., & Campbell, W. B. (1981). The pharmacologic alteration of renin release. *Pharmacological Reviews, 31,* 82–202.

Kobrin, I., Kardon, M. B., Trippodo, N. C., Pegram, B. L., & Frolich, E. D. (1985). Renal response to acute volume overload in conscious rats with atrial appendectomy. *Journal of Hypertension, 3,* 145–148.

Krakoff, L. R., & Eisenfeld, A. J. (1977). Hormonal control of plasma renin substrate (angiotensin). *Circulation Research, 41*(Suppl. 2), 43–46.

Kubo, S. H., Cody, R. J., Laragh, J. H., Prida, X. E., Atlas, S. A., Yuan, Z., & Sealey, J. E. (1985). Immediate converting-enzyme inhibition with intravenous enalapril in chronic congestive heart failure. *American Journal of Cardiology, 55,* 122–126.

LaChance, D., Garcia, R., Gutkowska, J., Cantin, M., & Thibault, G. (1986). Mechanisms of release of atrial natriuretic factor. I. Effect of several agonists and steroids on its release by atrial minces. *Biochemical and Biophysical Research Communications, 135,* 1090–1098.

Lang, R. E., Thoelken, H., Ganten, D., Luft, F. C., Ruskoaho, H., & Unger, T. H. (1985). Atrial natriuretic factor is a circulating hormone, stimulated by volume loading. *Nature, 314,* 264–266.

Laragh, J. H. (1985). Atrial natriuretic hormone. *New England Journal of Medicine, 313,* 1330–1340.

Laragh, J. H., & Sealey, J. E. (1973). The renin–angiotensin–aldosterone hormonal system and regulation of sodium, potassium, and blood pressure homeostasis. In J. Orloff & R. W. Berliner (Eds.), *Handbook of physiology: Renal physiology* (pp. 831–908). Baltimore, MD: Waverly Press.

Ledsome, J. R., Wilson, N., Courney, C. A., & Rankin, A. J. (1985). Release of atrial natriuretic peptide by atrial distension. *Canadian Journal of Physiology and Pharmacology, 63,* 739–742.

Luetscher, J. A., Cohn, A. P., Camargo, C. A., Dowdy, A. J., & Callaghan, A. M. (1963). Aldosterone secretion and metabolism in hyperthyroidism and myxedema. *Journal of Clinical Endocrinology, 23,* 873–880.

Maack, T., Camargo, M. J. F., Kleinert, H. D., Laragh, J. H., & Atlas, S. A. (1985). Atrial natriuretic factor: Structure and functional properties. *Kidney International 27,* 607–615.

Manning, P. T., Schwartz, D., Katsube, N. C., Holmberg, S. W., & Needleman, P. (1985). Vasopressin-stimulated release of atriopeptin: Endocrine antagonists in fluid homeostasis. *Science, 229,* 395–397.

Matsuo, H., & Nakazato, H. (1987). Molecular biology of atrial natriuretic peptides. *Endocrinol. Metabol. Clinics of North America, 16,* 43–61.

McKenzie, J. K., & Clements, J. A. (1974). Simplified radioimmunoassay for serum aldosterone utilizing increased antibody specificity. *Journal of Clinical Endocrinology and Metabolism, 38,* 622–627.

Menard, J., Guyenne, T. T., Corvol, P., Pau, B., Simon, D., & Roncucci, R. (1985). Direct immunometric assay of active renin in human plasma. *Journal of Hypertension, 3*(Suppl. 3), S275–S278.

Michener, M. L., Gierse, J. K., Seetharam, R., Fok, K. F., & Needleman, P. (1986). Proteolytic processing of atriopeptin prohormone. *Molecular Pharmacology, 30,* 552–557.

Morganti, A., Sealey, J. E., Lopez-Ovejero, J., Pickering, T. G., & Laragh, J. H. (1979). The substitutive role of ACTH in supporting aldosterone response to headup tilt during acute renin suppression in patients with essential hypertension. *Hypertension, 1,* 130–135.

Morton, J. J., Semple, P. F., Waite, M. A., Brown, J. J., Lever, A. F., & Robertson, J. I. S. (1976). Estimation of angiotensin I and II in the human circulation by radioimmunoassay. In H. Antoniades (Ed.), *Hormones in human blood* (pp. 607–642). Cambridge, MA: Harvard University Press.

Needleman, P., Adams, S. P., Cole, B. R., Currie, M. G., Geller, D. M., Michener, M. L., Saper, C. B., Schwartz, D., & Standaert, D. G. (1985). Atriopeptins as cardiac hormones. *Hypertension, 7,* 469–482.

Ng, K. K. F., & Vane, J. R. (1968). Fate of angiotensin I in the circulation. *Nature, 218,* 144–150.

Nussberger, J., Brunner, D. B., Waeber, B., & Brunner, H. R. (1985). True versus immunoreactive angiotensin II in human plasma. *Hypertension, 70,* I-1–I-7.

Nussberger, J., Brunner, D. B., Waeber, B., & Brunner, H. R. (1988). In vitro renin inhibition to prevent generation of angiotensins during determination of angiotensin I and II. *Life Sciences, 42,* 1683–1688.

Ondetti, M. A., & Cushman, D. W. (1982). Enzymes of the renin–angiotensin system and their inhibitors. *Annual Review of Biochemistry, 51,* 283–308.

Phillips, M. I., & Stenstrom, B. (1985). Angiotensin II in rat brain comigrates with authentic angiotensin II in high pressure liquid chromatography. *Circulation Research, 56,* 212–219.

Preibisz, J. J., Sealey, J. E., Aceto, R. M., & Laragh, J. H. (1982). Plasma renin activity measurements: An update. *Cardiovascular Reviews and Reports, 3,* 787–804.

Quirion, R., Dalpe, M., deLean, A., Gutkowska, J., Cantin, M., & Genest, J. (1984). Atrial natriuretic factor (ANF) binding sites in brain and related structures. *Peptides, 5,* 1167–1172.

Raine, A. E., Erne, P., Murgisser, E., Mueller, F. B., Bolli, P., Burkart, F., & Buhler, F. R. (1986). Atrial natriuretic peptide and atrial pressure in patients with congestive heart failure. *New England Journal of Medicine, 315,* 533–537.

Rascher, W., Tulassay, T., & Lang, R. E. (1985). Atrial natriuretic peptide in plasma of volume overloaded children with chronic renal failure. *Lancet, 2,* 303–305.

Re, R. N. (1984). Cellular biology of the renin–angiotensin systems. *Archives of Internal Medicine, 144,* 2037.

Sagnella, G. A., Markandu, N. D., Shore, A. C., & MacGregor, G. A. (1985). Effects of changes in dietary sodium intake and saline infusion on immunoreactive atrial natriuretic peptide in human plasma. *Lancet, 2,* 1208–1210.

Sala, C., Camargo, M. J. F., Laragh, J. H., Aceto, R. M., Cody, R. J., & Atlas, S. A. (1987). Circulating peptides derived from the human atrial natriuretic factor (ANF) precursor. *Clinical Research, 35,* 605a (Abstract).

Sala, C., Pecker, M., Laragh, J. H., Mueller, F. B., Epstein, M., Cody, R., & Atlas, S. A. (1987). Relationship of endogenous or exogenous ANF to plasma cGMP levels in humans. 2nd World Congress on Biologically Active Peptides, p. 192 (Abstract).

Schiffrin, E. L., & Genest, J. (1983). Tonin–angiotensin II system. In J. Genest, O. Kuchel, P. Hamet, & M. Cantin (Eds.), *Hypertension* (2nd ed., pp. 309–320). New York: McGraw–Hill.

Schwartz, D., Geller, D. M., Manning, P. T., Siegel, N. R.,

Fok, K. F., Smith, C. E., & Needleman, P. (1985). Ser-Leu-Arg-Arg-atriopeptin III: The major circulating form of atrial peptide. *Science, 229,* 397–400.

Sealey, J. E. (1981). Measurement of the hormones of the renin system in hypertensive patients. *Clinical Biochemistry, 14,* 273–281.

Sealey, J. E., Atlas, S. A., & Laragh, J. H. (1980). Prorenin and other large molecular weight forms of renin. *Endocrine Reviews, 1,* 365–391.

Sealey, J. E., Bühler, F. R., Laragh, J. H., Manning, E. L. & Brunner, H. R. (1972). Aldosterone excretion: Physiologic variations in man measured by radioimmunoassay or double isotope dilution. *Circulation Research, 31,* 367–378.

Sealey, J. E., Gerten-Banes, J., & Laragh, J. H. (1972). The renin system: Variations in man measured by radioimmunoassay or bioassay. *Kidney International, 1,* 240–253.

Sealey, J. E., Moon, C., Laragh, J. H., & Alderman, M. (1976). Plasma prorenin: Cryoactivation and relationship to renin substrate in normal subjects. *American Journal of Medicine, 61,* 731–738.

Sealey, J. E., Moon, C., Laragh, J. H., & Atlas, S. A. (1977). Plasma prorenin in normal, hypertensive and anephric subjects and its effect on renin measurements. *Circulation Research, 40*(Suppl. 1), 41–45.

Sealey, J. E., White, R. P., Laragh, J. H., & Rubin, A. L. (1977). Plasma prorenin and renin in anephric patients. *Circulation Research, 41*(Suppl. 2), 17–21.

Shenker, Y., Sider, R. S., Ostafin, E. A., & Grekin, R. J. (1985). Plasma levels of immunoreactive atrial natriuretic factor in healthy subjects and in patients with edema. *Journal of Clinical Investigation, 76,* 1684–1698.

Shiono, S., Nakao, K., Morii, N., Yamada, T., Itoh, H., Sakamoto, M., Sugawara, A., Saito, Y., Katsuura, G., & Imura, H. (1986). Nature of atrial natriuretic polypeptide in rat brain. *Biochemical and Biophysical Research Communications, 135,* 728–734.

Skeggs, L. T., Dorer, F. E., Kahn, J. R., Lentz, K. E., & Levine, M. (1981). Experimental renal hypertension: The discovery of the renin–angiotensin system. In R. L. Soffer (Ed.), *Biochemical regulation of blood pressure* (pp. 3–38). New York: Wiley.

Skinner, S. L. (1967). Improved assay methods for renin concentration and activity in human plasma. Methods using selective denaturation of renin substrate. *Circulation Research, 20,* 391–402.

Skofitsch, G., Jacobowitz, D. M., Eskay, R. L., & Zamir, N. (1985). Distribution of atrial natriuretic factor-like immunoreactive neurons in brain. *Neuroscience, 16,* 917–948.

Soffer, R. L. (1981). Angiotensin-converting enzyme. In R. L. Soffer (Ed.), *Biochemical regulation of blood pressure* (pp. 123–164). New York: Wiley.

Sonnenberg, H., & Veress, A. T. (1984). Cellular mechanism of release of atrial natriuretic factor. *Biochemical and Biophysical Research Communications, 124,* 443–449.

Stockigt, J. R., Collins, R. D., & Biglieri, E. G. (1971). Determination of plasma renin concentration by angiotensin I immunoassay. *Circulation Research, 28/29*(Suppl. II), 175–189.

Tait, J. F., Tait, S. A. S., Little, B., & Laumas, K. R. (1961). The disappearance of 7-H^3-d-aldosterone in the plasma of normal subjects. *Journal of Clinical Investigation 40,* 72–80.

Thibault, G., Lazure, C., Schiffrin, E. L., Jutkowska, J., Chartier, L., Garcia, R., Seidah, N. G., Chretien, M., Genest, J., & Cantin, M. (1985). Identification of a biologically active circulating form of rat atrial natriuretic factor. *Biochemical and Biophysical Research Communications, 130,* 981–986.

Tigerstedt, R., & Bergman, P. G. (1898). Niere and Kreislauf. *Skandinavisches Archiv fuer Physiologie, 8,* 223–271.

Ulick, S., Laragh, J. H., & Lieberman, S. (1958). The isolation of a urinary metabolite of aldosterone in urine. *Transactions of the Association of American Physicians, 71,* 225–235.

Veress, A. T., & Sonnenberg, H. (1984). Right atrial appendectomy reduces the renal response to acute hypervolemia in the rat. *American Journal of Physiology 247 (R16),* R610–R613.

Waldman, S., Rapoport, R. M., & Murad, F. (1984). Atrial natriuretic factor selectively activates particulate guanylate cyclase and elevates cyclic GMP in rat tissues. *Journal of Biological Chemistry, 259,* 14332–14334.

Williams, G. H., Cain, J. P., Dluhy, R. G., & Underwood, R. H. (1972). Studies in the control of plasma aldosterone concentration in normal man. I. Response to posture, acute and chronic volume depletion, and sodium loading. *Journal of Clinical Investigation, 51,* 1731–1742.

Yamaji, T., Ishibashi, M., Nakaoka, H., Imataka, K., Amano, M., & Fujii, J. (1985). Possible role for atrial natriuretic peptide in polyuria associated with paroxysmal atrial arrhythmias. *Lancet, 1,* 1211.

Yamaji, T., Ishibashi, M., & Takaku, F. (1985). Atrial natriuretic factor in human blood. *Journal of Clinical Investigation, 76,* 1705–1709.

Yamaji, T., Ishibashi, M., Sekihara, H., Takaku, F., Nakaoka, H., & Fujii, J. (1986). Plasma levels of atrial natriuretic peptide in primary aldosteronism and essential hypertension. *Journal of Clinical Endocrinology and Metabolism, 63,* 815–818.

Yandle, T. G., Richards, A. M., Nicholls, M. G., Cuneo, R., Espiner, E. A., & Livesey, J. H. (1986). Metabolic clearance rate and plasma half life of alpha-human atrial natriuretic peptide in man. *Life Sciences, 38,* 1827–1833.

Ambulatory Monitoring

Section Editor: Thomas G. Pickering

Recent technological developments in ambulatory monitoring have made possible cardiovascular measurements in field studies, and correlation of these measures with behavioral factors. In this section some of the more important aspects of this field are reviewed. In Chapter 16 Pickering reviews the technical aspects of ambulatory monitoring, and emphasizes that a number of physiological variables can be monitored, not only the electrocardiogram (ECG) and blood pressure. Some of the factors which may influence cardiovascular variables, such as changes in physical and mental activity and in the external environment, are briefly discussed, as are the relative roles of intrinsic sources of variation such as circadian and ultradian rhythms. If the information obtained from such ambulatory recordings made in uncontrolled settings is to be generalizable, it is important to know how reproducible they are. The rationale for such studies lies in the fact that they can give a reliable measure both of the average level of the variables being measured and of their variability over prolonged periods of time. The need to be able to relate laboratory and field studies is also reviewed.

In Chapter 17 Kligfield reviews the applications of ambulatory ECG monitoring. This was first in-

troduced nearly 25 years ago, and although it has become standard practice for the clinical evaluation of arrhythmias, it has been surprisingly little used in behavioral studies. He describes the technical aspects of available recorders, such as whether all or only selected portions of the monitored data are stored, and he also gives a useful survey of rhythm abnormalities to be expected in clinically healthy subjects of different ages. The occurrence, classification, and prognosis associated with ventricular premature contractions are also reviewed. In addition, there are sections on the relationship between symptoms and arrhythmias and on "silent" myocardial ischemia.

Harshfield, Hwang, Blank, and Pickering review the technical aspects of noninvasive ambulatory blood pressure recording in Chapter 18. This includes a description of the available instrumentation, and calibration and validation procedures. The available technology leaves a lot to be desired, and none of the recorders will give accurate readings in every subject. Characteristics of subjects in whom the procedures are likely to be unsuccessful are reviewed, and emphasis is placed on proper training of both subjects and the technicians who make the recordings.

Techniques are also available for sampling blood and urine in ambulatory subjects, as discussed by Dimsdale in Chapter 19. Timed urine samples can be used, provided that the sampling interval is relatively long, i.e., several hours. Although a choice of techniques for taking blood

Thomas G. Pickering • Department of Medicine, Cardiovascular Center, The New York Hospital–Cornell Medical Center, New York, New York 10021.

samples is available, the most widely used is the Cormed pump which can take venous blood samples automatically, but which in its present form cannot take multiple samples.

The correlation of behavior and cardiovascular variables during ambulatory monitoring requires that the subjects keep diaries of their activities, and this subject is reviewed by Chesney and Ironson in Chapter 20. This is in effect a form of self-monitoring, the consequences of which have been extensively studied in the past, but as yet not applied to the design of diaries. Thus, although subjects are often asked to take part in normal daily activities while wearing a monitor and keeping a diary, the measurement procedures and the way in which they are presented to the subjects may themselves influence the subjects' behavior. Diary content should ideally include factors such as the subjects' environment, behavior, and mood, but the diary should not be too complex, and neutral points in response scales should be avoided.

Finally, in Chapter 21 Clark, Denby, and Pregibon discuss some general problems of data analysis of ambulatory recordings. Sources of variability include individual differences in pressure (or other variables being analyzed), diurnal variations, differences due to physical and mental activity, and artifactual readings. The basic technique recommended is modeling, where the observed data are regarded as the sum of the variables predicted by the model plus the residuals. Graphical display of the data is emphasized, which is advantageous both for fitting the model and for identifying outliers. In general, a series of linear models is tested, ranging from overly simple to more complex ones. Examination of the residuals provides information as to the extent of the model's inaccuracy.

CHAPTER 16

Ambulatory Monitoring
Applications and Limitations

Thomas G. Pickering

The study of behavior has traditionally focused on two areas: (1) laboratory-based studies where the experimental situation can be rigidly controlled, and (2) field-based studies typified by ethologists' observations of naturally occurring behavioral patterns. For the study of the role of behavior in causing or modifying human cardiovascular disease, both approaches are desirable. The former approach enables studies to be carried out under highly standardized conditions, but may be of questionable relevance to what goes on in real life. The latter approach has in the past suffered from limitations imposed by the difficulty of monitoring cardiovascular variables in free-ranging subjects. The development of ambulatory monitoring techniques has added a new dimension to these investigations, and enables a precise comparison between behavior and physiological variables in subjects who are engaged in their normal daily activities.

The new dimension is time. There is a dynamic component to cardiovascular disease, which cannot be adequately explored by measurements made on a single occasion. Thus, whereas coronary artery disease can be regarded as a relatively fixed level of obstruction in the coronary arteries which takes years to develop, sudden cardiac death, which is one of the commonest endpoints, may occur in a matter of seconds, and the events that lead up to it may be very different from those that cause deposition of the atheromatous plaque. Similarly, whereas the type A behavior pattern is often considered to be stable over time, with identifiable antecedents apparent in early childhood, its physiological components can only be demonstrated by measuring changes occurring during periods of behavioral challenge (Matthews & Haynes, 1986).

There are two ways in which measurements made over prolonged periods of time by ambulatory monitoring may enhance the evaluation of cardiovascular disease. First, conventional measurements made at a single moment may give a misleading impression of the variable in question. Thus, in the case of blood pressure the clinic measurement process may itself change the pressure, leading to the phenomenon of "white coat" hypertension, i.e., hypertension that is only seen in the clinic environment. Second, ambulatory monitoring provides the opportunity to observe changes occurring in natural situations which may be difficult to reproduce in the clinic or laboratory. For many people, their work may be a major source of stress in their lives, and there is a growing body of evidence to indicate that occupational stress may be a risk factor for cardiovascular disease (Alfredson, Karasek, & Theorell, 1982). Both blood pres-

Thomas G. Pickering • Department of Medicine, Cardiovascular Center, The New York Hospital–Cornell Medical Center, New York, New York 10021.

sure (Harshfield, Pickering, Kleinert, Blank, & Laragh, 1982) and the frequency of ventricular premature contractions (Orth-Gomer, Hogstedt, Bodin, and Söderholm, 1986; Pickering, Johnston, & Honour, 1978) tend to be highest during the working hours. The mechanisms underlying such phenomena can only be adequately assessed by field studies.

Techniques of Ambulatory Monitoring

Although blood pressure is the variable that has attracted most attention among psychologists, it is only one of a number of variables that could be monitored, and in the next few years we are likely to see the introduction of multichannel recorders which can monitor several channels at the same time. In general, ambulatory monitoring can be divided into two types—"dry" and "wet." The former includes recording of any physiological variable that can be detected noninvasively as an electrical signal. Examples include blood pressure, heart rate, electrocardiogram (ECG), respiration, body movement, and electroencephalogram (EEG). Figure 1 shows a four-channel ambulatory

recording of ECG, EEG, and eye movements from an ambulatory study investigating changes of arrhythmias during sleep (Pickering *et al.*, 1978). Although ECG monitoring was the first type to be introduced, and is a standard cardiological diagnostic procedure, it has found surprisingly few applications in behavioral studies. In part, this may be because the emphasis has been on the detection of transient arrhythmias, rather than the quantitative analysis of heart rate changes, but a number of recent developments, such as spectral analysis of heart rate to identify sympathetic and parasympathetic components, and the recognition of silent ischemia in patients with coronary heart disease, suggest that this situation may change in the future. The techniques of blood pressure monitoring are reviewed by Pickering and Blank (this volume).

"Wet" monitoring includes invasive sampling of venous blood for measurement of biochemical or hormonal changes (see Dimsdale, this volume). This technique is still in its infancy, and at present can only be used for relatively short periods of an hour or so. Blood is continually withdrawn from a venous catheter; because currently available models have a single storage tube, it is only possible to obtain values that are integrated over a defined

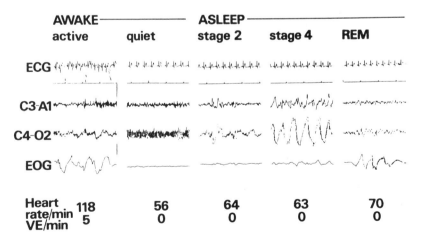

Figure 1. Ambulatory recordings of ECG, EEG, and eye movements (EOG) at different levels of arousal. The four channels are, from above: ECG, EEG (leads C3-A1 and C4-O2), and EOG. During activity, ventricular extrasystoles (VE) are present on the ECG channel, and movement and elec-

tromyographic activity are present on EEG channels. During quiet wakefulness, alpha rhythm is evident on EEG (C4-O2). During REM (rapid eye movement) sleep, note bursts of eye movement and "sawtooth" waves on upper channel of EEG. From Pickering *et al.* (1978).

period of time, as opposed to a series of discrete measurements.

At present, the most widely used technique is with recorders that store the data that have been monitored, either on tape or in solid-state memory. For blood pressure, most recorders store the processed data (e.g., systolic, mean, and diastolic pressures) rather than the raw data (e.g., Korotkoff sounds or oscillometric pulsations). Although this enables more readings to be stored, it limits the amount of editing that can be done to detect artifacts. An alternative method of ambulatory monitoring uses radiotelemetry, which has the advantages of being able to observe the data as they are monitored (as done in ECG telemetry units in most hospitals), and also of not requiring bulky data storage systems to be carried by the subjects. Its main disadvantage is the limitation imposed by the distance over which the signals can be transmitted. A spectacular example of this technique was provided by the work of Van Citters and Franklin (1969), who implanted flowmeters and arterial pressure monitors in Alaskan sled dogs, and studied changes of heart rate and blood pressure while they were pulling sleds across the snow. Systolic blood pressure increased from 130 mm Hg at rest, to 300 mm Hg during exercise.

The Possible Importance of the Variability of Blood Pressure and Heart Rate versus the Average Level

In the cases of both ECG and blood pressure monitoring, the rationale usually given for their clinical relevance is that they provide a more valid estimate of the average level of arrhythmias in the former case, and of blood pressure in the latter, than measurements made at a single point in time. Thus, there is extensive evidence to indicate that the average frequency of ventricular premature contractions (VPCs) in patients who have already survived a myocardial infarction may be an important predictor of future risk (Ruberman, Weinblatt, Goldberg, Frank, & Shapiro, 1977; Mukharji et al., 1984). Because the occurrence of VPCs is spo-

radic, their frequency can only be accurately assessed by prolonged monitoring.

With blood pressure it is not yet conclusively established that prolonged monitoring provides a better measure of risk than isolated readings taken in the clinic, but there are several lines of circumstantial evidence suggesting that this may prove to be the case. First, clinic measurements provide a rather imprecise estimate of the average 24-h level of pressure (Pickering, Harshfield, Devereux, & Laragh, 1985); second, several studies have shown that target organ damage is more closely related to ambulatory than to clinic pressures (reviewed by Pickering & Devereux, 1987), and two prospective studies have found that ambulatory pressures may be better predictors of morbid events than are clinic pressures (Perloff, Sokolow, & Cowan, 1983; Mann, Millar-Craig, & Raftery, 1985).

Although the role of the average level of blood pressure in the hypertensive disease process is easy to accept, ambulatory monitoring also offers the possibility of studying the relevance of the variability of pressure. It is theoretically possible that at least three components of blood pressure could contribute to vascular damage: first, the average, or integrated, level of pressure; second, the peaks of pressure might also contribute; and third, the shape of the individual pressure waveform could be a factor, since the rate of rise of pressure is a determinant of the physical stress placed on the arterial wall (Palmer, 1981; O'Rourke, 1985). So far, there is little direct evidence to implicate blood pressure variability. Animal studies have been few, although a number have shown that blood pressure variability can be increased by baroreceptor denervation without much effect on the average level of pressure (Cowley, Liard, & Guyton, 1973), but there has been little investigation into the effects of this on vascular damage.

It is commonly assumed that transient changes of blood pressure are mediated mainly via the sympathetic nervous system. Studies of spontaneous blood pressure variability, however, using intermittent noninvasive measurements, have shown that sympathetic blockade (with either α or β blockers) does not reduce such variability, whereas parasympathetic blockade does (Clement, De Pue, Jordaens, & Padret, 1985). Such variability is largely due to the effects of respiration on blood pressure.

For heart rate, there is some recent evidence that variability may be an independent predictor of sudden death in susceptible patients (Klieger, Miller, Bigger, Moss, and the Multicenter Post-infarction Group, 1987; Magid *et al.*, submitted). This has been attributed to defective parasympathetic control of the heart.

Whatever the relative importance of the average level versus the variability of these factors in determining cardiovascular damage, ambulatory monitoring has the potential of giving a better measure of them than measurements made over shorter periods of time.

Factors Influencing Cardiovascular Variables during Everyday Life

A large number of activities have been identified which are likely to exert a significant influence on cardiovascular variables that are studied by ambulatory monitoring. Most of the published studies have dealt with blood pressure, but their findings are in many cases likely to apply to heart rate as well.

If the effects of environmental stimuli and changes in physical activity are minimized, the profile of blood pressure during the day becomes relatively flat, with a fall of about 20% occurring during sleep (Athassaniadis, Drayer, Honour, & Cranston, 1969). In selected groups of patients, blood pressure may actually increase during sleep. These include patients with idiopathic orthostatic hypotension (Mann, Altman, Raftery, & Bannister, 1983), preeclampsia (Redman, Beilin, & Bonnar, 1976), and cardiac transplants (Reeves, Shapiro, Thompson, & Johnson, 1986). It has also been shown that diurnal blood pressure changes are less pronounced in hospitalized patients than in patients studied in their natural environment (Young, Rowlands, Stallard, Watson, & Littler, 1983). Both the average level of blood pressure and its variability are reduced during periods of bed rest as compared to periods of physical activity (Watson, Stallard, & Littler, 1979). Some of the

more relevant activities influencing the changes of blood pressure and other variables that might be detected by ambulatory monitoring are briefly reviewed below; they are divided into physical and mental activities, although obviously there is considerable overlap.

Physical Activity

Blood pressure, heart rate, and plasma norepinephrine are usually at their maximum during intense physical exercise, and at their lowest level during sleep (Watson, Hamilton, Reid, & Littler, 1979). The position of the subject is also important. Large increases of pressure and heart rate are also seen during another form of exercise, sexual intercourse (Littler, Honour, & Sleight, 1974b). Transient changes occur during micturition and defecation (Littler, Honour, & Sleight, 1974a). Laboratory studies by Lynch's group have shown that talking is also a potent pressor stimulus; the cardiovascular changes depend both on physical factors such as the rate of talking (Friedman, Thomas, Kulick-Ciuffo, Lynch, & Suginahara, 1982), and on psychological factors such as the size of the audience (Thomas *et al.*, 1984).

Ingestion

Most of the studies investigating the effects of ingested substances have been carried out in the laboratory, but their results may in most cases be extrapolated to the field. For 3 h after a meal, there is an increase of heart rate, a decrease of diastolic pressure, and little change of systolic pressure (Lipsitz, Nyquist, Wei, & Rowe, 1983). Smoking a cigarette raises both heart rate and blood pressure for about 15 min (Cellina, Honour, & Littler, 1975). Alcohol may increase heart rate, with small but variable effects on blood pressure in normal subjects (Orlando, Aronow, Cassidy, & Prakash, 1976; Gould, Zahir, DeMartino, & Gomprecht, 1971). Caffeine can increase blood pressure, plasma catecholamines, and renin, but not heart rate (Robertson *et al.*, 1978), although these changes are diminished in people who use caffeine regularly (Izzo, Ghosal, Kwong, Freeman, & Jaenike, 1983). It is likely that other factors such as dietary sodium intake may influence blood pressure variations during ambulatory monitoring (Ambrosioni, Costa, & Borghi, 1982), although little direct information is available concerning this.

Mental Activity

At least two studies have reported some correlation between self-rated mental "stress" or "arousal" and blood pressure during noninvasive ambulatory monitoring (Dembroski & Mac-Dougall, 1984; Schmieder et al., 1985). We have found levels of blood pressure to be higher when people are at work than when they are at home (as shown in Figure 2), which we attributed to mental rather than physical factors, because most of our subjects had sedentary jobs (Harshfield et al., 1982; Pickering, Harshfield, Kleinert, Blank, & Laragh, 1982).

A study using ambulatory heart rate monitoring of surgeons showed that the average rate while operating was 121/min, and in some cases went as high as 150/min (Foster, Evans, & Hardcastle, 1978); an example is shown in Figure 3. Such rates might be maintained for periods of half an hour or longer; the same level of heart rate during physical activity (bicycling) could only be maintained for

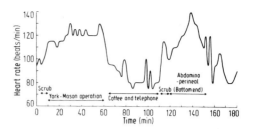

Figure 3. Heart rate measured by ambulatory ECG monitoring in a surgeon while performing two operations, with a period of relaxation in between. From Foster *et al.* (1978).

less than 10 min. The tachycardia was abolished by β-adrenergic blockade. Marked heart rate increases have also been reported while driving a car in city traffic (Taggart, Gibbons, & Somerville, 1969).

Mood has also been reported to be a potent determinant of blood pressure during ambulatory monitoring. We have found that self-reported levels of anger, anxiety, and happiness are correlated with pressure: systolic pressure decreased as the intensity of happiness increased, and diastolic pressure increased with the intensity of anxiety (James, Yee, Harshfield, Blank, & Pickering, 1986). A number of other factors may be expected to influence blood pressure changes during ambulatory monitoring, although they have not yet been studied in this context. They include both genetic (family history of hypertension) and environmental factors (e.g., seasonal variations, noise, and crowding).

Circadian and Ultradian Rhythms

Many of the physiological and biochemical variables that can be evaluated by ambulatory monitoring are normally subject to characteristic patterns of diurnal variation. Thus, heart rate and blood pressure tend to be lowest during the night; plasma catecholamines also decrease, whereas cortisol and renin both peak during the night (reviewed by Pickering, 1980). An important question is whether these rhythms are determined by changes in physical activity and the sleep–wakefulness cycle, or by an underlying circadian rhythm. The

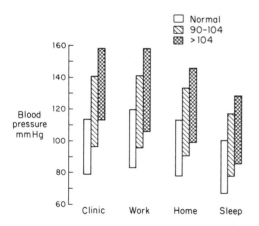

Figure 2. Average blood pressures in four different situations (clinic, work, home, and sleep) measured by ambulatory monitoring in three groups of subjects: normal pressure, diastolic pressure between 90 and 104 mm Hg, and diastolic greater than 104. Upper limit of each bar indicates systolic pressure, lower limit diastolic.

changes of blood pressure seem to be largely of the former type: when subjects remain awake all night, there is little or no fall of blood pressure (Stumpe et al., 1976). In subjects who sleep, there is an immediate increase of blood pressure on awakening, although some workers have claimed that there is a gradual increase in the early hours of the morning while the subject is still asleep (Millar-Craig, Bishop, & Raftery, 1978). This may, however, be a reflection of the fact that blood pressure is lowest during stages 3 and 4 of sleep, which occur mostly during the early hours of the night (Bristow, Honour, Pickering, & Sleight, 1969). Thus, there is no very convincing evidence for a true circadian rhythm of blood pressure.

There is a marked diurnal variation in the occurrence of transient myocardial ischemia (ST segment depression) during ECG monitoring in patients with coronary artery disease (Campbell et al., 1986), the majority of the episodes occurring between 6 a.m. and noon. A number of studies have also shown that attacks of variant (spontaneous) angina show a diurnal pattern, occurring most commonly in the early morning hours (Waters, Miller, Bouchard, Bosch, & Theroux, 1984). Sudden cardiac death is also commonest between 7 and 9 a.m. (Willich et al., 1986).

Body temperature, and to a much lesser extent heart rate, does show a true circadian rhythmicity (Mills, 1966). Thus, if the sleep–wakefulness cycle is suddenly reversed, the rhythm of body temperature may be out of phase with the activity cycle for several days, whereas heart adjusts very rapidly. As Kleitman (1963) wrote, "although under the normal routine of living there is a complete parallelism between the body temperature and heart-rate 24 hour curves, the former is a true rhythm, resisting a change once established, whereas the latter is a periodicity coupled with the schedule of meals, activity, and sleep." Plasma cortisol and urinary electrolyte excretion are also subject to circadian rhythms.

Circadian rhythms normally have a periodicity of approximately 24 h, but there may also exist ultradian rhythms, which have a periodicity of approximately 90 min. These were first described for rapid eye movement (REM) sleep (Aserinsky & Kleitman, 1953), but may also be apparent during

the day. Thus, a study using continuous monitoring of heart rate, blood pressure, and cardiac output in conscious dogs showed a 90-min periodicity for all three (Shimada & Marsh, 1979). It was concluded that the rhythm was due to phasic variations in the level of sympathetic drive to the heart, because this periodicity of both pressure and heart rate can be suppressed by clonidine (Livnat, Zehr, & Broten, 1984). The amplitude of this ultradian rhythm of blood pressure may actually exceed the amplitude of the circadian rhythm in dogs.

It is not known to what extent ultradian rhythms of heart rate and blood pressure exist in humans. It seems reasonable to suppose that they do, but they might not be readily detectable in studies of free-ranging individuals, because they would be obscured by extraneous stimuli.

Can the Effects of Factors Influencing Diurnal Variations of Cardiovascular Variables Be Quantified?

In the past, analyses of ambulatory recordings of heart rate and blood pressure have typically expressed the data in terms of the mean level plus an overall measure of variability. Although this approach provides much useful information, students of behavior want to quantify the effects of specific activities or moods on such variables. In the case of blood pressure, we were interested to see how much of the overall variance could be accounted for by changes of activity (Clark et al., 1987). We found that accounting for the average effect of 15 commonly occurring activities (including sleep) on blood pressure (using the patient's clinic pressure as a covariate) accounted for 41% of systolic and 36% of diastolic variance. Time of day was a less important determinant of blood pressure. This type of modeling approach is reviewed by Clark, Denby, and Pregibon (Chapter 21, this volume).

Although these modeling techniques can account for a sizable portion of the overall variation of blood pressure or other variables, obviously only a first approximation is obtained. Thus, the idea that the effects of each activity can be represented by a single coefficient is clearly an oversimplification, because the intensity of any activity may vary, and individual subjects will have different pressure responses to the same activity, e.g., from differences in baroreflex sensitivity (Conway, Boon, Davies, Vann Jones, & Sleight, 1984). Furthermore, it is not clear to what extent the effects of one activity "carry over" to another. Thus, we are currently exploring the hypothesis that blood pressures measured at home in the evening are higher if the subject has been to work earlier in the day, as compared to being at home all day.

What Is the Reproducibility of Data Obtained from Ambulatory Monitoring?

Since the activities of an individual undergoing ambulatory monitoring are usually relatively uncontrolled, it might be anticipated that the reproducibility of such data might be lower than for corresponding data collected in the laboratory. However, several studies have shown that the reproducibility of ambulatory blood pressure is quite high (Mann, Millar-Craig, Balasubramanian, Cashman, & Raftery, 1980; Jacob des Combes, Porchet, Waeber, & Brunner, 1984; Weber, Drayer, Wyle, & DeYoung, 1982); in our own study we found correlation coefficients of 0.93 and 0.87 for systolic and diastolic ambulatory pressures measured on two occasions separated by 2 weeks, 0.96 and 0.93 for home pressures, and 0.97 and 0.85 for clinic pressures (James, Pickering, Yee, Harshfield, & Laragh, 1988).

Several studies have shown that the reproducibility of VPCs is relatively low (Winkel, 1978; Calvert, Lown, & Gorlin, 1979), so that multiple recordings are needed to obtain valid data.

In contrast to the good reproducibility of the average level of blood pressure, the reproducibility of blood pressure variability as measured by indirect recorders is low (Weber *et al.*, 1982; James *et al.*, 1988). This implies that blood pressure variability measured in this way is not a reliable variable to be correlated with others such as cardiovascular reactivity.

Some Problems Imposed by Intermittent versus Continuous Readings

Ideally, one would like to have continuous recordings for all the variables being measured. At present, this can be achieved for all the physiological variables that can be monitored except blood pressure, unless it is monitored invasively. For noninvasive blood pressure monitoring, which is the only form likely to find wide application, it is practical to obtain readings no more than about once every 10 min. It is therefore important to know the extent to which such intermittent sampling affects the interpretation of the true changes that are taking place. At least two studies (DiRienzo, Grassi, Pedotti, & Mancia, 1983; Llabre, Ironson, Spitzer, & Schneiderman, 1988), have shown that sampling every 30 min can give an accurate estimate of the mean level of pressure over 24 h. In contrast, blood pressure monitoring for periods of a few hours a day cannot provide a reliable estimate of the 24-h average (DiRienzo *et al.*, 1985). What such sampling cannot do, however, is estimate the true variability of blood pressure. Such variability includes oscillations of relatively high frequency (e.g., respiratory variations of blood pressure), of intermediate frequencies (ultradian rhythms, if they exist in humans), plus less predictable oscillations imposed by mood and activity. When the sampling frequency is less than the respiratory frequency, this oscillation of pressure will appear as random variability.

Comparison of Cardiovascular Responses to Reactivity Testing in the Laboratory and in Everyday Life

Laboratory tests of the cardiovascular response to physical or mental stress have been used for many years for the diagnosis of cardiovascular disease. The best known example of this is the exercise stress test used to diagnose coronary artery disease. The rationale is that abnormalities that are not present in the resting condition may be exposed during periods of stress. Interpretation of the results is in this case relatively simple, because it has been proven that ST segment changes in the ECG provoked by stress usually imply coronary artery disease.

Ambulatory ECG monitoring in such patients may reveal episodes of ST depression (silent ischemia) which are important predictors of clinical outcome (Gottlieb, Weisfeldt, Ougang, Mellitus, & Gerstenblith, 1986). There is generally a good correlation between the detection of ischemic ST changes by treadmill exercise testing and by ambulatory monitoring (Wolf, Tzivoni, & Stern, 1974). It is of interest that ST changes detected in everyday life typically occur at a lower heart rate than when provoked by exercise testing, suggesting that such episodes could be due in part to coronary artery spasm as opposed to increased myocardial oxygen demand (Schang & Pepine, 1977), which is the predominant mechanism of ischemia during exercise testing. Thus, in this particular instance, a combination of field and laboratory studies suggests that different mechanisms may be involved in different circumstances.

A similar analogy is often used to justify the use of laboratory psychological "stress tests" in hypertension. The analogy with exercise stress testing does not hold, however, because it is not at all clear what, if anything, an "abnormal" test means in this context. There are two possible ways in which such testing could be of value in evaluating patients with hypertension. First, it has been proposed that hyperreactivity of blood pressure to a laboratory stress test implies hyperreactivity in everyday life. Second, it could be that hyperreactivity is a predictor of future hypertension or cardiovascular morbid events. This idea was first proposed by Hines and Brown (1933) but is still unproven.

While the relevance of reactivity testing in hypertension remains unclear, the role of ambulatory monitoring is conceptually easier to accept, although conclusive evidence of its clinical role in evaluating patients remains lacking. It does, however, provide the possibility of testing the hypothesis that hyperreactivity diagnosed by laboratory testing can be observed in everyday life. So far there are little published data on this point, although in our own study we did not find good correlations between reactivity measured by three commonly used laboratory tests (mental arithmetic, playing a video game, and a standard treadmill exercise test) and ambulatory blood pressure (Harshfield *et al.*, 1988). One of the problems in attempting such correlations is the quantification of reactivity in everyday life. If the level of generalizability were very high, one might expect a close correlation between reactivity to laboratory tests and the overall level of blood pressure variability measured over 24 h. Such a finding might, paradoxically, be of relatively little interest to behaviorists, because the mechanism responsible for it would most likely not be psychological. Since blood pressure responses in everyday life are determined at least as much by physical as by mental activity, an increased level of 24-h blood pressure variability is likely to reflect a nonspecific increase of response to any stimulus, without any particularly behavioral connotations. Two mechanisms by which increases of both reactivity and 24-h variability might occur are a diminished sensitivity of the baroreflexes, and an exaggerated vasoconstrictor response to adrenergic stimulation.

Another, more practical problem with trying to relate reactivity to overall blood pressure variability is that, as we have seen above, it may not be possible to obtain a reliable measure of variability from intermittent recordings.

There are other problems as well. One is that the activities of individuals are likely to vary during the period of ambulatory recordings, so that differences in blood pressure or heart rate variability may be due to differences in activity rather than reactivity. Finally, there is the problem of defining a baseline level for measuring reactivity. There is considerable dispute as to how this should be measured even for the laboratory tests, and the problems with ambulatory recordings are correspondingly greater. One solution is to use the pressures measured during a period of at-home relaxation, and to relate the pressures during other activities to them. In this way one can draw up a table of the effects of commonly occurring activities on blood pressure as shown in Table 1.

If a more restricted view is taken of the generalizability of laboratory reactivity testing to blood pressure variability in everyday life, it should be possible to relate changes occurring during specific laboratory tests to changes during specific everyday activities of a similar nature. An example where this was done is a recently published study by Matthews, Manuck, and Saab (1986), who found a correlation between the blood pressure response to mental arithmetic where the answers were verbalized, and making a public speech. No correlations were seen with two other laboratory tests of reactivity. These results suggest that while some generalization of laboratory tests to everyday life may occur, it is relatively limited.

An alternative approach to relating laboratory and field studies, which has so far received little attention, is to make observations in the field and attempt to replicate them in the more controlled laboratory setting so that the factors contributing to the observed changes can be evaluated. One such example is the study of surgeons' heart rates while operating, described above (Foster *et al.*, 1978). There is no way in which this response could have been predicted from laboratory reactivity testing.

Once the tachycardia in the operating room was observed, however, it was appropriate to determine whether it could be explained on the basis of physical activity. The fact that it was possible to exercise only for a relatively short period of time at that heart rate demonstrates that some other explanation must be sought, presumably psychological rather than physical.

A potential example to be studied by this approach would be the differences between blood pressure measured at home and at work. For people who have jobs which involve standing much of the time, but who may be seated much of the time while at home, it would be possible to determine whether the higher pressures at work are due to psychological or physical factors by designing laboratory tests that replicate the differences in physical activity between the two situations, while maintaining the psychological factors constant.

Future Applications

The technology of ambulatory monitoring is evolving at a rapid pace. The first-generation blood pressure monitors were bulky, inconvenient, and technically not very reliable. They also may make embarrassing sounds during cuff inflation, so that they may actually elevate blood pressure in some subjects. The second-generation recorders are smaller and quieter, and are much more acceptable to the subjects wearing them. What is needed ultimately, however, is a noninvasive beat-to-beat blood pressure monitor, which would not require a cuff (and bulky battery-operated pump to inflate it), and which would also be able to obtain an accurate measure of blood pressure variability.

Another technological advance will be the ability to record several channels of data simultaneously. This is already possible with some recorders, but not with the commonly used blood pressure devices. One of the problems besetting investigators of the behavioral aspects of cardiovascular functions is the extent to which observed changes are due to physical as opposed to mental activity. The ability to monitor physical activity (e.g., by accelerometers) simultaneously

Table 1. Average Changes of Blood Pressure (mm Hg) Associated with 15 Commonly Occurring Activities[a]

Meetings	+20.2	+15.0
Work	+16.0	+13.0
Transportation	+14.0	+ 9.2
Walking	+12.0	+ 5.5
Dressing	+11.5	+ 9.7
Chores	+10.7	+ 6.7
Telephone	+ 9.5	+ 7.2
Eating	+ 8.8	+ 9.6
Talking	+ 6.7	+ 6.7
Desk work	+ 5.9	+ 5.3
Reading	+ 1.9	+ 2.2
Business (at home)	+ 1.6	+ 3.2
Television	+ 0.3	+ 1.1
Relaxing	0	0
Sleeping	−10.0	− 7.6

[a]Changes are shown relative to blood pressure while relaxing.

with heart rate and blood pressure would be an enormous advantage in resolving this issue.

Even with the existing technology, there is a potential gold mine of information waiting to be explored. Epidemiologists have so far made little use of ambulatory monitoring, although a limited amount of ECG and blood pressure monitoring is being conducted by the Framingham survey. As these techniques are more widely used to study disease states, there will be an increasing need for data obtained by ambulatory monitoring in normal subjects. At present, this need is most pressing in the case of blood pressure.

Since coronary heart disease and hypertension are the two major conditions of interest to specialists in cardiovascular behavioral medicine, it is likely that most of the future applications will be in these areas, although there are a number of other conditions such as panic disorder and depression where autonomic disturbances might be studied by ambulatory monitoring. Numerous studies have compared the cardiovascular reactivity of Type A and B subjects in the laboratory, but there is a glaring lack of information as to whether these differences can also be detected in field studies. In hypertension, it is likely that ambulatory monitoring will become a standard technique for the evaluation of any form of treatment, whether pharmacological or behavioral, as well as for the evaluation of the need for treatment. Although it has been shown that emotional changes can acutely alter blood pressure, the big question in behavioral hypertension research is whether or not psychological factors can contribute to sustained elevations of pressure. Ambulatory monitoring studies could help to resolve this issue.

References

Alfredson, L., Karasek, R., & Theorell, T. (1982). Myocardial infarction risk and psychosocial work environment: An analysis of the male Swedish working force. *Social Science and Medicine, 16,* 463–467.

Ambrosioni, E., Costa, F. V., & Borghi, C. (1982). Effects of moderate salt restriction on intralymphocytic sodium and pressor response to stress in borderline hypertension. *Hypertension, 4,* 789.

Aserinsky, E., & Kleitman, N. (1953). Regularly occurring periods of eye motility, and concomitant phenomena, during sleep. *Science, 118,* 273–274.

Athassaniadis, D., Drayer, G. J., Honour, A. J., & Cranston, W. I. (1969). Variability of automatic blood pressure measurements over 24 hour period. *Clinical Science, 36,* 147–156.

Bristow, J. D., Honour, A. J., Pickering, T. G., & Sleight, P. (1969). Cardiovascular and respiratory changes during sleep in normal and hypertensive subjects. *Cardiovascular Research, 3,* 476–487.

Calvert, A., Lown, B., & Gorlin, R. (1979). Ventricular premature beats and anatomically defined coronary heart disease. *American Journal of Cardiology, 39,* 627–633.

Campbell, S., Barry, J., Rebecca, G. S., Rocco, M. B., Nabel, E. G., Wayne, R. R., & Selwyn, A. P. (1986). Active transient myocardial ischemia during daily life in asymptomatic patients with positive exercise tests and coronary artery disease. *American Journal of Cardiology, 57,* 1010–1016.

Cellina, G. U., Honour, A. J., & Littler, W. A. (1975). Direct arterial pressure, heart rate, and electrocardiogram during cigarette smoking in unrestricted patients. *American Heart Journal, 89,* 18–25.

Clark, L. A., Denby, L., Pregibon, D., Harshfield, G. A., Pickering, T. G., Blank, S., & Laragh, J. H. (1987). A quantitative analysis of the effects of activity and time of day on the diurnal variations of blood pressure. *Journal of Chronic Diseases, 40,* 671–681.

Clement, D. L., De Pue, N., Jordaens, L. J., & Padret, L. (1985). Adrenergic and vagal influences on blood pressure variability. *Clinical and Experimental Hypertension A7* (2&3), 159–166.

Conway, J., Boon, N., Davies, C., Vann Jones, J., & Sleight, P. (1984). Neural and humoral mechanisms involved in blood pressure variability. *Journal of Hypertension, 2,* 203–208.

Cowley, A. M., Liard, J. F., & Guyton, A. C. (1973). Role of the baroreceptor reflex in daily control of arterial blood pressure and other variables in dogs. *Circulation Research, 32,* 564.

Dembroski, T. M., & MacDougall, J. M. (1984). Validation of the Vita-Stat automated noninvasive ambulatory blood pressure recording device. In J. A. Herd, A. M. Gotto, P. G. Kaufmann, & S. M. Weiss (Eds.), *Cardiovascular instrumentation* (NIH Publication No. 84-1654, pp. 55–57).

DiRienzo, M., Grassi, G., Pedotti, A., & Mancia, G. (1983). Continuous vs. intermittent blood pressure measurements in estimating 24-hour average blood pressure. *Hypertension, 5,* 264–269.

DiRienzo, M., Parati, G., Pomidossi, G., Veniani, M., Pedotti, A., & Mancia, G. (1985). Blood pressure monitoring over short day night times cannot predict 24-hour average blood pressure. *Journal of Hypertension, 3,* 343–349.

Foster, G. E., Evans, D. F., & Hardcastle, J. D. (1978). Heart rates of surgeons during operations and other clinical activities and their modification by oxprenolol. *Lancet, 2,* 1323–1325.

Friedman, E., Thomas, S. A., Kulick-Ciuffo, D., Lynch, J. J.,

& Suginahara, M. (1982). The effects of normal and rapid speech on blood pressure. *Psychosomatic Medicine, 44,* 545–553.

Gottlieb, S. O., Weisfeldt, M. L., Ougang, P., Mellitus, E. D., & Gerstenblith, G. (1986). Silent ischemia as a marker for early unfavorable outcomes in patients with unstable angina. *New England Journal of Medicine, 314,* 1214–1219.

Gould, L., Zahir, M., DeMartino, A., & Gomprecht, R. F. (1971). The cardiac effects of a cocktail. *Journal of the American Medical Association, 218,* 1799–1802.

Harshfield, G. A., Pickering, T. G., Kleinert, H. D., Blank, S., & Laragh, J. H. (1982). Situational variation of blood pressure in ambulatory hypertensive patients. *Psychosomatic Medicine, 44,* 237–245.

Harshfield, G. A., James, G. D., Schlussel, Y., Yee, L. S., Blank, S. G., & Pickering, T. G. (1988). Do laboratory tests of blood pressure reactivity predict blood pressure variability in real life? *American Journal of Hypertension, 1,* 168–174.

Hines, E. A., & Brown, G. E. (1933). A standard test for measuring the variability of blood pressure: Its significance as an index of the prehypertensive state. *Annals of Internal Medicine, 7,* 209.

Izzo, J. L., Ghosal, A., Kwong, T., Freeman, R. B., & Jaenike, J. R. (1983). Age and prior caffeine use alter the cardiovascular and adrenomedullary responses to oral caffeine. *American Journal of Cardiology, 52,* 769–773.

Jacob des Combes, B., Porchet, M., Waeber, B., & Brunner, H. R. (1984). Ambulatory blood pressure recordings: Reproducibility and unpredictability. *Hypertension, 6,* C110–115.

James, G. D., Yee, L. S., Harshfield, G. A., Blank, S. G., & Pickering T. G. (1986). The influence of happiness, anger, and anxiety on the blood pressure of borderline hypertensives. *Psychosomatic Medicine, 48,* 502–508.

James, G. D., Pickering, T. G., Yee, L. S., Harshfield, G. A., & Laragh, J. H. (1988). The reproducibility of ambulatory, home, and clinic blood pressures in normotensive and borderline hypertensive subjects. *Hypertension, 11,* 545–549.

Kleitman, N. (1963). *Sleep and wakefulness* (p. 182). Chicago: University of Chicago Press.

Klieger, R. E., Miller, J. P., Bigger, J. T., Moss, A. J. and the Multicenter Post-infarction Group. (1987). Decreased heart rate variability and its association with increased mortality after acute myocardial infarction. *American Journal of Cardiology, 59,* 256–262.

Littler, W. A., Honour, A. J., & Sleight, P. (1974a). Direct arterial pressure, pulse rate, and electrocardiogram during micturition and defecation in unrestricted man. *American Heart Journal, 88,* 205–210.

Littler, W. A., Honour, A. J., & Sleight, P. (1974b). Direct arterial pressure, heart rate, and electrocardiogram during human coitus. *Journal of Reproduction and Fertility, 40,* 321–331.

Lipsitz, L. A., Nyquist, R. P., Wei, J. Y., & Rowe, J. W. (1983). Postprandial reduction in blood pressure in the elderly. *New England Journal of Medicine, 309,* 81–83.

Livnat, A., Zehr, J. E., & Broten, T. P. (1984). Ultradian oscillations in blood pressure and heart rate in free-running dogs. *American Journal of Physiology, 246,* R817–R824.

Llabre, M. M., Ironson, G. H., Spiker, S. B., & Schneiderman, N. (1988). How many blood pressure measurements are enough? An application of generalizability theory to blood pressure reliability. *Psychophysiology, 25,* 97–106.

Magid, N. M., Martin, G. J., Kehoe, R. F., Zheutlin, T. A., Myers, G. A., Eckberg, D. L., Barnett, P. S., Weiss, J. S., Lesch, M., & Singer, D. H. (submitted). Diminished heart rate variability in patients with sudden cardiac death.

Mann, S., Millar-Craig, M. W., Balasubramanian, V., Cashman, P. M. M., & Raftery, E. B. (1980). Ambulant blood pressure: Reproducibility and the assessment of interventions. *Clinical Science, 59,* 497–500.

Mann, S., Altman, D. G., Raftery, E. B., & Bannister, R. (1983). Circadian variation of blood pressure in autonomic failure. *Circulation, 68,* 477–483.

Mann, S., Millar-Craig, M. W., & Raftery, E. B. (1985). Superiority of 24-hour measurement of blood pressure over clinic values in determining prognosis in hypertension. *Clinical and Experimental Exp. Hypertension, A7*(2 & 3), 279–281.

Matthews, K. A., & Haynes, S. G. (1986). Type A behavior pattern and coronary disease risk: Update and critical evaluation. *American Journal of Epidemiology, 123,* 923–960.

Matthews, K. A., Manuck, S. B., & Saab, P. G. (1986). Cardiovascular response of adolescents during a naturally occurring stressor and their behavioral and psychophysiological predictors. *Psychophysiology, 23,* 198–209.

Millar-Craig, M. W., Bishop, C. N., & Raftery, E. B. (1978). Circadian variation of blood-pressure. *Lancet, 1,* 795–798.

Mills, J. N. (1966). Human circadian rhythms. *Physiological Reviews, 46,* 128–171.

Mukharji, J., Rude, R. E., Poole, W. K., Gustafson, N., Thomas, L. J., Strauss, H. W., Jaffee, A. S., Muller, J. E., Roberts, R., Raabe D. S., Croft, C. H., Passamani, E., Braunwald, E., & Willerson, J. T. (1984). Risk factors for sudden death after acute myocardial infarction: Two-year follow-up. *American Journal of Cardiology, 54,* 31–36.

Orlando, J., Aronow, W. S., Cassidy, J., & Prakash, R. (1976). Effect of ethanol on angina pectoris. *Annals of Internal Medicine, 84,* 652–655.

O'Rourke, M. F. (1985). Basic concepts for the understanding of large arteries in hypertension. *Journal of Cardiovascular Pharmacology, 7,* S14–S21.

Orth-Gomer, K., Hogstedt, C., Bodin, L., & Söderholm, B. (1986). Frequency of extrasystoles in healthy male employees. *British Heart Journal, 55,* 259–264.

Palmer, R. F. (1981). Vascular compliance and pulsatile flow as determinants of vascular injury. In J. H. Laragh, F. R. Bühler, & D. W. Seldin (Eds.), *Frontiers in hypertension research* (pp. 396–400). Berlin: Springer-Verlag.

Perloff, D., Sokolow, M., & Cowan, R. (1983). The prognostic value of ambulatory blood pressure. *Journal of the American Medical Association, 249,* 2792–2798.

Pickering, T. G. (1980). Sleep, circadian rhythms, and cardiovascular disease. *Cardiovascular Review Reports, 1,* 37–46.

Pickering, T. G., & Devereux, R. (1987). Ambulatory monitoring of blood pressure as a predictor of cardiovascular risk. *American Heart Journal, 114,* 925–928.

Pickering, T. G., Johnston, J., & Honour, A. J. (1978). Comparison of the effects of sleep, exercise, and autonomic drugs on ventricular extrasystoles, using ambulatory monitoring of ECG and EEG. *American Journal of Medicine, 65,* 575–583.

Pickering, T. G., Harshfield, G. A., Kleinert, H. D., Blank, S., & Laragh, J. H. (1982). Blood pressure during normal daily activities, sleep, and exercise: Comparison of values in normal and hypertensive subjects. *Journal of the American Medical Association, 247,* 992–996.

Pickering, T. G., Harshfield, G. A., Devereux, R. B., & Laragh, J. H. (1985). What is the role of ambulatory blood pressure monitoring in the management of hypertensive patients? *Hypertension, 7,* 171–177.

Redman, C. W. G., Beilin, L. J., & Bonnar, J. (1976). Reversed diurnal blood pressure rhythm in hypertensive pregnancies. *Clinical Science and Molecular Medicine, 51,* 687s–689s.

Reeves, R. A., Shapiro, A. P., Thompson, M. E., & Johnson, A. M. (1986). Loss of nocturnal decline in blood pressure after cardiac transplantation. *Circulation, 73,* 401–408.

Robertson, D., Frolich, J. C., Carr, R. K., Watson, J. T., Hollifield, J. W., Shand, D. G., & Oates, J. A. (1978). Effects of caffeine on plasma renin activity, catecholamines and blood pressure. *New England Journal of Medicine, 298,* 181–186.

Ruberman, W., Weinblatt, E., Goldberg, J. E., Frank, C. W., & Shapiro, S. (1977). Ventricular premature beats and mortality after myocardial infarction. *New England Journal of Medicine, 297,* 750–757.

Schang, S. J., & Pepine, C. J. (1977). Transient asymptomatic S-T segment depression during daily activity. *American Journal of Cardiology, 39,* 396–402.

Schmieder, R., Rüddel, H., Langewitz, W., Neus, J., Wagner, O., & von Eiff, A. W. (1985). The influence of monotherapy with oxprenolol and nitrendipine on ambulatory blood pressure in hypertensives. *Clinical and Experimental Hypertension, A7,* 445–454.

Shimada, S. G., & Marsh, D. J. (1979). Oscillations in mean arterial blood pressure in conscious dogs. *Circulation Research, 44,* 692–700.

Stumpe, K. O., Kolloch, R., Vetter, H., Gramann, W., Krück, F., Ressel, C., & Higuchi, M. (1976). Acute and long-term studies of the mechanism of action of beta-blocking drugs in lowering blood pressure. *American Journal of Medicine, 60,* 853–856.

Taggart, P., Gibbons, D., & Somerville, W. (1969). Some effects of motor car driving on the normal and abnormal heart. *British Medical Journal, 4,* 130–134.

Thomas, S. A., Friedman, E., Lottes, L. S., Gresty, S., Miller, C., & Lynch, J. J. (1984). Changes in nurses' blood pressure and heart rate while communicating. *Research in Nursing and Health, 7,* 119–126.

Van Citters, R. L., & Franklin, D. L. (1969). Cardiovascular performance of Alaska sled dogs during exercise. *Circulation Research, 24,* 33–42.

Waters, D. D., Miller, D. D., Bouchard, A., Bosch, X., & Theroux, P. (1984). Circadian variation in variant angina. *American Journal of Cardiology, 54,* 61–64.

Watson, R. D. S., Hamilton, C. A., Reid, J. L., & Littler, W. A. (1979). Changes in plasma norepinephrine, blood pressure and heart rate during physical activity in hypertensive man. *Hypertension, 1,* 34–346.

Watson, R. D. S., Stallard, T. J., & Littler, W. A. (1979). Influence of once-daily administration of β-adrenoceptor antagonists on arterial pressure and its variability. *Lancet, 1,* 1210–1213.

Weber, M. A., Drayer, J. I. M., Wyle, F. A., & De Young, J. L. (1982). Reproducibility of the whole-day blood pressure pattern in essential hypertension. *Clinical and Experimental Hypertension, A4*(8), 1377–1390.

Willich, S., Rocco, M., Tofler, G., Stone, P., Muller, J., & Levy, D. (1986). Circadian frequency distribution of sudden cardiac death: The Framingham heart study. *Circulation, 74*(Suppl. II), II-268.

Winkel, R. A. (1978). Antiarrhythmic drug effect mimicked by spontaneous variability of ventricular ectopy. *Circulation, 57,* 1116.

Wolf, E., Tzivoni, D., & Stern, S. (1974). Comparison of exercise tests and 24-hour ambulatory electrocardiographic monitoring in detection of ST-T changes. *British Heart Journal, 36,* 90–95.

Young, M. A., Rowlands, D. B., Stallard, T. H., Watson, R. D. S., & Littler, W. A. (1983). Effect of environment on blood pressure: Home versus hospital. *British Medical Journal, 286,* 1235–1236.

CHAPTER 17

Ambulatory Electrocardiographic Monitoring
Methods and Applications

Paul Kligfield

Introduction

Heart rate and rhythm, even in clinically normal subjects, can exhibit a wide range of daily variability as the body responds to changes in physical exertion, emotional state, and neurohumoral tone. Obviously, a standard electrocardiogram (ECG), which records the electrical activity of the heart during the course of several seconds with the subject at rest, provides limited information regarding the response of the heart to daily activity. However, the development of methods for the continuous recording and analysis of the ECG over prolonged periods of ambulatory activity can provide physiologic insight into cardiovascular responsiveness (Kligfield, 1984).

Continuous electrocardiographic recording of ambulatory subjects has evolved over the past 25 years from early work in radiotelemetry and signal processing by Holter (1961), whose method identi-

Adapted from Kligfield, P. (1984). Clinical applications of ambulatory electrocardiography. *Cardiology, 71,* 69–99.

Paul Kligfield • Division of Cardiology, Department of Medicine, The New York Hospital–Cornell Medical Center, New York, New York 10021.

fied changes in rate and rhythm by cycle-length-dependent superimposition of electrocardiographic complexes with a 60-fold ratio of playback to recording speed. Within several years, Gilson, Holter, and Glasscock (1964) were able to report observation of simple arrhythmias, brief changes in electrocardiographic morphology, and a range of artifacts in 65 otherwise apparently normal subjects. Early association of transient arrhythmias with symptoms was found by Corday *et al.* (1965) in 36 of 286 patients studied with 10-h continuous recordings. Despite initial enthusiasm for the use of ambulatory electrocardiography in the diagnosis of ischemia, practical and theoretical limitations of early recording and analysis equipment were emphasized by Hinkle, Meyer, Stevens, and Carver (1967).

Advancing technology soon made it practical to acquire and store greater than 6–12 h of rhythm data on a lightweight, portable, battery-powered tape recorder. The advantage of longer, 24-h continuous electrocardiographic monitoring, to include a normal sleep cycle, for fully characterizing highly sporadic and variable ambulatory supraventricular and ventricular arrhythmias was demonstrated by Lopes, Runge, Harrison, and Schroeder (1975). Even further improved sensitivity for detecting ventricular ectopy with more prolonged periods of up to 48 h of recording (Kennedy, Chandra, Sayther, & Carasis, 1978) is consistent with evolving recognition of the striking spontaneous and activity-related variability of ventricular arrhythmias (Pickering, Johnston, & Honour, 1978; Winkle, 1978). Practical considerations, however, have made 24-h continuous recordings in ambulatory populations the most widely used compromise.

Ambulatory electrocardiography is currently used to correlate transient symptomatic events with the ECG, and as an increasingly important predictive base for assessing cardiovascular risk in a variety of conditions. In addition, this method has become important for the assessment of therapeutic intervention in cardiovascular disease, and rhythm profiles are increasingly incorporated into clinical descriptions of both normal and abnormal population groups. Several reviews and texts are available for further clinical perspective (Bleifer, Bleifer, Hansmann, Sheppard, & Karpamn, 1974; Iyengar, Castellanos, & Spence, 1971; Kennedy, 1981; Moss, 1980; Winkle, 1980, 1981).

Clinical Applications of Ambulatory Monitoring

Current clinical applications of ambulatory electrocardiographic monitoring are summarized in Table 1. Ambulatory recording is based on the observation that significant electrocardiographic findings are commonly sporadic, so that a standard 12-lead ECG taken during an asymptomatic period may not detect changes in rhythm or configuration

Table 1. Applications of Ambulatory Electrocardiography

To assess the relationship of symptoms to underlying rhythm and repolarization
To profile rate and rhythm in specfic clinical circumstances
To detect sporadic asymptomatic cardiac events
To predict cardiovascular risk
To evaluate therapeutic intervention
To profile populations with cardiac disease
To derive pathophysiologic insights into disease mechanism

that occur during transient symptomatic or other asymptomatic periods (Kennedy, 1981; Winkle, 1981). Ambulatory electrocardiography requires that a sensitive and specific method be available for identifying these qualitative and quantitative abnormalities from a large body of acquired data. The more efficient and convenient this process, the better. Qualitative ambulatory electrocardiographic findings can often be correlated with transient symptoms and may suggest therapeutic intervention. Quantitative electrocardiographic data, on the other hand, are generally required for the prediction of risk and for the assessment of the success or failure of therapeutic intervention.

Qualitative rhythm changes, such as the occurrence of sinus pauses or ventricular tachycardia, are often sought as an explanation for otherwise unexplained dizziness or syncope and for documentation of symptomatic palpitation. Repolarization changes may also be examined in the evaluation of transient episodes of chest pain, particularly when incompletely associated with effort provocation and potentially related to coronary artery spasm, and for the assessment of "silent" ischemia. Qualitative findings may influence therapeutic decisions, even in the absence of definitely related symptoms, as may occur when paroxysmal atrial fibrillation is found in patients with otherwise unexplained systemic embolic events or when transient advanced atrioventricular block is discovered in a patient with progressive conduction tissue disease.

For profiling arrhythmias in various diseases and for the prediction of risk from ambulatory electrocardiographic signs, quantitative analysis of rhythm is essential. By way of example, both the frequency and complexity of ventricular premature complexes have been used to estimate the likelihood of developing a first manifestation of ischemic heart disease (Chiang, Perlman, Ostrander, & Epstein, 1969; Chiang, Perlman, Fulton, Ostrander, & Epstein, 1970; Desai, Hershberg, & Alexander, 1973; Hinkle, Carver, & Stevens, 1969; Rodstein, Wolloch, & Gubner, 1971), and ventricular arrhythmias have also been clearly documented as predictors of sudden death after myocardial infarction (Bigger, Heller, Wenger, & Weld, 1978; Coronary Drug Project Research

Group, 1973; Kotler, Tabatznik, Mower, & Tominaga, 1973; Moss, Schnitzler, Green, & DeCamilla, 1971; Moss *et al.*, 1975; Moss, Davis, DeCamilla, & Bayer, 1979; Ruberman, Weinblatt, Goldberg, Frank, & Shapiro, 1977; Ruberman *et al.*, 1981; Schulze, Strauss, & Pitt, 1977; Vismara, Vera, Foerster, Amsterdam, & Mason, 1977). Assessment of therapeutic intervention also requires quantitative analysis of the ambulatory ECG, and appreciation of periodic variability of arrhythmias (Winkle, 1978) is essential to judge, for example, whether a medication has substantially decreased the number or complexity of ventricular premature complexes.

An additional application of ambulatory electrocardiography is the acquisition of correlative data that can be used to profile specific clinical circumstances. For example, ambulatory monitoring has been used to quantify rate and rhythm changes in patients with panic disorder during asymptomatic intervals and during episodes of panic, partial panic, and anxiety (Shear *et al.*, 1987). This approach assures collection of data during sporadically occurring events, without a major effect of procedural intervention on alteration of the event itself. Ambulatory monitoring also allows derivation of heart rate variability indices that can be related to autonomic tone (Berger, Akselrod, Gordon, & Cohen, 1986; O'Brien, O'Hare, & Corrall, 1986; Smith & Smith, 1981), with potential applications to the study of neurophysiologic mechanisms in health and disease.

Methodologic Considerations

The most commonly used ambulatory electrocardiographic recording and analysis systems are later-generation computer-assisted descendants of the original Holter method (Holter, 1961; Gilson *et al.*, 1964). These currently scan at up to 240 times real-time, using simultaneous visual complex superimposition, visual cycle-length display, audio transformation of cycle-length variation, and computer sorting and storage of interval and configuration data to identify arrhythmias and changes in morphology (Kennedy, 1981). As "full

disclosure" analysis systems, these allow all electrocardiographic data to be printed on paper for visual inspection and validation as needed. Advances in computer-based signal analysis and data reduction have led to increasingly widespread use of "real-time" devices (Mark & Ripley, 1985) that generate summaries of heart rate, rhythm, and repolarization variability with time, often without "full disclosure." These systems can markedly simplify data processing, but it must be emphasized that these recorders can obviously be no more accurate or reliable than the often erratic electrocardiographic signals they receive.

With "full disclosure" monitoring systems, it is rather simple, but time-consuming, to validate the presence of individual rhythm or repolarization abnormalities by printout and analysis of selected electrocardiographic strips. Although false-positive interpretations, due to artifact or to misclassification of aberrant, wide complexes as ventricular rather than supraventricular in origin, may be eliminated by this type of screening, it is far more difficult to achieve a comparable level of confidence regarding potential false-negative inferences. How, in effect, can one ever be certain that the absence of recognition means that a sporadic electrocardiographic sign has not occurred?

One approach to this problem, using "full disclosure" systems, has been the rapid printing of the entire recording in a compressed format. This allows visual review of all electrocardiographic complexes on paper, with identification of areas of apparent irregularity allowing retrieval of a standard rhythm strip for more detailed analysis. Although this technology can reduce false-negative interpretations, it is limited by the high cost of the light-sensitive, silver-based paper needed for efficient production of the small complex printout, and also limited by poor frequency response and poor reproduction of P wave morphology.

In this regard, it is apparent that compression of data by "real-time" recorders that continuously analyze rhythm and configuration, but only store detected abnormalities, raises significant uncertainty regarding false-negative conclusions. Since no retrieval and review of presumably normal data may be available, these devices generally are dependent on their programming accuracy and may be otherwise inflexible regarding data analysis. Other real-time devices allow sampled rhythm strips to be retrieved. This same problem affects intermittent recorders, which may be triggered by the patient during infrequent symptoms or may be preprogrammed to periodically sample rates and rhythms. In the case of patients with infrequent symptoms, this type of device may be of qualitative diagnostic value, although the initiation of an arrhythmia may be missed if a long enough delay loop is not present, and loss of consciousness during serious arrhythmias may interfere with the triggering of recording in some cases.

Quantification of morphologic changes, such as ST segment depression, is strongly dependent on additional technical characteristics of ambulatory monitoring devices. Practical and theoretical early limitations of recording equipment were discussed by Hinkle et al. (1967), and a recent study by Bragg-Remschel, Anderson, and Winkle (1982) has examined the effect of the frequency response characteristics of several systems on the accuracy of analysis of repolarization. Although current recommendations of the American Heart Association call for low- and high-frequency cutoffs at -3 dB of 0.05 and 100 Hz for standard electrocardiography (Pipberger et al., 1975), these criteria are not uniformly met in equipment used for ambulatory recording and playback (Bragg-Remschel et al., 1982). Therefore, ST segment shifts suggestive of ischemia, when dissociated from symptoms or when occurring in unlikely subjects, must be interpreted in the context of the frequency response of the equipment in use. New frequency-modulated or digital recorders have improved the accuracy of repolarization data.

Cardiac Rhythm in Clinically Normal Subjects

In general, heart rate in clinically normal subjects is faster during periods of wakefulness, and increases during physical exertion and episodes of emotional stress. Commonly seen disorders of impulse formation such as ventricular premature complexes (VPCs), potentially related to changes in sympathetic tone and circulating levels of cate-

cholamines, are often more frequent during wakeful hours of the day. In contrast, heart rate is generally slower during sleep, which is also occasionally associated with periods of slower intracardiac conduction, potentially related to changes in vagal tone and withdrawal of sympathetic stimulation.

Ambulatory electrocardiography has been widely used to study the prevalence of disorders of impulse formation and impulse conduction in specific populations. Quite clearly, the interpretation of arrhythmias in individuals and in groups of patients with ischemic heart disease (Califf, Burks, Behar, Margolis, & Wagner, 1977; Califf et al., 1982; Johnson et al., 1982; Ruberman et al., 1980; Ryan, Lown, & Horn, 1975), mitral valve prolapse (DeMaria, Amsterdam, Vismara, Neumann, & Mason, 1976; Kramer, Kligfield, Devereux, Savage, & Kramer-Fox, 1984; Savage et al., 1983; Winkle et al., 1975), cardiomyopathy (Bjarnason, Hardarson, & Jonsson, 1982; Canedo, Frank, & Abdulla, 1980; Holmes, Kubo, Cody, & Kligfield, 1985; McKenna, Chetty, Oakley, & Goodwin, 1980; McKenna, England, et al., 1981; McKenna, Harris, et al., 1981), and other specific types of heart disease (Hindman, Last, & Rosen, 1973; Hochreiter, Niles, Devereux, Kligfield, & Borer, 1986; Isaeff, Gaston, & Harrison, 1972) depends on an understanding of the prevalence of rhythm findings in clinically normal populations.

Data bearing on cardiac rhythm in apparently normal populations are available for newborn infants, healthy children, male medical students, young women, working adults, and active elderly people. Several important trends and observations emerge from these studies. Most obvious is the extraordinarily high prevalence of potentially significant arrhythmias present in ambulatory subjects of all ages. Also apparent is a shift in the type of prevalent arrhythmia that accompanies aging. These data are summarized in Table 2.

In presumed normal infants and children, Southall et al. (1980; Southall, Johnston, Shinebourne, & Johnston, 1981) have demonstrated a high prevalence of episodic sinus pauses and periods suggesting various forms of sinus exit block, with occasional periods of AV junctional escape rhythms during sinus bradycardia. Despite such findings in

Table 2. Prevalence of Disorders of Impulse Formation and Conduction in Clinically Normal Populations, by Age (in Percent)

Population group/reference	Sinus pauses Sinus block	SB with AVJ escape	2° AVB	Any APCs	Any VPCs	VPC couplets	VT	Early cycle VPCs
Infants								
Southall et al. (1980)	72	20	—	14	0	0	0	0
Children								
Southall et al. (1981)	65	45	3	21	1	0	0	—
Young men								
Brodsky et al. (1977)	50	22	6	56	50	2	2	6
Young women								
Sobotka et al. (1981)	34	4	4	64	54	0	2	4
Working adults								
Clarke et al. (1976)	—	10	2	—	73	13	2	2
Hinkle et al. (1969)	1	—	1	76	62	—	3	—
Savage et al. (1983)	—	—	—	89	68	15	—	—
Elderly								
Glasser et al. (1979)	0	0	0	100	100	23	0	
Camm et al. (1980)	0	4	1	37	69	6	6	
Kantelip et al. (1986)	10	0	0	100	96	8	2	

approximately two-thirds of children, the prevalence of atrial ectopy was found to be low, and ventricular ectopy vanishingly uncommon. Among young male medical students (Brodsky, Wu, Denes, Kanakis, & Rosen, 1977) and young women (Sobotka, Mayer, Bavernfeind, Kanakis, & Rosen, 1981), sinus pauses and apparent SA block have been found in up to one-half of otherwise normal subjects. Both atrial and ventricular ectopy were present in over half of these healthy young adults, with VPC couplets found in 1%, ventricular tachycardia found in 2%, and early cycle VPC forms found in 5% of this population.

Among working adults (Hinkle et al., 1969; Clarke, Shelton, Hamer, Tayler, & Venning, 1976), in contrast to younger subjects, sinus pauses and periods suggesting SA block appear to be less prevalent, while over two-thirds have atrial and ventricular ectopy. More complex forms of ventricular ectopy were noted by Hinkle et al. (1969) in some of these subjects, including a 13% prevalence of VPC couplets and 3% prevalence of ventricular tachycardia. Although some subjects included in this series of working men were in fact independently shown to have ischemic heart disease, complex ventricular ectopy was by no means confined to this subset. Indeed, Savage et al. (1983) found VPC couplets or runs in 15% of recently examined Framingham subjects (mean age 44 years) without clinical or echocardiographic evidence of cardiopulmonary disease.

In evaluating ambulatory rhythms of the elderly, it is even more difficult to assure normality. However, in clinically well older populations (Camm, Evans, Ward, & Martin, 1980; Glasser, Clark, & Applebaum, 1979; Kantelip, Sage, & Duchene-Marullaz, 1986), sinus pauses and block have been exceedingly rare, while atrial and ventricular arrhythmias are common. Glasser et al. (1979) found VPC couplets in nearly one-fourth of a group of apparently healthy people aged 60–84, all of whom had simple VPCs during 24 h of recording, whereas Camm et al. (1980) found a lower VPC couplet prevalence of 4% but observed a 6% prevalence of asymptomatic ventricular tachycardia in elderly subjects.

Even allowing for potential error caused by inhomogeneity of these populations, several important trends appear when the prevalence of arrhythmias is examined in relationship to age (Table 2). Sinus pauses, various forms of sinus exit block, and marked sinus bradycardia with AV junctional escape rhythms are common in childhood and through young adulthood, but become very uncommon in middle and advanced age. Although far less common, moderately advanced sporadic AV node conduction delay also appears to decrease with aging. On the other hand, ectopic disorders of impulse formation can be seen to clearly increase with age, so that VPCs, which are extraordinarily uncommon in children, are rather an expected finding in adults and are quite common in the elderly.

Since age is such an important factor in determining the prevalence of specific arrhythmias in an apparently normal population, it is obvious that rhythm analysis of populations with specific diseases requires comparison with age-matched controls. If this source of bias is not considered, it becomes easy to conclude that an arrhythmia is a feature of a specific disease, rather than a characteristic of the population in which the disease occurs.

Another potential source of selection bias in profiling assumed normal populations is the effect of symptoms on the likelihood of being tested. If a subject presents with palpitations and has ventricular ectopy documented by ambulatory electrocardiography, and subsequently no organic cardiac disease can be found, should this individual be included as representative of the normal population? Clearly not, unless the symptoms were also representative of the normal population, since this would skew our perception of true arrhythmia prevalence. Although this type of error does not significantly affect the population studies referred to above, failure to assume unbiased sampling is a great problem in acquiring appropriate control subjects for ambulatory rhythm studies. This same type of bias, in which symptoms cause selection for testing, also affects the validity of rhythm profiling in specific disease conditions.

Age trends themselves, however, may also be affected by occult selection bias. For example, among the apparently normal infants and children with marked sinus pauses and sporadic sinus exit

block may be some ultimately lost to various forms of sudden death. Conversely, symptomatic or asymptomatic adults with these same findings may well be excluded from analysis of clinically normal groups, either because disease has been defined or has been presumed. Similarly, although VPCs or even complex forms need not be precise markers for disease, their higher prevalence in older populations might partially reflect the higher likelihood of occult cardiac disorder in these subjects.

Ventricular Arrhythmias in Heterogeneous Populations

Several long-term observational studies have been performed that bear on the significance of ventricular arrhythmias in heterogeneous populations. These studies have confirmed the increasing prevalence of ventricular ectopy that is associated with aging and have also linked VPCs with sudden death in some cases when important underlying heart disease is present. The Tecumseh study (Chiang et al., 1969; Chiang, Perlman, Fulton, Ostrander, & Epstein, 1970) demonstrated a higher risk of development of coronary artery disease and subsequent sudden death among adult subjects with VPCs, after adjustment for age. In the Equitable Life study (Rodstein et al., 1971), excess mortality in the presence of VPCs occurred only in subjects with underlying disease and was highest in those with rated heart disease. Age- and disease-matched cohorts with VPCs reported by the Lahey Clinic (Desai, Hershberg, & Alexander, 1973) demonstrated higher mortality only in patients with cardiac disease, with greatest risk concentrated in the post-myocardial infarction subgroup.

Hinkle et al. (1969) examined ambulatory recordings in a prospectively followed group of nearly 300 working adult men. Over 60% of these subjects were found to have ventricular ectopy, which most commonly consisted of single and infrequent VPCs. Yet nearly 9% of the group had frequent VPCs, defined as more than 10 per 1000 normal beats, and sequential VPCs were found in nearly 13% of these men, with self-limited ventricular tachycardia in 3%. Over a 6-year period, cardiac deaths were found to be directly associated with VPC density, rising from a relative risk of 0.3 with no VPCs to 3.6 with greater than 10 per 1000 VPCs. This risk exceeded the 1.9 relative risk of coronary death independently associated with VPC couplets, and, curiously, no deaths occurred in the small group of men with ventricular tachycardia.

Of course, in this heterogeneous ambulatory population, some subjects had independent evidence of ischemic heart disease and were clearly a high-risk subset, while others were quite normal. Both VPCs and complex forms were indeed more common in those otherwise at high risk (Hinkle *et al.*, 1969), heralding later observations from homogeneously ischemic populations that the prognostic value of ventricular ectopy is highly dependent on the functional severity of underlying disease (Borer *et al.*, 1980; Ryan *et al.*, 1975; Schulze *et al.*, 1977). On the other hand, Kennedy *et al.* (1985) have demonstrated an absence of adverse cardiac events during longitudinal study of a large group of subjects with complex arrhythmias, but with no detectable underlying heart disease. These observations suggest that while arrhythmias may be symptomatic of structural heart disease, they are usually prognostically benign in otherwise normal subjects.

Classification and Grading of Ventricular Arrhythmias

In order to derive prognostic value from analysis of ventricular arrhythmias, a stratification of risk features must be established to link distinct ambulatory electrocardiographic findings with clinical outcome. Progress toward this fundamental requirement has been difficult and controversial, since varying approaches to qualitative and quantitative analysis of arrhythmias are available.

Distinct electrocardiographic features of ventricular arrhythmias include estimates of VPC frequency, grading of VPC complexity, and classification of VPC forms. In different clinical situations, these qualitative and quantitative features of arrhythmias may be independent or related variables, and their sensitivity and specificity for predicting a clinical outcome will vary. Clinical outcomes, in turn, vary from the ultimate development of disease within heterogeneous populations to the occurrence of morbid events within homogeneous, diseased populations. In view of varying sensitivity and specificity, there is no inherent reason why one system of arrhythmia analysis need be optimal, or even appropriate, for assessing all types of clinical outcome, since the predictive value of any rhythm finding depends on the prevalence of disease or outcome in the population under study (Diamond & Forrester, 1979). For analysis of ventricular arrhythmias, VPC frequency, VPC complexity, and VPC forms may all be relevant in different clinical settings. Both the grading systems of Hinkle *et al.* (1969) and Lown and co-workers (Calvert, Lown, & Gorlin, 1977; Lown & Wolf, 1971; Lown, Calvert, Armington, & Ryan, 1975; Lown, Graboys, 1977) are in current use, and it is relevant to briefly review the types of populations from which these classifications evolved.

Among middle-aged men, some but not all of whom had independent evidence of ischemic heart disease, Hinkle *et al.* (1969) found that the incidence of subsequent sudden death was directly related to mean VPC density, the VPC frequency normalized per thousand beats. Although a significant increase in subsequent 6-year mortality was found among subjects with greater than 10 VPC/1000 beats, no additional independent risk was apparent in subjects with bigeminy, multiform VPCs, VPC couplets, or even in subjects with brief runs of ambulatory ventricular tachycardia.

It must be noted that among the 301 working men in this study, only 10 had definite evidence of prior myocardial infarction at the time of initial evaluation, while 29 others had independent evidence of probable prior infarction or additional angina. Most mortality occurred in this distinctly "high-risk" subset of the total population, and in this subset sequential VPCs and VT were clearly associated with a greater-than-expected incidence of sudden death. Yet in this heterogeneous population, enough "low-risk" subjects also had complex VPC forms independent of VPC frequency, so that the resulting overall predictive value of complex forms for sudden death was poor. The role of population heterogeneity in leading to this conclusion is again emphasized, and these results remain valuable for evaluation of ambulatory men, but need not apply to the evaluation of more homogeneous populations where established disease is an entry requirement.

Greater weighting of ventricular arrhythmia complexity is the distinctive basis of the Lown grading system. Emphasis on VPC complexity is based on attempts to apply early coronary care unit experience to the prediction of sudden death in ambulatory populations. As originally proposed by Lown and Wolf (1971), a hierarchical progression of VPC complexity, which is only partially structured at its lower end by VPC frequency, was hypothesized to correlate with increasing risk of sudden death in patients with ischemic heart disease. The grading system incorporates the following VPC classification: grade 0, no VPCs; grade 1, unifocal VPCs < 30/h; grade 2, unifocal VPCs > 30/h; grade 3, multiform VPCs; grade 4a, VPC couplets; grade 4b, VPC triplets or runs of VT; grade 5, early cycle VPCs.

Within the hierarchy of seven Lown grades, three grades of either absent or "simple" VPCs are partitioned by frequency only, and contain no multiform, sequential, or early cycle ectopy, while four grades of "complex" VPCs are partitioned independent of frequency. Clinical studies of risk stratification after myocardial infarction have commonly separated patients into those with "simple" (grades 0–2) and those with "complex" (grades 3–5) ventricular ectopy (Moss et al., 1979; Ruberman et al., 1977; Schulze et al., 1977). Although arbitrary, this separation does indeed correlate with broad, but far from perfect, prognostic trends in some types of homogeneous populations.

Problems with this approach involve both the hierarchy of grading itself and the division of grades into "simple" and "complex" groups. In the Lown grading system, a patient is classified according to the highest applicable mutually exclusive grade, each of which supersedes theoretically lower-risk subsets. Thus, a patient with frequent, multiform VPCs and several VPC couplets would typically be classified as only grade 4a. According to the hierarchical risk hypothesis, another patient with infrequent, unifocal VPCs and just one VPC couplet would also be classified as grade 4a and assigned to the same risk group, despite obvious major differences in VPC frequency and configuration. Furthermore, just one early cycle VPC is sufficient to assign a subject to a high-risk subset, even if no other ectopy is present.

Perhaps most important, the hierarchical grading system obscures any potentially significant prognostic contribution of a lower grade rhythm. For example, consider a situation in which most subjects with early cycle VPCs also had VPC couplets. Further, suppose that in this situation, couplets, not early cycle forms, ultimately proved to be of greatest predictive accuracy. Because of the mutual exclusivity of the grading system, the early cycle VPCs would be incorrectly associated with the clinical outcome. Similarly, if multiformity of VPCs or repetitive forms were common in patients with frequent VPCs, the independent contribution of VPC frequency might be lost in hierarchical grading, and any potential prognostic value of VPC frequency might be lost in the concept of complexity.

Therefore, the relationship of VPC frequency and VPC complexity requires closer examination. It has been generally recognized that subjects with frequent ventricular ectopy also tend to have a high prevalence of associated complex ectopy, as observed by Hinkle et al. (1969) in ambulatory working men and also found among specific populations of patients surviving myocardial infarction (Ruberman et al., 1977), with hypertrophic cardiomyopathy (Savage et al., 1979), and with mitral valve prolapse (Winkle et al., 1975). But it is also apparent that complex ventricular ectopy can occur in subjects without associated frequent VPCs, as observed by Savage et al. (1979) among patients with hypertrophic cardiomyopathy and by Meyerburg et al. (1980) in survivors of out-of-hospital cardiac arrest. While clearly the patient population characteristics of these latter studies make complex ectopy predictable, Messineo, Al-Hani, and Katz (1981) have recently reported a 50–60% prevalence of complex VPCs, including a 25% prevalence of VPC couplets or VT, among unselected patients with otherwise infrequent VPCs.

Yet reliance on standard Lown grading to identify high-risk patients based on complexity of VPCs alone assumes that no independent risk can be inferred from VPC frequency, since patients are placed into mutually exclusive hierarchical grades. Emphasis on complexity of ventricular ectopy further implies that clinical outcome is accurately predicted within homogeneous study populations using this grading system. However, Bigger and Weld (1981) have emphasized the marked heterogeneity of the "complex" Lown grades 3 through 5 which in effect comprise 30 subgroups even when only one partition value for VPC frequency is used (30 VPCs/h). In 400 patients evaluated after myocardial infarction, the best predictors of death were found to be both VPC frequency and sequential VPCs, and a very-high-risk subset was identified from the combination of these features. Furthermore, stratification of mortality risk within Lown grade 5 (early cycle VPCs) was extreme, ranging from 9% among patients with infrequent VPCs and no other "complex" features, to as high as 59% when frequent VPCs and other complex patterns also occurred (Bigger & Weld, 1981).

In addition, the longitudinal evaluation of postinfarction patients by Ruberman et al. (1981) suggests that among "complex" VPC forms, bigeminal and multiform VPCs (where multiform VPCs but not bigeminal VPCs comprise Lown grade 3) confer significantly lower 5-year risk of sudden death (13%) than do more advanced Lown grades of complex forms (25%). Indeed, the sudden death risk with multiform and bigeminal VPCs was found to be similar to the risk associated with simple VPCs alone (12%). These observations suggest that reliance on traditional Lown grade "complex" forms to identify high-risk subsets, at least in the postinfarction population, will result in marked prognostic heterogeneity. These data further suggest that frequency and grading techniques can provide complementary prognostic information for a variety of clinical outcomes.

As noted by Bigger and Weld (1981) with particular reference to early cycle VPCs (Lown grade 5), these observations are of great importance in the design of therapeutic trials in the postinfarction population. Since substantial heterogeneity of risk clearly exists among presumed "high-risk" population subsets identified by VPC complexity alone,

potential harm to low-risk patients included in intervention trials must be weighed, and the effect of these patients on assessing the results of intervention must be considered.

Spontaneous Variability of Ventricular Arrhythmias

Quantitative assessment of therapeutic intervention by ambulatory electrocardiography has been widely applied to the study of antiarrhythmic drug efficacy, and most specifically to the evaluation of VPC suppression (Bigger, Giardina, Perel, Kantor, & Glassman, 1977; De Soyza et al., 1982; DiBianco et al., 1982; Hodges et al., 1982; Krone, Miller, Kleiger, Clark, & Oliver, 1981; Rocchini, Chun, & Dick, 1981; Velebit, Podrid, Lown, Cohen, & Graboys, 1982; Woosley et al., 1979). Accurate inference from these studies requires appreciation of several statistical phenomena that also bear on interpretation of sampled correlative data in individuals. Of primary importance is the marked spontaneous variability in day-to-day VPC frequency that occurs in monitored subjects even in the absence of therapy. From an understanding of the magnitude of spontaneous variability of VPC frequency, criteria for successful therapeutic intervention can be established. Such criteria, in turn, depend both on underlying VPC frequency and on the duration of ambulatory monitoring used to assess ventricular ectopy. And, finally, statistical comparison of mean VPC frequencies in different populations, or in one population before and after treatment, requires appropriate methods of data analysis.

In order to establish whether a quantitative change in an observed arrhythmia is due to therapeutic intervention, the range of variability of rhythm findings with time in the absence of intervention must be appreciated. Morganroth et al. (1978) examined spontaneous variability of VPCs in consecutive 24-h ambulatory ECGs from 15 patients with frequent ventricular ectopy. The extent of hourly spontaneous variation was found to be 48%, while day-to-day variation was 23%, so that attribution of reduction in ventricular ectopy to intervention based on two 24-h recordings was calculated to require a greater than 83% decrease in VPC frequency.

Using linear regression analysis in 21 patients to compare baseline and placebo VPC frequencies, Sami *et al.* (1980) calculated that a 65% reduction of VPCs was required to establish antiarrhythmic efficacy with 95% confidence. Differences from the conclusions of Morganroth *et al.* (1978) were attributed to different methods of analysis of variance and to alternative statistical assumptions. In addition, the percent reduction in VPCs required to demonstrate antiarrhythmic efficacy was found to vary inversely with VPC frequency, so that the 65% reduction required to demonstrate efficacy when VPCs exceed a baseline of 20/h becomes as high as 90–100% reduction required when only 2–3 VPCs/h are present before intervention (Sami *et al.*, 1980).

Winkle, Gradman, Fitzgerald, and Bell (1978) also observed considerable spontaneous variability of VPC frequency between two 24-h control periods in 16 patients undergoing evaluation of the antiarrhythmic efficacy of propranolol, procainamide, and quinidine. Although the mean change in VPC frequency for the group as a whole was quite small (−12%), the range of variability extended from +198% to −91%, with nearly one-third of the patients demonstrating greater than 50% spontaneous reduction in VPCs during the second control period. With shorter monitoring periods, nearly two-thirds of patients in another series (Winkle, 1978) demonstrated greater than 50% spontaneous VPC reduction, a finding of great significance in evaluating the results of acute drug intervention studies.

An additional problem beyond spontaneous variability in assessing the VPC response to drug intervention is the choice of statistical methods used for analysis of data. Quite commonly, the paired Student's *t*-test is used to evaluate the significance of the difference between mean VPC frequencies before and after therapy. This test, however, is based on the underlying assumption that the VPC frequency in the populations under study is approximately normally distributed about the mean (Colton, 1974), both before and after intervention. However, VPC frequencies are generally quite broadly distributed, with ranges among patients under study often extending over several orders of magnitude, from tens to tens of thousands per 24-h period. In this setting, a nonparametric test may be more appropriate for comparison, and statistical inference may be more accurate when based on log transformation, signed rank, or rank sum methods (Colton, 1974).

Prognostic Value of Ventricular Arrhythmias in Patients with Heart Disease

Studies to evaluate the prognostic value of ventricular ectopy have been performed in homogeneous, ischemic populations composed of survivors of myocardial infarction (Bigger *et al.*, 1978; Coronary Drug Project Research Group, 1973; Kotler *et al.*, 1973; Moss *et al.*, 1971, 1975, 1979; Ruberman *et al.*, 1977, 1981; Schulze *et al.*, 1977; Vismara *et al.*, 1977) and patients with angina pectoris (Califf *et al.*, 1977, 1982; Johnson *et al.*, 1982; Ruberman *et al.*, 1980; Ryan *et al.*, 1975). Observations in these populations support the early findings of the Lahey Clinic study that excess mortality among cardiac patients with VPCs is largely found in the postinfarction subset (Desai *et al.*, 1973). Although it has become quite clear from these data that frequent and complex ventricular ectopy are important predictors of sudden death after myocardial infarction, it is increasingly apparent that mortality is also highly dependent on the functional level of ischemic impairment.

The independent risk conferred by variably complex ventricular ectopy above and beyond the effect of ventricular dysfunction after myocardial infarction requires clarification. All sudden death reported by Schulze *et al.* (1977) occurred in the subset of patients with both complex VPCs on 24-h ambulatory electrocardiography and poor left ventricular function by radionuclide evaluation of ejection fraction. Multivariate analysis by Ruberman *et al.* (1981) has suggested that the presence of complex VPCs is the strongest independent risk factor for sudden death (relative risk 2.3). The presence of VPCs remains an important risk factor after discriminant analysis by Luria, Knoke, Wachs, and Luria (1979) while less significant after multivariate analysis by Bigger *et al.* (1978), although in both studies VPCs may be dependent on underlying ventricular dysfunction. Indeed, Borer *et al.* (1980) found a modest, but significant, correlation between resting left ventricular ejection fraction determined by radionuclide cineangiography and the complexity of VPCs detected by ambulatory electrocardiography. Further, Taylor *et al.* (1980) found that previous infarction and low ejection fraction are the strongest primary predictors of mortality, and that late-phase complex ventricular arrhythmias added no additional independent prognostic information when evaluated by stepwise discriminant analysis.

In addition to its application in the study of ischemic heart disease, ambulatory electrocardiography has also been used to evaluate arrhythmias in some forms of cardiomyopathy (Bjarnason *et al.*, 1982; Canedo *et al.*, 1980; Holmes *et al.*, 1985; McKenna *et al.*, 1980; McKenna, England, *et al.*, 1981; McKenna, Harris, *et al.*, 1981), valvular disease (DeMaria *et al.*, 1976; Kramer *et al.*, 1984; Savage *et al.*, 1983; Winkle *et al.*, 1975), and conduction disorders (Hindman *et al.*, 1973; Isaeff *et al.*, 1972). As applied to nonischemic populations, such studies may profile arrhythmia prevalence, correlate arrhythmias with symptoms or signs of disease, predict disease outcome based on specific findings, or evaluate specific treatment.

It is particularly difficult to ensure adequate control subjects for these types of investigations because of arrhythmia variability with age and because of the important problem of selection bias. The potential error in failing to age-match control populations has already been discussed, and is obvious from a brief examination of Table 2. Less obvious, but perhaps even more significant, is the potential error introduced by selection bias. When specific symptoms such as palpitation, or specific signs such as ventricular ectopy on routine evaluation, lead to recognition of an underlying disorder, such patients may well skew the prevalence of recognized arrhythmia when they are incorporated into a series supposedly representative of the disease. Inclusion of subjects with symptoms or signs in whom no underlying disease can be found into a supposedly normal group may similarly increase arrhythmia prevalence among controls. But perhaps most important, exclusion of subjects with any symptoms or signs from control populations may well erroneously decrease arrhythmia prevalence. In this context, it is not unpredictable that an older population of symptomatic patients with recognized disease might be found to have a higher prevalence of arrhythmia than a younger, asymptomatic control subset, even if arrhythmias were not an independent feature of the disease.

Sudden death occurring during ambulatory electrocardiography has been reported by several groups (Denes, Gabster, & Huang, 1981; El-Sherif *et al.*, 1976; Gradman, Bell, & DeBusk, 1977; Hinkle *et al.*, 1977; Nikolic, Bishop, & Singh, 1982), with potentially fatal arrhythmias often, but not invariably, associated with complex or early cycle ventricular ectopy in patients with ischemic or myopathic hearts. Other instances of arrhythmic death have been associated with late-cycle VPCs, particularly in patients with prolonged QT intervals.

It is apparent that behavioral factors can influence sudden death in man. Hinkle (1981) found that 88% of arrhythmic deaths among a large, prospectively followed cohort of employed men occurred while the subjects were awake; activities associated with autonomic effects on the heart were involved in half of these fatalities. The role of vagal, sympathetic, and related behavioral mechanisms in experimental arrhythmogenesis is well reviewed by Saini and Verrier in another section of this volume. Inferences regarding autonomic tone derived from quantitative evaluation of ambulatory electrocardiographic recordings may provide further understanding of these complex interactions.

As classified by Hinkle and Thaler (1982), arrhythmic death without prior circulatory collapse occurs commonly as a terminal event when heart disease is the primary cause of the final illness. Present more typically is ischemic heart disease or other types of cardiomyopathy leading to congestive heart failure (Holmes *et al.*, 1985; Nikolic *et al.*, 1982), although potentially lethal arrhythmias may be seen in the localized disorder of arrhythmogenic right ventricular dysplasia (Dungan, Gardon, & Gillette, 1981; Palileo *et al.*, 1982). Recurrence of potentially fatal arrhythmias is more common when unassociated with acute myocardial infarction (Schaffer & Cobb, 1975), a finding consistent with the prognostic ambiguity of early, as opposed to late phase, infarction arrhythmias (Vismara *et al.*, 1977).

Hemodynamic profiles of patients resuscitated from out-of-hospital cardiac arrest reveal reduced cardiac index and ejection fraction in the majority, but normal left ventricular function in as many as one-third of this group (Meyerburg *et al.*, 1980). Ambulatory electrocardiography in 144 survivors of prehospital ventricular fibrillation reported by Weaver, Cobb, and Hallstrom (1982) revealed multiform ventricular ectopy in over 75%, VPC couplets or triplets in over 50%, and nonsustained ventricular tachycardia in nearly 10%. Subsequent sudden death was most accurately predicted by frequent multiform VPCs, bigeminy or trigeminy, and sequential forms, but not by frequency of simple VPCs alone. The apparent importance of VPC complexity in predicting recurrent, potentially fatal arrhythmias is also seen in the observation by Graboys, Lown, Podrid, and DeSilva (1982) that abolishing both ventricular tachycardia and early cycle VPCs with antiarrhythmic drugs reduces sudden death. As has been observed in postinfarction patients, poor prognosis after resuscitation is also predicted by poor left ventricular function (Ptacin, Tresch, Soin, & Brooks, 1982).

Evaluation of the Relationship of Symptoms to Arrhythmias

Since dizziness, syncope, palpitation, and chest pain are commonly sporadic in occurrence, and brief in duration, association of symptoms with transient disorders of rhythm or with repolarization changes is a common goal of ambulatory electrocardiography. However, data bearing on the causal relationship of arrhythmias to symptoms, and to transient alterations of consciousness most specifically, are conflicting.

Qualitative brief rhythm abnormalities often found in symptomatic patients include variant forms of the sick sinus syndrome (Crook, Cash-man, Stott, & Raftery, 1973; Easley & Goldstein, 1970; Ferrer, 1973; Rubenstein, Schulman, Yurchak, & DeSanctis, 1972), such as sinus pauses or the marked sinus overdrive suppression that may follow a brief burst of supraventricular tachycardia, transient high-grade AV block, brief ventricular tachycardia, and occasional examples of pacemaker dysfunction (Phillips & Kligfield, 1983). Although characteristic repolarization abnormalities accompanying effort angina are generally detectable by exercise provocation according to standard protocols, these may also be found with chest pain during ambulatory recording. In addition, in the relatively rare situations where sporadic chest pain related to pure coronary artery spasm is not inducible by laboratory exercise, rather dramatic evidence of transmural ischemia may occasionally be detected. Several studies have suggested good correlation between arrhythmias and sporadic alteration of consciousness. Abdon (1981) examined the ambulatory ECGs in over 100 elderly subjects, and found evidence of sinus node dysfunction, AV block, significant bradycardia, or tachyarrhythmia in nearly half of a subset with prior dizziness or syncope, contrasted with just 6% of the subset with no previous symptoms. Arrhythmias were detected in just over half of a group of 55 patients studied with 24-h ambulatory electrocardiography by Lipski *et al.* (1976) because of syncope, dizziness, or palpitations. Most commonly noted were marked sinus bradycardias, comprising half the arrhythmias, which usually occurred at night and were not of certain relationship to patient symptoms. But approximately one-quarter of the total group had arrhythmias or likely symptomatic association, such as sinus arrest, bradycardia–tachycardia variation, atrial fibrillation with rapid ventricular response, and ventricular tachycardia.

Although it is quite clear that ambulatory electrocardiography can in this way reveal underlying arrhythmias in patients with dizziness and syncope (Boudoulas, Schaal, Lewis, & Robinson, 1979; 1976; Jonas, Klein, & Dimant, 1977; McHenry, Toole, & Miller, Van Durme, 1975), establishment of a cause-and-effect relationship rather than simple association requires either documentation of coincidence or, less convincingly, demonstration of a significant excess prevalence of potentially symptomatic arrhythmia in the population studied. Improvement of chronic symptoms by effective specific therapy of observed bradyarrhythmias or tachyarrhythmias (Levin, 1976; Tzaivoni & Stern, 1975; Walter, Reid, & Kass Wenger, 1970) argues presumptively in favor of a cause-and-effect relationship between rhythm and symptom. Quite clearly, demonstration of normal rhythm during typical symptoms excludes an arrhythmic basis for the patient's complaint, but it is also apparent that absence of arrhythmia during an asymptomatic period is hardly proof of normality.

Uncertainty regarding a conclusive association of symptoms and arrhythmia is seen in the study of Goldberg, Raftery, and Cashman (1975), which demonstrated highly variable atrial and ventricular dysrhythmias, including several dramatic individual episodes of advanced AV block and asystole, in nearly three-quarters of a group of ambulatory patients with dizziness, syncope, or palpitations. However, no attempt was made to correlate symptoms occurring during the recording with specific rhythms, and in the absence of control subjects, attribution of symptoms to arrhythmias, except to the extreme bradyarrhythmias shown, must be considered presumptive.

Among patients with otherwise unexplained dizziness or syncope, the difficulty in attributing symptoms to even apparently major arrhythmias occurring during ambulatory recording was highlighted by Clark, Glasser, and Spoto (1980), who noted no difference in the types of rhythms recorded in patients with or without symptoms occurring during study. Also noted was the rare occurrence of symptoms and arrhythmias in this series. Another striking example of the potential problems associated with attributing symptoms to only possibly related significant rhythm disorders is the demonstration of Dhingra *et al.* (1974) of orthostatic hypotension and seizure, rather than transient advanced heart block, as a relatively common cause of syncope among patients with chronic conduction tissue disease expressed as bifascicular block.

The often striking discrepancy between patient symptoms and arrhythmias detected by ambulatory electrocardiography was well illustrated by Zeldis, Levine, Michelson, and Morganroth (1980). Presenting complaints of syncope, dizziness, palpitations, dyspnea, and chest pain occurred in just under half the recordings of 371 patients, but when symptoms did occur, only about one-quarter could be explained by the ECG, so that overall, about one recording in eight in this series successfully correlated symptoms with an arrhythmia.

However, the lack of association of potentially significant arrhythmias during 24-h recording with concurrent symptoms by no means excludes their relationship at other times. Abdon, Johansson, and Lessem (1982) found that over two-thirds of patients with a significant arrhythmia during an initially asymptomatic period of recording could later be shown to have the same arrhythmia during symptoms. In this population, "significant" arrhythmias were found to be various expressions of the sick sinus syndrome, atrial tachycardias, advanced AV block, and frequent or complex ventricular ectopy.

Evaluation of Symptomatic and Asymptomatic Myocardial Ischemia

The application of ambulatory electrocardiography to the evaluation of myocardial ischemia requires consideration of several potentially limiting factors. First, the sensitivity of standard laboratory exercise electrocardiography for the detection of significant obstructive coronary artery disease is relatively poor, ranging in most centers from 60 to 70% (Bartel, Behar, Peter, Orgain, & Kong, 1974; Goldschlager, Selzer, & Cohn, 1976). Second, the generally higher specificity of exercise electrocardiography, which approximates 90%, still results in significant false-positive diagnoses in otherwise normal subjects. Third, application of even a highly specific test to a population with a low prevalence of disease leads to major predictive error and tends to produce fewer true-positive than false-positive test results (Diamond & Forrester, 1979; Rifkin & Hood, 1977). And, finally, the frequency response of recording and playback equipment must be adequate for accurate representation of repolarization (Balasubramanian, Lahiri, Green,

Stott, & Raftery, 1980; Bragg-Remschel, Anderson, & Winkle, 1982; Stern & Tzivoni, 1972).

Of 50 patients with chest pain studied with coronary angiography by Stern, Tzivoni, and Stern (1975), 31 had greater than 60% coronary obstruction of one or more vessels. In this population, ST segment shifts of 1 mm or T wave inversion on ambulatory electrocardiography were highly sensitive (90%) but less specific (79%) for identifying significant coronary obstruction. Although overall predictive accuracy in this study was good, it is essential to consider the major effect that the 21% false-positive rate would have on populations with a lower prevalence of ischemic disease. Simple calculation from these data demonstrates that in a population with a 10% prevalence of disease, identification of coronary artery disease by repolarization changes detected on ambulatory recording would result in twice as many false-positive as true-positive test responses. Of course, this accuracy would be improved by incorporating other clinical data such as the quality of pain, sex, and age (Diamond & Forrester, 1979).

Substantially lower sensitivity (62%) and specificity (61%) of ambulatory electrocardiography for detecting coronary artery disease were found by Crawford et al. (1978) in 70 patients with chest pain suggestive of ischemia and normal standard ECGs. The false-positive findings in these studies are similar to the 16% postural repolarization changes reported by Lachman, Semler, and Gustafson (1965) and the 30% prevalence of transient T wave inversion found among normal men by Armstrong, Jordan, Morris, and McHenry (1982). However, using frequency-modulated ambulatory recordings, Deanfield, Ribiero, Oakley, Krikler, and Selwyn (1984) found that while 36% of asymptomatic, clinically normal subjects demonstrated upsloping ST segment depression during rapid heart rates, only 2% had the horizontal or downsloping ST segment depression that is characteristically associated with myocardial ischemia. Differences among these studies may be explained in part by patient selection and by recording methodology.

On the other hand, specificity is far less an influence on predictive accuracy in populations with high disease prevalence. Allen, Gettes, Phalan, and Avington (1976) reported the absence of symptoms during nearly two-thirds of episodes of ST depression among patients with angina and positive exercise ECGs, an observation confirmed by Cecchi et al. (1983) and Schang and Pepine (1977). These findings suggest that in some situations, the ambulatory ECG may be more sensitive than anginal symptoms for the detection of ischemia. Improved predictive accuracy of ambulatory electrocardiographic repolarization changes in homogeneously diseased populations is also seen in the patients admitted to a coronary care unit because of unstable angina as reported by Biagini et al. (1982). In this group, only 12% of episodes of ST segment elevation, ST segment depression, or T wave alteration were associated with symptoms, and coronary injection during asymptomatic transient repolarization abnormalities demonstrated spontaneous coronary spasm in six of eight patients. Since coronary artery tone is influenced by autonomic innervation, these observations suggest a potential role of behavioral factors in the pathophysiology of angina pectoris. Asymptomatic, or "silent" ischemia detected by continuous electrocardiographic recording has been found in additional recent studies of patients with unstable angina to be more common than previously suspected and to be associated with a higher risk of advanced coronary obstruction and unfavorable clinical outcome (Gottlieb, Weisfeldt, Ouyang, Mellits, & Gerstenblith, 1986; Johnson et al., 1982). But the high pretest likelihood of severe disease in these populations must be emphasized.

References

Abdon, N.-J. (1981). Frequency and distribution of long-term ECG-recorded cardiac arrhythmias in an elderly population. *Acta Medica Scandinavica, 209,* 175–183.

Abdon, N.-J., Johansson, B. W., & Lessem, J. (1982). Predictive use of 24-hour electrocardiography in suspected Adams–Stokes syndrome: Comparison with cardiac rhythm during symptoms. *British Heart Journal, 47,* 553–558.

Allen, R. D., Gettes, L. S., Phalan, C., & Avington, M. D. (1976). Painless ST-segment depression in patients with angina pectoris: "Correlation with daily activities and cigarette smoking. *Chest, 69,* 467–473.

Armstrong, W. F., Jordan, J. W., Morris, S. N., & McHenry, P. L. (1982). Prevalence and magnitude of S-T segment and

T wave abnormalities in normal men during continuous ambulatory electrocardiography. *American Journal of Cardiology, 49,* 1638–1642.

Balasubramanian, V., Lahiri, A., Green, H. L., Stott, F. D., & Raftery, E. G. (1980). Ambulatory ST segment monitoring: Problems, pitfalls, solutions, and clinical application. *British Heart Journal, 44,* 419.

Bartel, A. G., Behar, V. S., Peter, R. H., Orgain, E. S., & Kong, Y. (1974). Graded exercise stress tests in angiographically documented coronary artery disease. *Circulation, 49,* 348–356.

Biagini, A., Mazzei, M. G., Carpeggiani, C., Testa, R., Antonelli, R., Michelassi, C., L'Abbate, A., & Maseri, A. (1982). Vasospastic ischemic mechanism of frequent asymptomatic transient ST-T changes during continuous electrocardiographic monitoring in selected unstable angina patients. *American Heart Journal, 103,* 13–20.

Bigger, J. T., & Weld, F. M. (1981). Analysis of prognostic significance of ventricular arrhythmias after myocardial infarction: Shortcomings of Lown grading system. *British Heart Journal, 45,* 717–724.

Bigger, J. T., Giardina, E. G. V., Perel, J. M., Kantor, S. J., & Glassman, A. H. (1977). Cardiac antiarrhythmic effect of imipramin hydrochloride. *New England Journal of Medicine, 296,* 206–208.

Bigger, J. T., Heller, C. A., Wenger, T. L., & Weld, F. M. (1978). Risk stratification after acute myocardial infarction. *American Journal of Cardiology, 42,* 202–210.

Bjarnason, L., Hardarson, T., & Jonsson, S. (1982). Cardiac arrhythmias in hypertrophic cardiomyopathy. *British Heart Journal, 48,* 198–203.

Bleifer, S. B., Bleifer, D. J., Hansmann, D. R., Sheppard, J. J., & Karpamn, H. L. (1974). Diagnosis of occult arrhythmias by Holter electrocardiography. *Progress in Cardiovascular Diseases, 16,* 569–599.

Borer, J. S., Rosing, D. R., Miller, R. H., Stark, R. M., Kent, K. M., Bacharach, S. L., Green, M. V., Lake, C. R., Cohen, H., Holmes, D., Donohue, D., Baker, W., & Epstein, S. E. (1980). Natural history of left ventricular function during 1 year after acute myocardial infarction: Comparison with clinical, electrocardiographic and biochemical determinations. *American Journal of Cardiology, 46,* 1–12.

Boudoulas, H., Schaal, S. F., Lewis, R. P., & Robinson, J. L. (1979). Superiority of 24-hour outpatient monitoring over multi-stage exercise testing for the evaluation of syncope. *Journal of Electrocardiology, 12,* 103–108.

Bragg-Remschel, D. A., Anderson, C. M., & Winkle, R. A. (1982). Frequency response characteristics of ambulatory ECG monitoring systems and their implications for ST segment analysis. *American Heart Journal, 103,* 20–31.

Brodsky, M., Wu, D., Denes, P., Kanakis, C., & Rosen, K. M. (1977). Arrhythmias documented by 24 hour continuous electrocardiographic monitoring in 50 male medical students without apparent heart disease. *American Journal of Cardiology, 39,* 390–395.

Califf, R. M., Burks, J. M., Behar, V. S., Margolis, J. R., & Wagner, G. S. (1977). Relationships among ventricular arrhythmias, coronary artery disease, and angiographic and electrocardiographic indicators of myocardial fibrosis. *Circulation, 57,* 725–732.

Califf, R. M., McKinnis, R. A., Burks, J., Lee, K. L., Harrell, F. E., Behar, V. S., Pryor, D. B., Wagner, G. S., & Rosati, R. A. (1982). Prognostic implications of ventricular arrhythmias during 24 hour ambulatory monitoring in patients undergoing cardiac catheterization for coronary artery disease. *American Journal of Cardiology, 50,* 23–31.

Calvert, A., Lown, B., & Gorlin, R. (1977). Ventricular premature beats and anatomically defined coronary heart disease. *American Journal of Cardiology, 39,* 627–634.

Camm, A. J., Evans, K. E., Ward, E. D., & Martin, A. (1980). The rhythm of the heart in active elderly subjects. *American Heart Journal, 99,* 598–603.

Canedo, M. I., Frank, M. J., & Abdulla, A. M. (1980). Rhythm disturbances in hypertrophic cardiomyopathy: Prevalence, relation to symptoms and management. *American Journal of Cardiology, 45,* 848–855.

Cecchi, A. C., Dovellini, E. V., Marchi, F., Pucci, P., Santoro, G. M., & Fazzini, P. F. (1983). Silent myocardial ischemia during ambulatory electrocardiographic monitoring in patients with effort angina. *Journal of the American College of Cardiology, 1,* 934–939.

Chiang, B. N., Perlman, L. V., Ostrander, L. D., & Epstein, F. H. (1969). Relationship of premature systoles to coronary heart disease and sudden death in the Tecumseh epidemiologic study. *Annals of Internal Medicine, 70,* 1159–1166.

Chiang, B. N., Perlman, L. V., Fulton, M., Ostrander, L. D., & Epstein, F. H. (1970). Predisposing factors in sudden cardiac death in Tecumseh, Michigan: A prospective study. *Circulation, 41,* 31–37.

Clark, P. I., Glasser, S. P., & Spoto, E. (1980). Arrhythmias detected by ambulatory monitoring: Lack of correlation with symptoms of dizziness and syncope. *Chest, 77,* 722–725.

Clarke, J. M., Shelton, J. R., Hamer, J., Tayler, S., & Venning, G. R. (1976). The rhythm of the normal human heart. *Lancet, 2,* 508–512.

Colton, T. (1974). *Statistics in medicine* (pp. 219–227). Boston: Little, Brown.

Corday, E., Bazika, V., Lang, T.-W., Pappelbaum, S., Gold, H., & Bernstein H. (1965). Detection of phantom arrhythmias and evanescent electrocardiographic abnormalities. *Journal of the American Medical Association, 193,* 417–421.

Coronary Drug Project Research Group; prepared by Tominaga, S., & Blackburn, H. (1973). Prognostic importance of premature beats following myocardial infarction: experience in the Coronary Drug Project. *Journal of the American Medical Association, 223,* 1116–1124.

Crawford, M. H., Mendoza, C. A., O'Rourke, R. A., White, D. H., Boucher, C. A., & Gorwit, J. (1978). Limitations of continuous ambulatory electrocardiogram monitoring for detecting coronary artery disease. *Annals of Internal Medicine, 89,* 1–5.

Crook, B. R. M., Cashman, P. M. M., Stott, F. D., & Raftery,

E. B. (1973). Tape monitoring of the electrocardiogram in ambulant patients with sinoatrial disease. *British Heart Journal, 35,* 1009–1013.

Deanfield, J. E., Ribiero, P., Oakley, K., Krikler, S., & Selwyn, A. P. (1984). Analysis of ST-segment changes in normal subjects: Implications for ambulatory monitoring in angina pectoris. *American Journal of Cardiology, 54,* 1321–1325.

DeMaria, A. N., Amsterdam, E. A., Vismara, L. A., Neumann, A., & Mason, D. T. (1976). Arrhythmias in the mitral valve prolapse syndrome: Prevalence, nature, and frequency. *Annals of Internal Medicine, 84,* 656–660.

Denes, P., Gabster, A., & Huang, S. K. (1981). Clinical, electrocardiographic and follow-up observations in patients having ventricular fibrillation during Holter monitoring: Role of quinidine therapy. *American Journal of Cardiology, 48,* 9–16.

Desai, D. C., Hershberg, P. L., & Alexander, S. (1973). Clinical significance of ventricular premature beats in an outpatient population. *Chest, 64,* 564–569.

De Soyza, N., Shapiro, W., Chandraratna, P. A. N., Aronow, W. S., Laddu, A. R., & Thompson, C. H. (1982). Acebutolol therapy for ventricular arrhythmia: A randomized, placebo-controlled, double-blind study. *Circulation, 65,* 1129–1133.

Dhingra, R. C., Denes, P., Wu, D., Chuquimia, R., Amat-Y-Leon, F., Wyndham, C., & Rosen, K. M. (1974). Syncope in patients with chronic bifascicular block: Significance, causative mechanisms, and clinical implications. *Annals of Internal Medicine, 81,* 302–306.

Diamond, G. A., & Forrester, J. S. (1979). Analysis of probability as an aid in the clinical diagnosis of coronary-artery disease. *New England Journal of Medicine, 300,* 1350–1358.

DiBianco, R., Fletcher, R. D., Cohen, A. I., Gottdiener, J. S., Singh, S. N., Katz, R. J., Bates, H. R., & Sauerbrunn, B. (1982). Treatment of frequent ventricular arrhythmia with encainide: Assessment using serial ambulatory electrocardiograms, intracardiac electrophysiologic studies, treadmill exercise tests, and radionuclide cineangiographic studies. *Circulation, 65,* 1134–1147.

Dungan, W. T., Gardon, A., & Gillette, P. C. (1981). Arrhythmogenic right ventricular dysplasia: A cause of ventricular tachycardia in children with apparently normal hearts. *American Heart Journal, 102,* 754–750.

Easley, R. M., & Goldstein, S. (1970). Sino-atrial syncope. *American Journal of Medicine, 50,* 166–176.

El-Sherif, N., Myerburg, R. J., Scherlag, B. J., Befeler, B., Aranda, J. M., Castellanos, A., & Lazzara, R. (1976). Electrocardiographic antecedents of primary ventricular fibrillation: Value of the R-on-T phenomenon in myocardial infarction. *British Heart Journal, 38,* 415–422.

Ferrer, M. I. (1973). The sick sinus syndrome. *Circulation, 47,* 635–641.

Gilson, J. S., Holter, N. J., & Glasscock, W. R. (1964). Clinical observations using the electrocardiocorder–AVSEP continuous electrocardiographic system: Tentative standards and typical patterns. *American Journal of Cardiology, 14,* 204–217.

Glasser, S. P., Clark, P. I., & Applebaum, H. J. (1979). Occurrence of frequent complex arrhythmias detected by ambulatory monitoring: Findings in an apparently healthy asymptomatic elderly population. *Chest, 75,* 565–568.

Goldberg, A. D., Raftery, E. B., & Cashman, P. M. M. (1975). Ambulatory electrocardiographic records in patients with transient cerebral attacks or palpitation. *British Medical Journal, 4,* 569–571.

Goldschlager, N., Selzer, A., & Cohn, K. (1976). Treadmill stress tests as indicators of presence and severity of coronary artery disease. *Annals of Internal Medicine, 85,* 277–286.

Gottlieb, S. O., Weisfeldt, M. L., Ouyang, P., Mellits, E. D., & Gerstenblith, G. (1986). Silent ischemia as a marker for early unfavorable outcomes in patients with unstable angina. *New England Journal of Medicine, 314,* 1214–1219.

Graboys, T. B., Lown, B., Podrid, P. J., & DeSilva, R. (1982). Long-term survival of patients with malignant ventricular arrhythmia treated with antiarrhythmic drugs. *American Journal of Cardiology, 50,* 437–443.

Gradman, A. H., Bell, P. A., & DeBusk, R. F. (1977). Sudden death during ambulatory monitoring: Clinical and electrocardiographic correlations: report of a case. *Circulation, 55,* 210–211.

Hindman, M. C., Last, J. H., & Rosen, K. M. (1973). Wolff–Parkinson–White syndrome observed by portable monitoring. *Annals of Internal Medicine, 79,* 654–663.

Hinkle, L. E. (1981). The immediate antecedents of sudden death. *Acta Medica Scandinavica, 210,*(Suppl. 651), 207–217.

Hinkle, L. E., & Thaler, H. T. (1982). Clinical classification of cardiac deaths. *Circulation, 65,* 457–464.

Hinkle, L. E., Meyer, J., Stevens, M., & Carver, S. T. (1967). Tape recordings of the ECG of active men: Limitations and advantages of the Holter–Avionics instruments. *Circulation, 36,* 752–765.

Hinkle, L. E., Carver, S. T., & Stevens, M. (1969). The frequency of asymptomatic disturbances of cardiac rhythm and conduction in middle-aged men. *American Journal of Cardiology, 24,* 629–650.

Hinkle, L. E., Argyros, D. C., Hayes, J. C., Robinson, T., Alonso, D. R., Shipman, S. C., & Edwards M. E. (1977). Pathogenesis of an unexpected sudden death: Role of early cycle ventricular premature contractions. *American Journal of Cardiology, 39,* 873–879.

Hochreiter, C., Niles, N., Devereux, R. B., Kligfield, P., & Borer, J. S. (1986). Mitral regurgitation: Relationship of non-invasive right and left ventricular performance descriptors to clinical and hemodynamic findings and to prognosis in medically and surgically treated patients. *Circulation, 73,* 900–912.

Hodges, M., Haugland, J. M., Granrud, G., Conard, G. J., Asinger, R. W., Mikell, F. L., & Krejci, J. (1982). Suppression of ventricular ectopic depolarizations by flecainide acetate, a new antiarrhythmic agent. *Circulation, 65,* 879–884.

Holmes, J., Kubo, S. H., Cody, R. J., & Kligfield, P. (1985).

Arrhythmias in ischemic and nonischemic dilated cardiomyopathy: Prediction of mortality by ambulatory electrocardiography. *American Journal of Cardiology, 55,* 146–151.

Holter, N. J. (1961). New method for heart studies. *Science, 134,* 1214–1220.

Isaeff, D. M., Gaston, J. H., & Harrison, D. C. (1972). Wolff–Parkinson–White syndrome: Long-term monitoring for arrhythmias. *Journal of the American Medical Association, 222,* 449–453.

Iyengar, R., Castellanos, A., & Spence, M. (1971). Continuous monitoring of ambulatory patients with coronary disease. *Progress in Cardiovascular Diseases, 13,* 392–404.

Johnson, S. M., Mauritson, D. R., Winniford, M. D., Willerson, J. T., Firth, B. G., Cary, J. R., & Hillis, L. D. (1982). Continuous electrocardiographic monitoring in patients with unstable angina pectoris: Identification of high-risk subgroup with severe coronary disease, variant angina, and/or impaired early prognosis. *American Heart Journal, 103,* 4–12.

Jones, S., Klein, I., & Dimant, J. (1977). Importance of Holter monitoring in patients with periodic cerebral symptoms. *Annals of Neurology, 1,* 470–474.

Kantelip, J.-P., Sage, E., & Duchene-Marullaz, P. (1986). Findings on ambulatory electrocardiographic monitoring in subjects older than 80 years. *American Journal of Cardiology, 57,* 398–401.

Kennedy, H. L. (1981). *Ambulatory electrocardiography, including Holter recording technology.* Philadelphia: Lea & Febiger.

Kennedy, H. L., Chandra, V., Sayther, K. L., & Carasis, D. G. (1978). Effectiveness of increasing hours of continuous ambulatory electrocardiography in detecting maximal ventricular ectopy: Continuous 48 hour study of patients with coronary heart disease and normal subjects. *American Journal of Cardiology, 42,* 925–930.

Kennedy, H. L., Whitlock, J. A., Sprague, M. K., Kennedy, L. J., Buckingham, T. A., & Goldberg, R. J. (1985). Long-term follow-up of asymptomatic healthy subjects with frequent and complex ventricular ectopy. *New England Journal of Medicine, 312,* 193–197.

Kligfield, P. (1984). Clinical applications of ambulatory electrocardiography. *Cardiology, 71,* 69–99.

Kotler, M. N., Tabatznik, B., Mower, M. M., & Tominaga, S. (1973). Prognostic significance of ventricular ectopic beats with respect to sudden death in the late post-infarction period. *Circulation, 47,* 959–966.

Kramer, H. M., Kligfield, P., Devereux, R. B., Savage, D. D., & Kramer-Fox, R. (1984). Arrhythmias in mitral valve prolapse: Effect of selection bias. *Archives of Internal Medicine, 144,* 2360–2364.

Krone, R. J., Miller, J. P., Kleiger, R. E., Clark, K. W., & Oliver, G. C. (1981). The effectiveness of antiarrhythmic agents on early-cycle premature ventricular complexes. *Circulation, 63,* 664–669.

Lachman, A. G., Semler, J. H., & Gustafson, R. H. (1965). Postural ST-T wave changes in the radioelectrocardiogram simulating myocardial ischemia. *Circulation, 31,* 557–563.

Levin, E. B. (1976). Use of the Holter electrocardiographic monitor in the diagnosis of transient ischemic attacks. *Journal of the American Geriatrics Society, 24,* 516–521.

Lipski, J., Cohen, L., Espinoza, J., Motro, M., Dack, S., & Donoso, E. (1976). Value of Holter monitoring in assessing cardiac arrhythmias in symptomatic patients. *American Journal of Cardiology, 37,* 102–107.

Lopes, M. G., Runge, P., Harrison, D. C., & Schroeder, J. S. (1975). Comparison of 24 versus 12 hours of ambulatory ECG monitoring. *Chest, 67,* 269–273.

Lown, B., & Graboys, T. B. (1977). Management of patients with malignant ventricular arrhythmias. *American Journal of Cardiology, 39,* 910–918.

Lown, B., & Wolf, M. (1971). Approaches to sudden death from coronary heart disease. *Circulation, 44,* 130–142.

Lown, B., Calvert, A. F., Armington, R., & Ryan, M. (1975). Monitoring for serious arrhythmias and high risk of sudden death. *Circulation, 51/52*(Suppl. III), 189–198.

Luria, M. H., Knoke, J. D., Wachs, J. S., & Luria, M. A. (1979). Survival after recovery from acute myocardial infarction: Two and five year prognostic indices. *American Journal of Medicine, 67,* 7–14.

Mark, R. G., & Ripley, K. L. (1985). Ambulatory ECG monitoring: Real-time analysis versus tape scanning systems. *MD Computing: Computers in medical practice, 2,* 38–50.

McHenry, L. C., Toole, J. F., & Miller, H. S. (1976). Long-term EKG monitoring in patients with cerebrovascular insufficiency. *Stroke, 7,* 264–269.

McKenna, W. J., Chetty, S., Oakley, C. M., & Goodwin, J. F. (1980). Arrhythmia in hypertrophic cardiomyopathy: Exercise and 48 hour ambulatory electrocardiographic assessment with and without beta adrenergic blocking therapy. *American Journal of Cardiology, 45,* 1–5.

McKenna, W. J., England, D., Doi, Y. L., Deanfield, J. E., Oakley, C., & Goodwin, J. F. (1981). Arrhythmia in hypertrophic cardiomyopathy. I. Influence on prognosis. *British Heart Journal, 46,* 168–172.

McKenna, W. J., Harris, L., Perez, G., Krikler, D. M., Oakley, C., & Goodwin, J. F. (1981). Arrhythmia in hypertrophic cardiomyopathy. II. Comparison of amiodarone and verapamil in treatment. *British Heart Journal, 46,* 173–178.

Messineo, F. C., Al-Hani, A. J., & Katz, A. M. (1981). The relationship between frequent and complex ventricular ectopy during 24 h ambulatory electrocardiographic monitoring. *Cardiology, 68,* 91–102.

Meyerburg, R. J., Conde, C. A., Sung, R. J., Mayorga-Cortes, A., Mallon, S. M., Sheps, D. S., Appel, R. A., & Castellanos, A. (1980). Clinical, electrophysiologic and hemodynamic profile of patients resuscitated from prehospital cardiac arrest. *American Journal of Medicine, 68,* 568–576.

Morganroth, J., Michelson, E. L., Horowitz, L. N., Josephson, M. E., Pearlman, A. S., & Dunkman, W. B. (1976). Limitations of routine long-term electrocardiographic monitoring to assess ventricular ectopic frequency. *Circulation, 58,* 408–414.

Moss, A. J. (1980). Clinical significance of ventricular arrhythmias in patients with and without coronary artery disease. *Progress in Cardiovascular Diseases, 23,* 33–52.

Moss, A. J., Schnitzler, R., Green, R., & DeCamilla, J. (1971). Ventricular arrhythmias 3 weeks after acute myocardial infarction. *Annals of Internal Medicine, 75,* 837–841.

Moss, A. J., DeCamilla, J., Mietlowski, W., Greene, W. A., Goldstein, S., & Locksley, R. (1975). Prognostic grading and significance of ventricular premature beats after recovery from myocardial infarction. *Circulation, 51/52*(Suppl. III), 204–210.

Moss, A. J., Davis, H. T., DeCamilla, J., & Bayer, L. W. (1979). Ventricular ectopic beats and their relation to sudden and nonsudden cardiac death after myocardial infarction. *Circulation, 60,* 998–1003.

Nikolic, G., Bishop, R. L., & Singh, J. B. (1982). Sudden death recorded during Holter monitoring. *Circulation, 66,* 218–225.

O'Brien, I. A. D., O'Hare, P., & Corrall, R. J. M. (1986). Heart rate variability in healthy subjects: Effect of age and the derivation of normal ranges for tests of autonomic function. *British Heart Journal, 55,* 348–354.

Palileo, E. V., Ashley, W. W., Swiryn, S., Bauernfeind, R. A., Strasberg, B., Petropoulos, A. T., & Rosen, K. M. (1982). Exercise provocable right ventricular outflow tract tachycardia. *American Heart Journal, 104,* 185–193.

Phillips, P. L., & Kligfield, P. (1983). Myopotential interference with unipolar pacemakers: Recognition and detection by ambulatory electrocardiography. *Cardiovascular Reviews and Reports, 4,* 1185–1190.

Pickering, T. G., Johnston, J., & Honour, A. J. (1978). Comparison of the effects of sleep, exercise and autonomic drugs on ventricular extrasystoles, using ambulatory monitoring of electrocardiogram and electroencephalogram. *American Journal of Medicine, 65,* 575–583.

Pipberger, H. V., Arzbaecher, R. C., Berson, A. S., Briller, S. A., Brody, D. A., Flowers, N. C., Geselowitz, D. B., Lebeschkin, E., Oliver, G. C., Schmitt, O. H., & Spach, M. (1975). Recommendations for standardization of leads and of specifications for instruments in electrocardiography and vector-cardiography. Report of the Committee on Electrocardiography, American Heart Association. *Circulation, 52,* 11.

Ptacin, M. J., Tresch, D. D., Soin, J. S., & Brooks, H. L. (1982). Evaluation of postresuscitation left ventricular global and segmental function by radionuclide ventriculography in sudden coronary death survivors of prehospital cardiac arrest: Correlation to subsequent short-term prognosis. *American Heart Journal, 100,* 54–56.

Rifkin, R. D., & Hood, W. B. (1977). Bayesian analysis of electrocardiographic exercise stress testing. *New England Journal of Medicine, 297,* 681–686.

Rocchini, A. P., Chun, P. O., & Dick, M. (1981). Ventricular tachycardia in children. *American Journal of Cardiology, 47,* 1091–1097.

Rodstein, M., Wolloch, L., & Gubner, R. S. (1971). Mortality study of the significance of extrasystoles in an insured population. *Circulation, 44,* 617–625.

Rubenstein, J. J., Schulman, C. L., Yurchak, P. M., & DeSanctis, R. W. (1972). Clinical spectrum of the sick sinus syndrome. *Circulation, 46,* 5–13.

Ruberman, W., Weinblatt, E., Goldberg, J. D., Frank, C. W., & Shapiro, S. (1977). Ventricular premature beats and mortality after myocardial infarction. *New England Journal of Medicine, 14,* 750–757.

Ruberman, W., Weinblatt, E., Goldberg, J. D., Frank, C. W., Shapiro, S., & Chaudhary, B. S. (1980). Ventricular premature complexes in prognosis of angina. *Circulation, 61,* 1172–1178.

Ruberman, W., Weinblatt, E., Goldberg, J. D., Frank, C. W., Chaudhary, B. S., & Shapiro, S. (1981). Ventricular premature complexes and sudden death after myocardial infarction. *Circulation, 64,* 297–305.

Ryan, M., Lown, B., & Horn, H. (1975). Comparison of ventricular ectopic activity during 24-hour monitoring and exercise testing in patients with coronary heart disease. *New England and Journal of Medicine, 292,* 224–229.

Sami, M., Kraemer, H., Harrison, D. C., Houston, N., Shimasaki, C., & DeBusk, R. F. (1980). A new method for evaluating antiarrhythmic drug efficacy. *Circulation, 62,* 1172–1179.

Savage, D. D., Seides, S. F., Maron, B. J., Myers, D. J., & Epstein, S. E. (1979). Prevalence of arrhythmias during 24-hour electrocardiographic monitoring and exercise testing in patients with obstructive and nonobstructive hypertrophic cardiomyopathy. *Circulation, 59,* 866–875.

Savage, D. D., Levy, D. L., Garrison, R. J., Castelli, W. P., Kligfield, P., Devereux, R. B., Anderson, S. J., Kannel, W. B., & Feinleib, M. (1983). Mitral valve prolapse in the general population, part 3: dysrhythmias. The Framingham Study. *American Heart Journal, 106,* 582–586.

Schaffer, W. A., & Cobb, L. A. (1975). Recurrent ventricular fibrillation and modes of death in survivors of out-of-hospital ventricular fibrillation. *New England Journal of Medicine, 293,* 259–262.

Schang, S. J., Jr., & Pepine, C. J. (1977). Transient asymptomatic S-T segment depression during daily activity. *American Journal of Cardiology, 39,* 396–402.

Schulze, R. A., Strauss, H. W., & Pitt, B. (1977). Sudden death in the year following myocardial infarction: Relation to ventricular premature contractions in the late hospital phase and left ventricular ejection fraction. *American Journal of Medicine, 62,* 192–199.

Shear, M. K., Kligfield, P., Devereux, R. B., Hashfield, G., Polan, J., Frances, A., Mann, J., & Pickering, T. G. (1987). Cardiac rate and rhythm in panic disorder patients. *American Journal of Psychiatry, 144,* 633–637.

Smith, S. E., & Smith, S. A. (1981). Heart rate variability in healthy subjects measured with a bedside computer-based technique. *Clinical Science, 61,* 379–383.

Sobotka, P. A., Mayer, J. H., Bauernfeind, R. A., Kanakis, C., & Rosen, K. M. (1981). Arrhythmias documented by 24-hour continuous ambulatory electrocardiographic monitoring in young women without apparent heart disease. *American Heart Journal, 101,* 753–758.

Southall, D. P., Richards, J., Mitchell, P., Brown, D. J., Johnston, P. G. B., & Shinebourne, E. A. (1980). Study of cardiac rhythm in healthy newborn infants. *British Heart Journal, 43,* 14–20.

Southall, D. P., Johnston, F., Shinebourne, E. A., & Johnston, P. G. B. (1981). 24-hour electrocardiographic study of heart rate and rhythm patterns in population of healthy children. *British Heart Journal, 45,* 281–291.

Stern, S., & Tzivoni, D. (1972). The reliability of the Holter–Avionics system in reproducing the ST-T segment. *American Heart Journal, 84,* 427–428.

Stern, S., Tzivoni, D., & Stern, Z. (1975). Diagnostic accuracy of ambulatory ECG monitoring in ischemic heart disease. *Circulation, 52,* 1045–1049.

Taylor, G. J., Humphries, J. O., Mellits, E. D., Pitt, B., Schulze, R. A., Griffith, L. S. C., & Achuff, S. C. (1980). Predictors of clinical course, coronary anatomy and left ventricular function after recovery from acute myocardial infarction. *Circulation, 62,* 960–970.

Tzivoni, D., & Stern, S. (1975). Pacemaker implantation based on ambulatory ECG monitoring in patients with cerebral symptoms. *Chest, 67,* 274–278.

Van Durme, J. P. (1975). Tachyarrhythmias and transient cerebral ischemic attacks. *Annotations, 89,* 538–540.

Velebit, V., Podrid, P., Lown, B., Cohen, B. H., & Graboys, T. B. (1982). Aggravation and provocation of ventricular arrhythmias by antiarrhythmic drugs. *Circulation, 65,* 886–894.

Vismara, L. A., Vera, Z., Foerster, J. M., Amsterdam, E. A., & Mason, D. T. (1977). Identification of sudden death risk factors in acute and chronic coronary artery disease. *American Journal of Cardiology, 39,* 821–828.

Walter, B. F., Reid, S. D., & Kass Wenger, N. (1970). Transient cerebral ischemia due to arrhythmia. *Annals of Internal Medicine, 72,* 471–474.

Weaver, W. D., Cobb, L. A., & Hallstrom, A. P. (1982). Ambulatory arrhythmias in resuscitated victims of cardiac arrest. *Circulation, 66,* 212–218.

Winkle, R. A. (1978). Antiarrhythmic drug effect mimicked by spontaneous variability of ventricular ectopy. *Circulation, 57,* 1116–1121.

Winkle, R. A. (1980). Ambulatory electrocardiography and the diagnosis, evaluation, and treatment of chronic ventricular arrhythmias. *Progress in Cardiovascular Diseases, 23,* 99–128.

Winkle, R. A. (1981). Current status of ambulatory electrocardiography. *American Heart Journal, 4,* 757–770.

Winkle, R. A., Lopes, M. G., Fitzgerald, J. W., Goodman, D. J., Schroeder, J. S., & Harrison, D. C. (1975). Arrhythmias in patients with mitral valve prolapse. *Circulation, 52,* 73–81.

Winkle, R. A., Gradman, A. H., Fitzgerald, J. W., & Bell, P. A. (1978). Antiarrhythmic drug effect assessed from ventricular arrhythmia reduction in the ambulatory electrocardiogram and treadmill test: Comparison of propranolol, procainamide and quinidine. *American Journal of Cardiology, 42,* 473–480.

Woosley, R. L., Kornhauser, D., Smith, R., Reele, S., Higgins, S. B., Nies, A. S., Shand, D. G., & Oates, J. A. (1979). Suppression of chronic ventricular arrhythmias with propranolol. *Circulation, 60,* 819–827.

Zeldis, S. M., Levine, B. J., Michelson, E. L., & Morganroth, J. (1980). Cardiovascular complaints: Correlation with cardiac arrhythmias on 24-hour electrocardiographic monitoring. *Chest, 78,* 456–462.

CHAPTER 18

Research Techniques for Ambulatory Blood Pressure Monitoring

Gregory A. Harshfield, Chun Hwang, Seymour G. Blank, and Thomas G. Pickering

Introduction

The technique of ambulatory blood pressure and heart rate monitoring allows the behavioral scientist to directly assess the physiological impact of normal psychological functioning rather than relying on inferences based upon laboratory studies or self-reports. Just as any other technique, it requires knowledge, patience, practice, and attention to detail. In this chapter we try to provide the user with insights we have gained through our experience over the last eight years. We also try to provide the novice user with a background in ambulatory blood pressure and heart rate monitoring and suggest ways in which the use of the technique can be expanded.

Instrumentation

The first ambulatory blood pressure and heart rate unit was developed by Stott and his colleagues (Bevan, Honour, & Stott, 1969). The Oxford Medilog recorder (Oxford Instruments, Oxford, U.K.) is an invasive system which requires the subject to have a small catheter in his or her arm throughout the recording procedure. The invasive nature of the unit has severely limited its use and therefore it will not be discussed in detail in this chapter. There are currently nine automatic noninvasive ambulatory blood pressure and heart rate recording systems available: the Remler M2000 (Remler, San Francisco, CA); the Spacelabs 5200 and 90202 (Spacelabs, Seattle, WA); Pressurometer II, III, and IV (Del Mar Avionics, Irvine, CA); the Accutracker (Suntech, Chapel Hill, NC); the ABPM-630 (Colin Medical Instruments, South Plainfield, NJ); and the Applause (Diagnostic Medical Instruments, Syracuse, NY). There are several important considerations to take into account prior to the purchase of a system. These will be discussed briefly along with our experiences where appropriate. The discussion will remain as general as possible rather than focusing on specific systems now available.

Gregory A. Harshfield • Department of Pediatrics, University of Tennessee, Memphis, Tennessee 38103.   *Chun Hwang* • Hypertension Center, Department of Medicine, Charles R. Drew Postgraduate Medical School, Los Angeles, California 90059.   *Seymour G. Blank and Thomas G. Pickering* • Department of Medicine, Cardiovascular Center, The New York Hospital–Cornell Medical Center, New York, New York 10021.

Accuracy

Validation studies have been performed on the Remler M2000. In one study on 12 normotensives (Waeber, Jacot-des-Combes, Porchet, & Brunner, 1984), correlations of 0.95 for systolic and 0.85 for diastolic pressure were found between readings obtained by the recorder and a human observer. In addition, ''most'' of the readings were within ± 4mm Hg. In another study of 35 subjects (Fitzgerald, O'Callaghan, McQuaid, O'Malley, & O'Brian, 1982), correlations of 0.98 for systolic and 0.97 for diastolic pressure were found.

The validation data on the Spacelabs 5200 are less extensive. In our study (Harshfield, *et al.*, 1984) on 48 subjects, we found a correlation between the recorder and a technician of 0.97 for systolic and 0.95 for diastolic pressure. In a more recent study (Light, Obrist, & Cobeddu, 1988) on 27 subjects, the median correlation was 0.83 for systolic and 0.77 for diastolic pressure. There has been one preliminary validation study performed on the Spacelabs 90202 (Santucci, Steiner, Zimbler, James, & Pickering, 1988). A total of 27 normotensive and hypertensive subjects were studied. There was an average difference between the observer and the 90202 of + 1.1 mm Hg for systolic and −2.5 mm Hg for diastolic pressure. The correlations between the observer and the 90202 were 0.98 for systolic and 0.96 for diastolic pressure.

Several validation studies have now been performed on the Del Mar Avionics PII and PIII recorders which use an identical system for the determination of blood pressure. The major difference between the two systems is that the PII connects to a Holter monitor for the simultaneous collection of ECG (and thus requires a Holter scanner to decode) while the PIII has built-in solid-state data storage. All of the validation studies have produced similar results. (These models may now be somewhat outdated, but this information may be of value to an investigator who will be able to obtain a system at a reduced rate or for historical interest since most studies published to date have used these systems.) In our validation study, we (Harshfield, Pickering, & Laragh, 1979) compared

30 blood pressure readings obtained by the PII with readings obtained by a technician using a mercury column and stethoscope on 15 different individuals during rest for a total of 450 readings. We found an overall correlation of 0.99 for systolic pressure and 0.94 for diastolic pressure. Correlations for individual subjects ranged from 0.64 to 0.97 for systolic pressure and 0.50 to 0.91 for diastolic pressure. We also found an overall correlation of 0.95 for systolic and 0.86 for diastolic pressure while the subject walked in place. We lost 30% of our recordings as the result of equipment failure and the unit worked on approximately 80% of the individuals attempted. A study by Corsi *et al.* (1983) on ten subjects found a similar range in correlations between the recorder and a technician: 0.41 to 0.93 for systolic and 0.41 to 0.81 for diastolic pressure.

We have recently performed an extensive validation study on the Del Mar Avionics PIV (Harshfield, Hwang, & Grim, in press). We tested the equipment on a total of 109 individuals according to the standards of the Association for the Advancement of Medical Instrumentation (1986). The subjects consisted of 59 males and 50 females; 59 were hypertensive and 50 normotensive. The subjects ranged in age from 15 to 85 years old (mean 37.9 ± 15). Weight ranged from 45 to 118kg (mean 78.8 ± 40) and midbrachial arm circumference from 20 to 40 cm (mean 29.8 ± 4). Three seated blood pressures were recorded by two trained observers using a double stethoscope and the PIV recorder, for a total of 327 readings. The PIV was able to obtain readings in 77% of the subjects tested. Of these, 81% of the systolic and 79% of the diastolic readings were within +4 mm Hg of the average of the two observers.

Three recent validation studies have been performed on the Suntech Accutracker. One study compared values obtained by the Accutracker during 199 determinations on 18 subjects with values obtained simultaneously by a clinician using a mercury column and stethoscope on the same arm (White, Schulman, McCabe, & Nardone, in press). The subjects ranged in systolic pressure between 90 and 200 mm Hg and diastolic pressure between 50 and 110 mm Hg. Correlations between the clinician and the Accutracker were 0.98 and 0.91 for systolic and diastolic pressure, respectively. The Accutracker diastolic readings were slightly lower than those obtained by the clinician. In the second study (Nelson, Weber, & Murphy, 1988), 215 blood pressure determinations obtained on 24 subjects were compared. Correlations were 0.89 and 0.86 for systolic and diastolic pressure, respectively. The Accutracker overestimated systolic pressure by 1.7 mm Hg and underestimated diastolic pressure by 1.9 mm Hg. Subjects were excluded from both studies if the initial values obtained by the Accutracker deviated by greater than 5 mm Hg from those obtained by the technician. The third study compared readings obtained by the Accutracker and intra-arterial pressure levels in 12 subjects as well as with stethoscopic auscultatory determinations in 27 normotensive and hypertensive subjects (Light, *et al.*, 1988). They found high correlations between the Accutracker and intraarterial readings, with a median correlation of 0.90 for systolic and 0.92 for diastolic blood pressure. The correlations with stethoscopic readings were 0.93 for systolic and 0.88 for diastolic blood pressure. They also found that the systolic pressures obtained by the Accutracker were consistently too high and the diastolic pressures were occasionally too low.

We are not aware of any validation studies to date for either the ABPM-630 or the Applause. We also are not aware of any studies which have checked the accuracy of the heart rate data obtained with any of the recording systems. From our experience, this has been for two related reasons: (1) the major focus has always been blood pressure because of its clinical relevance and (2) there is not enough time to do everything you would like to do! However, it is now becoming increasingly clear that heart rate, taken in conjunction with blood pressure, is an important variable which deserves greater attention.

It is clear from the above studies that proper attention has not been given to the validation of equipment. This is especially true for units available for purchase by the general public. We take this opportunity to recommend the adoption of the AAMI standards (1986) for equipment validation

and encourage investigators to perform and report these studies. These standards specify that data be obtained on at least 85 subjects with a range in age from 15 to 80 years old, a range in blood pressure of 100–200 mm Hg systolic and 60–110 mm Hg diastolic. Values obtained by the recorder must be compared to those of two observers using a double stethoscope.

Performance

It is unrealistic at this stage to expect ambulatory blood pressure and heart rate recorders to perform without breakdowns over an extended period of time. The performance of the different recorders varies considerably based on a variety of factors. First, performance is related to the length of time the unit has been available. For example, the early Del Mar Avionics recorders had a breakdown rate in our hands of one in every three recordings, as did the original ICR recorders (Harshfield *et al.*, 1984). Following extensive field experience with these units, the manufacturers reduced the failure rates significantly to approximately 5–10% for both units. A second factor affecting performance is equipment maintenance and care. It must be remembered that these units are sophisticated electronic devices which are subjected to a great deal of abuse. It is important to have the units serviced on a regular basis and the accompanying cables, etc. checked on a routine basis (perhaps daily). The third factor which affects performance are the conditions under which the units are operated. Recorders which are subjected to the rigors of manual labor and subways cannot be expected to last as long as units worn in an academic setting or used only under laboratory conditions. A final factor which affects performance in a more general sense is the ability of the manufacturer to service the units and provide loaners during the interim. This has been a major problem in the past.

Features

Features of the units that are currently available are summarized in Table 1, and are described below in general terms which will also be applicable to the new units coming out on the market.

Table 1. A Comparison of the Features of the Automatic Noninvasive Blood Pressure Recorders

Feature	Remler M2000	Avionics PII	Avionics PIII	Avionics PIV	Spacelabs 5200	Spacelabs 90202	Suntech Accutracker	Colin ABPM-630	DMI Applause
Method of blood pressure determination	Auscultatory	Auscultatory	Auscultatory	Auscultatory	Auscultatory/oscillometric	Oscillometric	Auscultatory	Auscultatory/oscillometric	Photoplethysmography
Criteria for rejection of artifactual readings	Hand edit	Systolic 50-255	Same as PII	Same as PII	No sound detected	No sound detected	Readings flagged	Readings flagged	None
Mode of data storage	Magnetic tape	Magnetic tape	Solid state	Solid state	Solid state	solid state	Solid state	Solid state	Solid state
Model of data retrieval	Decoder	Holter scanner printer	Microcomputer printer	Microcomputer printer	Microcomputer modem	Microcomputer modem	Microcomputer	Microcomputer printer	Printer
Power requirements	Hand inflate	Rechargeable battery pack	Rechargeable battery pack	Two 9-volt batteries	Six C-cell batteries	Four C-cell batteries	Rechargeable battery pack	CO_2 cartridge	9-volt battery
Dimensions	—; .7 kg	6×22×14.5 cm; 2.23 kg	8×22×14.5 cm; 2 kg	3.5×10×17.5; 1 kg	5.5×21×11.5 cm; 1.89 kg	14.5×8.6×3.9 cm; .36 kg	13.5×5×11.5 cm; 1.34 kg	29×20×12 cm; 4 kg	15×10×3 cm; .24 kg
Simultaneous EKG	No	Yes	No	Yes	No	Yes	No	No	No
EKG gating	No	Yes	Yes	Yes	No	No	Yes	No	No
Automatic activation	Self	Yes	Yes	Yes	Yes	Yes	Yes	Yes	Yes
Timing intervals		2, 7.5, 15 30 min	Same as PII	Programmable	Programmable	Programmable	Programmable	Programmable	Programmable
Manual activation	Yes	Yes	Yes	Yes	Yes	Yes	Yes	Yes	Yes
Stand-by control	—	Yes	Yes	No	No	No		No	No
Display on/off	—	Yes	Yes	Yes	Yes	Yes	Yes	Yes	Yes
Calibration mode	Yes	Yes	Yes	Yes	No	No	Yes	Yes	Yes
Sensitivity switch		Yes	Yes	Yes	No	No	No	No	No
Patient compatibility	Poor	Poor	Moderate	Very good	Good	Very good	Good	Very good	Very good

Method of Blood Pressure and Heart Rate Determination

Ambulatory recorders generally use either the auscultatory or oscillometric techniques for blood pressure determination. With the auscultatory technique, a transducer (microphone) is placed over the brachial artery. The cuff is then inflated 20–30 mm Hg above the previous systolic determination (or some preset level on the initial determination) and deflates at a set rate of 2–3 mm Hg/s. The Avionics units determine systolic pressure following the detection of three consecutive sounds, the first of which is designated as systolic. It then determines diastolic pressure by tracking four heartbeats following the cessation of sound, the first of which is designated as diastolic. The Spacelabs 5200 unit also designates systolic pressure as the first sound following the appearance of three consecutive sounds. It then drops a designated level in pressure and "searches" for diastolic pressure. If the unit is unable to detect diastolic pressure, it reinflates and determines pressure using the oscillometric technique. The oscillometric technique does not require the placement of a transducer directly on the subject's arm; instead a cuff is placed on the subject's arm, inflated and then deflated. Mean blood pressure is determined by detecting oscillations in the blood pressure cuff which are produced by the pulsations of the artery. The Suntech unit uses the auscultatory method and stores each Korotkoff sound, determining systolic and diastolic pressure using a pattern recognition algorithm. The ABPM-630 determines blood pressure using both the auscultatory and oscillometric methods, and displays both. The Applause uses a finger cuff photoplethysmography technique in which blood flow is detected beneath the finger cuff and referenced back to blood pressure obtained on the arm in the standard manner during a calibration procedure.

The heart rate data are obtained in a variety of ways. Some units derive heart rate from ECG gating leads while other units derive it from the pulsations obtained by the pressure transducer or the pulsations transmitted through the blood pressure cuff. In any event the heart rate is obtained during the blood pressure determination. This is prefera-

ble because it provides a measure of heart rate at the same time as the blood pressure. However, the heart rate measure might be artificially influenced by the blood pressure measurement process.

Calibration

Calibration is the most important feature of an ambulatory blood pressure and heart rate recorder. Not all recorders work on everyone. The only way to determine if a unit does work on a particular individual is by calibrating it on that individual. This is essential. The ease of calibration is also an important factor. The Avionics and Suntech units allow the technician to deflate the unit in the calibration mode facilitating auscultation of the Korotkoff sounds. The Spacelabs units do not, which makes it quite difficult to hear the calibration Korotkoff sounds. As stated previously, we do not have experience with the other units. None of the units allow calibration of the heart rate data.

Artifact Rejection

Each of the units has its own criteria for automatic rejection, or flagging of artifactual blood pressure and heart rate readings. This is done either at the time of measurement or during data reduction. It is quite important for the unit to retain every reading for artifact rejection by the experimenter at a later time. With today's technology there is no absolute way of determining if an individual reading is "accurate" or "artifactual." Questionable readings usually fall into one of two categories: (1) readings which have pulse pressures (the difference between systolic and diastolic pressure) which are either very large or very small and (2) readings of systolic or diastolic pressure which are either exceptionally high or low relative to readings prior to and following the reading in question. We have used three different post hoc methods to cope with the problem: (1) examination of each reading by a trained technician who either accepts or rejects the reading based on his/her experience in blood pressure measurement as well as the activity of the subject at the time of the reading (Harshfield et al., 1984); (2) applying an algorithm to the group data (pulse pressure < 0.41 × diastolic pressure – 17 for diastolic pressures between 60 and 150 mm Hg), which was derived by consensus of a group of experienced investigators as representing valid blood pressure readings (Pickering, Harshfield, Kleinert, Blank, & Laragh, 1982); and (3) applying an algorithm to the group data which rejects readings based upon the level of both systolic and diastolic pressure during the performance of specific activities, which was derived from the analysis of blood pressures during these activities in several hundred subjects (Clark *et al.*, 1987). None of these methods have proven completely satisfactory and there is always a possibility of eliminating "real" but unusual readings. We would like to encourage manufacturers in the future to store the Korotkoff signals which would allow investigators to check the Korotkoff signal pattern of each questionable value, as the Remler system now does.

Once again, little to no attention has been paid to rejection of artifactual heart rate data.

Automatic Operation/Manual Activation

It is important for the recorder to have automatic and manual operation capability. Automatic activation allows the experimenter to collect data while the subject is not "thinking" about the blood pressure and heart rate. The subject's participation in the process could easily affect the readings in two ways. First, the reading may be "artificially" elevated because the thought of having one's blood pressure taken can produce a pressor response and elevation in heart rate in many individuals, particularly hypertensives (Pickering *et al.*, 1982). Second, the blood pressure and heart rate reading may be "artificially" low because the subject relaxes to some extent while stopping his/her activity to take a measurement. The manual mode, on the other hand, allows for the collection of data during predetermined activities, allowing for more "experimental control" over data collection

Simultaneous ECG and ECG Gating

Some of the units use a three-lead ECG system to gate the timing of the pulses to prevent artifac-

tual readings. The recorder detects an ECG signal and then opens a window at a preset time and samples signals from the transducer. This gating helps ensure the readings are "real" and not due to sources of artifact such as muscle movement or environmental noises. The use of a simultaneous ECG lead system has both positive and negative aspects. On the positive side, the ECG system will lessen the number of "artifactual" readings in most patients as well as provide for more accurate heart rate data. On the negative side, the ECG system in patients with extensive arrhythmias or pacemakers will result in more artifactual readings. It also requires additional technician time in setting up the patient and increases patient discomfort due to the placement of ECG leads on the chest.

Standby Mode

There are periods during a recording in which you may not want blood pressure and heart rate determinations to be taken. During these periods it is necessary to deactivate the unit. For example, current recorders do not provide accurate readings while the subject is driving, riding on a subway, jogging, and so forth. The unit will detect the excessive movement or vibrations, interpret these as pressure pulses, and pump up to excessive pressure levels trying to get above systolic pressure. This can be uncomfortable and, in the case of driving, dangerous. Another example is during sleep. Many subjects find it impossible to sleep with the recorders pumping intermittently. As a result, the pressures and heart rates do not represent true sleep values which can lead to misinterpretation of the data. It is our general impression this occurs in about 30% of the subjects tested (and about 90% of their spouses!), although the more recent smaller, quieter units do seem better in this regard.

Calibration

Proper calibration is often overlooked but is *essential*. This is particularly true in ambulatory studies for two reasons: First, although the recorders will provide readings on everyone, the readings are not accurate on approximately 20% of the individuals attempted and these individuals should be excluded from the research studies and from clinical evaluation with an ambulatory device. (This will be discussed in detail later.) Second, it can be quite difficult to determine if 5–10% of the readings per recording period are valid. Calibration data will give the investigator some knowledge on which to base data rejection. Unfortunately, few investigators currently provide calibration information or refer to such in their publications.

Training Personnel

We have trained 15 technicians on five different ambulatory recording systems—the Del Mar Avionics Ambulatory PII, PIII, and PIV, and the Spacelabs recorders. As with any technique, the key to proficiency is practice. The rate of successful calibrations for three technicians trained at New York Hospital–Cornell Medical Center was 35–40% on their first 50 patients. Following this "learning period" all three had a success rate of approximately 80%. We found the same to be true of trainees at the King/Drew Medical Center. Based on these figures, we recommend that technicians train on 30–50 subjects prior to collection of data, and that these trial subjects vary according to the parameters set forth in the section below on patient characteristics.

The training procedures themselves are also quite important for successful recordings. First, the individual doing the training should have considerable familiarity with ambulatory blood pressure monitoring techniques on a practical level. There are many "tricks of the trade" which simply cannot be passed on through written descriptions or over the phone. It is worth the investment to send someone to an active lab or bring someone in from an active lab to teach the technique. Second, the trainee should be well versed in the auscultatory method of blood pressure measurement. We often consider blood pressure an easy variable to measure with little intraobserver variability. This is not true. Data now show a high incidence of terminal digit bias even among professionals (Grim, Grim, Klimazewski, & Wolde-Tsadik, 1985). We recommend the trainee be checked

against the recorder and also against the trainer using the double stethoscope technique, with the visual blood pressure display out of the sight of the trainee. Third, the trainee should be taught how to troubleshoot the equipment both in the lab and by telephone. Ambulatory recorders are susceptible to frequent malfunctions and breakdowns due to the conditions under which they are operated. Many of the malfunctions can be corrected by the subject while he or she is wearing the recorder, thus preventing the loss of valuable data. Others can be corrected by the technician once the recorder is returned to the laboratory, minimizing downtime. Fourth, the technician needs to be trained in the care and maintenance of the equipment, which also reduces malfunctions and downtime.

Subject Characteristics

As indicated above, the current ambulatory blood pressure recorders function on about 80% of the general population. The other 20% have physiological, pathological, and psychological characteristics which prevent a successful recording.

Biotype

The greatest difficulties are presented by obese individuals during both the calibration and the recording periods. Among these we have more difficulty with shorter obese individuals for several reasons. First, it is difficult to find a good location to place the transducer. Second, it is difficult to accurately auscultate the Korotkoff sounds which are weakened due to the thick adipose tissue layer. Third, it is difficult to place the blood pressure cuff in the proper position on the arm so that the pressure inside the cuff is distributed equally due to the significant difference between proximal arm circumference and distal arm circumference (see Figure 1). Fourth, although a large size cuff should be used for accurate measurements, not all manufacturers make the large size cuffs.

We attempted to quantify the relationship between biotype and accuracy of blood pressure measurements in our recent validation study of the Avionics PIV recorder referred to previously. Using the average difference between the readings

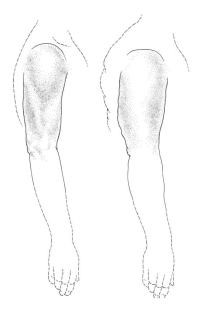

Figure 1. The differences in anatomy between the right upper extremities of an individual of normal biotype (left) and one of obese biotype (right), in lateral view. Note the significant difference between proximal arm circumference and distal arm circumference in the obese person when compared to the normal person.

obtained with the recorder and those obtained by the experimenters as a measure of the unit's accuracy, we found significant positive correlations between weight and accuracy for systolic ($r = 0.56$) and diastolic pressure ($r = 0.52$). This indicated that as weight increased, so did the difference between the recorder and the observers. We did not, however, find significant correlations between midarm circumference and the accuracy of the PIV units for either systolic ($r = 0.09$) or diastolic pressure ($r = 0.025$). There are better standardized anthropometric methods to study biotype than the two we employed. These include measures of skin thickness (including subcutaneous tissue) and circumferences on several different parts of the body. We recommend in future studies the assessment of biotype of an individual with these standardized anthropometric techniques.

Gender

Gender differences are also important. Young athletic males with muscular arms usually have

relatively small amounts of fat tissue on their body and thus have strong brachial artery pulses. These individuals have a greater percentage of inaccurate readings although it would seem they would be ideal for recordings. We observed in a number of these individuals that the hypertrophied medial portion of the bicep muscle was extended over the brachial artery, creating a barrier between the artery and transducer. We had better readings in these individuals when we placed the transducer slightly lower than the usual position, placing it right above the elbow joint. We also had more difficulty with obese female patients than with obese male patients. We found that the difference in arm circumference between the proximal and distal part of the arm was greater in females than males, creating difficulties in adjusting the cuff properly over the arm as illustrated in Figures 1 and 2.

Age

Age is another factor which affects the operation of ambulatory blood pressure monitors. As people age, their skin wrinkles and loses turgor. The vascular bed of the dermis decreases cellular nutrition, ultimately resulting in reduction of collagen and elastic fiber and also resulting in the reduction of subcutaneous tissue along with skeletal muscles

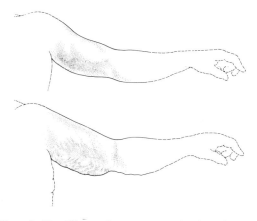

Figure 2. The difference between a normal and an obese person's arm in the horizontal position. The presence of excessive fat tissue gives the obese arm a pendulous shape. This arm type is more common among the middle-aged obese female population.

which are responsible for sustaining adjacent vessels, nerves, and so forth. The brachial artery itself also suffers and becomes stiffer and less compliant due to atherosclerosis. It also becomes more mobile due to the hypotrophy of adjacent sustaining tissues. These changes observed with the aging process result in lax skin which easily slides over the aged deep anatomic structures such as the atherosclerotic brachial artery and atrophied skeletal muscles. The progression of the aging process ultimately results in a pendulous shape arm (see Figure 3) which is due to the complete lack of consistency of soft anatomic structures. This phenomenon is more common among female patients and creates difficulty in keeping the transducer in the ideal position.

We examined age as a factor in our study on the Avionics PIV. As one would expect, we had more difficulty during the calibration procedures and a higher frequency of inaccurate readings during recordings in the geriatric population. To quantitate these observations, we correlated the accuracy of the recorder (see above) with age and found positive correlations of 0.33 for systolic and 0.40 for diastolic pressure, indicating that as age increased so did the discrepancy between readings obtained by the observers and the recorder.

Pathology

It is known that several diseases may affect the physiology of the arm in a direct or indirect manner. We analyzed our PIV calibration data in terms of a relationship between the diseased state and accuracy of the recorders and found a correlation

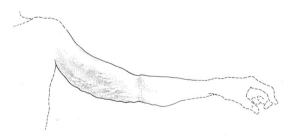

Figure 3. The elderly person's arm. The changes of the left upper extremity due to aging result in a pendulous arm with wrinkled skin.

between duration of hypertension and accuracy of the recorder of $r = 0.34$ for systolic and $r = 0.42$ for diastolic pressure. We also had difficulty during the calibration procedure and had a high rate of unsuccessful recordings in patients who had any type of arrhythmia. Among aged individuals, the most common type of arrhythmia is a premature ventricular contraction (PVC). The PVC is an abnormal contraction of the heart due to an abnormal electric pulse originating from the ventricles and usually occurs between two normal physiological contractions. The PVC causes inaccurately high diastolic readings. A possible explanation for this is that the PVC is usually followed by a compensatory pause of electromechanical activity of the heart, consequently creating a significant gap, which the recorders interpret as diastolic pressure. Another possible explanation is that the pulse pattern generated by the PVC is not the same pattern generated by the normal pulse, creating an unusual signal to the transducer. The function and accuracy of the monitors on these individuals depends on the frequency of the PVCs and also on the mechanism the device uses to detect diastolic pressure. Another type of arrhythmia which deserves comment is atrial fibrillation. We had two hypertensive patients with atrial fibrillation and on both occasions we were not able to calibrate the PIV units.

Among young individuals, the most common cause of an irregular pulse is sinus arrhythmias. This condition is normally a fluctuation of heart rate that is synchronous with the respiratory cycle. The pulse accelerates slightly on inspiration and slows on expiration. The variation of the heart rate during the respiratory cycle differs among individuals and can be accentuated by hyperventilation. It usually does not cause inaccurate readings except in extreme cases and under the influence of accentuating factors such as hyperventilation. We had one person with severe sinus arrhythmias diagnosed by ECG and we were not able to calibrate the PIV unit.

An auscultatory gap is a silence that separates two consecutive Korotkoff sounds when a normal contraction of the heart has actually occurred. This phenomenon tends to occur when there is venous distension or reduced velocity of arterial flow into the arm. Korotkoff sound sensitizing techniques such as handgrip exercises or elevation of the arm before inflation of the cuff help to temporarily overcome this phenomenon but are not practical for the 24-h recordings. As far as we are aware, there are no data on the prevalence of this condition in a normal or hypertensive population. Our data suggest that it can be either a transient or a permanent phenomenon depending on the individual and can lead to an inaccurately high diastolic reading.

Personality

The success of ambulatory blood pressure recording depends in part on the patient's psychological state. Patients who are very anxious or hyperreactive have a high percentage of unsuccessful recordings. The major technical problem with such patients is incomplete relaxation of the arm during the blood pressure determination, due either to reflexive contraction of the arm in response to cuff inflation or to a generalized increase of muscular tone. As described previously, the transducer measures systolic and diastolic pressure by searching for the appearance and disappearance of the sound frequency generated by the Korotkoff signal. Unfortunately, the frequency is similar to that produced by a skeletal muscle contraction. Consequently, the transducer is not able to differentiate between the two, resulting in artifactual readings.

Medication

There is the possibility that different classes of antihypertensive medication may influence the accuracy and functioning of ambulatory blood pressure recorders. It seems reasonable to hypothesize that sympatholytic agents might affect the pressure waveform in a much different way than a diuretic, converting enzyme inhibitor or calcium channel blocker. We are not aware of any studies which have systematically investigated this possibility.

Procedures

We recommend that at least three readings be taken with the normal auscultatory technique (stethoscope) prior to calibration. This will give

the experimenter an idea of the ''quality'' of the Korotkoff sounds (e.g., the loudness of the sounds, the presence of an auscultatory gap, arrhythmias) and also will give the experimenter an idea of the pressor effect of the recorder per se.

As stated above, most currently available monitors use Korotkoff sounds to determine blood pressure. Consequently, their accuracy depends on the sensitivity of the transducer and the intensity of the Korotkoff sounds. The sensitivity of the transducer can be adjusted on some units during the setup procedure but the intensity of the Korotkoff sounds depends on both transducer placement and the physiology of the patient's arm. The best way to place the transducer over the artery is to find the strongest brachial pulse using the palpitation technique and place the center of the transducer directly over it. The ideal site is a small anatomical area located in the anteromedial face in the distal part of the arm where the brachial artery runs closest to the skin surface. The best anatomical reference to define this area is the intersection between the end of the medial border of the bicep muscle and the elbow joint. We place the transducer 1–1.5 cm above the elbow joint to give the subject more freedom to flex the arm and on the nondominant arm to minimize interference with the patient's normal daily activities.

The actual calibration procedures are dictated by the goals of the study. We will give a few examples of projects we are or have been involved in to demonstrate this point. Many of our studies at Cornell were directed at determining the clinical significance of ambulatory blood pressure recordings. In these studies we were primarily interested in a measure of blood pressure at work and at home. Most of our subjects were middle- to upper-middle-class individuals with sedentary jobs. Therefore (at the time) we found it was sufficient to collect calibration data in the seated position. The subjects came to the Hypertension Center on the day of testing and were seated in a comfortable chair. The recorder was attached to the subject and calibration readings obtained simultaneously by the recorder and a technician using a mercury column and a stethoscope. Our criterion for a successful calibration was five consecutive readings which differed between the recorder and the technician by less than 5 mm Hg. If we were not able to obtain five successive "good" readings we made the necessary adjustments in the transducer placement or sensitivity levels until our criterion was met. No further testing was performed on the subject if this was not possible.

Some of our studies at Drew have taken a similar approach, examining such variables as genetic factors and black/white differences in ambulatory blood pressure patterns. We have expanded our protocol in these studies to include calibration readings in the standing and reclining positions. (This has led to the unfortunate discovery that, although the recorders work while the subject is seated, they may not work while the subject is reclining.) In other studies we have taken a more structured approach because we are interested in examining the responses to normal activities with specific physical or psychological demands. In these studies we also obtain calibration readings during a physical stress test (mental arithmetic). This allows us to determine if the recorder will work during tasks with these demands and also provides "anchor points" for the individual for activities with similar demands throughout the recording period. We have also decreased the number of readings we take per condition from five to three when using the Avionics recorders, having discovered in over 700 subjects that once the recorder was applied correctly it continued to provide accurate values throughout the calibration procedure. We initially recalibrated the equipment upon the subject's return to the clinic on the following day. We found in our first 200 patients using the Avionics recorders that, without exception, if the recorder was applied correctly and did not malfunction it remained in calibration throughout the 24 h. If the unit was not applied correctly, as during the technician's learning phase, we found the unit came back out of calibration up to 50% of the time. This may not be true of other units, however, which flip-flop between methods of blood pressure determination. For example, the Spacelabs unit uses both the auscultatory and the oscillometric methods for blood pressure determination. Because this unit has not been subjected to the validation procedures that the Avionics units have, we examined the calibrations in detail in 80

subjects. We found that only 42 of the 80 subjects met our original calibration criterion of five consecutive readings within 5 mm Hg. A closer examination of the calibration readings showed that 17% of the first readings, 9% of the second readings, 11% of the third readings, 7% of the fourth readings, and 4% of the fifth readings did not meet the 5 mm Hg criterion. Given the inherent difficulties with the oscillometric technique, we assume the "bad" readings occur when this technique is used. We have no information on any of the other recording systems but suggest quite strongly that all new units be rechecked upon the subject's return.

Recordings

Patient Training

One of the keys to a successful ambulatory blood pressure and heart rate recording is the training and education of the subject. You are totally dependent on the subject to accurately collect the data. Greater involvement of the subject in the study will increase the likelihood of successful recordings. It is important to recognize that you are going to put the subject through a potentially difficult experience over the next 24 h. Wearing the recorder will attract a great deal of attention which the subject might not desire or be accustomed to along with minimal embarrassment, to say the least.

It is very helpful to begin the education process prior to the study. During the initial contact we show the subjects the recorder they will be wearing and describe its operation. Even with today's smaller, quieter recorders, many subjects are initially hesitant though they can usually be persuaded to participate in the study. We also discuss the purpose of the study (which may not be appropriate in some studies) and show the subjects how they can benefit from participating. We do this by referring to the risks of hypertension and demonstrating the extreme variability of blood pressure. We then tell them what kind of clothing to wear for the recording and provide them with some written material which further explains the value of the procedure both to the particular research project and to themselves.

Calibration of the recorders can be quite awkward for the subjects so we talk to them as much as possible during the procedure. We tell them of interesting results we have found in our studies and interesting 24-h profiles we have seen in the past. We tell them the range in pressures they are likely to see and how to deal with "artifactual" readings. Following calibration we explain our diary collection procedure in detail. We give them examples of the kind of information we are looking for and *stress* the fact that the recordings are virtually useless without this information. We also provide them with the name and phone number of someone who can be reached 24 h a day for questions and difficulties. The subjects are fully debriefed upon their return the following day. This involves going over their diaries and readings, which most subjects are quite eager to talk about. The subjects are also provided with a "preliminary" report which consists of a printout and graphic display of their readings.

Sampling Intervals

The sampling procedures are dictated by the design of the study. Most groups have chosen to use time sampling, obtaining a reading every 7.5 min. A study by Mancia's group in ten hospitalized patients (Di Rienzo, Grassi, Pedotti, & Mancia, 1983) showed that a 10-min sampling interval was sufficient to obtain blood pressure values which were similar to the circadian fluctuations which were obtained by continuous intraarterial measurements.

Our studies at Cornell took a behavioral approach to blood pressure patterns. We used a combination of fixed time sampling and behavioral sampling procedures. In these studies we obtained a blood pressure reading once every 15 min during the day and 30 min at night. In addition, the subjects were requested to initiate additional readings each time they changed activities as well as when they were curious about their blood pressure. Our choice of a 15-min sampling period during the day was dictated by the number of readings we could obtain with corresponding diary information. More

frequent intervals severely interfered with the collection of the diary information. We chose a 30-min sleep cycle for two reasons. First, we found that many of our subjects were able to get into deep sleep in the 30 min the recorder did not activate. Once into this stage the recorder often did not bother them during the night. This significantly increased the number of sleep recordings when compared to using a 15-min sampling period. Second, activity changes, which have been the focus of our research, are generally somewhat limited during the sleep period.

A third possibility not yet utilized is behavioral sampling, which is dealt with in detail by Chesney and Ironson (this volume).

Uses of Ambulatory Blood Pressure Monitoring

The technique of ambulatory blood pressure and heart rate monitoring has thus far been used primarily in clinical research in hypertension. This has been dictated by two factors: the cost of the equipment and the desire of many researchers for control over the collection of data. This is now changing. First, the new systems have brought the cost of the equipment into the affordable range of most laboratories. Second, and most important, has been a growing realization that data obtained under laboratory conditions often do not reflect cardiovascular, biochemical, and other functioning under natural conditions.

Hypertension

Ambulatory blood pressure monitoring has thus far been primarily used in the area of clinical hypertension, focusing on the question of who to treat and who not to treat. This has led to at least three important clinical findings to date. First, blood pressure varies considerably throughout a normal day, changing by as much as 70 mm Hg for systolic and 40 mm Hg for diastolic pressure (Littler, Honour, Sleight, & Stott, 1972). Researchers have long suspected this to be the case, but simply did not have the technology to demonstrate it until the development of ambulatory blood pressure re-corders. Second, ambulatory blood pressure mea-surements have greater predictive value than do casual blood pressure measurements. Sokolow and colleagues in a pioneering study demonstrated (Sokolow, Werdegar, Keim, & Hinman, 1966) that ambulatory blood pressures were more closely related to indices of target organ damage than were casual blood pressure measurements. These find-ings have now been confirmed by many authors (Rowlands et al., 1981; Drayer, Weber, & De-Young, 1983; Devereux et al., 1983). In the only follow-up study to date on 1076 patients over a 5-year period, Perloff, Sokolow, and Cowan (1983) showed that patients with ambulatory pressures higher than clinic pressures had a higher incidence of mortality than did individuals with ambulatory blood pressures lower than clinic pressures. Third, a percentage of "hypertensives" actually are not hypertensive but only show a pressor response to the clinic situation. In a group of 178 "patients" with a diastolic pressure between 90 and 104 mm Hg in the clinic, we found that 25% had both nor-mal systolic and diastolic pressure at work, 21% were normal at home, and 32% were in the normal range during sleep (Pickering, Harshfield, De-vereux, & Laragh, 1985). Normal was defined as the 90th percentile for 42 normotensive volunteers.

These clinical studies have also provided impor-tant clues into the etiology of hypertension, es-pecially from the point of view of the behavioral scientist. In our studies we have repeatedly shown that blood pressure varies according to the situa-tional demands in which the measurement is ob-tained, with elevated pressure in the clinic and at work, a decrease at home, and a further decrease during sleep (Harshfield, Pickering, Kleinert, Blank, & Laragh, 1982). We have also found that not all patients show this pattern, with about 10% of patients showing higher blood pressures at home than at work (Harshfield, Pickering, Blank, & Laragh, 1986). In addition, we have shown that blood pressure patterns are influenced by person-ality factors (Thailer, Friedman, Harshfield, Kleinert, & Pickering, 1982) as well as environ-mental factors (Pickering, Harshfield, & De-vereux, 1984). For example, in a recent study we assessed the level of domestic stress experienced by the subject and found that individuals who ex-perience pathological levels of stress similar to lev-els experienced by individuals undergoing marital or family therapy also show consistently elevated pressures throughout the day (VanUum et al., 1986).

The assessment of the effectiveness of anti-hypertensive treatment has been another use for ambulatory blood pressure monitoring in hyperten-sion. For example, Jacot-des-Combes, Brunner, Waeber, Porchet, and Biollaz (1984) performed a retrospective analysis of 200 patients, 55 of whom received no medication, 28 β-blocker therapy, 42 diuretic therapy, and 75 both β-blocker and diuret-ic therapy. They found comparable levels of aver-age blood pressure between the groups coupled with comparable levels of blood pressure vari-ability reflected by differences in range (the aver-age of the three highest readings minus the three lowest readings), standard deviation, and blood pressure pattern. A second study by Palma and Codina (1985) investigated the effects of metoprolol on ambulatory blood pressure patterns in 20 patients. They found that a 100 mg dose was effective in reducing overall 24-h blood pressure in 80% of the subjects but did not influence the blood pressure pattern. The addition of diuretics in the other 20% achieved the same effects. A third study by Waeber et al. (1986) compared the antihyper-tensive effect of enalapril, a converting enzyme inhibitor, and diltiazem, a calcium entry blocker. They found no differences in the response to the two drugs. Both lowered the average 24-h blood pressure. In still another study, Hornung, Jones, Gould, Sonecha, and Raftery (1986) compared the responses to verapamil, a slow calcium channel inhibitor, and propranolol, a β-blocker. They also found that both drugs lowered ambulatory blood pressures similarly.

Psychological/Psychiatric Disorders

A second, almost untapped use of ambulatory blood pressure and heart rate monitoring is in the study of sympathetic nervous system activity in the etiology of psychiatric/psychological disorders. The work by Shear and colleagues (Shear et al., 1983) with panic disorder patients can serve as a model for other investigators. The question in this study was whether panic disorder patients show sympathetic hyperresponsivity to daily life events which in turn trigger panic attacks. Panic attacks are characterized by a combination of several of the following symptoms: dyspnea, palpitations, chest pain or discomfort, choking sensations, dizziness, feelings of unreality, hot or cold flashes, sweating, faintness, trembling, and fear of dying. In this study they compared the blood pressure and heart rate patterns of 28 patients with panic disorder to 41 normals. The ambulatory recordings revealed that not only do panic disorder patients not show a generalized hyperresponsivity throughout a normal day, but blood pressure responses during actual panic attacks were not even among the highest readings the individuals reached during the day. This approach can certainly be extended to the other disorders in which the sympathetic nervous system may play an etiological role, such as other anxiety and affective disorders as well as bipolar disorder, schizophrenia, and borderline personality disorder.

The technique may also be used to detect the *source* of psychological stress in a variety of both "physical" and "psychological" disorders such as hypertension, cancer, diabetes, and depression. For example, Lynch found that an individual shows sudden elevations in blood pressure when discussing "controversial" topics even though the person is not aware the topic is controversial (Lynch, 1985). This suggests the person is showing innate fight/flight responses to topics which are totally below the conscious level of the individual. In other words, the responses can give a "window" into the individuals' inner consciousness of which they are not aware.

Alternatives

Ambulatory blood pressure and heart rate monitoring provides unique information which cannot be obtained in any other way. Depending on the goals of the study, however, alternative procedures can be considered.

Home Recordings

One alternative which is often proposed is self-recording of blood pressure and heart rate at home. This is a reasonable cost-effective alternative if the experimenter is looking for a measure of an individual's overall level of blood pressure and heart rate which is not influenced by the pressor response often associated with the clinic. In a sample of 93 subjects we found good correlations between blood pressures collected over a 3-week period at home using conventional techniques and a 24-h blood pressure recording, with $r = 0.67$ for systolic pressure and $r = 0.76$ for diastolic pressure. Home readings are not a suitable alternative in studies in which it is important to also get a measure of variability. We found that the home blood pressures consistently overestimated the 24-h blood pressures (Kleinert *et al.*, 1984) because the home pressure did not include the 24-h variability introduced by elevated readings during the work situation and reduced readings during the sleep period. This would argue for obtaining readings during the work situation as well as at home. In addition, it is not possible to get a measure of reactivity during normal conditions.

Laboratory Measurements

A second alternative to ambulatory blood pressure and heart rate measurements are measurements obtained during laboratory testing. This again is suitable if one is interested in obtaining an overall estimate of an individual's level of pressure for a prolonged period of time, such as work. McKinney *et al.* (1985) found a correlation between playing a video game and blood pressure at work of 0.69 for systolic and 0.49 for diastolic pressure. Correlations between the video game pressure and blood pressure at home were 0.53 for systolic and 0.50 for diastolic pressure. Similar correlations were also found between the pressures obtained during a reaction time task and the cold pressor test and blood pressure at work and at home. Values of blood pressure during the laboratory tasks were always greater than values at work or at home. Smaller correlations were found between casual blood pressure measurements and pressures at work and home.

We have recently extended this association to mental arithmetic and treadmill exercise tests. However, we found the casual pressures predicted the ambulatory pressures just as well as the task-induced pressures (Harshfield, James, *et al.,* 1988). We, as did McKinney *et al.,* also found that the laboratory tasks did not provide a measure of reactivity which generalizes to functioning under normal activities. This is an important point. In both of these studies, blood pressure responses during the laboratory tasks did not predict blood pressure changes during the day. In our study, we looked at the association between changes in blood pressure to the laboratory tasks and changes in blood pressure from work to home, home to sleep, and awake to sleep and found correlations ranging from 0.00 to 0.06. We also found similar levels of correlation coefficients between changes in blood pressure during laboratory tasks and changes to a variety of specific activities ranging from walking to watching television to performing normal business tasks. There are at least three explanations to account for these results. An inspection of our data shows that the changes seen during the performance of the laboratory tasks were invariably much greater than the changes seen during the day. As a result we ended up correlating differences of 30 mm Hg during the video game task with differences of 4 mm Hg from work to home or during business activities. Second, there is a large degree of individual differences in the blood pressure responses both to the laboratory tasks and during the day. Third, and most important, the laboratory tasks are conceptually different from the tasks an individual engages in during a normal day and thus produce different physiological responses.

Miscellaneous

Pressor Responses

One of the questions often asked about ambulatory blood pressure monitoring is whether subjects experience a pressor response during a blood pressure measurement as they often do when a physician is taking their pressure. A recent study by Parati, Pomidossi, Casadei, and Mancia (1985) suggests they do not. In this study, 22 hospital inpatients were connected to the Oxford Medilog intraarterial blood pressure recorder for a 2-h period. During this time, blood pressure readings were also obtained automatically with a semiautomatic blood pressure recorder (Spacelabs 901) which obtained readings at 2-min intervals for the 2-h period. The period just prior to, during, and after the automatic inflations were compared and showed no evidence of an alerting response. It is our general impression that the subjects do, however, show a pressor response during the first hour of the recording period, but seem to adapt to the process by the second hour.

Sleep Data

A second question often asked is whether wearing the recorder influences the sleep readings. A study by Parati, Pomidossi, Casadei, Malaspina, *et al.* (1985) suggests that the Spacelabs unit does not. In this study on ten hospitalized subjects, sleep blood pressure recordings obtained by the Oxford Medilog recorder in combination with the Spacelabs unit were identical to sleep recordings obtained with the Oxford Medilog system alone. They caution that these findings might differ with different units. Recent data by Palatini, Sperti, and Cordone (1985) using the Del Mar Avionics units suggest that they are right. They found in 15 patients that the blood pressures obtained with the Avionics units during sleep did not predict pressures obtained with the intraarterial system. The Avionics units showed higher readings. It is our experience that sleep readings are affected in some individuals but not in others.

Conclusion

In conclusion, the relatively new technique of noninvasive ambulatory blood pressure and heart rate monitoring offers the behavioral scientist a means of testing hypotheses concerning the impact of day-to-day psychological functioning on the disease process. With this opportunity, however, comes an increased need for attention to equipment function and performance. Furthermore, ambulatory monitoring requires the development of new experimental strategies which are appropriate for testing in natural settings.

References

AAMI Standard. (1986). Association for the Advancement of Medical Instrumentation.

Bevan, A. T., Honour, A. J., & Stott, F. D. (1969). Direct arterial pressure reading in unrestricted man. *Clinical Science, 36,* 329–344.

Clark, L. A., Denby, L., Pregibon, D., Harshfield, G. A., Pickering, T. G., Blank, S. G., & Laragh, J. H. (1987). A data-based method for bivariate outlier detection: Application to automatic blood pressure recording devices. *Psychophysiology, 24,* 119–125.

Corsi, V., Germano, G., Apploloni, A., Cavarella, M., Zorzi, A., & Calcagnini, G. (1983). Fully automated ambulatory blood pressure in the diagnosis and therapy of hypertension. *Clinical Cardiology, 6,* 143–150.

Devereux, R. B., Pickering, T. G., Harshfield, G. A., Kleinert, H. D., Denby, L., Clark, L., Pregibon, D., Jason, M., Sachs, I., Borer, J. S., & Laragh, J. H. (1983). Left ventricular hypertrophy in patients with hypertension: Importance of blood pressure responses to regularly recurring stress. *Circulation, 68*(3), 470–476.

Di Rienzo, M., Grassi, G., Pedotti, A., & Mancia, G. (1983). Continuous vs. intermittent blood pressure measurements in estimating 24 hour average blood pressure. *Hypertension, 5*(2), 264–269.

Drayer, J. M., Weber, M. A., & DeYoung, J. L. (1983). BP as a determinant of cardiac left ventricular muscle mass. *Archives of Internal Medicine, 143,* 90–92.

Fitzgerald, D. J., (O'Callaghan, R., McQuaid, K., O'Malley, K., & O'Brian, E. (1982). Accuracy and reliability of two indirect ambulatory blood pressure recorders: Remler M2000 and Cardiodyne Sphygmolog. *British Heart Journal, 48,* 572.

Grim, C. E., Grim, C. M., Klimazewski, D. L., & Wolde-Tsadik, G. (1985). An audiovisual system for monitoring quality control in blood pressure observers. *CV Epidemiology Newsletter, 37,* 50.

Harshfield, G. A., Pickering, T. G., & Laragh, J. H. (1979). A validation study of the Del Mar Avionics Ambulatory Blood Pressure System. *Ambulatory Electrocardiography, 1,* 7–12.

Harshfield, G. A., Pickering, T. G., Blank, S., Lindahl, C., Stround, L., & Laragh, J. H. (1984). Ambulatory blood pressure monitoring: Records, applications, and analysis. In M. A. Weber & J. I. M. Drayer (Eds.), *Ambulatory blood pressure monitoring* (pp. 1–7). Dannstadt: Steinhopff-Verlag.

Harshfield, G. A., Pickering, T. G., Blank, S., & Laragh, J. H. (1986). How well do casual blood pressures reflect ambulatory blood pressures? In G. Germano (Ed.), *Blood pressure recording in the clinical management of hypertension* (pp. 50–54). Rome: Edizion Pozzi.

Harshfield, G. A., James, G. D., Schlussel, Y., Yee, L. S., Blank, S. G., & Pickering, T. G. (1988). Do laboratory tests of blood pressure reactivity predict blood pressure changes during everyday life? *American Journal of Hypertension, 1,* 168–174.

Harshfield, G. A., Hwang, C., & Grim, C. E. (in press). A validation study of the Del Mar Avionics Pressurometer IV according to AAMI guidelines. *Journal of Hypertension.*

Hornung, R. S., Jones, R. I., Gould, B. A., Sonecha, T., & Raftery, E. B. (1986). Twice daily verapamil for hypertension: A comparison with propranolol. *American Journal of Cardiology, 57,* 93D–98D.

Jacot-des-Combes, B., Brunner, H., Waeber, B., Porchet, M., & Biollaz, J. (1984). Blood pressure variability in ambulatory hypertensive patients: Effect of beta-blocking agents and/or diuretics. *Journal of Cardiovascular Pharmacology, 6,* 263–266.

Kleinert, H. D., Harshfield, G. A., Pickering, T. G., Devereux, R., Sullivan, P., Mallory, W., & Laragh, J. H. (1984). What is the value of home blood pressure measurement in patients with mild hypertension? *Hypertension, 6*(4), 574–578.

Light, K. C., Obrist, P. A. & Cubeddu, L. X. (1988). Evaluation of a new ambulatory blood pressure monitor (Accutracker 102): Laboratory comparisons with direct arterial pressure, stethoscopic auscultatory pressure, and readings from a similar monitor (Spacelabs model 5200). *Psychophysiology, 25*(1), 107–116.

Littler, W. A., Honour, A. J., Sleight, P., & Stott, F. D. (1972). Continuous recording of direct arterial pressure and electrocardiogram in unrestricted man. *British Medical Journal, 3,* 76–78.

Lynch, J. J. (1985). *The language of the heart.* New York: Basic Books.

McKinney, M. E., Miner, M. H., Ruddel, H., McIlvain, H. E., Witte, II., Buell, J., & Eliot, R. (1985). The standardized mental stress protocol: Test-retest reliability and comparison with ambulatory blood pressure monitoring. *Psychophysiology, 22*(4), 453–463.

Nelson, K. S., Weber, R. R., & Murphy, M. B. (1988). Evaluation of the Suntech Accutracker, a noninvasive ambulatory blood pressure recorder. *American Journal of Hypertension, 1,* 1215–1235.

Palatini, G., Sperti, L., & Cordone, P. (1985). Reliability of indirect blood pressure monitoring for the evaluation of hypertension. *Clin Exp Theory Prac,* 437–443.

Palma, J. L., & Codina, J. (1985). Ambulatory monitoring of blood pressure and arrhythmias by non-invasive methods in hypertensive patients treated with metoprolol. *Clinical and Experimental Theory and Practice, A7,* 365–369.

Parati, G., Pomidossi, G., Casadei, R., Malaspina, D., Colombo, A., Ravogli, A., & Giuseppe, M. (1985). Ambulatory blood pressure monitoring does not interfere with the hemodynamic effects of sleep. *Journal of Hypertension, 3(Suppl. 2),* S107–S109.

Parati, G., Pomidossi, G., Casadei, R., & Mancia, G. (1985). Lack of alerting reactions to intermittent cuff inflations during noninvasive blood pressure monitoring. *Hypertension, 7*(4), 597–601.

Perloff, D., Sokolow, M., & Cowan, R. (1983). The pronostic value of ambulatory blood pressure. *Journal of the American Medical Association, 249,* 2793–2798.

Pickering, T. G., Harshfield, G. A., Kleinert, H. D., Blank, S., & Laragh, J. H. (1982). Comparisons of blood pressure during normal daily activities, sleep, and exercise in normal and hypertensive subjects. *Journal of the American Medical Association, 247,* 992–996.

Pickering, T. G., Harshfield, G. A., & Devereux, R. B. (1984). Ambulatory monitoring of blood pressure: The importance of blood pressure during work. In M. A. Weber & J. I. M. Drayer (Eds.), *Ambulatory blood pressure monitoring* (pp. 193–197). Dannstadt: Steinhopff-Verlag.

Pickering, T. G., Harshfield, G. A., Devereux, R. B., & Laragh, J. H. (1985). What is the role of ambulatory blood pressure monitoring in the management of hypertensive patients? *Hypertension, 7*(2), 171–177.

Pickering, T. G., James, G. D., Boddie, C., Harshfield, G. A., Blank, S. G., & Laragh, J. H. (1988). How common is white coat hypertension? *Journal of the American Medical Association, 259,* 225–228.

Rowlands, D. B., Ireland, M. A., Glover, D. R., McLeay, R. A. B., Stallard, R. A. B., & Littler, W. A. (1981). The relationship between ambulatory blood pressure and echocardiographically assessed left ventricular hypertrophy. *Clinical Science, 61*(Suppl.), 101s–103s.

Santucci, S., Steiner, D., Zimbler, M., James, G. D., & Pickering, T. G. (1988). A validation study of the Spacelabs 90202 and 5200 ambulatory bloodpressure monitors. Presented at the American Soc of Hypertension, June, 1988.

Shear, M. K., Harshfield, G. A., Polan, J., Mann, J., & Frances, A. (1983). Autonomic function in panic disorder patients. *Psychophysiology, 20,* 470.

Sokolow, M., Werdegar, D., Keim, H. K., & Hinman, A. T. (1966). Relationship between level of blood pressure measured casually and by portable recorders and severity of complications in essential hypertension. *Circulation, 34,* 279–298.

Thailer, S. A., Friedman, R., Harshfield, G. A., Kleinert, H. D., & Pickering, T. G. (1982). Blood pressure variability in hypertension: Are physiological factors important? *Circulation, 66,* 11–36.

VanUum, K. E., Harshfield, G. A., Thailer, S. A., Clarkin, J. F., Pickering, T. G., James, G. D., & Friedman, R. F. (1986). Domestic discord and blood pressure responses during the day. *Society for Behavioral Medicine.*

Waeber, B., Jacot-des-Combes, B., Porchet, M., & Brunner, H. (1984), Accuracy, reproducibility and usefulness of ambulatory blood pressure recording obtained with the Remler system. In M. A. Weber & J. I. M. Drayer (Eds.), *Ambulatory blood pressure monitoring* (pp. 65–69). Dannstadt: Steinhopff-Verlag.

Waeber, B., Bidiville, J., Nussberger, G., Nussberger, J., Waeber, B., Porchet, M., & Brunner, H. R. (1986). Ambulatory blood pressure monitoring during long-term treatment of hypertensive patients with enalapril. Abstract presented at the International Society of Hypertension.

White, W. B., Schulman, P., McCabe, E. J., & Nardone, M. (in press). Clinical validation of the Accutracker ambulatory blood pressure monitor. *American Society of Clinical Pharmacology and Therapy,*

CHAPTER 19

Methods for Ambulatory Monitoring of Blood and Urine

Joel E. Dimsdale

Introduction

Most laboratory chemistries are obtained at the doctor's office or at the hospital. Such settings are efficient because of the presence of trained personnel and proximity to the medical laboratory. Furthermore, such studies are appropriate because most clinical chemistries focus on the overall level of a compound in blood or urine and are less oriented toward sampling a compound that fluctuates substantially over the day.

However, there are indications for studying compounds that do not remain at a constant level but react in dynamic fashion to certain stimuli. There are pulsatile secretory bursts of many compounds, and the amplitude of such bursts may be related to various disease states. As a result, sampling must occur repeatedly to detect this sort of dynamic hormonal activity. If there were techniques for ambulatory blood sampling, study of such compounds would be facilitated.

The major impetus for deriving ambulatory collection techniques in behavioral cardiovascular research is to observe physiology under behaviorally

appropriate conditions. Investigators are studying the physiological response to a panoply of stressors. To a certain extent, this research may be done experimentally in the laboratory; alternatively, it can be accomplished through naturalistic observation of the subject's physiology in his/her free-ranging environment. In the latter circumstance, the chemistry sampling essentially resembles "wet Holter monitoring" (Dimsdale, 1983, 1984a) in that it allows one to sample physiology under widely differing conditions, not just under the rigorously controlled physiology manifested in a medical setting. Some work suggests that, at least for plasma catecholamines, ambulatory samples reveal a rather different perspective on sympathoadrenomedullary activity than do samples obtained in the laboratory (Dimsdale, 1983, 1984b).

Indications

There are diverse indications for ambulatory collection of blood and urine. Some indications are primarily economical, some are in terms of convenience, and some are of more theoretical importance. With the advent of sophisticated insulin delivery systems for diabetes, it is of increasing importance to sample blood glucose levels throughout the day. This can be accomplished in a hospital

Joel E. Dimsdale • Department of Psychiatry, University of California, San Diego Medical Center, San Diego, California 92103.

setting at substantial cost and considerable patient inconvenience. Another drawback to such hospital monitoring is that the diet and physical activity imposed in such a setting may not be a good reflector of the patients' glucose physiology in their normal ambulatory settings. Thus, some technique for obtaining ambulatory blood samples repeatedly over the course of the day would be useful both in caring for hard-to-manage diabetic patients, and for revealing insights into the fundamental physiology of diabetes.

Numerous hormones such as luteinizing hormone and cortisol are secreted in a pulsatile fashion (see Kuhn, this volume). For this reason, reliance on an isolated blood sample for these hormones is ill-founded. Instead, one needs repeated blood samples with careful documentation of the time of sampling. Recently, this approach has not only revealed underlying pathophysiological abnormalities, but also suggested treatment. In Kallmann's syndrome, there is anosmia, combined with an underlying failure in sexual maturity, both being caused presumably by a hypothalamic deficit (Males, Townsend, & Schneider, 1973). Through the careful study of patients in a clinical research center setting, investigators have learned that Kallmann's syndrome patients have a markedly decreased frequency of pulses of gonadotropin-releasing hormone (GnRH). Using this knowledge, Hoffman and Crowley (1982) have demonstrated normal sexual maturation and fertility in such patients when they receive long-term episodic pulses of GnRH via an ambulatory infusion pump. Like the blood glucose studies discussed earlier, this work depends on careful repeated monitoring of blood GnRH levels. Such monitoring is usually performed in a hospital setting at substantial inconvenience and cost to the patient or to research grants.

The explosion in neuroendocrinology has led to a state whereby we simply do not know the range of physiological response of many new neuroendocrine factors. Because of the substantial cost and inconvenience of long-term sampling of subjects in a hospital setting, work has been slow to accumulate on the reactivity of many newly discovered hormones. Ambulatory monitoring techniques could potentially facilitate such research. There are some beginning observations on plasma catecholamines and cortisol in ambulatory subjects at their work setting. Rose, Jenkins, and Hurst (1978) examined cortisol responses among air traffic controllers. Dimsdale and Moss (1980) tracked plasma catecholamines in young doctors while they were presenting cases at formal academic conferences. In the initial minutes of speaking, both norepinephrine and epinephrine increased significantly. However, epinephrine was particularly sensitive to the anxiety of the situation, in most cases tripling (in one case, increasing tenfold) over baseline levels.

Alternative Techniques for Measurement in Ambulatory Settings

The bulk of this chapter discusses techniques for collecting blood samples in ambulatory settings. Urine sampling is also of interest. Studies of urinary sodium excretion, for instance, are of clear interest because of their relevance to blood pressure regulation. Urine samples are also advantageous because they reflect a longer time interval and thus may represent an index of tonic hormonal activity. However, numerous factors such as posture and diet affect urine concentrations and, for some compounds, the true physiological implications of a urinary hormonal level are far from clear. Urine collections have many problems in common with blood sampling. Like blood sampling, urine sampling must consider the preservation and stability of the compound in urine. Urine pH, preservatives, and temperature are relevant considerations for studies of compounds such as catecholamines (see Ziegler, this volume).

However, the major problems in urine collection are more a function of urine volume. If one is interested in studying response to a stimulus that lasts for at least 30 min, one has a chance of obtaining an adequate urine volume. However, it is not possible to obtain a sufficient void volume over a briefer interval of time. Prior to the urine sample of interest, the patient must empty the bladder and discard the urine. The subsequent bladder contents would then represent the clinical intervention with the patient. Particularly with short collection intervals of less than an hour, one runs the risk of not obtaining a complete bladder void, and thus obtaining a highly distorted sample measurement. One can, of course, volume load the patient, but that in itself alters substantially renal performance and may distort some findings (Liedtke & Duarte, 1980).

In obtaining repeated blood samples, there are basically four techniques which can be used in ambulatory subjects:

1. Repeated venipuncture: Certainly this is the most familiar way of obtaining blood samples. It has the advantage of being simple and inexpensive. However, subjects do not appreciate repeated venipunctures. In addition, for most rapid-acting hormones such as catecholamines and renin, the act of venipuncture alone causes a pulse in hormonal activity, such that what one really is measuring is the response to venipuncture as opposed to the imposed experimental intervention (Kopin, Lake, & Ziegler, 1978).

2. The next most familiar technique for obtaining repeated sampling consists of an indwelling catheter coupled to a heplock. With careful positioning and anchoring of the catheter, there is minimal discomfort because only one venipuncture is required. Reasonable volumes of blood can be withdrawn on a moment's notice. The disadvantages are that for some compounds such as free fatty acids, the continuous infusion of heparin into the patient can distort the underlying physiology (Shepherd & Champion, 1980). Furthermore, a laboratory assistant must accompany the patient and perform the necessary catheter flushing and blood withdrawal. This is not a technique that can be used by subjects on their own.

3. A third technique and one that has been little used in cardiovascular behavioral medicine research, relies on an Ulster Microlance Device (VWR Scientific). The device uses a spring-loaded lancet to make a small, standardized stick into the skin. A microsample of blood is then collected through a capillary tube. This device is extremely portable and inexpensive. Subjects can obtain small-volume blood samples on themselves without the necessity of having a laboratory assistant present. It is, of course, uncomfortable to go through repeated sticks, but the device is probably less uncomfortable than undergoing repeated manual sticks. Furthermore, the volume of blood obtained is sufficient for studies such as hematocrit and RIAs that require small volumes (cortisol), but too small a volume to be useful for compounds such as catecholamines where larger sample volumes are required.

4. The fourth technique, and that which I will discuss at greatest length, involves continuous sampling, as opposed to intermittent sampling, through an indwelling catheter. Two technological developments make this a useful technique for behavioral cardiovascular research. Small peristaltic pumps on the order of $3 \times 3 \times 1\frac{1}{2}$ inches can be readily carried by subjects. Second, chemists discovered that tridodecylmethylammonium chloride (TEDMAC) is a compound that binds heparin. When the internal catheter wall is coated with TEDMAC and the catheter flooded with heparin prior to insertion, blood can be withdrawn essentially continuously by virtue of the slow leaching of heparin from the catheter wall into the catheter lumen (Kowarski, Thompson, Migeon, & Blizzard, 1971). No heparin enters the patient; however, the catheter is essentially anticoagulated for many hours. This felicitous combination allows the subject to have one venipuncture, and yet to be completely ambulatory for many hours without the requirement for repeated heparin flushing of the catheter. The TEDMAC–heparin loses its anticoagulant properties slowly so that, in our experience, it is reliable for 6 h.

We know of only one manufacturer of a pump for this purpose, Dakmed, Inc. of Buffalo, New York. The manufacturer has a number of pumps, all of similar external dimensions; however, the various models are capable of pumping at somewhat different flow ranges. As will be discussed below, most behavioral cardiovascular researchers would require the high-speed pump, which is capable of blood withdrawal of up to about 2 ml/min (Figure 1).

Catheter Considerations with the Cormed Pump

The technique of ambulatory blood withdrawal is a simple idea, but one that brings with it certain peculiar problems. Obviously, one can infuse into a vein of small caliber. However, one runs into difficulties in continuously withdrawing blood from small veins because the vein tends to collapse around the lumen of the catheter. Furthermore, through bad fortune, one occasionally positions the catheter at the site of a valve in the veins. For these reasons, the more proximal the catheter placement, the more reliable is the blood withdrawal.

Although TEDMAC is not a patented substance, it is not practical to manufacture catheters for human use in the laboratory because of sterility concerns. There is one manufacturer, Dakmed, Inc., that pretreats and sterilizes catheters appropriate for human study. The manufacturer has two types of catheters, an intracath and a butterfly. The intracath is tedious to insert, but may be advantageous for ambulatory studies because the catheter is threaded about 6 inches proximal to the site of venipuncture, and thus the vein is of larger caliber. In using the intracath, the best site for insertion is directly into the antecubital vein. There is no problem with the movement of the joint at the elbow if the catheter is appropriately anchored.

The butterfly catheter is very easy to use and is clearly preferable for any laboratory studies. Because of its more distal location, however, the butterfly is probably more susceptible to closing off of the catheter because of movement artifact in ambulatory subjects. One can partially deal with this problem by adding an armboard at the site of catheter insertion.

Both catheters would be improved if there were a three-hole tip as opposed to a one-hole tip. The three-hole tip would decrease the likelihood of shutting off blood flow due to a collapse of the vein

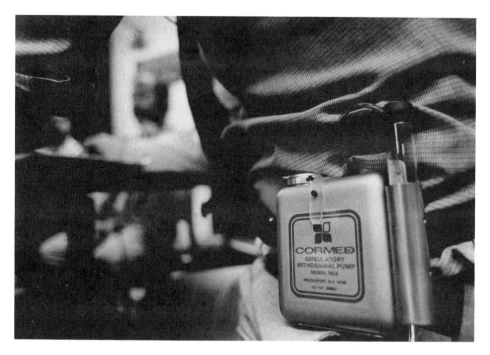

Figure 1. Cormed ambulatory withdrawal pump and blood collection tube in place on a volunteer's waist.

around the tip or due to the tip's brushing up against a valve in the vein. Unfortunately, no one makes such a TEDMAC-treated three-hole catheter.

Just prior to use, the catheter is flushed with approximately 1 ml of 10,000 unit heparin. The catheter is then connected to the peristaltic blood withdrawal pump and inserted into the subject. A disadvantage of the system is that it is impossible to obtain an instantaneous rapid blood withdrawal. The pump withdraws blood continuously; its fastest rate is about 2 ml/min. It is too tedious a process to remove the catheter from the pump, withdraw blood from the catheter into a syringe, and then reinsert the catheter into the pump. In addition, one risks clotting in the line if the column of blood in the catheter stops moving, even briefly. Efforts to jerry-rig a three-way stopcock have been disappointing because of problems of coagulation at the stopcock.

Setting Rate of Withdrawal of the Cormed Pump

The blood withdrawal pumps can be set to withdraw blood at differing rates. In most protocols, there are intervals of time during which one is not interested in sampling blood. By setting the pump to a low speed, one can minimize blood loss under those circumstances. However, in the standard model, it is not easy to change the rate of withdrawal quickly. The manufacturer has an option of a simple switch, allowing blood to be withdrawn at either a high or a low rate of withdrawal for a given pump size. The provision of this optional switch makes the pump a far more useful device.

The pump allows considerable flexibility. The withdrawal rates are readily determined depending on the study design. First, one needs to consider the pulsatility of the compound under study. Related to this is the consideration of the compound's half-life in blood. A further consideration is the compound's thermal stability once it leaves the body and is exposed to room air. Next, one must consider the assay requirements in terms of plasma volume needed.

Finally, one must consider the appropriate total blood loss to the patient participating in the protocol. The pumps work like the veritable sorcerer's

apprentice. They are quiet, slow, and persistent. Yet, over the course of several hours, a pump withdrawing blood at the rate of 1 ml/min will yield a substantial blood loss.

For most behavioral cardiovascular research, it is advantageous to withdraw blood at the rate of 1–2 ml/min, and to integrate the blood samples over a 2- to 5-min interval of time. This will generate a sufficient volume for assay and, furthermore, this time interval is physiologically appropriate, particularly for rapidly responding hormones. For hormones that are slower to respond or for assays that require only small amounts of blood, one could select a slower pump and collect continuously miniscule amounts of blood integrated in one collection tube for an interval of about an hour.

Fractional Collection

The final component of this ambulatory blood withdrawal system involves its fractional collector or lack of same. The device merely pours blood into an anticoagulated blood collection tube. At appropriate intervals, the tube must be switched, and a new tube inserted. This is a simple process that can be done with one hand; it involves less manipulation than a heplock flush and sample collection. A motivated subject can readily insert a new tube without needing a laboratory assistant. However, it is not quite accurate to view this process as effortless.

There need be no concern about sending a patient with a butterfly catheter out of the hospital unaccompanied by a chaperone. The patient, at any time, can turn off the pump; however, in that eventuality, the catheter would clot. If the protocol calls for an accompanying laboratory assistant, this can be done easily with little obtrusiveness on the subject. We have, for instance, had an assistant switch tubes in public speakers before large audiences.

However, it would clearly be preferable if a portable fractional collector could be interfaced with the pump. We know of two efforts to derive a portable fractional collector. D. H. Vandercar (personal communication) developed a cluster of modified plastic disposable syringes attached to a common manifold. As blood leaves the pump and enters the first syringe, it forces up the modified plunger of the syringe until the plunger encounters a string which, in turn, triggers the blood to enter the second syringe, and so forth. There are some preliminary models of this device and it appears useful, if somewhat cumbersome. It can certainly readily accommodate five, or perhaps more, blood collection tubes, each corresponding to a given interval of time. Dimsdale and Hilger have been attempting to apply autoanalyzer techniques to their fractional collector. The portion of the catheter distal to the pump is a long coil. As new blood enters the catheter, the earlier collected blood is merely pushed back farther into the coil. Introduction of a time spacer into the catheter, either air or immiscible liquid, marks off time. This can be accomplished by piggybacking an additional pump into the system. This concept remains on the drawing board without having been tested.

Particularly for rapid sampling, i.e., on the order of every 3–5 min, a portable fractional collector is needed before one can confidently state that the unit is entirely self-sufficient. Otherwise, the unit works best in a laboratory setting or ambulatory setting when the patient is attended by a laboratory assistant. The assistant, however, need do only minimal intervention with the subject.

In the preceding paragraphs, I alluded to the fact that the hormone's thermal stability needs to be considered. Compounds such as catecholamines and renin degrade at room temperature rapidly (see Ziegler, this volume; Atlas, this volume). For this reason, it is important to place the collection tube on ice rather quickly. Some compounds, however, may degrade so rapidly that the transit time in the catheter makes the technique of questionable value. In an ambulatory setting, various dry chemical coolant pouches can be placed around the blood collection tubes to keep them chilled. If the compound under study requires special preservatives, these can be added in advance to the blood collection tubes themselves.

Conclusion

For a number of reasons, obtaining blood and/or urine from patients in their normal ambulatory en-

vironments is of value. Problems of modesty, inconvenience, and comfort have a large impact on the acceptability of ambulatory monitoring techniques. There are already adequate bioengineering devices to obtain such sampling. The fundamental requirement in applying such a technique is to consider the physiology of the hormone under study. Such considerations will then guide the sampling details.

References

Dimsdale, J. (1983). Wet holter monitoring: Techniques for studying plasma responses to stress in ambulatory subjects. In T. Dembroski, T. Schmidt, & G. Blumchen (Eds.), *Biobehavioral bases of coronary heart disease.* Basel: Karger.

Dimsdale, J. (1984a). Techniques for collecting blood samples in the field and in the laboratory. In J. Herd, A. Gotto, P. Kaufmann, & S. Weiss (Eds.), *Cardiovascular instrumentation: Applicability of new technology to biobehavioral research.* Bethesda: NIH.

Dimsdale, J. (1984b). Generalizing from laboratory studies to field studies of human stress physiology. *Psychosomatic Medicine, 46,* 463–469.

Dimsdale, J., & Moss, J. (1980). Short-term catecholamine response to psychological stress. *Psychosomatic Medicine, 42,* 493–497.

Hoffman, A., & Crowley, W. (1982). Induction of puberty in men by long-term pulsatile administration of low-dose gonadotropin-releasing hormone. *New England Journal of Medicine, 307,* 1237–1241.

Kopin, I., Lake, C., & Ziegler, M. (1978). Plasma levels of norepinephrine. *Annals of Internal Medicine, 88,* 671–680.

Kowarski, A., Thompson, R., Migeon, C., & Blizzard, R. (1971). Determination of integrated plasma concentrations and true secretory rates of human growth hormone. *Journal of Clinical Endocrinology, 32,* 356–360.

Liedtke, R., & Duarte, C. (1980). Laboratory protocols and methods for the measurement of glomerular filtration rate and renal plasma flow. In C. Duarte (Ed.), *Renal function tests: Clinical laboratory procedures and diagnosis.* Boston: Little, Brown.

Males, J., Townsend, J., & Schneider, R. (1973). Hypogonadotropic hypogonadism with anosmia—Kallmann's syndrome. *Archives of Internal Medicine, 131,* 501–507.

Rose, R., Jenkins, C., & Hurst, M. (1978). *Air traffic controller health change study.* Boston: Boston University School of Medicine.

Shepherd, G., & Champion, M. (1980). Simple method for repeated blood sampling. *Lancet, 1,* 740–741.

CHAPTER 20

Diaries in Ambulatory Monitoring

Margaret A. Chesney and Gail H. Ironson

Ambulatory monitoring equipment frees the clinician and research scientist from the confines of the clinic and laboratory settings and permits the assessment of physiological parameters in the natural environment. There is increasing evidence that ambulatory monitoring provides a more representative assessment of an individual's functioning than that afforded by standard clinic and laboratory measurements. Moreover, ambulatory monitoring is an opportunity to study interactions between physiological functioning and characteristics of the individual's environment or behavior. These interactions are of interest because they may shed light on the marked variability in physiological measurements that is often observed. To examine these interactions, it is necessary to record information about the subject's behavior and environment at the time ambulatory physiological measurements are made. Typically, the subject records this information in a diary throughout the monitoring period.

This chapter will focus on the use of diaries in ambulatory monitoring of blood pressure. Diaries are being used in conjunction with monitoring of other physiological parameters, such as heart rate, and conditions including angina and silent is-

chemia, but the emphasis in this chapter will be on blood pressure monitoring because it is the parameter on which the most work has been done. First, after a brief introduction to the use of diaries in ambulatory blood pressure monitoring studies, a background discussion of the use of self-monitoring in behavioral medicine and its implications for ambulatory monitoring applications will be presented. Second, the content and design of diaries as they have been and are currently used in ambulatory monitoring of blood pressure will be described. Third, considerations relevant to the logistics of diary design and instructions to subjects will be discussed. Fourth, validity of diary data will be presented as an important issue to be considered, followed by a section on the use of diary data in analysis. The chapter will conclude with recommendations for the use of diaries in ambulatory monitoring of blood pressure and suggestions for future directions in research and practice with ambulatory monitoring diaries.

Self-Monitoring in Behavioral Medicine: Implications for Ambulatory Monitoring

The importance of diaries in conjunction with ambulatory monitoring became apparent when it was established that variability in blood pressure can be behaviorally induced (see Harshfield *et al.*,

Margaret A. Chesney • Department of Epidemiology, School of Medicine, University of California at San Francisco, San Francisco, California 94143. *Gail H. Ironson* • Department of Psychiatry and Behavioral Sciences, Stanford University Medical Center, Stanford, California 94305.

this volume). This recognition pointed out the necessity of developing a strategy for tracking such potential behavioral influences. For example, knowing that a subject is carrying a heavy object when blood pressure is being assessed will cause the clinician or researcher to view a resulting diastolic blood pressure (DBP) of 105 mm Hg quite differently from a similar blood pressure taken at rest.

The form taken by ambulatory monitoring diaries evolved with practice in the research setting. The earliest diaries consisted of log sheets on which subjects were instructed to record "significant events" occurring at the time of blood pressure measurement. A hypothetical example of such a log is presented in Figure 1. With use, problems with the log sheets—including subjects' variability in compliance and in the extent of detailed information provided—became apparent. In reaction to these problems, researchers developed more structured diaries that inquired about specific behaviors thought to be related to blood pressure variability. An example of one such diary is shown in Figure 2. The specific content of diaries in use today will be discussed in the next section of this chapter. What is important at this point is that the evolution of the use of diaries in conjunction with ambulatory monitoring appears to have occurred independently of the literature on self-monitoring in behavioral medicine discussed below.

Self-monitoring of behavior has played a major role in research and treatment in behavioral medicine for some time. Often labeled self-observation or self-recording, this procedure involves individuals' systematically recording aspects of their behavior and physical symptoms, as well as events surrounding each instance of measurement across time. This procedure is not new. Thoresen and Mahoney (1974) reported that Benjamin Franklin had a detailed method of recording his behavior in 13 areas or "virtues" he wished to increase. More recently, self-monitoring has been used in the behavioral treatment of a wide variety of health-related problems (Kazdin, 1974; McFall, 1977; Nelson, 1977). Patients have self-recorded physical symptoms and behavioral events in the management of pain (Sjoden, Bates, & Nyren, 1983), sleep disorders (Lawrence, 1982), cigarette smoking (Orleans & Shipley, 1982), stress (Roskies *et al.*, 1986), and psychophysiological disorders (Blanchard, 1981; Ward & Chesney, 1985). In these applications, subjects typically keep written records of the occurrence of target variables (e.g., headache pain), events before and after target variables, mood states accompanying the target variables, and characteristics of the environmental context surrounding the target variables.

The experience gained from the use of self-monitoring in behavioral medicine has implications for the use of diaries in ambulatory monitoring.

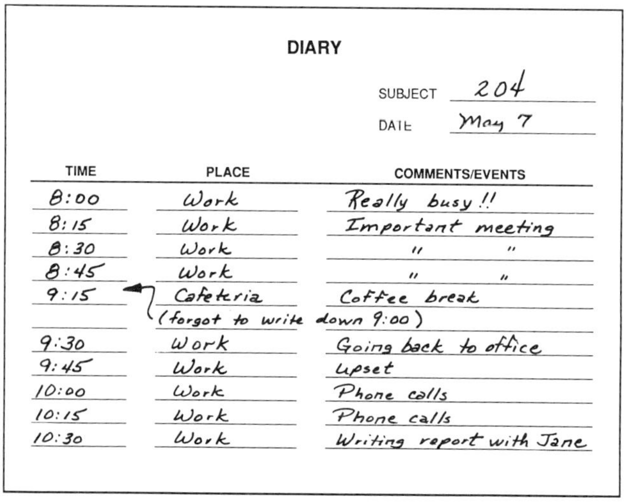
DIARY

SUBJECT 204

DATE May 7

TIME	PLACE	COMMENTS/EVENTS
8:00	Work	Really busy !!
8:15	Work	Important meeting
8:30	Work	" "
8:45	Work	" "
9:15	Cafeteria	Coffee break
	(forgot to write down 9:00)	
9:30	Work	Going back to office
9:45	Work	upset
10:00	Work	Phone calls
10:15	Work	Phone calls
10:30	Work	Writing report with Jane

Figure 1. Hypothetical example of an early ambulatory monitoring diary.

Time of Reading: _____ AM
                                           PM

1. Posture <u>During</u> This Reading (circle only one):

    Reclining   Sitting   Standing   Walking
        1   2   3   4

2. Activities During <u>Last 5 Minutes</u> Preceding This Reading
   (circle all that apply):

    Reclining   Sitting   Standing   Walking
        1   2   3   4

    Running or   Physical   In Moving   Laughing
    Climbing   Exertion   Automobile   or Coughing
        5   6   7   8

3. Persons Talked With During Last 5 Minutes Preceding
   This Reading (circle all that apply):

      None   Friend   Family   Stranger
        1   2   3   4

                                             2 or More
     Client   Boss   Coworker   People
        5   6   7   8

4. Tension Level During Last 5 Minutes Preceding This
   Reading (circle only one):

     Very   Very
    Relaxed   Relaxed   Tense   Tense
        1   2   3   4

5. Anger Level During Last 5 Minutes Preceding This
   Reading (circle only one):

                 Slightly
    Neutral   Irritated   Irritated   Angry
        1   2   3   4

6. Products Consumed <u>Since</u> Last Reading (circle all
   that apply):

                 Caffeinated   Alcoholic   Tobacco
      None   Beverage   Beverage   Product
        1   2   3   4

     Small   Salad or   Full   Medication
     Snack   Sandwich   Meal   or Drug
        5   6   7   8

Comment: _____

Figure 2. Example of a more recent diary for ambulatory blood pressure monitoring. Source: G. Black, M. Hecker, A. Kremer, and M. Ward, Department of Behavioral Medicine, SRI International, Menlo Park, CA.

Two implications in particular will be discussed here: how self-monitoring *per se* influences the behavior being measured, and how compliance to self-monitoring can be enhanced.

Reactive Effects of Self-Monitoring

The self-recording by individuals of their own behavior has been shown to change the behaviors under observation (Kazdin, 1974). This potentially dramatic effect of self-monitoring, known as "reactance," is perhaps best illustrated by controlled treatment studies in which self-monitoring served as the control condition with which behavioral treatment approaches were compared. These comparisons have shown that for some behaviors, self-monitoring alone is as effective as direct treatment strategies, or *more* effective (Ciminero, Nelson, & Lipinski, 1977). Thus, self-monitoring diaries have come to be seen by some as integral components of therapeutic interventions (Lawrence, 1982; Romanczyk, 1974). Awareness of the reactive effects of monitoring is important in that their existence implies that an unbiased assessment of behavior and the environment is not possible. An alternative to self-monitoring is behavioral observation by others, but research has shown that, to the extent that the subject is aware of this observation, this method also may lead to changes in behavior (Hartman & Wood, 1982). Unobstrusive behavioral observation is another alternative to self-monitoring but is considered unethical in many research settings.

The probability that self-monitoring will produce significant changes in behavior is influenced by a number of factors. Recognizing the importance of these factors and attending to them can minimize their effect on self-monitoring in conjunction with ambulatory monitoring. One such factor is the positive or negative valence assigned to the behavior being monitored (Kanfer, 1970). For example, for the obese hypertensive individual, recording high-calorie food intake would have a negative valence, whereas the opposite would be the case for an anorexic individual. Research has shown that the direction of reactive change is in the desired direction and the magnitude of the reactive change is related to the strength of the valence. A second factor influencing reactive changes is the "set" or expectation given to the individual with regard to characteristics of the behaviors being observed (Nelson, Lipinski, & Black, 1976). For example, if subjects are instructed to expect variability in mood, such variability is more likely to be recognized and reported (Kazdin, 1974). Third, the presence of specific goals set for the behavior being recorded influences performance of the behavior. For example, subjects given a concrete goal to increase physical activity to a frequency of three times per week are more likely to show increases in physical activity than subjects given the vague goal of "increasing activity." In developing diaries and protocols, attention should be given to the importance that monitoring-induced changes in the behavior under study may have for clinical or research application. Then the diary and associated protocol, including the instructions given to the subject, could be de-

signed to control reactive effects. In general, however, it is necessary to recognize that these effects cannot be avoided and that the self-reports provided in the diaries will be subject to some degree of bias.

Enhancing Compliance

The self-monitoring literature has shown that compliance to monitoring and accuracy of monitoring are enhanced if the diary has a low "response cost" to the subject. This implies that diaries should be utilitarian and require little of the subject's time. Diaries that are onerous in their "response cost" have been shown to result in noncompliance, subversion, or withdrawal from research or treatment protocols (Condiotte & Lichtenstein, 1981). Another factor that can enhance compliance to self-monitoring diaries is acknowledging *all* data collected, indicating to subjects that the data collected have both value and meaning (Orleans & Shipley, 1982). Expectation of accuracy checks has also been shown to increase accuracy (Evans, Hansen, & Mittlemark, 1977). Finally, critical reviews of the self-monitoring literature conclude that accuracy and compliance are also influenced by providing subjects with a thorough demonstration of the diary's use, emphasizing the importance of honesty in data recording, and indicating that successful and complete monitoring will result in an award (Ciminero *et al.*, 1977).

The development of diaries for use in ambulatory monitoring appears to have occurred without consideration of the implications for controlling reactive effects and enhancing compliance discussed in this section. Instead, there has been a trend toward increasing the detail regarding the behavioral and environmental context at the time of measurements and not toward gathering specific data to test hypotheses or address research questions. Unfortunately, little of this detailed information has been incorporated in the published literature on ambulatory blood pressure monitoring, probably at least in part because of a lack of consideration for design and psychometric issues, which will be discussed in the next section.

Diary Content and Design

Content

Compared with the technological advances in ambulatory blood pressure monitors, methods of behavioral monitoring have been crude. Content coverage has typically included questions about the subject's environment, behavior, and mood, as well as control variables. Environmental variables typically included are *place* (e.g., home, work, car) and *social situation* (e.g., alone, with others). Behavioral variables often recorded are the subject's *physical position* (e.g., sitting, standing) and *physical activity* (e.g., running, walking). *Mood states* often recorded include happy, sad, angry, and tense. Control variables are other factors that are thought to affect cardiovascular functioning and thus may need to be taken into account. These include cigarette smoking, medications taken, caffeine and alcohol intake, and food consumed.

Many other variables could be included within each of the three content areas. For the environment, questions concerning physical properties such as noise and temperature could be asked. For the subject's behavior, questions could cover specific activities of interest, such as writing reports or reading. For the subject's mood, questions could address boredom or energy level. For the control variables, as well, factors such as time since last meal or the need to void may be appropriate. In addition to the three content areas, others may be relevant to blood pressure monitoring, such as physical symptoms (e.g., pain, headache, illness), which have rarely been included.

Although, as noted above, the content covered in the diary can be expanded, it is important to add variables systematically, selecting those areas that are directly relevant to the research questions at hand. If a research question involved blood pressure monitoring in angina patients, for example, one would want to include in a diary questions covering whether a patient is having chest pain at the time of blood pressure measurement; the quality of the pain; its severity, duration, and location; whether the patient is resting or active; what emotions are elicited by the pain; and whether the pa-

tient is angry or feels under stress at the time. As another example, if a study were to involve bus drivers at work, the diary might include questions as to whether the driver is on schedule, whether the bus is stuck in traffic, whether it's raining or snowing, and whether the customer who just got on the bus is argumentative, and questions assessing the driver's current perception of job stress and satisfaction. The fact that many of these content areas are not covered by the diaries currently in use points out the importance of not merely taking a diary "off the shelf."

In conjunction with a needed focus on the research question at hand, data collected by diaries are strengthened if certain conceptual issues are addressed *a priori*. Among these is the need to decide whether diary items should assess the subject's *evaluation* of an event or whether they should focus on obtaining a *description* of the event. For an item assessing environment, an answer indicating that the subject was "driving a car" would be considered descriptive, whereas "stuck in traffic" would be considered evaluative. Another important conceptual issue that must be addressed *a priori* is the frame of reference subjects are to consider in responding to diary items. For example, an item about noise levels can be given (1) an absolute frame of reference in terms of decibels, (2) a relative frame of reference involving criteria drawn from common experience (e.g., as loud as a train whistle), or (3) a personal frame of reference (e.g., "average compared to a typical week"). The selection of the most appropriate frame of reference should be consistent with the research design. Yet another conceptual issue involves the extent of specificity desired in the item. For example, asking subjects to indicate whether they are feeling positive or negative is a more general mood question than asking subjects the extent to which they are feeling relaxed, happy, anxious, or sad. The time frame is still another conceptual issue. An advantage of ambulatory monitoring is that it allows one to study transient changes in physiology. Therefore, it is important to instruct patients to consider specific time frames around each measurement so that the behavioral variable's period of assessment coincides with that of the physiological variable. Also, with regard to time, an important conceptual issue and design consideration is the selection of the most appropriate sampling strategy. For example, blood pressure can be sampled to occur at fixed time intervals or to coincide with specific behavioral events. The selection of sampling strategy is typically based on the research questions under study.

In conclusion, it is suggested that selection of diary content be driven by the research questions, including but not limited to the subject's environment, behavior, and mood, as well as control variables. Moreover, it is suggested that consideration be given to important conceptual issues, including whether diary items should be evaluative or descriptive, what the appropriate frame of reference is, whether items should be specific or general, whether items should reflect a certain time frame, and what the appropriate sampling strategy is. In addition to structured items, it is also recommended that ambulatory monitoring diaries provide a space for comments by the subject. Subjects are instructed to use this space to record any additional information that is not covered specifically by the diary but that they believe to be important.

Design and Psychometric Issues

Diaries can be considered psychometric instruments recording samples of behavior. As such, several psychometric issues are relevant, including the definition of items to assess variables, the design of items with mutually exclusive and exhaustive response categories, and the advantages and disadvantages of including a neutral point in items with multiple-point (Likert-style) response scales. Although these issues will be discussed below with specific reference to ambulatory monitoring, fuller expositions of these topics are available (Anastasi, 1982; Edwards, 1957; Guilford, 1954; Guion, 1965; Nunnally, 1978; Smith, Kendall, & Hulin, 1969).

Item Design

The initial step in designing a diary involves converting the variables to be assessed into items. Within each item, unidimensional, mutually ex-

clusive, and exhaustive categories should be used. For example, to assess mood, some diaries have separate items for each mood state such as depression (see Figure 3, items 1 and 2). Other diaries assess mood with one item (see Figure 3, item 3). The former set of items assesses mood with mutually exclusive and exhaustive categories. The latter item is multidimensional; that is, it measures more than one mood state and these mood states overlap. Thus, a subject who is feeling *both* tense and angry will select only one of the mood states to report, forcing the assumption that the subject is only feeling the one mood state.

When multidimensional items are used, the data can be dealt with in one of two ways. First, the multidimensional item can be considered as a set of separate items if the subject is instructed to circle all of the response options that apply (rather than circling only one, as in Figure 3, item 3). Then each separate response can be analyzed as a dichotomous yes (if circled) or no (if not circled) variable. Second, the separate responses can be grouped so that any responses within the group result in a certain score. Thus, the mood item could be given a dichotomous score for positive or negative mood. Circling one or more mood states, such as calm, happy, or hopeful, would produce a single score representing a "positive mood." Conversely, subjects indicating any of the other moods (e.g., tense, depressed, or angry) would be given a score for "negative mood." The former approach presumes that the subjects were given the appropriate instructions, whereas the latter approach sacrifices considerably information. In general, dichotomous items do not provide the psychometric strength and statistical power that unidimensional items with multiple response categories do. Either multidimensional solution thus is less satisfactory than designing, in advance, items with unidimensional, mutually exclusive and exhaustive response categories for each variable of interest.

The assessment of social situation (i.e., who is present when blood pressure measurements are made) provides another example of the problem of having multidimensional items. Many diaries include one item to assess social situation (see item 4 in Figure 3). If the subject is in a group of several people, circling one response category will not ac-

| 1. **Depressed** | No ☐ ☐ ☐ ☐ ☐ Yes |

| 2. **Depression level**
(circle one) | Not at all
depressed | A little
depressed | Moderately
depressed | Very
depressed |

3. **Mood** *(circle one)*	Happy	Hopeful
	Angry	Tense
	Calm	Sad

4. **Social situation** *(circle one)*	Alone	With superior
	With spouse	With co-worker(s)
	With family member(s)	With friend(s)

5. **Social situation**

How many people are you with? ☐☐

Who are these people?
(circle all that apply)

Spouse	Subordinate(s)
Family member(s)	Friend(s) (other than boss, superior, or co-worker)
Superior(s)	
Co-worker(s)	Stranger(s)

| 6. **Mood**
(circle one) | Very
relaxed | Moderately
relaxed | A little
relaxed | Not at all
relaxed |

| 7. **Mood**
(circle one) | Sad | Neutral | Happy |

| 8. **Mood**
(circle one) | Sad | Happy |

Figure 3. Successful and unsuccessful strategies for design of diary items.

curately characterize the situation. A solution would be to ask two questions (as in item 5 in Figure 3): the first to assess the number of people present and the second to identify these people.

In summary, it is suggested that for each variable, an item or set of related items be designed to have a unidimensional framework, with responses that are mutually exclusive and exhaustive. If a multidimensional item must be included, the subject should be directed to circle each response option that applies (not just one). Then each option can be considered as a separate unidimensional, dichotomous (yes/no) item. To determine whether items are unidimensional or multidimensional, they can be inspected, pilot-tested, or submitted to more precise scaling methods (Edwards, 1957).

Neutral Points in Response Scales

Many variables of interest in ambulatory blood pressure monitoring involve various levels of intensity. For example, subjects can be asked to indicate the extent to which they feel relaxed on a multiple-point scale ranging from "very relaxed" to "not at all relaxed." Within each item, a decision must be made regarding the number of categories to include and whether or not a neutral point is necessary. With regard to the number of categories, the rating scale literature indicates that four or more categories is sufficient to ensure adequate reliability. An illustration of a mood question with four response categories is given in item 6 in Figure 3. If the number of observations in each category is insufficient and the item is unidimensional, adjacent categories can be combined. Thus, if insufficient numbers of observations in each of the four categories in item 6 in Figure 3 were available, categories 1 and 2 and categories 3 and 4 could be combined for analysis.

The decision concerning the inclusion of a neutral point can have consequences in the analysis and interpretation of the resulting data. Item 7 in Figure 3 is a mood question that has a neutral point, whereas item 8 does not. The neutral point here allows respondents to indicate that they are neither happy nor sad. From a conceptual standpoint, it may be preferred to force respondents to choose a nonneutral response because there is a tendency for subjects to overreport the neutral position. Such forced choices can be accomplished by phrasing the item to ask which choice most closely describes their current mood, for example. There is some question as to whether a numerically intermediate or "neutral" response is in fact "neutral." In the context of job satisfaction, for example, when subjects are given a choice of responding to a question with "Yes," "No," or "Don't Know," the supposedly neutral "Don't Know" has been found to be a negative response (Smith *et al.,* 1969). There may be situations, however, in which a neutral or intermediate point is appropriate. In such situations, consideration should be given to providing subjects with a definition of, criteria for, and the expected frequency of the use of the neutral point. Consideration should

also be given to selecting the words that optimally capture the intent of the item. For example, the adjective "content" might be preferred to "neutral" for assessing an intermediate point between "happy" and "sad" moods.

The use of a neutral point must also be considered from a statistical point of view. In the context of diaries, a comparison between blood pressure and the three moods listed in item 7 (i.e., happy, neutral, and sad) would require that each subject have a blood pressure measured under each mood condition (a requirement of a within-subjects design). Thus, including the neutral point will result in more missing data (i.e., subjects without recordings in all three moods) than if subjects are forced to choose between happy and sad. The advantage of having less missing data when the neutral point is not included must be balanced against the greater power for detecting a relationship between mood and blood pressure that may result if the neutral point is included and adequate numbers of observations in each mood are available. Given these considerations, it is recommended that the neutral point be used only if there is specific interest in the neutral response and if the sample is large enough to withstand the impact of attrition due to missing data.

Logistics of Diary Design and Instructions

In addition to determining the content and design of items, there are important considerations for the design of the diary itself. In this section, issues regarding diary design and the instructions given to subjects for use of the diary will be addressed.

The self-monitoring literature discussed in the first section of this chapter has implications for the diary design. Specifically, research in self-monitoring has indicated that compliance is hampered when the monitoring task is inconvenient, time-consuming, and otherwise onerous. Therefore, the number of questions asked should be kept to a minimum. As noted before, it is recommended that the decision to include a question be based on research and clinical issues of interest rather than on a desire to be all-inclusive. Convenience, and thus compliance, can be enhanced by simplifying the subject's recording task. For example, it is more convenient to circle response options or code numbers than it is to write in responses. Moreover, strategies for recording data that are more convenient for the subject are often more convenient for computer data entry. Van Egeren and Madarasmi (n.d.), for example, have subjects complete the diary entries on computer cards by darkening spaces that are optically scanned for direct data entry. Their computer card is presented in Figure 4.

The physical design of the diary should also be such that it is convenient for the subjects. The diary should be portable and small enough to fit in a purse or pocket, or in a space on the monitor if one is provided. One investigator attaches a pencil to the diary to further enhance convenience. As another aspect of convenience, the diary also provides a useful place to put information about operating the monitor and what to do if problems are encountered.

The instructions given to subjects about the use of the diary can improve the quality and completeness of the data collected and enhance compliance. As discussed previously, self-monitoring research has shown that compliance is enhanced if subjects are told that the data they are collecting are of value and meaning (Orleans & Shipley, 1982). This message can be conveyed through careful instruction of the subjects on the rationale for the diary, procedures for its completion, the timing of the diary entries in relation to blood pressure measurements, and the definition of the terms used in the diary. Pointing out that the diary is likely to show a link between activity and blood pressure changes may also enhance cooperation, considering the self-monitoring research finding that accuracy checks increase compliance. The instructions should also indicate that all diary entries will be used. Providing subjects with feedback reflecting use of the diary information they collected is also likely to increase cooperation for later monitoring.

The manner in which the instructions for the diary are given can influence the likelihood that monitoring will lead to behavioral changes. For example, subjects could be told to expect variability in moods (or other variables) assessed by the diary. Self-monitoring research indicates that

this instruction is likely to increase the variability of moods reported (Kazdin, 1974). This factor and others that have been shown to influence reactance may be incorporated into the instructions. Decisions as to the advisability of including such elements in the instructions in order to influence reactance should be based on the objectives of the ambulatory blood pressure monitoring.

Subjects can be instructed to engage in a certain set of prescribed behaviors during the monitoring period. This procedure is a departure from the typical use of diaries to record naturally occurring events. Prescribing certain activities would help circumvent the problem of insufficient parallel data collected across subjects. The diary could be used to verify that the subject complied with the request or to actually remind or prompt the subject to perform the prescribed behavior.

One efficient way to train subjects in the use of the diary is to have them complete an entry when blood pressure measurements are made during instrumentation and calibration, i.e., before the subjects leave the clinic or laboratory wearing the monitor.

Validity of Ambulatory Monitoring Diaries

To the extent that diaries are psychometric instruments and are used to provide important data, the issue of validity needs to be considered. There are three types of validity: content, construct, and criterion validity. Content validity addresses the question of whether the diary measures what was intended. Do the questions in the diary adequately sample the universe of questions that can and should be asked? The methods to establish this validity include, but are not limited to, content-analyzing self-monitoring logs for features not attended to in the diary, interviewing subjects, accompanying subjects throughout their day, and having others describe the subjects' environment and behavior.

Construct validity and criterion validity are more difficult to establish. Several approaches are feasible and could yield important information.

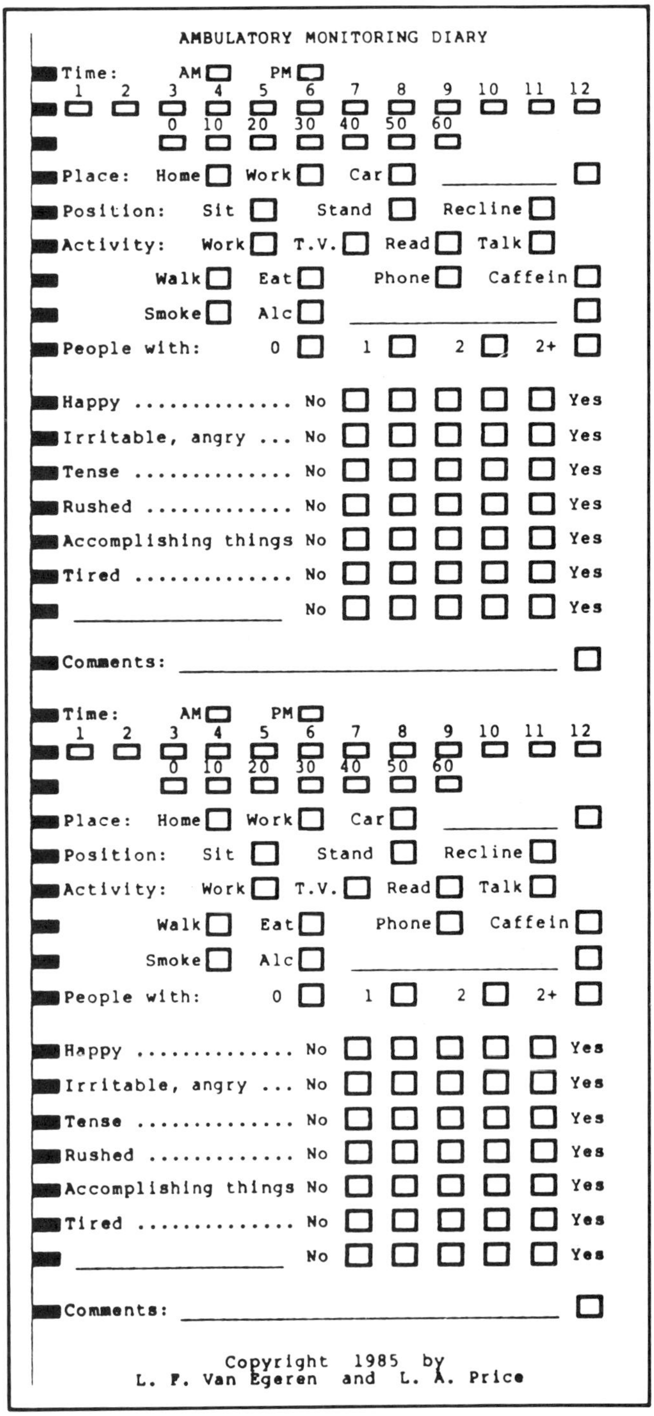

AMBULATORY MONITORING DIARY

Time: AM ☐ PM ☐
1 2 3 4 5 6 7 8 9 10 11 12
0 10 20 30 40 50 60

Place: Home ☐ Work ☐ Car ☐ ________ ☐
Position: Sit ☐ Stand ☐ Recline ☐
Activity: Work ☐ T.V. ☐ Read ☐ Talk ☐
Walk ☐ Eat ☐ Phone ☐ Caffein ☐
Smoke ☐ Alc ☐ ____________ ☐
People with: 0 ☐ 1 ☐ 2 ☐ 2+ ☐

Happy .... No ☐ ☐ ☐ ☐ ☐ Yes
Irritable, angry ... No ☐ ☐ ☐ ☐ ☐ Yes
Tense .... No ☐ ☐ ☐ ☐ ☐ Yes
Rushed .... No ☐ ☐ ☐ ☐ ☐ Yes
Accomplishing things No ☐ ☐ ☐ ☐ ☐ Yes
Tired .... No ☐ ☐ ☐ ☐ ☐ Yes
____________ No ☐ ☐ ☐ ☐ ☐ Yes

Comments: ____________ ☐

Time: AM ☐ PM ☐
1 2 3 4 5 6 7 8 9 10 11 12
0 10 20 30 40 50 60

Place: Home ☐ Work ☐ Car ☐ ________ ☐
Position: Sit ☐ Stand ☐ Recline ☐
Activity: Work ☐ T.V. ☐ Read ☐ Talk ☐
Walk ☐ Eat ☐ Phone ☐ Caffein ☐
Smoke ☐ Alc ☐ ____________ ☐
People with: 0 ☐ 1 ☐ 2 ☐ 2+ ☐

Happy .... No ☐ ☐ ☐ ☐ ☐ Yes
Irritable, angry ... No ☐ ☐ ☐ ☐ ☐ Yes
Tense .... No ☐ ☐ ☐ ☐ ☐ Yes
Rushed .... No ☐ ☐ ☐ ☐ ☐ Yes
Accomplishing things No ☐ ☐ ☐ ☐ ☐ Yes
Tired .... No ☐ ☐ ☐ ☐ ☐ Yes
____________ No ☐ ☐ ☐ ☐ ☐ Yes

Comments: ____________ ☐

Figure 4. Computer card used by Van Egeren to record diary data. Copyright 1985 by L. F. Van Egeren and L. A. Price; used with permission.

First, diaries typically assess various mood states with one item, whereas in other research protocols entire scales (e.g., Spielberger's State/Trait Anxiety questionnaire) are used to measure these constructs. It would be possible to have subjects complete a diary entry including the diary's standard assessment of mood at a time when they are given other scales that have been validated as measures of various mood states. Then responses on the diary could be correlated with responses on the scales. A strategy to validate activity would be to correlate diary responses with activities that are known and can be predicted (e.g., regularly occurring activities, such as punching a time clock).

One question relevant to measurement in any setting is the extent to which the act of measuring changes the behavior. This potential problem of reactance was discussed in the first section on self-monitoring literature. In a general way, this reactance can be investigated by a pilot study contrasting occasions when blood pressure is assessed with and without the diary and when the diary is completed with and without blood pressure assessment. This pilot study design would provide answers to two questions: Is blood pressure the same with and without the diary? Is the diary the same with and without blood pressure measurements? In summary, it is suggested that attention be paid to issues of validity and that feasible methods for checking on the validity of diaries are available.

Use of Diary Data in Analyses

Diary data have not been included in the majority of published papers on ambulatory blood pressure monitoring. The reasons include problems in the design of diaries with multidimensional and overlapping categories, as well as problems with data reduction. When these difficulties have been surmounted, two additional problems in analysis are likely to be encountered: the failure to control for confounding variables (i.e., variables that should have been included as control variables) and problems of missing data encountered when attempting to analyze data in the context of a within-subjects design. In this section we illustrate both points by addressing the question of whether blood pressure

at work is higher than blood pressure at home because of differences in physical position.

Confounding Variables

The measurement of blood pressure is likely to be confounded by several variables. It is therefore important to decide in advance what variables should be included in the diary as control variables so that they are available for subsequent analyses. For example, it is well documented that place (work versus home versus clinic) is associated with blood pressure differences (Pickering, Harshfield, Kleinert, Blank, & Laragh, 1982). In addition, position (upright versus supine) is also strongly associated with blood pressure. Blood pressure is higher during activities performed while walking or standing than during those performed while sitting or lying down (Gellman et al., 1986), although the process of rising from a supine position to a standing position tends to be associated with a drop in systolic blood pressure level (Gomella, Braen, & Olding, 1983). Thus, position may be a variable that confounds blood pressure differences observed between places such as home and work. To determine whether a potential confound exists, one could first examine whether there is a relationship between the potentially confounding variable (e.g., position) and the independent variable (e.g., place). This examination would address the question whether subjects are more likely to be sitting at home and standing at work. If this examination reveals a relationship between the confounding variable (or covariate) and the independent variable, then the covariate needs to be taken into account in the analysis. Whether this need is addressed through matching or analysis of covariance is beyond the scope of this chapter (see Cohen and Cohen, 1975, for a discussion). The important point is that potential covariates should be identified beforehand and included in the diary.

In addition to position, other potentially confounding variables in ambulatory blood pressure monitoring include medications, beverages consumed (e.g., caffeine, alcohol), activities (e.g., sleeping, relaxation, exercise), age, location (e.g., home, work), and mood (Southard et al., 1986). Other points that must be considered in determining appropriate analytic strategies are that an individual's blood pressure measurements are not independent and are influenced by the time of day.

Losing Data in the Context of a Within-Subjects Design

Analysis of ambulatory blood pressure data often employs a within-subjects design. In this analytic strategy, data obtained on the same subject under separate conditions are compared. For example, one such design would compare blood pressures assessed at home and at work on the same subjects. To enhance the likelihood that the comparison can be made, subjects probably would be asked to wear the monitor both at home and at work. As additional variables come into consideration, such as the confounding variables mentioned in the preceding section, missing data become a problem. An analysis comparing home and work pressures and controlling for position requires that blood pressures be available on each of the subjects in all the situations under study: at home and at work while sitting and standing. The extent to which missing data can present problems when diary information is considered in the analysis is illustrated by a recent study in which approximately half of the subjects did not have readings in all four of the possible observation combinations of work, home, sitting, and standing. This problem becomes magnified when additional variables are involved, as would be the case if blood pressure comparisons were to be made in three settings: work, home, and car. In this example, an analysis comparing blood pressures in the three settings and controlling for position is likely to encounter a missing-data problem of significant proportions. Any analysis based on group means calculated with different subjects in each condition would be invalid since it does not meet the assumptions of either a within- or between-subjects design. Furthermore, recent analyses suggest that, to obtain reliable measurements, several observations in each setting are necessary (Llabre, Ironson, Spitzer, & Schneiderman, n.d.).

One alternative to this problem was discussed in the sections on logistics of diary design and instructions to the subjects. Specifically, the instructions to the subjects could emphasize the importance of obtaining blood pressure readings in a number of key conditions. This strategy, although providing parallel data, is inconsistent with the concept of ambulatory monitoring of behavior as it would occur spontaneously in the natural setting. An alternative strategy would be to seek large enough samples to allow for the expected missing data.

Outliers

Certain general statistical issues assume special importance when viewed in the context of diary data; primary among these is determining whether an aberrant blood pressure reading is an outlier and should be excluded from analysis. An outlier is an observation that seems discordant with some type of pattern. There are two ways in which an outlier can occur that are relevant here.* In one case, a mistake is made in the reading, i.e., the ambulatory blood pressure monitor malfunctions. In the other case, a "true" rare deviation has been observed. The manner in which outliers are treated in the analysis should ideally depend on the cause; unfortunately, it is not possible to know the cause with certainty. For example, physical activity affects blood pressure and also increases the likelihood of machine malfunction. Thus, if an ambulatory monitor always malfunctions while taking blood pressures when subjects are driving, it would be difficult to estimate blood pressure while driving. To make decisions about outliers, many researchers consult the subject's diary to see whether any of the known causes of malfunction (e.g., driving an automobile) were present at the time of the reading. This information is then used to decide whether to consider the blood pressure assessment in the analysis. Although this practice may seem reasonable at this stage of the "science" of ambulatory monitoring, it does introduce bias and should be reported when data are published. To avoid this problem and to eventually have data on blood pressure in environments or

---

*A third way in which an outlier can occur is specification of an incorrect model. For a discussion of model selection in outlier analysis, see Clark et al. (n.d.).

during activities that may lead to spurious assessments, it would be desirable to conduct pilot studies in the field to attempt to establish normative data against which data collected with ambulatory monitors could be compared.

Summary

Diaries represent a method of tracking potential behavioral influences on physiological variables. This chapter has reviewed several considerations to keep in mind when designing and implementing such a system, in order to maximize the potential benefits of diaries.

In designing the diary, it is important to focus on questions covering specific hypotheses of interest rather than merely to take a diary off the shelf or limit measurement to areas already covered in existing diaries, such as environmental, behavioral, and control variables. Potential covariates, such as place and position, and control variables. Potential covariates, such as place and position, should be identified and measured. If possible, items should be unidimensional with mutually exclusive and exhaustive categories. Additional conceptual issues to be addressed when designing items include use of the neutral point, focus on evaluation or description, specificity, time frame, and frame of reference. Finally, to enhance compliance, the number of questions should be kept to a minimum and the physical design should be as convenient as possible to yield a low response cost.

Directions given to the participant are of vital importance; the self-monitoring literature suggests that they may influence both reactive effects and compliance. Such instructions might include emphasizing the value of the data being collected, the importance of getting blood pressure and diary entries in key settings (or, alternatively, oversampling diary readings corresponding to high blood pressure values), setting expectations with respect to variability in behavior or mood, setting expectations of accuracy checks and feedback, and including an actual demonstration of diary use.

Some areas of needed research were noted. These include research on how self-monitoring influences the behavior being measured, validation of diary responses versus other established measures or objective data, and collection of normative data to aid in outlier identification and interpretation.

Future Directions

To date, ambulatory monitoring of physiological parameters and behavior has greatly enhanced opportunities for assessment in cardiovascular behavioral medicine. The future can be expected to produce further developments in two areas: the use of ambulatory monitoring for the assessment of physiological parameters in addition to blood pressure and heart rate and the application of new technological developments to improve ambulatory monitoring equipment and capabilities.

The research and clinical advantages made evident by ambulatory blood pressure monitoring are encouraging investigators to explore other uses of this technology. These new applications include assessment of physiological parameters requiring invasive methods, such as plasma catecholamines (see Dimsdale, this volume). Extension of ambulatory monitoring technology will undoubtedly continue in the future and will generate new diaries for the assessment of activities—diaries that are appropriate for the parameters being measured and the research and clinical objectives of the measurements.

Ambulatory monitoring and the assessment of daily activities in studies of silent ischemia illustrate this trend. Ambulatory electrocardiographic (Holter) monitoring with a diary for the assessment of anginal pain revealed that approximately two-thirds of ischemic episodes are asymptomatic (Tzivoni, Gavish, Benhorin, Keren, & Stern, 1986). This finding has important clinical implications. Specifically, it indicates that evaluating the severity of ischemic disease based on the presence of anginal pain may result in underestimates. Ambulatory monitoring has also been enlisted in studies of silent ischemia to investigate whether there are environmental or behavioral correlates of ischemic episodes. With a diary used in conjunction with electrographic monitoring, Tzivoni *et al.* (1986) observed that ischemia is more frequent during daily activities than during stress. Previously, Schang and Pepine (1977) recorded 2826 hours of electrographic monitoring of 20 patients with coronary heart disease. Using a simple diary, they concluded that the majority of ischemic episodes occurred at rest or during light activity, not during the stress of treadmill exercise. More recently, electrographic monitoring in conjunction with a diary for level of mental and physical activities in a study of 21 patients with coronary heart disease again showed transient ischemia to be most common during activities demanding mental arousal and not physical exertion (Rebecca *et al.*, 1986). Although ambulatory monitoring research on silent ischemia has just begun, the potential benefits are already evident with results that are providing important information for clinical management of the disease. In the future, other clinical conditions, such as left ventricular dysfunction or coronary spasm, are likely to become candidates for the use of ambulatory monitoring.

Regardless of the physiological parameter under study, the capabilities of ambulatory monitoring equipment will benefit from technological advances in bioengineering hardware and software and in telecommunications. Among these developments will be devices that regularly or continuously monitor for a specific pattern of physiological changes and alert subjects to complete diary entries when these changes are detected. The Q-med Star device for electrographic monitoring is an example of such a ''smart'' monitor.

The technological advances seen in the monitor hardware are likely to extend into the realm of ambulatory monitoring diaries. For example, the technology exists to simplify data entry with touch-sensitive key pads, including automatic recording of time by internal semiconductor clock chips. Cellular technology and other advances in telemetry and telecommunications offer new strategies for recording behavior in conjunction with physiological monitoring. These advances will enhance accuracy as well as minimize the reactance involved in self-monitoring of behavior by reducing the inconvenience of completing pencil-and-paper diaries, and by automatic recording of certain activities and behaviors, such as speech and physical activity. A likely result of these more convenient, efficient, and technologically sophisti-

cated diaries will be the development of a standard set of programmed diary items that will be used across studies and the capability to tailor an additional ancillary set of items for specific clinical or research applications.

The two future trends suggested above will coincide and promote one another. The search for and adaptation of technological advances will be spurred on by application of ambulatory monitoring to additional physiological parameters, both individually and simultaneously. Concurrently, technological advances in bioengineering and communications will promote new and broader applications of ambulatory monitoring to cardiovascular behavioral medicine.

References

Anastasi, A. (1982). *Psychological testing* (5th ed.). New York: Macmillan Co.

Blanchard, E. B. (1981). Behavioral assessment of psychophysiologic disorders. In D. H. Barlow (Ed.), *Behavioral assessment of adult disorders* (pp. 239–270). New York: Guilford Press.

Ciminero, A. R., Nelson, R. O., & Lipinski, D. P. (1977). Self-monitoring procedures. In A. R. Ciminero, K. S. Calhoun, & H. E. Adams (Eds.), *Handbook of behavioral assessment: Self-monitoring procedures* (pp. 195–232). New York: Wiley.

Clark, L. A., Denby, L., Pregibon, D., Harshfield, G. A., Pickering, T. G., Blank, S., & Laragh, J. H. (n.d.). *A data based method for bivariate outlier detection: Application to automatic blood pressure recording devices.* Unpublished paper, AT&T Bell Laboratories, Murray Hill, NJ.

Cohen, J., & Cohen, P. (1975). *Applied multiple regression/correlation analysis for the behavioral sciences.* New York: Erlbaum.

Condiotte, M. M., & Lichtenstein, E. (1981). Self-efficacy and relapse in smoking cessation programs. *Journal of Consulting and Clinical Psychology, 49,* 648–659.

Edwards, A. L. (1957). *Techniques of attitude scale construction.* New York: Appleton–Century–Crofts.

Evans, R. I., Hansen, W. B., & Mittlemark, M. B. (1977). Increasing the validity of self-reports of smoking behavior in children. *Journal of Applied Psychology, 62,* 521–523.

Gellman, M., Ironson, G., Spitzer, S., Keenan, M., Schneiderman, N., & Weidler, D. (1986, November). *Ambulatory blood pressure as a function of race, gender, place, and mood.* Paper presented at the American Heart Association meeting, Dallas.

Gomella, L. G., Braen, G. R., & Olding, M. J. (1983). *Clinician's pocket reference* (4th ed.). Norwalk, CT: Appleton.

Guilford, J. P. (1954). *Psychometric methods* (2nd ed.). New York: McGraw–Hill.

Guion, R. M. (1965). *Personnel testing.* New York: McGraw–Hill.

Hartman, D. P., & Wood, D. D. (1982). Observational methods. In A. S. Bellack, M. Hersen, and A. E. Kazdin (Eds.), *International handbook of behavior modification and therapy* (pp. 109–138). New York: Plenum Press.

Kanfer, F. (1970). Self-monitoring: Methodological limitations and clinical application. *Journal of Consulting and Clinical Psychology, 35,* 148–152.

Kazdin, A. E. (1974). Reactive self-monitoring: The effects of response desirability, goal setting, and feedback. *Journal of Consulting and Clinical Psychology, 42,* 704–716.

Lawrence, P. S. (1982). Behavioral assessment of sleep disorders. In F. J. Keefe & J. A. Blumenthal (Eds.), *Assessment strategies in behavioral medicine* (pp. 197–221). New York: Grune & Stratton.

Llabre, M. M., Ironson, G. H., Spitzer, S. B., & Schneiderman, N. (n.d.). *How many blood pressure measurements is enough? An application of generalizability to the study of blood pressure reliability.* Unpublished paper, University of Miami.

McFall, R. M. (1977). Parameters of self-monitoring. In R. B. Stuart (Ed.), *Behavioral self-management: Strategies, techniques, and outcome* (pp. 196–214). New York: Brunner/Mazel.

Nelson, R. O. (1977). Methodological issues in assessment via self-monitoring. In J. D. Cone & R. P. Hawkins (Eds.), *Behavioral assessment: New directions in clinical psychology* (pp. 217–240). New York: Brunner/Mazel.

Nelson, R. O., Lipinski, D. P., & Black, J. L. (1976). The relative reactivity of external observations and self-monitoring.. *Behavior Therapy, 7,* 314–321.

Nunnally, J. C. (1978). *Psychometric theory* (2nd ed.). New York: McGraw–Hill.

Orleans, C. S., & Shipley, R. H. (1982). Assessment in smoking cessation research: Some practical guidelines. In F. J. Keefe & J. A. Blumenthal (Eds.), *Assessment strategies in behavioral medicine* (pp. 261–317). New York: Grune & Stratton.

Pickering, T. G., Harshfield, G. A., Kleinert, H. D., Blank, S., & Laragh, J. H. (1982). Blood pressure during normal activities, sleep and exercise: Comparison of values in normal and hypertensive subjects. *Journal of the American Medical Association, 247,* 992–996.

Rebecca, G. S., Wayne, R. R., Campbell, S., Rocco, M., Nabel, E., Barry, J., & Selwyn, A. P. (1986, March). *Transient ischemia in coronary disease is associated with mental arousal during daily life.* Paper presented at the 35th Annual Scientific Session, American College of Cardiology, Atlanta.

Romanczyk, K. (1974). Self-monitoring in the treatment of obesity: Parameters of reactivity. *Behavior Therapy, 5,* 531–540.

Roskies, E., Seraganian, P., Oseasohn, R., Hanley, J. A., Collu, R., Martin, N., & Smilga, C. (1986). The Montreal type A intervention project: Major findings. *Health Psychology, 5,* 45–69.

Schang, S. J., & Pepine, C. J. (1977). Transient asymptomatic S-T segment depression during daily activity. *American Journal of Cardiology, 39,* 396–402.

Sjoden, P. O., Bates, S., & Nyren, O. (1983). Continuous self-recording of epigastric pain with two rating scales: Compliance, authenticity, reliability, and sensitivity. *Journal of Behavioral Assessment, 5,* 327–344.

Smith, P. C., Kendall, L. M., & Hulin, C. L. (1969). *The measurement of satisfaction in work and retirement.* Chicago: Rand McNally.

Southard, D. R., Coates, T. J., Kolodner, K., Parker, F. C., Padgett, N. E., & Kennedy, H. L. (1986). Relationship between mood and blood pressure in the natural environment: An adolescent population. *Health Psychology, 5,* 469–480.

Thoresen, C. E., & Mahoney, M. J. (1974). *Behavioral self-control.* New York: Holt, Rinehart & Winston.

Tzivoni, D., Gavish, A., Benhorin, J., Keren, A., & Stern, S. (1986). Myocardial ischemia during daily activities and stress. *American Journal of Cardiology, 58,* 47B–50B.

Van Egeren, L., & Madarasmi, S. (n.d.). *A computerized diary for ambulatory blood pressure monitoring.* Unpublished paper, Michigan State University.

Ward, M. M., & Chesney, M. A. (1985). Diagnostic interviewing for psychophysiological disorders. In M. Hersen & S. M. Turner (Eds.), *Diagnostic interviewing* (pp. 261–285). New York: Plenum Press.

CHAPTER 21

Data Analysis of Ambulatory Blood Pressure Readings

Before p Values

L. A. Clark, L. Denby, and D. Pregibon

Introduction

The nature of ambulatory blood pressure (BP) monitoring is such that exploratory data analysis is both useful and necessary. In any study using ambulatory monitoring there are many sources of uncontrolled variability, including individual levels of BP, individual diurnal patterns of BP, individual physical activity patterns, individual mental activity (psychological) patterns, and artifactual readings. Failure to properly account for these sources of variation will typically obscure real effects in the data and can bias the estimates of the effects of primary interest. In this chapter we report our experience with the exploratory analysis which should precede the calculation of p values. Our experience has been primarily with large samples. When the sample size is large, computing resources can be severely strained and statistical significance (via a p value) takes a backseat to practical significance. We do not discuss the interpretation of significance tests in any detail but refer readers to the discussions by Ware, Mosteller, and Ingelfinger (1986) and Royall (1986).

Classical statistical methods rely on a thorough appreciation of the sources of variability giving rise to the data. Typically this is done using unverifiable assumptions. Our approach reflects the current trend in data analysis that one should use methods which not only address questions of interest, but also allow unsuspected phenomena to be discovered. The basic paradigm we use is

$$\text{Data} = \text{Fit} + \text{residual}$$

where *fit* is some tentative description of the data, and *residual* is the difference between the data and its tentative description. The data analysis strategy which we use relies on successively *removing* structure from the data (by fitting), and carefully analyzing the residuals to determine whether the current description (*fit*) is adequate or not. Our presentation downplays the fitting process itself and emphasizes the analysis of residuals. Thus, for example, rather than concentrate on the analysis of variance table which summarizes what we did fit, we focus our attention on the residuals to determine whether what we did not fit is important.

The basic tools are graphical in nature. The primary disadvantage of graphical procedures is that they may appear to lack objectivity in contrast to

L. A. Clark, L. Denby, and D. Pregibon • AT&T Bell Laboratories, Murray Hill, New Jersey 07974.

numerical summaries and so-called test statistics. Our view is that both numerical and graphical procedures have their place in data analysis, but that graphical procedures should be used first so that the numerical procedures can be most effective. Uncritical application of standard numerical methods, without careful checking of assumptions that underlie them, can easily lead to erroneous results. This chapter is organized to reflect this view, drawing on examples to illustrate the use of graphical displays in all phases of analysis. The data upon which the examples are based are drawn entirely from studies we have been involved with in collaboration with The Hypertension Center at New York Hospital.

Premodeling

Our emphasis in this chapter is on modeling BP monitoring data. It is important to remember that any model fitting method can only be relied on if the data they are applied to make sense. They cannot distinguish good readings from bad readings, nor whether certain segments of the study group are qualitatively different than the rest. The methods are merely algorithms, and as such, garbage-in will ultimately lead to garbage-out. We therefore recommend "getting a feel for the data" prior to formal modeling. By this we mean displaying the data in a variety of ways with the aim of: identifying unusual BP readings, identifying unusual values of other measured variables, understanding the relationship between the other measured variables, and understanding the relationship between BP and the other measured variables. Identification of unusual readings is recommended for two reasons: if these readings are artifacts, including them in our models can lead to seriously biased estimates of the effects of interest; and if they are genuine, they are important in their own right for gaining insight into the determinants of BP. Understanding the relationship between the other measured variables serves to highlight peculiarities in their joint distribution and also the extent of the dependencies between them. If two variables are closely related, the data may not contain enough information to

provide distinct estimates of their individual effects. Thus, in the modeling stage, only one of these measured variables or some single composite quantity should be included in the models. Understanding the relationship between BP and the other measured variables is in fact the motivation for modeling, and any simple relationships that can be uncovered prior to formal modeling will make the job of residual analysis much easier.

Identification of unusual BP readings usually proceeds by graphically displaying the systolic and diastolic readings. Histograms are convenient summaries of these distributions, examples of which are given in Figure 1. Depending on the amount of data and the heterogeneity of the study group, pooling across subjects may or may not be appropriate. But at the premodeling stage we are primarily looking for gross outliers and pooling is usually performed. If the study group is known to be heterogeneous, an adjustment for this may be useful before pooling, even if the adjustment may be crude. For example, one can subtract each subject's 24-h mean pressure or the mean clinic pressure from the readings prior to plotting. The fact that both of these adjustments may be biased is not critical since at this stage we are interested in finding gross outliers only. In the next section we describe a less-biased way of adjusting for heterogeneity.

Outliers are readings which occur in the extremes, or tails, of the distribution. As an objective aid to interpreting the display, cutpoints are usually specified so that readings beyond these points are regarded as outliers. So, for example, if x and y denote a systolic and diastolic reading respectively and s_x and s_y the corresponding standard deviations, then any reading not satisfying

$$\bar{x} - 2s_x < x < \bar{x} + 2s_x$$
$$\bar{y} - 2s_y < y < \bar{y} + 2s_y \tag{1}$$

is an outlier in the sense that it is far from the mean of one or both of the marginal distributions.

A problem with looking at the distributions of systolic and diastolic pressures separately is that an obvious artifact, say a reading of 100/99 mm Hg,

Figure 1. The data are 917 BP measurements of 15 ambulatory subjects (Clark *et al.*, 1987a) with mild untreated hypertension taken by an automatic recorder at 15-min intervals. The readings were taken over a consecutive 24-h period starting and ending with a calibration of the device in the clinic. The recorder could be manually initiated by the subject to obtain additional readings or could be turned off by the subject for a period of time. The subjects were instructed to follow their usual daily activity pattern, and in addition, to maintain a diary describing the activity and position at the time of each reading. Panel a displays the histogram of

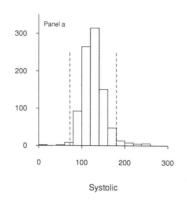
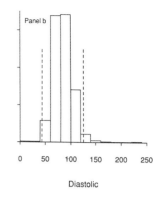

the systolic readings ($\bar{x} = 126.48$ and $S_x = 27.15$) and panel b the diastolic readings ($\bar{y} = 84.67$ and $S_y = 20.59$). Both distributions exhibit slight asymmetry. The dashed lines define the boundaries of the outlier detection rule of equation (1). There are 38 systolic and 29 diastolic readings outside the boundaries. This corresponds to 4 and 3% of the systolic and diastolic readings, respectively.

will not be identified since neither a systolic reading of 100 mm Hg nor a diastolic reading of 99 mm Hg is unusual. Systolic pressure does not vary independently of diastolic pressure and there exists a demonstrable positive correlation between the two. Separate assessment of their marginal distributions fails to take this correlation into account. This can be rectified by considering two new variables, x^* and y^*, that are derived from x and y as follows:

$$x^* = \frac{x}{s_x} - \frac{y}{s_y}, \qquad y^* = \frac{x}{s_x} + \frac{y}{s_y} \qquad (2)$$

The new variables x^* and y^* are uncorrelated and amenable to the same type of analysis as x and y including graphical display (Figure 2). Any readings not satisfying

$$\bar{x}^* - 2s_{x^*} < x^* < \bar{x}^* + 2s_{x^*}$$
$$\bar{y}^* - 2s_{y^*} < y^* < \bar{y}^* + 2s_{y^*} \qquad (3)$$

are outliers in the sense that they are far from the mean of one or both of the marginal distributions of x^* and y^*.

An alternative graphical display to aid in the detection of outliers is a scatterplot of systolic versus diastolic readings. Outliers correspond to readings which occur in the extremes, or tails, of

the bivariate distribution. Figure 3 provides an example.

The rules for outlier identification given above can be displayed graphically as an enhancement to the basic scatterplot. The rules given in (1) define a rectangular region centered at $(\bar{x}, \bar{y})$. The rules given in (3) define a parallelogram-shaped region centered at $(\bar{x}, \bar{y})$. Readings falling outside these regions violate one or the other of these rules. For highly correlated data, the improvement provided by the second of these is readily apparent (Figure 4).

A further refinement of this method for identifying outliers while accommodating correlation employs an elliptical region centered at $(\bar{x}, \bar{y})$ (Clark *et al.*, 1987a). The differences lie in the borderline readings which would normally be examined in any case.

Unusual values of the other measured variables can be identified either marginally or by using the device described above for pairs of variables which are highly correlated. A multivariate outlier detection rule is given by Healy (1968) but unfortunately no simple graphical display is available. Indeed, when there are many variables under consideration, current technology forces us to inspect pairwise relationships between them rather than dealing directly with their multivariate distribution. A convenient and useful way of displaying all possi-

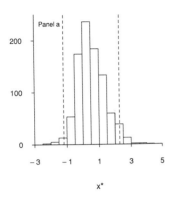
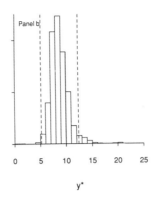

Figure 2. The data are the same as those described in the legend of Figure 1. Using the formulas given in equation (2), panel a displays the histogram of x^* ($\bar{x}^* = 0.54$ and $S_{x^*} = 0.86$) and panel b, y^* ($\bar{y}^* = 8.76$ and $S_{y^*} = 1.8$). Both distributions are reasonably symmetric. The dashed lines define the boundaries of the outlier detection rule of equation (3). There are 40 x^* and 36 y^* readings outside the boundaries. This corresponds to about 4% of the readings in both cases.

ble scatterplots of p variables is to arrange them in a scatterplot matrix (Cleveland, 1985, p. 98). The entry in the ith row and the jth column of the scatterplot matrix is the scatterplot of variable i versus variable j. Scanning across rows or columns of the scatterplot matrix allows one to quickly assess the relationship of each variable to all other variables.

A low-tech way to view the joint distribution of three variables is by starting with a scatterplot of two of them, and encoding the remaining variable

in the plotting symbol. This works particularly well if the third variable is discrete (takes on only a few distinct values). For example, a scatterplot of systolic versus diastolic pressures can be enhanced by plotting an "H" or "N" to denote the subject's designation as hypertensive or normal, or plotting a "T" or "C" to denote the subject's designation as treatment or control. Figure 5 provides an example.

A scatterplot is also useful for displaying the nature and extent to dependencies between two variables. A least-squares line or a scatterplot

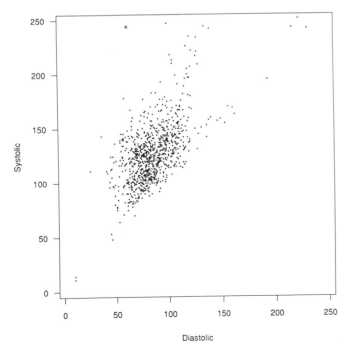

Figure 3. The data are the same as those described in the legend of Figure 1. The scatterplot displays the bivariate distribution of systolic and diastolic readings. The distribution is quite irregularly shaped but a positive correlation ($r = 0.625$) between the systolic and diastolic pressures is apparent. Several readings in the upper region of the plot are somewhat far removed from the others.

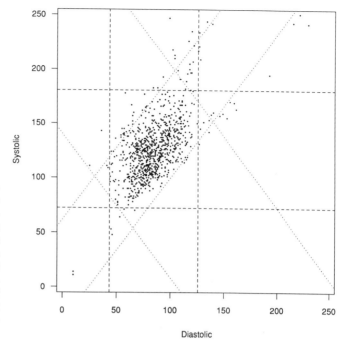

Figure 4. The data are the same as those described in the legend of Figure 1. This is the scatterplot of Figure 3 with two regions superimposed. The rectangular one parallel with the axes is given by equation (1) and the other one is given by equation (3). The 42 points outside the rectangle violate the outlier detection rules of equation (1); the 73 points outside the parallelogram violate the outlier detection rules of equation (3). They are outliers in the sense that they are far from the mean of the bivariate distribution of systolic and diastolic readings.

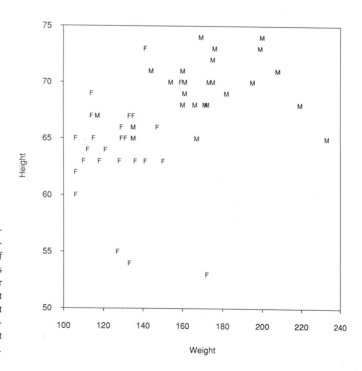

Figure 5. The data are height and weight measurements for 25 males and 25 females involved in the study described in the legend of Figure 7. This is a scatterplot of height versus weight with the plotting character ''F'' for females and ''M'' for males. Note that height and weight are moderately correlated for most of the subjects but that there are a few individuals (e.g., the three females less than 5 feet tall at the bottom of the plot) who are outliers.

smooth (Collomb, 1981) can be superimposed on the plot to help assess any apparent trend. The former is simply a single equation of the form

$$y = a + bx$$

whereas the latter can be viewed as a "moving" least-squares line

$$y = a_k + b_k x$$

where the coefficients a_k and b_k are determined from the x–y pairs in the kth window. Figure 6 illustrates the idea. One can put both the least-squares line and the scatterplot smooth on the same plot to assess the linearity of the smooth curve.

Lineplots are useful for displaying the salient features of the joint distribution of a continuous variable and a categorical variable. A lineplot displays the mean, standard deviation, and any data values outside two standard deviations of the continuous variable, for each value of the categorical variable. Alternatively, one could display the histograms of the continuous variable for each value of the categorical variable. The lineplot condenses

some of this detail and allows assessment, at a glance, of the level and variability of the continuous variable over the entire range of the categorical variable. It is particularly useful if the categorical variable is ordinal in nature, say corresponding to successive hours in the day, but this is not a requirement of the display. Figure 7 provides an example.

Modeling Methodology

In this section we discuss models that are useful in understanding the mechanisms generating the level and variability of BP monitoring data. In doing so, we do not really believe that the models we are using are "correct" in any strict sense of the word. All models are wrong, but some are *useful*. In exploratory analyses of the type we are advocating, the usefulness of any particular model is based on how well it summarizes the data at hand for the purpose of satisfying the objectives of the study.

We will downplay as much as possible the details of model fitting since this information is discussed

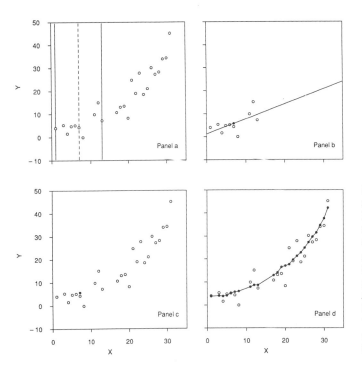

Figure 6. These graphs show how a *scatterplot smooth* is computed using the "moving" least-squares line technique. Panels a–c illustrate the computations at x_6. In panel a the solid lines highlight a window of 10 data points symmetrically situated around x_6. Panel b shows the least-squares line fitted to the 10 points in the window. The value of the line at x_6, $\hat{y}_6$, is the smoothed estimate of y_6, highlighted in panels b and c by the solid circle. These three steps are repeated for each point on the plot resulting in the curve traced out by the solid circles in panel d.

Figure 7. The data are 8730 BP measurements from 190 subjects being evaluated for mild hypertension at The Hypertension Center of The New York Hospital–Cornell Medical Center (Clark *et al.*, 1987b). The readings were taken over a consecutive 24-h period starting and ending with a calibration of the device in the clinic. The subjects wore the recorder on a day when they did not go to work. They were instructed to follow their usual daily activity pattern and, in addition, to maintain a diary describing the activity and position at the time of each reading. This figure shows the diastolic pressure readings adjusted by the subject clinic means versus hour of the day. The hourly averages (solid circles) ± 2 S.D. (whiskers) are plotted versus the corresponding hour of the day. Points outside these intervals are plotted individually. The variation in means appears to vary according to the hour of the day, with pressures being lowest in early morning and reaching a high near midday. A smooth decline throughout the day is marred by a slight increase near 1800 h, followed by a steady decline to early morning lows.

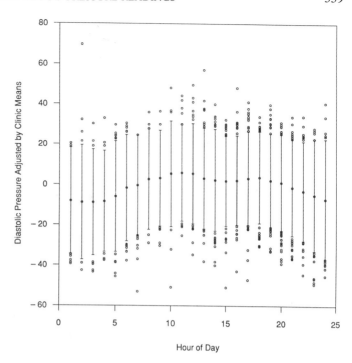

in standard textbooks. Instead we will emphasize data analysis strategy and graphical techniques to assess and enhance the modeling process.

The level of an ambulatory BP reading is related to many factors, some of which are controlled while others are uncontrolled. Controlled factors are those which are under the control of the researcher and typically refer to some intervention such as prescribed medication. Uncontrolled factors are those which are not under the control of the researcher, such as the subject's "baseline" BP level, the time of day, or what the subject was doing at the time of the reading.

In the formative stages of understanding the determinants of ambulatory BP, all effects are treated as equally important. As experience with ambulatory monitoring broadens and we learn which uncontrolled sources of variation matter and which do not, researchers will concentrate on the effects of the controlled or design factors. To avoid seriously biased estimates of these effects, we must still take into account those sources of uncontrolled variability that do matter. This can be accomplished by postulating a model which includes all sources of variability and jointly estimating their

effects. We do not distinguish between so-called *random* and *fixed* effect models. For exploratory analysis the distinction is neither relevant nor important.

We use a model in which the factors are additively related to BP level. For each subject the model is of the form

$$BP = Diurnal + ambulatory + treatment + error$$
$$(4)$$

where each term represents the effect of one source of variability. The *diurnal* effect accounts for the so-called circadian rhythm of BP (Halberg, Halberg, Halberg, & Halberg, 1984; Millar-Craig, Bishop, & Raftery, 1978; Millar-Craig, Mann, Balasubramanian, & Raftery, 1978). The *ambulatory* effect represents the anecdotal information that subjects record throughout the monitoring period. The *treatment* effect refers to the controlled design factors, such as whether or not a drug is administered. The *error* term represents the inaccuracy of the hypothesized model. In the ideal situation where the model adequately represents the data, the errors then represent random variability. If the model is not adequate, the errors represent the composite bias resulting from missing important sources of variability, incorrect functional form for an explanatory variable, or contributions from nonadditivity.

The above model is quite general and we demonstrate this in two ways. First, each effect can be modeled in a variety of ways. If the effect is qualitative, as opposed to quantitative, it is usually represented by separate constants for each qualitative level. Thus, if the *ambulatory* effect captures the position of the subject at the time the reading was recorded, say standing, sitting, and lying down, then the model allows three constants to capture the *ambulatory* effect. If the effect is quantitative, say obtained by counting or by measurement, a variety of representations are possible. The simplest is to model the effect linearly, possibly after reexpression to another scale. For example, if the amount x of an administered drug is being used to quantify the treatment effect, then simple relationships of the form

$$\text{Treatment} = \alpha + \beta x$$

or

$$\text{Treatment} = \alpha + \beta \log(x)$$

are commonly used. When the exact form of the dependence between BP level and a continuous variable is unknown, the effect can be captured by discretizing the variable into distinct classes. Separate constants can then be used to model the effect as though it were qualitative rather than quantitative. For example, consider the variable t, representing the time of day when the reading was recorded. A typical representation of the diurnal effect is a sinusoid,

$$\text{Diurnal} = \alpha + \beta \sin(\omega t) + \gamma \cos(\omega t)$$

An alternative is

$$\text{Diurnal} = \begin{cases} f_1 & \text{if } 2400\text{ h} < t \le 0100\text{ h} \\ f_2 & \text{if } 0100\text{ h} < t \le 0200\text{ h} \\ \vdots & \vdots \\ f_{24} & \text{if } 2300\text{ h} < t \le 2400\text{ h} \end{cases}$$

where the different values $\{f_i\}$ represent the hourly dependence of BP on time of day. Yet another alternative, intermediate between the sinusoid and the step function induced by the discretization, is the representation of the diurnal effect by

$$\text{Diurnal} = s(t), \qquad s \text{ smooth and periodic in } t$$

This corresponds more closely to our current understanding of diurnal variation without committing ourselves to an explicit functional form such as a sinusoid which may be woefully inadequate. Below we describe how such a representation can be fitted to data.

The second way to illustrate the generality of model (4) is to consider its application to a heterogeneous study group. If data are abundant, it may be reasonable to model some of the effects separately for each subject while the others are assumed constant. Thus, the model can be generalized to

$$\text{BP}(i) = \text{Diurnal}(i) + \text{ambulatory} + \text{treatment} + \text{error}, \qquad i = 1, \ldots, n$$

where the *ambulatory* and *treatment* effects are common across all n subjects but the *diurnal* effect, often used for adjustment, is subject-specific. The paper by Marler, Jacob, Lehoczky, and Shapiro (1988) provides an example. This model, although relevant in most situations, may be impractical to fit in cases where data are limited. An alternative is to model each subject's diurnal effect with a common shape, say an arbitrary but smooth dependence on time, but allow the overall BP level of each subject to account for between-subject differences. In the notation of model (4) we have

$$\text{BP}(i) = \text{Baseline}(i) + \text{diurnal} + \text{ambulatory} + \text{treatment} + \text{error}, \qquad i = 1, \ldots, n$$

Although this model oversimplifies the true relationship between BP and time of day, it could model sparse data quite well if the ambulatory effects are detailed enough to account for the heterogeneity of the study group.

The effects can be made specific to groups of

subjects rather than individual subjects. So, for example, if we let g denote the label of the group that subject i belongs to, we could formulate the model

$$BP\ (i,g) = \text{Diurnal}\ (i) + \text{ambulatory} + \text{treatment}\ (g) + \text{error}, \qquad i=1, \ldots, n$$

whereby each subject's diurnal pattern is distinct and their daily activity patterns the same, but that certain subgroups of the study group respond differently to treatment than others. This might be the case if upon entry into the study, each subject was classified as having mild or severe hypertension.

Other generalizations of the basic model equation will be appropriate in different situations. Our objective here is to give a flavor for the different ways these generalizations can be made and no attempt at completeness is suggested.

The basic tools needed to fit models of this type are analysis of variance (ANOVA) if all the effects are measured by categorical variables, analysis of covariance (ANCOVA) if some of the effects are measured on a continuum, or linear regression if all the effects are measured on continua. Linear regression algorithms must also be used to fit ANOVA and ANCOVA models in unbalanced designs. The details of fitting these models can be found in most standard statistics textbooks such as Snedecor and Cochran (1967) and Draper and Smith (1981).

Specialized techniques are required for fitting the arbitrary smooth functional dependence discussed above. See Collomb (1981) for an extensive bibliography. The simplest is obtained using a scatterplot smoother. The "moving" least-squares line (Figure 6) is a particular case of the general method. The appropriateness of the fitted function can be determined graphically by superimposing the fitted curve on the scatterplot. Inspection of this plot may indicate a parametric form for the curve which can be subsequently fitted and compared for its closeness to the nonparametric curve that was fit.

If one needs to fit a curvilinear relationship to one or more variables (say the diurnal effect) and there are other effects to be estimated in model (4), one can use the backfitting algorithm of Hastie and Tibshirani (1986). This is an iterative method which at each step of the iteration uses a scatterplot smoother to fit a smooth function of the dependence of BP on the variable of interest. Several fits for diurnal variation are compared in Figure 8.

The art of statistical modeling is similar to that of detecting artifacts, namely a problem of identification. As we have tried to illustrate above, there are many possible models from which to choose. On the basis of experience, the data at hand, and the study goals, the statistical modeler hopes to narrow the field to a few contenders. We reemphasize that models are not to be treated as truth *per se*, but rather as useful approximations thereof. In this regard, the most useful models must be detailed enough to describe the data accurately, yet simple enough to understand, and broad enough to generalize to other related data. The trick is to consider a *family* of models, defined in a hierarchical fashion ranging from overly simple models to overly complicated models. The representations we used above for the *diurnal* effect provide an illustration of such a family. The task of model identification takes place within the chosen family. Of course, the family may have to be broadened at some stage if the initial range is found to be too restrictive, but this is natural and with experience, the right range will suggest itself. On the other hand, it will also become apparent if the range is too large, especially with limited data where no hope of discriminating between complex relationships will be possible although one would really like to do so. The researcher can fit these models sequentially to the data starting with either the simplest or the most complicated and at each step use techniques such as those discussed in the next section to compare the two fits.

Residual Analysis

Prior to fitting models, we use plots of BP readings to look for extreme values and for preliminary assessment of the extent and nature of the dependence of BP on the various sources of variability. Both during and after model fitting, residuals take the place of the original BP readings in the plots. In a way, one can think of the residuals as the

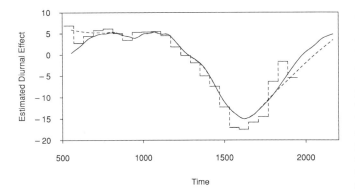

Figure 8. The data are 3164 BP measurements of 27 subjects obtained in a study of reproducibility of BP monitoring data. Two sets of readings were taken, each over a consecutive 24-h period starting and ending with a calibration of the device in the clinic. This figure compares three fits for diurnal variation. The step function shows the 24 hourly estimate when the continuous time values are discretized into 24 hourly values and an ANOVA model with main effects of baseline pressure and diurnal variation is fitted to the data. This model uses 24 degrees of freedom for describing diurnal variation. The step function can be compared with the fit (dashed line) assuming circadian rhythm is a continuous and smooth function of time. This model uses 8.8 degrees of freedom for describing diurnal variation. Note that the two fits are quite close. The one based on the scatterplot smoother is more parsimonious since it uses about 15 fewer degrees of freedom. The solid curve represents a further restriction to periodic functions obtained using a circular smoother (McDonald, 1986) in estimating the time component. The difference between a circular and a noncircular smoother is that the circular smoother wraps the data. In other words, to estimate the value for the last data reading in the recording period it uses a weighted average of observations at the start of the recording period as well as at the end of the recording period. This ensures that estimated readings are invariant to the time when the subjects started the 24-h recording session. This is also useful in eliminating the end effect biasing that occurs with noncircular smoothers. Comparing this fit to the one obtained with the noncircular smoother, we see that it is close to that of the noncircular smoother except at the ends of the interval where we see that the former one gives a smooth transition for the fitted function from the times at the end of the interval to those at the beginning of the interval. The fit based on the circular smoother uses 8.1 degrees of freedom to estimate the diurnal effect.

original readings *adjusted* for the sources of variability included in the model. In the ideal situation where we have identified and fitted the true (but unknown) model, the residuals should be totally free of structure and represent random variation alone. To the extent that the model is incorrect, the residuals contain the clues as to the nature and extent of the model's inaccuracy.

One must be open-minded when it comes to the analysis of residuals since there are a variety of ways in which the model may be wrong. We may have the correct form of the model but due to some artifactual readings, the estimated effects may be seriously biased and thus spoil any conclusions. Or the data may be valid but the form of the model inaccurate, as would be the case of using linear relationships when curvilinear ones are required. Or a major source of variability may be missing from the model, as in the case with a missing interaction effect among the covariates. In other cases the analysis of residuals can aid in simplifying a model without undue loss of model accuracy, e.g., perhaps a parametric representation could be used in place of a nonparametric smooth.

Whether interest centers on determining the

nature or the extent of model inadequacies, graphical displays of residuals are the key to discovery. We now give some examples of using graphical techniques to validate models for BP monitoring data.

A scatterplot of residuals from the model fitted to the systolic BP readings against the residuals from the model fitted to the diastolic BP readings is useful in detecting bivariate outlying observations, i.e., readings that exhibit marked lack of fit to the model. This is the analogue of the scatterplot of diastolic BP readings against the systolic BP readings used in the premodeling phase. Although both scatterplots are used primarily for the same purpose, the difference is that the residuals represent *adjusted* readings, and as such, are more directly comparable than the original (unadjusted) readings. Both plots are necessary, however, since without prescreening the original readings for artifacts, the fitted model can result in residuals which hinder rather than help in the identification of outliers. Figure 9 is an example of a scatterplot of bivariate residuals corresponding to the same readings as Figure 3.

An effective graphical display to illustrate the

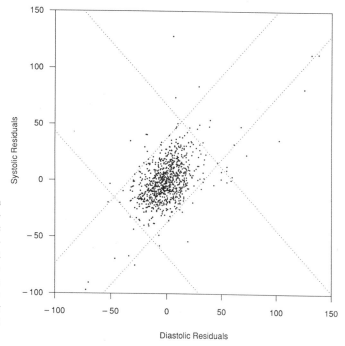

Figure 9. The data of Figure 3 are fitted with an analysis of covariance model with baseline pressure and activity as the main effects and clinic pressure as the covariate. This figure is a scatterplot of the bivariate residual pressures from fitting this model to these data. The parallelogram-shaped region given by equation (3) is superimposed. The 56 readings outside this region are outliers in the sense that they are far from their bivariate mean value after adjustment for subject baseline BP level and activity.

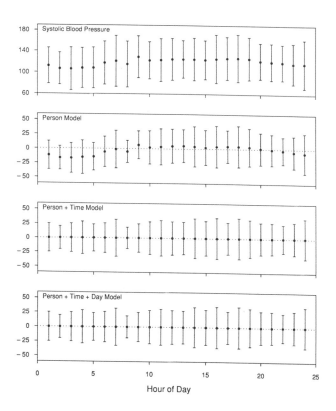

Figure 10. The data are those described in the legend to Figure 8. The figure displays the original data and residuals from successively more complex models as displayed in a four-panel plot. In each plot the hourly average (solid circle) ± 2 S.D. (whiskers) are plotted versus the corresponding hour of the day. The top panel displays the original BP data. The second shows the effect of subtracting average clinic pressure for each subject. The dependence on time of day is still visible. The third shows the effect of including time of day in the model. Note that the residuals become tighter and that the time dependence has been effectively eliminated. The last panel shows the effect of including the day that the recording was taken. This is the effect of interest in this study. The fact that there is little change from the previous panel reinforces the hypothesis of no day effect.

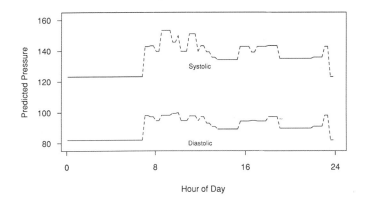

Activities by time of day for a prototype day

Time	Activity	Time	Activity
10–10:15 a.m.	Clinic	6–7 p.m.	Eating (H)
10:15–11 a.m.	Transportation (O)	7–10 p.m.	TV (H)
11–11:45 a.m.	Chores (O)	10–11 p.m.	Reading (H)
11:45–noon	Transportation (O)	11–11:30 p.m.	Dressing (H)
noon–12:30 p.m.	Eating (H)	11:30 p.m.–7 a.m.	Sleeping (H)
12:30–1 p.m.	Desk Work (H)	7–7:30 a.m.	Dressing (H)
1–1:30 p.m.	Reading (H)	7:30–8 a.m.	Eating (H)
1:30–3:30 p.m.	Relaxing (H)	8–8:30 a.m.	Transportation (O)
3:30–4:30 p.m.	Chores (H)	8:30–9:30 a.m.	Walking (O)
4:30–5 p.m.	Talking (H)	9:30–10 a.m.	Shopping (O)
5–6 p.m.	Chores (H)	10–10:15 a.m.	Clinic

Figure 11. The predicted 24-h systolic and diastolic pressures for an individual with a clinic pressure of 150/100 mm Hg and the activity profile. The predicted values are based on an analysis of covariance model fitted to the data of Figure 7 using the mean clinic pressure as the covariate and estimating the main effects of baseline pressure, location (H = home and O = other), and activity.

effect of successively adding more terms to a model is obtained using a series of aligned lineplots. Figure 10 illustrates the basic idea whereby the original data and residuals from successively more complex models are displayed in a four-panel plot.

A thorough residual analysis will result in a "final" model which can be displayed in a variety of ways. For a chosen subject and some specified typical daily profile, an annotated timeplot summarizes the results of modeling (Figure 11).

Computing Requirements

The type of analysis that we are advocating is similar to detective work; we are searching for clues, in observed data, that ultimately bear upon an increased understanding of hypertension. We do not see that a fixed recipe of analysis will suffice in any study and suggest that improvisation is more closely suited to our needs. This means that we must not only have an arsenal of *tools* at our disposal, but also the ability to *forge* new tools as we see fit. In many cases the new tools can be quite simple, such as a modification of a standard graphical display. In other cases they may require new algorithms and their subsequent software implementation.

Thus, what we envisage as important is an *interactive computing environment* that has adequate built-in numerical and graphical tools and is extensible to allow for additional tools to be added as they are required. The system should be interactive primarily to increase throughput, and reduce analyst time. It also encourages a type of *what-if* analysis whereby the analyst can quickly look at the consequences of some particular decision when alternatives are available. By *environment* we mean a system which not only provides the numerical and graphical tools which the analysis requires, but also *data management* facilities and other various tools such as text editors and word processing facilities. These must be integrated, or otherwise much analyst time must be devoted to getting the data in a form with which to apply the tools and extract results.

There are many commercially available statistical analysis programs which meet these needs to varying degrees. We are not in a position to critique these since most are hardware-specific and we have inadequate experience on the full range of PCs, micros, minis, and mainframes in current use. Rather, in the paragraph that follows, we give an overview of the facilities we currently use so that readers can see how we solved the integration problems identified above.

We currently do all of our work under the Unix™ operating system running on a time-shared Vax™ 11/750 microcomputer. The computer is configured with 6 megabytes of memory and has a 474-megabyte disk. This much memory and storage is not needed for most applications. We use an AT&T Teletype 5620 bitmapped terminal which communicates to the host computer over the Datakit™ local area network. This terminal provides us with high-resolution graphics (800 × 1024) and a *windowing* facility which permits us to simultaneously carry on a variety of tasks in a natural and unobtrusive fashion. A Laserwriter™ printer is also on the network which allows us to get quality hard copy of graphics, program listings, data listings, and reports. The principal software tool we use is the S system (Becker & Chambers, 1984). It uses the Unix file system for data base management and provides a host of statistical and graphical functions which comprise our basic toolbox of techniques. The system is extendable in two different ways, via *macros* and *functions*. The former are just collections of ordinary expressions in the language which combine to do a certain composite task. The latter requires writing in a special language, a somewhat tedious but useful way to proceed when the desired procedure will be used extensively.

References

Becker, R.A., & Chambers, J. M. (1984). *S: An interactive environment for data analysis and graphics*. Belmont, CA: Wadsworth.

Clark, L. A., Denby, L., Pregibon, D., Harshfield, G. A., Pickering, T. G., Blank, S., & Laragh, J. H. (1987a). A data based method for bivariate outlier detection: Application to automatic blood pressure recording devices. *Psychophysiology, 24,* 119–125.

Clark, L. A., Denby, L., Pregibon, D., Harshfield, G. A., Pickering, T. G., Blank, S., & Laragh, J. H. (1987b). A quantitative analysis of the effects of activity and time of day on the diurnal variations of blood pressure. *Journal of Chronic Diseases, 40,* 671–681.

Cleveland, W. S. (1985). *The elements of graphing data*. Belmont, CA: Wadsworth.

Collomb, G. (1981). Estimation Non-Parametrique de la Regression: Revue Bibliographique. *International Statistics Review, 49,* 75–94.

Draper, N. R., & Smith, H. (1981). *Applied regression analysis*. New York: Wiley.

Halberg, F., Halberg, E., Halberg, J., & Halberg, F. (1984). Chronobiologic assessment of human blood pressure variation in health and disease. In M. A. Weber & J. I. M. Drayer (Eds.), *Ambulatory blood pressure monitoring* (pp. 137–156). Berlin: Springer-Verlag.

Hastie, T., & Tibshirani, R. (1986). Generalized additive models (with discussion). *Statistical Science, 1,* 297–318.

Healy, M. J. R. (1968). Multivariate normal plotting. *Applied Statistics, 17,* 157–161.

Marler, M. A., Jacob, R. G., Lehoczky, J. P., & Shapiro, A. P. (1988). The statistical analysis of treatment effects in 24-hour ambulatory blood pressure recordings. *Statistics in Medicine, 7,* 697–716.

McDonald, J. A. (1986). Periodic smoothing of time series. *SIAM Journal of Scientific and Statistical Computing, 7,* 665–688.

Millar-Craig, M. W., Bishop, C. N., & Raftery, E. B. (1978). Circadian variation of blood pressure. *Lancet, 1,* 795.

Millar-Craig, M. W., Mann, S., Balasubramanian, V., & Raftery, E. G. (1978). Blood pressure circadian rhythm in essential hypertension. *Clinical Science and Molecular Medicine, 55,* 391s.

Royall, R. M. (1986). The effect of sample size on the meaning of significance tests. *American Statistician, 40,* 313–315.

Snedecor, G. W., & Cochran, W. G. (1967). *Statistical methods* (6th ed.). Ames: Iowa State University Press.

Ware, J. H., Mosteller, F., & Ingelfinger, J. A. (1986). P values. In J. C. Bailar, III, & F. Mosteller (Eds.), *Medical uses of statistics*. Waltham, MA: NEJM Books.

Laboratory Tasks, Procedures, and Nonpsychometric Subject Variables

Section Editor: Neil Schneiderman

Cardiovascular and hormonal responses to behavioral stimuli in the laboratory have often been investigated as possible markers or contributing factors in the pathogenesis or expression of cardiovascular disorders. Although there is considerable value in examining hemodynamic and hormonal function in persons at rest, important new information can be obtained when subjects are also exposed to behavioral tasks in the laboratory. Thus, for example, several investigators have observed that normotensive subjects with hypertensive parents reveal greater blood pressure responses to difficult mental challenges than do the normotensive offspring of normotensive parents (e.g., Falkner, Onesti, Angelakos, Fernandes, & Langman, 1979; Hastrup, Light, & Obrist, 1982). More recently, Ditto (1986) reported that the sons of hypertensive parents showed greater systolic blood pressure responses than did the sons of normotensive parents to mental arithmetic and to the Stroop test, but not to an isometric handgrip task.

Psychophysiologic experimentation in the laboratory offers opportunity for comprehensive measurement and precise stimulus control in a dynamic situation, but the results of such studies need to be interpreted cautiously. One reason for this is that different tasks, procedures used in presenting these

tasks, study populations, and individual differences within subject populations all can produce large main effects. A second reason for interpreting the role of psychophysiologic experiments cautiously is that the variables just described have a large potential for interaction. A third reason for urging caution is that distinctions that are conceptually useful in one framework (e.g., active versus passive coping) may not be as useful in another. Thus, for example, mental arithmetic may be described as an active coping task as opposed to the cold pressor test which involves passive coping. The two tasks, however, can also be contrasted in terms of a psychologic versus physical dimension, β-adrenergic versus α-adrenergic activation, or the absence versus presence of a physical pain stimulus.

The eight chapters that comprise this section explore the laboratory tasks, procedures, and nonpsychometric subject variables that have been shown to influence psychophysiologic reactivity in the laboratory. Psychometric subject variables, which also can influence psychophysiologic reactivity, are discussed in Section V. Meaningful interpretation of the outcome of psychophysiologic laboratory experiments is dependent on a grasp of the issues involved in the selection of laboratory tasks and procedures and in the analysis of subject variables.

In Chapter 22, which deals with psychophysiologic strategies in laboratory research, Schneiderman and McCabe discuss the nature of

Neil Schneiderman • Behavioral Medicine Research Center, Department of Psychology, University of Miami, Coral Gables, Florida 33124.

the tasks employed. Distinctions are made between responses to physical versus emotional stressors and between responses to active coping versus passive/inhibitory/vigilance behavioral tasks. Schneiderman and McCabe also discuss the extent to which reactivity findings in the laboratory generalize to nonlaboratory settings.

Manuck, Kasprowicz, Monroe, Larkin, and Kaplan in Chapter 23 then discuss psychophysiologic reactivity as a dimension of individual differences. Receiving particular attention in this chapter are: (1) the temporal stability of individual differences in psychophysiologic reactivity, (2) the reproducibility of these individual differences under varying stimulus conditions, and (3) the generalization of individual differences in physiologic responses from laboratory evaluations to measurements obtained in the field. Consideration of these issues is preceded by a discussion of the quantitative expression of individual differences in reactivity particularly in regard to the use of ''difference'' or ''change'' scores as opposed to ''residualized'' scores.

The social context of laboratory and field studies in cardiovascular behavioral medicine is described by Krantz and Ratliff-Crain in Chapter 24. These authors review the social interaction and instructional factors that influence outcomes in studies of psychophysiologic and behavioral responses to stressors. Several relatively subtle components of the total experimental situation are discussed, including the methods by which subject consent is obtained, ''demand characteristics'' and experimenter bias, and the way in which study descriptions are presented to subjects prior to the experimental session. This chapter also considers the underlying characteristics of commonly used tasks that determine the intensity of subjects' responses. These characteristics include task difficulty, level of challenge, harassment, competition, incentives, and instructions.

The next two chapters each deal with hemodynamic assessment and pharmacologic manipulations in laboratory task situations. In Chapter 25 DeQuattro and Lee discuss the hemodynamic adjustments that occur in response to physical stressors including isotonic and isometric exercise as well as the cold pressor test. This chapter also

discusses the effects of antihypertensive drug therapies upon the responses to exercise and cold stimuli. In Chapter 26 Julius examines the manner in which hemodynamic assessment and pharmacologic probes are used as tools to analyze cardiovascular reactivity in behavioral medicine research. As Julius points out, measurement of systemic and regional hemodynamics can provide important information about qualitative differences (e.g., in renal blood flow, sodium retention, forearm blood flow) between normotensives and hypertensives that are not necessarily reflected in the overall magnitude of blood pressure responses. Julius also discusses how the examination of hemodynamic responses to pharmacologic probes can shed some light on the complex interactions that occur among central efferent autonomic discharges, receptor properties, and end organ responsiveness.

The remaining three chapters in this section deal with subject variables that influence psychophysiologic reactivity in behavioral medicine experiments. In Chapter 27 Light examines the effects of age, family history of hypertension, blood pressure status, diabetes, obesity, and aerobic fitness upon reactivity. Anderson in Chapter 28 discusses ethnic differences in resting and stressor-induced cardiovascular and humoral reactivity. Finally, Chapter 29 by Saab describes differences in cardiovascular and neuroendocrine responses to challenge in male and female subjects. It is clear from these last three chapters that careful attention has to be paid to subject variables if we are to interpret meaningfully the outcomes of psychophysiologic reactivity experiments in cardiovascular behavioral medicine.

References

Ditto, B. (1986). Parental history of essential hypertension, active coping, and cardiovascular reactivity. *Psychophysiology, 23,* 62–70.

Falkner, B., Onesti, G., Angelakos, E. T., Fernandes, M., & Langman, C. (1979). Cardiovascular response to mental stress in normal adolescents with hypertensive parents. *Hypertension, 1,* 23–30.

Hastrup, J. L., Light, K. C., & Obrist, P. A. (1982). Parental hypertension and cardiovascular response to stress in healthy young adults. *Psychophysiology, 19,* 615–622.

CHAPTER 22

Psychophysiologic Strategies in Laboratory Research

Neil Schneiderman and Philip M. McCabe

Psychophysiologic laboratory research has begun to play an important role in the study of biobehavioral aspects of cardiovascular regulation and putative disease processes. Progress has been made both in specifying task characteristics (e.g., psychological versus physical stressors; active coping versus passive tasks) and in defining the experimental context of these tasks (e.g., instructions; experimenter effects; sociocultural factors; social interactions). Nevertheless, discrepant findings often occur between ostensibly similar experiments, in part because important differences in task characteristics have not always been recognized.

Several investigators have reported that normotensive subjects with hypertensive parents reveal greater blood pressure responses to difficult mental challenges than do the normotensive offspring of normotensive parents (e.g., Falkner, Onesti, Angelakos, Fernandes, & Langman, 1979; Hastrup, Light, & Obrist, 1982; Jorgensen & Houston, 1981; Manuck, Giordani, McQuaid, & Garrity, 1981). In contrast, other investigators have not confirmed this finding (Hohn *et al.*, 1983; Obrist, Light, James, & Strogatz, 1987; Reming-

ton, Lambarth, Moser, & Boobler, 1960). One explanation offered for the disparity in results has been in terms of the differences in experimental tasks used (Obrist, 1981). This hypothesis has received support from the findings of Hastrup *et al.* (1982), who reported that the normotensive sons of hypertensive parents showed greater systolic pressure responses to a reaction time task involving threat of shock, but not to a cold pressor test. Similarly, Ditto (1986) found that the sons of hypertensive parents showed greater systolic blood pressure responses than did the sons of normotensive parents to mental arithmetic and the Stroop test, but not to an isometric handgrip task.

The importance of adequately classifying tasks in order to understand differences in responsivity between groups can also be seen in comparisons that have been made between normotensives and borderline hypertensives. Nestel (1969) reported that borderline hypertensives reveal greater systolic and diastolic blood pressure increases and larger catecholamine responses than do normotensives while performing tasks such as puzzle-solving. Steptoe, Melville, and Ross (1984) also found that borderline hypertensives show greater heart rate, pulse transit time, and diastolic pressure responses while performing a Stroop test or playing a video game, but not while passively watching a stressful film. Similarly, Bohlin *et al.* (1986) observed that borderline hypertensives revealed

Neil Schneiderman and Philip M. McCabe • Behavioral Medicine Research Center, Department of Psychology, University of Miami, Coral Gables, Florida 33124.

greater systolic responses than did normotensives during a self-paced arithmetic task, but not during an externally paced task.

Because the Type A behavior pattern has been identified as a possible risk factor for coronary heart disease (Rosenman *et al.*, 1975), numerous studies have compared the psychophysiologic responses of Type A and B individuals to a variety of behavioral challenges. Krantz and Manuck (1984) examined 37 of these studies and found that in 26 of them, Type A's revealed greater reactivity than did B's during behavioral challenges on at least one of several cardiovascular or endocrine measures. The most frequent A/B differences observed were in terms of systolic blood pressure responses. Positive results were most often obtained in studies that used Type A-relevant challenges such as time-urgent active coping tasks or competition. In contrast, A/B differences have rarely been found to occur in response to passive tasks or to those predominantly involving physical stressors (e.g., cold pressor test; exercise). Interactions have been reported between the A/B dimension and variables such as harassment (Diamond *et al.*, 1984), fitness level (Lake, Suarez, Schneiderman, & Tocci, 1985), level of challenge instructions (Dembroski, MacDougall, Herd, & Shield, 1979), and unpredictable noise distraction (Weidner & Matthews, 1978).

The studies just cited examined cardiovascular and/or neurohormonal responses to behavioral stimuli in the laboratory as possible markers and/or contributing factors in the pathogenesis or expression of cardiovascular disorders. Current evidence suggests that the magnitude and specificity of these cardiovascular and endocrine responses are influenced by a number of variables. These variables include the nature of the behavioral task and its context, the past experiences of the individual (e.g., learning, habituation), personality factors such as perceptual or response styles, and various constitutional factors. Responsiveness may also be influenced by exogenous substances including the ingestion of sodium, caffeine, alcohol, tobacco smoke, and medications.

The present chapter discusses some of the strategies used in psychophysiologic laboratory research. Among the issues covered are the nature of the tasks employed, their advantages and limitations, and the extent to which reactivity findings in the laboratory generalize to nonlaboratory settings. The chapter concludes with a discussion of strategies that could facilitate our understanding of relationships between psychophysiologic experiments and our knowledge of cardiovascular regulation.

Situational Stereotypy

Situational stereotypy refers to the extent to which different situations elicit stereotypically distinct patterns of physiological and hormonal responses (Lacey, 1967). Mason (1975), for instance, found that heat, cold, exercise, and food deprivation stressors each led to a different profile of hormonal response, and that in the absence of psychological threat, corticosteroid production did not increase.

Responses to Active Coping versus Passive/Inhibitory/Vigilance Behavioral Tasks

While various stressors may elicit different responses, the central nervous system appears to be organized to produce integrated responses rather than single, isolated response changes (Hilton, 1975). Animals confronted with an aversive situation, for example, tend to reveal one pattern of autonomic reactivity if appropriate coping responses are being attempted, but another pattern if coping responses seem unavailable.

The former pattern is called the defense reaction (Abrahams, Hilton, & Zbrozyna, 1960; Cannon, 1929; Hess, 1957); it includes increased striate muscle activity, vasodilation in skeletal muscle, heart rate, cardiac output, and blood pressure. The second pattern, which occurs during aversive situations in which an active coping pattern does not seem available to the organism, includes increased vigilance, total peripheral resistance, blood pressure, and other manifestations of sympathetic nervous system activity accompanied by decreased skeletal movement and vagally mediated bradycardia (Adams, Bacelli, Mancia, & Zanchetti, 1968; Anderson & Tosheff, 1973).

The defense reaction or active coping response has been demonstrated during fight or flight (Adams *et al.,* 1968) or during active avoidance conditioning (Langer, Obrist, & McCubbin, 1979). In contrast, the pattern of autonomic responses associated with the lack of effortful, active coping possibilities has been demonstrated in the time period immediately preceding instrumental avoidance conditioning sessions in dogs (e.g., Anderson & Tosheff, 1973), and in the anticipation of fighting in cats (e.g., Adams *et al.,* 1968).

A pattern of responses that appears to be somewhat similar to the defense reaction has also been demonstrated albeit in attenuated form during the performances of tasks that are less obviously aversive, but which nevertheless involve active coping. The responses to mental arithmetic, for example, which is one such task, include increases in heart rate, systolic blood pressure, and forearm vasodilation (e.g., Brod, 1963; Williams *et al.,* 1975, 1982). In contrast, the responses to more passive sensory intake tasks have been shown to be associated with forearm vasoconstriction (Williams *et al.,* 1975, 1982).

Table 1 lists some of the terms that have been used to distinguish two presumed patterns of reactivity and their associated responses. These two dichotomous patterns have been demonstrated in animal experiments that used aversive stimulation and elicited sympathetic nervous system activation. To the extent that the constellation of responses is usually much less complete in the human experimental laboratory, however, it may be misleading to use the same labels to classify the outcome of both animal and human experiments.

The problem may not be insurmountable in situations classified as *mental work, active coping,* or the *defense reaction,* in which the component responses can all be increased along an intensity dimension. Thus, when harassment is included in a mental arithmetic task (e.g., Brod, 1963), the full constellation of responses can be elicited.

In contrast, during tasks in the human laboratory that are said to involve *vigilance, passive coping,* or *sensory intake,* the full constellation of responses observed in aversive animal experiments is not seen (e.g., Williams *et al.,* 1982). Moreover, when the intensity dimension is increased in human experiments either by harassment or by instructions during a vigilance/sensory intake task, the obtained pattern of cardiovascular responses tends in part to resemble the pattern obtained during the defense reaction. Thus, in human experiments that lead to pronounced sympathetic nervous system activation but in which an active coping response is not apparent, we are more likely to see

Table 1. Two Patterns of Reactivity and Their Components

Patterns of reactivity	
Defense reaction	Aversive vigilance
Active coping	Inhibitory coping
Active avoidance	Passive avoidance
Go	No go
Mental work	_____
Aerobic exercise	_____

Component responses	
Blood pressure increase	Blood pressure increase
Primarily systolic	Primarily diastolic
Skeletal muscle vasodilation	Skeletal muscle vasoconstriction
Tachycardia	Bradycardia
Increased cardiac output	Increased peripheral resistance
Increased β_1-adrenergic activity	Increased α-adrenergic activity
Decreased vagal tone	Increased vagal tone
	Accentuated antagonism

a mixed pattern of cardiovascular responses than the pattern of responses described under *aversive vigilance* or *passive coping* in Table 1.

Response Modulation and Mixed Patterns of Response

Some researchers have emphasized the distinction between sensory intake and mental work (Williams *et al.*, 1975)—and this distinction may be valid. Nevertheless, it is difficult to conceptualize a psychological task that does not involve both sensory intake and mental work although the proportion of each may vary among tasks.

Another distinction that is often made in the human psychophysiologic literature is between active and inhibitory or passive coping. Occasionally the distinction is a source of confusion because investigators do not further distinguish between passive coping and conservation-withdrawal (or learned helplessness). In the case of passive coping (e.g., passive avoidance), the individual may be engaging in concomitant preparation for action that could lead to either a mixed pattern (i.e., a combination of responses seen on both sides of Table 1) or even the pattern of responses seen during active coping.

In general, aerobic exercise, the defense reaction, mental work under conditions of harassment, and participation in a stressful interview all represent instances in which individuals actively attempt to cope with the environment. Under such circumstances a person is likely to become sympathetically aroused with an increase in heart rate and cardiac output. At relatively low levels of stimulation the increase in cardiac output could be due to a decrease in vagal tone at the heart, but at higher levels the increase in cardiac output would clearly be due to increases in cardiac β-adrenergic activity.

There are a number of factors that appear to be able to modulate the active coping pattern in humans, including such contextual factors as predictability, controllability, effortfulness, novelty, competition, harassment, task duration, incentives, task instructions, and the presence or absence of other people in the same room. The exact manner in which these variables influence the active coping

pattern is unknown, because most studies that have manipulated these variables have measured only blood pressure and/or heart rate. Nevertheless, some of these studies are suggestive.

Steptoe (1983) has reviewed a number of psychophysiologic studies, which suggest that effort and uncertainty can exert independent effects that may sum algebraically to determine final cardiovascular responses. Making a task criterion impossible to achieve, thereby encouraging a passive rather than an active coping strategy, can reduce cardiovascular responsiveness to either aversive (Obrist *et al.*, 1978) or appetitive (Light & Obrist, 1983) contingencies. Conversely, interpersonal competition (Light, 1981) and harassment during competition (Diamond *et al.*, 1984) have been shown to enhance cardiovascular reactivity.

There is some suggestive evidence that individual differences may play an important role in whether an active coping pattern or a more mixed response pattern is elicited by a particular task. For example, Morrison, Bellack, and Manuck (1985) reported that assertive hypertensives responded to a role play test with increased pulse pressure that was mostly due to an increase in systolic blood pressure. In contrast, unassertive hypertensives responded to the role play test with decreased pulse pressure, which was due to a relatively larger increase in diastolic relative to systolic pressure. Interestingly, assertive subjects did not differ from unassertive subjects in their physiologic responses to cognitive challenges. The results suggest that in a social situation in which competence may be seen as an issue, assertive individuals may tend to show an active coping pattern, whereas unassertive individuals may show a more mixed response pattern.

We have observed an interaction in reactivity between race and gender in our laboratory, which may also be related to a differential elicitation of patterns (Tischenkel, Gellman, Nelesen, & Schneiderman, 1986). In this study, cardiovascular and hormonal reactivity were examined in black and white, male and female subjects during a number of tasks. Interestingly, in response to the Type A structured interview and a video game, white males and black females revealed greater heart rate and plasma epinephrine reactivity than either black males or white females, while reliable differences in blood pressure elevations were not observed.

Although not yet subjected to empirical test, the results suggest that the white males and black females may have responded to the behavioral stressors with increases in cardiac output, whereas the white females and black males may have been more likely to respond with a mixed pattern that included a somewhat greater increase in total peripheral resistance. It is conceivable that racial differences in vascular reactivity may have interacted with other variables, since in a recent study comparing responses to the placement of an ice pack on the foreheads of black and white males, Anderson, Muranaka, Williams, and Lane (1985) found that the blacks exhibited significantly greater increases in systolic and diastolic blood pressure and forearm vascular resistance, but not a significant difference in heart rate.

Not only hemodynamic factors vary between laboratory tasks; neuroendocrine variables do as well. According to Frankenhaeuser (1983), different patterns of catecholamine and cortisol responsiveness can occur during stressful tasks as a function of particular combinations of effort and distress. Thus, according to Frankenhaeuser, effort without distress (e.g., exercise; playing a video game) is associated with elevated catecholamines and a suppression of cortisol secretion; effort with distress is accompanied by an elevation of both catecholamines and cortisol; and distress without effort (e.g., situations making an individual feel helpless) is associated with elevated cortisol. Frankenhaeuser's conclusions are based on laboratory and field studies in which urinary hormones were excreted in situations that varied in terms of predictability and control (e.g., Collins & Frankenhaeuser, 1978; Frankenhaeuser, 1983; Frankenhaeuser et al., 1978).

Responses to Physical versus Emotional Stressors

As previously noted, cardiovascular and hormonal responses to laboratory stressors can be examined in terms of whether or not an active coping task is employed. These responses can also be ex-amined in terms of whether the stressor is primarily physical or emotional. In general, the experimental evidence indicates that relative to normotensives, borderline hypertensives reveal exaggerated blood pressure responses to psychological stressors such as mental arithmetic (Bohlin et al., 1986), the Stroop test (Ditto, 1986), and puzzle-solving (Nestel, 1969) but not to isometric handgrip (Ditto, 1986), dynamic exercise (Julius & Conway, 1968), or tilt (Sannerstedt, Julius, & Conway, 1970). This suggests that patients with borderline hypertension do not suffer from a generalized blood pressure dysregulation that is manifested as a state of exaggerated responsiveness to all stimuli (Julius, Weder, & Hinderliter, 1986).

Although the preponderance of evidence suggests that physical stressors do not distinguish between normotensives and borderline hypertensives, there is some evidence that reactivity to the cold pressor test (Wood, Sheps, Elveback, & Schirger, 1984) or exercise (Dlin, Hannew, Silverberg, & Oded, 1983; Franz, 1980) can predict future hypertension although this has not been a universal finding (Eich & Jacobsen, 1967; Harlan, Osborne, & Gabiel, 1964).

The inconsistent findings concerning the cold pressor test may in part be due to the task having important psychological as well as physical aspects. Thus, while immersing a limb in ice water is predominantly an α-adrenergic maneuver that tends to elicit pronounced vasoconstriction, it is also a pain stimulus with important psychological concomitants. The psychophysiologic impact of the stimulus can vary as a function of the duration of the stimulus, prior experiences of a subject, the general experimental context, or specific task instructions. Experimental evidence exists, for instance, that highly challenging instructions can lead to pronounced β-adrenergic activity during the cold pressor test (Dembroski et al., 1979; Ruddel et al., 1984). Such findings suggest a need for caution in interpreting responses to tasks intended as purely physical stressors.

Evidence also exists that subjects shown to be high heart rate reactors during a cold pressor test produced the greatest changes in heart rate, systolic and diastolic blood pressures, ventricular ejection time, cardiac output, and rate–pressure product during a subsequent reaction time task (Lovallo, Pincomb, & Wilson, 1986). The results suggest that under certain conditions, heart rate may be a relatively stable trait that can generalize between what are generally thought to be passive versus active and physical versus psychological tasks. It would therefore seem important to identify modulators (e.g., family history of hypertension) that may impact upon more than one class of stressor.

To the extent that the circulatory and metabolic adjustments of exercise are ultimately directed toward providing optimal blood flow and oxygen transport to working muscles, bicycle erogometry or treadmill testing would seem to be useful in attempts to separate environmental from perceptual processes. When the performance of a Stroop task was superimposed upon dynamic exercise, however, heart rate was shown to increase without a further increase in oxygen consumption (Siconolfi, Garber, Baptist, Cooper, & Carleton, 1984). This suggests that emotional factors can interact with the exercise demands of a situation to determine circulatory responses.

Aerobic fitness, of course, has been associated with decreased heart work during exercise. Fit people show smaller increases in heart rate at a given work load and in general can do more myocardial work with greater cardiac efficiency than can sedentary individuals (Astrand & Rodahl, 1977). Such findings have encouraged research to determine whether aerobic fitness can modulate cardiovascular responses to psychological stressors. The data thus far are mixed, but do not yet present compelling evidence that aerobic fitness *per se* can serve as a buffer against cardiovascular reactivity to psychological stressors (see Dimsdale, Alpert, & Schneiderman, 1986; Schneiderman & Pickering, 1986, for reviews). One conceivable reason for the inconsistency of results reported is that many studies have used preexisting groups of fit versus unfit subjects and have thus confounded the effects of aerobic fitness with life-style, attitudes toward exercise, and various selection biases. In addition, studies of exercise reactivity need to take into account more traditional considerations including age, percentage of body fat, resting blood pressure

and heart rate, maximal oxygen uptake, smoking, and family history of hypertension.

Sympathoinhibitory Responses

Thus far, the blood pressure and hormonal responses that have been described can be related primarily to activation of the sympathetic nervous system. In contrast, there is also a separate class of responses that appears to be *sympathoinhibitory,* and is characterized by neurohormonal and blood pressure decreases. These responses, often subsumed under the rubric of *relaxation,* are thought to be integrated hypothalamic responses that result in generalized decreases in sympathetic activity (Benson, 1975; Benson, Beary, & Carol, 1974) as well as parasympathetic activation (McCabe, Schneiderman, Winters, Gentile, & Teich, 1988). In general, relaxation responses consist of cardiovascular, hormonal, and behavioral changes which contrast with those seen during active coping. Originally described as the ''trophotropic response'' by Hess (1957), this integrated pattern of responses also can be elicited by discrete hypothalamic stimulation (Hess, 1957; Ban, 1966; McCabe *et al.,* 1988).

In humans, the primary methods used to elicit relaxation responses are progressive muscular relaxation (Davidson, Winchester, Taylor, Alderman, & Ingels, 1979), meditation (Benson, Dryer, & Hartley, 1978; Hoffman *et al.,* 1982), autogenic relaxation (Luthe & Schultz, 1969), and biofeedback-assisted relaxation (McGrady, Yonker, Tan, Fine, & Woerner, 1981; Patel, Marmot, & Terry, 1981). These techniques, in general, produce some cardiovascular and hormonal responses that are opposite to those responses seen during stressful tasks. Relaxation training has been reported to decrease cardiac output and stroke volume (Lantzsch & Drunkenmolle, 1975), myocardial contractility (Davidson *et al.,* 1979), blood pressure (McGrady *et al.,* 1981), catecholamines (Davidson *et al.,* 1979), adrenocortical hormones (McGrady *et al.,* 1981; Patel *et al.,* 1981), and plasma renin (Patel *et al.,* 1981). It should be mentioned, however, that several studies have failed to show significant decreases in one or more of these responses as a function of relaxation (e.g., McGrady *et al.*, 1981; Pollack, Weber, Case, & Laragh, 1977). It has been suggested that specific hemodynamic/hormonal responses may vary depending on the nature of the task (e.g., type of meditation), subject characteristics, or whether acute or chronic changes are measured (Jacob & Chesney, 1986).

There is accumulating evidence that relaxation training may produce reliable and clinically relevant reductions in blood pressure in patients with essential hypertension (Patel & North, 1975; Patel, 1975; Taylor, Farquhar, Nelson, & Agras, 1977; Bali, 1979; Brauer, Horlick, Nelson, Farquhar, & Agras, 1979; McGrady *et al.*, 1981; Patel *et al.*, 1981; Southam, Agras, Taylor, & Kraemer, 1982; Crowther, 1983). Although the results of these studies are encouraging, a well-controlled, full-scale clinical trial has not been undertaken.

Because relaxation responses consist of cardiovascular/hormonal decreases, it may be possible to attenuate sympathetic reactivity by pitting the sympathoinhibition of relaxation against stimuli that elicit cardiovascular/hormonal increases. Several studies, in humans and animals, have used operant conditioning techniques to attenuate cardiovascular responses to exercise (Goldstein, Ross, & Brady, 1977; Perski, Engel, & McCroskery, 1982), handgrip (Clemens & Shattock, 1979), cold pressor (Reeves & Shapiro, 1982; Victor, Mainardi, & Shapiro, 1978), or electrical stimulation of the brain (Joseph, Quilter, & Engel, 1982). In our laboratory, we have recently begun a series of experiments in rabbits that are examining the extent to which responses mediated by the sympathetic nervous system can be attenuated by classical conditioning. By pairing a tone with electrical stimulation of the lateral hypothalamus, we can elicit a conditioned response that consists of decreases in heart rate, blood pressure, and motor activity. This conditioned relaxation response is then elicited during concomitant procedures that produce sympathetic activation (e.g., peripheral tail shock). By pitting the conditioned activation of the CNS pathways mediating bradycardia/depressor responses against activation of the CNS pathways mediating the sympathetic responses to imperative stimuli, we are studying the manner by

which the CNS permits relaxation training and similar procedures to counteract sympathetically mediated responses to stressful stimuli.

Generalizability of Laboratory Reactivity Findings

Numerous studies have examined cardiovascular and/or neurohormonal responses to behavioral stimuli in the laboratory as possible markers and/or contributing factors in the pathogenesis or expression of cardiovascular disorders. For example, it now seems clear that normotensive subjects with hypertensive parents reveal greater blood pressure responses to psychological tasks involving active coping than do the normotensive offspring of normotensive parents. The extent to which the exaggerated reactivity is a marker for subsequent hypertension remains to be determined, but promises to provide an important line of inquiry.

Studies that have shown that borderline hypertensives reveal greater hemodynamic and hormonal responses to psychological tasks involving active coping are beginning to provide information about the expression of cardiovascular disorders and interesting clues about pathogenesis.

Some regulatory disorders such as hypertension have traditionally been assessed under basal conditions at either one or a few points in time. To the extent that this approach has been successful, sophisticated cardiovascular and hormonal measures taken with the patient at rest in the clinic are clearly useful. But just as the glucose tolerance test and the exercise stress test have been able to provide important information that cannot be obtained by measurement under static conditions, the active coping psychological tasks described in this chapter have begun to provide useful new information.

Standardized psychophysiologic experimentation in the laboratory offers the advantages of comprehensive measurement and precise stimulus control, but tends to be artificial and somewhat removed from the ongoing, continuous adjustments that occur in ordinary daily life. Thus, there is a need to relate the comprehensive findings observed in tightly controlled laboratory experiments to cardiovascular and hormonal adjustments that occur in more natural settings.

Psychophysiologic laboratory studies by their nature tend to focus on acute, relatively transitory changes in physiologic responses. The outcome of some of these studies, such as the finding that borderline hypertensive subjects tend to show exaggerated responses to psychologically relevant stimuli requiring active coping, appears to be interesting and important. Findings such as these have led to the hypothesis that recurring stressors can elicit repeated, transitory increases in blood pressure that ultimately may result in established hypertension. The conceptual framework for such thinking has been provided by Folkow (1982). According to Folkow, repeated pressor episodes cause hypertrophy of the media in the arterioles. This, in turn, causes the arteriolar walls to encroach on the lumen, thereby increasing resistance to flow.

Although the preceding argument appears to be plausible, clinical data suggest that blood pressure variability *per se* is not a predictor of hypertensive vascular damage (Sokolow, Werdegar, Kain, & Hinman, 1966). In addition, a fair number of animal studies that have used recurrent central (Folkow & Rubinstein, 1966) or peripheral nervous system electrical stimulation (Liard *et al.*, 1975), or central deafferentation of the baroreceptors (Talman, Alonso, & Reis, 1980) to produce recurrent pressor episodes have failed to produce instances of sustained hypertension.

An interesting study by Anderson and Tosheff (1973) suggests that it may be important to assess not only what is happening during episodes of recurrent active coping, but also what is happening between these episodes. Briefly, Anderson and Tosheff examined the cardiovascular responses of dogs during daily 1-h sessions of unsignaled shock-avoidance as well as during the 1 h preceding the avoidance task when the animals were kept in a restraint harness within the experimental chamber. The investigators found that once the avoidance contingency was initiated, heart rate and cardiac output increased substantially. Anderson and Tosheff also found, however, that blood pressure became elevated in the 1 h preceding avoidance sessions and that this elevation was due to an increase in total peripheral resistance.

Findings such as those reported by Anderson and Tosheff suggest that it may be important to examine not only the phasic responses that individuals make to recurrent psychophysiologic stressors, but also the more tonic cardiovascular and hormonal adjustments that individuals make between acute, recurrent stressful episodes. Some indication of the nature of these long-term cardiovascular adjustments can be made using ambulatory circulatory monitoring and by assessing urinary catecholamines and cortisol.

Generalization between the Laboratory and More Naturalistic Settings

Several studies have examined the relationship between acute physiologic activity in the laboratory and blood pressure measurements made in more naturalistic settings. A study by McKinney *et al.* (1985), for instance, found that systolic blood pressure recorded at work correlated $r = 0.49$ with casual systolic blood pressure recorded during an office visit, but 0.57, 0.61, and 0.69 with systolic blood pressure recorded in response to a cold pressor test, a reaction time test, or the playing of a video game, respectively. In an earlier study, Manuck, Corse, and Winkelman (1979) reported that systolic blood pressure recorded during a frustrating cognitive task predicted both peak systolic blood pressure level and the variability of systolic blood pressure taken during the usual occupational activities of working professionals. Heart rate responses to a mental arithmetic task have also been shown to predict heart rate and blood pressure measurements recorded immediately before a midterm exam (Krantz & Manuck, 1984). Still another study reported that systolic blood pressure recorded during mental arithmetic, but not during a cold pressor test, differentiated "office hypertensives" from "nonresponders" (Giardi, Blanchard, Andrasik, & McCoy, 1984).

We have examined the relationship between blood pressure reactivity in the laboratory and blood pressure obtained both at home and at work in 119 normotensive black and white males and females (Ironson, Gellman, Spitzer, Llabre, Pasin,

Weidler, & Schneiderman, in press). Laboratory tasks consisted of the Type A structured interview, a video game, stationary bicycle exercise, and a cold pressor test.

Several of the laboratory tasks showed significant zero-order Pearson product correlations with ambulatory blood pressure. These correlations were invariably better for blood pressure responses at work than they were for responses at home. The correlations for blood pressure at work with resting blood pressure in the laboratory were $r = 0.69$ for systolic and $r = 0.77$ for diastolic pressures. Correlations between systolic blood pressure recorded at work and during laboratory tasks were 0.56, 0.57, 0.44, and 0.21 for responses to the video game, structured interview, cold pressor test, and dynamic exercise, respectively.

When we subjected our data to stepwise multiple regression analyses, we found that resting blood pressure in the laboratory was the best predictor of ambulatory blood pressure, obtained either at home or at work. Systolic blood pressure during the interview, however, added significantly to the prediction of systolic blood pressure at work beyond what was predicted by resting systolic blood pressure alone. Although blood pressure responses to the video game also had initially high zero-order correlations with ambulatory systolic and diastolic blood pressure, these did not contribute a significant proportion of unique variance in the regression analyses, presumably because the blood pressure responses to the video game shared a good deal of variance with the baseline.

Systolic blood pressure during the video game predicted systolic blood pressure better for whites than for blacks. In contrast diastolic blood pressure during the cold pressor test predicted ambulatory diastolic blood pressure better for blacks than for whites. Although the exact bases for these differences are not known, they suggest that blacks may be more sensitive to sources of α-adrenergic stimulation and that whites may be more reactive to β_1 adrenergic stimulation.

The finding that blood pressure responses to laboratory tasks can be related to ambulatory blood pressure measures is likely to be important because several studies have reported relationships between field measurements of blood pressure and subsequent hypertension (Rose, Jenkins, & Hurst, 1978) and the complications of hypertension (Devereux et al., 1982; Perloff, Sokolow, & Cowan, 1983; Pickering, Harshfield, Devereux, & Laragh, 1985; Sokolow et al., 1966; Sokolow, Werdegar, Perloff, Cowan, & Brenenstuhl, 1970). Moreover, these studies have pointed out that ambulatory measurements add important information beyond that obtained by casual blood pressure readings in the clinic. For example, Devereux et al. found that ambulatory blood pressure in the workplace was more highly correlated with echocardiographically documented left ventricular hypertrophy than were blood pressure readings taken at home or casually in a physician's office.

Psychophysiologic Strategies

In this chapter we have begun to describe a basic psychophysiologic strategy for cardiovascular behavioral medicine research. This strategy involves the comprehensive assessment of cardiovascular and hormonal functions while the individual is at rest, perturbation of these functions by well-chosen, standardized laboratory manipulations, and comparison of psychophysiologic responses in the laboratory to adjustments that occur in more naturalistic settings such as at home or work. Within this context, psychosocial assessments can be used to link individual differences to such variables as task reactivity in the laboratory and psychophysiologic adjustments in the workplace.

Control Levels

Most psychophysiologic experiments assess reactivity against resting control levels or baselines that are not truly basal. These control levels can vary as a function of time of day, posture of the subject, level of sleep or wakefulness, previous substance ingestion, familiarity with the laboratory and experimenters, characteristics of the informed consent form, and so forth. Because of these variations, it is better to think of baselines in terms of control levels rather than in terms of a true basal state.

For the purposes of classifying subjects as normotensive or hypertensive, it is probably best to use a known standard such as the procedure recommended by the American Heart Association (Kirkendall, Feinleib, & Mark, 1980), thereby remaining consistent with the extant literature. At the same time it should be recognized that having one's blood pressure taken in the clinic is itself a behavioral task that is likely to change the blood pressure from a previous control level. It is for this reason that most investigators make some effort to habituate the subject to the experimental situation.

In our studies we usually conduct psychophysiologic laboratory experiments after the subject has visited the laboratory several times and is familiar with the experimenters. The subject is asked to sit quietly in a recliner chair for 30 min, while the blood pressure cuff automatically inflates every 2 min. We have found that hemodynamic variables such as heart rate and blood pressure will stabilize within 30 min even after insertion of a venous catheter used to collect blood for hormone analyses.

In many experiments it is desirable to use multiple tasks. Under these conditions it is important to be able to recapture baselines. Table 2 shows blood pressure and heart rate baselines of 40 normotensive subjects equally divided by race and gender. In this experiment the initial resting baseline always preceded the Type A structured interview, and the remaining tasks (cold pressor test, stationary bicycle exercise, video game) were given in random order at 20-min intervals. The exercise level in this study was fairly low (65% of maximum heart rate); with more rigorous exercise it is necessary to present this task last or to use a much longer intertask interval to recapture baseline.

In experiments in which cortisol responses as well as hemodynamic and catecholamine re-

sponses are being assessed, intertask baseline intervals may also have to be extended. In contrast to hemodynamic responses, which occur within seconds, and catecholamine responses, which occur within a few minutes, cortisol responses are best seen after 20–30 min (Orth *et al.*, 1983; see also Kuhn, this volume).

Table 2 indicates that control baseline levels were successfully recaptured for blood pressure but not for heart rate when four tasks were given over a 2-h period. Significant differences did not occur across intertask control levels for plasma epinephrine or norepinephrine (not shown) or as a function of race or gender (not shown). Debriefing of the subjects suggested that the slight increase in heart rate across the session was associated with subjects becoming fatigued during the course of the 2-h experiment. Based on findings such as those shown in Table 2, which we have since replicated several times, we have chosen to use the initial resting baseline taken after 30 min as the control level for our experiments.

An alternative procedure for obtaining a control level has been used by Obrist (1981). Briefly, he and his colleagues obtain their resting baseline on a day following experimental stressors. In comparing this baseline with our own 30-min initial baseline procedure, we have found little difference in obtained control levels of heart rate and blood pressure. We prefer our own 30-min initial resting baseline procedure, however, primarily because we wish to keep electrode placements constant and because we want to limit the number of venous catheter insertions required to draw blood for hormonal analyses. In more recent studies, Obrist and colleagues preferred to obtain baselines during the same sessions in which the laboratory challenges were given for reasons that are similar to ours (e.g., Obrist *et al.*, 1987).

Table 2. Baseline Comparisons

	Initial resting baseline	Pre cold pressor	Pre bike	Pre game	Post relaxation	*p*
SBP (mm Hg)	111	112	112	111	111	ns
DBP (mm Hg)	63	65	65	69	66	ns
HR (beats/min)	63	68	65	68	69	<0.001

In our experiments, blood pressure is initially recorded with a mercury sphygmomanometer three times after the subject has been seated for 5 min. After being seated for another 20 min, an 18-gauge heparinized butterfly catheter (Kowarski–Cormed Thromboresistant Needle and Tubing Set) is inserted into a forearm vein and attached to a small portable peristaltic pump (Cormed ML6). This device, by adjustment of flow rate, allows us to obtain continuous integrated blood samples. The three rates we use are 5.0, 2.5, and 0.2 ml/min. During measurement periods, we collect blood in EDTA tubes at a flow rate of 5.0 ml/min. Throughout the remainder of the session, the pump is set at 0.2 ml/min. In all, we collect a little less than 200 ml of blood from each subject.

Choice of Tasks

The selection of tasks, of course, depends on the purposes of the investigators, but in most psychophysiologic experiments, at least one psychologically relevant active coping task will be employed. Such tasks may include an electronic video game (Diamond et al., 1984); a mental arithmetic task, such as counting backwards by serial sevens (Brod, Fencl, Hejl, & Jirka, 1959); cognitive problems such as the Stroop color-word test (Manuck & Proietti, 1982); a reaction time task (Obrist et al., 1978); structured interviews, such as the one used to assess Type A (MacDougall, Dembroski, & Krantz, 1981); public speaking (Dimsdale & Moss, 1980); or competitive card games (Lake et al., 1985). Provided that sufficient incentive, challenge, or ego-threat (e.g., harassment) is involved, the preceding tasks will elicit increases in plasma catecholamines as well as the kinds of hemodynamic responses shown on the left side of Table 1.

The exact choice of psychologically relevant active coping tasks may depend on various factors. If the experimenters are attempting to relate cardiovascular reactivity to a particular psychosocial dimension such as hostility, for instance, they may prefer to use a task likely to elicit frustration and annoyance (e.g., mirror-star tracing with harassment) rather than a non-anger-inducing task. If even small movements are likely to introduce ar-

tifacts into physiologic recordings, the investigators may choose a task that allows the subject to remain immobile. In drug studies incorporating a within-subject design, tasks may be chosen for which there are either alternate forms, or the response characteristics can be shown to be stable across repeated testing. Unfortunately, little published data exist concerning the effects of test–retest stability of psychophysiologic responses.

In some experiments the experimenters may wish to compare responses elicited by psychological versus physical stressors. For example, it has been shown that children of hypertensive parents reveal exaggerated blood pressure responses to psychological stressors such as a shock-avoidance reaction time task but not to a cold pressor test (Hastrup et al., 1982). In conducting such experiments, it is important to recall, however, that such comparisons appear to confound several dimensions. For example, the two tasks not only differ across the psychological versus physical stimulus dimension, but also in terms of being an active coping versus a passive task, and the extent to which β_1-adrenergic and α-adrenergic activity is elicited. Fortunately, Hastrup et al. were well aware of these issues, and the literature indicates that borderline hypertensives have exaggerated blood pressure responses to a wide range of psychological stressors including mental arithmetic (Bohlin et al., 1986), the Stroop test (Ditto, 1986), and puzzle-solving (Nestel, 1969) as well as the reaction time task. In contrast, it has been shown that borderline hypertensive typically fail to show exaggerated pressor responses not only to the cold pressor test but also to other physical stressors such as isometric handgrip (Ditto, 1986), dynamic exercise (Julius & Conway, 1968), or tilt (Sannerstedt et al., 1970).

Response Measures

Because the physiologic adjustments that an individual stressor elicits consist of an integrated pattern of responses, it is important to select judiciously a sufficient number of response measures to allow for the response pattern and its variation to be identified. Under ideal conditions, it would be desirable to assess the electrocardiogram, cardiac output and its determinants, blood pressure, peripheral resistance, and blood flow in different vascular beds as well as the status of the heart and coronary arteries. Usually, it is not possible to assess all of these variables in psychophysiologic experiments, and compromises are necessary. Increasingly, however, noninvasive cardiovascular instrumentation is becoming available that permits the assessment of the patterns of responses described in this chapter. For example, noninvasive instrumentation is currently available that permits the evaluation not only of heart rate and blood pressure, but also of changes in cardiac output, peripheral resistance, vasodilation or vasoconstriction in skeletal muscle, cerebral blood flow, left ventricular function, or cardiac vagal tone (for reviews, see Schneiderman & Pickering, 1986; Larsen, Schneiderman, & Pasin, 1986; Wilson *et al.*, this volume). The technical advances that have recently been made in terms of cardiovascular instrumentation and hormonal assessment, are having a profound effect on the psychophysiologic strategies that have begun to be adopted in cardiovascular behavioral medicine research.

Conclusions

We have attempted in this chapter to provide the outline for a basic psychophysiologic strategy that is already proving to be useful in research in cardiovascular behavioral medicine. This strategy includes comprehensive evaluation of cardiovascular and hormonal functions while the individual is at rest, perturbation of these functions by standardized laboratory manipulations, and comparison of physiologic adjustments at rest, during laboratory tasks, and in field settings. Individual differences obtained as a function of control level, laboratory tasks, and particular naturalistic settings can then be analyzed in terms of psychosocial, nutritional, metabolic, and/or physical status variables.

To the extent that the CNS appears to be organized to produce integrated adjustments rather than single, isolated response changes, it is important to select appropriate response measures that allow basic adjustment patterns to be identified. It is also necessary to select tasks that will adequately challenge the organism so that the dynamic aspects of these adjustments can be studied.

In the section on situational stereotypy, we discussed the kinds of laboratory tasks that have typically been used in psychophysiologic laboratory experiments. One distinction we made was between physical and psychological stressors. Another distinction of interest was between tasks that seemed to involve mental work, active coping, or the defense reaction on the one hand, and vigilance, passive coping, or sensory intake on the other.

When different tasks are used in the same study, they are likely to differ in terms of more than one dimension. Mental arithmetic and the cold pressor test, for instance, not only are qualitatively different in terms of an active versus passive coping distinction, but also in terms of psychological versus physical characteristics. Moreover, to at least some degree, virtually all tasks involve both physical and psychological demands. Mental arithmetic tasks, for example, typically involve speaking, which necessitates cardiorespiratory adjustments. Similarly, the cold pressor test, a handgrip dynamometer task, and submaximal treadmill exercise all involve emotional factors that can influence hormonal and cardiovascular adjustments.

It may not be possible to interpret quantitatively the differences in cardiovascular adjustments obtained between tasks solely in terms of active versus passive coping or physical versus psychological stimulus characteristics, because laboratory tasks typically differ across more than a single dimension. At the same time, when used appropriately, these distinctions can be conceptually useful. For example, the experimental evidence indicates that relative to normotensives, borderline hypertensives reveal exaggerated blood pressure responses to a whole gamut of psychological stressors (e.g., Bohlin *et al.*, 1986; Ditto, 1986; Nestel, 1969), but not to a variety of physical ones (e.g., Ditto, 1986; Julius & Conway, 1968; Sannerstedt *et al.*, 1970). As previously mentioned, this has led to the conclusion that patients with borderline hypertension do not suffer from a generalized blood pressure dysregulation that is manifested as a state of exaggerated responsiveness to all stimuli (Julius *et al.*, 1986). It would thus appear that the use of primarily psychological and primarily physical stressors in the same experiment can provide a useful tool for distinguishing generalized dysregulations (e.g., narrowing of arterioles) from other processes.

We have outlined in this chapter a psychophysiologic strategy that is proving useful in cardiovascular behavioral medicine research. To the extent that it involves concomitant analyses of control levels of adjustment, responses to a variety of laboratory tasks, and adjustments made under field conditions, it permits us to gain a comprehensive view of the relationships that exist between behavior and cardiovascular regulation. The strategy does pose some risks, however, because erroneous inferences can be made, generalizations can be drawn too broadly, and superficial similarities or differences can easily be misinterpreted. To minimize such risks, it is necessary for us to specify stimulus–response relationships as precisely as possible and to use comprehensive measurement strategies that can allow us to identify response patterns and their variations adequately. We must also be cautious in our inferences and avoid jargon (e.g., active coping; sensory intake; defense reaction) when generalizing across tasks and situations that obviously differ along multiple dimensions.

References

Abrahams, V. C., Hilton, S. M., & Zbrozyna, A. (1960). Active muscle vasodilation produced by stimulation of the brain stem: Its significance in the defense reaction. *Journal of Physiology, 154,* 491–513.

Adams, D. B., Bacelli, G., Mancia, G., & Zanchetti, A. (1968). Cardiovascular changes during naturally elicited fighting behavior in the cat. *American Journal of Physiology, 216,* 1226–1235.

Anderson, C. E., & Tosheff, J. (1973). Cardiac output and total peripheral resistance changes during preavoidance periods in the dog. *Journal of Applied Physiology, 34,* 650–654.

Anderson, N. B., Muranaka, M., Williams, R. B., & Lane, J. D. (1985). Peripheral vasoconstriction in response to cold stress in black and white males. *Psychophysiology, 22,* 582 (Abstract).

Astrand, P. O., & Rodahl, K. (1977). *Textbook of work physiology* (2nd ed.). New York: McGraw-Hill.

Bali, L. R. (1979). Long term effect of relaxation on blood pressure and anxiety levels in essential hypertensive males: A controlled study. *Psychosomatic Medicine, 41,* 637–646.

Ban, T. (1966). The septo-preoptico-hypothalamic system and its autonomic function. In T. Tokizane & J. P. Schade (Eds.), *Progress in brain research: Correlative neurosciences. Part A. Functional mechanisms.* Amsterdam: Elsevier.

Benson, H. (1975). *The relaxation response.* New York: Morrow.

Benson, H., Beary, J. F., & Carol, M. P. (1974). The relaxation response. *Psychiatry, 37,* 37–46.

Benson, H., Dryer, T., & Hartley, L. H. (1978). Decreased VO_2 consumption during exercise with elicitation of the relaxation response. *Journal of Human Stress, 4,* 38–42.

Bohlin, G., Eliason, K., Hjemdahl, P., Klein, K., Fredrikson, M., & Frankenhaeuser, M. (1986). Personal control over work place—circulatory, neuroendocrine and subjective responses in borderline hypertension. *Journal of Hypertension, 4,* 295–305.

Brauer, A., Horlick, L. F., Nelson, B., Farquhar, J. U., & Agras, W. S. (1979). Relaxation therapy for essential hypertension: A Veterans Administration outpatient study. *Journal of Behavioral Medicine, 2,* 21–29.

Brod, J. (1963). Hemodynamic basis of acute pressor reactions and hypertension. *British Heart Journal, 25,* 227–245.

Brod, J., Fencl, V., Hejl, Z., & Jirka, G. (1959). Circulatory changes underlying blood pressure elevation during acute emotional stress (mental arithmetic) in normotensive and hypertensive subjects. *Clinical Science, 23,* 339–349.

Cannon, W. R. (1929). *Bodily changes in pain, hunger, fear and rage* (2nd ed.). New York: Appleton.

Clemens, W. J., & Shattock, R. J. (1979). Voluntary heart rate control during static muscular effort. *Psychophysiology, 16,* 327–332.

Collins, A., & Frankenhaeuser, M. (1978). Stress responses in male and female engineering students. *Journal of Human Stress, 4,* 23.

Crowther, J. H. (1983). Stress management training and relaxation imagery in the treatment of essential hypertension. *Journal of Behavioral Medicine, 6,* 169–187.

Davidson, D. M., Winchester, M. A., Taylor, C. B., Alderman, E. A., & Ingels, N. B. (1979). Effects of relaxation therapy on cardiac performance and sympathetic activity in patients with organic heart disease. *Psychosomatic Medicine, 41,* 303–309.

Dembroski, T. M., MacDougall, J. M., Herd, J. A., & Shield, J. L. (1979). Effects of level of challenge on pressor and heart rate responses in Type A and B subjects. *Journal of Applied Social Psychology, 9,* 208.

Devereux, R., Pickering, T., Harshfield, G., Denby, L., Clark, L., Kleinert, H., Pregibon, D., Borer, J., & Laragh, J. (1982). Does home blood pressure improve prediction of change in patients with hypertension? *Circulation, 66*(Suppl. II), II-63.

Diamond, E. L., Schneiderman, N., Schwartz, D., Smith, J. C., Vorp, R., & Pasin, R. D. (1984). Harassment, hostility, and Type A as determinants of cardiovascular reactivity during competition. *Journal of Behavioral Medicine, 7,* 171.

Dimsdale, J. E., Alpert, B. S., & Schneiderman, N. (1986). Exercise as a modulator of cardiovascular reactivity. In K.

A. Matthews, S. M. Weiss, T. Detre, T. M. Dombroski, B. Falkner, S. B. Manuck, & R. B. Williams (Eds.), *Handbook of stress, reactivity, and cardiovascular disease* (pp. 365–384). New York: Wiley.

Ditto, B. (1986). Parental history of essential hypertension, active coping, and cardiovascular reactivity. *Psychophysiology, 23*(1), 62–70.

Dlin, R. A., Hannew, N., Silverberg, D., & Oded, B.-O. (1983). Follow-up of normotensive men with exaggerated blood pressure response to exercise. *American Heart Journal, 106,* 316–320.

Eich, R. H., & Jacobsen, E. C. (1967). Vascular reactivity in medical students followed for 10 years. *Journal of Chronic Disease, 20,* 583–592.

Falkner, B., Onesti, G., Angelakos, E. T., Fernandes, M., & Langman, C. (1979). Cardiovascular response to mental stress in normal adolescents with hypertensive parents. *Hypertension, 1,* 23.

Folkow, B. (1982). Physiological aspects of primary hypertension. *Physiological Review, 62,* 347–503.

Folkow, B., & Rubinstein, E. H. (1966). Cardiovascular effects of acute and chronic stimulation of the hypothalamic defense area in the rat. *Acta Physiologica Scandinavia, 68,* 48–57.

Frankenhaeuser, M. (1983). The sympathetic–adrenal and pituitary–adrenal response to challenge: Comparison between the sexes. In T. M. Dembroski, T. H. Schmidt, & G. Blumchen (Eds.), *Biobehavioral bases of coronary heart disease.* Basel: Karger.

Frankenhaeuser, M., Rauste-von Wright, M., Collins, A., von Wright, J., Sedvall, G., & Swahn, L. G. (1978). Sex differences in psychoneuroendocrine reactions to examination stress. *Psychosomatic Medicine, 40,* 334.

Franz, I. W. (1980). Ergometrische Untersuchungen zur Beurteilung der Grenzwerthypertonie. *Therapiewoche, 30,* 7857.

Giardi, R. J., Blanchard, E. B., Andrasik, F., & McCoy, G. C. (1984). Psychological dimensions of "office hypertension." *Biofeedback and Self-Regulation, 9,* 106 (Abstract).

Goldstein, D. S., Ross, R. S., & Brady, J. V. (1977). Biofeedback heart rate training during exercise. *Biofeedback and Self-Regulation, 2,* 107–126.

Harlan, W. J., Jr., Osborne, R. K., & Gabiel, A. (1964). Prognostic value of the cold pressor test and the basal blood pressure: Based on an eighteen year follow-up study. *American Journal of Cardiology, 13,* 683.

Hastrup, J. L., Light, K. C., & Obrist, P. A. (1982). Parental hypertension and cardiovascular response to stress in healthy young adults. *Psychophysiology, 19,* 615–622.

Hess, W. R. (1957). *Functional organization of the diencephalon.* New York: Grune & Stratton.

Hilton, S. M. (1975). Ways of viewing the central nervous control of the circulation—old and new. *Brain Research, 87,* 213.

Hoffman, J. W., Benson, H., Arns, P. A., Stainbrook, G. L., Landsberg, L., Young, J. B., & Gill, A. (1982). Reduced sympathetic nervous system responsivity associated with the relaxation response. *Science, 215,* 191–192.

Hohn, A. R., Riopel, D. A., Keil, J. E., Loadhott, C. B., Margolius, H. S., Haluszka, P. V., Privitera, P. J., Webb, J. G., Medley, E. S., Schuman, S. H., Rubin, M. I., Pantell, R. H., & Braunstein, M. L. (1983). Childhood familial and racial differences in physiologic and biochemical factors related to hypertension. *Hypertension, 5,* 56–70.

Ironson, G., Gellman, M., Spitzer, S., Llabre, M., Pasin, R., Weidler, D., & Schneiderman, N. (in press). Predicting home and work blood pressure measurements from resting baselines and laboratory reactivity in black and white Americans. *Psychophysiology.*

Jacob, R. G., & Chesney, M. A. (1986). Psychological and behavioral methods to reduce cardiovascular reactivity. In K. A. Matthews, S. M. Weiss, T. Detre, T. M. Dembroski, B. Falkner, S. B. Manuck, & R. B. Williams (Eds.), *Handbook of stress, reactivity, and cardiovascular disease* (pp. 417–457). New York: Wiley.

Jorgensen, R. S., & Houston, B. K. (1981). Family history of hypertension, gender, and cardiovascular reactivity and stereotypy during stress. *Journal of Behavioral Medicine, 4,* 1975.

Joseph, J. A., Quilter, R. E., & Engel, B. T. (1982). Changes in hippocampal rhythmic slow activity during instrumental cardiovascular conditioning. *Physiology and Behavior, 28,* 653–659.

Julius, S., & Conway, J. (1968). Hemodynamic studies in patients with borderline blood pressure elevation. *Circulation, 38,* 282–288.

Julius, S., Weder, A. B., & Hinderliter, A. L. (1986). Does behaviorally induced blood pressure variability lead to hypertension? In K. A. Matthews, S. M. Weiss, T. Detre, T. M. Dembroski, B. Falkner, S. B. Manuck, & R. B. Williams (Eds.), *Handbook of stress, reactivity, and cardiovascular disease* (pp. 71–84). New York: Wiley.

Kirkendall, W. M., Feinleib, M., & Mark, A. L. (1980). American Heart Association recommendations for human blood pressure determination by sphygmomanometer. *Circulation, 62,* 1146–1155.

Krantz, D. S., & Manuck, S. B. (1984). Acute psychophysiologic reactivity and risk of cardiovascular disease: A review and methodologic critique. *Psychological Bulletin, 96,* 435.

Lacey, J. I. (1967). Somatic response patterning and stress: Some revisions of activation theory. In M. H. Applcy & R. Trumble (Eds.), *Psychological stress* (p. 14). New York: Appleton–Century–Crofts.

Lake, B. W., Suarez, E., Schneiderman, N., & Tocci, N. (1985). The Type A behavior pattern, physical fitness, and psychophysiological reactivity. *Health Psychology, 4,* 169.

Langer, A. W., Obrist, P. A., & McCubbin, J. A. (1979). Hemodynamic and metabolic adjustments during exercise and shock avoidance in dogs. *American Journal of Physiology. Heart and Circulatory Physiology, 5,* H225.

Lantzsch, W., & Drunkenmolle, C. (1975). Kreislaufanalytische untersuchungen bei patienten mit essentieller hypertonie wahrend der ersten und zweiten standardubung des autogenen trainings. *Psychiatric Clinician, 8,* 223–228.

Larsen, P., Schneiderman, N., & Pasin, R. D. (1986). Physiological bases of cardiovascular psychophysiology. In M. Coles, E. Donchin, & S. Porges (Eds.), *Psychophysiology: Systems, processes and applications* (pp. 122–165). New York: Guilford.

Liard, J. F., Tarazi, R. C., Ferrario, C. M., & Manger, W. M. (1975). Hemodynamic and humoral characteristics of hypertension induced by prolonged stellate ganglion stimulation in conscious dogs. *Circulation Research, 36,* 455.

Light, K. C. (1981). Cardiovascular responses to effortful active coping: Implications for the role of stress in hypertension development. *Psychophysiology, 18,* 216.

Light, K. C., & Obrist, P. A. (1983). Task difficulty, heart rate activity, and cardiovascular responses to an appetitive reactive time task. *Psychophysiology, 20,* 301–312.

Lovallo, W. R., Pincomb, G. A., & Wilson, M. F. (1986). Predicting response to a reaction time task: Heart rate reactivity compared with Type A behavior. *Psychophysiology, 23,* 648–656.

Luthe, W., & Schultz, J. H. (1969). *Autogenic therapy: II. Medical application.* New York: Grune & Stratton.

MacDougall, J. M., Dembroski, T. M., & Krantz, D. S. (1981). Effects of types of challenge on pressor and heart rate responses in Type A and B women. *Psychophysiology, 18,* 1–9.

Manuck, S. B., & Proietti, J. (1982). Parental hypertension and cardiovascular response to cognitive and isometric challenge. *Psychophysiology, 19,* 481–489.

Manuck, S. B., Corse, C. D., & Winkelman, A. (1979). Behavioral correlates for individual differences in blood pressure reactivity. *Journal of Psychosomatic Research, 23,* 281–288.

Manuck, S. B., Giordani, B., McQuaid, K. J., & Garrity, S. J. (1981). Behaviorally-induced cardiovascular reactivity among sons of reported hypertensive and normotensive parents. *Journal of Psychosomatic Research, 25,* 261.

Mason, J. W. (1975). A historical view of the stress field: Part II. *Journal of Human Stress, 1,* 22–36.

McCabe, P. M., Schneiderman, N., Winters, R. W., Gentile, C. G., & Teich, A. (1988). Learned aspects of cardiovascular regulation. In R. Ader & A. Baum (Eds.), *Perspectives in behavioral medicine* (Vol. 6; pp. 1–23). Hillside, NJ: Lawrence Erlbaum.

McGrady, A. V., Yonker, R., Tan, S. Y., Fine, T. H., & Woerner, M. (1981). The effect of biofeedback assisted relaxation training on blood pressure and selected biochemical parameters in patients with essential hypertension. *Biofeedback and Self-Regulation, 6,* 343–353.

McKinney, M. E., Miner, M. H., Ruddel, H. McIlvain, H. E., Witte, H., Buell, J. C., Eliot, R. S., & Grant, L. B. (1985). The standardized mental stress protocol: Test–retest reliability and comparison with ambulatory blood pressure monitoring. *Psychophysiology, 22,* 453.

Morrison, R. L., Bellack, A. S., & Manuck, S. B. (1985). Role of social competence in borderline essential hypertension. *Journal of Consulting and Clinical Psychology, 53*(2), 248.

Nestel, P. J. (1969). Blood pressure and catecholamine excretion after mental stress in labile hypertension. *Lancet, 1,* 692.

Obrist, P. A. (1981). *Cardiovascular psychophysiology.* New York: Plenum Press.

Obrist, P. A., Gaebelein, C. T., Teller, E. S., Langer, A. W., Grignolo, A., Light, K. C., & McCubbin, J. A. (1978). The relationship among heart rate, carotid dp/dt and blood pressure in humans as a function of the type of stress. *Psychophysiology, 15,* 102.

Obrist, P. A., Light, K. C., James, S. A., & Strogatz, D. S. (1987). Cardiovascular responses to stress. I. Measures of myocardial response and relationships to high resting systolic pressure and parental hypertension. *Psychophysiology, 24,* 65–78.

Orth, D. N., Jackson, R. V., DeCherney, G. S., DeBold, C. R., Alexander, A. N., Island, D. P., Rivier, J., Rivier, C., Speiss, J., & Vale, W. (1983). Effects of ovine synthetic corticotropin releasing factor: Dose response of plasma adrenocorticotropin and cortisol. *Journal of Clinical Investigation, 71,* 587–595.

Patel, C. (1975). Twelve month follow-up of yoga and biofeedback in the management of hypertension. *Lancet, 1,* 62–64.

Patel, C., & North, W. R. S. (1975). Randomized controlled trial of yoga and biofeedback in the management of hypertension. *Lancet, 2,* 93–95.

Patel, C., Marmot, M. G., & Terry, D. J. (1981). Controlled trial of biofeedback aided behavioral methods in reducing mild hypertension. *British Medical Journal, 282,* 2005–2008.

Perloff, D., Sokolow, M., & Cowan, R. (1983). The prognostic value of ambulatory blood pressures. *Journal of the American Medical Association, 249,* 2792.

Perski, A., Engel, B. T., & McCroskery, J. H. (1982). The modification of elicited cardiovascular responses by operant conditioning of heart rate. In J. T. Cacioppo & R. E. Petty (Eds.), *Perspectives in cardiovascular psychophysiology.* New York: Guilford Press.

Pickering, T. G., Harshfield, G. A., Devereux, R. B., & Laragh, J. H. (1985). What is the role of ambulatory blood pressure monitoring in the management of hypertensive patients? *Hypertension, 7*(2), 171.

Pollack, A. A., Weber, M. A., Case, D. B., & Laragh, J. H. (1977). Limitations of transcendental meditation in the treatment of essential hypertension. *Lancet, 1,* 71–72.

Reeves, J. L., & Shapiro, D. (1982). Heart rate biofeedback and cold pressor pain. *Psychophysiology, 19,* 393–403.

Remington, R. D., Lambarth, B., Moser, M., & Boobler, S. E. (1960). Circulatory reactions to normotensive and hypertensive subjects and of the children of normotensive and hypertensive parents. *American Heart Journal, 59,* 58–70.

Rose, R., Jenkins, C., & Hurst, M. (1978). *Air traffic controller health change study.* Boston University School of Medicine.

Rosenman, R. H., Brand, R. J., Jenkins, C. D., Friedman, M., Strauss, R., & Wurm, M. (1975). Coronary heart disease in the Western Collaborative Group Study: Final follow-up experience of 8½ years. *Journal of the American Medical Association, 233,* 872–877.

Ruddel, H., McKinney, M., Buell, J. C., & Eliot, R. S. (1984). Reliabilitat S—Cold pressor test. *Herz Medizineo, 7,* 39–43.

Sannerstedt, R., Julius, S., & Conway, J. (1970). Hemodynamic response to tilt with beta-adrenergic blockade in young patients with borderline hypertension. *Circulation, 42,* 1057–1064.

Schneiderman, N., & Pickering, T. G. (1986). Cardiovascular measures of physiologic reactivity. In K. A. Matthews, S. M. Weiss, T. Detre, T. M. Dombroski, B. Falkner, S. B. Manuck, & R. B. Williams (Eds.), *Handbook of stress, reactivity, and cardiovascular disease* (pp. 145–186). New York: Wiley.

Siconolfi, S. F., Garber, C. E., Baptist, G. D., Cooper, F. S., & Carleton, R. A. (1984). Circulatory effects of mental stress during exercise in coronary artery disease patients. *Clinical Cardiology, 7,* 441.

Sokolow, M., Werdegar, D., Kain, H., & Hinman, A. (1966). Relationships between level of blood pressure measured casually and by portable recorder and severity of complications in essential hypertension. *Circulation, 34,* 279.

Sokolow, M., Werdegar, D., Perloff, D., Cowan, R., & Brenenstuhl, H. (1970). Preliminary studies relating recorded blood pressures to daily life events in patients with essential hypertension. In M. Koster, H. Musaph, & P. Visser (Eds.), *Psychosomatics in essential hypertension.* Basel: Karger.

Southam, M. A., Agras, W. S., Taylor, C. B., & Kraemer, H. C. (1982). Relaxation training: Blood pressure during the work day. *Archives of General Psychiatry, 39,* 715–717.

Steptoe, A. (1983). Stress, helplessness and control: The implications of laboratory studies. *Journal of Psychosomatic Research, 27*(5), 361.

Steptoe, A., Melville, D., & Ross, A. (1984). Behavioral response demands, cardiovascular reactivity and essential hypertension. *Psychosomatic Medicine, 46,* 33.

Talman, W. T., Alonso, D. R., & Reis, D. J. (1980). Impairment of baroreceptor function and chronic lability of arterial pressure produced by lesions of A2 catecholamine neurons of rat brain: Failure to evolve into hypertension. In P. Sleight (Ed.), *Arterial baroreceptors in hypertension* (pp. 448–454). London: Oxford University Press.

Taylor, C. B., Farquhar, J. W., Nelson, E., & Agras, W. S. (1977). Relaxation therapy and high blood pressure. *Archives of General Psychiatry, 34,* 339–342.

Tischenkel, N., Gellman, M., Nelesen, R., & Schneiderman, N. (1986). Behavioral factors affecting blood pressure in blacks. *Cardiovascular Disease Epidemiology Newsletter, 315.*

Victor, R., Mainardi, A., & Shapiro, D. (1978). Effects of biofeedback and voluntary control procedures on heart rate and perception of pain during the cold pressor test. *Psychosomatic Medicine, 40,* 216–225.

Weidner, G., & Matthews, K. A. (1978). Reported physical symptoms elicited by unpredictable events and the Type A coronary-prone behavior pattern. *Journal of Personality and Social Psychology, 36,* 213.

Williams, R. B., Bittker, T. E., Buchsbaum, M. S., & Wynne, L. C. (1975). Cardiovascular and neurophysiologic correlates of sensory intake and rejection. I. Effect of cognitive tasks. *Psychophysiology, 12,* 427–433.

Williams, R. B., Lane, J. D., Kuhn, C. M., Melosh, W., White, A. R., & Schanberg, S. M. (1982). Physiological and neuroendocrine response patterns during different behavioral challenges: Differential hyperresponsivity of Type A men. *Science, 218,* 483.

Wood, D. L., Sheps, S. G., Elveback, L. R., & Schirger, A. (1984). Cold-pressor test as a predictor of hypertension. *Hypertension, 6,* 301.

CHAPTER 23

Psychophysiologic Reactivity as a Dimension of Individual Differences

Stephen B. Manuck, Alfred L. Kasprowicz, Scott M. Monroe,
Kevin T. Larkin, and Jay R. Kaplan

Studies of hemodynamic and neuroendocrine reactions to behavioral stimuli comprise a substantial portion of laboratory research in cardiovascular behavioral medicine. It is widely thought that exaggerated physiologic responses to psychological challenge, or stress, may be implicated in the etiology or clinical expression of certain cardiovascular disorders, including coronary heart disease and essential hypertension (Manuck & Krantz, 1986). As described in the previous chapter, behaviorally elicited physiologic reactions vary in their magnitude and patterning, in part, as a function of the nature of the eliciting stimuli (i.e., stimulus specificity). It is also well established that individuals exposed to the same experimental stimulus exhibit marked variability in cardiovascular and neuroendocrine responses. The present chapter addresses several issues relating to the latter phenomenon, individual differences in psychophysiologic reac-

tivity. Considered specifically are three attributes of individual differences that have significance for current hypotheses linking cardiovascular and neuroendocrine reactivity to aspects of cardiovascular disease: (1) the temporal stability of individual differences in psychophysiologic reactivity; (2) the reproducibility of these individual differences under varying stimulus conditions; and (3) the generalization of individual differences in physiologic responses from laboratory evaluations to measurements obtained in field (or natural) settings. Consideration of these issues is preceded by a discussion of common aspects of protocols used in psychophysiologic assessment, as well as of related matters regarding the quantitative expression of individual differences in reactivity.

Assessment of Psychophysiologic Reactivity

In laboratory investigations, physiologic parameters of interest are typically recorded during subjects' exposure to discrete experimental challenges, or stressors. The actual stimuli employed are quite variable, including aversive stimulation, such as immersion of a limb in cold water (the "cold press-

Stephen B. Manuck, Alfred L. Kasprowicz, and Scott M. Monroe • Department of Psychology, University of Pittsburgh, Pittsburgh, Pennsylvania 15260.   *Kevin T. Larkin* • Department of Psychology, West Virginia University, Morgantown, West Virginia 26506.   *Jay R. Kaplan* • Department of Comparative Medicine, Bowman Gray School of Medicine, Wake Forest University, Winston-Salem, North Carolina 27109.

or'' test), challenges of an interpersonal nature, and most commonly, the performance of difficult or frustrating cognitive and psychomotor tasks (e.g., mental arithmetic; reaction time). Physiologic measurements are ordinarily obtained throughout the period of stimulus presentation (i.e., one to several minutes; occasionally, a half-hour or more). To some researchers, the maximum value observed during stimulus presentation (e.g., the peak heart rate or blood pressure) is of greatest interest, though most investigators simply calculate the mean of all values obtained or examine successive intervals of measurement separately (e.g., by minutes). At present, it is not clear that the varying information provided by these different computational procedures is of practical significance, except perhaps where subjects' reactions may be expected to show rapid habituation over time or an idiosyncratic temporal patterning.

The psychophysiologic ''response'' of the individual is often expressed as the difference between physiologic states recorded during such ''stimulus'' periods and comparative observations made under ''baseline'' conditions. To the extent possible, the baseline measurements are obtained in an environment free of notable behavioral stimuli and during periods of inactivity. Because the attachment of recording instruments is itself likely to have an arousing effect upon subjects, baseline assessments are typically preceded by a period of relative quiet during which individuals may adapt to the laboratory setting. Although published reports often do not include information on adaptation intervals, it is probable that most investigators employ periods ranging from 5 to 15 min or, alternatively, await several successive measurements demonstrating that the physiologic variables of interest have stabilized (see Hastrup, 1986, for a discussion of heart rate baseline variability as a function of the adaptation interval). Where subjects are to be exposed to especially provocative stressors (e.g., electric shock), an accurate determination of basal physiologic states may not be feasible in the same recording session at which experimental stimuli are presented, due to anticipatory arousal. In these instances, adequate assessment of baseline values may require that additional recordings be made on a separate occasion,

during which no experimental tasks are presented and subjects are informed that only resting physiologic measurements will be recorded (Obrist, 1981). Finally, when continuous or repeated blood samples are to be collected, as for measurement of plasma catecholamine or cortisol concentrations, adaptation intervals of 30 min or more may be advisable due to the stress associated with venipuncture and insertion of an indwelling catheter.

Some confusion surrounds the appropriate quantitative expression of psychophysiologic ''reactivity,'' particularly among studies of individual differences in cardiovascular and neuroendocrine response characteristics. Consider, for example, the frequently reported ''difference,'' or ''change'' score. For a given physiologic parameter, this value reflects the deviation from baseline that is associated with a particular subject's exposure to a specific experimental challenge. Hence, one individual may respond during a common laboratory task such as ''mental arithmetic'' (e.g., serial subtraction) with a 25 beat per min (bpm) acceleration of heart rate, whereas in the same situation a second subject's heart rate may increase by 15 bpm. If we examine *only* the change score, we are tempted to conclude that the first subject is substantially more ''reactive'' than the second, at least for heart rate and under these stimulus conditions.

Now, let us say that the baseline heart rate of the first individual is 60 bpm, and that of the second, 75 bpm. The subject with the lower baseline therefore achieved a heart rate of 85 bpm during mental arithmetic, and the subject with the higher baseline a heart rate of 90 bpm. In view of the differing baselines, it may be asked whether the more elevated heart rate of the second subject during the experimental stressor was due, in part, to the fact that his resting heart rate was also somewhat elevated—and conversely, it may be asked whether or not the larger change score of the first subject was due in part to the fact that his prestimulus heart rate was relatively lower. In fact, for any group of individuals exposed to a common stimulus or laboratory task, there will often be found a significant correlation between baseline and task-related measurements. Across individuals, then, measurements made during stress periods may be predicted, in part, from preceding baseline values.

Frequently, there is also a significant correlation between baseline values and change scores, this correlation sometimes (but not always) reflecting an inverse association between baseline and change in accordance with the so-called "law of initial values" (Wilder, 1957). Because correlations of baseline measurements with both task values and arithmetic change scores are rarely, if ever, perfect, individuals' physiologic states during periods of stimulus presentation exhibit residual variability that cannot be accounted for by a knowledge of baseline values alone. It is this residual variability that might best be considered as capturing variability indicative of the psychophysiologic "reactivity" of individuals.

Some of the foregoing points are illustrated in Figure 1. Depicted there are the data of 24 young adults whose heart rates were recorded at baseline and during performance of the Stroop color-word

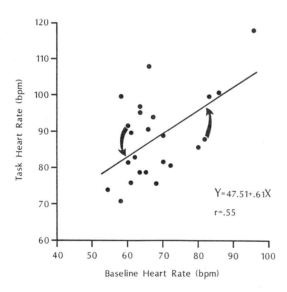

Figure 1. Heart rate (in beats per minute) on baseline (abscissa) and at peak elevation during task performance (ordinate) in 24 young adults. Note that while there is a substantial correlation between baseline and task measurements, the actual (or observed) task heart rates vary appreciably about the plotted regression line. The deviation of actual from predicted values is termed the "residual." An expression of the individual's physiologic response independent of baseline influences is captured by the residual; this value is commonly referred to as a residualized, or baseline-free, change score.

interference test (a distinctly frustrating cognitive task). The actual data are taken from the index cases of a previously reported study of psychophysiologic reactivity among monozygotic and dizygotic twin pairs (Shapiro, Nicotero, Sapira, & Scheib, 1968). Among these subjects, heart rates averaged 68.1 bpm on baseline and 88.9 bpm (at peak elevation) during task performance. Note that there is a substantial positive correlation ($r = 0.55$) between heart rates recorded under these two conditions, as higher baselines tend to predict higher task values. Still, the actual task-related heart rates of individuals are rather widely distributed around the line of regression (i.e., relative to values that would be predicted from individuals' baseline measurements alone). The difference between the actual heart rate observed during the challenge and the heart rate value predicted for a given subject from the regression equation is commonly termed the residual, or "error of prediction." The residual reflects (in this instance) the extent to which an individual's actual heart rate during task performance was either greater or less than the expected value predicted from a knowledge of the same subject's baseline heart rate and of the overall association between baseline and task values for the group as a whole. This score—the task response with baseline influences statistically removed—is sometimes referred to as a "residualized" or baseline-free change score.

Thus, the residualized change score provides one means of quantifying idiosyncratic physiologic responses to behavioral stimuli, while separating the numerical expression of such responses from the concomitant influences of baseline differences among individuals. It may be noted that while there is no correlation (by definition) between baseline and residualized changes, in the example above the correlation between baseline heart rates and arithmetic change scores was moderate and inverse ($r = -0.39$). In the authors' own experience, negative correlations of this magnitude are encountered relatively infrequently, so that the simple "difference" measure often provides an index of some comparability to the covariance-adjusted (residualized) change score. Because this is not always the case, however, it is important to keep in mind that simple difference scores and residualized changes can yield distributions of some discrepancy.

Of course, in employing psychophysiologic assessments, the clinical researcher is not necessarily interested in evaluating a "pure," baseline-free response characteristic of the individual. The manner in which psychophysiologic measurements are quantified should therefore be dictated by the objectives of the investigator. If individual differences in behaviorally induced physiologic *reactivity* are of specific concern, though, the investigator should apply quantitative techniques that are aimed at removing the influence (if any) of differing baseline values on response measures. In our own work employing an animal model, for instance, we are interested in determining if an association exists between heart rate and the coronary artery atherosclerosis of cholesterol-fed cynomolgus monkeys (*Macaca fascicularis*) (e.g., Manuck, Kaplan, & Clarkson, 1983). To examine this relationship, we assess the heart rates of experimental animals under baseline conditions, as well as during monkeys' exposure to a standardized laboratory stressor. In one study we observed that among monkeys housed in small social groups subject to periodic reorganization, atherosclerosis correlated modestly (albeit nonsignificantly) with baseline heart rate measurements ($rho = 0.28$); a somewhat stronger relationship existed between atherosclerosis and residualized heart rate changes related to our experimental stressor ($rho = 0.41$, $p < 0.07$). Because the absolute values of heart rate observed under stress convey information pertaining to both the baseline characteristics of the animals and their response propensities, it is not surprising that these measurements yield the greatest overall association with lesion extent ($rho = 0.46$, $p < 0.05$). The latter correlation provides the strongest numerical answer to our question: is there a relationship between heart rate (however assessed) and severity of diet-induced atherosclerosis in animals housed under these experimental conditions? Yet, having partitioned the baseline and response parameters and examined these values separately, we can also address questions regarding the *relative* association between coronary artery atherosclerosis and heart rate measurements

recorded under differing environmental circumstances.

However quantified, the variability of subjects' physiologic reactions to experimental challenges is primarily of interest in cardiovascular behavioral medicine as a potential expression of a broader construct of individual differences in psychophysiologic reactivity. It is reasonable to assume, for example, that the exaggerated heart rate or pressor responses that some subjects experience when performing a frustrating psychomotor task reflect a stable, or enduring, characteristic of these individuals. Similarly, if the distribution of idiosyncratic reactions to one experimental task or challenge cannot be replicated under other stimulus conditions, it would be difficult to conclude that the variability of observed responses (as on the first task) defines a robust phenomenon of individual differences. Finally, many hypotheses regarding the clinical significance of psychophysiologic reactivity presume that response differences among individuals are not simply a laboratory phenomenon, but find expression as well in subjects' physiologic reactions to the naturally occurring events of daily life.

The remaining sections of this chapter deal briefly and in turn with each of these matters— namely, the reproducibility of behaviorally elicited physiologic responses over time and across varying experimental stimuli, and the generalization of laboratory assessments to measurements recorded in field settings. The following discussions are intended less as reviews of existing literature, however, than as illustrations of general points germane to the conceptualization of psychophysiologic reactivity as a dimension of individual differences.

Temporal Stability of Individual Differences

To date, few investigators have examined the reproducibility of psychophysiologic responses over multiple experimental sessions, and most published data are restricted to cardiovascular measurements (principally heart rate and blood pressure). The available studies generally report test–retest correlations among subjects exposed to the same experimental stimuli on two separate occasions. Intersession intervals vary widely, from a few days to several years, although most studies involve retest intervals of 3 months or less. Summarized in Table 1 are the results of 12 investigations, as related to the temporal stability of heart rate and blood pressure reactions to common laboratory stressors. The experimental stimuli presented to subjects are typical of those used in psychophysiologic studies, including psychomotor challenges (e.g., reaction time, video games), cognitive tasks (e.g., serial subtraction, problems in concept formation), and, occasionally, the cold pressor test. Note that the subject samples employed in these investigations are of variable ages, ranging from preadolescent children to middle-aged adults. While some studies involve males and females, most are comprised of males only.

The majority of studies failed to report baseline measurements or the stability of baseline assessments across testing sessions. Where the latter values are reported, however, baseline evaluations of heart rate and blood pressure tend to correlate significantly over time. Yet, the magnitude of these associations is not overwhelming (the retest coefficients are generally less than 0.75), indicating that differences in the physiologic states of individuals under ostensibly uniform conditions of minimal stimulation (i.e., at rest) are only partially reproducible on repeated laboratory testing. The extent to which this is due to investigators' failure to provide a truly stimulus-free environment during baseline measurement or, alternatively, to preexperimental influences on heart rate and blood pressure (e.g., effects of recent events or fluctuations in mood) that may extend into the period of laboratory assessment is unknown. Interestingly, where reported (Arena, Blanchard, Andrasik, Cotch, & Myers, 1983; Faulstich *et al.*, 1986; Giordani, Manuck, & Farmer, 1981; Lacey & Lacey, 1962; Matthews, Rakaczky, Stoney, & Manuck, 1987; McKinney *et al.*, 1985), the absolute values of heart rate and blood pressure recorded during task periods frequently yield test–retest correlations of

about the same or greater magnitude than those obtained for baseline measurements.

Almost uniformly, the quantification of physiologic reactions to laboratory stressors among studies listed in Table 1 involves calculation of a simple change score—the arithmetic difference between baseline and task values. The between-session correlations based on these scores vary appreciably across studies, though in most instances the coefficients are statistically significant. For heart rate, the majority of data collections reveal correlations in the range of 0.67–0.91, indicating that changes from baseline for subjects' heart rate responses to the experimental tasks were reasonably stable across testing sessions. While systolic blood pressure reactions show a similar, if somewhat weaker, reproducibility over time, the generally small between-session correlations for changes in diastolic blood pressure suggest that individual differences on this response parameter are of questionable reliability. Unfortunately, many of the studies that present weaker findings are also more difficult to interpret, due to: (1) examination of relatively small samples (Arena *et al.*, 1983; Rombouts, 1982) and (2) an absence of information regarding either the magnitude of heart rate and blood pressure responses elicited by the experimental tasks or the degree of response habituation that may have occurred between the first and later testing sessions (e.g., Arena *et al.*, 1983; Faulstich *et al.*, 1986; McKinney *et al.*, 1985). It would not be surprising, for example, if tasks failing to evoke a marked cardiovascular response overall, or to elicit a response of similar magnitude when presented on subsequent occasions (e.g., owing to familiarity or acquisition of skill), also failed to generate reproducible distributions of individual difference. In the latter regard, it is noteworthy that several investigations demonstrating strong between-session correlations employed, at follow-up, either novel tasks (e.g., Glass, Lake, Contrada, Kehoe, & Erlanger, 1983; Lovallo, Pincomb, & Wilson, 1986; Manuck & Garland, 1980) or the same tasks presented in a novel form (Giordani *et al.*, 1981; Manuck & Schaefer, 1978); an effect of such procedures may have been to mitigate, in part, habituation of phys-

Table 1. Temporal Stability of Individual Differences in Heart Rate and Blood Pressure Responses to Behavioral Stimuli[a]

Reference	Subjects	Interval between assessments	Tasks	Intersession correlations (r) (*p > 0.05)			Comments and additional analyses
				HR	SBP	DBP	
Lacey and Lacey (1962)	N: 20 male (m); 17 female (f) Age: 74–209 months at initial assessment	4 years	Cold pressor				Baseline and task values based on peak values, adjusted for age and sex. Change scores adjusted for initial values.
			Baseline	0.56	0.20*	0.16*	
			Task values	0.79	0.59	0.71	
			Baseline-free Δ	0.44	0.75	0.75	
Manuck and Shaefer (1978)	N: 42 m Age: young adult	1 week	Concept formation	HR	SBP	DBP	"Reactors" and "nonreactors" defined as extreme thirds of session 1 change score distributions for each variable. Session 2 HR, SBP, and DBP changes differed significantly between groups. Baselines did not differ between groups.
			Baseline	Not reported			
			Arithmetic Δ	0.69	0.68	0.46	
Manuck and Garland (1980)	N: 19 m Sample derived from Manuck and Schaefer (1978)	13 months	Session 1: Concept formation Session 2: Concept formation, mental arithmetic	HR	SBP	DBP	"Reactors" and "nonreactors" defined by year 1 median split of combined week 1 and 2 change score distributions for each variable. Year 2 HR and SBP, but not DBP, changes differed significantly between groups. Baselines did not differ between groups.
			Baseline	Not reported			
			Arithmetic Δ				
			Concept formation	0.81	0.63	0.24*	
			Concept formation (year 1) with mental arithmetic	0.69	0.32*	0.23*	
Giordani et al. (1981)	N: 34 m Age: M = 101.9 months (SD = 7.95)	1 week	Concept formation	HR			"High" and "low" reactors defined by median split of session 1 change score distribution. Session 2 HR changes differed significantly between groups. Baselines did not differ between groups.
			Baseline	0.65			
			Task values	0.74			
			Arithmetic Δ	0.77			
Rombouts (1982)	N: 14 m; 10 f Age: M = 31.6 years, all patients with cardiovascular symptoms	2–3 days	Mental arithmetic, sentence forming, landscaping viewing, arithmetic under time pressure, stressful imagery	HR			Sixteen patients received unspecified medication.
			Baseline	Not reported			
			Arithmetic Δ				
			Mental arithmetic	0.70			
			Other tasks	Not reported			

Glass et al. row group — HR

	HR	

Study 1

N: 13 m; 18 f
Age: M = 25 years

2–3 days

Each of the following paired with word task: relaxation, mental arithmetic, counting objects, digit span

	HR	
	Males	Females
Baseline	Not reported	
Arithmetic Δ		
Relaxation	0.30*	0.50
Arithmetic	−0.23*	0.75
Counting	0.35*	0.74
Digit span	0.10*	0.85

Glass et al. (1983)

N: 56 m
Age: 25–29 years, M = 41.6 years

2 months

Session 1: Mental arithmetic
Session 2: Modified Stroop color word test

	HR	SBP	DBP
Baseline	Not reported		
Arithmetic Δ — Session 1 SBP With Session 2:	0.45	0.69	0.47

"High" and "low" reactors defined as extreme thirds of session 1 SBP change score distribution. Session 2 changes in HR, SBP and DBP differed significantly between groups. Baselines did not differ between groups.

Arena et al. (1983)

N: 6 m; 9 f
Age: M = 21.9 years

Session
1–2: 1 day
1–3: 7 days
1–4: 27 days

Mental arithmetic, stressful imagery, cold pressor

(HR only)

	Session Comparisons		
	1–2	1–3	1–4
Baseline	0.66	0.43	0.06*
Task values			
Mental arithmetic	0.53	0.56	0.30*
Stressful imagery	0.79	0.50	0.34*
Cold pressor	−0.10*	0.54	0.56
Arithmetic Δ			
Mental arithmetic	0.43*	0.52	0.21*
Stressful imagery	0.52	0.02*	−0.10*
Cold pressor	0.26*	0.62	0.43*
Percent Δ			
Mental arithmetic	0.52	0.54	0.20*
Stressful imagery	0.49	0.06*	0.07*
Cold pressor	0.33*	0.63	0.23*

Carroll et al. (1984)

N: 42 m
Age: 18–25 years

1 week

Unsignaled reaction time, video game

	HR
Baseline	Not reported
Arithmetic Δ	
Reaction time	0.69
Video game	0.80

Reported change scores to be independent of baseline values.

N: 24 f
Age: 17–38 years

13–14 days

Video game

	HR
Baseline	Not reported
Arithmetic Δ	0.91

Reported change scores to be independent of baseline values.

(continued)

Table 1. (Continued)

Reference	Subjects	Interval between assessments	Tasks		Intersession correlations (r) (*p > 0.05)			Comments and additional analyses
					HR	SBP	DBP	
McKinney et al. (1985)	N: 60 m Age: M = 45.1 years	3 months	Videogame, choice reaction time, cold pressor	Baseline				
				Sitting	0.74	0.56	0.72	
				Supine	0.70	0.50	0.42	
				Task values				
				Video game	0.58	0.70	0.72	
				Reaction time	0.57	0.62	0.56	
				Cold pressor	0.45	0.62	0.66	
				Arithmetic Δ				
				Video game	0.36	0.48	0.36	
				Reaction time	0.38	0.46	0.15*	
				Cold pressor	0.23*	0.39	0.48	
					HR	SBP	DBP	
Faulstich et al. (1986)	N: 48 m and f Age: young adult	2 weeks	Mental arithmetic, history quiz, handgrip, cold pressor	Baseline				
				Mental arithmetic	0.73	0.62	0.70	
				History quiz	0.58	0.52	0.62	
				Handgrip	0.77	0.36	0.51	
				Cold pressor	0.69	0.57	0.64	
				Task values				
				Mental arithmetic	0.72	0.58	0.51	
				History quiz	0.60	0.46	0.70	
				Handgrip	0.73	0.67	0.74	
				Cold pressor	0.66	0.55	0.56	
				Arithmetic Δ				
				Mental arithmetic	0.59	0.27*	0.21*	
				History quiz	0.22*	-0.01*	0.06*	
				Handgrip	0.30	0.44	0.40	
				Cold pressor	0.50	0.46	0.23*	
					HR		MAP	
Lovallo et al. (1986)	N: 28 Age: 21–35 years	1 year	Session 1: Unavoidable shock and noise (passive coping), avoidable shock and noise (active coping) Session 2: Cold pressor	Baseline	Not reported		Not reported	Change scores based on 10-sec. peak responses to each task. "High" and "low" HR reactors during cold pressor defined by median split of change score distribution. HR, SBP, and DBP differed significantly between groups during active coping but not during passive coping tasks. Baselines did not differ between groups.
				Task values				
				Arithmetic Δ				
				Cold pressor with active coping	0.65		0.49	
				Cold pressor with passive coping	0.53		0.38	

					HR	SBP	DBP	Intersession correlations adjusted for baseline differences (partial correlations).
Matthews et al. (1987)	N: 18 f Age: M = 14.2 years	10 months	Mental arithmetic, mirror image tracing, handgrip	Baseline	0.80	0.79	0.52	
				Task values				
				Mental arithmetic	0.49	0.48	0.43*	
				Image tracing	0.55	0.26*	0.73	
				Handgrip	0.44*	0.48	0.28*	
				Mean of three tasks	0.65	0.53	0.55	
				Arithmetic Δ				
				Mental arithmetic	0.40*	0.36*	−0.18*	
				Image tracing	0.58	−0.18*	0.83	
				Handgrip	0.07*	0.32*	0.10*	
				Mean of three tasks	0.60	0.17*	0.30*	
	N: 18 m Age: M = 10.4 years	41 months	Session 1: Videogame Session 2: Mental arithmetic, mirror image tracing, handgrip	Baseline	0.58	0.69	0.37*	Intersession correlations adjusted for baseline differences (partial correlations).
				Task values Videogame (Session 1) with:				
				Mental arithmetic	0.67	0.51	0.35*	
				Image tracing	0.66	0.67	0.52	
				Handgrip	0.73	0.74	0.49	
				Mean of three tasks	0.74	0.69	0.62	
				Arithmetic Δ Videogame (Session 1) with:				
				Mental arithmetic	0.21*	0.04*	0.30*	
				Image tracing	0.40*	0.28*	0.45*	
				Handgrip	0.82	0.38*	0.37*	
				Mean of three tasks	0.68	0.32*	0.54	

[a]Nonsignificant intersession correlations are identified by an asterisk; all other correlations are statistically significant for at least $p < 0.05$.

iologic reactions that would otherwise have occurred across testing sessions.

As noted, arithmetic change scores were computed to describe the reactivity of individuals in nearly all studies cited in Table 1. However, some investigators do report the absence of a significant correlation in their samples between baseline values and calculated change scores (Carroll, Turner, Lee, & Stephenson, 1984; Glass *et al.*, 1983). In these instances, it is presumed that arithmetic changes did not share appreciable variance with baseline measurements. It should be cautioned, though, that with small sample sizes a moderate correlation between baseline and change may exist but elude significance (and possibly the investigator's concern) due to limited statistical power.

In still other studies, the stability of individual differences has been examined among discrete subgroups of subjects partitioned according to the initial magnitude of their responses to behavioral challenge. For example, we observed that young adult males who were identified as either "high" or "low" heart rate or systolic blood pressure reactors by their responses to a difficult cognitive task differed significantly in their reactions to the same task 1 week later, and to both the same and a similar task on additional follow-up after 13 months. Importantly, the high and low reactive groups did not differ on corresponding baseline measurements (Manuck & Schaefer, 1978; Manuck & Garland, 1980). The reproducibility of response differences among similarly differentiated groups of more and less reactive individuals, at least for heart rate and systolic blood pressure, has also been reported by other investigators and for a broader range of subject populations (Carroll *et al.*, 1984; Giordani *et al.*, 1981; Glass *et al.*, 1983; Lovallo *et al.*, 1986).

In summary, there is preliminary evidence that the differences observed among individuals on some measures of behaviorally elicited cardiovascular response are consistent across different occasions of testing. Available studies are few in number, however, and frequently entail observations derived from relatively small samples. At present, there is also little information regarding the temporal stability of individual differences on other physiologic parameters of interest to psycho-

physiologists, particularly plasma measurements of catecholamine and cortisol response. Another limitation of current data pertains to the retest intervals employed by most investigators. With few exceptions, follow-up testing has been conducted within a few months of participants' initial evaluations; thus, it is not known whether variability in responses to behavioral stimuli are reproducible over relatively protracted intervals, such as years or decades. In the future, it will be important also to examine more heterogeneous subject populations and to extend observations to pertinent patient samples. The latter point, in particular, is relevant to current hypotheses linking heightened psychophysiologic reactivity to the clinical sequelae of hypertension or coronary artery disease (Manuck & Krantz, 1986).

Finally, on a more conceptual note, it is possible that the temporal stability of psychophysiologic responses in itself constitutes a meaningful dimension of individual differences. For instance, some people may exhibit cardiovascular and neuroendocrine reactions of greater or lesser magnitude with considerable reliability across repeated testing sessions, whereas other individuals may show a more variable responsivity over time. If so, an adequate assessment of psychophysiologic response characteristics may require multiple observations. This situation would be analogous in some respects to the clinical evaluation of hypertension, which similarly requires repeated measurements at successive office visits to discriminate stable and fluctuating (labile) elevations of blood pressure. Also, if the reproducibility of psychophysiologic reactivity is variable among individuals, it should perhaps not be surprising that test–retest correlations such as those reported in Table 1 are rarely of impressive magnitude: those subjects who show an inconsistent pattern of response will necessarily reduce the strength of temporal association observed across two occasions of measurement in an otherwise unselected group of individuals.

Intertask Consistency

In the previous chapter, Schneiderman and Mc-Cabe described a number of task parameters that influence subjects' cardiovascular and neuroendocrine responses, such as the availability of coping behaviors, differing attentional demands, and the propensity of a stimulus to elicit varying emotional reactions. The fact that stimulus attributes exert a potent influence on psychophysiologic response suggests that the "reactivity" of individuals may also vary under differing task conditions. Yet, it is assumed by many investigators—if not explicitly, then tacitly through use of single-task protocols—that individual differences in psychophysiologic reactivity (1) generalize from one stimulus to another and (2) do not vary as a function of task influences on the overall magnitude or patterning of observed responses. If distributions of idiosyncratic physiologic response are reproducible across stimuli, of course, appreciable intertask correlations should be seen among studies employing more than one experimental challenge. Unfortunately, few investigators have reported such correlations and those who have describe relationships limited primarily to heart rate and blood pressure.

For example, Obrist (1981) contrasted subjects' reactions to three laboratory stimuli that may be considered either aversive or arousing, but which had somewhat different hemodynamic effects. One task, shock avoidance, exerted a strong β-adrenergic influence on cardiac performance; the two other stimuli, the cold pressor test and a pornographic film, had less pronounced cardiac effects, but evoked a substantial vascular response. Among the 56 young adult males exposed to this protocol, individuals falling within the upper and lower quartiles of the distribution of heart rate responses during shock avoidance showed mean elevations of 57 and 9 bpm, respectively. These clearly differentiated groups differed also in the magnitude of their heart rate responses to the cold pressor test (33 versus 13 bpm) and film (23 versus 5 bpm). Moreover, correlations of all subjects' heart rate reactions across the three experimental stimuli were significant and in the range of +0.53 to +0.58. Correlations of systolic pressor responses recorded during the same tasks were significant as well and of similar magnitude ($r = +0.49$ to $+0.75$). Thus, persons who showed differing heart rate and systolic blood pressure reactions during

one behavioral stressor (shock avoidance) tended to differ also when exposed to two other, relatively dissimilar stimuli.

Depending upon the types of attentional demands placed on subjects (Lacey, Kagan, & Lacey, 1963), bidirectional heart rate responses can be elicited in laboratory experiments. Deceleration of heart rate frequently accompanies subjects' performance of tasks requiring vigilance, or attentiveness to an external stimulus (sensory intake), while heart rate tends to increase when subjects are exposed to tasks of a cognitive, or "mental," nature. (The latter are situations which necessitate concentration and, hence, rejection of irrelevant sensory information.) Interestingly, people who differ in the magnitude of their heart rate responses during sensory rejection tasks exhibit parallel, albeit somewhat smaller, differences when performing sensory intake tasks. In one study, Bunnell (1982) identified two groups of subjects on the basis of their heart rate reactions to mental arithmetic (a prototypic "rejection" task); the mean heart rate responses of the groups were +17.5 and −0.8 bpm, respectively. During an auditory reaction time task (sensory intake), heart rate reactions of the same groups averaged +2.3 and −4.8 bpm ($p < 0.01$). Hence, individuals whose heart rates failed to increase during mental arithmetic showed expected cardiac deceleration during sensory intake, while the most reactive subjects during mental arithmetic actually exhibited a slight increase in heart rate when performing the reaction time task. A similar relationship was observed by Lawler (1980), who compared phasic (second-by-second) heart rate responses to a sensory intake task among subjects who had also been identified as either high or low heart rate responders during mental arithmetic. The high responders showed increases in heart rate on performance of a "tone" identification task, whereas low heart rate reactive subjects exhibited cardiac deceleration under the same stimulus conditions.

In our laboratory, we recently examined the consistency of heart rate and blood pressure reactions across three experimental stressors: a frustrating psychomotor task (tracing the outline of a star guided only by the design's mirror image) and two cognitive challenges (mental arithmetic and problems in concept formation). Intertask correlations employing baseline-free (residualized) change scores yielded coefficients in the range of $+0.57$ to $+0.82$ for heart rate, $+0.49$ to $+0.63$ for systolic blood pressure, and $+0.49$ to $+0.57$ for diastolic blood pressure. However, not all investigators report comparable correlations among subjects' cardiovascular responses to different experimental tasks. McKinney *et al.* (1985), for instance, exposed middle-aged males to three laboratory stimuli—the cold pressor test and two psychomotor challenges (a video game and a choice reaction time task). Subjects' heart rate responses to the two psychomotor tasks (also adjusted for baseline influences) covaried more strongly with each other ($r = +0.58$) than did responses to either task with heart rate reactions observed during the cold pressor test (r's $= +0.22$ and $+0.32$). Subjects' diastolic blood pressure responses also correlated more highly between the video game and reaction time tasks ($r = +0.54$) than between either of the psychomotor challenges and cold pressor (r's $= +0.29$ and $+0.35$). Corresponding correlations for systolic blood pressure were more consistent across comparisons, ranging from $+0.51$ to $+0.60$. In another study, Carroll *et al.* (1984) observed that while heart rate responses of young adult males to two psychomotor challenges—again, a video game and reaction time task—correlated significantly ($r = +0.43$) on one occasion of measurement, the magnitude of this association declined substantially (to $+0.24$) when the experimental protocol was readministered 1 week later.

The foregoing observations discourage speculation that there exists an underlying or unitary dimension of individual differences in psychophysiologic reactivity which is expressed independently of concomitant stimulus characteristics. From an assessment perspective, therefore, it is unlikely that the use of any one experimental challenge will permit adequate evaluation of the psychophysiologic response characteristics of individuals. Instead, such evaluation may require the construction of a battery of test stimuli, sampling across a variety of task variables known to affect cardiovascular and neuroendocrine responses. In this regard, recall our previous suggestion that individuals may differ in the degree to

which they exhibit temporal stability of psychophysiologic reactions. Consistency of response across varying task conditions may also differ substantially among individuals, and thereby represent yet another conceptually meaningful individual difference. Hence, some persons may show exaggerated pressor reactions to all stimulus presentations, while others may reveal a more selective pattern of responses; in turn, it may be the uniformly hyperreactive individual who is of greatest interest in relation to cardiovascular risk and prediction of disease endpoints. The frequent report that hypertensive patients are more likely than normotensives to exhibit a stereotypic, or stimulus-independent hyperresponsivity of blood pressure when exposed to a broad range of laboratory tasks and challenges (Engel & Bickford, 1961; Fredrikson *et al.*, 1985), for example, is consistent with such speculation.

Lab-to-Field Generalization

If idiosyncratic physiologic reactions to standardized behavioral stressors reflect a robust construct of individual differences, we might also expect these response differences to generalize beyond the laboratory setting. Moreover, insofar as the reactivity of individuals is defined by physiologic responses to stimuli of a behavioral, or psychological nature, such generalization would predictably emerge during naturally occurring events that possess at least some parallel, psychologically salient features. In this regard, Matthews, Manuck, and Saab (1986, and unpublished observations) have examined adolescents' cardiovascular reactions to performance challenges in the laboratory (e.g., mental arithmetic) as predictors of heart rate and blood pressure measurements recorded in the interval surrounding subjects' presentation of a regularly scheduled, tenth-grade classroom "speech." To demonstrate that relationships between individuals' physiologic states in the two stimulus contexts (laboratory and classroom) were plausibly associated with corresponding behavioral attributes of these situations, additional (control) measurements were obtained at the same time of day on a separate occasion, when subjects were not scheduled for classroom presentation. Illustrated in Figure 2 are mean values of heart rate and systolic blood pressure, as seen immediately preceding (measures 1 and 2) and following subjects' presentations, as well as at the subsequent non-speech-day ("Control") recording; all measurements were obtained while subjects were in a seated position. The two groups depicted in Figure 2 were comprised of students who had shown baseline-adjusted heart rate responses of greater or lesser magnitude across a series of laboratory stressors (i.e., high versus low heart rate reactors). Statistical analyses showed that the high heart rate reactors had significantly greater heart rate and systolic blood pressure before and after their classroom presentations when compared to low reactive subjects, but that the two groups did not differ reliably on non-speech-day (control) measurements. These data are therefore consistent with the hypothesis that laboratory-assessed cardiovascular reactivity generalizes to measurements obtained during natu-

rally occurring events. It is also noteworthy that the investigators here were assured an opportunity to address this hypothesis, as a circumstance of "probable" generalization (the classroom speech) was selected in advance of data collection and because the event selected involved an experience common to all of the participants.

Unfortunately, in most attempts to address the generalization issue, field measurements are obtained without knowledge of the corresponding behavioral states and activities of the subject. This is a particular difficulty in studies of ambulatory blood pressure monitoring, where successive measurements often occur at intervals dictated by available cycling times of the investigator's ambulatory recorder. What is lost here is the experimenter's ability to identify readings that are coincident with events of psychological significance (i.e., the context in which generalization would be predicted). Also lost is the opportunity to examine these values apart from recordings obtained at times of behavioral "irrelevance," or to account for the concomitant influences of extraneous factors such as postural adjustments, movement, or proximity to meals. Some of the shortcomings of ambulatory measurements may be ameliorated through use of mood and activity diaries that are filled out at the time of each measurement, or, as described in the previous chapter, by partitioning data sets in relation to the "ecology" of daily activities (e.g., work, home, sleep). In the latter regard, however, it must be appreciated that individual experiences vary even in environmental contexts of great uniformity; "work" is not of necessity a stressful stimulus, nor does "home" provide a setting of benign respite and emotional support for every individual. Hence, while it may be useful to aggregate measurements within periods that tend to correspond with varying activity patterns, it is potentially misleading (and in a substantial proportion of individual cases, surely inaccurate) to attribute psychological import *per se* to different portions of the day.

Other considerations bearing on the generalization of individual differences in psychophysiologic reactivity are both statistical and conceptual in nature. On the statistical side, the magnitude of any association observed between laboratory and field

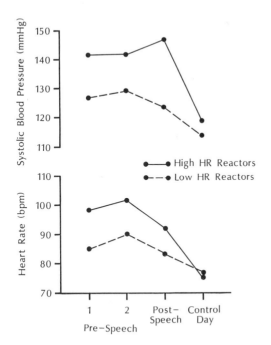

Figure 2. Mean heart rate and systolic blood pressure measurements of "high" and "low" heart rate reactors prior to and following presentation of a classroom speech, and on a separate occasion ("Control Day") when subjects were not scheduled for presentation.

measurements is constrained by the reliability of assessment achieved in both settings. For purposes of illustration, let us assume that for a given stimulus or class of stimuli there exists a construct of individual differences in behaviorally elicited systolic blood pressure reactivity that is associated with a "true" value or score for each subject (Sre*) and that there also exists a "true" distribution of systolic blood pressure values prevailing during working hours of the day (as seen among individuals wearing ambulatory recorders) (Samb*). (Admittedly, we have just argued that ambulatory measurements alone, without knowledge of concomitant psychological and environmental variables, provide an inadequate vehicle to test hypotheses regarding the generalization of reactivity; for the moment, however, these reservations will be set aside in order to simplify our example.)

Let us now say that in the sample under study, we have assessed subjects' systolic blood pressure reactivity by use of a single laboratory challenge, such as mental arithmetic. For each subject, the systolic response observed on presentation of this task (Sre) reflects a combination of the true reactivity of the individual and some degree of error (Sre* + e). The reliability with which the true construct (Sre*) is assessed under these conditions may be estimated from the correlation ($r_{Sre_1Sre_2}$) between measurements obtained on different occasions (retest) or by subjects' exposure to two or more ostensibly comparable stimuli (alternate forms). As Cohen and Cohen (1983) note, the reliability coefficient expresses the proportion of the measure's variance associated with the true construct that is available for correlation with other variables of interest—the latter in this case being ambulatory blood pressure measurements. For this example, then, let us say that the reliability of our measurement of systolic blood pressure reactivity is 0.70 (a rather generous estimate in view of earlier discussions in this chapter).

Of course, reliability is a matter of equal interest in relation to our ambulatory recordings. McKinney *et al.* (1985) reported a test–retest correlation ($r_{Samb_1Samb_2}$) of 0.60 for the mean of systolic blood pressure measurements obtained during working hours in a sample that we will identify, for convenience, as comparable to our own. Psy-chometric theory predicts that where reliability of measurement departs from unity on one or both variables under study, the correlation of "obtained" scores on these variables will tend to underestimate the association which actually exists between the unobservable, "true" scores. For example, if there exists a true correlation of 0.50 between systolic blood pressure reactivity and the mean of work-associated systolic blood pressure measurements, and if our evaluation of each of these variables involves a single assessment with reliabilities as indicated above, we will not expect our own data to reveal a correlation of these parameters exceeding 0.32 (where $r_{SreSamb} = r_{Sre*Samb*} \sqrt{r_{Sre_1Sre_2}r_{Samb_1Samb_2}}$ (Cohen & Cohen, 1983). Thus, the limited reliability of assessments in this area, whether of reactivity or of field measurements (or both), severely restricts the investigator's ability to detect significant lab-to-field generalization.* This is especially problematic for opportunistic studies that capitalize on the availability of interesting, but small clinical samples. In these instances, the investigator should attempt to minimize error variance through *repeated* administration of carefully constructed, multitask protocols and by collection of ambulatory data on more than one day of recording. It is likely that less serious attempts to enhance the reliability of psychophysiologic measurements will only foster proliferation of a weak and inconclusive literature.

A more conceptual consideration concerns the manner in which generalization of laboratory-assessed reactivity may occur. Several models of this process have been delineated. One possibility is that the variability of cardiovascular and neuroendocrine states in the laboratory experience recapitulates "real life." For example, individuals who exhibit large physiologic reactions to labora-

---

*An extension of this point concerns computation of the arithmetic difference score. Recall that this measure is a composite of (1) the baseline measurement and (2) values obtained during task (stimulus) periods. As discussed previously, neither baseline nor task-related measurements are without elements of unreliability. The unreliability of the constituent variables is therefore compounded when calculating the arithmetic change score, a fact which constrains this measure's ability to yield significant relationships with other variables of interest.

tory stressors (hyperreactors) may also show heightened responses to daily events of a similarly stressful nature; conversely, persons who exhibit little reactivity in the laboratory (hyporeactors) may experience small or only moderate physiologic responses to naturally occurring events. Thus, the daily experience of the hyperreactor—if it involves exposure to significant behavioral challenges, or stress—may be characterized by repeated episodes, or occurrences, of acute physiologic reactivity that are mimicked by responses exhibited in the laboratory.

We have previously described this particular form of laboratory-to-life relationship as the recurrent activation model (Manuck & Krantz, 1984). The stylized drawing in Figure 3 illustrates predictions predicated on this model for a prototypic hyperreactor and hyporeactor (the upper and lower panels, respectively). (Although heart rate is depicted on the ordinate as the physiologic measure of interest, any other commonly recorded response parameter, such as plasma epinephrine concentration or blood pressure, may be substituted.) The daily lives of these two individuals are accompanied, as described above, by recurrent episodes

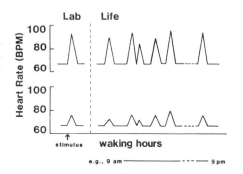

RECURRENT ACTIVATION MODEL

Figure 3. Stylized figure depicting the generalization to nonlaboratory settings of individual differences in laboratory-assessed heart rate reactivity, as predicted by the "recurrent activation model." The upper and lower panels illustrate responses of a prototypic hyperreactor and hyporeactor, respectively. Depicted on the left ("Lab") are subjects' heart rate responses to a standardized behavioral stimulus (or stressor) in the laboratory. Illustrated on the right ("Life") are the predicted heart rate responses of these individuals to naturally occurring events in daily life. (See text.) From Manuck and Krantz (1984); used by permission.

of reactivity which resemble closely subjects' physiologic reactions to the laboratory stressor. Because precipitating environmental events encountered outside the laboratory are also likely to differ in their intensity, subjects' corresponding physiologic responses may vary in magnitude; nevertheless, the model stipulates that an ordered relationship among individuals is retained across stimuli in their natural life context.

An important assumption of the recurrent activation model is that the laboratory-derived baseline measurement denotes a representative state of the organism. It follows, then, that challenges experienced during the course of subjects' daily activities will give rise to transient episodes of reactivity, which may be thought of as acute deviations from a common baseline. Yet, the substantial effort most investigators expend to achieve a truly stimulus-free environment just for purposes of baseline recording suggests that such resting measurements may represent, in fact, the more anomalous states of the individual. That is, levels of physiologic activity approximating the laboratory baseline may be seen relatively infrequently in daily life, or at least infrequently over the preponderance of waking hours in which individuals are engaged in significant, ongoing activities (e.g., work demands, interactions with other people). In contrast, it may be the reactive state of the organism, as observed in the laboratory assessment, that correlates best with levels of physiologic activity experienced most frequently in daily life. If so, individual differences in psychophysiologic reactivity would be more predictive of physiologic states prevailing throughout the waking, active hours of the day than they are of transient episodes of acute arousal. This relationship, which we have labeled the prevailing state model, is illustrated in Figure 4.

These two formulations—recurrent activation and prevailing states—present contrasting models of the generalization of psychophysiologic reactivity, with respect to which available findings unfortunately provide little clarification. Previously described data relating adolescents' relative heart rate reactivity to heart rate and systolic blood pressure measurements during public speaking (Figure 2), for instance, may appear to support predictions based on the recurrent activation model. Recall

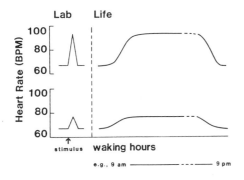

PREVAILING STATE MODEL

Figure 4. Stylized figure depicting the generalization to non-laboratory settings of individual differences in laboratory-assessed heart rate reactivity, as predicted by the "prevailing state model." The upper and lower panels illustrate responses of a prototypic hyperreactor and hyporeactor, respectively. Depicted on the left ("Lab") are subjects' heart rate responses to a standardized behavioral stimulus (or stressor) in the laboratory. Illustrated on the right ("Life") are the predicted heart rate responses of these individuals to naturally occurring events in daily life. (See text.) From Manuck and Krantz (1984); used by permission.

that high and low heart rate reactive groups differed substantially in recordings made around the time of subjects' classroom presentations, but were comparable on measurements taken at the same time of day on a separate, but more benign occasion. Yet, because recordings were not obtained over longer intervals preceding and following the students' presentations, it is unclear whether the heightened cardiovascular arousal of high heart rate reactive subjects on the "speech" day describes a phenomenon of minutes or of hours, i.e., whether these measurements (the only recordings available) reflect a period of transient or more protracted elevation of heart rate and blood pressure. Due to the limited interpretation that may be applied to these findings (as well as to other data reported in this literature), it awaits further research to determine whether one of the two models presented above, or, indeed, some other formulation of lab–life relationships, best describes the generalization of psychophysiologic reactivity. To this end, however, more clearly articulated hypotheses regarding the potential nature of such generalization should provide useful guidelines for the collection of pertinent data.

Summary Comment

The purpose of this chapter has been to identify several issues relevant to the conceptualization of psychophysiologic reactivity as a dimension of individual differences. Considered first were matters bearing on the quantification of behaviorally elicited physiologic reactions, and, in particular, the problem of divorcing the numerical expression of these responses from the concomitant influences of baseline differences among individuals. We next discussed the stability of individual differences in psychophysiologic reactivity, both temporally and across varying stimulus conditions. A relatively limited literature demonstrates statistically significant, but only modest, relationships between individual differences in cardiovascular reactions measured at different points in time or on presentation of different experimental stimuli. These imperfect associations suggest, in turn, that the consistency of physiologic reactions seen on retesting and under differing task conditions may itself vary among individuals. Thus, the relative magnitude of response exhibited by some persons when exposed to laboratory tasks or stressors may be highly reproducible, while others' reactions may vary appreciably over time or as a function of differing test stimuli. If so, it is likely that "true" distributions of idiosyncratic cardiovascular and neuroendocrine reactivity are inadequately captured through single-task protocols administered on a single occasion of measurement. These considerations suggest as well that current hypotheses linking an exaggerated psychophysiologic responsivity to cardiovascular disease and disease pathogenesis may be germane only to a limited subset of persons composed of stereotypically hyperreactive individuals.

The final issue addressed in this chapter concerned the generalization of individual differences in reactivity from laboratory assessments to measurements obtained in natural (or field) settings. This is a largely unexplored question, which nonetheless is likely to receive substantial attention in the future due to the advent of new technologies for ambulatory physiologic recording. Our comments on this topic were limited to methodological and statistical concerns that may hamper the demonstration of true associations between laboratory and field measurements, and to delineation of conceptual models describing possible forms that the generalization of reactivity may take. We noted that the expression of an individual's reactivity in "real life" logically presumes exposure to an eliciting stimulus, as it does in the laboratory; this suggests that measurement of physiologic states accompanying subjects' experiences of similar, or uniformly stressful, life events should permit reasonable tests of the generalization of reactivity. If such data collection is not feasible, then individuals' affective experiences and social environments must be measured with enough sensitivity to permit plausible identification of the idiosyncratic behavioral correlates, if any, of ambulatory or field recordings. Among other recommendations following from our previous discussions are: (1) that physiologic measurements be obtained with sufficient frequency to describe the time course of any "response" that may be associated with particular events or activities and (2) that all reasonable efforts be made to reduce the appreciable error variance which frequently characterizes both laboratory and field measurements. Finally, regarding our suggestion that temporal and intertask consistency of physiologic responses may represent an additional dimension of individual differences, it may be appropriate to extend measurements of psychophysiologic reactivity in the future to include the use of multitask protocols that are presented at two or more laboratory sessions.

ACKNOWLEDGMENT. Preparation of this chapter was supported, in part, by grants HL-29028, HL-35221, and HL-40962.

References

Arena, J. G., Blanchard, E. B., Andrasik, F., Cotch, P., & Myers, P. (1983). Reliability of psychophysiological assessment. *Behaviour Research and Therapy, 21,* 447–460.

Bunnell, D. E. (1982). Autonomic myocardial influences as a factor determining inter-task consistency of heart rate reactivity. *Psychophysiology, 19,* 442–448.

Carroll, D., Turner, J. R., Lee, H. J., & Stephenson, J. (1984). Temporal consistency of individual differences in cardiac response to a video game. *Biological Psychology, 19,* 81–93.

Cohen, J., & Cohen, P. (1983). *Applied multiple regression/correlation analysis for the behavioral sciences* (2nd ed.). Hillsdale, NJ: Erlbaum.

Engel, B. T., & Bickford, A. F. (1961). Response-specificity: Stimulus–response and individual–response specificity in essential hypertensives. *Archives of General Psychiatry, 5,* 478–489.

Faulstich, M. E., Williamson, D. A., McKenzie, S. J., Duchmann, E. G., Hutchenson, K. M., & Blouin, D. C. (1986). Temporal stability of psychophysiological responding: A comparative analysis of mental and physical stressors. *International Journal of Neuroscience, 30,* 65–72.

Fredrikson, M., Danielson, T., Engel, B. T., Frisk-Holmberg, M., Strom, G., & Sundin, O. (1985). Autonomic nervous system function and essential hypertension: Individual response specificity with and without beta adrenergic blockage. *Psychophysiology, 22,* 167–174.

Giordani, B., Manuck, S. B., & Farmer, J. F. (1981). Stability of behaviorally-induced heart rate changes in children after one week. *Child Development, 52,* 533–537.

Glass, D. C., Lake, C. R., Contrada, R. J., Kehoe, K., & Erlanger, L. R. (1983). Stability of individual differences in physiologic responses to stress. *Health Psychology, 4,* 317–342.

Hastrup, J. L. (1986). Duration of initial heart rate assessment in *Psychophysiology:* Current practices and implications. *Psychophysiology, 23,* 15–18.

Lacey, J. I., & Lacey, B. C. (1962). The law of initial value in the longitudinal study of autonomic constitution: Reproducibility of autonomic responses and response patterns over a four year interval. *Annals of the New York Academy of Sciences, 98,* 1257–1290, 1322–1326.

Lacey, J. I., Kagan, J., & Lacey, B. C. (1963). The visceral level: Situational determinants and behavioral correlates of autonomic response patterns. In P. H. Knapp (Ed.), *Expression of emotions in man.* New York: International University Press.

Lawler, K. A. (1980). Cardiovascular and electrodermal response patterns in heart rate reactive individuals during psychological stress. *Psychophysiology, 17,* 464–470.

Lovallo, W. R., Pincomb, G. A., & Wilson, M. F. (1986). Heart rate reactivity and type A behavior as modifiers of physiological response to active and passive coping. *Psychophysiology, 23,* 105–112.

Manuck, S. B., & Garland, F. N. (1980). Stability of individual differences in cardiovascular reactivity: A thirteen month follow-up. *Physiology and Behavior, 24,* 621–624.

Manuck, S. B., & Krantz, D. S. (1984). Psychophysiologic reactivity in coronary heart disease. *Behavioral Medicine Update, 6,* 11–15.

Manuck, S. B., & Krantz, D. S. (1986). Psychophysiologic reactivity in coronary heart disease and essential hypertension. In K. A. Matthews, S. B. Weiss, T. Detre, T. M. Dembroski, B. Falkner, S. B. Manuck, & R. B. Williams (Eds.), *Handbook of stress, reactivity, and cardiovascular disease.* New York: Wiley–Interscience.

Manuck, S. B., & Schaefer, D. C. (1978). Stability of individual differences in cardiovascular reactivity. *Physiology and Behavior, 21,* 675–678.

Manuck, S. B., Kaplan, J. R., & Clarkson, T. B. (1983). Behaviorally induced heart rate reactivity and atherosclerosis in cynomolgus monkeys. *Psychosomatic Medicine, 45,* 95–108.

Matthews, K. A., Manuck, S. B., & Saab, P. G. (1986). Cardiovascular responses of adolescents during a naturally occurring stressor and their behavioral and psychophysiological predictors. *Psychophysiology, 23,* 198–209.

Matthews, K. A., Rakaczky, C. J., Stoney, C. M., & Manuck, S. B. (1987). Are cardiovascular responses to behavioral stressors a stable individual difference variable in childhood? *Psychophysiology, 24,* 464–473.

McKinney, M. E., Miner, M. H., Ruddel, H., McIlvain, H. E., Witte, H., Buell, J. C., Eliot, R. S., & Grant, L. B. (1985). The standardized mental stress protocol: Test–retest reliability and comparison with ambulatory blood pressure monitoring. *Psychophysiology, 22,* 453–463.

Obrist, P. A. (1981). *Cardiovascular psychophysiology.* New York: Plenum Press.

Rombouts, R. (1982). The reproducibility of cardiovascular reactions during cognitive tasks. *Activitas Nervosa Superior,* Suppl. 3(Pt. 2), 283–294.

Shapiro, A. P., Nicotero, J., Sapira, J., & Scheib, E. T. (1968). Analysis of the variability of blood pressure, pulse rate and catecholamine responsivity in identical and fraternal twins. *Psychosomatic Medicine, 47,* 90 (Abstract).

Wilder, J. (1957). The law of initial values in neurology and psychiatry: Facts and problems. *Journal of Nervous and Mental Diseases, 125,* 73–86.

CHAPTER 24

The Social Context of Stress and Behavioral Medicine Research

Instructions, Experimenter Effects, and Social Interactions

David S. Krantz and Jeffrey Ratliff-Crain

In studies of stress, factors such as the context of the research situation, and subtle variations in the instructions presented can have significant effects on resulting psychological, behavioral, and physiological responses. Specifically, both laboratory and field psychophysiology studies involve procedural elements, from the obtaining of informed consent to payment for participation, that can be significant sources of error variance that remain even if the most stringent experimental controls are instituted. This chapter will address potential sources of bias in research that are associated with the social context in which studies are conducted.

This chapter will also consider psychological characteristics of stress tasks that influence the intensity of physiological responses they produce. There is considerable evidence that the effects of physical stressors depend strongly on psychological factors, and that specific types of stressors can produce rather specific patterns of responses (Mason, 1971; Elliott & Eisdorfer, 1982; Williams,

1985). There are numerous ways of dimensionalizing the tasks and stimulus situations that produce different patterns of bodily responses. However, implicit in the description of a stressor as *psychological* is that the individual's response to a challenging or stressful stimulus depends on the way that stimulus is interpreted or appraised, the context in which that stimulus occurs, and the personal resources available for coping (Cohen *et al.,* 1982; Lazarus, 1966). A body of research demonstrates that if situations are viewed as harmful, threatening, or noxious, they can produce substantial physiological responses (Lazarus, 1966; Mason, 1971). Conversely, when conditions are designed to change the demands of a stressor, or to reduce the psychological threat that might be engendered by potentially aversive procedures, they may produce smaller, and perhaps only minimal physiological responses and/or behavioral reactions (Lazarus, 1966).

The focus of this review will be on social interaction and instructional factors that influence outcomes in studies of psychophysiological and behavioral responses to stress. First, subtle components of the overall experimental situation will be discussed, including such factors as the method of

David S. Krantz and Jeffrey Ratliff-Crain • Department of Medical Psychology, Uniformed Services University of the Health Sciences, Bethesda, Maryland 20814.

obtaining informed consent, "demand characteristics" and experimenter bias, study descriptions given to subjects prior to the session, and manipulation checks. Next will be considered the underlying characteristics of commonly used tasks that determine the intensity of subjects' responses in psychophysiological studies. These characteristics include the difficulty of the tasks, the level of challenge, harassment, competition, incentives, and instructions.

The Structure of the Experimental Situation

Experimentation with humans involves a set of ritualized, standard procedures including the signing of the consent form, reimbursement for participation, and/or a description of the study given to participating subjects. Each of these procedures occurs in a social-psychological context, and depending on how these procedures are conducted, can exert subtle influences on the behavior of subjects.

Informed Consent

Subjects participate in experiments for several reasons: interest in advancing science, monetary incentives, credit in psychology classes, or hopes of gaining information about themselves. All subjects are given a document to read and sign at the beginning of a study; this document describes what the study is about, what they can expect during the session, and the risks and benefits of the study to them. There is also usually an explicit statement that their participation is voluntary, and that they can therefore withdraw from the study at any time without penalty. Guidelines will differ from institution to institution concerning how explicitly the affirmation of the subject's right to withdraw is presented.

Clearly, one of the intended effects of the informed consent procedure is to provide the subject with a degree of control over aspects of the experimental procedure. However, research on stress has demonstrated that the predictability of the stressor and subjects' perceptions about whether they are able to control the stressor (e.g., modify its out-

come) constitute important mediators of stress responses. Perceived control may be defined as the felt ability to escape, avoid, or modify threatening stimuli (Glass & Singer, 1972; Seligman, 1972). Predictability is the ability to anticipate a particular stimulus. In general, the greater the perceived controllability of a stressor, the less harmful are the effects on the organism. The work of Seligman (1972), for example, suggests that a psychological state of helplessness results when individuals encounter aversive events about which they can do nothing. Research by Glass and Singer (1972) demonstrates that exposure to noise and other stressors that subjects believe cannot be controlled, results in aftereffects in the form of impaired cognitive performance, appearing after the stress is over. By giving subjects even the *perception* of control over the stressor (e.g., by telling them they could press a button to terminate the stress), these aftereffects could be avoided.

Informed consent procedures, as outlined by Federal human subjects guidelines, make it clear to subjects that they can discontinue their participation in any experiment without penalty, thereby giving subjects the perception that they have control over the stressors used in the research. In studies that were performed before implementation of Federal guidelines at one institution in the Midwest, investigators were able to successfully replicate Glass and Singer's (1972) aftereffects of exposure to uncontrollable noise. However, in stress studies that were performed subsequent to these consent guidelines, this effect could not be obtained. A study by Gardner (1978) demonstrated that Federal human subjects guidelines could influence the data obtained in environmental stressor research. Gardner conducted an experiment on two groups of subjects treated identically except that one group gave informed consent and the other did not. Results supported the view that informed consent can prevent the emergence of negative aftereffects of noise and other stressors. Therefore, excessive attention to the consent provisions of human use guidelines can create a psychological atmosphere so free that it interferes with the conduct of stress research.

The amount of control that is imparted by a consent form obviously depends on how that consent form is worded. Subjects can be informed generally about their ability to withdraw from a study when they initially volunteer, with little additional attention directed to the voluntary nature of the procedure when the study actually begins. Given the importance of the construct of personal control in determining responses to stress, the manner in which informed consent is obtained and the amount of information that subjects receive about the study deserve the attention of the researcher as a possible source of experimental bias.

Human consent procedures vary in the amount of information they present to subjects, the precise information presented being determined by the risk to subjects (whether physiological or psychological), and what human subjects review committees define as adequately informed consent (Smith, 1976). If insufficient information is given about what is going to happen during the experimental session, a feeling of uncertainty may be created for the subject. If too much information is provided in a study involving use of aversive stimuli, this may mitigate some of the effect of the manipulations (see above). Furthermore, Silvia, Street, and Baum (1986) demonstrated that when subjects were uncertain about the aversiveness of an impending stressful film portraying surgical procedures, they showed anticipatory increases in cardiovascular responses while waiting for the task to begin that were as great or greater than produced by the task itself.

What would be the possible effects of added uncertainty caused by lack of information? Studies manipulating subjects' level of uncertainty about a stressor indicate that the more uncertainty, the more reactivity to the stressor and the more reactivity during the prior anticipatory period (Elliott, 1966; Silvia *et al.*, 1986). As noted above (Silvia *et al.*, 1986), when too much detailed information is provided, this may reduce anticipatory physiological reactions during the period subjects are waiting, and while viewing the stressful stimulus that follows. Thus, a careful balance of information must be provided to subjects in stress studies to avoid these potential pitfalls.

Manipulation Checks

Researchers who employ experimental operations that are *psychological* in nature often have subjects answer several written or interview questions to determine how experimental manipulations were perceived by subjects. For example, in a study designed to determine the effects of stressful tasks of several difficulty levels on psychophysiological reactions, questions may be asked such as "How difficult did you perceive the task(s) to be?" or "How much effort did you exert on the tasks?" These "checks on the manipulations" function to determine if the experimental operations were perceived as the experimenter intended, and thus whether the manipulations were successful in inducing the intended psychological states in subjects. Additional benefits of such questions are that they allow the experimenter to correlate the subjects' rated psychological state with physiological and behavioral outcomes.

In the event that an experimental manipulation did not work, the researcher can, using the manipulation check items and the dependent variables, perform an *internal* analysis of the data (see Carlsmith, Ellsworth, & Aronson, 1976). For example, suppose the researcher desires to study the effect of making subjects anxious on anticipatory neuroendocrine responses to a stressful event, and assigns subjects randomly to two experimental treatments designed to create high and low anxiety. However, suppose the manipulations did not induce anxiety in all the anxiety-treatment subjects as intended, but the researcher had the foresight to provide a separate measure to determine if some subjects were made anxious by the manipulation. In such a circumstance, the researcher can reanalyze the data using subjects' responses on the manipulation check as a substitute for the independent variable in the study (Carlsmith *et al.*, 1976). This is an internal analysis. It should be noted that although this procedure can be used as a means for exploratory testing of a hypothesis, an internal analysis is not an adequate substitute for an effective experimental manipulation in which subjects are randomly assigned to treatments.

If manipulation checks are given at the conclusion of the study, it is quite possible that subjects are responding based on their behavior during the entire study, rather than solely according to their perceptions of the manipulation. To get around this problem, manipulation checks are often taken after the manipulation, but prior to the measurement of the dependent variable. This practice of utilizing manipulation checks has been criticized (Kidd, 1976) on the grounds that taking a manipulation check before measuring the impact of a treatment on a dependent variable introduces unwanted error variance into the procedure. Kidd (1976) argued that the act of filling out a manipulation check questionnaire is an experience that can mediate or even cause observable differences in the dependent measure. Suggested solutions include (1) abandoning the use of checks entirely, (2) counterbalancing the taking of manipulation checks so that in any one study, half the subjects receive the checks before the dependent measure, and the other half afterwards. (3) Another solution is to create manipulation check groups analogous to control groups in an ordinary experiment (Kidd, 1976). In retrospect, each researcher must weigh the possible benefits of use of manipulation checks against an assessment of the bias or experimental error they may introduce.

Social–Psychological Source of Bias: Experimenter Bias and Demand Characteristics

In addition to the level of information provided to the subject, the social situation of being in a study has the potential of introducing factors that further complicate how subjects may react to experimental manipulations. Two kinds of social–psychological bias can intrude into the research setting. These sources of bias are related but different, and arise from (1) the "demand characteristics" of the experimental situation itself (Orne, 1962), and (2) the unintentional influence of the experimenter (Rosenthal, 1966).

Demand Characteristics

As described by Aronson and Carlsmith (1968), the demand characteristics problem is closely related to the placebo problem in medical research. Subjects are aware that they are in an experimental situation and that certain behaviors are expected of them. Thus, subjects may be reacting to their interpretations of the behaviors the experimental setting is supposed to elicit, rather than to the experimental operations themselves. This is either done

by the subject to make a good impression or out of a desire to "help" the experimenter by verifying the experimental hypothesis (Aronson & Carlsmith, 1968; Riecken, 1962; Rosenberg, 1965). It is also conceivable that other subjects may act to disconfirm what is expected, by behaving contrary to what is expected. There is, apparently, little evidence for this type of behavior, but considerable evidence that subjects attempt to put themselves in the best possible light (Aronson & Carlsmith, 1968). Thus, in studies where conscious attempts by subjects to "verify" a hypothesis may bias results, the experimenter must take special precautions to conceal in some way the true purpose of the study lest the subject act to confirm the hypothesis (Aronson & Carlsmith, 1968).

An interesting study by Orne (1962) set out to find a set of experimental operations that would lead experimental subjects to refuse to cooperate, and found that this was difficult to accomplish. A set of boring and meaningless psychological tasks was designed, and it was found that subjects who agreed to participate in an experiment would perform these tasks for hours with little overt signs of hostility. Similar evidence for the docility of subjects in experimental settings has been found by others (Milgram, 1963).

Subjects' general expectancies about the study situation and setting can also influence their reactions to experimental manipulations in studies of stress (Blom & Craighead, 1974; Aronson & Carlsmith, 1968). For example, subjects led to believe that they were undergoing a test of fear exhibited greater signs of anxiety than those led to believe that they were in a study testing their ability to simulate relaxation therapy.

Can subjects' expectations about an experimental situation directly affect psychophysiological responses? There is some evidence that this is, in fact, possible. In a study of the physiological effects of placebos, Sternbach (1964) gave three sets of instructions in a "drug" experiment, during which subjects swallowed a pill. It was stated that one kind of pill would relax the stomach, that a second placebo pill would have no effect, and that a third pill was a stimulant in the stomach. In actuality, in all three pills were encapsulated magnets that were used to monitor gastric activity. Results indicated that most of the subjects showed significant differences in stomach contractions in the directions predicted by the instructions presented. In another study, in a condition where random biofeedback for altering heart rate was given, the experimenter's instructions to increase or decrease heart rate led to significantly better heart rate control (London & Schwartz, 1980).

Aronson and Carlsmith suggest that perhaps the best solution is to follow the medical placebo model by devising manipulations that appear essentially identical to subjects in all conditions, just as placebos are visually identical to active drugs. By such means, attempts by the subject to surmise the experimenter's hypothesis cannot have a systematic effect on the results of the study and will simply have the effect of increasing error variance. Another obvious solution is to remove the experiment from the context of the laboratory and to conduct a naturalistic or field experiment. While this latter solution will make some difference, the well-known "Hawthorne effect" (Roethlisberger & Dickson, 1939) suggests that even in a naturalistic setting, the cooperativeness of subjects can be a serious impediment to research. The Hawthorne studies investigated the effects of lighting conditions on workers' performance in a factory and showed that just the fact that the workers were being studied affected their performance, perhaps because they felt that at last the management cared about them.

Experimenter Bias

Experimenters differ from one another on such characteristics as their level of experience, personality, and gender, all of which can interact with certain experimental manipulations. One study (McGuigan, 1963) examined whether different experimenters would obtain differing results in a learning experiment conducted with similar groups of subjects. Diverse results were obtained among the various experimenters.

Numerous examples have been presented from the fields of psychology and other sciences which show how researchers can, in very subtle and inadvertent ways, bias data to support their hypotheses (Rosenthal, 1966; Wilson, 1952). Rosenthal and colleagues (Rosenthal, 1966) conducted a series of studies involving the introduction of contradictory

hypotheses to samples of experimenters. The studies revealed that the experimenters obtained from human subjects data that were biased in the direction of the "false" hypothesis. Even more dramatic results were obtained in experiments involving learning in rats (Rosenthal & Fode, 1963).

The Rosenthal paradigm used to illustrate the operation of experimenter bias has been criticized as being one that *invites bias* and exaggerates the operation of experimenter effects in research. That is because in these studies, each experimenter ran only one experimental condition—thus making it different from the usual laboratory study (Aronson & Carlsmith, 1968). Nevertheless, whether such effects are prevalent or not, it is important to implement techniques for eliminating this kind of inadvertent bias.

The usual technique that is suggested is some form of blinding of the experimenter. A more extreme measure is to keep the research assistant blind to experimental hypotheses, and/or to eliminate all personal contact between researcher and subject by using taped instructions (Rosenthal, Persinger, Vikan Kline, & Mulry, 1963). Some have argued that an intelligent experimenter would still form hypotheses about the study, and that avoiding experimenter contact can lessen the impact of certain experimental manipulations (Aronson & Carlsmith, 1968). A less extreme solution is to allow the experimenter to know the true hypothesis but to keep him/her ignorant of the specific experimental condition that the subject is in, and to tape some but not all of the delivered instructions or to use closed-circuit television to preserve impact.

In sum, this portion of the chapter has discussed social and procedural characteristics of the experimental situation, other than experimental manipulations themselves, that can influence the behavior of subjects. In the remainder of this chapter, we direct our attention to ways that experimental manipulations can be presented by the stress researcher that can alter or intensify subjects' reactions to the setting.

Effects of Race and Sex of Experimenter

Another social–psychological source of potential bias are the effects of the interaction between the race and sex of the experimenter and those of the subject. Although such effects have received relatively little attention, there are data to suggest that experimenter sex and race may be important.

Experimenter Race

Murphy, Alpert, and Moes (1985) found that heart rate responses during a video game were higher when subjects were paired with an experimenter of the same race. Blood pressure responses showed the same general pattern, but were not as consistently different. In an earlier study, Fisher and Kotses (1973) found that white subjects showed a slower decrease in the magnitude of galvanic skin responses (GSR) over the experimental session when paired with a black experimenter. There were no experimenter race differences in basal GSR levels in this study.

Experimenter Sex

With regard to experimenter sex effects, at least one study has shown that this factor can also have an influence in psychophysiological research. Fisher and Kotses (1974) examined experimenter and subject sex effects on the skin conductance response. They found that male subjects paired with a female experimenter showed higher basal skin conductance levels and a more rapid decrease in basal skin conductance levels over trials in the session. With regard to the magnitude of GSR to noise bursts, all subjects in the female experimenter condition failed to habituate.

Other effects of experimenter gender are possible, although as yet unproven. For example, it is conceivable that subjects participating in a competitive task may put forth either more or less effort to perform well when paired with a different-sex experimenter than with a same-sex experimenter. There is also the question as to the effects on psychophysiological responses of competing against a same- or different-sex experimenter.

In sum, since relatively few studies have directly looked at the effects of experimenter race and sex on various psychophysiological measures, it seems premature to describe specific effects of particular experimenter–subject combinations.

However, it is appropriate to conclude that the social-psychological effects of experimenter sex and race can add to error variance or have a systematic and perhaps unwanted effect.

Experimental Manipulations That Determine Intensity of Responding in Psychophysiological Studies

Considerable attention in recent years has been addressed to the study of psychophysiological reactivity (responsiveness) to psychological stress (see Krantz & Manuck, 1984). Numerous psychological stressors and tasks are employed in this research, and effort has been directed to identifying the dimensions of stressors that alter the intensity and patterning of cardiovascular and neuroendocrine responding. The intensity of a subject's responses to an experimental task can be increased or decreased by varying the task instructions or the task characteristics according to a number of criteria. For example, increasing the positive or negative incentives for task performance, increasing the level of challenge in task instructions, and increasing the subjects' level of engagement/involvement in the experimental situation can heighten physiological responses. Often these motivational dimensions overlap one another and covary in manipulations of experimental situations.

Level of Difficulty of the Experimental Task

Studies that have independently manipulated task difficulty have found that this variable does have an effect on subjects' blood pressure and heart rate responses. It appears that the maximal physiological responses are produced by tasks that are seen as sufficiently difficult to put effort into, but not so difficult that subjects will give up on them.

One explanation for this effect (Obrist *et al.*, 1978) is that tasks that elicit "active effortful coping" are thought to elicit a β-adrenergic pattern of cardiovascular responding characterized by increased heart rate and systolic blood pressure. For example, Obrist *et al.* (1978) found differences in cardiovascular reactions between easy and moderately difficult conditions where subjects responded to avoid shock. Here, it was hypothesized and found that a difficult criterion would be associated with greater effort and therefore with larger and more sustained increases in heart rate and systolic blood pressure compared to either a very easy or impossible reaction time criterion. However, Light and Obrist (1983) found somewhat different results using a reaction time task in which earning money was contingent upon performance (see below).

Responding to control a difficult stressor may have different cardiovascular consequences than responding to control an easy stressor. Manuck and colleagues (Manuck, Corse, & Winkelmen, 1979) studied the effects of coping on blood pressure reactions to tasks that were either difficult or easy. They found that when working on a difficult task, responding to control an aversive stimulus led to greater cardiovascular reactions. However, when working on an easy task, there were no heightened cardiovascular reactions associated with coping.

Whether the subject's cardiovascular reactions vary in direct proportion to the value or amount of incentive applied, has not been examined directly (see Manuck *et al.*, 1979). It is clear, however, that most studies only present subjects with a single level of task difficulty. Therefore, some populations of subjects may find specific tasks more difficult than others and may react physiologically more or less strongly to them. Ideally, tasks being considered for use in studies of cardiovascular reactivity should be carefully piloted so that they are at a moderate level of difficulty for the subject population being studied.

Performance Incentives

The inclusion of performance incentives can also affect the magnitude of cardiovascular responses to a stressor. Both positive and negative task incentives for doing well are often utilized in psychophysiological studies. A study of the effects of paying subjects two cents for each success on a task versus giving subjects feedback only, found that the monetary incentive was necessary for the task to cause an increase in heart rate (Fowles, Fisher, & Tranel, 1982). A comparison of two studies from Obrist's laboratory (Light & Obrist, 1983; Obrist *et al.*, 1978) indicates that using positive incentives (such as working to win money), and negative incentives (e.g., working to avoid shock) can produce different patterns of cardiovascular reactivity on certain tasks. Positive incentives led to differences between impossible and other tasks in diastolic blood pressure and no differences in heart rate, but negative incentives led to heart rate, but not diastolic differences between the tasks.

Another type of incentive that can influence the magnitude of psychophysiological responses to a task is the subject's perception of a contingency between performance on the task and the presentation of aversive stimuli. Obrist *et al.* (1978) proposed and demonstrated that when subjects perceive the ability to avoid shock by responding appropriately, this led to more active effortful coping and greater heart rate and systolic blood pressure responses to a task. Another study (Contrada *et al.*, 1982) also found that subjects who were not told that they could avoid shock and loud noise did not react as much physiologically to a reaction time task as subjects who believed that doing well on the task prevented the aversive stimuli.

It is likely, however, that the effects of providing a contingency depend on whether subjects perceive the task as difficult or easy. As noted in a study described in the section on task difficulty, Manuck *et al.* (1979) found that when subjects felt there was a contingency between their performances and receiving aversive stimuli, a greater systolic blood pressure response was produced when the task was moderately difficult. When the task was easy, contingent and noncontingent conditions both produced a similar, lesser systolic blood pressure response.

In sum, studies using negative incentives have demonstrated that if receipt of aversive stimuli is contingent on task performance, a greater level of reactivity will occur if subjects are actively engaged in coping to escape or avoid the stressor. However, this occurs only if the task is at least moderately difficult, but not so difficult that subjects will give up on it.

Challenge, Harassment, and Competition

The level of challenge perceived to be involved in an experimental task refers to how demanding the subject perceives that task to be. Challenge is a psychological dimension that overlaps with many other dimensions, and is related to such factors as the type of incentive used (e.g., positive or negative), the difficulty of the task, whether competition is used as a motivator, or whether the subject is being evaluated in the experimental situation. A common technique employed by experimenters to heighten level of challenge is to deliver a demanding instruction set for the tasks to be performed.

The use of instructions to manipulate challenge is illustrated by a study (Dembroski, MacDougall, Herd, & Shields, 1979) that varied the level of challenge given to subjects prior to a cold pressor test. "High-challenge" instructions, delivered in a crisp tone of voice, informed subjects of the difficulty of the cold pressor task and the need for willpower, whereas "low-challenge" instructions described the task as routine. Results indicated only minimal differences between Type A and B subjects in the low-challenge situation, and larger and statistically reliable differences in the high-challenge situation.

Harassment by the experimenter is a usual component of commonly used mental stress tasks, such as when subjects are told to count backwards as quickly as possible, being reminded in a crisp voice to go faster and be more accurate (e.g., Brod, Fencl, Heil, & Jirka, 1959). Similar harassing statements have been used to heighten the reactivity to other types of cognitive and psychomotor tasks (e.g., Glass, Lake, Contrada, Kehoe, & Erlanger, 1983). It is not clear whether harassment heightens physiological reactivity because it increases the level of challenge or because it heightens emotions such as anger.

Looking closely at the Dembroski et al. (1979) manipulation, this study appeared to entail not only a heightened challenge but also concomitant increases in the subjects' level of task involvement, overall incentive to perform well, perceptions of task difficulty, and so on. Therefore, the precise psychological factors that led to Type A–B differences in reactivity or that made the task so

effective are not clear. Explicit and even subtle variations in these and other aspects of experimental instructions can make certain tasks effective elicitors of heightened physiological responses or can act to reveal or obscure individual differences in cardiovascular reactivity (see Houston, 1983; Krantz, Manuck, & Wing, 1986).

Competition

A social–psychological manipulation that can elicit physiological reactivity in subjects is the use of competition. Competition can be between the subject and a machine (MacDougall et al., 1983), or between the subject and a confederate or another subject (Glass, Krakoff, Contrada, Hilton, Kehoe, Mannucci, Collins, Snow, & Elting, 1980; Van Egeren, 1979). To keep the level of competition standardized and controlled, competition has generally been created between subjects and either machines or confederates. Competition can also be used together with other manipulations, such as incentives and harassment, to elicit large-magnitude changes in physiological responding.

Cardiovascular responses in competitive situations are of interest because competitiveness is a putative etiological factor in cardiovascular disorders. Individuals obviously bring to the laboratory different propensities for competition. Some subjects will treat any situation as a competitive one, whereas others will be reluctant to compete (e.g., Dembroski et al., 1979). This is illustrated by a study (Glass et al., 1980) that investigated the effects of competition with and without harassment on reactivity in Type A and B subjects. The investigators found that Type A's working against a harassing competitor showed greater heart rate and systolic blood pressure responses compared to Type B's and Type A's not being harassed. Thus, this study manipulation revealed that for Type A's, hostile competition was necessary to produce heightened cardiovascular and neuroendocrine responses.

A study by Van Egeren (1979) examined cardiovascular changes during a game that involved both cooperation and competition (mixed-motive game). Male and female subjects played against a male confederate who employed either a cooperative or competitive strategy. Results indicated that females had higher heart rate responses than males during play against a competitive strategy, and males had higher responses during play against a cooperative strategy. Van Egeren suggested that in this study, males seemed to find play against a cooperative strategy, during which they won, more "stimulating" than play against a competitive program, during which they lost. Males and females may have approached the competitive game differently, with males focused more on winning and females focused more on their chances of losing. However, since competitive situations have been shown to elicit large cardiovascular reactions in males (Glass *et al.*, 1980), the failure to find this in Van Egeren's (1979) study may be an anomaly.

Summary

This chapter has reviewed potential sources of bias in stress research that are associated with the social context in which studies are conducted. Considered were such standard experimental procedures as obtaining informed consent, demand characteristics and experimenter bias, and the possible effects of manipulation checks. We have noted that the behavioral and psychophysiological effects of stressors depend on psychological factors such as the amount and nature of the information provided and the subject's understanding of these events. Routine components of experimental tasks may therefore have a significant impact in studies of stress.

This chapter has also reviewed psychological and social dimensions of commonly used stress manipulations in psychophysiological studies that determine the intensity of subjects' physiological responses. Included here are characteristics such as the difficulty of the tasks, the level of challenge, harassment, and competition presented to the subject, and the specific instructions and incentives to motivate performance. Often these motivational dimensions overlap with one another and covary in experimental manipulations. Once again, even subtle variations in these dimensions of tasks and instructions can act to bring out or conceal individual differences in physiological reactivity to stress.

ACKNOWLEDGMENTS. Preparation of this chapter was assisted by NIH Grant HL-31514 and USUHS Grant R07233.

References

Aronson, E., & Carlsmith, J. M. (1968). Experimentation in social psychology. In G. Lindzey & E. Aronson (Eds.), *Handbook of social psychology* (2nd ed., pp. 1–80). Reading, MA: Addison–Wesley.

Blom, B. E., & Craighead, W. E. (1974). The effects of situational and instructional demand on indices of speech anxiety. *Journal of Abnormal Psychology, 83*(6), 667–674.

Brod, J., Fencl, V., Heil, Z., & Jirka, J. (1959). Circulatory changes underlying blood pressure elevation during acute emotional stress in normotensive and hypertensive subjects. *Clinical Science, 18,* 269–279.

Carlsmith, J. M., Ellsworth, P. L., & Aronson, E. (1976). *Methods of research in social psychology.* Reading, MA: Addison–Wesley.

Cohen, F., Horowitz, M., Lazarus, R., Moos, R., Robins, L., Rose, R., & Rutter, M. (1982). Panel report on psychosocial assets and modifiers of stress. In G. Elliott & C. Eisdorfer (Eds.), *Stress and human health* (pp. 147–288). Berlin: Springer.

Contrada, R. J., Glass, D. C., Krakoff, L. R., Krantz, D. S., Kehoe, K., Isecke, W., Collins, L., & Elting, E. (1982). Effects of control over aversive stimulation and type-A behavior on cardiovascular and plasma catecholamine response. *Psychophysiology, 19,* 408–419.

Dembroski, T. M., MacDougall, J. M., Herd, J. A., & Shields, J. C. (1979). Effect of level of challenge on pressor and heart rate responses in type A and B subjects. *Journal of Applied Social Psychology, 9,* 209–228.

Elliott, G. R., & Eisdorfer, C. (Eds.). (1982). *Stress and human health.* Berlin: Springer.

Elliott, R. (1966). Reaction time and heart rate as a function of magnitude of incentive and probability of success: A replication and extension. *Journal of Experimental Research in Personality, 1,* 174–178.

Fisher, L. E., & Kotses, H. (1973). Race differences and experimenter race effect in galvanic skin response. *Psychophysiology, 10,* 578–582.

Fisher, L. E., & Kotses, H. (1974). Experimenter and subject sex effects in the skin conductance response. *Psychophysiology, 11,* 191–196.

Fowles, D. C., Fisher, A. E., & Tranel, D. T. (1982). The heart beats to reward: The effect of monetary incentive on heart rate. *Psychophysiology, 19,* 506–513.

Gardner, G. T. (1978). Effects of federal human-subjects regulations on data obtained in environmental stressor research. *Journal of Personality and Social Psychology, 36,* 628–634.

Glass, D. C., & Singer, J. E. (1972). *Urban stress: Experiments on noise and social stressors.* New York: Academic Press.

Glass, D. C., Krakoff, L. R., Contrada, R., Hilton, W. F., Kehoe, K., Mannucci, E. G., Collins, C., Snow, B., & Elting, E. (1980). Effect of harassment and competition upon cardiovascular and plasma catecholamine responses in Type A and Type B individuals. *Psychophysiology, 17*(5), 453–463.

Glass, D. C., Lake, C. R., Contrada, R. J., Kehoe, K., & Erlanger, C. R. (1983). Stability of individual differences in physiological responses to stress. *Health Psychology, 2,* 317–341.

Houston, B. K. (1983). Psychophysiological responding and the type-A behavior pattern. *Journal of Research in Personality, 17,* 22–39.

Kidd, R. F. (1976). Manipulation checks: Advantage or disadvantage. *Representative Research in Social Psychology, 7,* 160–165.

Krantz, D. S., & Manuck, S. B. (1984). Reactivity and cardiovascular disease. *Psychological Bulletin, 96,* 435–464.

Krantz, D. S., Manuck, S. B., & Wing, R. (1986). Psychological stressors and task variables as elicitors of reactivity. In K. A. Matthews, S. M. Weiss, T. Detre, T. M. Dembroski, B. Falkner, S. B. Manuck, & R. B. Williams (Eds.), *Handbook of stress, reactivity, and cardiovascular disease.* New York: Wiley.

Lazarus, R. S. (1966). *Psychological stress and the coping process.* New York: McGraw–Hill.

Light, K. C., & Obrist, P. A. (1983). Task difficulty, heart rate, and cardiovascular responses to an appetitive reaction time task. *Psychophysiology, 20,* 301–312.

London, M. D., & Schwartz, G. E. (1980). The interaction of instruction components with cybernetic feedback effects in the voluntary control of human heart rate. *Psychophysiology, 17,* 437–443.

MacDougall, J. M., Dembroski, T. M., Slaats, S., Herd, J. A., & Eliot, R. S. (1983). Selective cardiovascular effects of stress and cigarette-smoking. *Journal of Human Stress, 9*(3), 13–21.

Manuck, S. B., Corse, C. D., & Winkelmen, P. A. (1979). Behavioral correlates of individual differences in blood pressure reactivity. *Journal of Psychosomatic Research, 23,* 281–288.

Mason, J. (1971). Re-evaluation of the concept of nonspecificity in stress theory. *Journal of Psychiatric Research, 8,* 323–333.

McGuigan, F. J. (1963). The experimenter: A neglected stimulus object. *Psychological Bulletin, 60,* 421–428.

Milgram, S. (1963). Behavioral study of obedience. *Journal of Abnormal and Social Psychology, 67,* 371–378.

Murphy, J. K., Alpert, B. S., & Moes, D. M. (1985). Race and reactivity: A neglected relationship. *Psychosomatic Medicine, 47*(1), 91.

Obrist, P. A., Gaebelein, C. J., Teller, E. S., Langer, A. W., Grignolo, A., Light, K. C., & McCubbin, J. A. (1978). The relationship among heart rate, carotid dP/dt and blood pressure in humans as a function of the type of stress. *Psychophysiology, 15,* 102–115.

Orne, M. (1962). On the social psychology of the psychological experiment. *American Psychologist, 17,* 776–783.

Riecken, H. W. (1962). A program for research on experiments in social psychology. In N. Washburne (Ed.), *Decision, values, and groups* (Vol. 2, pp. 25–41). Elmsford, NY: Pergamon Press.

Roethlisberger, F. J., & Dickson, W. J. (1939). *Management and the worker.* Cambridge, MA: Harvard University Press.

Rosenberg, M. J. (1965). When dissonance fails: On eliminating evaluation apprehension from attitude measurement. *Journal of Personality and Social Psychology, 1,* 28–42.

Rosenthal, R. (1966). *Experimenter effects in behavioral research.* New York: Appleton–Century–Crofts.

Rosenthal, R., & Fode, K. L. (1963). The effect of experimenter bias on the performance of the albino rat. *Behavioral Science, 8,* 183–189.

Rosenthal, R., Persinger, G. W., Vikan Kline, L., & Mulry, R. C. (1963). The role of the research assistant in the mediation of experimenter bias. *Journal of Personality, 31,* 313–335.

Seligman, M. E. (1972). Learned helplessness. *Annual Review of Medicine, 23,* 407.

Silvia, C., Street, S., & Baum, A. (1986). *Anticipation and certainty: Mediators of responding to a stressful event.* Unpublished manuscript, Uniformed Services University of the Health Sciences.

Smith, M. B. (1976). Some perspectives on ethical-political issues in social science research. *Personality and Social Psychology Bulletin, 2*(4), 445–453.

Sternbach, R. A. (1964). The effects of instructional sets on autonomic responses. *Psychophysiology, 1,* 67–72.

Van Egeren, L. F. (1979). Cardiovascular changes during social competition in a mixed motive game. *Journal of Personality and Social Psychology, 37,* 858–864.

Williams, R. B. (1985). Neuroendocrine response patterns and stress: Biobehavioral mechanisms of disease. In R. B. Williams (Ed.), *Perspectives on behavioral medicine: Vol. 2. Neuroendocrine control and behavior* (pp. 71–101). New York: Academic Press.

Wilson, E. B. (1952). *An introduction to scientific research.* New York: McGraw–Hill.

CHAPTER 25

Physical Stressors and Pharmacologic Manipulations
Neurohumoral and Hemodynamic Responses in Hypertension

Vincent DeQuattro and Debora De-Ping Lee

Muscular Effort and Neural Regulation of Hemodynamic Alterations

An Overview

Muscular work increases oxygen demand; as a result, changes in heart rate, stroke volume, cardiac output, and peripheral vascular resistance, enhance blood flow to the active muscle groups. Cardiac output and flow to the exercising muscles increase linearly, while resistance increases in vascular beds of resting muscles. Centers in the cerebral cortex are linked to cardiovascular regulation via the brain stem, and accommodate both isometric and isotonic exercise (Stone, Dormer, Foreman, Thies, & Blair, 1985). Further, afferent fibers from the exercising muscles are integrated to mediate central control of the circulation. The various components involved in cardiovascular control during exercise, including the "central command" concept, are indicated in Figure 1.

Exercise training may establish patterns of central neural control of cardiovascular regulation (Stone *et al.*, 1985) (Figures 1 and 2). Exercise training not only lowers heart rate response to submaximal work load, but daily exercise alters basal, central, and peripheral autonomic activity as well. There is evidence of central command alteration from studies of cardiovascular reflexes in response to volume load (Stone, 1977), a reduced incidence of sudden cardiac death in dogs (Billman, Schwartz, & Stone, 1984), and changes of human pressor responses to lower body negative pressure (Raven, Rohm-Young, & Blomqvist, 1984).

Rhythmic exercise of the forearm or leg muscles increases arterial pressure in proportion to the magnitude of exertion, as demonstrated by Alam and Smirk (1937). After circulation to the exercising limb is obstructed by a pneumatic cuff, the pressure rises prior to any sensation of pain (Shepherd, Blomqvist, Lind, Mitchell, & Saltin, 1981; Alam & Smirk, 1937). The blood pressure remains elevated when the exercise is stopped, and yet returns quickly to baseline values with deflation of

Vincent DeQuattro and Debora De-Ping Lee • Department of Medicine, University of Southern California School of Medicine, Los Angeles, California 90007.

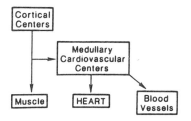

Figure 1. Diagrammatic representation of the concept of central command as the primary regulator of cardiovascular function during exercise. From Stone *et al.* (1985).

the cuff. Ergoreceptors, activated during muscle contraction, and pain receptors or nociceptors contribute to the blood pressure elevation. These afferents conduct below 15 m/s, and are thought to be nonproprioceptive high-threshold group III and IV, myelinated and unmyelinated afferents (Shepherd *et al.*, 1981) (Figure 3). The fibers enter the spinal cord via the dorsal routes and ascend via the spinothalamic tract into the brain stem, and most likely intersect into the lateral reticular nucleus. Thus, in humans, increased sympathetic and reduced vagal outflow regulate the cardiovascular response to isometric exercise, as integrated by cortical centers. These non-motor cortex stimuli may be related to arousal or emotion. We found enhanced pressor responses to isometric exercise

in patients with high anxiety and anger "in" (Sullivan, Procci, *et al.*, 1981a). Different muscle fibers appear to have different numbers and types of ergoreceptors.

During isometric exercise, there is an increase in cardiac output, left ventricular contractility, heart rate, and both systolic and diastolic blood pressure. Left ventricular end diastolic pressure is increased at greater than moderate work loads. An increase in heart rate is responsible chiefly for the increase in cardiac output. There is a restriction of blood flow to vascular beds outside the active muscle due to increased noradrenergic tone. The quantity of active muscle mass rather than the mode of contraction is the primary determinant of the hemodynamic response. Measurements during dynamic exercise activating 25, 50, and 75% of muscle mass during two-leg bicycle exercise showed a gradual transition of hemodynamic responses from a static to a dynamic pattern.

Both static and dynamic exercise produce an increase in heart rate and cardiac output. Systemic vascular resistance remains at the resting level when the active muscle mass is small, and in some circumstances mean arterial pressure increases in direct proportion to the increase in cardiac output. The increase in cardiac output above resting level is tightly coupled to the increase in systemic oxy-

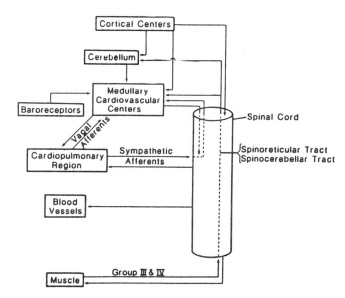

Figure 2. Schematic representation of current knowledge concerning the regulation of the cardiovascular system during exercise. Both central command and feedback loops are included. Heart, baroreceptors, and muscle compose the feedback loops in the peripheral system and the cerebellum for a central feedback loop. From Stone *et al.* (1985).

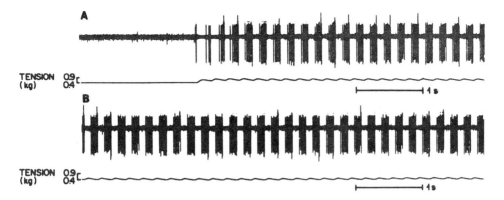

Figure 3. Stimulation of a group III afferent (conduction velocity 20.4 m/s) by rhythmic contraction of the muscle with 5-Hz stimulation of the ventral roots. (A) It should be noted that this afferent responded rapidly to the first contraction and to a small increase in muscle tension. (B) Section of record 25 s after the end of A. The group III afferent fiber was still responding vigorously. From Kaufman *et al.* (1984).

gen demand during isotonic exercise, irrespective of active muscle mass and intensity of the effort (Blomqvist, Lewis, Taylor, & Graham, 1981). In contrast, the increase in cardiac output during isometric exercise is disproportionately large relative to the increase in oxygen uptake. This is observed even at low intensities when the mechanical obstruction to flow is much less severe than during heavy static efforts (Asmussen & Hansen, 1981). There is a linear increase in left ventricular end diastolic pressure with increase in cardiac output during dynamic exercise involving large muscle groups, particularly noticeable in the upright position. Ejection fraction also increases and systolic volume decreases. Thus, there are both Starling effects and an enhanced contractile state. Changes in left ventricular end diastolic and end systolic dimension during static exercise are smaller. Both static and dynamic exercise induce vasoconstriction, but the increase in preload is larger during dynamic exercise due to the added effects of the muscle pump and a greater respiratory effort. The balance between afterload and contractile state is likely to be different in static and dynamic exercise. Heart rates during heavy exercise are usually much higher during dynamic exercise. The magnitude of the raised plasma catecholamines is evidence that sympathetic drive during dynamic exercise is much greater than during static exercise (Lewis *et al.,* 1980).

Isotonic (Dynamic) Exercise

Isotonic exercise is more natural for the human in terms of locomotion, requiring contraction and relaxation of opposing pairs of muscles. This form of exercise is usually upright and involved with antigravity reflexes as well. In addition to providing locomotion, the alternative relaxing and contraction of muscles, especially in the calf region, assists in venous return and promotes cardiac output. Pulse and blood pressure increase in direct relation to the oxygen requirement of the exercising muscles. Neurohumoral control regulates blood flow first by increasing cardiac output, second by dilating peripheral vasculature to exercising muscles, and further by increasing blood flow to the skin to reduce body heat elaborated during muscular work.

Treadmill exercise can determine physical conditioning and coronary blood flow indirectly via electrocardiographic and radionuclide techniques indicating effectiveness of coronary or collateral blood flow. Standard techniques include 3 min at each level to allow the individual to reach equilibrium at each work load. This technique may offer some advantages over the bicycle exercise test, in that some individuals are unfamiliar with or uncomfortable on a bicycle and cannot perform maximum exercise. Further, treadmill exercise does include a greater component of gravity as a stimulus in evoking hemodynamic and neurochemical responsiveness.

Bicycle versus Treadmill

Treadmill exercise requires the subject to run at a prescribed speed and grade. This is the most commonly used method of exercise testing in clinical medicine. The exercise depends on the number of muscle groups involved, and walking employs the largest number of muscle groups. Treadmill exercise requires less cooperation and motivation. The patient does not have to maintain a preset pedaling rate. This is difficult for people unfamiliar with the bicycle. For all these reasons, maximal heart rate achieved with treadmill exercise is significantly greater than that with bicycle ergometry. The chief disadvantage of treadmill exercise is the movement of the patient which makes electrocardiographic and physiologic parameter recording difficult during peak exercise. It also interferes with the use of stress echocardiography and radionuclides for angiography. This form of exercise is difficult for patients with peripheral vascular disease, arthritis, and other lower extremity problems. The equipment is noisy and requires additional room.

Protocols

The Bruce treadmill protocol is the most commonly used in clinical medicine (Bruce, 1971), although other protocols such as the Naughton are useful for patients with poor exercise tolerance such as those with congestive heart failure (Naughton & Haider, 1973). In normal subjects undergoing muscular exercise while pedaling a bicycle ergometer, oxygen consumption increases from an average of 152 to 477 ml/min per m^2 body surface area, heart rate from an average of 69 to 104 beats, and mean arterial pressure from 81 to 94 mm Hg. Others such as the Balke protocol may also be used in well-trained individuals, especially young people; this will be discussed later. In the Naughton protocol, each stage corresponds to one MET; a MET is a multiple of a person's basal metabolic oxygen consumption (Naughton & Haider, 1973).

Ergometry

On the other hand, in assessing hemodynamic changes to the stress of isotonic exercise, the seated patient provides the opportunity for more accurate blood pressure, hemodynamic, echocardiographic, electrocardiographic, and radionuclide assessments. Thus, position can be better secured during bicycle exercise and improve standardization of repetitive measures in the same individual. Further, it is easier to collect blood and administer pharmacologic and radionuclide agents to the exercising patient.

With this stress the patient pedals but otherwise can be relatively motionless. Supine exercise can also be performed with this equipment (Naughton & Haider, 1973). Further, radionuclide and echocardiographic studies may also be made in patients undergoing bicycle ergometry. In patients with coronary artery disease, left ventricular dysfunction may be characterized by globally reduced or regionally reduced contraction of ventricular chambers. Effects of drugs may also be quantitated. Of the two types of protocols, one requires constant-level exercise; the other requires the exercise to be performed in stages. While isometric exercise is performed at one level of stress, treadmill and bicycle ergometry involve graded protocols. In graded protocols, it is important to design the pattern of exercise so that the maximum heart rate can be achieved by the patient before fatigue and exhaustion. To reach physiological equilibrium, each stage should be approximately 3–5 min in duration.

For bicycle ergometry, the exercise is performed in the supine or upright position starting with work loads of approximately 25 W; each stage lasts for approximately 5 min, with increments of 25 w/stage.

Routine Monitoring

It is important to spend sufficient time with the patient to explain the procedure to be conducted. The patient should not have "stage fright" at the time the specific test is made. Further, care must be taken when it is performed so that endpoints of exercise are clearly defined and reproducible. The patient should be carefully monitored to ensure safety in a scientifically valid test. Routine monitoring for maximum exercise includes evaluation of the patient's condition, vital signs, and electrocardiogram (ECG). ECG monitoring is necessary for all maximum treadmill tests, and at least one lead should be monitored throughout the test.

ST Segment Changes

ECG criteria for ischemic responses are as follows: development of 1-mm horizontal or downsloping ST segment depression; slowly developing upsloping ST segment depression, which remains depressed at 1 and 1/2 mm, 80 ms after the J point of the QRS complex; 1-mm ST segment elevation in a lead without a significant Q wave at baseline, i.e., a prior myocardial infarction (Figure 4). Interpretation of exercise-induced ST segment depression is valid only when the resting ECG is reasonably normal. Preexisting ECG abnormalities, such as left bundle branch block, left ventricular hypertrophy, drugs, and electrolyte abnormalities preclude any interpretation of an exercise test. Exercise testing is a safe procedure; one mortality in 10,000 exercise tests has been reported (Rochmis & Blackburn, 1971). The prevalence of

ventricular tachycardia was 4 and 0.07% in patients with and without a clinical diagnosis of coronary artery disease, respectively (Milanes, Romero, Hultgren, & Shettigar, 1986).

Ischemia is produced when oxygen supply is exceeded by oxygen demand as determined by coronary perfusion. Heart rate and blood pressure are major determinants of oxygen demand. As a rule, patients should exercise until they have achieved at least 85% of their maximum predicted heart rate to ensure that oxygen demand has increased sufficiently. If a patient demonstrates no ST segment change, but fails to achieve this level of exercise, the test may be falsely labeled negative. In this situation, the test should be interpreted as a negative, but inadequate stress test.

Proper electrode placement is required to reduce artifacts. This may be obtained with adequate skin cleansing and special vests. To reduce motion artifacts, modified lead systems have been developed. The right and left arm electrodes are placed in the infraclavicular fossa, and the leg electrodes are placed midway between the costal margin and the iliac crest in the anterior axillary line. The precordial leads are placed in their standard position. The use of 12 leads increases the chance of detecting ischemic changes, although usually lead 5 will detect the majority of abnormalities. Lead 2 and

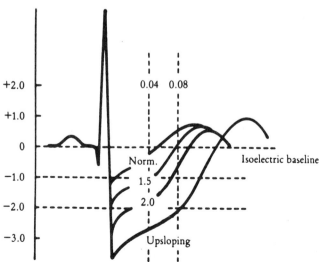

Figure 4. Types of junctional depression. From Stone and Cohn (1982).

AVF are also used frequently. Patients with deep ST segment depression are more likely to have severe coronary disease. Upsloping, horizontal, or downsloping ST segments are seen in patients with normal coronary angiography, approximately 32, 15, and 1% of the time, respectively (Goldschlager, Selzer, & Cohn, 1976). Proper selection of patients, correction of the underlying metabolic abnormalities, and discontinuation of certain drugs prior to testing are all important to obtain maximum information (Smith & Flowers, 1986).

The prognostic value of ST segment changes detected by means of exercise testing in identifying patients at increased risk of a coronary event has been demonstrated (Kennedy, 1981). Ellestad and Wan (1975) demonstrated that the development of ST segment depression at 1.5 mm during exercise predicted an incidence of new coronary events of 9.5% per year, compared with a rate of 1.7% per year in persons without this finding. This rate increased to 11.4% when ventricular ectopic beats were also found with the ST segment depression. St segment upsloping of 2 mm, 0.08 s after the J point, confirmed a similar coronary event rate of 9% per year. In other studies, ST segment depression was not necessarily associated with poor prognosis. This outcome may represent improved medical therapy for patients with ischemic heart disease (Podrid, Graboys, & Lown, 1981).

Ventricular Arrhythmias

With regard to ventricular arrhythmias during treadmill exercise, about 50% of normal adults will have such arrhythmias on a 24-h recording, with the incidence increasing to 75% on a 48-h tracing. Exercise-induced ventricular arrhythmias occur in 35–50% of normal middle-aged men. The incidence increases with age and with increased stress in exercise testing. Exercise-induced ventricular arrhythmias occur in 35–65% of coronary disease patients, with complex forms in 30%. Exercise-induced ventricular events *per se* have generally not been predictive of future cardiac events in patients with chronic coronary artery disease. However, in the presence of ischemic ST segment depression, they are predictive of significant multivessel coronary disease and impaired left ven-

tricular wall motion. In addition, they carry a two- to threefold greater risk of death over a 5-year period (Udall & Ellestad, 1977). Other conditions besides coronary artery disease, which produce both ventricular arrhythmias and ST segment changes, are mitral valve prolapse and hypertrophic cardiomyopathy (Vasilomanolakis & Kennedy, 1983). The treadmill responses predictive for the diagnosis of severe multivessel left main coronary artery disease are shown in Table 1 (Goldschlager, 1982).

Left Ventricular Function: Effects of Age

Left ventricular ejection fraction can also be performed during upright bicycle exercise using radionuclide or echocardiographic techniques. In a study by Port and co-workers, age did not appear to influence these indices (Port, Cobb, Coleman, & Jones, 1980). However, during exercise, ejection fraction was less than 0.60 in 45% of subjects over age 60, compared with 2% of younger subjects. In addition, with aging, there was a decline in the change of left ventricular ejection fraction with exercise. Wall motion abnormalities during

Table 1. Predictive Treadmill Test Response for Diagnosis of Severe Multivessel and/or Left Main Coronary Artery Disease[a]

Electrocardiographic
  ST segment response
    Downsloping
    Elevation
  ST segment depression exceeding 2.5 mm
  Serious ventricular arrhythmias occurring at low (120–130/min) heart rates
  Early onset (first 3 min) of ischemic ST segment depression or elevation
  Prolonged duration in the posttest recovery period ($\geq$8 min) of ischemic ST segment depression
Nonelectrocardiographic
  Low achieved heart rate ($\leq$120/min)
  Hypotension[b] ($\geq$10 mm Hg fall in systolic pressure)
  Rise in diastolic blood pressure ($\geq$110–120 mm Hg)
  Low achieved rate–pressure product ($\leq$15,000)
  Inability to exercise beyond 3 min

[a]From Goldschlager (1982).
[b]In the absence of antihypertensive medications or hypovolemia of any cause.

exercise occurred with increased frequency in patients age 50 and older. These age-related changes in older subjects were not associated with differences in end diastolic volume or blood pressure (Port *et al.*, 1980). In children, blood pressure increased during exercise with the greatest rise in systolic pressure occurring in the first minute (Kennedy, 1981). Thereafter, there was a more gradual increase in pressure until peak exercise was achieved. There was a progressively greater rise in systolic pressure with size and age, as illustrated by the progressively greater rise in peak pressures in these patients (Figure 5). Diastolic pressures tend to either remain constant or decrease during exercise. This results in a larger pulse pressure peak during exercise from the smallest to the largest children (Riopel, Taylor, & Hohn, 1979).

Neurohumoral Responses

Arterial norepinephrine level increased twofold and oxygen consumption increased an average of threefold over the resting values. Noradrenaline increased from 0.28 μg/liter to 0.46 μg/liter under these conditions (Chidsey, Harrison, & Braunwald, 1962). Patients with congestive heart failure and excessive augmentation of plasma norepinephrine during this exercise reflected an increased response of the sympathetic nervous system. This has implications for its importance as a supportive role in these patients (Chidsey *et al.*, 1962). In more recent studies, not only was there an increase in norepinephrine and epinephrine with each increasing work load for normal exercising subjects on bicycle ergometry, but immediately after the end of the work load, plasma norepinephrine and epinephrine levels soared over the maximum exercise achieved, probably coincident with a reduced cardiac output related to reduced venous return in the patients after exercise during the cool-down period (Dimsdale, Hartley, Guiney, Ruskin, & Greenblatt, 1984). In one subject, blood pressure dropped to 75 mm Hg systolic, and diastolic blood pressure was not obtainable. Catecholamines rose to 2756 pg/ml and norepinephrine to 7644 pg/ml. Thus, there is a peril of postexercise catecholamine excess in the hypotensive patient (Dimsdale *et al.*,

1984). Further, Jansson, Hjemdahl, and Kaijser (1982) discovered that diet also induced changes in sympathoadrenal activity during submaximal exercise in relation to the substrate utilized in human subjects. Exercise-induced increases in noradrenaline were more pronounced after a carbohydrate-poor diet than after a carbohydrate-rich diet at 25 min of exercise. It was concluded that when compared to a diet rich in carbohydrates, one that was poor in carbohydrates increased the relative contribution of fat to oxidative metabolism, and increased the sympathoadrenal response to exercise. These investigators thought that stimulation of the lypolysis by sympathetic nervous system mechanisms were of importance for substrate availability when the carbohydrate intake was low.

Exercise Training for Hypertension Therapy

Finally, the role of exercise in the routine treatment of hypertension is controversial. In several studies, regular supervised exercise has been shown to lower blood pressure in patients with both established and mild or borderline hypertension. Some studies in humans have revealed that regular physical activity lowers blood pressure. Although several studies are promising, and exercise seems to reduce sympathetic nervous system tone at rest (Black, 1979), the efficacy of regular exercise as part of routine antihypertensive therapy is under study. Chronic isometric exercise may help in lowering blood pressure, but no extensive studies are available, and on the contrary, there is evidence that such exercise, especially lifting heavy weights repeatedly, may be harmful (Black, 1979).

Isometric (Static) Exercise

Overview

Isometric exercise of the forearm muscles increases arterial pressure, while blood flow to the opposite forearm is augmented. Simultaneously, blood flow to the calf is usually unchanged. Thus, assessment of calculated vascular resistance reveals that the forearm vessels dilate while those of

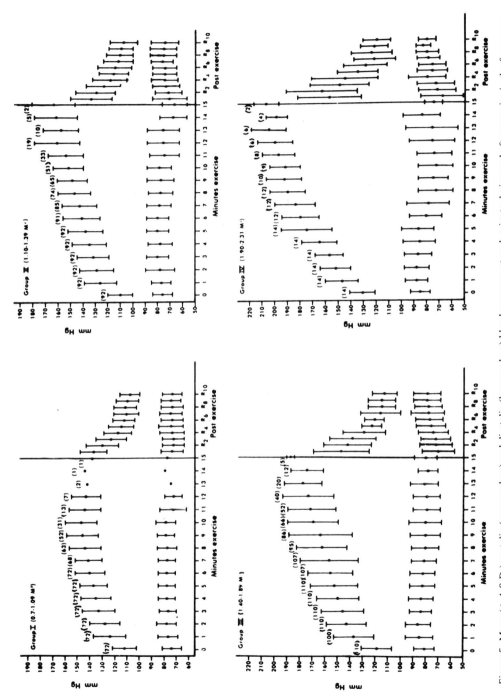

Figure 5. Mean (± 1 S.D.) systolic (upper values) and diastolic (lower values) blood pressures at each minute during and after exercise in the four groups. Numbers in parentheses indicate the number of subjects exercising at that minute. R values were obtained during the 10-min postexercise period. From Riopel *et al.* (1979).

the calf constrict (Eklund, Kaijser, & Knuttson, 1974). Bevegard and Shepherd's (1967) experiments demonstrate that where mental effort is required, forearm vessels, but not those of the calf, dilate presumably because of coadrenergic activation. Other stresses accompanied by mental effort, such as rhythmic exercise of the leg muscles, resistant breathing (Roddie & Shepherd, 1957; Rusch, Shepherd, Webb, & Vanhoutte, 1981), and coughing (Rusch et al., 1981), may trigger forearm dilator mechanisms which offset the normal vasoconstrictor response to isometric exercise.

Maximum handgrip exercise is an easy-to-teach, reproducible form of isometric exercise. The subject squeezes the device for a prescribed period of time, usually 2–3 min. Initially, maximum handgrip is determined by the average gauge reading after two or three attempts, each separated by 2–3 min rest. The subject is then asked to squeeze the handgrip at a specified tension, either 33 or 50% of his or her maximum, for 2–3 min; 33% of maximum is nearly equivalent to lifting a 30-lb weight. This procedure allows for easy sampling of both blood and hemodynamic measurements in the opposite extremity. The subject may fatigue during the 2- to 3-min period, and be unable to maintain tension for the latter one-half or one-third of the experiment. Another disadvantage of handgrip exercise is the associated pain and discomfort of the handgrip stress, which may alter the responses to the work load *per se*.

Static exercise involves sustained activity that changes muscle tension without altering muscle length. Examples are handgrip exercise, lifting weights, and pushing against immovable objects. Untreated hypertensives showed two distinct patterns of hemodynamic responses to isometric handgrip exercise (Ewing, Irving, Kerr, & Kirby, 1973). Systolic and diastolic blood pressures increased in all patients. However, one group responded with increased cardiac index and heart rate without change in systemic vascular resistance, while the second group showed increased vascular resistance with little or no change in cardiac index or rate. The patients in the latter group had left ventricular hypertrophy. In another study of hypertensive adolescents versus controlled subjects, although hypertensives had greater blood

pressure responses to isotonic exercise, there were no differences between controlled and hypertensive groups after isometric handgrip exercise (Fixler et al., 1979).

Hemodynamic, Neurohumoral Responses in Hypertensives

In one study, catecholamine responses to handgrip exercise were measured in coronary sinus, aorta, and femoral vein of patients undergoing cardiac catheterization. Norepinephrine levels were greatest in coronary sinus and least in femoral vein samples. On the other hand, epinephrine levels were greatest in aortic blood samples and least in femoral vein samples. Isometric handgrip exercise induced elevations of norepinephrine and epinephrine in every portion of the circulation. Increments of norepinephrine were 81, 54, and 67% of resting levels in coronary sinus, aorta, and femoral vein, respectively. Corresponding increments in epinephrine were 75, 71, and 70%. These studies demonstrate the universal response of sympathetic discharge in isometric exercise (Miura et al., 1976).

In our study of hypertensives and normotensives subjected to isometric handgrip stress for 3 min, the isometric stress produced significant increments of systolic and diastolic blood pressures of 5–10% and pulse rates of 8–15%, and which were of similar magnitude for both groups (Figure 6) (Sullivan, Schoentgen, et al., 1981). Norepinephrine increased approximately 33% in response to isometric handgrip exercise in both groups. There was a greater increase of epinephrine in hypertensives (80%) compared with normotensives (40%); the difference was not significant (Sullivan, Schoentgen, et al., 1981). However, primary hypertensives with anxiety scores above the 50th percentile, had increased noradrenaline and systolic blood pressure responses to isometric handgrip exercise compared to primary hypertensive patients with low anxiety scores, $p < 0.05$. Furthermore, subjects with a combination of increased anxiety scores and suppressed anger, had enhanced pressor response in systolic blood pressure after isometric handgrip, $p < 0.05$ (Sullivan, Procci, et al., 1981).

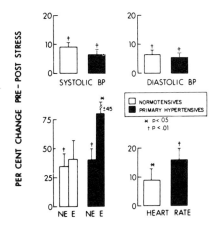

Figure 6. Effects of isometric stress on blood pressures, heart rate, and catecholamines. The increment in pressures, heart rate, and catecholamines was similar for both groups. From Sullivan, Schoentgen, *et al.* (1981).

Effects of Age

To compare the effects of isometric exercise on young and elderly subjects, Goldstraw and Warren (1985) compared isometric exercise performed by means of a handgrip strain gauge dynamometer while the subjects were lying supine. Each subject performed isometric exercise at 10, 20, and 30% of maximum voluntary contraction (MVC) on three separate occasions for each tension. Exercise of 20% MVC by both groups produced a heart rate and systolic and diastolic blood pressure that were significantly greater than those of the 10% exercise level. The heart rate similarity and systolic and diastolic blood pressure differential between young and elderly subjects at control and 10% MVC were maintained (Table 2). Exercise at 30% MVC showed insignificant heart rate changes for both groups when compared to 20% MVC. The systolic blood pressure rise in the young was significant; this was not so in the elderly. The diastolic pressure was greater for both groups. The variability of systolic blood pressure in both groups in response to exercise at 30% MVC was greater than during the controlled period. The variability of systolic blood pressure at 30% MVC was greatest in the elderly. Heart rate and diastolic blood pressure variability in the young was increased compared to

control; this was not so in the elderly. Analysis of data, with regard to time, demonstrates that old age does not alter the characteristic pattern of the response. The lowest rise of diastolic blood pressure in elderly subjects of this study was 15 mm Hg (Goldstraw & Warren, 1985). A study of diabetic patients suggested that a diastolic blood pressure rise of 10 mm Hg or less was indicative of damage to the autonomic nervous system (Ewing, Irving, Kerr, Wildsmith, & Clarke, 1974).

Cold Pressor Test— Hemodynamic/Neurohumoral Responses

The cold pressor test is the most commonly used noxious stimulus to elicit hemodynamic and neurochemical responses. The hand or arm is inserted into an ice bucket for 2–3 min. This technique requires little equipment and allows for repeated measures from the opposite arm. The influence of gravity may be removed by having the subject supine. There may be variable responses to pain, as well as to the temperature challenge.

The cold pressor test has long been employed for measuring reactivity of blood pressure in both normal and hypertensive subjects (Hines & Brown, 1936). Despite the early hope that vascular hyperreaction as measured by the cold pressor test would be predictive of future likelihood to develop hypertension, there has been no consensus that this is the case (Hines, 1940). The general responses of blood pressure have been in the range of +12/+10 mm Hg for systolic and diastolic blood pressure, respectively. Increment of heart rate has been only minor, 1 or 2 beats/min. The one unifying change in hemodynamics has been an increased peripheral resistance, which occurs during cold immersion. Generally, the increase has been on the order of 100% (Cuddy, Smulyan, Keighley, Markason, & Eich, 1966). There have been findings of increased catecholamines in plasma during cold pressor tests, especially norepinephrine. The range of increase has been on the order of 35–50%. Prior treatment with 1.5 mg of atropine i.v. prior to cold immersion resulted in a better correlation of the increment in

Table 2. Heart Rate and Systolic and Diastolic Blood Pressure in Young and Elderly Subjects in Response to Isometric Exercise at 10, 20, and 30% MVC[a,b]

| | Control | | | Isometric exercise | | | | | | | | |
| | | | | 10% MVC | | | 20% MVC | | | 30% MVC | | |
Subjects	HR (bpm)	SBP (mm Hg)	DBP (mm Hg)	HR (bpm)	SBP (mm Hg)	DBP (mm Hg)	HR (bpm)	SBP (mm Hg)	DBP (mm Hg)	HR (bpm)	SBP (mm Hg)	DBP (mm Hg)
Young (n = 12)												
Mean	69	116	66	72	122	70	84**	135**	82**	92	148**	91**
S.E.M.	2.2	2.3	1.8	1.8	2.1	1.8	4.0	3.3	2.5	5.5	3.1	2.4
Elderly (n = 12)												
Mean	64	134	72	68	146	78	77*	164**	90**	82	173	98*
S.E.M.	2.2	1.9††	1.8†	2.2	2.1††	2.1†	2.3	4.7††	2.6†	2.4	6.3††	2.5†

[a]From Goldstraw and Warren (1985).
[b]Daggers show the significance of the comparison of the values in young and elderly subjects. Asterisks show the significance of the comparison to the preceding contraction strength. †,*$p < 0.05$; ††,**$p < 0.01$.

norepinephrine with the increment of peripheral resistance (Cuddy *et al.*, 1966).

Because the hypertensive properties of cold were widely known, the cold pressor test was proposed as an index of vascular reactivity. Striking individual differences in responses to cold were observed by Hines. He divided subjects into hypo- and hyperreactors. On the other hand, much less is known about the effect of whole body immersion in cold water. In one study of subjects who were members of an "ice bear" club, blood pressures rose while subjects were waiting undressed in cold air from 146/84 to 175/90, but there was little further change in blood pressure after 1 min immersion when outside air temperature was 0°C and water temperature 1–2°C. Blood pressures returned to control values a few minutes after the short exposure to cold (Zenner, DeDecker, & Clement, 1980). Training did not change the response; similar responses were noted both in subjects used to cold exposure for 3 years or more and in untrained subjects. Although profound vasoconstriction of skin arteries would be expected to be a major mechanism of blood response to cold, systolic blood pressure increased much more than diastolic blood pressure in almost all subjects, suggesting an important role of cardiac output. Capacitance veins are known to react vigorously to cold, and play an important role in regulation of cardiac output in this phenomenon (Zenner *et al.*, 1980). In more recent studies of cold pressor test responsiveness, Eliasson (1984) found that 3 min of cold

pressor testing yielded increases of blood pressure of 30 mm Hg in normotensives, and increases in pulse rate of 5–10 beats/min. The increases in heart rate were similar in normotensives, borderline hypertensives, and essential hypertensives, being 14, 16, and 12 beats/min, respectively. The increases in noradrenaline were on the order of 90% over baseline, for both normotensive and hypertensive groups. The increases in noradrenaline were correlated with blood pressure increases in all groups, $r = 0.48$, $p < 0.001$ and $r = 0.39$, $p < 0.01$ respectively for systolic blood pressure and diastolic blood pressure in all patients. There were no correlations between increases in adrenaline and any of the circulatory variables during cold pressor testing.

Hemodynamic/Neurohumoral Responses to Exercise and Cold: Effects of Drug Therapy

β-Receptor Blockers

In the resting state, heart rate is controlled mainly by the vagal nerves, and the metabolic requirements of the tissue are approximately 20% of those at maximum exercise. β-Receptor blockade produces a small reduction in heart rate, an increase in systemic vascular resistance, and a small reduction in cardiac output. Changes in resistance are due to a constriction of the muscle resistance vessels.

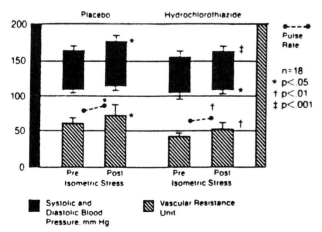

Figure 7. Blood pressure, peripheral vascular resistance, and pulse rate before and after isometric exercise in patients treated with hydrochlorothiazide or placebo. From DeQuattro *et al.* (1986).

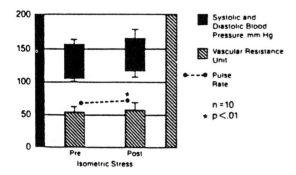

Figure 8. Blood pressure, peripheral vascular resistance, and pulse rate before and after isometric exercise in patients treated with guanadrel sulfate plus hydrochlorothiazide. From DeQuattro *et al.* (1986).

Blockade of β receptors in the forearm, with the β blocker propranolol, causes a slight reduction in forearm blood flow (Hartling, Noer, Svendsen, Clausen, & Trap-Jensen, 1980). In man after standing, there is a reduction in venous return due to a shift of blood from the cardiopulmonary region. Cardiopulmonary receptors play a major role in increasing sympathetic outflow to the heart, systemic resistance and capacitance vessels to the adrenal medulla and the JG cells of the kidney. Although stroke volume is reduced, there is an increase in heart rate and constriction of muscle, splanchnic, and renal resistance vessels. Further, there is an increase in splanchnic resistance and plasma renin activity. Angiotensin II is eventually increased to amplify the sympathetic mediated responses. Although β-blocking drugs attenuate the increase in heart rate and contractility and reduce renin and angiotensin II output, the net increase in sympathetic outflow mediates vasoconstriction, and postural hypotension does not occur.

During exercise, the increase in cardiac output is primarily due to an increase in heart rate, which follows a reduction in vagal activity and an increased sympathetic tone and release of norepinephrine and epinephrine to stimulate β_1 receptors of the sinus node and atrial ventricular node to both shorten refractory period and enhance myocardial contractility. Thus, adequate cardiac filling is permitted to maintain an increased ejection as heart rate increases. Arterial baroreceptors control total systemic vascular resistance during exercise. Although the response to β-adrenergic stimulation is increased with age, and cardiac contractility in heart rate increase is lessened, Starling mechanisms compensate because of an age-related increase in end diastolic volume and stroke volume (Rodeheffer *et al.*, 1984). After β blockade, heart rate is attenuated, and the maximum achievable is decreased to approximately 140 beats/min. Stroke volume increases by 10% more than the resting value. Thus, exercise conditioning is attenuated by β blockade (Marsh, Hiatt, Brammell, & Horwitz, 1983). During isometric exercise, β blockade had little net effect on the significant increase in systemic arterial pressure. However, the rise in cardiac output is less due to the blunted heart rate and contractility response. There is a compensatory increase in reflex constriction of systemic resistance vessels and increased peripheral resistance.

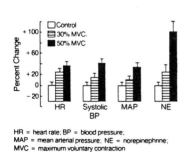

HR = heart rate; BP = blood pressure;
MAP = mean arterial pressure; NE = norepinephrine;
MVC = maximum voluntary contraction

Figure 9. Cardiovascular and norepinephrine responses to isometric handgrip exercise. From DeQuattro (1987).

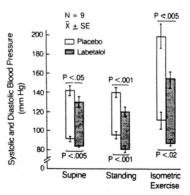

Figure 10. Effect of labetalol on systolic and diastolic blood pressure. From DeQuattro (1987).

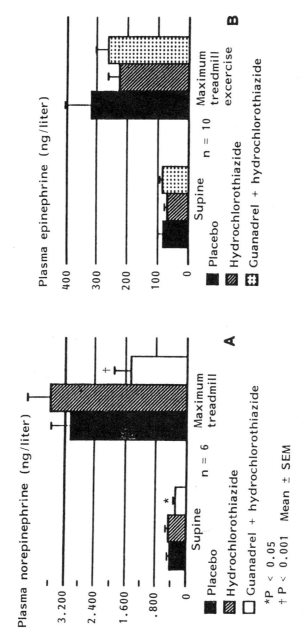

Figure 11. Effects of placebo, hydrochlorothiazide, and guanadrel plus hydrochlorothiazide on (A) plasma norepinephrine levels and (B) plasma epinephrine levels. From DeQuattro *et al.* (1986).

Diuretics and Adrenergic Blockade

Antihypertensive drugs alter both hemodynamic and neural responses of patients performing muscular exercise. In one study of patients with primary hypertension, hydrochlorothiazide lowered blood pressure and peripheral vascular resistance before and after isometric handgrip exercise at 30% MVC (Figure 7). The addition of the sympatholytic agent (neuronal reuptake blocker) guanadrel lowered both systolic and diastolic pressures when the patients performed isometric exercise (Figure 8). In another group of hypertensives we found that at 30 and 50% MVC there were significant elevations of heart rate, blood pressure, and plasma norepinephrine (Figure 9). The blood pressures (Figure 10) as well as heart rate and plasma renin activity were lower at baseline and the responses at 30% MVC were blunted by the α- and $\beta_{1,2}$-receptor blocker, labetalol (DeQuattro, 1987). Although labetalol blocked the receptors mediating the pressor response to handgrip exercise, the reflex of sympathetic nervous stimulation increased plasma norepinephrine. The rise of noradrenaline in plasma after handgrip was blunted by labetalol via β_2 blockade of presynaptic adrenergic modulation usually present during the exercise (DeQuattro, 1987).

Another class of sympatholytic agents, the α agonists, act centrally to neutralize sympathetic tone. Lofexidine, a clonidine-like α agonist, suppresses norepinephrine release and controls blood pressure of hypertensives before and during exercise at one-half maximum (Figure 11). The catecholamine and renin aldosterone responses to lofexidine therapy in these patients, both at rest and during exercise, are given in Figure 11. Only the catecholamine suppression was significant, suggesting the importance of the noradrenergic system in blood pressure elevation during isotonic exercise. The thiazide diuretics are effective in lowering blood pressure responses to maximum treadmill exercise (Table 3). However, they cause a slight reflex increase in sympathetic tone (Figure 11). The addition of either guanadrel or propranolol to their hydrochlorothiazide therapy improved blood pressure control and lowered heart rate (Figure 11). Blood pressure reduction with guanadrel sulfate was associated with a reduction

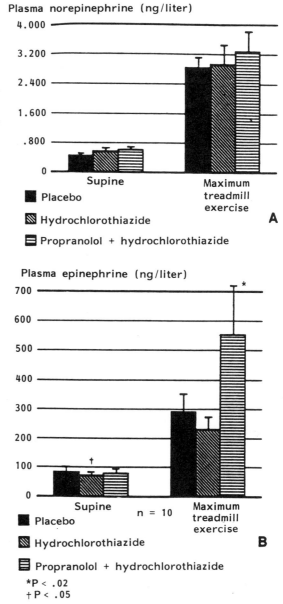

Figure 12. Effects of placebo, hydrochlorothiazide, and propranolol plus hydrochlorothiazide on (A) plasma norepinephrine levels and (B) plasma epinephrine levels. From DeQuattro *et al.* (1986).

in neural tone (Figure 11), whereas the pressure lowering after propranolol was related to unchanged norepinephrine and increased epinephrine in plasma (Figure 12). The latter changes might be explained by altered excretion or enhanced secretion of epinephrine after β blockade.

*Table 3. Effect of Adding Guanadrel or Propranolol on Blood Pressure and Pulse
of Hydrochlorothiazide-Treated Patients (Maximum Exercise)[a]*

	Guanadrel subgroup ($N = 10$)		Propranolol subgroup ($N = 10$)	
	Blood pressure (mm Hg)	Pulse (bpm)	Blood pressure (mm Hg)	Pulse (bpm)
Placebo	204/100	162	214/105	161
Hydrochlorothiazide	181**/91***	164	208/98*	161
Step 2 agent	158**/81**	132**	158**/88*	122***

[a]From DeQuattro (1987).
*$p < 0.05$, **$p < 0.01$, ***$p < 0.001$.

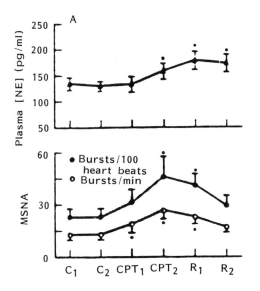

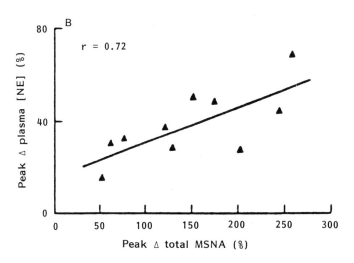

Figure 13. Comparison of plasma norepinephrine (NE) and muscle sympathetic nerve activity (MSNA) responses to the cold pressor test. (A) Simultaneous measurements of plasma NE and MSNA in ten subjects (mean ± S.E.; $p < 0.05$ compared with control) during 2 min each of control (C_1, C_2), cold pressor test R_2). The increases in plasma NE lagged behind the increases in MSNA by approximately 1 min. (B) Relationship between the peak responses (percentage increase) in plasma NE and in total MSNA to the cold pressor test in the ten subjects. There was a significant linear relationship between these variables ($y = 0.15$, $x = +17$; $r = 0.72$, $p < 0.05$). However, large increases in MSNA were associated with small changes in plasma NE. From Victor *et al.* (1987).

Studies of pressor and pulse rate responses of human subjects to the cold pressor test reveal the importance of both cardiac and muscle sympathetic nerve stimulation (Victor, Leimbach, Seals, Wallin, & Mark, 1987). The initial response to the cold stimulus is an increase in heart rate which can be blocked with propranolol. Later, the pressor response is related to increased firing of muscle sympathetic nerves as reflected by concomitant elevation of venous plasma norepinephrine (Figure 13).

Thus, antihypertensive agents which affect sympathetic nervous system function may have potent effects on the pressor responses to isotonic and isometric exercise and cold water immersion.

References

Alam, M., & Smirk, F. H. (1937). Observations in man upon a blood pressure raising reflex arising from the voluntary muscles. *Journal of Physiology (London), 89*, 372–383.

Asmussen, E., & Hansen, E. (1981). Uber den einflub statischer muskelarbeit auf atmung und kreislauf. *Skandinavisches Archiv fuer Physiologie 78*, 283–303.

Bevegard, B. S., & Shepherd, J. T. (1967). Regulation of the circulation during exercise in man. *Physiological Reviews, 47*, 178–213.

Billman, G. E., Schwartz, P. J., & Stone, H. L. (1984). The effects of daily exercise on susceptibility to sudden cardiac death. *Circulation, 69*, 1182–1189.

Black, H. R. (1979). Nonpharmacologic therapy for hypertension. *American Journal of Medicine, 66*, 837–842.

Blomqvist, C. G., Lewis, S. F., Taylor, W. F., & Graham, R. M. (1981). Similarity of the hemodynamic responses to static and dynamic exercise of small muscle groups. *Circulation Research, 48* (Suppl. I), I-87–I-92.

Bruce, R. A. (1971). Exercise testing of patients with coronary heart disease. *Annals of Clinical Research, 3*, 323.

Chidsey, C. A., Harrison, D. C., & Braunwald, E. (1962). Augmentation of the plasma nor-epinephrine response to exercise in patients with congestive heart failure. *New England Journal of Medicine, 267*, 650–654.

Cuddy, R. P., Smulyan, H., Keighley, J. F., Markason, C. R., & Eich, R. H. (1966). Hemodynamic and catecholamine changes during a standard cold pressor test. *American Heart Journal, 71*, 446–454.

DeQuattro, V. (1987). The effect of antihypertensive therapy on exercise tolerance. *Practical Cardiology* (Spec. Suppl.), 38–46.

DeQuattro, V., Foti, A., DeOrtiz, H. K., DeGrau, A., DeQuattro, E., & Allen, J. (1986). The comparative antihypertensive and cardiac effects of guanadrel sulfate and pro-pranolol during vigorous exercise. *Practical Cardiology* (Spec. Suppl.), 37–47.

Dimsdale, J. E., Hartley, L. H., Guiney, T., Ruskin, J. N., & Greenblatt, D. (1984). Postexercise peril. Plasma catecholamines and exercise. *Journal of the American Medical Association, 251*, 630–632.

Eklund, B., Kaijser, L., & Knuttson, E. (1974). Blood flow in resting (contralateral) arm and leg during isometric contraction. *Journal of Physiology (London), 240*, 111–124.

Eliasson, K. (1984). Borderline hypertension. Circulatory, sympathoadrenal and psychological reactions to stress. *Acta Medica Scandinavica, Supplementum, 692*, 7–90.

Ellestad, M. H., & Wan, M. K. C. (1975). Predictive implications of stress testing. Follow-up of 2700 subjects after maximum treadmill stress testing. *Circulation, 51*, 363–369.

Ewing, D. J., Irving, J. B., Kerr, F., & Kirby, B. J. (1973). Static exercise in untreated systemic hypertension. *British Heart Journal, 35*, 413–421.

Ewing, D. J., Irving, J. B., Kerr, E., Wildsmith, J. A. W., & Clarke, B. F. (1974). Cardiovascular responses to sustained handgrip in normal subjects and in patients with diabetes mellitus: A test for autonomic function. *Clinical Science and Molecular Medicine, 46*, 295–306.

Fixler, D. E., Laird, W. P., Browne, R., Fitzgerald, V., Wilson, S., & Vance, R. (1979). Response of hypertensive adolescents to dynamic and isometric exercise stress. *Pediatrics, 64*, 579–583.

Goldschlager, N. (1982). Use of the treadmill test in the diagnosis of coronary artery disease in patients with chest pain. *Annals of Internal Medicine, 97*, 383–388.

Goldschlager, N., Selzer, A., & Cohn, K. (1976). Treadmill stress tests as indicators of presence and severity of coronary artery disease. *Annals of Internal Medicine, 85*, 277–286.

Goldstraw, P. W., & Warren, D. J. (1985). The effect of age on the cardiovascular responses to isometric exercise: A test of autonomic function. *Gerontology, 31*, 54–58.

Hartling, O. J., Noer, I., Svendsen, T. L., Clausen, J. P., & Trap-Jensen, J. (1980). Selective and non-selective beta-adrenoceptor blockade in the human forearm. *Clinical Science, 58*, 279–286.

Hines, E. A., Jr. (1940). The significance of vascular hyperreaction as measured by the cold-pressor test. *American Heart Journal, 19*, 408.

Hines, E. A., Jr., & Brown, G. E. (1936). The cold pressor test for measuring the reactivity of the blood pressure: Data concerning 571 normal and hypertensive subjects. *American Heart Journal, 11*, 1.

Jansson, E., Hjemdahl, P., & Kaijser, L. (1982). Diet induced changes in sympatho-adrenal activity during submaximal exercise in relation to substrate utilization in man. *Acta Physiologica Scandinavica, 114*, 171–178.

Kaufman, M. P., Rybicki, K. J., Waldrop, T. G., & Mitchell, J. H. (1984). Effect on arterial pressure of rhythmically contracting the hind-limb muscles of cats. *Journal of Applied Physiology, 56*, 1265–1271.

Kennedy, H. L. (1981). Comparison of ambulatory electrocardiography and exercise testing. *American Journal of Cardiology, 47*, 1359–1365.

Lewis, S. F., Taylor, W. F., Graham, R. M., Schutte, J. E., Pettinger, W. A., & Blomqvist, C. G. (1980). Role of active muscle mass in adrenergic and hemodynamic exercise responses. *Circulation, 62* (Suppl. II), III-202.

Marsh, R. C., Hiatt, W. R., Brammell, H. L., & Horwitz L. D. (1983). Attenuation of exercise conditioning by low dose beta-adrenergic receptor blockade. *Journal of the American College of Cardiology, 3,* 551–556.

Milanes, J., Romero, M., Hultgren, H. N., & Shettigar, U. (1986). Exercise tests and ventricular tachycardia. *Western Journal of Medicine, 145,* 473–476.

Miura, Y., Haneda, T., Sato, T., Miyazawa, K., Sakuma, H., Kobayashi, K., Minai, K., Shirato, K., Honna, T., Takishima, T., & Yoshinaga, K. (1976). Plasma catecholamine levels in the coronary sinus, aorta, and femoral vein of subjects undergoing cardiac catheterization at rest and during exercise. *Japanese Circulation Journal, 40,* 929–934.

Naughton, J., & Haider, R. (1973). Methods of exercise testing. In J. P. Naughton & H. K. Hellerstein (Eds.), *Exercise testing and exercise training in coronary heart disease* (pp. 79–91). New York: Academic Press.

Podrid, P. J., Graboys, T. B., & Lown, B. (1981). Prognosis of medically treated patients with coronary-artery disease with profound ST segment depression during exercise testing. *New England Journal of Medicine, 305,* 1111–1116.

Port, S., Cobb, F. R., Coleman, R. E., & Jones, R. H. (1980). Effect of age on the response of the left ventricular ejection fraction to exercise. *New England Journal of Medicine, 303,* 1133–1137.

Raven, P. B., Rohm-Young, D., & Blomqvist, C. G. (1984). Physical fitness and cardiovascular response to lower body negative pressure. *Journal of Applied Physiology, 56,* 138–144.

Riopel, D. A., Taylor, A. B., & Hohn, A. R. (1979). Blood pressure, heart rate, pressure–rate product and electrocardiographic changes in healthy children during treadmill exercise. *American Journal of Cardiology, 44,* 697–704.

Rochmis, P., & Blackburn, H. (1971). Exercise tests. A survey of procedures, safety and litigation experience in approximately 170,000 tests. *Journal of the American Medical Association, 217,* 1061–1066.

Roddie, I. C., & Shepherd, J. T. (1957). The effects of carotid artery compression in man with special reference to changes in vascular resistance in the limbs. *Journal of Physiology (London), 139,* 377–384.

Rodeheffer, R. J., Gerstenblith, G., Becker, L. C., Fleg, J. L., Weisfeldt, M. L., & Lankatta, E. G. (1984). Exercise cardiac output is maintained with advanced age in healthy human subjects; cardiac dilation and increased stroke volume compensate for a diminished heart rate. *Circulation, 69,* 203–213.

Rusch, N. J., Shepherd, J. T., Webb, C. R., & Vanhoutte, P. M. (1981). Different behavior of the resistance vessels of the human calf and forearm during contralateral isometric exercise, mental stress, and abnormal respiratory movements. *Circulation Research, 48*(Suppl. I), I-118–I-130.

Shepherd, J. T., Blomqvist, C. G., Lind, A. R., Mitchell, J. H., & Saltin, B. (1981). Static (isometric) exercise. *Circulation Research, 48*(Suppl. I), I-179–I-188.

Smith, M. S., & Flowers, N. C. (1986). Pitfalls in recording and interpreting exercise stress tests. *Internal Medicine, 7,* 153–161.

Stone, H. L. (1977). Cardiac function and exercise training in conscious dogs. *Journal of Applied Physiology, 42,* 824–832.

Stone, H. L., Dormer, K. J., Foreman, R. D., Thies, R., & Blair, R. W. (1985). Neural regulation of the cardiovascular system during exercise. *Federation Proceedings, 44,* 2271–2278.

Stone, P. H., & Cohn, P. (1982). Exercise testing. In P. Cohn & J. Wynne (Eds.), *Diagnostic methods in clinical cardiology.* Boston: Little, Brown.

Sullivan, P., Procci, W. R., DeQuattro, V., Schoentgen, S., Levine, D., Van der Meulen, J., & Bornheimer, J. F. (1981). Anger, anxiety, guilt and increased basal and stress-induced neurogenic tone: Causes or effects in primary hypertension? *Clinical Science, 61,* 389s–392s.

Sullivan, P., Schoentgen, S., DeQuattro, V., Procci, W., Levine, D., Van der Meulen, J., & Bornheimer, J. (1981). Anxiety, anger, and neurogenic tone at rest and in stress in patients with primary hypertension. *Hypertension, 3*(Suppl. II), II-119–II-123.

Udall, J. A., & Ellestad, M. H. (1977). Predictive implications of ventricular premature contractions associated with treadmill stress testing. *Circulation, 56,* 985–989.

Vasilomanolakis, E. C., & Kennedy, H. L. (1983). Ambulatory electrocardiography and exercise testing in cardiac disease. *Practical Cardiology, 9,* 205–222.

Victor, R. G., Leimbach, W. N., Seals, D. R., Wallin, B. G., & Mark, A. L. (1987). Effects of the cold pressor test on muscle sympathetic nerve activity in humans. *Hypertension, 9,* 429–436.

Zenner, R. J., DeDecker, D. E., & Clement, D. L. (1980). Blood-pressure response to swimming in ice-cold water. *Lancet, 2,* 120–121.

CHAPTER **26**

Hemodynamic Assessment and Pharmacologic Probes as Tools to Analyze Cardiovascular Reactivity

Stevo Julius

Hemodynamic Assessment

The blood pressure and heart rate responses to a laboratory task are most frequently used to assess an individual's cardiovascular reactivity. Information from such observation is useful for general categorization and for the delineation of subgroups of hyper- and hyporesponders. Measurement of systemic and regional hemodynamics further complements reactivity studies by providing important information about qualitative differences which are not necessarily reflected in the overall magnitude of the blood pressure response. Hollenberg, Williams, and Adams (1981) engaged patients with borderline hypertension and normotensive control subjects in resolving Ravens progressive matrices. The blood pressure responses to this challenge were similar in both groups, but patients with borderline hypertension had a significant decrease of renal blood flow. This observation, that renal vasculature tends to overrespond to the mental stress, provided important inference as to how

behavioral factors might lead to hypertension. As Light, Koepke, Obrist, and Willis (1983) suggest, mental stress might cause excessive salt retention in patients with borderline hypertension. It is not difficult to visualize how sodium retention might lead to hypertension. Another example of the differential behavior of local vasculature was provided by Mark, Lawton, and Abboud (1975). They observed that chronic salt loading does not alter the mean blood pressure in borderline hypertensive and normotensive subjects, but the forearm vascular resistance in normotensive individuals decreased whereas in patients with borderline hypertension it increased.

The two examples above illustrate how study of regional vascular responses to laboratory tasks and physical challenges may provide new information. Measurement of systemic hemodynamics also can give new insights which could not be gathered from simple observations of blood pressure and heart rate responses to laboratory tasks or stressors. If patients with borderline hypertension are subjected to a number of physical stressors, such as low levels of dynamic exercise (Julius & Conway, 1968), isometric exercise (Sannerstedt & Julius, 1972), change of posture (Sannerstedt, Julius, & Conway, 1970), and blood volume ex-

---

Stevo Julius • Division of Hypertension, Department of Internal Medicine, University of Michigan Medical Center, Ann Arbor, Michigan 48109-0356.

pansion (Lund-Johansen, 1967), their blood pressure and heart rate responses are entirely similar to those of normal individuals. They start from a higher baseline pressure, but from that point on the increase of blood pressure is proportional to that for normotensive subjects. However, when one analyzes hemodynamic components of such responses, major qualitative differences emerge. Patients with borderline hypertension achieve the same blood pressure response with a lesser increase of the cardiac output and a greater increase of the vascular resistance (Julius, Pascual, Sannerstedt, & Mitchell, 1971). Patients with borderline hypertension have high resting cardiac output and their calculated peripheral resistance values are normal. It has been argued, however, that their resistance should be lower to accommodate the higher output and that, therefore, the resistance is relatively high, e.g., inappropriately adjusted to the flow (Widimsky, Fejfarova, & Fejfar, 1957). Whereas conceptually this was a sound analysis, the biologic significance of this statement was doubtful as one could not test the validity of the expectation that the resistance "should" be lower for the observed levels of cardiac output. A study of hemodynamic responses to stressors provided factual proof for what has been empirically suspected from the analysis of resting data: that the regulation of vascular resistance is abnormal in borderline hypertension (Julius *et al.*, 1971).

A further example of the usefulness of hemodynamic evaluation is found in the works of Obrist, Langer, Light, and Koepke (1983) and Williams (1986). They contend that blood pressure responses to a stressor, while quantitatively similar, are modulated by different hemodynamic patterns depending on the nature of the host–stressor interaction. Two distinct patterns are described. Pattern 1 is characterized by an elevation of cardiac output together with forearm vasodilation and is characteristic of stressors that elicit active effortful coping. Passive coping and vigilant behavior are more likely to elicit pattern 2: forearm vasoconstriction and an unchanged cardiac output.

Whereas much more work is needed to establish the specificity and reproducibility of these different hemodynamic pressor patterns, this line of inquiry clearly shows that a hemodynamic analysis

can provide more and qualitatively different information than the simple recording of the magnitude of the blood pressure response.

Acute Pharmacologic Probes

The "cardiovascular reactivity" to standardized laboratory stressors is the end product of complex interaction between the centrally efferent autonomic discharge, the receptor properties, and the end organ responsiveness. Acute hemodynamic responses to pharmacologic probes, albeit not perfectly, can shed some important light on these interactions.

Operational Definitions

Central Drive

This is the amount of efferent impulses through the autonomic nerves. For the sympathetics it is roughly approximated by the A-V norepinephrine difference across an organ. However, as indicated in other portions of this handbook, the A-V difference is also importantly dependent on blood flow, spillover rates, and neuronal reuptake of norepinephrine.

Receptor Properties

These include receptor number, receptor affinity, and receptor sensitivity. The number of receptors and their affinity can be measured in isolated cells or tissue homogenates, but the functional significance of these biochemical findings is rarely apparent. Receptor sensitivity is a functional definition acquired from dose–response curves of an organ to the specific agonist. Increased receptor sensitivity implies a lower threshold responsiveness and a shift of the dose response to the response axis.

Organ Responsiveness

Organ responsiveness depends on the intrinsic properties of the responding tissue. In the cardiovascular system this is determined by the intrinsic contractile properties of the smooth muscle and by the quantity and arrangement of structural non-contractile components in the heart and blood vessels. Organ responsiveness is usually assessed by responses to a number of pharmacologic agents which are chosen to produce the same organ effect, but through different receptors or different activation pathways.

Autonomic Tone

Autonomic tone is the end result of the interaction between central drive, receptor sensitivity, and the end organ responsiveness. It is assessed by the amount of cardiac (e.g., stroke volume and heart rate) or vascular (e.g., vascular resistance or venous capacitance) responses to a specific autonomic antagonist.

Methodologic Issues

Cardiac tone. The cardiac tone could be assessed by the response to cardioselective β-blocking agents combined with the response to parasympathetic blockade. α-Adrenergic receptors play little practical role as determinants of the cardiac autonomic tone. Extrapolation from the data on cardiac tone to the central sympathetic drive is facilitated by determination of the cardiac responsiveness to isoproterenol. However, to complete the picture it is important to have information on cardiac contractility since it in turn affects the overall response to isoproterenol.

Because of these complexities it is very important that experiments using pharmacologic probes to assess cardiac tone also include measurement of systemic hemodynamics. The assumption that changes in the heart rate always approximate changes in cardiac output is simply erroneous. Furthermore, β-adrenergic agonists directly affect peripheral vessels and elicit active reflex responses. Measurement of systemic hemodynamics is useful in unraveling these complex interactions. In the past we made claims that the chronotropic responsiveness of the heart to isoproterenol is decreased in borderline hypertension and could support this statement only by providing evidence that vascular resistance responses of patients and control sub-

jects to isoproterenol were similar (Julius *et al.*, 1975).

If the purpose of the experiment is to assess the cardiac autonomic tone, then only acute responses to drugs should be analyzed. Effects observed a few hours after initiation of the dosage, are complex and frequently unrelated to the pharmacologic action of the drug. Isoproterenol, for example, causes vasodilation, induces hormonal responses, and possibly alters receptor sensitivity so that the end result might be uninterpretable. Similar interpretative difficulties emerge with the use of β-blocking agents inasmuch as they initially decrease the cardiac output (Frohlich, Tarazi, Dustan, & Page, 1968), but later also alter plasma renin levels (Laragh, 1976), plasma volume (Julius, Pascual, Abbrecht, & London, 1972), and in about 50% of subjects also decrease blood pressure.

The sequence in which drugs are given is very important as the response to the second agent is inevitably affected by the first one. It is, therefore, necessary to rotate the sequence and analyze for a possible order effect.

Finally, to fully assess the cardiac autonomic tone, one needs information about the overall cardiac contractility. Should, for example, a group of patients respond to β-adrenergic blockade with a larger decrease of cardiac output, this could be indicative of a higher sympathetic drive to the heart, but it may also reflect increased cardiac contractility. Comparison of indices of cardiac performance (systolic and diastolic time intervals, ejection fraction, rate of fiber shortening) before and after blockade may resolve the issue. If sympathetic drive is enhanced, then patients should show increased myocardial contractility before blockade and after the blockade the contractility should become normal. Conversely, if decreased cardiac contractility is responsible for the finding, the resting contractility of the two groups might be comparable, but after blockade the patient group should manifest impaired contractility.

Resistance vessel tone. The basic tactic to assess vascular sympathetic tone involves intraarterial infusion of an antagonist and measurement of the flow in the organ. If one chooses the right dose, it is possible to elicit considerable response of the local vasculature while the systemic hemodynamics remain unaffected. Consequently, the flow is not affected by distant reflex or humoral changes and the observed effect is truly representative of the properties of the local vasculature. In theory, therefore, the response to an α_1 antagonist should represent the amount of postsynaptic sympathetic tone, and the response to norepinephrine assesses the vascular responsiveness to α-adrenergic stimulation. Such information on tone and responsiveness should provide sufficient basis to assess the sympathetic vascular drive. For example, if α-adrenergic responsiveness to norepinephrine is normal, changes of flow in response to an α-adrenergic blockade will be directly proportional to the central drive. In practice, when *different* responses are found in two groups of subjects, the issues are much more complicated. To illustrate the complexities it may be best to analyze a hypothetical situation. Let us assume that prazosin causes a larger vasodilation in a group of subjects. This could mean that α-adrenergic tone is enhanced. However, it is also possible that the nonspecific myogenic tone in the smooth muscle is increased and the enhanced response to prazosin reflects the tendency of the vascular smooth muscle to respond more vigorously to *all* vasodilating stimuli. Consequently, only if responses to a variety of unspecific vasodilators (nitroprusside, calcium antagonists, and angiotensin receptor antagonists) are normal can one claim specificity for the excessive prazosin response. Let us now assume that this had been done and the excessive response is specific for prazosin. This suggests that the regional vascular α-adrenergic drive is increased, but the finding is compatible with a *normal* drive if the α-adrenergic receptors are hyperresponsive. Thus, the next step is to assess the vascular responsiveness to an α-adrenergic agonist. If this is normal or decreased, one can safely assume that the excessive response to prazosin reflects increased central α-adrenergic drive to the vasculature.

Such a vigorous analysis of the regional responses to agonists and antagonists is necessary to understand human hypertension. Long-standing hypertension accentuates vascular responsiveness through the development of vascular smooth muscle hypertrophy. The hypertrophic vascular wall impinges on the lumen of the blood vessels, there-

by increasing the baseline vascular resistance. More importantly, the changed wall-to-lumen ratio renders the blood vessel hyperresponsive to pressor stimuli since the same degree of smooth muscle contraction causes a much higher resistance increase in a hypertrophic blood vessel (Folkow, 1982). This structural enhancement of vascular responses must be taken into consideration. The following are the criteria upon which one can determine whether the enhanced regional vascular responsiveness is due to structural factors. (1) Hypertrophic vessels offer more resistance to the flow during maximal vasodilation. This "minimal resistance" at maximal dilation (when all the myogenic tone is abolished) reflects the physical properties of the blood vessels. In the human forearm one can study such maximal vasodilation during reperfusion after 10 min of ischemic exercise. (2) The maximal resistance, e.g., response to the largest dose of a vasoconstrictor, is substantially increased. (3) The threshold dose to elicit a response is not altered. (4) The dose–response curve is steeper. (5) The blood vessels are hyperresponsive to a variety of different agonists.

Chronic Pharmacologic Probes

If all facets are properly analyzed, acute pharmacologic probes provide reasonably straightforward information. Unfortunately, during a chronic treatment the situation is much more complex. It is usually assumed that (1) patients showing a larger decrease of blood pressure to sympatholytic agents have "neurogenic" hypertension and (2) blood pressure variability is predominantly neurogenic and should, therefore, be preferentially influenced by sympatholytic agents. As will be seen, both these statements cannot be supported and the response to chronic antihypertensive treatment, while useful to select and define subgroups of patients, at best can only set agenda for further research to elucidate the prevailing pathophysiology of these subgroups.

Acute pharmacologic blockade shows that mild hypertensive patients with high renin levels suffer from a substantial increase of sympathetic cardiovascular tone (Esler, Julius, *et al.*, 1977). Such patients also respond well to β-adrenergic blockade (Esler, Zweifler, Randall, & DeQuattro, 1977). Consequently, the finding that a drug that interferes with enhanced sympathetic cardiac tone also preferentially lowers the blood pressure in these patients is reassuring and appears to complement the overall pathophysiologic picture. However, the specificity of this finding must be questioned. First, β-blocking agents are effective also in patients with low renin hypertension (Hollifield, Sherman, VanderZwagg, and Shand, 1976) who have low sympathetic tone (Esler *et al.*, 1976). Furthermore, it has been shown by Frohlich *et al.* (1968) that responders and nonresponders have similar initial levels of cardiac output and show similar initial declines of cardiac output. Though we do find a relationship between the magnitude of the initial decrease of cardiac output and the later fall in blood pressure (Colfer, Cottier, Sanchez, & Julius, 1984) we explain this relationship as reflecting total body autoregulation which is unrelated to an individual's starting sympathetic tone. Thus, a straightforward assumption—that since β-blockers lower the blood pressure, this proves that a group of patients has a "sympathetic cardiac component" in their hypertension—is not tenable.

Extrapolations from the responses to chronic drug treatment are particularly difficult since the blood pressure response to a drug is a dynamic process and is in part unrelated to the pharmacologic action of the drug. Let us take the example of a diuretic. The antihypertensive action of diuretics is correlated to their initial natriuretic and diuretic action; in patients with renal failure they are ineffective. However, the underlying hemodynamic pattern of the hypotensive response is changing (Conway & Lauwers, 1960). In the beginning the blood pressure fall is associated with a low cardiac output and a decreased plasma volume; however, after a few weeks the cardiac output and plasma volume return to normal levels. At that point the antihypertensive action of the diuretic shifts from the initial depression of output to a lowering of vascular resistance. The early mechanism seems to be directly related to diuresis, but the later adjustment of the vascular resistance cannot be explained by the pharmacologic action of diuretics. Consequently, it is not appropriate to

label diuretic-responsive patients as "volume" or "sodium" dependent; with equal justification they could be called "vasodilation-prone."

Issues are even further complicated since a chronic hypotensive response, to a large extent, depends on the magnitude of secondary counter-regulatory mechanisms. Failure to respond to direct vasodilators or sympatholytic agents is most frequently due to fluid retention and not to a failure to respond to the drug's specific antihypertensive mechanism (Dustan, Tarazi, & Bravo, 1972). Ibsen *et al.* (1979) showed that resistance to diuretics is due to the secondary, sympathetically mediated release of renin. Based on this, failure to respond to diuretics may represent either "sodium resistance" or "sympathetic compensatory hyperactivity." Similarly, failure to respond to centrally active sympatholytics such as methyldopa, gives little information about an individual's initial sympathetic tone and to a large degree is dependent on the individual's water and sodium balance.

When a response occurs in the course of antihypertensive treatment, its specificity is frequently dubious. For example, sympatholytic agents lower blood pressure in renovascular hypertension, where the pressure elevation is renin-dependent. Similarly in pheochromocytoma, the blood pressure elevation is due to the catecholamine release by the tumor, but clonidine, a centrally acting sympatholytic agent, lowers the blood pressure (Bravo, Tarazi, Fouad, Vidt, & Gifford, 1981).

These interpretive difficulties extend also to the issues of blood pressure variability and the specific influence sympatholytic agents might have on such variability. Since most of the blood pressure variability is caused by enhanced central cardiovascular drive, agents that decrease the CNS sympathetic discharge should also positively affect blood pressure variability. In a recent study we were unable to show such a specific effect of clonidine. Clonidine did lower the baseline blood pressure, but did not affect the blood pressure variability.

In summary, some hypertensive patients respond very well to central or peripheral sympatholytic agents, whereas the others respond to diuretics. Such patterns of blood pressure responsiveness cannot be simplified to mean that responders to sympatholytic agents have a "neurogenic" and responders to diuretics a "sodium-dependent" hypertension. Success of a class of compounds frequently depends on factors which are not related to their primary pharmacologic activity. Blood pressure responsiveness to a class of agents can at best characterize a subgroup of patients who lend themselves to further research, and set the research agenda to investigate the mechanism(s) which renders these patients responsive.

References

Bravo, E. L., Tarazi, R. C., Fouad, F. M., Vidt, D. G., & Gifford, R. W. (1981). Clonidine-suppression test: A useful aid in the diagnosis of pheochromocytoma. *New England Journal of Medicine, 305,* 623–626.

Colfer, H. T., Cottier, C., Sanchez, R., & Julius, S. (1984). Evidence for the autoregulatory theory of blood pressure reduction by beta-adrenoreceptor blocking agents in hypertension. *Hypertension, 6,* 145–151.

Conway, J., & Lauwers, P. (1960). Hemodynamic and hypotensive effects of long-term therapy with chlorothiazide. *Circulation, 21,* 21–27.

Dustan, H. P., Tarazi, R. C., & Bravo, E. L. (1972). Dependence of arterial pressure on intravascular volume in treated hypertensive patients. *New England Journal of Medicine, 286,* 861–866.

Esler, M., Zweifler, A., Randall, O., Julius, S., Bennett, J., & Rydelek, P. (1976). Suppression of sympathetic nervous function in low-renin essential hypertension. *Lancet, 2,* 115–118.

Esler, M., Julius, S., Zweifler, A., Randall, O., Harburg, E., Gardiner, H., & DeQuattro, V. (1977). Mild high-renin essential hypertension: Neurogenic human hypertension? *New England Journal of Medicine, 296,* 405–411.

Esler, M., Zweifler, A., Randall, O., & DeQuattro, V. (1977). Pathophysiologic and pharmacokinetic determinants of the antihypertensive response to propranolol. *Clinical Pharmacology and Therapeutics, 22,* 299–308.

Folkow, B. (1982). Physiological aspects of primary hypertension. *Physiological Reviews, 62,* 347–503.

Frohlich, E. D., Tarazi, R. C., Dustan, H. P., & Page, I. H. (1968). The paradox of beta-adrenergic blockade in hypertension. *Circulation, 37,* 417–423.

Hollenberg, N. K., Williams, G. H., & Adams, D. F. (1981). Essential hypertension: Abnormal renal vascular and endocrine responses to a mild psychological stimulus. *Hypertension, 3,* 11–17.

Hollifield, J. W., Sherman, K., VanderZwagg, R., & Shand, D. G. (1976). Proposed mechanisms of propranolol's antihypertensive effects in essential hypertension. *New England Journal of Medicine, 295,* 68–73.

Ibsen, H., Leth, A., Hollnagel, H., Kappelgaard, A. M.,

Damkjaer Nielsen, M., Christensen, N. J., & Giese, J. (1979). Renin angiotensin system and sympathetic nerve activity in mild essential hypertension: The functional significance of angiotensin II in untreated and thiazide treated hypertensive patients. *Acta Medica Scandinavica, 625*(Suppl.), 97.

Julius, S., & Conway, J. (1968). Hemodynamic studies in patients with borderline blood pressure elevation. *Circulation, 38,* 282–288.

Julius, S., Pascual, A. V., Sannerstedt, R., & Mitchell, C. (1971). Relationship between cardiac output and peripheral resistance in borderline hypertension. *Circulation, 43,* 382–390.

Julius, S., Pascual, A. V., Abbrecht, P., & London, R. (1972). Effect of beta-adrenergic blockade on plasma volume in human subjects. *Proceedings of the Society for Experimental Biology and Medicine, 140,* 982–985.

Julius, S., Randall, O. S., Esler, M. D., Kashima, T., Ellis, C. N., & Bennett, J. (1975). Altered cardiac responsiveness and regulation in the normal cardiac output type of borderline hypertension. *Circulation Research, 36–37*(Suppl. I), I-199–I-207.

Laragh, J. H. (1976). Biochemistry of the renin axis; prostaglandins, indomethacin and renin; angiotensin blockade; beta-blockers as antirenin drugs. *American Journal of Medicine, 60,* 733–736.

Light, K. C., Koepke, J. P., Obrist, P. A., & Willis, P. W. (1983). Psychological stress induces sodium and fluid retention in men at high risk for hypertension. *Science, 220,* 429–431.

Lund-Johansen, P. (1967). Hemodynamics in early essential hypertension. *Acta Medica Scandinavica, 482*(Suppl.), 1–105.

Mark, A. L., Lawton, W. J., & Abboud, F. M. (1975). Effects of high and low sodium intake on arterial pressure and forearm vascular resistance in borderline hypertension. *Circulation Research, 36–37*(Suppl. I), I-194–I-198.

Obrist, P. A., Langer, A. W., Light, K., & Koepke, J. P. (1983). Behavioral–cardiac interactions in hypertension. In D. S. Krantz, A. Baum, & J. E. Singer (Eds.), *Handbook of psychology and cardiovascular disorders & behavior:* Vol. 3. *Health.* Hillsdale, NJ: Erlbaum.

Sannerstedt, R., & Julius, S. (1972). Systemic haemodynamics in borderline arterial hypertension: Response to static exercise before and under the influence of propranolol. *Cardiovascular Research, 6,* 398–403.

Sannerstedt, R., Julius, S., & Conway, J. (1970). Hemodynamic response to tilt and beta-adrenergic blockade in young patients with borderline hypertension. *Circulation, 42,* 1057–1064.

Widimsky, J., Fejfarova, M. H., & Fejfar, Z. (1957). Changes of cardiac output in hypertensive disease. *Cardiologia, 31,* 381–389.

Williams, R. B. (1986). Patterns of reactivity and stress. In K. A. Matthews, S. M. Weiss, T. Detre, T. M. Dembroski, B. Falkner, S. B. Manuch, & R. B. Williams (Eds.), *Handbook of stress, reactivity and cardiovascular disease* (pp. 109–125). New York: Wiley–Interscience.

CHAPTER **27**

Constitutional Factors Relating to Differences in Cardiovascular Response

Kathleen C. Light

Introduction

It is a common observation in cardiovascular psychophysiology that individuals differ substantially in their physiological responses at rest and most dramatically during behavioral stressors. For example, one individual may show an increase in heart rate from 60 to 110 beats/min during a mental arithmetic task, while another person shows a much lesser change from 75 to only 80 beats/min. The reasons for these individual differences in response to the same behavioral event are not fully understood, although this topic has been and will continue to be a major research focus in this field. Nonetheless, a number of specific constitutional factors have been shown to contribute to these individual differences in important ways. These factors include age, gender, racial or ethnic group, family history of hypertension, early or borderline hypertension, diabetes, obesity, and aerobic fitness.

The purpose of this chapter is to review the research literature relating each of these factors (excepting gender and racial or ethnic group, which are reviewed in other chapters) to cardiovascular

disease and cardiovascular responses at rest and during stressors. Particular attention will be paid to possible physiological mechanisms that may mediate differences in response, and to possible explanations for any inconsistencies within the literature reviewed. Then, after reviewing and evaluating the available literature, suggested directions for future research to complement and extend the existing findings are described.

Age

The relationship between increasing age and higher levels of resting blood pressure is an established phenomenon in industrialized nations (for reviews, see Epstein & Eckoff, 1967; Kannel, 1976; Genest, LaRochelle, Kuchel, Hamet, & Cantin, 1983). Both mean blood pressure and the incidence of diagnosed hypertension increase from the early adult years throughout the life span. Nonetheless, on an individual basis, an increase in blood pressure with age after adulthood is reached is not a certain occurrence. Longitudinal studies monitoring blood pressure levels in the same individuals over two or three decades have documented that blood pressure levels were unchanged in as many as half the participants studied over this time span (Oberman, Lane, Harlan, Graybiel, &

Kathleen C. Light • Departments of Psychiatry and Physiology, University of North Carolina at Chapel Hill, Chapel Hill, North Carolina 27599.

Mitchell, 1967). In addition, in some nonindustrialized societies, increases in blood pressure with age are the exception rather than the rule (Page, 1980).

Within that subgroup of individuals whose blood pressures do rise in their adult years to reach levels conventionally used to demarcate established hypertension, most theories on etiology assume that the rise occurs slowly and gradually over a period of years. One theory that has influenced the direction of psychophysiological research hypothesizes that an early stage of essential hypertension characterized by a high cardiac output and normal vascular resistance evolves to a later stage in which the blood pressure elevation results from an increase in resistance, while cardiac output levels are now returned to normal. This theory was largely based on cross-sectional comparisons between young adults with borderline hypertension and older persons with mild established hypertension, although some longitudinal data supporting this position were obtained by Birkenhager, Schalekamp, Krauss, Kolsters, and Zaal (1972) and Lund-Johansen (1977). The strongest documentation is the 17-year follow-up of 29 untreated mild hypertensives reported by Lund-Johansen (1983) as a sequel to his original 10-year follow-up. Their resting blood pressures had increased so that only seven still had diastolic pressures less than 100 mm Hg. In terms of hemodynamic changes over time, after 17 years cardiac output levels had continued to decline, while peripheral resistance had progressively increased. Nonetheless, other studies have documented that resistance may be elevated in borderline hypertension in some cases even as soon as early adolescence (Uhari & Paavilainen, 1982). Thus, even though this transition process may sometimes occur, many experts are not convinced that it is true for all or most cases of hypertension. Finally, as detailed by Folkow (1982), the basic mechanisms responsible for this transition are still the subject of considerable theoretical controversy.

A distinct yet not unrelated theory on hypertension development hypothesizes that age-related increases in blood pressure may in part reflect reductions in the density and/or sensitivity of β-adrenergic receptors on the myocardium and the

vasculature. A decrease in density or sensitivity of myocardial β receptors would result in a reduction in heart rate and contractile force for the same level of sympathetic tone, thus lessening cardiac output. In terms of heart rate, the effect of reduced sympathetic receptor sensitivity with age would add to the slowing resulting from age-related decreases in intrinsic heart rate (i.e., the rate at which the denervated heart beats) (Jose, 1966). Concurrently, the reduction in sensitivity of the vascular β-receptors would lessen vasodilation resulting in an increase in total peripheral resistance, unless compensated for by an equivalent decrease in α-adrenergic receptor activity or sensitivity. These age-related changes in sympathetically mediated cardiovascular responses might be even more pronounced under conditions of heightened sympathetic activity, such as exercise and stress.

Cross-sectional studies supporting an age-related diminution of β-adrenoceptor-mediated responses to both agonists and antagonists are numerous (Lakatta, Gerstenblith, Angell, Shock, & Weisfeldt, 1974; Vestal, Wood, & Shand, 1979; Bertel, Buhler, Kiowski, & Lutold, 1980; Buhler et al., 1980; Dillon, Chung, Kelly, & O'Malley, 1980; Fleisch, 1980; van Brummelen, Buhler, Kiowski, & Amann, 1981). The hypothesis was supported for both vascular and myocardial receptors, and consistent evidence was obtained using animal models, hypertensive patients, and normotensive individuals. However, presumably in part to compensate for these sensitivity changes, circulating levels of catecholamines increase with age both at rest (Ziegler, Lake, & Kopin, 1976) and in response to stress (Palmer, Ziegler, & Lake, 1978).

These findings may account for observations that the cardiovascular response pattern to standardized stressors is different in young and older adults, with young adults showing greater heart rate increases and older adults showing greater blood pressure increases (Palmer et al., 1978; Powell, Milligan, & Furchtgott, 1981; Garwood, Engel, & Capriotti, 1982; Faucheux, Dupuis, Baulon, Lille, & Bourliere, 1983). Other studies have failed to confirm an association between increasing age and enhanced blood pressure reactivity to stressors, although the reduction in heart rate response was observed (Steptoe & Ross, 1981; Gintner, Hollandsworth, & Intrieri, 1986). One factor that may have contributed to these apparent inconsistencies is that different age ranges were used. Studies that did not include truly elderly subjects (over age 65) have generally failed to find any increase in blood pressure response with age. The lone exception (Palmer et al., 1978) used the cold pressor test rather than cognitive challenges, suggesting that the type of stressor is another factor that may help account for these differences.

Future psychophysiologic studies in this area should ideally include young, middle-aged, and elderly subject samples, and should employ a variety of stressors, including those evoking primarily increased α-adrenoceptor as well as increased β-adrenoceptor responses. Furthermore, with the increasing availability of impedance cardiography to permit noninvasive evaluation of stroke volume changes during stress, the ideal study should be able not only to evaluate heart rate and blood pressure response differences but also to obtain a full assessment of hemodynamic patterns, including cardiac output and total peripheral resistance changes. These studies might then be followed with additional research into the mechanisms of observed age-related changes in cardiovascular stress responses, including not just the sympathetic nervous system but also possible changes in parasympathetic response (Dauchot & Gravenstein, 1971), left ventricular afterload (Weisfeldt, 1980), factors affecting the working capabilities of cardiac muscle (Lakatta & Yin, 1982), and the vascular smooth muscle cell concentrations of free sodium and calcium (Buhler, 1983).

Family History of Hypertension

A positive family history of hypertension is well established as a risk factor for the development of essential hypertension (for reviews, see Feinleib, 1979; Rapp, 1983; Rose, 1986). Therefore, many researchers concerned with establishing the role of stress reactivity in hypertension development have attempted to document the relationship indirectly by demonstrating that offspring of hypertensive parents show enhanced cardiovascular responses to stressors. A number of these efforts have supported this hypothesis. In 1961, Shapiro first observed that systolic pressure responses were greater in individuals with versus without hypertensive relatives who were hypertensive during several stressors, such as painful injections, the cold pressor test, and the Stroop test. Subsequently, Falkner, Onesti, Angelakos, Fernandes, and Langman (1979) reported that normotensive adolescents with hypertensive parents showed greater heart rate and blood pressure increases during mental arithmetic than did age-mates with normotensive parents, although their blood pressure responses were not as great as in subjects with both borderline hypertension and hypertensive parents. Jorgensen and Houston (1981) similarly found that college students who reported that one parent was hypertensive showed greater heart rate and blood pressure responses to a number of difficult mental challenges as well as in anticipation of and during a digit recall task involving threat of shock. Likewise, Manuck and associates (Manuck, Giordani, McQuaid, & Garrity, 1981; Manuck & Proietti, 1982) found that male college students with hypertensive as compared with normotensive parents showed greater systolic pressure increases to mental tasks and the onset of a handgrip task, while diastolic pressure and heart rate responses did not differ. However, the combination of parental hypertension and high heart reactivity was associated with the most exaggerated blood pressure responses to stress.

In contrast, a number of other investigations have not obtained differences in cardiovascular stress responses between subjects with and without a family history of hypertension (e.g., Remington, Lambarth, Moser, & Hoobler, 1960; Hohn et al., 1983; Obrist, Light, James, & Strogatz, 1987). One explanation offered for the failure to obtain consistent group differences is that different stressors were employed in these studies. Obrist (1981) theorized that more individuals with a positive family history of hypertension may demonstrate myocardial sympathetic hyperreactivity, and so may show enhanced responses to stressors that tend to elicit increased myocardial sympathetic activity (tasks involving active coping/mental work) but not to stressors that elicit primarily increases in vascular sympathetic activity or decreases in parasympathetic activity (like the cold pressor test or isometric exercise). Consistent with this interpretation, Hastrup, Light, and Obrist (1982) found that among 102 normotensive young men, sons of hypertensive parents showed greater heart rate and systolic pressure increases than did sons of normotensive parents to a reaction time task involving threat of shock, but not to the cold pressor test. Also supporting this hypothesis are the results of Ditto (1986), who found that sons of hypertensive parents showed higher systolic responses to mental arithmetic and the Stroop test but not to an isometric handgrip task.

However, even though reactivity differences associated with family hypertension history have been less consistent with the cold pressor and isometric handgrip tasks, negative findings have also been obtained with responses to active coping tasks. For example, Obrist *et al.* (1987) were recently unable to replicate their previous findings of group differences in response to a reaction time task involving threat of shock using a large sample ($N = 183$) of male college students, although sons of hypertensive parents did show higher absolute levels of systolic pressure than did sons of normotensive parents both at rest and during stress. One probable factor behind these inconsistencies may be the multiple etiologies that are subsumed under the category of essential hypertension. Stress and high reactivity may contribute to only some of these forms. Thus, different samples of subjects may or may not exhibit robust relationships between parental hypertension and stress reactivity of the offspring, depending on the proportion of parents whose hypertension was stress-related. However, in addition, Obrist *et al.* (1987) cited the limitations involved in determining from medical histories whether parents are and will continue to be normotensive or hypertensive as the major factor behind the inconsistency of the relationship between parental history and cardiovascular stress reactivity. For college students, many normotensive parents range in age from 35 to 50, and a significant proportion of them may yet become hypertensive. Also, since the parents underwent blood pressure determinations in different

environments and by different physicians, who may differ in the criteria they require to designate a patient as hypertensive, there is considerable room for error variation in this classification. Even more subject to error are studies relying exclusively on reports by the sons or daughters to classify parents as normotensive or hypertensive, since the children may not be fully knowledgeable about their parents' medical status. This lack of knowledge is apparent in cases where the children do not live with both parents, a problem that is more common among lower-income families, but may occur even in intact families.

One solution for obtaining more accurate information on the parents' blood pressure status is represented by the efforts of Matthews, Manuck, and Saab (1986), who utilized the ambitious strategy of performing complete cardiovascular stress studies with both parents and their elementary and high school age children. When the parents have had their blood pressures assessed over a prolonged rest period under controlled conditions, a high degree of confidence in the comparability of blood pressure levels obtained across different individuals is achieved. However, since the conditions of assessment differ from those under which the clinical criterion of 140/90 was established, use of the peak percentiles within each age group (such as the highest 20%) to identify the hypertensive parents may be preferable to using a specific cutoff level. Since each parent will be compared only with those of similar ages in generating percentile rankings, this strategy also diminishes the concern over inappropriately assigning young parents who will become hypertensive later to the normotensive group. However, it does exclude from study the many hypertensives who are on drug treatment, unless they may be temporarily withdrawn from medications prior to the assessment.

Another strategy for dealing with the possible inconsistencies in the designation of hypertension across different physicians is to recruit for study the offspring of parents who share the same physician, or better still, who have all undergone full hypertension assessment under the same systematic program. Other alternatives are certainly possible (e.g., Ohlsson & Henningsen, 1982), and although all of them require additional effort and/or special cooperation with physicians, findings from studies employing these strategies are needed in order to strengthen the literature on cardiovascular stress reactivity and family history of hypertension.

Still another problematic issue in this literature is the concern over interpreting the familial influences on reactivity as genetic versus environmental. The clearest data relating to this issue are from comparisons of cardiovascular stress responses in monozygotic and dizygotic twins. McIlhany, Shaffer, and Hines (1975) demonstrated that intrapair differences in blood pressure responses to the cold pressor test were greater in dizygotic than in monozygotic adolescent twins. Shapiro, Nicotero, Sapira, and Scheib (1968) obtained similar findings for blood pressure responses to the Stroop test and an ischemic pain stimulus. In a more recent study, Hume (1973) reported that although intrapair correlations for heart rate responses to the cold pressor test did not differ between mono- and dizygotic pairs, monozygotic pairs showed much higher correlations in their finger pulse volume responses to this stressor. Altogether these findings suggest a strong genetic basis for cardiovascular stress reactivity, but correlations alone do not provide as effective an evaluation comparing genetic versus environmental models as do other forms of analysis. Carroll, Hewitt, Last, Turner, and Sims (1985) have argued that use of analysis of best fit to weighted least-squares models provides a better assessment of the relative contributions of genetic variation, shared family environment, and individual experience. Their model-fitting procedures supported the position that environmental factors alone cannot account for their obtained data on heart rate responses of subjects aged 16–24 to a challenging video game, and in fact the model closest to the actual data was a model that implicated genetic factors plus individual environmental factors, while minimizing the contribution of shared family environment. However, subsequent research by this same group (Sims, Hewitt, Kelly, Carroll, & Turner, 1986) indicated that the contribution of genetic factors to blood pressure responses appears to be less powerful in middle-aged than in young adults, while both individual and family environmental factors have a greater influ-

ence in determining heart rate responses of this older age group. These results are encouraging, and further efforts along these lines involving evaluation of cardiovascular responses other than heart rate to other stressors in twin pairs from different age groups are needed to expand this growing literature. A preliminary report by Rose, Grim, and Miller (1984), using five different stressors and multiple cardiovascular measures, is representative of the type of investigation that is still needed.

Early or Borderline Hypertension

Although some studies of cardiovascular stress reactivity in patients with established hypertension have shown that these individuals are more responsive to stress than are normotensives (e.g., Shapiro, Moutsos, & Krifcher, 1963), other studies, including the classic invasive studies by Brod, Fencl, and Jirka (1959), have found no differences between hypertensive and normotensive persons in cardiovascular stress responses. However, it has been asserted that once the hypertension is established, secondary adjustments to the pressure elevation may occur, making it more difficult to detect response differences that preceded and contributed to the development of the disorder. Therefore, there has been considerable attention paid to studying cardiovascular stress reactivity in persons with borderline hypertension, who have an increased risk of developing hypertension but who are assumed to show lesser secondary alterations in blood pressure control mechanisms.

The preponderance of evidence available indicates that persons with borderline hypertension do demonstrate exaggerated cardiovascular and neuroendocrine responses to certain stressors. Nestel (1969) reported greater systolic and diastolic pressure increases and greater catecholamine responses to a difficult puzzle-solving task in borderline hypertensives. Jern (1982) observed greater diastolic increases among borderline hypertensives during a mental arithmetic task. In two different studies, Drummond (1983, 1985) found that borderline hypertensive subjects showed greater blood pressure increases during mental arithmetic and postural change than did normotensive subjects, as well as showing greater heart rate increases during task instructions.

The type of stressor as well as the specific cardiovascular measures recorded influence whether borderline hypertensives and normotensives differ in their responses. Steptoe, Melville, and Ross (1984) found that borderline hypertensives show greater heart rate, pulse transit time, and diastolic pressure responses during active coping tasks (Stroop test and video game) but not a passive task (stressful film). Bohlin et al. (1986) found that borderline hypertensives showed greater systolic pressure responses than did normotensives during a self-paced arithmetic task, but the groups did not differ during a more stressful externally paced task. Interestingly, during a 25-min rest period after the tasks, diastolic pressure remained more elevated in the borderline hypertensive group.

Studies in children and adolescents (e.g., Falkner et al., 1979; Lawler & Allen, 1981) have likewise observed that individuals with marginally elevated resting blood pressure tend to be more reactive to stress. However, in general these investigations have used a different method for identifying borderline hypertension. While the studies using adult subjects have typically used blood pressure levels exceeding 140/90 or varying above and below this fixed criterion level to define borderline hypertension, almost no children meet this criterion and so the upper 5% of the blood pressure distribution for that age group is used instead as a cutoff point. This percentile-based definition of borderline hypertension lacks support from some clinicians, but it has distinct advantages in terms of making age-appropriate comparisons.

Another methodological issue that must be considered is that essentially all of the studies relating borderline hypertension to stress reactivity have used a few casual clinical determinations to classify their subjects as normotensive or hypertensive. When such casual determinations are used, it may be that a large proportion of the subjects identified as having elevated resting pressure are simply high reactors to stress whose true resting pressures are not elevated but who are responding to the nonspecific stressful characteristics associated with a clinical examination. Studies by Parati, Pomidossi, Casadei, and Mancia (1985, p. 600) where

blood pressure was recorded continuously using an indwelling catheter have shown that "systolic and diastolic blood pressures increase by an average of 27.0 and 14.0 mmHg respectively when patients undergo a first or second visit by a doctor and that the increases are 12.0 and 6.0 mmHg respectively when the visits are made by a nurse. . . ." Using the logical assumption that most individuals who tend to be high reactors will respond more greatly to the stress of a clinical visit, the use of clinical stethoscopic determinations to define borderline hypertension predetermines that an association will be observed between this trait and high cardiovascular reactivity to stress. The relationship to reactivity might be less robust if the subjects were classified according to blood pressure levels obtained under more controlled restful conditions.

This hypothesis was recently evaluated by Obrist et al. (1987) in a study involving over 180 male college undergraduates. First, two subsamples with elevated resting systolic blood pressure were identified: (1) those in the top 15% of the sample during three casual stethoscopic readings that preceded the stressors and (2) those in the top 15% of the sample after a 15-min rest obtained on a later day when no stressors were scheduled. The results indicated that these two subgroups did not include the same individuals. Also, while the group with high casual stethoscopic pressures did show greater heart rate and systolic pressure responses to a reaction time task and the cold pressor test than did the remaining 85% of the sample, the group with high resting pressures actually tended to show below-average cardiovascular increases during the stressors. These findings reinforce the interpretation that the stressfulness of the conditions under which borderline hypertension is defined is a critical determinant of whether this characteristic is related to high reactivity to laboratory stressors. Conversely, these findings reinforce previous findings that under usual clinical conditions, stethoscopic blood pressure determinations by health professionals constitute a stressor, and the predictive relationship between these readings and later development of hypertension may in part be due to the contribution of cardiovascular stress reactivity. This latter hypothesis was previously supported by the findings of Falkner, Kushner,

Onesti, and Angelakos (1981), demonstrating that borderline hypertensive adolescents who were high cardiovascular reactors to mental stress were more likely to develop fixed hypertension over the next 2–3½ years than were borderline hypertensive persons who showed lesser stress reactivity.

Diabetes

Diabetes mellitus, particularly the more severe form designated as insulin-dependent diabetes, is a powerful risk factor for myocardial infarction and other major cardiovascular disorders. Furthermore, diabetics frequently develop high blood pressure as well, and this combination of hypertension and diabetes carries an even greater risk of serious cardiovascular complications and mortality. Behavioral factors in the form of dietary intake clearly influence the blood glucose levels in both diabetics and nondiabetics. The role of other behavioral influences, such as life stresses, on blood glucose and other physiological responses in diabetics are less well understood.

Blood glucose levels have been found to be elevated in medical students anticipating an exam and surgical patients just before surgery (Sharda, Gupta, & Khuteta, 1975). Furthermore, there is evidence that a proportion of acute ketoacidosis crises in diabetics may have been triggered in part by a psychologically stressful event (Nabarro, 1965). Thus, until quite recently, the prevailing view among health professionals was that acute psychological stress universally leads to increases in blood glucose, particularly in diabetic patients. However, when the research literature was reviewed by Lustman, Carney, and Amado (1981), there appeared to be no firm support for this assumption and in fact there was some evidence that diabetics may show decreases in blood sugar following stress. Using a better controlled design, Carter, Gonder-Frederick, Cox, Clarke, and Scott (1985) evaluated blood glucose response to mental arithmetic (active) and noise (passive) stressors in insulin-dependent diabetics on two occasions 12 weeks apart. They found that the active arithmetic stressor led to greater changes in blood glucose than did the passive noise stressor. Both the direc-

tion and magnitude of change differed markedly among the individual patients, with some patients showing a hyperglycemic and others a hypoglycemic response, but these individual differences in stress responses were stable over time.

Stabler, Morris, et al. (1986) and Stabler, Surwit, et al. (1986) extended these findings on individual differences in diabetic patients in a study in which diabetic children were exposed to a competitive video game. They found that children identified by their teachers as Type A showed hyperglycemic responses to the stressor, while those classified as Type B showed hypoglycemic responses. Interestingly, both the Type A and Type B diabetic children showed similar elevations in heart rate and blood pressure responses during the task.

Cardiovascular responses to behavioral and physical stressors were evaluated in diabetics and nondiabetics with and without hypertension as long ago as 1963 by Shapiro, Moutsos, and Krifcher. The diabetic patients were found to show greater blood pressure increases to angiotensin infusion, intravenous saline injection, and the Stroop test, but were less responsive to the cold pressor test than was the nondiabetic normotensive group. These authors suggested that the increased response to angiotensin paired with the decreased cold pressor response reflected greater sympathetic denervation of arterioles which tends to increase the sensitivity of the understimulated sympathetic receptors to humoral influences. The modestly enhanced response to the saline injection and Stroop test might then be attributed to increased sensitivity of receptors to circulating catecholamines, even though the effects resulting from direct sympathetic innervation of vascular structures would be reduced.

More recently, investigators have begun to study cardiovascular responses to stress among different subgroups of diabetics, trying to assess what factors might influence why these responses, like blood glucose responses, varied widely across individuals. Kemmer et al. (1986) addressed the issue of individual differences in stress responses among diabetics by grouping their patients according to whether they were acutely in good or poor metabolic control, with the latter achieved by withholding their usual morning insulin. They found that blood glucose, heart rate, and blood pressure responses to mental arithmetic and public speaking stressors did not differ as a function of the acute state of metabolic control, but that plasma epinephrine responses to stress were greater in diabetics who had received insulin than in those who had not or in nondiabetic controls.

Kraemer (1985) addressed the issue of chronic metabolic control and reactivity in 56 adolescent diabetics, using the glycosylated hemoglobin test as an index. Her results showed that subjects chronically in poor control had higher blood glucose levels before and during a series of stressors, as well as a trend toward higher heart rate responses to the stressor. However, another factor, time since diagnosis, was even more strongly related to stress responses among these adolescents. Those subjects who had been diabetic for 7 years or more showed greater heart rate and blood pressure responses to the stressors, after covariance adjustment for age differences. These greater cardiovascular responses to stress could reflect changes that may contribute to the onset of an associated hypertension.

Cox et al. (1984) also used glycosylated hemoglobin to estimate long-term blood glucose control, and they found that this measure was related to the number of daily hassles experienced by their 50 adult diabetic patients, but not to Type A behavior. Unfortunately, no acute stress responses were evaluated in this study. However, they did obtain evidence that the patients themselves generally perceived life stressors to significantly affect their blood glucose control, and they obtained self-report data on emotional responses to stress that suggested that some stressors typically increase blood glucose while other stressors decrease it. No direct evidence confirming this suggestion is now available, but this is an interesting hypothesis for future research to address.

The physiological mechanisms which may mediate differences in cardiovascular responses at rest and during stress among diabetics are unclear, but in addition to the denervation–hypersensitivity hypothesis proposed by Shapiro et al. (1963), another potential mechanism is via the effects of insulin on the kidneys and on sympathetically medi-

ated vascular response. DeFronzo, Goldberg, and Agus (1976) have demonstrated that insulin increases tubular reabsorption of sodium by the kidneys, which could increase blood pressure by increasing blood volume and/or by enhancing vascular resistance responses to sympathetic stimulation. In addition, Young and Landsberg (1982) have reviewed evidence that dietary changes inducing altered insulin release led to corresponding changes in sympathetic activity even in nondiabetic patients and without evidence of hypoglycemia. They first detailed data from human and animal studies showing that decreased food intake leads to reduced blood pressure while increased ingestion of food or glucose produces a rise in plasma norepinephrine and increased blood pressure. Then, they cited their previous work using the glucose clamp technique together with 2 hr insulin and glucose infusions in order to separate the effects of these two factors. It was shown that increased glucose levels without increased insulin had no effect on norepinephrine or cardiovascular activity, while increased insulin led to pronounced signs of enhanced sympathetic activity. Clearly, this type of enhanced sympathetic activity could contribute to increased cardiovascular responses at rest and during stress, such as Kraemer (1985) observed in her diabetic subjects. Finally, another important study by Weidmann et al. (1979) in 17 diabetic patients with borderline hypertension revealed that these patients had an enhanced blood pressure increase to infusions of norepinephrine and angiotensin, replicating and extending Shapiro and associates' (1963) previous suggestion of increased adrenergic receptor sensitivity. These pressor responses (which may parallel responses to endogenous norepinephrine elicited by certain stressors) were attenuated following diuretic therapy which reduced previously elevated levels of exchangeable body sodium.

The study of physiological responses to stress in diabetics is a comparatively young area, and there are many directions which appear productive ones for future research. One direction is to employ Type A/B as a grouping factor in studies of blood glucose responses to stress in adults. Additionally, other personality factors (e.g., suppressed anger) may also be related to response patterns in diabetics. Another research direction would be to compare cardiovascular responses to stress in young borderline hypertensive versus diabetic patients, and to compare the effectiveness of β-receptor antagonists versus diuretic therapy in reducing the cardiovascular responses of the two diagnostic groups. Still another direction would be to use studies of stress-induced alterations in sodium and fluid excretion rates in animal models similar to those described by Koepke, Light, and Obrist (1983) and Koepke and DiBona (1985) comparing sodium and fluid retention in repeated studies with and without injection of insulin. These latter studies would reveal indications about mediating mechanisms, and would also have important implications for preventive intervention strategies. Finally, since biofeedback, relaxation training, and similar stress reduction training have been shown to improve glucose tolerance and aid in metabolic control in some diabetic patients (Fowler, Budzynski, & Vandenbergh, 1976; Seburg & DeBoer, 1980; Surwit & Feinglos, 1983), it is also important for future research to evaluate whether personality dimensions, acute stress reactivity measures, and measure of life hassles or stresses may, alone or in combination, be useful predictors of which patients may benefit most from this type of behavioral training.

Obesity

The association between obesity and hypertension is well established (Chiang, Perlman, & Epstein, 1969), and both characteristics are associated with a greater risk of coronary heart disease. The results of the Framingham Study indicated that obese individuals had eight times the risk of developing hypertension as did low and normal weight persons, while the risk of developing more severe cardiovascular disorders was ten times as great (Kannel, Brand, Skinner, Dawber, & McNamara, 1967). Furthermore, the relationship between obesity and hypertension is as true for children and adolescents as for adults (Berchtold, Jorgens, Finke, & Berger, 1981).

A number of different mechanisms have been proposed to explain why the obese tend to become

hypertensive. Most of these theories relate to sodium handling, or to the effects of insulin, or both. Excess sodium can contribute to hypertension by several mechanisms, including expansion of circulating blood volume and cardiac output, changes in the structure and reactivity of vascular smooth muscle cells to sympathetic activity, and enhancement of general sympathetic activity. One hypothesis is that sodium intake has increased along with caloric intake (Ellison et al., 1980). Another hypothesis is that the cellular sodium transport mechanisms are altered in the obese, leading to increased sodium concentration in the arteriolar smooth muscle cells (DeLuise, Blackburn, & Flier, 1980). Another hypothesis is that aldosterone secretion is maintained at inappropriately high levels in the obese, thus enhancing sodium retention (Hiramatsu, Yamada, Ichikawa, Izumiyama, & Nagata, 1981). Finally, a currently prominent hypothesis involves the increase in insulin levels that occurs in obesity. As previously described in the discussion of diabetes, increased circulating insulin has been shown to result in increased plasma norepinephrine and sympathetic myocardial activity, and also enhances renal sodium reabsorption (Young & Landsberg, 1982; DeFronzo et al., 1976). Furthermore, Pereda, Eckstein, and Abboud (1962) have shown that insulin injections could induce transient hypertension in dogs that was minimized following adrenergic or ganglionic blockade, confirming the role of the sympathetic nervous system in mediating insulin-related rises in blood pressure. Since many behavioral stressors have been shown to enhance α- and/or β-adrenergic activity, these observations are particularly exciting for researchers in cardiovascular behavioral medicine.

Even in the absence of concurrent hypertension, obesity necessarily induces a dramatic change in hemodynamic pattern. As described by Messerli (1986, pp. 378–379): "Any increase in body mass (be it adipose or muscular tissue) requires a higher cardiac output and expanded intravascular volume to meet the higher metabolic demands. . . . Since heart rate remains unchanged when a person becomes obese, the increase in cardiac output occurs by means of an expanded stroke volume . . . [and] the myocardium adapts by adding contractile elements. Thus, the myocardial mass increases and left ventricular hypertrophy of the eccentric type (wall thickening and chamber dilatation) ensues.'' Recently, MacMahon, Wilcken, and MacDonald (1986) demonstrated that weight reduction in young obese patients can reverse this left ventricular hypertrophy as well as reduce blood pressure. These researchers estimate that only 25% of the reduction in myocardial mass was associated immediately and directly with the change in body weight. They hypothesized that other important contributing factors included reductions in myocardial sympathetic activity, and lower plasma renin activity and aldosterone, each of which has individually been implicated in the development of left ventricular hypertrophy. The influence of sympathetic and neurohumoral factors on the myocardium may be even more pronounced during exposure to stressors, suggesting important opportunities for behaviorally oriented research.

In spite of this association between obesity and enhanced sympathetic activity, the literature on stress reactivity in obese subjects is extremely limited. The work by Falkner, Onesti, and Angelakos (1981) showing enhanced cardiovascular reactivity to mental arithmetic in adolescents with hypertensive parents mentioned that this group tended to be more obese than their age-mates with normotensive parents. Recent studies by Putnam and Rennert (1984) demonstrated that obese women tend to show phasic heart rate acceleration in response to visual stimuli that evoked predominantly deceleration in normal weight women, and that heart rate increases during mental arithmetic were greater among the obese sample.

There is obviously considerable room for further psychophysiologic investigations of stress responses to the obese. Furthermore, the possibility that sympathetic activity is enhanced in this diagnostic group strongly encourages such investigations. Among the many possibilities, it would be exciting to evaluate blood pressure, cardiac output, and peripheral resistance changes during several different types of stressors in obese and normal weight subjects, both with and without β- and/or α-adrenergic blockade. Also, since the obesity and borderline hypertension are associated in adolescents, it would be interesting to compare car-

diovascular responses to stress in obese normotensive versus obese borderline hypertensive versus normal weight subjects. Finally, studies varying dietary salt intake could be performed in obese and normal weight groups, and their cardiovascular stress responses after high, normal, and low sodium diets could be compared.

Aerobic Exercise/Fitness

It is well established that aerobic exercise training induces significant changes in myocardial function. The most commonly reported myocardial effect of training is a slowed resting heart rate. In addition, other effects reported following exercise training are increased stroke volume and increased maximal oxygen consumption. The mechanisms responsible for these myocardial adaptations have not been fully determined, but they include a reduction in resting sympathetic activity, an increase in parasympathetic activity, as well as a decrease in the intrinsic heart rate (see Scheuer & Tipton, 1977).

Resting blood pressure has been shown in cross-sectional studies to average 2–5 mm Hg lower in physically active versus inactive persons (see Siscovick, LaPorte, & Newman, 1985). Also, the incidence of hypertension is lower among persons who have been habitually more physically active and who are currently higher in physical fitness (Paffenbarger, Wing, Hyde, & Jung, 1983; Blair, Goodyear, Gibbons, & Cooper, 1984). In addition to helping to prevent hypertension, certain studies have documented that exercise training may be an effective treatment to reduce elevated blood pressure in some individuals (see Kenney & Zambraski, 1984). Reductions in blood pressure with training have been obtained in hypertensive adolescents (Hagberg et al., 1983) and in borderline hypertensives (Choquette & Ferguson, 1973; Kukkonen, Rauramaa, Voutilainen, & Lansimies, 1982). One recent study reported that training led to greater pressure reductions in individuals with high resting plasma catecholamines and that the magnitude of pressure reduction following training was directly correlated with reduction in catecholamine levels (Duncan, Hagan, Upton, Farr, &

Oglesby, 1983). It has also been reported that training leads to increased sensitivity to β-adrenergic stimulation, which may result from a general decrease in sympathetic activity (Krotkiewski *et al.*, 1983). Altogether, these findings suggest that cardiovascular changes resulting from exercise training in part reflect alterations in the function of the sympathetic nervous system.

A number of studies have investigated the hypothesis that aerobic exercise training may also be associated with a decrease in sympathetically mediated cardiovascular responses to behavioral stress. Hull, Young, and Ziegler (1984) observed that among persons older than 40, more fit subjects showed lesser diastolic pressure increases during several stressors, but no reduction in heart rate or systolic pressure increases. Furthermore, more and less fit subjects under age 40 did not differ in their cardiovascular reactivity. Other studies using young adults as participants also failed to demonstrate any differences in heart rate responses to stressful mental tasks in more fit versus less fit male subjects, although greater aerobic fitness was associated with more rapid recovery of heart rate following the tasks (Cantor, Zillman, & Day, 1978; Cox, Evans, & Jamieson, 1979; Sinyor, Schwartz, Peronnet, Brisson, & Seraganian, 1983). However, one study (Holmes & Roth, 1985) indicated that highly fit young women showed smaller heart rate responses to a memory challenge than did less fit women. Also, our laboratory (Light, Obrist, James, & Strogatz, 1987) recently observed that male college students reporting high levels of weekly aerobic exercise demonstrated lesser heart rate, systolic pressure, and preejection period responses to a pseudo-shock avoidance reaction time task than did low-exercise subjects, although responses to the cold pressor test did not differ reliably among exercise groups. Thus, both the age of the subjects and the nature of the stressor may be factors that help explain the inconsistencies in this area of research.

None of the previously described investigations directly compared the effects of an aerobic training program of known intensity and duration upon the stress responses of the same individuals. With only correlational data available, the relationship between exercise training and reduced cardiovascular stress reactivity cannot be firmly established. It is equally possible that those subjects who were more reactive to stress had chosen to avoid or reduce their exercise for reasons related to personality traits (e.g., Type A or high anger inhibition), time commitments, conditioned avoidance of any situation that evokes pressor responses, or other undefined factors. Recently, however, Sinyor, Golden, Steinert, and Seraganian (1986) completed an investigation evaluating heart rate responses to mental challenges in 38 men under age 30 before and after a 10-week period of either aerobic or weight training. Neither form of exercise training reduced heart rate responses during the stressors, but aerobic training was associated with faster heart rate recovery after the stressors. A previous study by Keller and Seraganian (1984) yielded a similar finding regarding recovery in electrodermal responses. However, these studies each employed only a single physiological measure, which limits their significance. Further investigations utilizing blood pressure and other cardiovascular measures when directly evaluating the effects of training on the stress responses of a broader class of subjects, including women, older men, and persons with borderline hypertension, are still needed. Studies in the latter group are particularly appropriate since borderline hypertension is associated with high cardiovascular stress reactivity and also because exercise training has been shown to reduce stress-induced hypertension in the borderline hypertensive rat model (Cox, Hubbard, Lawler, Sanders, & Mitchell, 1985). Also, whenever reductions in cardiovascular stress responses due to exercise training are documented, further studies using more direct evaluation of sympathetic mediation of responses (such as through use of sympathetic agonists and antagonists) are needed to verify whether these changes are a result of altered sympathetic nervous system function. Other physiological contributions should also be evaluated, including enhanced parasympathetic tone, changes in the vascular microcirculation, alterations in the control of body fluid volume and sodium balance, altered baroreceptor function, altered release of insulin, and modulation in the activity of the body's endogenous opiates (Kenney & Zambraski, 1984; Hutchins & Darnell, 1974). Another issue that should be addressed in future research is whether exercise training is associated with alterations in personality or behavioral traits, and whether such traits may be useful predictors of who is most likely to benefit from such a physical training program.

References

Berchtold, P., Jorgens, V., Finke, C., & Berger, M. (1981). Epidemioiogy of obesity and hypertension. *International Journal of Obesity, 5*, 1–7.

Bertel, O., Buhler, F. R., Kiowski, W., & Lutold, B. (1980). Decreased beta-adrenoceptor responsiveness as related to age, blood pressure and plasma catecholamines in patients with essential hypertension. *Hypertension, 2*, 130–138.

Birkenhager, W. H., Schalekamp, M. A. D. H., Krauss, X. H., Kolsters, G., & Zaal, G. A. (1972). Consecutive haemodynamic patterns in essential hypertension. *Lancet, 1*, 560–564.

Blair, S. N., Goodyear, N. N., Gibbons, L. W., & Cooper, K. H. (1984). Physical fitness and incidence of hypertension in healthy normotensive men and women. *Journal of the American Medical Association, 252*, 487–490.

Bohlin, G., Eliasson, K., Hjemdahl, P., Klein, K., Fredrikson, M., & Frankenhaeuser, M. (1986). Personal control over work pace—Circulatory, neuroendocrine and subjective responses in borderline hypertension. *Journal of Hypertension, 4*, 295–305.

Brod, J., Fencl, V., Hejl, Z., & Jirka, J. (1959). Circulatory changes underlying blood pressure elevation during acute emotional stress (mental arithmetic) in normotensive and hypertensive subjects. *Clinical Science, 18*, 269–279.

Buhler, F. R. (1983). Age and cardiovascular response adaptation. *Hypertension, 5*(Suppl. III), III-94–III-100.

Buhler, F. R., Kiowski, W., van Brummelen, P., Amann, F. W., Bertel, O., Landmann, R., Lutold, B. E., & Bolli, P. (1980). Plasma catecholamines and cardiac, renal and peripheral vascular adrenoreceptor-mediated responses in different age groups of normal and hypertensive subjects. *Clinical and Experimental Hypertension, 2*, 409–421.

Cantor, J. R., Zillman, D., & Day, K. D. (1978). Relationship between cardiorespiratory fitness and physiological responses to films. *Perceptual and Motor Skills, 46*, 1123–1130.

Carroll, D., Hewitt, J. K., Last, K. A., Turner, J. R., & Sims, J. (1985). A twin study of cardiac reactivity and its relationship to parental blood pressure. *Physiology and Behavior, 34*, 103–106.

Carter, W. R., Gonder-Frederick, L. A., Cox, D. J., Clarke, W. L., & Scott, D. (1985). Effect of stress on blood glucose in IDDM. *Diabetes Care, 8*, 411–412.

Chiang, B. N., Perlman, I. V., & Epstein, F. H. (1969). Over-weight and hypertension: A review. *Circulation, 39*, 403–421.

Choquette, C., & Ferguson, R. J. (1973). Blood pressure reduction in "borderline" hypertensives following physical training. *Canadian Medical Association Journal, 108*, 699–703.

Cox, D. J., Taylor, A. G., Nowacek, G., Holley-Wilcox, P., Pohl, S. L., & Guthrow, E. (1984). The relationship between psychological stress and insulin-dependent diabetic blood glucose control: Preliminary investigations. *Health Psychology, 3*, 63–75.

Cox, J. P., Evans, J. F., & Jamieson, J. L. (1979). Aerobic power and tonic heart rate responses to psychosocial stressors. *Personality and Social Psychology Bulletin, 5*, 160–163.

Cox, R. H., Hubbard, J. W., Lawler, J. E., Sanders, B. J., & Mitchell, V. P. (1985). Exercise training attenuates stress-induced hypertension in the rat. *Hypertension, 7*, 747–751.

Dauchot, P., & Gravenstein, J. S. (1971). Effects of atropine on the electrocardiogram in different age groups. *Clinical Pharmacology and Therapeutics, 12*, 274–280.

DeFronzo, R. A., Goldberg, M., & Agus, Z. S. (1976). The effects of glucose and insulin on renal electrolyte transport. *Journal of Clinical Investigation, 58*, 83–90.

DeLuise, M., Blackburn, C. L., & Flier, J. S. (1980). Reduced activity of the red cell sodium potassium pump in human obesity. *New England Journal of Medicine, 303*, 1017–1022.

Dillon, N., Chung, S., Kelly, J., & O'Malley, K. (1980). Age and beta-adrenoceptor-mediated function. *Clinical Pharmacology and Therapeutics, 37*, 769–772.

Ditto, B. (1986). Parental history of essential hypertension, active coping and cardiovascular reactivity. *Psychophysiology, 23*, 62–70.

Drummond, P. D. (1983). Cardiovascular reactivity in mild hypertension. *Journal of Psychosomatic Research, 27*, 291–297.

Drummond, P. D. (1985). Cardiovascular reactivity in borderline hypertensives during behavioral and orthostatic stress. *Psychophysiology, 22*, 626–628.

Duncan, J. J., Hagan, R. D., Upton, J., Farr, J. E., & Oglesby, M. D. (1983). The effects of an aerobic exercise program on sympathetic neural activity and blood pressure in mild hypertensive patients. *Circulation, 68*, II-285 (Abstract).

Ellison, R. C., Sosenko, J. M., Harper, G. P., Gibbons, J., Pratter, F. E., & Miettinen, O. S. (1980). Obesity, sodium intake and blood pressure in adolescents. *Hypertension, 2*(Suppl. I), I-78–I-82.

Epstein, F. H., & Eckoff, R. D. (1967). The epidemiology of high blood pressure—Geographic distributions and etiological factors. In J. Stamler, R. Stamler, & T. N. Pullman (Eds.), *The epidemiology of hypertension* (pp. 155–166). New York: Grune & Stratton.

Falkner, B., Onesti, G., Angelakos, E. T., Fernandes, M., & Langman, C. (1979). Cardiovascular response to mental stress in normal adolescents with hypertensive parents: Hemodynamics and mental stress in adolescents. *Hypertension, 1,* 23–30.

Falkner, B., Kushner, H., Onesti, G., & Angelakos, E. T. (1981). Cardiovascular characteristics in adolescents who develop hypertension. *Hypertension, 3,* 521–527.

Falkner, B., Onesti, G., & Angelakos, E. T. (1981). Effect of salt loading on the cardiovascular response to stress in adolescents. *Hypertension, 3* (Suppl. II), II-195–II-199.

Faucheux, B. A., Dupuis, C., Baulon, A., Lille, F., & Bourliere, F. (1983). Heart rate reactivity during minor mental stress in men in their 50s and 70s. *Gerontology, 29,* 149–160.

Feinleib, M. (1979). Genetics and familial aggregation of blood pressure. In G. Onesti & C. R. Klimt (Eds.), *Hypertension: Determinants, complications and intervention* (pp. 35–48). New York: Grune & Stratton.

Fleisch, J. H. (1980). Age-related changes in the sensitivity of blood vessels to drugs. *Pharmacology and Therapeutics, 8,* 477–487.

Folkow, B. (1982). Physiological aspects of primary hypertension. *Physiological Reviews, 62,* 347–504.

Fowler, J. E., Budzynski, T. H., & Vandenbergh, R. L. (1976). Effects of an EMG biofeedback relaxation program on the control of diabetes. *Biofeedback and Self-Regulation, 1,* 105–112.

Garwood, M., Engel, B. T., & Capriotti, R. (1982). Autonomic nervous system function and aging: Response specificity. *Psychophysiology, 10,* 378–385.

Genest, J., LaRochelle, P., Kuchel, O., Hamet, P., & Cantin, M. (1983). Hypertension in the elderly: Athero-arteriosclerotic hypertension. In J. Genest, O. Kuchel, P. Hamet, & M. Cantin (Eds.), *Hypertension: Physiopathology and treatment* (2nd ed., pp. 913–992). New York: McGraw–Hill.

Gintner, G. G., Hollandsworth, J. G., & Intrieri, R. C. (1986). Age differences in cardiovascular reactivity under active coping conditions. *Psychophysiology, 23,* 113–120.

Hagberg, J. M., Goldring, D., Ehsani, A. A., Heath, G. W., Hernandez, A., Schectman, K., & Holloszy, J. O. (1983). Effect of exercise training on the blood pressure and hemodynamic features of hypertensive adolescents. *American Journal of Cardiology, 52,* 763–768.

Hastrup, J. L., Light, K. C., & Obrist, P. A. (1982). Parental hypertension and cardiovascular response to stress in healthy young adults. *Psychophysiology, 19,* 615–622.

Hiramatsu, K., Yamada, T., Ichikawa, K., Izumiyama, T., & Nagata, H. (1981). Changes in endocrine activities relative to obesity in patients with essential hypertension. *Journal of the American Geriatrics Society, 29,* 25–30.

Hohn, A. R., Riopel, D. A., Keil, J. E., Loadhott, C. B., Margolius, H. S., Halushka, P. V., Privitera, P. J., Webb, J. G., Medley, E. S., Schuman, S. H., Rubin, M. I., Pantell, R. H., & Braunstein, M. L. (1983). Childhood familial and racial differences in physiologic and biochemical factors related to hypertension. *Hypertension, 5,* 56–70.

Holmes, D. S., & Roth, D. L. (1985). Association of aerobic fitness with pulse rate and subjective responses to psychological stress. *Psychophysiology, 22,* 525–529.

Hull, E. M., Young, S. H., & Ziegler, M. G. (1984). Aerobic fitness affects cardiovascular and catecholamine responses to stressors. *Psychophysiology, 21,* 353–360.

Hume, W. I. (1973). Physiological measures in twins. In G. Claridge, S. Canter, & W. I. Hume (Eds.), *Personality differences and biological variations: A study of twins* (pp. 87–114). Oxford: Pergamon Press.

Hutchins, P. M., & Darnell, A. E. (1974). Observation of a decreased number of small arterioles in spontaneously hypertensive rats. *Circulation Research, 34–35*(Suppl. I), I-161–I-165.

Jern, S. (1982). Psychological and hemodynamic factors in borderline hypertension. *Acta Medica Scandinavica Supplementum, 662,* 7–55.

Jorgensen, R. S., & Houston, B. K. (1981). Family history of hypertension, gender and cardiovascular reactivity and stereotype during stress. *Journal of Behavioral Medicine, 4,* 175–189.

Jose, A. D. (1966). Effect of combined sympathetic and parasympathetic blockade on heart rate and cardiac function in man. *American Journal of Cardiology, 18,* 476–478.

Kannel, W. B. (1976). Blood pressure and the development of cardiovascular disease in the aged. In F. I. Caird, J. L. C. Dall, & R. D. Kennedy (Eds.), *Cardiology in old age.* New York: Plenum Press.

Kannel, W. B., Brand, N., Skinner, J. J., Dawber, T. R., & McNamara, P. M. (1967). The relation of adiposity to blood pressure and development of hypertension. *Annals of Internal Medicine, 67,* 48–59.

Keller, S., & Seraganian, T. (1984). Physical fitness and autonomic reactivity to psychosocial stress. *Journal of Psychosomatic Research, 28,* 279–281.

Kemmer, F. W., Bisping, R., Steingruber, H. J., Baar, H., Hardtmann, F., Schlaghecke, R., & Berger, M. (1986). Psychological stress and metabolic control in patients with Type I diabetes mellitus. *New England Journal of Medicine, 314,* 1078–1084.

Kenney, W. K., & Zambraski, E. J. (1984). Physical activity in human hypertension: A mechanisms approach. *Sports Medicine, 1,* 459–473.

Koepke, J., & DiBona, G. (1985). High sodium intake enhances renal nerve and antinatriuretic responses to stress in spontaneously hypertensive rats. *Hypertension, 7,* 357–363.

Koepke, J., Light, K. C., & Obrist, P. A. (1983). Neural control of renal excretory function during behavioral stress in conscious dogs. *American Journal of Physiology, 245,* R251–R258.

Kraemer, D. (1985). Autonomic nervous system reactivity to stress in adolescent insulin-dependent diabetics. *Psychophysiology, 22,* 573–574 (Abstract).

Krotkiewski, M., Mandroukas, K., Morgan, L., William-Olsson, T., Feurle, G. E., von Schneck, H., Bjorntop, P., Sjostrom, L., & Smith, U. (1983). Effects of physical training on adrenergic sensitivity in obesity. *Journal of Applied Physiology, 55,* 1811–1817.

Kukkonen, K., Rauramaa, R., Voutilainen, E., & Lansimies, E. (1982). Physical training of middle-aged men with borderline hypertension. *Annals of Clinical Research, 14*(Suppl. 34), 139–145.

Lakatta, E. G., & Yin, F. C. P. (1982). Myocardial aging: Functional alterations and related cellular mechanisms. *American Journal of Physiology, 242,* H927–H941.

Lakatta, E. G., Gerstenblith, G., Angell, C. S., Shock, N. W., & Weisfeldt, M. L. (1974). Diminished ionotropic response of aged myocardium to catecholamines. *Circulation Research, 36,* 262–269.

Lawler, K. A., & Allen, M. T. (1981). Risk factors for hypertension in children: Their relationship to psychophysiological responses. *Journal of Psychosomatic Research, 23,* 199–204.

Light, K. C., Obrist, P. A., James, S. A., & Strogatz, D. (1987). Cardiovascular response to stress. II. Relationships to aerobic exercise patterns. *Psychophysiology, 24,* 79–86.

Lund-Johansen, P. (1977). Central haemodynamics in essential hypertension. *Acta Medica Scandinavica Supplementum, 606,* 35–42.

Lund-Johansen, P. (1983). Haemodynamics in early essential hypertension—still an area of controversy. *Journal of Hypertension, 1,* 209–213.

Lustman, P., Carney, R., & Amado, H. (1981). Acute stress and metabolism in diabetes. *Diabetes Care, 4,* 658–659.

MacMahon, S. W., Wilcken, D. E. L., & MacDonald, G. J. (1986). The effect of weight reduction on ventricular mass: A randomized controlled trial in young, overweight hypertensive patients. *New England Journal of Medicine, 314,* 334–339.

Manuck, S. B., & Proietti, J. M. (1982). Parental hypertension and cardiovascular response to cognitive and isometric challenge. *Psychophysiology, 19,* 481–489.

Manuck, S. B., Giordani, B., McQuaid, K. J., & Garrity, S. J. (1981). Behaviorally-induced cardiovascular reactivity among sons of reported hypertensive and normotensive parents. *Journal of Psychosomatic Research, 25,* 261–269.

Matthews, K. A., Manuck, S. B., & Saab, P. D. (1986). Predictors of cardiovascular responses to a naturally occurring stressor: Characteristics of the reactive adolescent during public speaking. *Psychophysiology, 23,* 198–209.

McIlhany, M. L., Shaffer, J. W., & Hines, E. A., Jr. (1975). Heritability of blood pressure: An investigation of 200 pairs of twins using the cold pressor test. *Johns Hopkins Medical Journal, 136,* 57–64.

Messerli, F. H. (1986). Cardiopathy of obesity: A not-so-Victorian disease. *New England Journal of Medicine, 314,* 378–380.

Nabarro, J. D. N. (1965). Diabetic acidosis: Clinical aspects. *Excerpta Medica International Congress Series, 84,* 545–557.

Nestel, P. J. (1969). Blood pressure and catecholamine excretion after mental stress in labile hypertension. *Lancet, 1,* 692–694.

Oberman, A., Lane, N. E., Harlan, W. R., Graybiel, A., & Mitchell, R. E. (1967). Trends in systolic blood pressure in the thousand aviator cohort over a twenty-four year period. *Circulation, 36,* 812–822.

Obrist, P. A. (1981). *Cardiovascular psychophysiology: A perspective* (pp. 141–181). New York: Plenum Press.

Obrist, P. A., Light, K. C., James, S. A., & Strogatz, D. S. (1987). Cardiovascular responses to stress. I. Measures of myocardial response and relationships to high resting systolic pressure and parental hypertension. *Psychophysiology, 24,* 65–78.

Ohlsson, O., & Henningsen, N. C. (1982). Blood pressure, cardiac output and systemic vascular resistance during rest, muscle work, cold pressor test and psychological stress: A study of male offspring from families with a history of essential hypertension for at least two generations. *Acta Medica Scandinavica, 212,* 329–336.

Paffenbarger, R. S., Wing, A. L., Hyde, R. T., & Jung, D. L. (1983). Physical activity and incidence of hypertension in college alumni. *American Journal of Epidemiology, 117,* 245–256.

Page, L. B. (1980). Hypertension and atherosclerosis in primitive and acculturating societies. In J. C. Hunt (Ed.), *Hypertension update: Mechanisms, epidemiology, evaluation and management* (pp. 1–12). Bloomfield, NJ: Health Learning Systems.

Palmer, G. J., Ziegler, M. G., & Lake, C. R. (1978). Response of norepinephrine and blood pressure to stress increases with age. *Journal of Gerontology, 33,* 482–487.

Parati, G., Pomidossi, G., Casadei, R., & Mancia, G. (1985). Lack of alerting reactions to intermittent cuff inflations during noninvasive blood pressure monitoring. *Hypertension, 7,* 597–601.

Pereda, S. A., Eckstein, J. W., & Abboud, F. M. (1962). Cardiovascular responses to insulin in the absence of hypoglycemia. *American Journal of Physiology, 202,* 249–252.

Powell, D. A., Milligan, W. L., & Furchtgott, E. (1981). Peripheral autonomic changes accompany learning and reaction time performance in older people. *Journal of Gerontology, 36,* 57–65.

Putnam, L. E., & Rennert, M. P. (1984). Effects of obesity on autonomic responding in a mental arithmetic task. *Psychophysiology, 21,* 594 (Abstract).

Rapp, J. P. (1983). Genetics of experimental and human hypertension. In J. Genest, O. Kuchel, P. Hamet, & M. Cantin (Eds.), *Hypertension: Physiopathology and treatment* (2nd ed., pp. 582–598). New York: McGraw–Hill.

Remington, R. D., Lambarth, B., Moser, M., & Hoobler, S. E. (1960). Circulatory reactions of normotensive and hypertensive subjects and of the children of normotensive and hypertensive parents. *American Heart Journal, 59,* 58–70.

Rose, R. J. (1986). Familial influences on cardiovascular reactivity to stress. In K. A. Matthews, S. M. Weiss, T. Detre, T. M. Dembroski, B. Falkner, S. B. Manuck, & R. B. Williams (Eds.), *Handbook of stress, reactivity and cardiovascular disease* (pp. 259–272). New York: Wiley.

Rose, R. J., Grim, C. E., & Miller, J. Z. (1984). Familial

influences on cardiovascular stress reactivity: Studies of normotensive twins. *Behavioral Medicine Update, 6,* 21–24.

Scheuer, J., & Tipton, C. M. (1977). Cardiovascular adaptations to physical training. *Annual Reviews of Physiology, 39,* 221–251.

Seburg, K. N., & DeBoer, K. F. (1980). Effects of EMG biofeedback on diabetes. *Biofeedback and Self-Regulation, 5,* 289–293.

Shapiro, A. P. (1961). An experimental study of comparative response of blood pressure to different noxious stimuli. *Journal of Chronic Diseases, 13,* 293–311.

Shapiro, A. P., Moutsos, S. E., & Krifcher, E. (1963). Patterns of pressor response to noxious stimuli in normal, hypertensive and diabetic subjects. *Journal of Clinical Investigation, 42,* 1890–1898.

Shapiro, A. P., Nicotero, J., Sapira, J., & Scheib, E. T. (1968). Analysis of the variability of blood pressure, pulse rate and catecholamine responsivity in identical and fraternal twins. *Psychosomatic Medicine, 30,* 506–520.

Sharda, S., Gupta, S. N., & Khuteta, K. P. (1975). Effects of mental stress on intermediate carbohydrate and lipid metabolism. *International Journal of Physiological Pharmacology, 19,* 2.

Sims, J., Hewitt, J. K., Kelly, K. A., Carroll, D., & Turner, J. R. (1986). Familial and individual influences on blood pressure. *Acta Geneticae Medicae et Gemellologiae, 35,* 7–21.

Sinyor, D., Schwartz, S. G., Peronnet, F., Brisson, G., & Seraganian, P. (1983). Aerobic fitness level and reactivity to psychosocial stress: Physiological, biochemical and subjective measures. *Psychosomatic Medicine, 45,* 205–217.

Sinyor, D., Golden, M., Steinert, Y., & Seraganian, P. (1986). Experimental manipulation of aerobic fitness and the response to psychosocial stress: Heart rate and self-report measures. *Psychosomatic Medicine, 48,* 324–337.

Siscovick, D. S., LaPorte, R. E., & Newman, J. M. (1985). The disease-specific benefits and risks of physical activity and exercise. *Public Health Reports, 100,* 180–188.

Stabler, B., Morris, M. A., Litton, J., Feinglos, M. N., & Surwit, R. S. (1986). Differential glycemic response to stress in Type A and B individuals with IDDM. *Diabetes Care, 9,* 550–552.

Stabler, B., Surwit, R. S., Lane, J. D., Morris, M. A., & Feinglos, M. N. (1986). Glycemic response to stress in children with insulin-dependent diabetes. *Psychophysiology, 23,* 463–464 (Abstract).

Steptoe, M., & Ross, A. (1981). Psychophysiological reactivity and the prediction of cardiovascular disorders. *Journal of Psychosomatic Research, 25,* 23–32.

Steptoe, A., Melville, D., & Ross, A. (1984). Behavioral response demands, cardiovascular reactivity and essential hypertension. *Psychosomatic Medicine, 46,* 33–48.

Surwit, R. S., & Feinglos, M. (1983). The effects of relaxation on glucose tolerance levels in diabetic persons. *Diabetes Care, 6,* 176–179.

Uhari, M., & Paavilainen, T. (1982). Haemodynamic changes in essential hypertension in young subjects. *Cardiology, 69,* 219–223.

van Brummelen, P., Buhler, F. R., Kiowski, W., & Amann, F. W. (1981). Age-related decrease in cardiac and peripheral vascular responsiveness to isoprenaline: Studies in normal subjects. *Clinical Science, 60,* 571–577.

Vestal, R. E., Wood, A. J. J., & Shand, D. G. (1979). Reduced beta-adrenoceptor sensitivity in the elderly. *Clinical Pharmacology and Therapeutics, 26,* 181–186.

Weidmann, P., Beretta-Piccoli, C., Keusch, G., Gluck, Z., Mujagic, M., Grimm, M., Meier, A., & Ziegler, W. H. (1979). Sodium-volume factor, cardiovascular reactivity and hypotensive mechanism of diuretic therapy in mild hypertension associated with diabetes mellitus. *American Journal of Medicine, 67,* 779–784.

Weisfeldt, M. L. (1980). Aging of the cardiovascular system. *New England Journal of Medicine, 303,* 1172–1174.

Young, J. B., & Landsberg, L. (1982). Diet-induced changes in sympathetic nervous system activity: Possible implications for obesity and hypertension. *Journal of Chronic Diseases, 35,* 879–886.

Ziegler, M. C., Lake, C. R., & Kopin, I. J. (1976). Plasma noradrenaline increases with age. *Nature, 261,* 333–335.

CHAPTER 28

Ethnic Differences in Resting and Stress-Induced Cardiovascular and Humoral Activity

An Overview

Norman B. Anderson

A Prologue on the Genetic and Social Diversity of U.S. Ethnic Groups

America's major ethnic groups—blacks, Asian Americans, Hispanics, and Native Americans—now constitute approximately 20% of the U.S. population. According to the most recent census information (Bureau of the Census, 1983), blacks represented 11.5%, Hispanics 6.4%, Asians 1.5%, and Native Americans 0.6% of the population in 1980. The recently released *Report of the Secretary's Task Force on Black and Minority Health* (1985) contains the most comprehensive summary to date on the chief contributors to mortality and morbidity among these ethnic groups. As for whites in the United States, cardiovascular diseases are among the primary causes of death in diseases between the majority population and

many minority groups. In many cases, ethnic groups suffer disproportionately higher rates of cardiovascular disease.

The research to be reviewed in this chapter on ethnic group differences in stress-induced physiological reactivity represents one approach aimed at understanding such disparities in health outcomes. Comparison research of this type has the potential to clarify the role of stress in cardiovascular disease of ethnic groups as well as whites (see Matthews *et al.*, 1986, for a review of the reactivity literature). When ethnic differences are observed, however, a difficulty arises in interpreting the meaning of such data. Watkins and Eaker (1986) have cautioned researchers against interpreting reactivity differences in terms of genetic differences. In summarizing this issue, Watkins and Eaker state that subjects' self-reports of racial or ethnic identification should not be viewed as indicative of specific underlying genetic characteristics. Indeed, the genetic composition of the U.S. black population contains a substantial proportion of Caucasian genes. Reed (1969) estimated that between 2 and 50% of the genes of the U.S. black population are derived from Caucasian ancestors. Thus, the ge-

Norman B. Anderson • Department of Psychiatry, Duke University Medical School, and Geriatric Research, Education, and Clinical Center, Veterans Administration Medical Center, Durham, North Carolina 27710.

netic characteristics of individuals who classify themselves as members of the same ethnic group may not be homogeneous. This lack of genetic homogeneity has prompted the view that the category "black" is primarily a sociological category (Cooper, 1984; Watkins & Eaker, 1986), which indicates exposure to certain common experiences (Washington & McLoyd, 1982).

At the same time, however, it should also be realized that ethnic group labels frequently group together individuals who have quite distinct social and cultural identities. For example, persons classified as "Hispanics" may be Mexican Americans, Puerto Ricans, or Cubans. "Asians" may be further classified as Japanese, Chinese, and Philippine. "Native Americans" include such groups as American Indians, Aleuts, Alaskan Eskimos, and native Hawaiians. These groups represent reasonably distinct populations that often differ in diet, diet, family and cultural institutions, socioeconomic status, genetic background, and geographic and age distribution.

The largest American ethnic group, black Americans, also shows considerable diversity. Valentine (1971) identified several black American subgroups: northern-urban U.S. blacks, southern-rural U.S. blacks, Anglo-African West Indians, French West Indians, Guyanese, Surinamers, West Africans, French Guianans, Louisiana Creoles, black Cubans, Panamanians, and black South Americans. Thus, while the majority of black Americans trace their ancestry to slaves brought to the continental United States directly from Africa, others are descendants of Africans who were held in the Caribbean and other locations.

The above prologue was intended to sensitize readers to one of the critical issues involved in the conduct and interpretation of ethnic group comparison research. As will be seen from the following review, ethnic group differences have been found on numerous physiological parameters. At this time, however, the meaning and origin of these differences, particularly in light of the genetic and social diversity between and within ethnic groups, represent one of the major challenges facing biomedical and biobehavioral researchers in this area. [See Anderson (in press) for a detailed discussion of this issue].

Outline of the Chapter

The purpose of this chapter is to provide an overview of research which has examined the influence of ethnicity on physiological processes relevant to cardiovascular functioning. The chapter is divided into five sections. Section one contains a summary of research on ethnic group differences in resting cardiovascular and humoral activity. This section includes information on physiological activity both in healthy subjects and in patients with cardiovascular disease—specifically, essential hypertension. Section two contains an overview of findings to date on ethnic group differences in physiological reactivity relevant to cardiovascular disease. Again, studies involving healthy and hypertensive subjects will be reviewed. In section three, the current state of knowledge concerning the variability *within* ethnic groups in stress-induced reactivity is addressed. Here, the focus is on the identification of individuals within an ethnic group who are potentially most at risk for cardiovascular disease due to exaggerated cardiovascular and humoral responses to stress. The chapter will conclude with a summary and integration of research findings followed by an outline of potential directions for future research.

Ethnic Group Differences in Resting Activity

Healthy Volunteers

Ethnic group differences in resting physiological activity relevant to cardiovascular functioning in healthy subjects have been the focus of a number of studies. The majority of these studies have compared black children with white children from infancy through adolescence on a number of cardiovascular indices. Several studies conducted by Schachter and associates (Schachter, Kerr, Wimberly, & Lachin, 1974; Schachter, Lachin, Kerr, Wimberly, & Ratey, 1976; Schachter, Lachin, & Wimberly, 1976) and others (Lee, Rosner, Gould, Lowe, & Kass, 1976) have found that black newborns, less than 6 months of age, have faster resting heart rates compared to white newborns.

Schachter et al. (1974) reported that in a sample of 78 black and 68 white newborns, heart rate measured on postnatal day 2 and 3 was on average significantly faster in black infants. In a subsequent study, Schachter, Lachin, and Wimberly (1976) replicated and extended this finding by showing that the faster heart rate of black infants was unrelated to parental socioeconomic status. Finally, Lee et al. (1976) found that at postnatal day 2 to 4, black newborns and newborns of Spanish-speaking parents had a mean pulse rate higher than that of white infants.

Among older children, current data suggest that black–white differences in heart rate are lessened or reversed (Schachter, Kuller, & Perfetti, 1984a; Shekelle, Liu, Raynor, & Miller, 1978; Voors, Webber, & Berenson, 1982). In a longitudinal study, Schachter et al. (1984a) measured heart rate shortly after birth (postnatal day 3) and again at 6, 15, 24, 36, 48, and 60 months of age in black and white subjects. Blacks were found to have the faster heart rates as newborns and at 6 months of age; from 15 to 60 months the ethnic group differences were no longer present. Shekelle et al. (1978) explored pulse rate in black and white children aged 6–11. A total of 6816 children (13.8% black) were studied using data collected by the National Health Examination Survey (NHES), a national probability sample. Black males and females had significantly lower heart rates regardless of age, family income, or region of the United States. The heart rate differences were not explicable by differences in systolic blood pressure, body surface area, body temperature, skinfold thickness, or grip strength. Using data from the Bogalusa Heart Study, Voors et al. (1982) examined differences in resting supine heart rate in black and white children aged 5–17. A small but reliable heart rate difference of 3–4 beats/min was found, with the lower rate being observed for the black children. This group effect was independent of age or sex.

Few studies have examined ethnic differences in heart rate using nonblack ethnic groups. One exception is a study by Levinson et al. (1985), who compared resting heart rate in four groups—black, white, Latino, and Oriental—from a sample of 4086 Chicago school children aged 5–10. For both boys and girls, blacks had significantly lower mean heart rate than the other three ethnic groups. Though not statistically significant, Oriental boys and girls tended to have faster heart rates than white and Latino children.

Studies of ethnic differences in heart rate among adults tend to indicate that the pattern of lower rates for black children continues into adulthood, but may disappear with increasing age. Persky, Dyer, Stamler, Shekelle, and Schoenberger (1979) examined mean heart rate in a sample of 30,786 adults (approximately 12% black) aged 18–64 who were screened as part of the Chicago Heart Association Detention Project in Industry. Among individuals aged 18–35, black males and females had lower heart rates than white males and females. These differences were not present in subjects 35 and older. Further, for persons aged 18–24, heart rates were also lower in black hypertensives compared to white hypertensives. Similarly, in the Evans County studies, black males aged 15–34 were also found to have significantly lower heart rates than white males of similar ages. This difference was not present in women or in older men (unpublished data cited in Persky et al., 1979).

The relationship between ethnicity and blood pressure in children has been explored fairly extensively. Unlike heart rate, however, the results for blood pressure have been inconsistent. Among infants, most studies find no ethnic group differences in blood pressure. In the Schachter, Kuller, and Perfetti (1984b) longitudinal study, neither systolic nor diastolic blood pressure differed between black and white children, as measured at birth and at 6, 15, 24, 36, 48, and 60 months of age. Though blood pressure tended to rise with age in both groups, the rise was somewhat faster among white children. Blood pressure did not vary with parental history of hypertension. Morrison et al. (1980) found no systolic or diastolic differences between black and white children aged 6–19. Negative findings have also been reported for infants (Lee et al., 1976; Schachter, Lachin, et al., 1976; Schachter, Lachin, & Wimberly, 1976) and for children 3–17 (Londe, Gollub, & Goldring, 1977; Roberts, 1978). Finally, Baron, Freyer, and Fixler (1986) conducted a study of blood pressure differences in black, white, and Mexican American children aged 13–19. They found no substantial ethnic differences in blood pressure between any of the groups. Similarly, Kilcoyne, Richter, and Alsup (1974) found no significant differences in the frequency distribution of blood pressure in three ethnic groups (black, Latin-American, white) attending a Harlem high school.

In contrast to the above studies reporting no ethnic differences in blood pressure in children, several studies have uncovered significant differences. However, the group with the higher pressure varies across studies. Harlan, Cornoni-Huntley, and Leaverton (1979) found that although the mean systolic pressures in black children aged 6–11 were lower compared to white children, the diastolic pressures were higher, particularly in males. No relationship was found for family income or urban/rural status. Goldring et al. (1977), in a study of 14- to 18-year-olds, found that white boys had significantly higher diastolic pressures at all ages and higher systolic pressures at all ages except 18, where there was no difference. Although no systolic pressure differences were found between black and white girls, white girls 14, 16, and 18 had higher diastolic pressures than black girls of the same ages. Several other studies, however, have demonstrated higher pressures in black children and adolescents. Kotchen, Kotchen, Schwertman, and Kuller (1974), reporting only systolic pressure, found that blacks aged 17–20 generally had higher pressures than whites. However, those blacks residing in an inner city and attending an inner city high school had higher pressures than blacks living in and attending a high school in a middle-class residential area. In their study comparing blood pressure in black, white, Latino, and Oriental children aged 5–10, Levinson et al. (1985) found that systolic and diastolic blood pressures were higher for the black and Oriental children. The differences were independent of age, weight, skinfold thickness, height, and season of measurement. Gutgesell, Terrell, and Labarthe (1981) studied blood pressure recorded in a primary care center in their sample of 2810 children aged 3–17, 49.2% of whom were of Spanish surname, 23.4% black, and 27.4% white. Black children had higher pressures than Spanish and white children.

A consistent finding in the epidemiological liter-ature is the higher resting blood pressure of healthy black adults compared to their white counterparts (Roberts & Rowland, 1981; Rowland & Roberts, 1982; Stamler, Rhomberg, et al., 1975; Stamler, Stamler, et al., 1975). Using data from the National Health and Nutrition Examination Survey (NHANES) obtained between 1971 and 1975, Roberts and Rowland (1981) found that systolic and diastolic blood pressure rose with age in both blacks and whites. The mean pressures, however, were generally higher in blacks. For males, the difference in systolic pressure ranged from 2.6 mm Hg at ages 25–34, to 12.6 mm Hg at ages 55–64; the range for diastolic was 3.3 mm Hg at ages 25–34, to 9.6 mm Hg at ages 55–64. A similar pattern of ethnic differences was observed in females. Mean systolic differences ranged from 5.6 mm Hg at 25–34 and 65–74, to 13.4 mm Hg at 35–44; for diastolic pressure the range was 4.6 mm Hg at 65–74, to 10.3 mm Hg at 35–44 (Roberts & Rowland, 1981).

While black Americans generally have higher resting blood pressure than whites, it should be remembered that there is currently considerable variability in blood pressure within the black population. Among blacks, blood pressure varies as a function of family history of hypertension (Hohn et al., 1983; Thomas et al., 1984), age (Anderson, 1988; Roberts & Rowland, 1981), obesity (Boyle, Griffey, Nichaman, & Talbert, 1967; Neser, Thomas, Semenya, Thomas, & Gillum, 1986), socioeconomic status (Hypertension Detection and Follow-up Program Cooperative Group, 1977; James, 1985), socioecologic stress (Harburg et al., 1973), stress coping style (Harburg et al., 1973; James, Hartnett, & Kalsbeek, 1983), and perhaps social support (Dressler, Dos Santos, and Viteri, 1986). Therefore, blood pressure level in blacks is not a monotonic phenomenon, but one which varies according to individual characteristics as well as environmental circumstances.

Several summaries are now available on blood pressure status in ethnic groups other than black Americans (Kumanyika & Savage, 1986a,b,c; U.S. DHEW, 1979). One of the few large-scale epidemiological studies which compared blood pressure in whites and Hispanics was the National Health and Nutrition Examination Survey I

(NHANES I). In the NHANES I, as reported by Kumanyika and Savage (1986a), systolic blood pressures of Spanish-American and Mexican-American men were similar to those of white men aged 18–44, but comparable to or higher than those of white men aged 45–74. Diastolic blood pressures of the Hispanic men were comparable to or lower than those of the white men. The blood pressures for white and Spanish/Mexican-American women were comparable. Data from the National Center for Health Statistics (Roberts & Maurer, 1977) indicate that in American Indian men, systolic and diastolic pressures were similar to those of white men for most age categories. The maximum difference between the groups was roughly 6 mm Hg systolic in the 65–74 age group (white group higher), and roughly 4 mm Hg diastolic in the 25–34 age group (whites higher). Among women, the data were more variable, in that the systolic pressures were higher in the Indians aged 25–34 and 45–54 (by roughly 4 and 7 mm Hg, respectively), but higher in the whites aged 35–44 and 65–74 (by approximately 5 and 6 mm Hg, respectively). The diastolic pressures of Indian and white women were more comparable, with the largest difference (4 mm Hg) occurring in the 65–74 age group (whites higher). Finally, although information on resting blood pressure of Asian Americans and whites is limited, there is some indication that resting blood pressure varies among the Japanese according to the geographic region in which they live. For example, Winkelstein, Kagan, Kato, and Sacks (1975) examined blood pressures of Japanese men residing in Japan, northern California, and Hawaii. Overall, the highest mean blood pressure was observed in those Japanese residing in California, followed by those residing in Japan, with the Hawaiian Japanese having the lowest pressure.

Ethnic differences among healthy individuals have also been explored on other physiological parameters related to cardiovascular disease, such as plasma norepinephrine and renin, lipoprotein cholesterol, dopamine-β-hydroxylase (DBH), and electrocardiographic abnormalities. Berenson, Voors, Webber, Dalferes, and Harsha (1979) studied a sample of 278 children aged 5–14, stratified into high, medium, and low diastolic groups. Regardless of blood pressure stratum or sex, black children had a lower percentage of body fat, lower plasma renin and serum DBH levels, and lower urine potassium excretion. Sodium excretion was equal across groups. In the high blood pressure stratum, black males had higher supine systolic blood pressure, lower heart rate, lower plasma renin, and lower 1-h glucose levels.

In adults, Sever, Peart, Meade, Davies, and Gordon (1979) compared blood pressure, plasma norepinephrine, and renin in a group of 62 white and 53 black factory workers. Blacks had generally higher systolic and diastolic blood pressures than whites. Although norepinephrine increased with age in both groups, levels did not differ between blacks and whites. Plasma renin, however, was 55% lower in blacks of both sexes compared to whites. Several studies of healthy adults have also found differences between blacks and whites in unstimulated plasma renin activity (Berenson, Voors, & Dalferes, 1979; Helmer & Judson, 1968; Hohn et al., 1983; Luft, Weinberger, & Grim, 1982), although others have not found such a difference (Kaplan et al., 1976; Luft, Grim, Higgins, & Weinberger, 1977). However, as will be reviewed shortly, it has been shown that under conditions of renin *stimulation*, blacks have consistently exhibited lower plasma renin activity than whites (Hohn et al., 1983; Luft et al., 1982; Kaplan et al., 1976).

Ethnic differences in electrocardiographic abnormalities have been the focus of a number of studies. Most notably, three large-scale epidemiological studies have investigated ethnic differences in electrocardiographic evidence of left ventricular hypertrophy (ECG-LVH), since this has been found to be associated with increased risk for CHD in the Framingham Study (Kannel, Gordon, Castelli, & Margolis, 1970). As reviewed in the *Report of the Secretary's Task Force on Black and Minority Health* (1986), studies have shown that ECG abnormalities are more common in blacks than whites of both sexes (Beaglehole et al., 1975; Riley, Oberman, Hurst, & Peacock, 1973; Savage, in press). For example, using Evans County data, Beaglehole et al. (1975) found that the prevalence of ECG-LVH was two or three times higher in blacks than whites after controlling for age, blood pressure, body habitus, activity level, and smoking. Similarly, data from the Birmingham Stroke Study (Riley *et al.*, 1973) indicated that the heightened R-wave amplitude in blacks was independent of blood pressure, history of treated hypertension, or history of angina pectoris or myocardial infarction. Although blacks apparently exhibit greater ECG abnormalities, it is at present unclear whether these abnormalities are as predictive of CHD in blacks as they are in whites. For example, Bartel *et al.* (1971) found that ECG abnormalities carried increased risk for CHD in white men, but not in black men. Black women had an increased CHD incidence only with left axis deviation.

Consistent black–white differences have been found in lipoprotein cholesterol (for review see Glueck, Gartside, Laskarzewski, Khoury, & Tyroler, 1984; Kumanyika & Savage, 1986d). Findings from several large-scale epidemiological studies suggest that black male children and adults have higher high-density lipoprotein (HDL) cholesterol levels and lower low-density lipoprotein (LDL) levels compared to white samples (Morrison *et al.*, 1979, 1981; Tyroler, Glueck, Christensen, & Kwiterovich, 1980; Tyroler *et al.*, 1975). In the Evans County study (Tyroler *et al.*, 1975), investigators compared HDL and LDL levels of 110 randomly selected black men with those of age-matched and total cholesterol-matched white men. Blacks had significantly higher HDL (by 11 mg/dl) but lower LDL cholesterol (by 6 mg/dl) than white men. Differences between black and white women on cholesterol values parallel those of men but are generally of lesser magnitude.

The above-mentioned cholesterol results parallel those of most other epidemiological studies, even after controls were introduced for age, Quetelet Index, and socioeconomic factors, though the range of socioeconomic levels has been somewhat limited. At least one study, however, the Framingham Minority Study (Wilson *et al.*, 1983), found that among college-educated men, HDL cholesterol was lower in blacks than whites, though the ratio of HDL to total cholesterol was similar.

In other ethnic groups, information on cholesterol is not as detailed, and comes generally from regional studies. Among Hispanics, data indicate that among lower SES persons, Mexican American males have higher age-adjusted serum cholesterol levels than non-Hispanic white men; levels are comparable for Mexican American and non-Hispanic white women (Friis, Nanjundappa, Pendergast, & Wesh, 1981; Kraus, Borhani, & Franti, 1980; Stern, Rosenthal, Haffner, Hazuda, & Franco, 1984). In comparing men in the Framingham Study (aged 45–64), Gordon, Garcia-Palmieri, Kagan, Kannel, and Schiffman (1974) found serum cholesterol levels to be approximately 15% lower among Hawaiian men compared to Framingham men. Another study found serum cholesterol levels at all ages to be lowest in Japanese men in Japan compared to those in Hawaii or in California (Nichaman *et al.*, 1975). Among American Indians, cholesterol levels are generally lower than in whites, though there are differences between Indian subgroups (Kumanyika & Savage, 1986b; Sievers, 1968).

Hypertensive Subjects

A number of studies have examined resting physiological differences between blacks and white in an attempt to account for the high morbidity rates of hypertension in blacks. These studies have been fewer in number than those utilizing normotensive populations. The vast majority of the studies of hypertensives have compared blacks with whites on factors such as norepinephrine (NE), plasma renin, and blood volume.

Plasma NE has been found to be elevated in many patients with essential hypertension (Goldstein, 1981), and is believed to play an etiological role in hypertension development in certain subgroups of patients (deChamplain, Cousineau, & Lapointe, 1980). Unfortunately, fewer comparisons of black and white hypertensives, or of black hypertensives with black normotensives on NE have been conducted. In his review of the literature, Goldstein (1983) found that only 8 of 78 studies comparing hypertensives with controls reported the ethnic makeup of the population. Of these, only one presented data separately by race (Sever, Peart, Davies, Turnbridge, & Gordon, 1979). Sever *et al.* did not find significant NE differences between black and white hypertensives, although black hypertensives showed an age-related increase in NE levels while the white hypertensives did not. Similarly, Lichtman and Woods (1967) did not find differences in NE between black hypertensives, black normotensives, or white normotensives.

As noted earlier, research on variations in unstimulated plasma renin activity in healthy populations as a function of ethnic group has been equivocal. With hypertensive subjects, however, the data are somewhat more consistent. As a group, black hypertensives have been shown to exhibit lower renin levels than white patients. It has been estimated that roughly 36–62% of black hypertensives have relatively suppressed renin levels as compared to 19–55% of white hypertensives (Gillum, 1979; Wisenbaugh et al., 1972). Age appears to be a crucial determinant of whether black–white differences in renin are observed. Brunner, Sealey, and Laragh (1973) found that for both black and white subjects, most hypertensives under age 30 exhibited low or normal renin values. In subjects over age 50, however, there was a significantly greater degree of low renin hypertension in the black population. Other researchers have shown that black hypertensives under age 40 have significantly higher plasma renin levels than black patients over age 40 (Grim et al., 1980).

The relationship between ethnic group, hypertension, and blood volume has been the focus of several projects (for review see Schachter & Kuller, 1984). Of the studies conducted on blood volume, two found ethnic group differences (Chrysant et al., 1979; Lilley, Hsu, & Stone, 1976) whereas two failed to do so (Messerli, Decarvalho, Christie, & Frohlich, 1979; Mitas, Holle, Levy, & Stone, 1979). Chrysant et al. (1979), using a sample of 35 black and 95 white hypertensives, determined the proportion of each group with expanded versus contracted plasma volume. It was found that 43% of the black subjects but only 21% of the white subjects were volume expanded; conversely, 57% of blacks but 79% of whites were volume contracted. Interestingly, no relationship was found between blood pressure or renin with either volume expansion or contraction in blacks; among whites, subjects with contracted volume had significantly higher arterial pressures and plasma renin activity. In contrast, Messerli et al. (1979) found no black–white differences in plasma volume, total blood volume, cardiac index, or total peripheral resistance.

One humoral system which has received comparatively little attention, but which could nonetheless be related to black–white blood pressure differences is the kallikrein–kinin system. Activity of this system, via secretion of renal kallikrein and ultimately kinin, produces both renal vasodilation and natriuresis (Warren & O'Connor, 1980). A deficiency in this mechanism has been hypothesized to play a role in the excessive hypertension rates in blacks (Warren & O'Connor, 1980). In support of this hypothesis, Levy, Lilley, Frigon, and Stone (1977) found that during unrestricted sodium ingestion, urinary kallikrein was greater in white normotensives than in black normotensives and hypertensives, or in white hypertensives. During restriction, all groups increased urinary kallikrein excretion, but the increase was blunted in the black hypertensives. It has been suggested that a deficient kallikrein–kinin system could explain the inhibited sodium excretion in blacks, and generally lower renin levels in older black hypertensives (Warren & O'Connor, 1980).

In summary, research on ethnic group differences of resting cardiovascular and humoral activity has produced a number of significant differences. Depending on the age group, blacks have been shown to have lower heart rates, higher blood pressure, higher levels of HDL and lower levels of LDL cholesterol, and more ECG abnormalities compared to whites.

Ethnic Group Differences in Reactivity

The research on racial group differences in response to laboratory stressors will be reviewed with reference to either healthy children or adults, or persons with essential hypertension. Studies which included both normotensives and hypertensives as subjects will be summarized in the section devoted to hypertensives. Several types of stressors were utilized in these studies, and may be broadly categorized as either physical (e.g., exercise, isometric handgrip, postural change, cold pressor, sodium loading) or psychosocial (e.g., mental arithmetic or aversive reaction time). This physical–psychosocial distinction is drawn only for organizational purposes, since many procedures contain both physical and psychosocial elements. Studies were categorized as either physical or psychosocial based upon the most salient feature of the stressor used. Studies which utilized both physical and psychosocial stressors will be reviewed in the section devoted to psychosocial stressors.

Children and Adolescents

Physical Stressors

Several studies of children and adolescents have exmined black–white differences in reactivity to physical stressors (Alpert, Dover, Booker, Martin, & Strong, 1981; Alpert et al., 1982; Berenson, Voors, Webber, et al., 1979; Hohn et al., 1983; Voors, Webber, & Berenson, 1980). Alpert et al. (1981) measured systolic blood pressure and heart rate responses in 184 black and 221 white subjects aged 6–15 during cycle ergometer testing at maximum work load. The racial differences were assessed with regard to age, sex, and four categories of body surface area (I–IV; IV = largest). Although no significant differences were observed between groups at rest, black males exhibited higher exercise-induced peak systolic blood pressures in the three largest body surface area groups, and greater change in systolic blood pressure across all body habitus groups. Black females showed greater peak systolic pressure at each level of body size, and greater systolic pressure changes from baseline in all but the largest body size group. Since no racial group differences were found in maximum heart rate, the authors speculated that the blood pressure differences were due to higher systemic vascular resistance in the blacks. Voors et al. (1980) examined cardiovascular responses of 278 male and female children aged 7–15, who were stratified by diastolic blood pressure (high, medium, and low). Stress procedures included

orthostasis (standing up from seated position), isometric handgrip, and the cold pressor test. Results showed that the black boys in the high diastolic blood pressure stratum exhibited higher resting and stress-induced systolic blood pressure *levels* during each of the tasks than any of the other race/sex groups. Diastolic blood pressure *changes* were greater in black children during orthostatic and cold pressor stress. White children generally had higher resting and stress-induced heart rate levels.

In one of the most comprehensive projects to date, Hohn et al. (1983) studied multiple physiological responses to a treadmill test in black and white children (aged 10–17) selected for the presence or absence of a family history of hypertension. Prior to exercise (prestress), blacks with a family history of hypertension had higher supine, seated, and standing systolic and diastolic blood pressures than blacks without such a family history. Family history blacks also had greater diastolic levels during maximum exercise than those without a family history of hypertension, as well as higher postexercise renin activity. Whites with and without a family history of hypertension did not differ from each other in blood pressure at any time. Comparisons of black and white subjects with a family history of hypertension revealed higher systolic and diastolic readings in the black subjects regardless of test period. No differences in blood pressure were detected between blacks and whites without a family history of hypertension.

Psychosocial Stressors

Two studies have compared reactivity to psychosocial challenges in black and white children and adolescents. Murphy, Alpert, Moes, and Somes (1986) examined cardiovascular responses to a video game in 213 healthy children and adolescents aged 6–18. In addition to investigating racial differences, the researchers also explored the effects of race of the experimenter (white versus black female). Results indicated that blacks exhibited significantly greater systolic and diastolic responses to the task compared to whites, regardless of gender. For male and female subjects, heart rate responses from baseline were more frequently significant when subjects were paired with a *same-*

race rather than a different-race experimenter. The interaction between subject race and experimenter race was not significant for the blood pressures. In a subsequent study, Murphy, Alpert, Walker, and Wiley (submitted for publication) replicated the finding of racial differences in systolic and diastolic blood pressure reactivity using a group of third-grade children (average age 9 years). Black children also had higher heart rate changes as well.

Normotensive Adults

Physical Stressors

Among adults, there have been comparatively few investigations of racial differences in response to physical manipulations. In a study by Anderson, Lane, Muranaka, Williams, and Houseworth (1988), blood pressure, heart rate, forearm blood flow, and forearm vascular resistance were measured during the application of an ice pack to the forehead of 10 black and 10 white males (aged 18–22). This maneuver has been shown to elicit a profound α-adrenergic peripheral vasoconstriction (Abboud & Eckstein, 1966). In response to the cold stimulus, blacks exhibited significantly greater increases in systolic and diastolic blood pressure, and forearm vascular resistance. Since no racial differences were observed in heart rate, the hyperreactivity among the blacks was interpreted as primarily vascular rather than cardiac. Venter, Joubert, and Strydom (1985) compared heart rate and blood pressure responses to the head-up tilt maneuver in 16 South African blacks and whites matched on age, sex, and body mass. Tilting from supine to 40°, and from 40° to 80°, caused significant increases in heart rate and diastolic pressure in both populations. Whites had higher systolic pressures than blacks when tilted to 80°. No significant heart rate or diastolic differences were observed. The authors hypothesized that racial differences in systolic response to tilting might be due to quantitative and/or qualitative differences in cardiac β_1 adrenoceptors.

Researchers at Indiana University have conducted an elegant series of studies on the effects on sodium loading in black and white adults (for review see Grim *et al.*, 1984; Luft, Grim, & Weinberger, 1985). To investigate the effects of volume expansion and contraction in males (Luft, Grim, Fineberg, & Weinberger, 1979; Luft, Grim, Higgins, & Weinberger, 1977), subjects were fed a 150 mEq/day sodium diet and given an intravenous infusion of 2 liters of normal saline (volume expansion). Sodium depletion was induced by a diet containing 10 mEq of sodium and three 40-mg doses of furosemide (volume contraction). Following sodium loading (expansion), blacks excreted significantly less sodium in urine than whites. In another study, blood pressure responses to six different levels of daily sodium intake (10, 300, 600, 800, 1200, 1500 mEq) were examined in black and white males (Luft, Rankin, *et al.*, 1979). At intakes of 600 mEq/day or greater, blacks showed consistently and significantly higher blood pressures than whites. No significant blood pressure differences were observed at the lower intake levels. Thus, while research has failed to demonstrate racial differences in sodium intake (Grim *et al.*, 1980), blacks may be more susceptible to its deleterious effects on blood pressure. Recently, Falkner, Kushner, Khalsa, Canessa, and Katz (1986) showed that following a sodium load, those blacks (aged 18–23) who were sodium-sensitive and had a parental history of hypertension exhibited a higher stress-induced MAP than the sodium-sensitive/negative parental history subjects. These findings suggest that the susceptibility to hypertension engendered by a positive parental history may interact with other risk factors such as sodium sensitivity to augment reactivity.

Psychosocial Stressors

Few studies have compared cardiovascular responses of normotensive blacks and whites to psychosocial stressors. In one recent study, Morrell, Myers, Shapiro, Goldstein, and Armstrong (in press) measured heart rate, blood pressure, and skin conductance responses to mental arithmetic in 34 black and 42 white normotensive males, selected for family history of hypertension. Blacks showed higher diastolic levels during the task; however, statistically covarying the baseline values removed the diastolic differences, and uncovered higher systolic levels in the white subjects. There were no significant interactions involving racial group and family history of hypertension. However, Anderson, Lane, Monou, Williams, and Houseworth (1988) found that during mental arithmetic, black normotensive males exhibited significantly *smaller* blood pressure and forearm blood flow responses than their white counterparts.

In a study of black and white normotensive females selected for parental history of hypertension, Anderson, Lane, Taguchi, and Williams (in press) examined cardiovascular responses to two stressors: mental arithmetic and the cold face stimulus. Blacks showed a slower diastolic blood pressure recovery from arithmetic and a greater systolic blood pressure response to the cold stimulus. Blacks also showed significantly greater emotional responses to the math task, as demonstrated by self-reported (via visual analogue scales) increases in anxiety, guilt, fear, and restlessness and decreases in alertness, relaxation, and happiness. In a similar study conducted with male subjects, neither race nor parental history of hypertension was related significantly to cardiovascular responses to either of the two stressors (Anderson, Lane, & Taguchi, 1988). However, there was a trend for blacks to exhibit a slower diastolic blood pressure recovery following arithmetic; a finding that parallels the results obtained in women. Additionally, the black males had significantly higher systolic and diastolic blood pressure levels before, during, and after the cold stimulus.

Hypertensive Adults

Physical Stressors

Two studies have compared black and white hypertensives with regard to reactivity to physical stressors. Rowlands *et al.* (1982) evaluated blood pressure and heart rate reactivity in 16 black and 16 white subjects (7 females in each group) with mild to moderate hypertension. In addition to gender, subjects were matched on age, blood pressure, and socioeconomic status. Tasks consisted of isometric handgrip, upright bicycle exercise, and the cold pressor test. No significant racial differences

in heart rate or blood pressure responses were obtained on any of the tasks.

Dimsdale, Graham, Ziegler, Zusman, and Berry (1987) infused NE in black and white normotensives and hypertensives maintained on two extremes of dietary sodium intake: 10 and 200 mEq/day. A highly significant dose–response relationship was found for NE dosage and blood pressure. Among hypertensives on the high-salt diet, blacks had steeper dose–response slopes than whites.

Psychosocial Stressors

Several recent studies have investigated racial differences in reactivity to psychosocial stressors among hypertensives, or those with casual elevated blood pressure. Fredrikson (1986) examined cardiovascular and noncardiovascular reactivity in three groups of black and white subjects: established hypertensives, borderline hypertensives, and normotensives. The task consisted of 16 signaled reaction time tasks where a 110-decibel white noise was delivered contingent upon poor performance, while measures of heart rate, blood pressure, respiration, skin conductance, and skin and muscle blood flow were obtained (muscle and skin vascular resistances were later calculated). Although resting cardiovascular activity was similar in black and white hypertensives and normotensives, heart rate and systolic pressure changes were smaller in black hypertensives and normotensives. Skin conductance changes were also attenuated in the black subjects. Additionally, muscle and skin vascular resistance increased during the task in black subjects irrespective of diagnosis, but not in the whites, suggesting enhanced vascular resistance among blacks.

In another study of black and white hypertensives, Nash, Jorgensen, Lasser, and Hymowitz (1985) examined heart rate and blood pressure responses of 98 black and white mild hypertensives (median age 48) to two challenging tasks: the video game PacMan and the Stroop color–word interference task. Although the authors found no significant race or gender effects on blood pressure, there was a significant heart rate effect. Black subjects, regardless of gender, exhibited smaller heart rate increases to the tasks. It was noted that the racial group differences could have been mediated by affective responding, since white subjects reported more task-related anxiety and frustration than blacks.

Schneiderman (1986) measured a variety of cardiovascular and humoral responses in black and white borderline hypertensives and normotensives to several challenging tasks (Type A interview, video game, bicycle ergometer, cold pressor test). Also assessed was ambulatory blood pressure at work and home. Black females and white males revealed greater epinephrine and heart rate reactivity to the tasks than black males or white females; this relationship was reversed for plasma renin reactivity. In an analysis of the predictability of home and work blood pressure based on the laboratory responses, Schneiderman found that the best predictor of home or work blood pressure was the laboratory baseline blood pressure; blood pressure during the video game added significantly to the prediction of work blood pressure. Among white subjects, the best *stress* predictor of ambulatory systolic blood pressure was the systolic pressure during the video game; in black subjects, diastolic response to the cold pressor test was the better predictor of ambulatory diastolic pressure.

Falkner, Kushner, Khalsa, and Katz (1987) examined the effects of sodium loading on cardiovascular responses to mental arithmetic in three groups of subjects: 45 representative blacks, who were selected from a larger group of participants in an epidemiological study; 45 borderline hypertensive blacks, who were also enrolled in the larger study; and 45 age- and gender-matched normotensive whites. Cardiovascular reactivity to mental arithmetic and tilting was measured before and after sodium loading. Following sodium loading, blacks showed the greatest increase in resting MAP, indicating greater sodium sensitivity. Black borderline hypertensives had the highest MAP *levels* at baseline and during stress, both before and after sodium loading; however, white subjects exhibited greater MAP *changes* from baseline to stress before and after the sodium intervention.

Light and associates have conducted perhaps the

most comprehensive assessment of black–white differences in stress reactivity. Cardiovascular and renal responses in black and white subjects, selected for normal or borderline systolic blood pressure, were examined in three studies. In one (Light, Obrist, Sherwood, James, & Strogatz, 1987), subjects were exposed to several stressors (cold pressor, noncompetitive reaction time, and competitive reaction time with and without money incentives), while a variety of cardiovascular parameters were assessed. Black borderline hypertensives were found to have greater increases in systolic pressure than their white counterparts to all four stressors. Heart rate and diastolic pressure responses to the active coping reaction time tasks were greater in the borderline hypertensive group than the normotensive group, but did not differ as a function of race. Absolute heart rate levels at rest and during stress were lower, however, in black subjects, especially in those with normal blood pressure.

In a second study, Light et al. (1986) investigated racial differences in physiologic responses with and without β blockade during a competitive reaction time task. Prior to blockade, cardiac output during stress increased significantly more in the hypertensives than in the normotensives, but the increases tended to be larger in the white hypertensives than in the black hypertensives. After β-adrenergic blockade, however, cardiac output fell more in the black subjects (both with and without borderline hypertension) and remained lower than in their white counterparts during stress. The authors noted that this finding suggested a lesser increase in β-adrenergic activity during the stressor in blacks, but a higher level of β-adrenergic activity at rest. Stress produced a significantly larger decrease in total peripheral resistance in whites than blacks prior to blockade (indeed, 40% of the blacks showed an *increase* in resistance). After β blockade, although all race–blood pressure groups exhibited an increase in peripheral resistance from preblockade (perhaps due to an unmasking of an α-adrenergic effect), this increase was significantly greater in the black borderline hypertensives.

In a final study, Light et al. (1986) examined renal and cardiovascular responses in 8 black and 8

white subjects under four conditions following sodium and water ingestion: (1) pretask rest, (2)
competitive task, (3) posttask rest 1, and (4) posttask rest 2. These procedures were repeated on a
second occasion with β blockade. Four primary
findings emerged. First, without blockade, renal
blood flow fell in both groups during stress, but
remained more depressed in blacks during the
posttask periods. With β blockade, it remained
equally depressed in whites and blacks. Second,
both with and without β blockade, blacks showed
a significantly greater drop in glomerular filtration
rate during the first posttask period. Third, blacks
had a tendency to excrete less fluid with or without
β blockade throughout the study and showed greater decreases in fluid excretion during the posttask
periods. Finally, while blacks and whites showed
similar stress-induced increases in systolic and diastolic blood pressure, the blood pressure of blacks
remained somewhat more elevated than whites
during posttask. Heart rate increased less in blacks
during stress without blockade.

The data thus far on racial differences in response to psychosocial stressors among hypertensive individuals have not clearly demonstrated a
propensity toward hyperreactivity in blacks relative to whites. While greater pressor responses in
blacks have occasionally been detected, in some
cases black hypertensives have been shown to have
lower cardiovascular responses than white hypertensives, especially in heart rate. Following the
next section on within-group differences, an attempt will be made to summarize and integrate the
findings to date on racial differences in reactivity
among both normotensives and hypertensives.

Within-Group Variability in Reactivity

As noted, there is considerable heterogeneity
among blacks in resting cardiovascular activity,
particularly in blood pressure. For example, as for
whites, blood pressure levels in blacks vary with
socioeconomic status, age, stress coping style,
obesity, and other factors. It is probable, then, that
the magnitude or pattern of cardiovascular responses to laboratory stressors also varies among
blacks. A substantial body of literature exists on
white samples pertaining to reactivity differences

in persons most at risk for cardiovascular disease
compared to those at reduced risk (e.g., male Type
As versus male Type Bs, or males with versus
those without a parental history of hypertension).
Besides the research summarized in the previous
section which compared blacks with and without
elevated blood pressure, a few studies have addressed individual differences in reactivity in
blacks. These are discussed below.

At least three studies have investigated reactivity differences in blacks as a function of Type A
behavior (Anderson, Lane, Muranaka, Houseworth, & Williams, 1986; Anderson, Williams, *et
al.*, 1986; Clark & Harrell, 1982). Although Type
A behavior has been shown not to predict hypertension in whites, its association with hypertension
(or coronary heart disease) in blacks has not been
determined. In a study of middle-aged black wom-
en, Anderson, Williams, *et al.* (1986) found Structured Interview-assessed Type A behavior to be
significantly associated with systolic and diastolic
blood pressure increases during the Structured Interview, but not during mental arithmetic—a relationship similar to that shown among white women
undergoing a challenging history quiz (Mac-
Dougall, Dembroski, & Krantz, 1981). Family
history of hypertension did not alone, nor in combination with Type A behavior, predict cardiovascular responses to either task. Anderson,
Lane, *et al.* (1986) completed a similar study in a
group of college-aged black females, adding forearm blood flow to the assessments of blood pressure and heart rate. In this study, Type A behavior
interacted with a parental history of hypertension,
such that among women with a positive parental
history, Type A scores were positively and significantly associated with systolic increases during the
Structured Interview. Among those without a parental history of hypertension, Type A scores were
negatively associated with systolic increases during the Interview. Watkins and Eaker (1986) cite a
study by Clark and Harrell (1982) which found a
significant positive correlation between Jenkins
Activity Survey-assessed Type A behavior and diastolic blood pressure reactivity in blacks.

As reviewed earlier, Hohn *et al.* (1983) found
cardiovascular and humoral hyperresponsivity in a
group of black children selected for family history

of hypertension. Among college-aged black women, however, Anderson, Williams, Lane, and Houseworth (1987) found that those with a family history of hypertension exhibited significantly smaller systolic blood pressure and forearm blood flow responses and moderately smaller diastolic responses than did their counterparts with a negative family history. Subsequent studies of parental history of hypertension effects on reactivity in blacks have generally failed to uncover group differences (Anderson, Lane, *et al.,* in press; Anderson, Lane, & Taguchi, 1988; Morrell *et al.,* in press).

The research on within-group differences in cardiovascular reactivity in blacks has not received the same attention as racial differences. This state of affairs is due in large part to the desire among researchers to understand why blacks have a higher rate of hypertension than whites—a desire that leads naturally to the study of racial differences in various parameters. However, it is clear that all blacks are not at risk for hypertension, and, as will be discussed in more depth in a later section, it might be more important to begin to explore differences in those blacks at enhanced risk for hypertension compared to those at reduced risk, rather than simply comparing blacks and whites.

Summary and Integration of Research Findings

This chapter has given an overview of research on racial group differences in resting and stress-induced cardiovascular activity. Consistent black–white differences have been found in resting heart rate, with black infants exhibiting faster rates than white infants—a difference that is diminished or reversed with advancing age. Resting blood pressure has been found to be higher among black adults, while the data on children are equivocal. Studies of racial differences in reactivity among normotensive children suggest that blacks may show greater blood pressure increases to physical procedures such as exercise, and perhaps psychosocial stressors as well. Black adults appear to be more sensitive to the effects of sodium, as indexed by their greater blood pressure response to sodium loading.

The role of black–white differences in stress reactivity as a potential mechanism for the higher rates of hypertension in blacks is emerging as an important field of investigation. Although no firm conclusions can be drawn at this time, two interesting trends have emerged from preliminary data and are deserving of mention. The first concerns the possibility of decreased cardiac reactivity in blacks compared to whites, and in blacks at risk for hypertension compared to those at reduced risk. Several studies have reported lower heart rate or cardiac output reactivity in blacks compared to whites to an aversive reaction time task (Fredrikson, 1986), a video game and the Stroop task (Nash *et al.,* 1985), mental arithmetic (Anderson, Lane, Monou, *et al.,* 1988), and during competitive and noncompetitive reaction time tasks (Light *et al.,* 1986). Anderson *et al.* (1987) found that black women at risk for hypertension had lower heart rates during mental arithmetic than those at reduced risk. If these findings are borne out in future studies, a question may arise as to the appropriateness of the β-adrenergic hyperreactivity hypothesis for the development of hypertension in blacks. That is, as discussed in the introduction, it has been hypothesized that excessive β-adrenergically-mediated cardiac output and heart rate responses to stress may ultimately produce sustained high blood pressure. Though speculative at this time, the failure to find exaggerated heart rate responses in blacks suggests that β-adrenergic influences may not underlie the higher rates of hypertension in blacks compared to whites. Indeed, there is some biomedical evidence supporting the idea that β-adrenergic factors may be less important in hypertension development in blacks than in whites. For example, studies have found lower plasma renin activity (Luft *et al.,* 1985) and decreased responsiveness to β-adrenergic blockade among black hypertensives (Hall, 1986), and lower resting heart rate in young black normotensive adults (Persky *et al.,* 1979) compared to their white counterparts. Clearly, more research is needed to clarify the appropriateness of the β-adrenergic reactivity hypothesis for understanding the development of hypertension in blacks.

A second trend suggests that blacks may show a propensity toward blood pressure reactivity mediated by peripheral vasoconstriction. Fredrikson (1986) reported that while muscular vascular resistance did not change during a reaction time task in white normotensives and hypertensives, it increased significantly in black groups. Anderson, Lane, Muranaka, *et al.* (1988) found that during the application of an ice pack to the forehead, blood pressure and forearm vascular resistance increased significantly more in black compared to white male normotensives. Finally, Light *et al.* (1986) found that during a competitive task following β-adrenergic blockade, black borderline hypertensives exhibited a significantly greater increase in total peripheral resistance than whites, suggesting perhaps the unmasking of a strong α-adrenergic effect in the blacks. These data are particularly interesting in light of pharmacological research showing the superior effect of labetolol (a combined α/β blocker) over propranolol (a β blocker) in reducing blood pressure in black hypertensives (Flamenbaum *et al.,* 1985). Thus, α-adrenergic hyperreactivity, as indexed by peripheral vasoconstriction, may prove to be an important contributor to elevated blood pressure in blacks.

Future Research Directions

There are numerous avenues for future research on ethnic group differences in reactivity. These avenues relate to both the nature of the experimental tasks and the characteristics of the subjects studied.

Subject Variables

Although the importance of ethnic group comparisons has been mentioned, it is equally critical to begin to address differences between individuals within the same ethnic group. As with many cardiovascular diseases such as hypertension, morbidity risk is not randomly distributed within the group. That is, within an ethnic group, some persons are more susceptible than others to certain conditions. Studies should be designed to address both ethnic differences and variations between members of the same group who might differ with respect to disease risk. An example of this type of

research are studies reviewed earlier by Fredrikson (1986), Light *et al.* (1986), and Schneiderman (1986) using black and white normotensives and borderline or established hypertensives. As a starting place, many of the factors shown to be predictive of *resting* cardiovascular activity may also be associated with *reactivity*. These include socioeconomic status, education or occupation, age, family history of disease, or marital status. Personality or behavioral factors should also be examined, such as John Henryism, anger suppression, Type A, and hostility. It should be noted, however, that whether any of these subject characteristics is associated with reactivity may depend on the nature of the experimental procedure. For example, one type of procedure may distinguish between people classified as either high or low in anger suppression, while another may not. Particularly when psychological constructs are under investigation, it is important to use tasks which are conceptually and theoretically relevant to the construct being studied (Houston, 1986).

Task Variables

Krantz, Manuck, and Wing (1986) have outlined several ways in which experimental tasks have been categorized. These include passive versus active coping, sensory intake versus mental work, emotional quality, level of personal control, effort versus distress, or the physical nature of the task. Some categories of tasks have been shown to elicit specific patterns of cardiovascular or hormonal adjustments. For example, an active coping task such as shock avoidance reaction time produces an increase in heart and blood pressure which is β-adrenergically mediated (Obrist, 1981). Conversely, a physical task such as the cold pressor test with nonchallenging instructions also produces a blood pressure increase, but which is mediated by α-adrenergic vasoconstriction (Andren & Hansson, 1981; Buell, Alpert, & McCrory, 1986). Further, other factors may be introduced into the experimental situation, such as pharmacological blockade or sodium intake (e.g., see Light *et al.,* 1986), which would serve to enhance or inhibit the effects of these procedures.

One direction for future research would be to

determine ethnic differences in reactivity to tasks known to produce specific patterns of physiological adjustment. In this way, if ethnic differences are observed, researchers would be somewhat closer to understanding the mechanisms which underlie the differences in reactivity. Similarly, pharmacological blockade procedures allow for the determination of underlying mechanisms in reactivity to certain tasks.

Finally, subject characteristics other than ethnic group may influence the degree of responsivity to certain types of tasks. For example, it is conceivable that two members of the same ethnic group will respond differently to a challenging mental arithmetic task if they differ in educational attainment. Moreover, it is at present unclear whether members of different ethnic groups perceive laboratory situations similarly, and the effects this might have on physiological responsivity. Therefore, researchers should be cognizant of the potential interactions of subject variables with task parameters, and assess subjects' subjective and emotional responses to laboratory procedures.

Conclusion

Research on ethnic group differences in resting cardiovascular and humoral activity has been an active area of investigation for a number of years, and has produced findings indicating differences and similarities in several physiological parameters. Conversely, research on ethnic differences in stress-induced reactivity has not enjoyed such a long history. However, research now beginning to emerge from several laboratories, using a variety of different approaches and subject populations, will provide an important foundation for future studies in this area. It is hoped that this research will contribute significantly to our understanding of biopsychosocial dimensions of cardiovascular diseases in ethnic groups.

References

Abboud, F. M., & Eckstein, J. W. (1966). Active reflex vasodilation in man. *Federation Proceedings, 25,* 1611–1617.
Alpert, B. S., Dover, E. V., Booker, D. L., Martin, A. M., &

Strong, W. B. (1981). Blood pressure response to dynamic exercise in healthy children—black versus white. *Journal of Pediatrics, 99,* 556–560.
Alpert, B. S., Flood, N. L., Strong, W. B., Dover, E. V., DuRant, R. H., Martin, A. M., & Booker, D. L. (1982). Responses to ergometer exercise in a healthy biracial population of children. *Journal of Pediatrics, 101,* 583–545.
Anderson, N. B. (in press). Racial differences in stress-induced cardiovascular reactivity and hypertension: Current status and substantive issues. *Psychological Bulletin.*
Anderson, N. B. (1988). Aging and hypertension in blacks: A multidimensional perspective. In J. Jackson (Ed.), *The black American elderly: Research on physical and psychosocial health* (pp. 190–214). Berlin: Springer.
Anderson, N. B., Lane, J. D., Muranaka, M., Houseworth, S. J., & Williams, R. B., Jr. (1986). Type A behavior, parental history of hypertension, and cardiovascular responses in young black women. *Psychophysiology, 23* (abstract), 423.
Anderson, N. B., Williams, R. B., Jr., Lane, J. D., Haney, T., Simpson, S., & Houseworth, S. J. (1986). Type A behavior, family history of hypertension, and cardiovascular responses among black women. *Health Psychology, 5,* 393–406.
Anderson, N. B., Williams, R. B., Jr., Lane, J. D., & Houseworth, S. J. (1987). Parental history of hypertension and cardiovascular responses in young black women. *Journal of Psychosomatic Research, 31,* 723–729.
Anderson, N. B., Lane, J. D., Monou, H., Williams, R. B., Jr., & Houseworth, S. J. (1988). Racial differences in cardiovascular responses to mental arithmetic. *International Journal of Psychophysiology, 6,* 161–164.
Anderson, N. B., Lane, J. D., Muranaka, M., Williams, R. B., Jr., & Houseworth, S. J. (1988). Racial differences in blood pressure and forearm vascular responses to the cold face stimulus. *Psychosomatic Medicine, 50,* 57–63.
Anderson, N. B., Lane, J. D., & Taguchi, F. (1988). Cardiovascular responses in young males as a function of race, parental hypertension, and type of stress (submitted for publication).
Anderson, N. B., Lane, J. D., Taguchi, F., & Williams, R. B., Jr. (in press). Race, parental history of hypertension, and patterns of cardiovascular reactivity in women. *Psychophysiology.*
Andren, L., & Hansson, L. (1981). Circulatory effects of stress in essential hypertension. *Acta Medica Scandinavica, 646,* 69–72.
Baron, A., Freyer, B., & Fixler, D. (1986). Longitudinal blood pressures in blacks, whites, and Mexican Americans during adolescence and early adulthood. *American Journal of Epidemiology, 123,* 809–817.
Bartel, A., Heyden, S., Tyroler, H., Tabesh, E., Cassel, J., & Hames, C. (1971). Electrocardiographic predictors of coronary heart disease. *Archives of Internal Medicine, 128,* 929–937.
Beaglehole, R., Tyroler, H., Cassel, J., Deubner, D. C., Bartel, A., & Hames, C. (1975). An epidemiological study of left ventricular hypertrophy in the biracial population of Evans County, Georgia. *Journal of Chronic Diseases, 28,* 554–559.

Berenson, G., Voors, A., & Dalferes, E. (1979). Creatinine clearance, electrolytes, and plasma renin activity related to the blood pressure of white and black children—The Bogalusa Heart Study. *Journal of Laboratory and Clinical Medicine, 93,* 535–548.

Berenson, G., Voors, A., Webber, L., Dalferes, E., Jr., & Harsha, D. (1979). Racial differences of parameters associated with blood pressure levels in children: The Bogalusa Heart Study. *Metabolism, 28,* 1218–1228.

Boyle, E., Jr., Griffey, W., Jr., Nichaman, M., & Talbert, C., Jr. (1967). An epidemiologic study of hypertension among racial groups of Charleston County, South Carolina: The Charleston Heart Study, Phase II. In J. Stamler, S. Stamler, & T. Pullman (Eds.), *The epidemiology of hypertension* (pp. 193–203). New York: Grune & Stratton.

Brunner, H., Sealey, J., & Laragh, J. (1973). Renin as a risk factor in essential hypertension: More evidence. *American Journal of Medicine, 52,* 175.

Buell, J., Alpert, B., & McCrory, W. (1986). Physical stressors as elicitors of cardiovascular reactivity. In K. Matthews, S. Weiss, T. Detre, T. Dembroski, B. Falkner, S. Manuck, & R. Williams, Jr. (Eds.), *Handbook of stress, reactivity, and cardiovascular disease* (pp. 127–144). New York: Wiley.

Bureau of the Census (1983, May). *General population characteristics: 1980* (supplementary report) (Chap. B, Vol. 1, Pt. 1). Washington, DC: U.S. Department of Commerce.

Chrysant, S., Danisa, K., Kem, D., Dillard, B., Smith, W., & Frohlich, E. (1979). Racial differences in pressure, volume and renin interrelationships in essential hypertension. *Hypertension, 1,* 136–141.

Clark, V., & Harrell, J. (1982). The relationship among Type A behavior, styles used in coping with racism, and blood pressure. *Journal of Black Psychology, 8,* 89–99.

Cooper, R. (1984). A note on the biologic concept of race and its application in epidemiologic research. *American Heart Journal, 108,* 715–723.

deChamplain, J., Cousineau, D., & Lapointe, L. (1980). Evidences supporting an increased sympathetic tone and reactivity in a subgroup of patients with essential hypertension. *Clinical and Experimental Hypertension, 2,* 359–377.

Dimsdale, J. E., Graham, R., Ziegler, M. G., Zusman, R., & Berry, C. C. (1987). Age, race, diagnosis, and sodium effects on the pressor response to infused norepinephrine. *Hypertension, 10,* 564–569.

Dressler, W., Dos Santos, J., & Viteri, F. (1986). Blood pressure, ethnicity, and psychosocial resources. *Psychosomatic Medicine, 48,* 509–519.

Falkner, B., Kushner, H., Khalsa, D. K., Canessa, M., & Katz, S. (1986). Sodium sensitivity, growth and family history of hypertension in young blacks. *Journal of Hypertension, 4,* S381–S383.

Falkner, B., Kushner, H., Khalsa, D. K., & Katz, S. (1987, March). The effect of chronic sodium load in young blacks and whites. In S. Weiss (Chair), *Biobehavioral factors affecting hypertension in blacks.* Symposium conducted at the annual meeting of the Society of Behavioral Medicine, Washington, DC.

Flamenbaum, W., Weber, M. A., McMahon, G., Materson, B., Albert, A., & Poland, M. (1985). Monotherapy with labetolol compared with propranolol: Differential effects by race. *Journal of Clinical Hypertension, 75,* 24–31.

Fredrikson, M. (1986). Racial differences in reactivity to behavioral challenge in essential hypertension. *Journal of Hypertension, 4,* 325–331.

Friis, R., Nanjundappa, G., Pendergast, T., & Wesh, M. (1981). Coronary heart disease mortality and risk among Hispanics and non-Hispanics in Orange County, California. *Public Health Reports, 96,* 418–422.

Gillum, R. (1979). Pathophysiology of hypertension in blacks and whites: A review of the basis of racial blood pressure differences. *Hypertension, 1,* 468–475.

Glueck, C., Gartside, P., Laskarzewski, P., Khoury, P., & Tyroler, H. (1984). High-density lipoprotein cholesterol in blacks and whites: Potential ramifications for coronary heart disease. *American Heart Journal, 108,* 815–826.

Goldring, D., Londe, S., Sivakoff, M., Hernandez, A., Britton, C., & Choi, S. (1977). Blood pressure in a high school population. I. Standards for blood pressure and the relation of age, sex, weight, height, and race to blood pressure in children 14 to 18 years of age. *Journal of Pediatrics, 91,* 884–889.

Goldstein, D. (1981). Plasma norepinephrine in essential hypertension: A study of the studies. *Hypertension, 3,* 48.

Goldstein, D. (1983). Plasma catecholamines & essential hypertension: An analytical review. *Hypertension, 5,* 86–99.

Gordon, T., Garcia-Palmieri, M., Kagan, A., Kannel, W., & Schiffman, J. (1974). Differences in coronary heart disease in Framingham, Honolulu and Puerto Rico. *Journal of Chronic Diseases, 17,* 328–344.

Grim, C., Luft, F., Miller, J., Meneely, G., Batarbee, H., Hames, C., & Dahl, K. (1980). Racial differences in blood pressure in Evans County, Georgia: Relationship to sodium and potassium intake and plasma renin activity. *Journal of Chronic Diseases, 33,* 87–94.

Grim, C., Luft, F., Weinberger, M., Miller, J., Rose, R., & Christian, J. (1984). Genetic, familial, and racial influences on blood pressure control systems in man. *Australian and New Zealand Journal of Medicine, 14,* 453–457.

Gutgesell, M., Terrell, G., & Labarthe, D. (1981). Pediatric blood pressure: Ethnic comparisons in a primary care center. *Hypertension, 3,* 39–46.

Hall, W. D. (1985). Pharmacologic therapy of hypertension in blacks. In W. D. Hall, E. Saunders, & N. Shulman (Eds.), *Hypertension in blacks: Epidemiology, pathophysiology, and treatment* (pp. 182–208). Chicago: Year Book.

Harburg, E., Erfurt, J., Hauenstein, L., Chape, C., Schull, W., & Schork, M. (1973). Socioecological stress, suppressed hostility, skin color, and black–white blood pressure: Detroit. *Journal of Chronic Diseases, 26,* 595–611.

Harlan, W., Cornoni-Huntley, J., & Leaverton, P. (1979). Blood pressure in childhood: The National Health Examination Survey. *Hypertension, 1,* 559–565.

Helmer, O., & Judson, W. (1968). Metabolic studies on hypertensive patients with suppressed plasma renin activity not due to hyperaldosteronism. *Circulation, 38,* 965–976.

Hohn, A., Riopel, D., Keil, J., Loadhold, C., Margolius, H., Halushka, P., Privitera, P., Webb, J., Medley, E., Schuman, S., Rubin, M., Pantell, R., & Braunstein, M. (1983). Childhood familial and racial differences in physiologic and biochemical factors related to hypertension. *Hypertension, 5*, 56–70.

Houston, B. (1986). Psychological variables and cardiovascular and neuroendocrine reactivity. In K. Matthews, S. Weiss, T. Detre, T. Dembroski, B. Falkner, S. Manuck, & R. Williams, Jr. (Eds.), *Handbook of stress, reactivity, and cardiovascular disease* (pp. 207–229). New York: Wiley.

Hypertension Detection and Follow-up Program Cooperative Group (1977). Race, education and prevalence of hypertension. *American Journal of Epidemiology, 106*, 351–361.

James, S. (1985). Psychosocial and environmental factors in black hypertension. In W. D. Hall, E. Saunders, & N. Shulman (Eds.), *Hypertension in blacks: Epidemiology, pathophysiology, and treatment* (pp. 132–143). Chicago: Year Book.

James, S., Hartnett, S., & Kalsbeek, W. (1983). John Henryism and blood pressure differences among black men. *Journal of Behavioral Medicine, 6*, 259–278.

Kannel, W., Gordon, T., Castelli, W., & Margolis, J. (1970). Electrocardiographic left ventricular hypertrophy and risk of coronary heart disease: The Framingham Study. *Annals of Internal Medicine, 84*, 639–645.

Kaplan, N., Kem, D., Holland, O., Kramer, N., Higgins, J., & Gomez-Sanchez, C. (1976). The intra-venous furosemide test: A simple way to evaluate renin responsiveness. *Annals of Internal Medicine, 84*, 639–645.

Kilcoyne, N., Richter, R., & Alsup, P. (1974). Adolescent hypertension. I. Detection and prevalence. *Circulation, 50*, 758.

Kotchen, J., Kotchen, T., Schwertman, N., & Kuller, L. (1974). Blood pressure distributions of urban adolescents. *Journal of Epidemiology, 99*, 315–324.

Krantz, D., Manuck, W., & Wing, R. (1986). Psychological stressors and task variables as elicitors of reactivity. In K. Matthews, S. Weiss, T. Detre, T. Dembroski, B. Falkner, S. Manuck, & R. Williams, Jr. (Eds.), *Handbook of stress, reactivity, and cardiovascular disease* (pp. 85–107). New York: Wiley.

Kraus, J., Borhani, N., & Franti, C. (1980). Socioeconomic status, ethnicity, and risk of coronary heart disease. *American Journal of Epidemiology, 111*, 407–414.

Kumanyika, S., & Savage, D. (1986a). Ischemic heart disease risk factors in Hispanic Americans. *Report on the Secretary's Task Force on Black and Minority Health.* Vol. IV, Pt. 2, pp. 393–412. U.S. Department of Health and Human Services.

Kumanyika, S., & Savage, D. (1986b). Ischemic heart disease risk factors in American Indians and Alaska Natives. *Report on the Secretary's Task Force on Black and Minority Health.* Vol. IV, Pt. 2, pp. 445–473. U.S. Department of Health and Human Services.

Kumanyika, S., & Savage, D. (1986c). Ischemic heart disease risk factors in Asian/Pacific Islander Americans. *Report on*

the Secretary's Task Force on Black and Minority Health. Vol. IV, Pt. 2, pp. 415–441. U.S. Department of Health and Human Services.

Kumanyika, S., & Savage, D. (1986d). Ischemic heart disease risk factors in black Americans. *Report on the Secretary's Task Force on Black and Minority Health.* Vol. IV, Pt. 2, pp. 229–343. U.S. Department of Health and Human Services.

Lee, Y., Rosner, B., Gould, J., Lowe, E., & Kass, E. (1976). Familial aggregation of blood pressure of newborn infants and their mothers. *Pediatrics, 58*, 727–729.

Levinson, S., Liu, K., Stamler, J., Stamler, R., Whipple, I., Ausbrook, D., & Berkson, D. (1985). Ethnic differences in blood pressure and heart rate of Chicago school children. *American Journal of Epidemiology, 122*, 366–377.

Levy, S., Lilley, J., Frigon, R., & Stone, R. (1977). Urinary kallikrein and plasma renin activity as determinants of renal blood flow. *Journal of Clinical Investigation, 60*, 129.

Lichtman, M., & Woods, J. (1967). Catecholamine excretion in young white and Negro males with normal and elevated blood pressure. *Journal of Chronic Diseases, 20*, 119–128.

Light, K. C., Obrist, P. A., Sherwood, A., James, S., & Strogatz, D. (1987). Effects of race and marginally elevated blood pressure on cardiovascular responses to stress in young men. *Hypertension, 10*, 555–563.

Light, K., Sherwood, A., Obrist, P., James, S., Strogatz, D., & Willis, P. (1986, August). Comparisons of cardiovascular and renal responses to stress in black and white normotensive and borderline hypertensive men. In N. Anderson (chair), *Biobehavioral aspects of hypertension in blacks: Current findings.* Symposium conducted at the meeting of the American Psychological Association, Washington, DC.

Lilley, J., Hsu, L., & Stone, R. (1976). Racial disparity of plasma volume in hypertensive man. *Annals of Internal Medicine, 84*, 707.

Londe, S., Gollub, S., & Goldring, D. (1977). Blood pressure in black and in white children. *The Journal of Pediatrics, 90*, 93–95.

Luft, F., Grim, C., Fineberg, N., & Weinberger, M. (1979). Effects of volume expansion and contraction in normotensive whites, blacks, and subjects of different ages. *Circulation, 59*, 653–650.

Luft, F., Grim, C., Higgins, J., Jr., & Weinberger, M. (1977). Differences in response to sodium administration in normotensive white and black subjects. *Journal of Laboratory and Clinical Medicine, 90*, 555–562.

Luft, F., Grim, C., & Weinberger, M. (1985). Electrolyte and volume homeostasis in blacks. In W. D. Hall, E. Saunders, & N. Shulman (Eds.), *Hypertension in blacks: Epidemiology, pathophysiology, and treatment* (pp. 115–131). Chicago: Year Book.

Luft, F., Rankin, L., Block, R., Weyman, A., Williams, L., Murray, R., Grim, C., & Weinberger, M. (1979). Cardiovascular and humoral responses to extremes of sodium intake in normal black and white men. *Circulation, 60*, 697–706.

Luft, F., Weinberger, M., & Grim, C. (1982). Sodium sensitivity and resistance in normotensive humans. *American Journal of Medicine, 72,* 726–736.

MacDougall, J., Dembroski, T., & Krantz, D. (1981). Effects of types of challenge on pressor and heart rate responses in Type A and B women. *Psychophysiology, 18,* 1–9.

Matthews, K., Weiss, S., Detre, T., Dembroski, T., Falkner, B., Manuck, S., & Williams, R., Jr. (Eds.) (1986). *Handbook of stress reactivity and cardiovascular disease.* New York: Wiley.

Messerli, R., Decarvalho, J., Christie, B., & Frohlich, E. (1979). Essential hypertension in black and white subjects: Hemodynamic findings and fluid volume states. *The American Journal of Medicine, 67,* 27–31.

Mitas, J., Holle, R., Levy, S., & Stone, R. (1979). Racial analysis of the volume–renin relationship in human hypertension. *Archives of Internal Medicine, 139,* 157–160.

Morrell, M. A., Myers, H., Shapiro, D., Goldstein, I., & Armstrong, M. (in press). Cardiovascular reactivity to psychological stressors in black and white normotensive males. *Health Psychology.*

Morrison, J., deGroot, I., Kelley, K., Mellies, M., Khoury, P., Edwards, B., Lewis, D., Lewis, A., Fiorelli, M., Heiss, G., Tyroler, H., & Glueck, C. (1979). Black–white differences in plasma lipids and lipoproteins in adults: The Cincinnati Lipid Research Clinic Population Study. *Preventive Medicine, 8,* 34–39.

Morrison, J., Khoury, P., Mellies, M., Kelley, K., Horvitz, R., & Glueck, C. (1981). Lipid and lipoprotein distributions in black adults. The Cincinnati Lipid Research Clinic Population Study. *Journal of the American Medical Association, 245,* 939–942.

Morrison, J., Khoury, P., Laskarzewski, P., Garatside, P., Moore, M., Heiss, G., & Glueck, C. (1980). Hyperalphalipoproteinemia in hypercholesterolemic adults and children. *Translantic Association of American Physicians, 93,* 230–243.

Murphy, J., Alpert, B., Moes, D., & Somes, G. (1986). Race and cardiovascular reactivity: A neglected relationship. *Hypertension, 8,* 1075–1083.

Murphy, J., Alpert, B. S., Walker, S. S., & Wiley, E. (submitted for publication). Race and reactivity: A replication.

Nash, J., Jorgensen, R., Lasser, N., & Hymowitz, N. (1985, March). *The effects of race, gender, and task on cardiovascular reactivity in unmedicated, mild hypertensives.* Presented at the Sixth Annual Meeting of the Society of Behavioral Medicine, New Orleans.

Neser, W., Thomas, J., Semenya, K., Thomas, D., & Gillum, R. (1986). Obesity and hypertension in a longitudinal study of black physicians: The Meharry Cohort Study. *Journal of Chronic Diseases, 39,* 105–113.

Nichaman, M., Hamilton, H., Kagan, A., Grier, R., Sacks, S., & Syme, S. (1975). Epidemiologic studies of coronary heart disease and stroke in Japanese men living in Japan, Hawaii, and California: Distribution of biochemical risk factors. *American Journal of Epidemiology, 102,* 491–501.

Obrist, P. (1981). *Cardiovascular psychophysiology: A perspective.* New York: Plenum Press.

Persky, V., Dyer, A., Stamler, J., Shekelle, R., & Schoenberger, J. (1979). Racial patterns of heart rate in an employed adult population. *American Journal of Epidemiology, 110,* 274–280.

Reed, T. (1969). Caucasian genes in American Negroes. *Science, 165,* 762–768.

Report of the Secretary's Task Force on Black and Minority Health (1985). Vol. I. U.S. Department of Health and Human Services.

Report of the Secretary's Task Force on Black and Minority Health (1986). Vol. IV, Pt. 1, pp. 23–24. U.S. Department of Health and Human Services.

Riley, C., Oberman, A., Hurst, D., & Peacock, P. (1973). Electrocardiographic findings in a biracial, urban population: The Birmingham Stroke Study. *Alabama Journal of Medical Science, 10,* 160–170.

Roberts, J. (1978). *Cardiovascular conditions of children and youths.* Series 11, No. 135.

Roberts, J., & Maurer, K. (1977). *Blood pressure levels of persons 6–74 years, United States, 1971–74.* DHEW Publication No. (HRA) 77–1648. Series 11, No. 203.

Roberts, J., & Rowland, M. (1981). *Hypertension in adults 25–74 years of age:* United States, 1971–75. DHEW Publication No. (PHS) 81-1671. Series 11, No. 221.

Rowland, M., & Roberts, J. (1982). *Blood pressure levels and hypertension in persons ages 6–74 years: United States, 1976–80.* DHHS Publication No. (PHS) 82-1250.

Rowlands, D., DeGivanni, J., McLeay, R., Watson, R., Stallard, T., & Littler, W. (1982). Cardiovascular response in black and white hypertensives. *Hypertension, 4,* 817–820.

Savage, D. (in press). Echocardiographic assessment of cardiac anatomy and function in black and white hypertensive subjects. In R. Williams (Ed.), *Textbook of ethnic medicine.*

Schachter, J., Kerr, J., Wimberly, F., & Lachin, J. (1974). Heart rate levels of black and white newborns. *Psychosomatic Medicine, 36,* 513–524.

Schachter, J., & Kuller, L. (1984). Blood volume expansion among blacks: An hypothesis. *Medical Hypotheses, 14,* 1–19.

Schachter, J., Kuller, L., & Perfetti, C. (1984a). Heart rate during the first five years of life: Relation to ethnic group (black or white) and to parental hypertension. *American Journal of Epidemiology, 119,* 554–563.

Schachter, J., Kuller, L., & Perfetti, C. (1984b). Blood pressure during the first five years of life: Relation to ethnic group (black or white) and to parental hypertension. *American Journal of Epidemiology, 119,* 541–553.

Schachter, J., Lachin, J., Kerr, J., Wimberly, F., & Ratey, J. (1976). Heart rate and blood pressure in black newborns and in white newborns. *Pediatrics, 58,* 283–287.

Schachter, J., Lachin, J., & Wimberly, F. (1976). Newborn heart rate and blood pressure: Relation to race and to socioeconomic class. *Psychosomatic Medicine, 38,* 390–398.

Schneiderman, N. (1986, August). Race, gender, and reactivity in the Miami minority hypertension project. In N. Anderson (Chair), *Biobehavioral aspects of hypertension in blacks: Current findings.* Symposium conducted at the annual meeting of the American Psychological Association, Washington, DC.

Sever, P., Peart, W., Davies, I., Turnbridge, R., & Gordon, D. (1979). Ethnic differences in blood pressure with observations on noradrenaline and renin. 2. A hospital hypertensive population. *Clinical and Experimental Hypertension, 1,* 745.

Sever, P., Peart, W., Meade, T., Davies, I., & Gordon, D. (1979). Ethnic differences in blood pressure with observations on noradrenaline and renin. 1. A working population. *Clinical and Experimental Hypertension, 1,* 733–744.

Shekelle, R., Liu, S., Raynor, W., & Miller, R. (1978). Racial difference in mean pulse rate of children aged six to eleven years. *Pediatrics, 61,* 119–121.

Sievers, M. (1968). Serum cholesterol levels in Southwestern American Indians. *Journal of Chronic Diseases, 21,* 107–115.

Stamler, J., Rhomberg, P., Schoenberger, J., Shekelle, R., Dyer, A., Shekelle, S., Stamler, R., & Wannamaker, J. (1975). Multivariate analysis of the relationship of seven variables to blood pressure: Findings of the Chicago Heart Association Detection Project in Industry, 1967–1972. *Journal of Chronic Diseases, 28,* 527–548.

Stamler, J., Stamler, R., Rhomberg, P., Dyer, A., Berkson, D., Reedus, W., & Wannamaker, J. (1975). Multivariate analysis of the relationship of six variables to blood pressure: Findings from Chicago community surveys, 1965–1971. *Journal of Chronic Diseases, 28,* 499–525.

Stern, M., Rosenthal, M., Haffner, S., Hazuda, H., & Franco, L. (1984). Differences in the effects of sociocultural status on diabetes and cardiovascular risk factors in Mexican Americans: The San Antonio Heart Study. *American Journal of Epidemiology, 120,* 834–851.

Thomas, J., Semenya, K., Neser, W., Thomas, D., Green, D., & Gillum, R. (1984). Precursors of hypertension in black medical students: The Meharry Cohort Study. *Journal of the National Medical Association, 76,* 111–121.

Tyroler, H., Glueck, C., Christensen, B., & Kwiterovich, P. (1980). Plasma high-density lipoprotein cholesterol: Comparisons in black and white populations. *Circulation, 62*(Suppl. 4), 99–107.

Tyroler, H., Hames, C., Krishnan, I., Heyden, S., Cooper, C., & Cassel, J. (1975). Black–white differences in serum lipids and lipoprotein in Evans County. *Preventive Medicine, 4,* 541–549.

U.S. DHEW (1979). *Selected vital statistics for Indian health service areas and service units, 1972–1977.* DHEW Publication No. (HSA) 79-1005.

Valentine, C. (1971). Deficit, difference and bicultural models of Afro-American behavior. *Harvard Educational Review, 41,* 137–157.

Venter, C., Joubert, P., & Strydom, W. (1985). The relevance of ethnic differences in haemodynamic responses to the head-up tilt manoeuvre to clinical pharmacological investigations. *Journal of Cardiovascular Pharmacology, 7,* 1009–1010.

Voors, A., Webber, L., & Berenson, G. (1980). Racial contrasts in cardiovascular response tests for children from a total community. *Hypertension, 2,* 686–694.

Voors, A., Webber, L., & Berenson, G. (1982). Resting heart rate and pressure–rate product of children in a total biracial community: The Bogalusa Heart Study. *American Journal of Epidemiology, 116,* 276–286.

Warren, S., & O'Connor, D. (1980). Does a renal vasodilator system mediate racial differences in essential hypertension? *The American Journal of Medicine, 69,* 425–429.

Washington, E., & McLoyd, V. (1982). The external validity of research involving American minorities. *Human Development, 25,* 324–339.

Watkins, L., & Eaker, E. (1986). Population and demographic influences on reactivity. In K. Matthews, S. Weiss, T. Detre, T. Dembroski, B. Falkner, S. Manuck, & R. Williams, Jr. (Eds.), *Handbook of stress, reactivity, and cardiovascular disease* (pp. 85–107). New York: Wiley.

Wilson, P., Savage, D., Castelli, W., Garrison, R., Donahue, R., & Feinleib, M. (1983). HDL-cholesterol in a sample of black adults. The Framingham Minority Study. *Metabolism, 32,* 328–332.

Winkelstein, W., Kagan, A., Kato, H., & Sacks, S. (1975). Epidemiologic studies of coronary heart disease and stroke in Japanese men living in Japan, Hawaii, and California: Blood pressure distributions. *American Journal of Epidemiology, 102,* 502–513.

Wisenbaugh, P., Garst, J., Hull, C., Freedman, R., Matthews, D., & Hadady, M. (1972). Renin, aldosterone, sodium and hypertension. *American Journal of Medicine, 52,* 175.

CHAPTER 29

Cardiovascular and Neuroendocrine Responses to Challenge in Males and Females

Patrice G. Saab

Increasing attention has been given to the role that physiological response to behavioral challenges, i.e., stressors, may play in the development of cardiovascular disease (see Matthews *et al.*, 1986). Behavioral stressors typically evoke notable cardiovascular and neuroendocrine responses. To date, preliminary evidence from the literature on both Type A behavior pattern (TABP) and essential hypertension implicates the role of behaviorally induced sympathetically mediated cardiovascular and neuroendocrine responses to mildly challenging stressors in the subsequent development of disease (for a thorough review, see Krantz & Manuck, 1984).

For the purposes of the present discussion, reactivity refers to challenge (stressor)-induced levels or changes from baseline. The objective of this chapter is to evaluate the literature that pertains to sex differences in reactivity. The review of the reactivity literature is limited to individuals who are presumed to be normotensive and healthy. First, sex differences in cardiovascular disease and

hypertension are discussed. Second, resting baseline cardiovascular and neuroendocrine activity in males and females is reviewed. Third, the literature directly comparing reactivity of males and females in both laboratory and field settings is presented. Fourth, the relationship among TABP, sex, and reactivity is examined. Fifth, the influence of menstrual cycle phase and menopausal status on reactivity is considered. The final section discusses recommendations for future work.

Sex Differences in Cardiovascular Disease and Hypertension

Cardiovascular disease is the leading cause of death in the United States (Stamler, 1975). There are marked differences for men and women in cardiovascular disease incidence, especially prior to older age. Data from the Framingham cohort reveal that the relative risk for cardiovascular disease is 4.5 for men prior to age 35, narrowing to 2.7 at age 50, 1.5 in the early 60s, and 1.1 in the late 70s (Kannel, Hjortland, McNamara, & Gordon, 1976). Although the incidence for the sexes be-

Patrice G. Saab • Department of Psychology, University of Miami, Coral Gables, Florida 33124.

comes more comparable in the late 50s, inspection of age-specific rates suggests that rates for women are similar to those of men approximately 10 years younger (Kannel *et al.,* 1976).

A sex differential is also apparent for prevalence of hypertension, a risk factor for cardiovascular disease. Prior to age 55, the prevalence of clinical hypertension is substantially greater among men than women. By the mid-60s to 70s, however, rates of hypertension are somewhat greater among women. Age-adjusted rates for black adults are approximately two times greater than those for white adults (Stamler, 1975).

While the etiology for the sex differential in cardiovascular disease and hypertension is unknown, some have speculated that sex hormone status plays a role (Berkson, Stamler, & Cohen, 1964; von Eiff, Plotz, Beck, & Czernik, 1971). It has been hypothesized that the diminution of ovarian function with menopause may account for the eventual narrowing of disease rates between men and women. It is known that a whole host of changes accompany menopause. For example, in contrast to premenopausal women, postmenopausal women have higher levels of circulating estrone, relative to the more biologically active estradiol (Emmens & Martin, 1964; Stout, 1982). Estrogens impact upon several risk factors for cardiovascular disease. Both estradiol and estrone are positively related to weight (Phillips, 1978). The lipid picture also changes with menopause. Prior to menopause, women have less total cholesterol, triglycerides, and low-density lipids (LDL) but greater high-density lipids (HDL) than age-matched males (McConathy & Alaupovic, 1981). With menopause, there is an increase in total serum cholesterol and LDL. One hypothesized mechanism to account for the protective effect of estrogens was the possible influence on the metabolism of lipids and lipoproteins. Administration of conjugated estrogens to menopausal women does not necessarily restore the premenopausal lipid profile (McConathy & Alaupovic, 1981). There is evidence, however, that estrogens not in combination with progesterone may increase HDL and decrease LDL (Bush & Barrett-Connor, 1985).

Furthermore, most of the available estrogens after menopause are synthesized by the adrenals, in contrast to the ovaries. Interestingly, there is some evidence to suggest that certain estrogens may have adrenergic actions. Wasilewska and associates (Wasilewska, Kobus, & Bargiel, 1980) cited evidence indicating that estrogens may increase norepinephrine (NE) in the synaptic vesicle. Likewise, there are data suggesting that estrone is responsive to adrenal cortical stimulation and can be influenced by stress (Klaiber *et al.,* 1982). While the implication of these findings is unclear, data regarding estrogen and cardiovascular risk have accumulated.

Inspection of male to female age-specific death rates for arteriosclerotic diseases illustrates that the narrowing of the sex differential is concomitant with the age of menopause in several populations (e.g., Tracy, 1966). The purported relationship between menopause and cardiovascular disease incidence has been explored in the Framingham cohort (Kannel *et al.,* 1976). It was hypothesized that if menopause did confer added risk, age-matched groups of premenopausal and postmenopausal women would differ in the incidence of cardiovascular disease (Kannel *et al.,* 1976). Though the number of events was small over the 20-year follow-up period, postmenopausal women less than 55 years old were at two times greater risk (rates expressed in person-years) than their premenopausal counterparts. In fact, both natural and surgical menopausal women were at substantial risk. Marked differences in male to female risk were obtained when men (40–54 years) were compared to age-matched premenopausal and postmenopausal women. Relative to premenopausal women, the relative risk for men ranged from 4.5 to 9.5. However, compared to postmenopausal women, the relative risk for men extended from only 1.5 to 2.5. It is noteworthy that menopause is not accompanied by significant change in weight, blood glucose, blood pressure, or vital capacity, though there is prospective evidence for a change in serum cholesterol (Hjortland, McNamara, & Kannel, 1976). The advantage for women, however, is absent when diabetics are evaluated. Other established risk factors apparently do not account for the discrepancy between the sexes (Kannel *et al.,* 1976).

Preliminary work has also been done on sex differences in vascular physiology (Freedman, Sabharwal, & Desai, 1986). This line of research is relevant since it addresses the issue of specific mechanisms that might account for cardiovascular-related differences between males and females. In response to α-adrenergic receptor and β-adrenergic receptor agonists, young women displayed evidence of diminished peripheral vascular sympathetic receptor sensitivity. This finding has been interpreted as reflecting decreased sensitivity and/or density of sympathetic receptors. Evidence is conflicting as to whether sex hormones might account for the decreased sensitivity in adrenergic vascular receptors in women (Freedman *et al.*, 1986).

Given the sex differential in cardiovascular disease and hypertension, it is compelling to consider whether the same pattern is paralleled in physiological responses to behavioral challenge. Augmented challenge-induced physiological responsivity is hypothesized to be a marker for eventual disease. Evidence that groups at high risk for cardiovascular disease and hypertension demonstrate heightened reactivity would provide further support for the influence of physiological as well as behavioral factors in the development of cardiovascular disease.

Baseline Cardiovascular and Neuroendocrine Activity in Males and Females

Prior to examining whether any sex differences in reactivity exist, it is critical to review differences in baseline parameters. Inspection of baseline values is relevant since such differences could, in part, explain challenge-induced sex differences in physiological responding.

Data from the Health and Nutrition Examination Survey of 1971–1974, surveying blood pressure (BP) levels of individuals aged 6–74 years, reveal that sex differences in BP are age-related. Prior to age 15, boys and girls display comparable systolic blood pressure (SBP) and diastolic blood pressure (DBP) levels. From 18 to 44 years, however, mean SBP levels are 4.4–9 mm Hg higher for men than women. This disparity in casual SBP narrows to 3.6 mm Hg between men and women 45–54 years of age. The trend reverses in the mid to late 50s when the casual SBP of women exceeds that of men by 3.4 mm Hg. Systolic blood pressure continues to increase in women, so that a 5.6 mm Hg difference between women and men is apparent for those in their 60s and 70s. Similarly, average DBP levels are 4.9–6.2 mm Hg greater in men than women from ages 18 to 54 years. By the mid 50s, comparable DBP levels are characteristic of men and women (National Center for Health Statistics, 1977).

Dissimilarity for heart rate (HR) is frequently observed. Heart rate is higher in children than adults (Gasul, Arcilla, & Lev, 1966), and among adults, higher in females than males (e.g., Bell, Davidson, & Scarborough, 1968). The size of the heart is among the factors that influence HR. On the average, the hearts of adult males are larger than adult females (300 versus 250 g). As HR is generally faster in smaller organisms (Prosser, 1973), the HR of a woman is often faster than that of a man.

Developmental changes in urinary cathecholamine metabolites have been examined in diverse age groups, ranging from neonates to adults (e.g., Cuche, Kuchel, Barbeau, & Genest, 1975; Dalmaz & Peyrin, 1982; Johansson & Post, 1974). Accurate determination of catecholamine levels necessitates collection under relatively standard conditions, such as abstinence from substances or activities that influence catecholamine responses. Daily urine samples collected from males and females revealed that NE and epinephrine (E) output levels were substantially greater in neonate females than males, but that E was lower in adult females than males when values were expressed as micrograms per 24 h. When data were adjusted for urine output and weight, adult sex differences in E did not persist (Dalmaz & Peyrin, 1982). Similar results for transformed urinary catecholamine output levels were obtained from employed men and women sampled monthly in order to ascertain seasonal influences on excretion under routine work conditions (Johansson & Post, 1974). Taken together, the findings of Dalmaz and Peyrin (1982) and Johansson and Post (1974) support the need to adjust for factors that may account for purported sex differences in urinary catecholamines.

Postural influences on resting urinary catecholamines in men and women have likewise been considered (Cuche *et al.*, 1975). During recumbency, NE was significantly greater in normotensive women than men. Upright posture decreased the dopamine/NE ratio in both sexes. In the same study, the influence of menstrual phase on catecholamine excretion was evaluated in two women, reported to be normally cycling. Multiple 24-h urine during the first 14 days and the last 14 days of a 28-day cycle was collected. Catecholamine responses during both halves of the cycle were similar (Cuche *et al.*, 1975).

Fluctuations in physiological activity across the menstrual cycle are controversial. Dividing the cycle in half, as in the Cuche *et al.* (1975) study, is an imprecise way to evaluate potential changes in resting values associated with changes in female steroid hormones. Precision in identifying the menstrual phases that accompany characteristic hormonal surges is requisite. Catecholamines have been systematically studied by collecting daily or every other day samples for a minimum of one cycle (e.g., Goldstein, Levinson, & Keiser, 1983; Lamprecht, Matta, Little, & Zahn, 1974; Patkai, Johansson, & Post, 1974; Zacur, Tyson, Ziegler, & Lake, 1978; Zuspan & Zuspan, 1973) or even less frequent samples (e.g., Kobus, Wasilewska, & Bargiel, 1979, cited in Wasilewska *et al.*, 1980). Findings across studies are inconsistent. Excreted E remained relatively stable across the cycle (e.g., Goldstein *et al.*, 1983; Patkai *et al.*, 1974) or elevated during the luteal phase (Kobus *et al.*, 1979, cited in Wasilewska *et al.*, 1980), while excreted NE remained constant (Patkai *et al.*, 1974) or significantly increased during the luteal phase of the cycle (Goldstein *et al.*, 1983; Kobus *et al.*, 1979, cited in Wasilewska *et al.*, 1980; Zuspan & Zuspan, 1973).

Plasma catecholamine activity is characterized by equally mixed results. When plasma NE and dopamine were collected every other day, no relationship to endocrine changes regulating the menstrual cycle was apparent (Zacur *et al.*, 1978). Likewise, no cycle-related fluctuations in plasma dopamine-β-hydroxylase (DBH), a catalyst for the

transformation of dopamine to NE, were reported (Lamprecht *et al.*, 1974; Zacur *et al.*, 1978). In contrast, when daily samples were obtained, plasma NE was lowest during the menses and the follicular phase, and greatest during the luteal phase, whereas plasma E and dopamine showed no phase-related fluctuations when samples were collected at least 20 min after venipuncture (Goldstein *et al.*, 1983). Plasma E and NE have also been reported to increase around the period of the luteinizing hormone surge associated with ovulation (Zuspan & Zuspan, 1973). In the latter case, it is more likely that the findings reflect enhanced sympathetic responding due to venipuncture, as it appears the samples were taken immediately after venipuncture, without an adequate intervening sampling interval.

The lack of consistency in the baseline findings may, in part, be accounted for by the variability in methods and lack of standard procedures across studies. Even within the same study, it is clear that urinary and plasma catecholamine assays do not yield similar results (e.g., Goldstein *et al.*, 1983). This is not unexpected since plasma catecholamines have a substantially shorter half-life, whereas urinary catecholamines reflect a longer-acting process and are responsive to an accumulation of events. Furthermore, methods of assay varied across studies. Methods include radioenzymatic assays (Zacur *et al.*, 1978), high-performance liquid chromatography with electrochemical detection (Goldstein *et al.*, 1983), and fluorometry (Patkai *et al.*, 1974; Zuspan & Zuspan, 1973). Variability existed with regard to whether substances and activities that influence catecholamines were controlled. In some studies, women were requested to either avoid conditions in the morning that affect catecholamines, such as physical activity, caffeine, alcohol, and medication (e.g., Patkai *et al.*, 1974), or to abstain from caffeine and nicotine throughout the course of the study (e.g., Goldstein *et al.*, 1983). On occasion, no mention was made of any attempts to control the above factors (e.g., Zacur *et al.*, 1978; Zuspan & Zuspan, 1973).

Evaluation of the menstrual cycle literature is further complicated by the lack of consistency in the manner that the menstrual cycle was divided up into phases. This was not accomplished in exactly the same manner across studies. Additionally, sample sizes were limited and based on as few as two subjects (e.g., Cuche *et al.*, 1975; Zuspan & Zuspan, 1973). This unfortunately limits confidence in the generalizability of the data.

Nonetheless, it appears that the modal finding involves elevated NE at some period during the latter half of the menstrual cycle (Goldstein *et al.*, 1983; Kobus *et al.*, 1979, cited in Wasilewska *et al.*, 1980; Zuspan & Zuspan, 1973). Caution, however, should be exercised in concluding that there is more sympathetic influence during these periods. The findings suggest that a potential for baseline differences across the menstrual cycle exists. When comparing resting catecholamine activity of women to other women or to men, variability might be reduced by controlling the influence of menstrual phase. This could be accomplished by evaluating women during a common phase of their cycle.

In conclusion, men and women vary consistently on certain resting baseline parameters (i.e., SBP, DBP, and HR) but inconsistently on others (i.e., catecholamines) used to index reactivity. Elevated BP in men under 60 and greater HR in women can function as important determinants of whether sex differences in responsivity to behavioral challenge exist. To judge whether there are sex differences in responsivity, it is necessary to control for baseline differences that appear, as well as other factors that might affect resting activity, e.g., age and weight/body mass, and for women, menstrual phase. Such precautions would enhance confidence that physiological responses to challenge are a function of response to challenge rather than due to differences apparent at rest. In the next sections, challenge-induced responsivity in males and females is examined.

Neuroendocrine Responses to Stress in Males and Females

The majority of work that has considered the influence of the sexes on neuroendocrine responsivity to challenge has been done by Frankenhaeuser and her colleagues (e.g., Collins &

Frankenhaeuser, 1978; Forsman & Lindblad, 1983; Frankenhaeuser, Dunne, & Lundberg, 1976; Frankenhaeuser, von Wright, Collins, von Wright, Sedvall, & Swahn, 1978; Johansson, 1972; Johansson & Post, 1974; Johansson, Frankenhaeuser, & Magnussen, 1973; Lundberg & Frankenhaeuser, 1980; Rauste-von Wright, von Wright, & Frankenhaeuser, 1981), though other investigators (e.g., Aslan, Nelson, Carruthers, & Lader, 1981; Davidson, Vandongen, Rouse, Beilin, & Tunney, 1984; Tennes & Kreye, 1985) have also contributed to this literature. Participants, who vary over a wide range of ages, have been studied in laboratory as well as field settings. Challenges ranged from scheduled scholastic examinations to venipunctures to mildly challenging tasks such as the Stroop Color Word Test (SCWT).

The impact of the stress of an achievement test on cortisol excretion and self-report of test anxiety, was studied in young school-aged children, i.e., second-graders (Tennes & Kreye, 1985). Morning cortisol samples, collected over normal school days and achievement test days, were averaged separately to obtain representative ''control'' and ''test'' values. Test levels were not related to self-reports of anxiety. Cortisol levels were substantially greater on test days relative to control days. Cortisol responsivity, however, did not distinguish the sexes. Since some investigators hypothesize that female sex hormones attenuate stress reactions (von Eiff *et al.*, 1971) and others suggest that sex differences in socialization patterns can account for sex differences in stress responses (Frankenhaeuser, 1983), the findings are not surprising. By virtue of their age, the children were unlikely to be subject to differential hormonal influences. Likewise, limited school experience may not have afforded boys and girls the opportunities to learn different ways to react to achievement stress that might influence physiological responding to this type of challenge.

Sex differences in catecholamine excretion emerged in response to laboratory challenge and academic examinations in older school-aged children (Johansson, 1972; Frankenhaeuser *et al.*, 1978). Sixth-grade boys and girls excreted substantially more E to a demanding arithmetic task that was designed to approximate usual academic activities, than to a neutral film. The active arithmetic task was associated with higher E levels in boys when body mass was controlled (Johansson *et al.*, 1973). For boys, the E response was negatively correlated with previous self-reports of apprehension regarding school work. Superficially, it appeared as if boys displayed physiological evidence of anxiety without accompanying subjective evidence of anxiety. Since assessment of state anxiety was not accomplished, the relationship between anxiety elicited by the stress of the arithmetic task, designed to approximate an everyday challenge, and the excretion of E, is uncertain in this sample.

However, in a high school sample, boys reported less discomfort before and during a matriculation examination than girls (Frankenhaeuser *et al.*, 1978). Relative to a typical school day (10 days postexamination) the examination significantly increased cortisol and NE (weight-adjusted) in the adolescent males. In contrast, the examination was associated with elevated weight-adjusted E and MOPEG, a metabolite of circulating catecholamines, in adolescent males and females, relative to the control day. In a reanalysis of these data (Rauste-von Wright *et al.*, 1981), E levels and change from control levels in females were negatively related to reported satisfaction following the test.

In contrast to the boys, a notable number of girls did not exhibit E increases. The subsample of nonresponding females was described as more traditional and was reputed to resemble the sample of males, in terms of their increased satisfaction on the exam, and higher values on the self-esteem measures (Rauste-von Wright *et al.*, 1981). No effort, however, was made to categorize female responders. These findings are intriguing since they suggest that socialization impacts on an observed sex difference in response to achievement stress and on differences between female responders and nonresponders to stress. Additional valuable information pertaining to this issue would have been available had the authors compared the neuroendocrine responses of the remaining 18 female responders with the 18 male responders (eliminating one male who did not react), to ascertain whether differences in reactivity existed between these groups when responders were examined.

The authors concluded that females physiologically cope more effectively with a psychologically demanding achievement-oriented situation than do males (Frankenhaeuser et al., 1978; Rauste-von Wright et al., 1981), but their psychological coping may be less efficient. This interpretation is appealing. It must be noted, however, that these conclusions are based on correlations that are problematic, given the sample size relative to the number of comparisons made.

Mixed support for sex differences in neuroendocrine responses was found in college-aged students who participated in laboratory challenges (Collins & Frankenhaeuser, 1978; Frankenhaeuser et al., 1976; Myrstern et al., 1984; Lundberg & Frankenhaeuser, 1980). In order to determine whether sex differences were a function of biological or social learning factors, male and female university students majoring in engineering, a male-dominated profession, were studied (Collins & Frankenhaeuser, 1978). Women in this study were presumed to represent a nontraditional sample, as they were assuming a male work role model. As found in earlier studies (Frankenhaeuser et al., 1978; Johansson et al., 1973), the stress-induced E level for males was substantially higher than that achieved by females, though it was noted that the sex difference was attenuated. This is relevant since both men and women showed significant increases in E from baseline conditions. Although the stressor elevated the HR of men and women, relative to the control condition, women were more responsive on this parameter, both in terms of level and change from baseline during stress. Perhaps because both groups responded with augmented physiological responses to stress in one parameter, albeit different ones, there were no differences in report of effort or in performance. The authors suggested that the women in this sample responded differently than women in previous studies since they represented a ''masculine behavior pattern or lifestyle'' (Collins & Frankenhaeuser, 1978, p. 47). However, undertaking a major in engineering is not equivalent to assuming a masculine life-style. The women were actually consistent in that they displayed less E reactivity to stress. Classification on the basis of sex-role assessments would have provided an alternative procedure to identify traditional and nontraditional groups of women.

The influence of sex-role orientation, as indexed by the Bem Sex Role Inventory, on HR and BP responses to behavioral (mental achievement stress) and physical (tilt) challenge was studied by Myrstern and her colleagues (Myrstern et al., 1984). College women had higher resting HR and college men had higher resting SBP. Heart rate, SBP, and DBP increases to psychological and physical stress were evoked in men and women. Significant interactions between gender and sex role were reported for HR and DBP. Feminine women had the highest stress-induced HR and DBP levels among the women, while feminine men had the lowest HR among the men. Undifferentiated status was associated with high-stress HR among men and low-stress HR among women. The results suggest that sex-role orientation may mediate cardiovascular stress responses in men and women in different ways. The findings are not consistent with the HR findings reported by Collins and Frankenhaeuser (1978), since presumed "masculine" women did not differ from "masculine" men in terms of HR. The two studies, however, differ on important features, specifically the stressors used and the selection of groups. Caution should also be taken in interpreting the findings of Myrstern and colleagues (Myrstern et al., 1984), since the representativeness of the sample was limited by group size, the failure to adjust for baseline sex differences in the analyses, as well as the lack of clarity regarding the sampling of the resting baseline parameters. Furthermore, it appears that the behavioral stress BP sample was actually a recovery sample as BP was taken after, but not during, the five challenging tasks.

College men and women have not consistently differed in neuroendocrine stress responses (Frankenhaeuser et al., 1976; Lundberg & Frankenhaeuser, 1980). In men, mean E stress levels, adjusting for baseline, were significantly greater than control levels, but men and women did not differ in their E, NE, HR, or psychological responses to stress (venipuncture and SCWT) (Frankenhaeuser et al., 1976). Although the study sample was quite small, positive findings have been reported with samples of identical size (e.g., Forsman & Lindblad, 1983), suggesting that the power was within range to determine a difference if it existed.

In fact, no effects were reported in a demographically similar, but substantially larger sample (Lundberg & Frankenhaeuser, 1980). In the Lundberg and Frankenhaeuser (1980) study, students were exposed to five stressors [vigilance, time estimation, reaction time (RT), SCWT, and movies] over two sessions. Different tasks were associated with augmented catecholamine and/or cortisol responses. Conceptually, the pattern of neuroendocrine responsivity was considered to reflect the differential capacities of the tasks to evoke effort without distress (sympathetic–adrenal response) or effort with distress (pituitary–adrenal response). Neuroendocrine and psychological stress responses of men and women were not significantly different, although the authors noted that the men tended to excrete more E.

Support for sex differences in neuroendocrine stress responses have also been sought in nonstudent groups. Examining older groups or nonstudent groups would help to understand whether the findings reported above generalize and would provide information about the specificity of responding to student groups. Employed men in their 20s to 40s responded to the stress of an intelligence test, personality questionnaire, and medical history inventory with a greater E response than women counterparts. Men and women did not differ in their catecholamine responses to routine work-related activities sampled at regular intervals over the course of a year (Johansson & Post, 1974). These results are notable since they indicate that sex differences in E responsivity to an achievement stress are not limited to an academic population.

Other laboratories have also evaluated neuroendocrine responses to stressors in young (22–35 years) and older (50–67 years) men and women (Aslan et al., 1981). Participants were exposed to the stress of the SCWT and venipuncture during one session, and to a relaxation session. Relative to relaxation, the stress-induced excreted E was greater for all groups but the young women. Relaxation levels of the young women exceeded stress levels, suggesting enhanced responsiveness to the relaxation situation. NE was elevated only in the elderly subjects. Sex differences in excretion were found among the younger subjects for E and among the older subjects for NE. Unfortunately, the direction of stated differences were not consistently reported. Furthermore, there is no information as to whether pre- or postsession values were used in the analyses. There is also no evidence that the elevated relaxation values, that exceeded stress values, were statistically examined. In addition, other physiological and self-report parameters, that reflected increases during the stress relative to the relaxation condition, were apparently not analyzed by sex.

Neuroendocrine studies of stress-induced responses in men and women are not limited to the sampling of urinary catecholamines and cortisol. In a carefully designed and well-executed study, the influence of mental stress on plasma catecholamines and on baroreceptor-mediated cardiovascular responses was examined in male and female laboratory personnel and medical students (Forsman & Lindblad, 1983). Measurement of HR, BP, and plasma catecholamines occurred at regular and frequent intervals during the pretest, control, stress, and poststress periods. Heart rate and SBP levels, not associated with neck suction, were significantly greater during stress (SCWT) than during the control condition. Although men had a higher SBP stress-related change from baseline than did women, sex differences were not obtained for stress cardiovascular levels. A sex difference was found for E. Epinephrine stress responses of men were substantially greater than those exhibited by women.

This study (Forsman & Lindblad, 1983) involved a comprehensive assessment of cardiovascular, neuroendocrine, as well as subjective responses to stress and nonstress periods and was quite complete. This methodology provides valuable information about acute short-term fluctuations, not possible with urinary catecholamine

measures or with BP taken only before or after stressors, characteristic of earlier studies (e.g., Aslan et al., 1981; Collins & Frankenhaeuser, 1978; Frankenhaeuser et al., 1976, 1978; Johansson, 1972; Johansson & Post, 1974; Johansson et al., 1973; Lundberg & Frankenhaeuser, 1980). The presence of the sex difference in E responding is particularly salient in this context as the subjects were medical personnel who would be likely to experience less discomfort in this setting (corroborated by self-report) and perhaps would be more likely to experience attenuated responses relative to a more naive sample.

The plasma catecholamine findings of Forsman and Lindblad (1983) were partially replicated in a subsequent report in which different sampling procedures and stressors were used (Davidson et al., 1984). Nonmedical personnel in their mid-20s to 40s participated as subjects. They were studied in the supine position during resting baselines and during three of the four stressors (sustained isometric handgrip at 30% maximal grip, serial subtractions, cold pressor, and standing). Blood pressure, HR, and blood was sampled before and after each stressor but not during the tasks as Forsman and Lindblad (1983) had done. Resting E was greater in men while resting NE was greater in women. Immediately following stress, NE levels were significantly augmented for women for all tasks but handgrip. Likewise, immediate poststress E levels were substantially higher for men in all tasks but standing, in which E was elevated in women. Cardiovascular responses also showed a divergent pattern for men and women. SBP was elevated during rest and immediately posttask for men, while HR was greater during rest and immediately posttask for women.

The Davidson study (Davidson et al., 1984) is useful as a starting point to underscore methodological features that distinguish and/or characterize the literature reviewed above. Control variables, group composition, consumption behaviors, menstrual influences, and baseline assessments are worthy of mention. The findings of the Davidson study are at variance with the majority of research that has not reported heightened stress-induced NE levels in women (Collins & Frankenhaeuser, 1978;

Forsman & Lindblad, 1983; Frankenhaeuser *et al.*, 1976, 1978; Johansson & Post, 1974; Lundberg & Frankenhaeuser, 1980). Catecholamine and cardiovascular sex differences during stress that are present during rest have been reported by other researchers. With few exceptions (e.g., Davidson *et al.*, 1984; Lundberg & Frankenhaeuser, 1980), however, adolescent and adult studies corrected for weight in the analyses of neuroendocrine sex differences (Aslan *et al.*, 1981; Collins & Frankenhaeuser, 1978; Frankenhaeuser *et al.*, 1976, 1978; Forsman & Lindblad, 1983; Johansson *et al.*, 1973; Johansson & Post, 1974). Since females, on the average, weigh less than males, considering weight in analyses of neuroendocrine as well as cardiovascular sex differences, would clarify whether purported sex differences might be explained by other characteristics, like weight or body mass.

Across studies, males and females have typically been matched on certain salient features like age and/or educational/occupational status. The homogeneous sample composition in the Davidson study (Davidson *et al.*, 1984) is unique by comparison and worthy of comment. Their sample was composed of Mormons and Seventh Day Adventists. The two religious groups share similar diets and do not ingest alcohol, nicotine, or caffeine, substances known to affect neuroendocrine and cardiovascular responses. In other work, homogeneous groups, such as nonsmokers, were occasionally selected for study (e.g., Frankenhaeuser *et al.*, 1976). Typically, participants are asked to refrain from such substances as well as medications having neuroendocrine or cardiovascular influences (e.g., Aslan *et al.*, 1981; Collins & Frankenhaeuser, 1978).

On occasion, the influence of food intake on physiological parameters was controlled by providing fasting subjects with breakfast, prior to participation (e.g., Collins & Frankenhaeuser, 1978; Myrstern *et al.*, 1984). In some cases, the factors were statistically controlled (e.g., Johansson & Post, 1974); or data were collected to determine if groups differed in their pattern of usage (e.g., Frankenhaeuser *et al.*, 1978). Rarely has compliance to directions about abstinence been as-

sessed (e.g., Myrstern *et al.*, 1984). This situation is noteworthy since sex differences in certain consumptive patterns have been reported (e.g., Schlaadt & Shannon, 1986). Therefore, adequate ascertainment about such factors is necessary to facilitate understanding of purported sex differences in responding.

The issue of menstrual cycle influences on the mediation of sex differences in stress-induced neuroendocrine responding was not addressed by any of the aforementioned studies. Even when menstrual cycle data and information regarding oral contraceptive usage were collected, they were not taken into consideration in the analyses (e.g., Frankenhaeuser *et al.*, 1978). There is evidence from the menstrual cycle studies reviewed below suggesting that stress responses for menstruating females are attenuated when evaluation is at different phases of the cycle for members of the group. This situation is further compounded by conducting stress and control evaluations during different phases of the menstrual cycle (e.g., Aslan *et al.*, 1981; Collins & Frankenhaeuser, 1978; Frankenhaeuser *et al.*, 1976, 1978). Given the plurality of evidence suggesting elevated neuroendocrine baseline responding in the latter half of the cycle (see the section Baseline Cardiovascular and Neuroendocrine Activity in Males and Females), more attention to menstrual influences appears warranted.

The use of separate stress and baseline sessions, however, has served as a control for circadian influences on neuroendocrine activity (Aslan *et al.*, 1981; Collins & Frankenhaeuser, 1978; Frankenhaeuser *et al.*, 1976, 1978; Lundberg & Frankenhaeuser, 1980; Tennes & Kreye, 1985). An appealing methodological feature of the Lundberg and Frankenhaeuser (1980) study was its inclusion of a separate baseline day during which multiple urine samples were taken. Over the course of the morning, E increased while NE and cortisol decreased. In a separate study (Forsman & Lindblad, 1983), the opposite pattern emerged for baseline plasma samples taken on the same day as stress samples. These observations suggest the importance of considering the timing of stress-related data over several hours, in order to determine if presumed stress-related neuroendocrine responses are actually different from baseline or if they reflect diurnal influences.

Overall, the neuroendocrine literature examining sex differences in physiological responses to stress in healthy individuals is intriguing. Taken together, the data are more suggestive than definitive. Among the ten studies reviewed, when a sex difference in neuroendocrine reactivity emerged (Collins & Frankenhaeuser, 1978; Forsman & Lindblad, 1983; Frankenhaeuser et al., 1978; Johansson et al., 1973; Johansson & Post, 1974), males were more reactive than females in all but one case (Davidson et al., 1984). More specifically, for E stress responses, four reports reflect heightened E response to stress in males relative to females, whether or not psychological and behavioral responses were equivalent (Collins & Frankenhaeuser, 1978; Forsman & Lindblad, 1983; Johansson et al., 1973; Johansson & Post, 1974), and four reports reflect no sex difference in E responsivity (Davidson et al., 1984; Frankenhaeuser et al., 1976, 1978; Lundberg & Frankenhaeuser, 1980). For NE, one report supports heightened reactivity for men (Frankenhaeuser et al., 1978) and one supports such reactivity for women (Davidson et al., 1984), and four studies do not report any sex difference in NE responsivity (Forsman & Lindblad, 1983; Frankenhaeuser et al., 1976; Johansson & Post, 1974; Lundberg & Frankenhaeuser, 1980). With regard to cortisol responses, one study indicates that males are more responsive to stress than females (Frankenhaeuser et al., 1978) and two studies did not find any sex differences (Tennes & Kreye, 1985; Lundberg & Frankenhaeuser, 1980). The lack of consistency in stress procedures may be a factor in understanding the discrepant results and is discussed in subsequent sections. It is also likely that larger samples may serve in potentiating the trends typically seen in the data. More recent findings regarding plasma values, that are particularly sensitive and informative about acute changes, are promising, and have value in studies of sex differences in laboratory-based challenge (e.g., Davidson et al., 1984; Forsman & Lindblad, 1983). The methodological issues germane to the discussion of sex differences and neuroendocrine responsivity also apply to cardiovascular responsivity discussed below.

Cardiovascular Responses to Stress in Males and Females

A body of literature examining stress-related sex differences in cardiovascular responsivity has also accumulated. This research has followed two directions: (1) comparison of males and females, without regard to individual difference variables (e.g., Awaritefe & Kadiri, 1982; Baldwin & Clevenger, 1980; Frey & Siervogel, 1983; Gackenbach, 1982; Graham, Cohen, & Shavonian, 1966; Hastrup & Light, 1984; Liberson & Liberson, 1975; Van Egeren, 1979); and (2) comparison of males and females, along the TABP dimension (e.g., Frankenhaeuser, Lundberg, & Forsman, 1980; Holmes, Solomon, & Rump, 1982; Lawler, Allen, Critcher, & Standard, 1981; Manuck, Craft, & Gold, 1978). Since a substantial amount of work has investigated the interaction between sex and TABP on physiological responsivity, this literature is discussed in a subsequent section. Although the preponderance of research has been done with college-aged men and women, grade school children as well as individuals in their 60s have also been compared. Studies have primarily been laboratory-based, but field studies have also been conducted. The two lines of research are discussed below.

Laboratory Studies

Laboratory-based studies have employed a variety of stressors to elicit augmented cardiovascular responses to challenge in men and women. Challenges include dyadic mixed-motive games, cognitive puzzles, delivered shock, and shock avoidance. For example, cardiovascular responses to a modified mixed-motive game yielded results for sex, contingent on random assignment of men and women college students to competitive or cooperative strategies (Van Egeren, 1979). Analysis of averaged HR prior to the trials revealed a significant interaction for sex and strategy: competition was associated with increased anticipatory, and decision-making HR, as well as decreased feedback HR for women. For men, cooperation was associated with highest HR. It is interesting to note that

TABP, as indexed by the Jenkins Activity Survey (JAS), and endorsement of being action-oriented to confront life stress was positively related to elevated HR during the mixed-motive game. As noted by the author (Van Egeren, 1979), the external validity of the findings is limited to cooperation and competition with male partners, only. It is conceivable that pairing with a woman confederate may have elicited a different pattern of responding from the male and female participants. Nonetheless, the study is relevant since it suggests that different challenges elicit augmented cardiovascular responses from men and women.

Cardiovascular responses to a cognitive challenge requiring visual-spatial organization were examined in a multigenerational study in healthy normotensive male and female relatives of an adult hypertensive male (Frey & Siervogel, 1983). Extensive cardiovascular assessment was accomplished during resting prestress baseline and during the brief 30-s stressor, i.e., one age-appropriate matrix from Raven's progressive matrices. For children (< 18 years) and for adults (≥ 18 years), males and females did not differ in age or on resting BP. During stress, left ventricular ejection time was significantly decreased in men and women, but the preejection period/left ventricular ejection time ratio was elevated in women. For men, forearm blood flow was attenuated. An interaction for sex with age indicated that HR during stress increased for men to a greater degree than women. The mean stress HR level achieved by adult men, however, was equivalent to the baseline HR obtained by women.

Several studies compared physiological responses of men and women to more aversive procedures (Graham et al., 1966; Hastrup & Light, 1984; Jorgensen & Houston, 1981; Liberson & Liberson, 1975). For example, age-matched groups of healthy adult men and women underwent physiological assessment during rest and shock (Liberson & Liberson, 1975). Significant sex differences were obtained for SBP and respiration. Resting SBP and levels immediately after shock were higher for men than women, while resting respiration rates were greater in women than men. DBP and HR levels did not discriminate the groups.

HR did, however, discriminate men and women during shock avoidance discrimination learning (Graham et al., 1966). Female nursing students were stressed, either during the luteal phase or during the follicular phase of their menstrual cycle. No differences in physiological responses to the threat of shock emerged between the women evaluated during the follicular and luteal phases. These women were compared to a group of men who had completed identical procedures as part of an earlier study. Overall, the physiological response patterns of the men and women to the conditioning trials differed even though their behavior was comparable. Men responded with enhanced galvanic skin response levels and women responded with elevated HR levels.

While women responded with enhanced cardiovascular responding in the Graham study (Graham et al., 1966), this study is somewhat problematic from a reactivity perspective. There was no evidence that any assessment of baseline functioning was made. Despite the obvious limitations, the study warrants attention since it considered the influence of menstrual phase as a possible mediator of challenge-induced physiological responses in a sex comparison. The salience of this attempt is underscored by the fact that control for menstrual phase has been virtually absent from the reactivity literature comparing men and women.

The exception is a recent investigation by Hastrup and Light (1984). Young college men and college women, not using oral contraceptives, were studied. Half of the women completed the stress assessment during their follicular phase while the remaining half were assessed during their luteal phase. Stress assessment included shock avoidance RT and cold pressor. For women, resting sessions were held in the luteal and follicular phase. For men, scheduling of the resting sessions was matched to the intervening intervals for women. Reactivity results were specific to stressor and to group. Although baseline HR was identical, the RT elicited substantially greater HR increases from men than from follicular phase women. Luteal phase women did not differ from men or from follicular phase women in HR reactivity. In contrast, SBP levels during baseline were substantially elevated during rest as well as during tasks for men, relative to both groups of women. Again, RT elicited greater SBP responses from men relative to follicular phase women. Luteal phase women also showed a substantially greater response than follicular phase women, but again, did not differ from men. No group baseline or stress differences emerged for DBP or to the cold pressor task.

The findings of Hastrup and Light (1984) are interesting since they imply that all tasks are not equally capable of eliciting sex differences in physiological responding. Furthermore, the findings suggest that menstrual phase may mediate the sex differences and responses to tasks. Although follicular and luteal phase women did not differ on baseline measures, luteal phase women, like men, responded with substantially greater SBP responses to RT than follicular phase women. This finding suggests that hormonal fluctuations may influence reactivity to certain challenges. A logical extension of this investigation would involve studying the same women in both phases of the mentrual cycle in order to discern whether their standing, relative to men in terms of reactivity, is affected by the cycle phase.

An exception to the enhanced systolic responsivity of males to shock challenge was reported by Jorgensen and Houston (1981). Cardiovascular responses were examined across several different challenges: shock avoidance RT, SCWT, serial subtractions, and digits backwards. College men and women did not differ in their challenge-induced SBP, DBP, or HR. However, the SBP of women with a family history of hypertension was greater than that of women without a family history, across stressors.

Field Studies

Field studies, examining BP and HR responses in men and women to naturally occurring stressors, such as competition, examinations, and class presentations, have also been conducted (Awaritefe & Kadiri, 1982; Baldwin & Clevenger, 1980; Gackenbach, 1982). Gackenbach (1982) demonstrated that, among collegiate swimmers, SBP prior to competition was higher in men than women (controlling for level prior to practice). Men also reported substantially lower state anxiety and hostility relative to women. These findings are

interesting for two reasons. First, they support Frankenhaeuser's (1983) contention that men are more physiologically responsive in achievement-oriented situations then women and that women respond with more evidence of psychological distress. Second, the findings demonstrate that physiological differences to challenge are evident among individuals who presumably have comparable levels of fitness.

Methodologically, the Gackenbach (1982) study shares a limitation with the examination study conducted by Awaritefe and Kadiri (1982). Description of procedures (Awaritefe & Kadiri, 1982; Gackenbach, 1982) suggests that only two BP measurements were taken for each subject, clearly not in accord with usual procedures where multiple blood pressures are taken. Nonetheless, in two separate studies with similar designs, comparable findings were obtained. Men endorsed significantly more trait anxiety and responded with substantially higher SBP levels over the examination and control assessments (Awaritefe & Kadiri, 1982). Preexamination SBP and DBP levels were significantly, though not markedly, greater than the control assessment. Since the difference between the two assessments was slight, ranging from 4 to 7 mm Hg, and the control assessment always occurred after the stress assessment, it is conceivable that the diminution in BP from test to control assessment might be a function of habituation and familiarity with the BP assessment procedures. This raises the possibility that the final examination in physiology was not physiologically arousing to the Nigerian students. The self-reported state anxiety, reported by the men prior to the examination, supported this observation. State anxiety was negatively correlated with SBP and DBP in men, though positively correlated for women (for a complete discussion of the influence of race and gender on reactivity, see N. Anderson, this volume).

Heart rate elicited by real-life challenge, i.e., public speaking, was also studied (Baldwin & Clevenger, 1980). Male and female pairs were matched on resting HR (within 7 bpm) and one member of each pair was randomly assigned to either the full classroom or small audience condition for presentation of a 3-min impromptu speech. HR assessment was accomplished via telemetry and baseline HR was recorded 1 week later. The small audience condition was most effective in eliciting HR changes from the subjects. Average HR change from baseline to speaking was appreciably higher for women than men (+40 bpm versus +26.5 bpm) across both speech conditions. These findings (Baldwin & Clevenger, 1980) are noteworthy as they suggest that women respond with augmented HR reactivity to a social-evaluative challenge.

Laboratory and field cardiovascular studies as a group lack some of the controls characteristic of the neuroendocrine studies discussed earlier. With the exception of one study reporting oral contraceptive usage patterns (Hastrup & Light, 1984), no information about exclusionary medication with potential cardiovascular consequences was provided. In no case were instructions about, or assessment of, stimulant and depressant (i.e., caffeine, nicotine, and alcohol) usage reported (Awaritefe & Kadiri, 1982; Baldwin & Clevenger, 1980; Frey & Siervogel, 1983; Gackenbach, 1982; Graham et al., 1966; Hastrup & Light, 1984; Jorgensen & Houston, 1981; Liberson & Liberson, 1975; Van Egeren, 1979). Likewise, subject description was frequently inadequate and acknowledgment of health status was typically lacking (Awaritefe & Kadiri, 1982; Baldwin & Clevenger, 1980; Frey & Siervogel, 1983; Gackenbach, 1982; Graham et al., 1966; Hastrup & Light, 1984; Jorgensen & Houston, 1981; Van Egeren, 1979). Frequently, no report of or control for body mass or weight was made in the sex-related analyses (e.g., Awaritefe & Kadiri, 1982; Baldwin & Clevenger, 1980; Frey & Siervogel, 1983; Hastrup & Light, 1984; Jorgensen & Houston, 1981; Liberson & Liberson, 1975; Van Egeren, 1979). This is particularly of concern when baseline differences were present (e.g., Hastrup & Light, 1984).

The laboratory and field studies share some notable similarities. To illustrate, augmented HR responses were characteristic of women confronted with a competitive challenge, as well as men in a cooperative challenge (Van Egeren, 1979); a cognitive puzzle (Frey & Siervogel, 1983); a social-evaluative stressor (Baldwin & Clevenger, 1980); and a shock avoidance task (Graham et al., 1966); but not with shock stimulation (Liberson & Liberson, 1975) or shock avoidance RT (Hastrup &

Light, 1984; Jorgensen & Houston, 1981). Likewise, increased SBP responses were characteristic of men prior to a medical school examination (Awaritefe & Kadiri, 1982) and prior to a swim competition (Gackenbach, 1982), and on occasion during shock-related procedures (Hastrup & Light, 1984; Liberson & Liberson, 1975).

Overall, a mixed picture for sex differences in cardiovascular responsivity emerges for the studies reviewed in this and the previous section. Of the 11 studies which evaluated HR, heightened HR responding was characteristic of men in three studies (Davidson et al., 1984; Frey & Siervogel, 1983; Hastrup & Light, 1984), and of women in three studies (Baldwin & Clevenger, 1980; Collins & Frankenhaeuser, 1978; Graham et al., 1966). An interaction of sex and condition on HR responding appeared in one study (Van Egeren, 1979), and in four studies there were no differences in HR responding for men and women (Forsman & Lindblad, 1983; Frankenhaeuser et al., 1976; Jorgensen & Houston, 1981; Liberson & Liberson, 1975). More consistent patterns are apparent for BP responding. Not one study of the eight that evaluated BP responding reflected any difference between males and females in DBP responding (Awaritefe & Kadiri, 1982; Davidson et al., 1984; Forsman & Lindblad, 1983; Frey & Siervogel, 1983; Gackenbach, 1982; Hastrup & Light, 1984; Jorgensen & Houston, 1981; Liberson & Liberson, 1975). For SBP responding, five studies (Awaritefe & Kadiri, 1982; Davidson et al., 1984; Gackenbach, 1982; Hastrup & Light, 1984; Liberson & Liberson, 1975) of the eight studies indicated that men were more systolically reactive than women.

It is necessary to note that the ratios reported above are not representative of all the cardiovascular reactivity research that has examined the influence of sex. In the next section, additional data on the influence of TABP on physiological responding are reviewed.

Type A, Sex, and Physiological Responsivity

As noted above, the other line of literature that has studied males and females has done so by determining the influence of TABP and sex on physiological reactivity to challenge. Children and adults have been studied. Previous research concentrating on males has typically found Type As to be more physiologically responsive to stress than Type Bs, despite similarities in resting activity (for a review see Houston, 1986). Another relevant body of literature has compared the responses of Type A and B females.

Male and Female Studies

Sixth-grade boys and girls were examined by Lawler and her colleagues (Lawler et al., 1981). TABP designations were made using the Bortner Type A scale and the Matthews Youth Test for Health (MYTH). Girls had higher HR levels than boys across tasks and rest. Type A and B findings were not consistent for the Bortner and the MYTH. Overall, Bortner Type As had higher HR at the beginning of the word task. There were no sex-related differences associated with the Bortner. Only MYTH Type A girls differed from Type B girls in their heightened SBP increases during that task. MYTH Type A and B boys and girls displayed different HR response patterns. Type A boys and Type B boys and girls had substantially higher stress and rest HR than Type A girls. Type A girls had the greater stress-induced HR increase. These findings are interesting since they suggest that, among presumably prepubescent children classified with the MYTH, Type A girls were more responsive to stress than Type B girls. Type A boys also had a greater mean HR than Type B boys.

The adult literature examining the influence of sex and TABP has employed the JAS (e.g., Frankenhaeuser et al., 1980; Holmes et al., 1982) and the Vickers (Manuck et al., 1978) as classification instruments. Holmes and associates (Holmes et al., 1982) monitored HR during rest, digit symbol substitution, and a two-step exercise task. An effect for TABP on HR across periods was obtained for the cognitive challenge. Post hoc analyses revealed that residualized HR levels were comparable for Type A and B women and Type A men. Type B men had the lowest values. HR levels were also higher for women than men at the end of exercise (Holmes et al., 1982).

The results of the Holmes study (Holmes et al., 1982) suggest that adult male and female Type A–B groups respond differentially to certain behavioral challenges. This was further supported by Manuck and his colleagues (Manuck et al., 1978) who found no main effects for sex on challenge-induced systolic responses. During challenge, however, Type A men had substantially higher SBP than Type B men. There were no Type A–B differences for women.

Urinary catecholamine and cortisol and HR responses to a choice RT task were also evaluated in a sample of Type A and B men and women (Frankenhaeuser et al., 1980). Although the Type As and Bs differed behaviorally, there were no differences in their physiological response to the purported achievement challenge. Challenge HR and catecholamine levels were substantially greater while cortisol levels were substantially lower than those obtained during a subsequent baseline session. Men responded with greater challenge-induced E change and reported substantially more effort than women. The findings (Frankenhaeuser et al., 1980) are discrepant with those of Holmes (Holmes et al., 1982) in that a main effect for A–B status was not obtained for HR. Instead, a main effect for sex was found for urinary E.

The findings of Frankenhaeuser (Frankenhaeuser et al., 1980), Holmes (Holmes et al., 1982), and Manuck (Manuck et al., 1978) show little parallel. The lack of consistency appears to be attributable to methodological differences between the studies. Although all participants were college students, the manner in which they were classified as Type A–B varied across studies. It is well documented that concordance for Type A measures varies (Matthews, 1982). Second, dissimilar physiological parameters were recorded. Third, there was a drastic difference in tasks across studies. For example, Holmes (Holmes et al., 1982) employed a brief sensorimotor integration task and exercise task, while a difficult visual conceptual task, with monetary incentive, was used by Manuck (Manuck et al., 1978). By contrast, Frankenhaeuser's (Frankenhaeuser et al., 1980) RT task was incredibly lengthy. As suggested by Holmes (Holmes et al., 1982), the Type A–B sex groups seemed to respond differentially to tasks, across studies (Frankenhaeuser et al., 1980; Holmes et al., 1982;

Manuck *et al.*, 1978). A fourth difference was the concerted effort made by Frankenhaeuser and her colleagues (Frankenhaeuser *et al.*, 1980) to control for diurnal influences and the effects of substances that influence physiological responding to stress. To this end, only nonsmokers were recruited, and instructions to abstain from substances with stimulant or depressant effects were made. Finally, across all three studies, weight was not controlled (Frankenhaeuser *et al.*, 1980; Holmes *et al.*, 1982; Manuck *et al.*, 1978). This is most relevant for the interpretation of the neuroendocrine findings of Frankenhaeuser (Frankenhaeuser *et al.*, 1980).

Female Studies

Insight into the relationship between TABP and reactivity can also be obtained by inspection of the TABP literature examining reactivity differences in women. Across studies, TABP classification has been accomplished with the Structured Interview (SI) (e.g., MacDougall, Dembroski, & Krantz, 1981; Lawler, Schmied, Mitchell, & Rixse, 1984), the JAS (e.g., Anderson, Williams, & Lane, 1981; Lane, White, & Williams, 1984; Lawler, Rixse, & Allen, 1983; Lawler & Schmied, 1986; Lawler *et al.*, 1984; MacDougall *et al.*, 1981; Stoney, Langer, & Gelling, 1986), and the Framingham Type A scale (MacDougall *et al.*, 1981). To date, all studies have been laboratory based. (For a complete discussion of the TABP literature in black women, the reader is referred to N. Anderson, this volume.)

The issue of task (stressor/challenge) relevance was addressed by MacDougall and his colleagues (MacDougall *et al.*, 1981). In the first of two studies presented, no cardiovascular differences were obtained for the SI designated groups challenged with cold pressor and choice RT. In the second study, a large sample of college women were monitored during procedures judged to be more challenging and relevant to the women: (1) SI, (2) oral history quiz, and (3) choice RT with monetary incentive. Main effects for TABP status were limited to SBP. Type A women had higher baseline SBP and systolic increases to the two interpersonally demanding tasks (SI and quiz), even when baseline levels and caffeine consumption were covaried. Type A women also performed better on

the quiz and RT tasks than Type B women. No relationships were found between the other measures of Type A (JAS and Framingham Type A scale) and the physiological responses in either study.

MacDougall's findings (MacDougall *et al.*, 1981) underscore the importance of selecting tasks relevant to the group under study. This issue is critical when considering sex differences in reactivity. Certain types of tasks may be more involving or engaging than others to the groups being evaluated. The findings suggest that it is worthwhile to study the impact of specific types of tasks on sex-related responses.

It is imperative to note, however, that the systolic effects for the interpersonally challenging oral history quiz were not replicated by Lawler and Schmied (1986). The cardiovascular responses of Type A and B college women did not differ at rest or during tasks (oral history quiz and SCWT). Family history of hypertension did not interact with TABP, but was associated with higher resting SBP. The methodological differences between the two reports (Lawler & Schmied, 1986; MacDougall *et al.*, 1981) might explain the discrepant findings. First, different procedures were used to make Type A classifications: Lawler and Schmied (1986) used extreme scores on the JAS, whereas MacDougall *et al.* (1981) reported effects with the SI categorizations. This is especially noteworthy since no correlations were found for the JAS and physiological responses in the MacDougall *et al.* study. Second, the final sample size of the Lawler and Schmied (1986) study is half that of the MacDougall *et al.* (1981) study. Third, the order of the challenges was held constant in MacDougall *et al.*, whereas the presentation was counterbalanced in Lawler and Schmied. Fourth, MacDougall *et al.* statistically controlled for caffeine consumption, but no mention was made of this or other factors that might influence cardiovascular responses in Lawler and Schmied.

Lawler and Schmied's (1986) findings, however, partially replicated the results of Lane and colleagues (Lane *et al.*, 1984) who found no differences in physiological responses to serial subtraction with incentive, among college women who scored at the extremes on the JAS, in opposition to their previous findings with men (Williams *et al.*, 1982). In contrast to Lawler and Schmied's (1986) report, family history status interacted with TABP. Type As with a positive family history, had a substantially greater HR response and fight–flight (i.e., increased HR, BP, and forearm blood flow) response to the task than Type As with a negative family history. Among the individuals with a family history, Type As had a greater HR response than Type Bs.

It is important to note that the prevalence of self-reported family history of hypertension in this sample (Lane *et al.*, 1984) was 28%. This indicates that the family history analyses were based on few subjects. The failure to replicate the findings of Williams *et al.* (1982) may, as Lane *et al.* point out, be partly attributable to the methodological differences in the studies. The Williams *et al.* study differed in three important aspects. First, the procedures were more lengthy. Second, procedures to sample plasma neuroendocrine responses were implemented. Third, TABP classification was accomplished using the combination of the SI and the JAS. Group designations based on this procedure would be different than categorization based on either method alone. Also, in the female study (Lane *et al.*, 1984), there was no evidence that substances that influence cardiovascular responses were controlled.

Both the SI and the JAS were used in one study to separately classify college women along the TABP dimension (Lawler *et al.*, 1984). The sample was composed of women from "traditional" and "nontraditional" female majors. All subjects completed the reactivity and SI and questionnaire assessment. Heart rate and BP were recorded during rest and three tasks: complex math (subject paced), Raven's matrices with time pressure, and Raven's matrices, experimenter paced, faster than previous task. Type A and B groups, based on either the JAS or the SI, did not differ on the basis of cardiovascular levels or change from baseline.

Additional effort was taken to form "maximally" different TABP groups (Lawler *et al.*, 1984). One group was composed of nontraditional majors, who espoused nontraditional values and were designated Type A on both the JAS and the SI. The second group was composed of women in traditional majors, who espoused traditional values

and were Type B on the JAS and either A_2 or B on the SI. The composition of the nontraditional group is problematic, given its purpose, since it included Type A women as defined by the SI. Nonetheless, the traditional and nontraditional groups did not differ in their cardiovascular responses to stress. It is plausible that the lack of differences was task related. Since the SI was administered, it would have been interesting had it been used as a reactivity task in order to compare the response of the women to an interpersonal challenge and to attempt to replicate the findings of MacDougall (MacDougall *et al.*, 1981).

The above findings diverge from the results of an earlier study using identical reactivity procedures with older women, ranging in age from 25 to 55 years (Lawler *et al.*, 1983). The sample was composed of employed professional women and nonemployed women. The groups had similar educational backgrounds, marital status, and health histories (the groups were said to be equivalent on cardiovascular history, but it is not clear whether all women were healthy or normotensive). Using only extreme scores on the JAS, all employed women were designated Type A. Unemployed women received Type A and B classifications. Employed Type As had substantially greater HR levels across rest and the tasks. However, when rest HR was covaried in the analyses of HR change, group differences were eliminated. Covarying rest DBP, stress-induced DBP change was substantially greater among the nonemployed Type As. Secondary analyses were also completed on the subsample of nonemployed women in order to control for the effects of employment on TABP status. Nonemployed Type As had substantially lower HR during rest, but achieved comparable levels during tasks. When the appropriate baselines were covaried, group effects for HR change and DBP change were eliminated. In contrast, nonemployed Type As did respond to the tasks with greater SBP increases than nonemployed Type Bs.

This finding is particularly relevant since it suggests that women older than college age respond differentially to cognitive challenge. Lawler's findings (Lawler *et al.*, 1983) are interesting for two reasons. They suggest that career-oriented women display enhanced diastolic responding to tasks that tap math and visual-spatial skills, presumably skills in which males excel (although precluded by the sample limitations, it would have been very informative to have compared Type A and B professional women). In addition, nonemployed Type A and B women showed the pattern of responding often seen with men: Type As being more systolically reactive to the behavioral challenge. However, conclusions should be regarded as tentative given the group sizes used in each of the comparisons. With the exception of the employed women, sample sizes were quite small and less likely to adequately represent the population they were purported to.

In addition to the age of the sample, the Lawler et al. (1983) study differs from other TABP studies with women, since women were studied during days 5–23 of their menstrual cycle. This is likely to have eliminated potential menstrual and premenstrual phase influences on reactivity. In a recent study with college-aged women (Stoney et al., 1986), the effects of menstrual cycle phase on reactivity in JAS-determined A and B women (extreme scorers) were more carefully examined. Only healthy undergraduate women, who reported normal menstrual cycles and who had not used oral contraceptives in the past 6 months, served as subjects. The Type A and B women were evaluated during rest, exercise, and video (threat of shock) stress, once during their self-reported follicular phase and once during their self-reported luteal phase. There were no TABP status nor menstrual cycle phase differences in reactivity to the psychological or physical challenge. Menstrual cycle phase differences were limited to baseline HR, which was higher during the luteal phase. It is noteworthy that the women responded to behaviorally induced stress with HR in excess of the metabolic demands, a pattern known to be characteristic of men. Since males were not included in this study, it is unknown whether the magnitude of the response was comparable between men and women. It was also noteworthy that minute-by-minute HR and SBP stayed elevated throughout the 15-min stressors. Possible reasons for null effects include the following: (1) use of the JAS to categorize TABP groups, (2) reliance on self-report of menstrual cycle without confirmation regarding the onset of later periods, and (3) failure to use an interpersonal challenge that was effective in eliciting differences in college-aged women. It was also unclear whether the order of the reactivity assessment was counterbalanced across phases. This is relevant since repeated exposure to the identical procedures is likely to result in a habituation of the physiological response.

With some notable exceptions, the methodological limitations of this TABP and sex literature are similar to those of the literature reviewed in earlier sections. Only three studies reported attempts to control for the impact of substances that influence physiological responding (Frankenhaeuser et al., 1980; MacDougall et al., 1981; Stoney et al., 1986). Overall, little information about health or other baseline characteristics was provided. Also there typically was no control for factors such as weight or cardiovascular baseline differences in the analyses when indicated.

Furthermore, the TABP and sex literature is inconsistent as pertains to TABP classification procedures, stress procedures, and findings. The SI, the standard for Type A assessment, was included in only two studies (Lawler et al., 1984; MacDougall et al., 1981). Less frequently used instruments such as Vickers, Bortner, and MYTH were each used in one study (Lawler et al., 1981; Manuck et al., 1978). By far the most commonly used measure was the JAS, employed in eight investigations (Frankenhaeuser et al., 1980; Holmes et al., 1982; Lane et al., 1984; Lawler et al., 1983, 1984; Lawler & Schmied, 1986; MacDougall et al., 1981; Stoney et al., 1986).

In sum, in all but two cases (Lawler et al., 1981, 1983), college-aged students were studied. TABP status differences were obtained in sixth-graders (Lawler et al., 1981) and women in their 20s to 50s, as a function of employment (Lawler et al., 1983). Main effects for TABP were not observed in seven reports (Frankenhaeuser et al., 1980; Holmes et al., 1982; Lane et al., 1984; Lawler et al., 1984; Lawler & Schmied, 1986; Manuck et al., 1978; Stoney et al., 1986), but were evident in two investigations (Lawler et al., 1981; MacDougall et al., 1981). Interactions between sex and TABP were apparent in three studies (Lawler *et al.*, 1981; Holmes *et al.*, 1982; Manuck *et al.*, 1978). Differences have emerged for HR (Lawler *et al.*, 1981, 1983; Holmes *et al.*, 1982), SBP (Lawler *et al.*, 1981, 1983; MacDougall *et al.*, 1981; Manuck *et al.*, 1978), and DBP (Lawler *et al.*, 1983). In two cases, main effects for sex were obtained: men had a higher E response to a lengthy choice RT task (Frankenhaeuser *et al.*, 1980); and women had a substantially greater HR response at the end of exercise (Holmes *et al.*, 1982). For women, only one study supported heightened SBP reactivity for Type As relative to Type Bs (Mac-Dougall *et al.*, 1981). The latter study is unique, as it stressed the women with interpersonal challenges and categorized the groups with the SI. With the exception of one other study that presented an interpersonal challenge but used the JAS (Lawler & Schmied, 1986), the remaining investigations employed tasks that involved exercise or visual, mathematical, conceptual, or spatial skills. The TABP and sex findings appear to be influenced by the manner in which TABP is classified, the type of challenge used, and the age of the individuals under study.

Menstrual Phase and Physiological Responsivity

As alluded to in the preceding discussion, consideration of the literature examining stress-induced reactivity as a function of menstrual cycle phase is requisite from a methodological perspective. It is important to determine whether menstrual cycle phase reliably affects reactivity to stress. Information from such studies could help clarify interpretation of the sex and physiological responsivity literature. It may be that responsivity varies across the menstrual cycle, i.e., is augmented in certain phases relative to others. Consequently, purported sex differences may be modulated by phase.

Neuroendocrine (Abplanalp, Livingston, Rose, & Sandwisch, 1977; Collins, Eneroth, & Landgren, 1985; Marinari, Leshner, & Doyle, 1976; Wasilewska *et al.*, 1980), and cardiovascular (Carroll, Turner, Lee, & Stephenson, 1984; Hastrup & Light, 1984; Little & Zahn, 1974; Polefrone &

Manuck, 1988; Stoney *et al.*, 1986; von Eiff *et al.*, 1971) responses to challenge have been studied across the menstrual cycle in purportedly normally menstruating women, free from oral contraceptives. With the exception of the Hastrup and Light (1984) paper, phase-related reactivity research has not addressed the issue of sex differences *per se* (e.g., Abplanalp *et al.*, 1977; Carroll *et al.*, 1984; Collins *et al.*, 1985; Garrett & Elder, 1984; Ladisich, 1977; Little & Zahn, 1974; Stoney *et al.*, 1986; Polefrone & Manuck, 1988; von Eiff *et al.*, 1971; Wasilewska *et al.*, 1980).

Menstrual cycle-related physiological responses have been evaluated during the menses (Abplanalp *et al.*, 1977; Little & Zahn, 1974; Garrett & Elder, 1984), follicular phase (Carroll *et al.*, 1984; Collins *et al.*, 1985; Hastrup & Light, 1984; Little & Zahn, 1974; Polefrone & Manuck, 1988; Stoney *et al.*, 1986), ovulatory phase (Abplanalp *et al.*, 1977; Collins *et al.*, 1985; Garrett & Elder, 1984; Little & Zahn, 1974; Marinari *et al.*, 1976; Wasilewska *et al.*, 1980), luteal phase (Carroll *et al.*, 1984; Collins *et al.*, 1985; Hastrup & Light, 1984; Little & Zahn, 1974; Polefrone & Manuck, 1988; Stoney *et al.*, 1986; von Eiff *et al.*, 1971; Ladisich, 1977; Garrett & Elder, 1984), and premenstrually (Garrett & Elder, 1984; Ladisich, 1977; Little & Zahn, 1974; Marinari *et al.*, 1976; Wasilewska *et al.*, 1980).

Premenstrual and ovulatory catecholamine excretion under rest and stress conditions (completing logical puzzles with knowledge of results) was investigated in healthy women in their early 20s and 30s (Wasilewska *et al.*, 1980). At rest, urinary catecholamines were elevated in the premenstrual, relative to the ovulatory phase. Only stress-excreted E was elevated over rest values in the premenstrual phase, whereas stress-excreted E and NE were greater than rest levels during the ovulatory phase. Plasma DBH did not differ across the phases, in stress or at rest.

In a recent study (Collins *et al.*, 1985) the findings of Wasilewska and colleagues (Wasilewska *et al.*, 1980) were partially replicated in a demographically similar sample. Comparably aged healthy women, with normal menstrual cycles, who were free from oral contraceptives were evaluated in the follicular, ovulatory, and luteal phases of two consecutive menstrual cycles. Six evaluations using the same stressors were completed for each subject. Catecholamines were sampled after three stressors (SCWT, mental arithmetic, and video game) and a poststress relaxation baseline. A significant effect for phase on reactivity was found only for the stress catecholamine levels during the first cycle. Although this finding apparently was not subjected to post hoc analyses, inspection of the means reveals levels were highest during the luteal phase, followed by the ovulatory and follicular phases. No effects for phase were found for HR, SBP, DBP, or cortisol. Unfortunately, the report lacks appropriate pairwise mean comparisons. Interactions involving cardiovascular parameters and cycle were reported but not probed, making interpretation difficult.

From a reactivity perspective, the excreted catecholamine phase differences elicited by stress in the Collins study (Collins et al., 1985) are noteworthy since they occurred despite repeated assessment with identical procedures, albeit only during the first cycle. The six repeated exposures to the same stressors probably contributed to habituation of responding, resulting in no phase effects for SBP, DBP, and HR. Lack of cardiovascular stress responses in a within-subject design is consistent with other reports (e.g., Carroll et al., 1984; Little & Zahn, 1974; Stoney et al., 1986).

The lack of phase effect for excreted cortisol was previously reported for plasma cortisol (Abplanalp et al., 1977). Determinations of plasma cortisol and human growth hormone were made several times per week for a complete menstrual cycle in healthy, normally menstruating women. One half of the women participated in a stressful 30-min interview during their menses while the remaining women participated during what was assumed to be the periovulatory period. No relationship between cortisol reactivity to the interview and menstrual cycle phase emerged. Unfortunately, hormonal markers revealed that the periovulatory interviews were not held at the appropriate point in time for approximately 50% of the women in that condition. Thus, menses phase women were not actually being compared with periovulatory women, but with women who were either follicular, periovulatory, or luteal. This situation underscores the need for reliable phase determinations.

With two notable exceptions (Hastrup & Light, 1984; Polefrone & Manuck, 1988), the preponderance of research exploring phase effects on cardiovascular responses to stress have used within-subject designs (Collins et al., 1985; Carroll et al., 1984; Little & Zahn, 1974; Stoney et al., 1986; von Eiff et al., 1971). Methods have varied across the within-subject design studies. For example, Little and Zahn (1974) evaluated presumably healthy women during rest and challenge (listening to tones, RT, and time estimation) for 6 days per week across one complete cycle. No significant task-induced cardiovascular differences occurred across the cycle; only resting differences were obtained. Increased resting HR was characteristic of the luteal phase and increased resting HR variability distinguished the preovulatory phase. Given the fact that few subjects were examined on at least 24 occasions, it is likely that the repeated assessment promoted habituation of responding. Even very challenging tasks would not be likely to maintain their potency with numerous exposures.

Similar stress response findings were obtained in protocols where women were tested only twice: (1) during the follicular phase and (2) during the luteal phase (Carroll et al., 1984; Stoney et al., 1986). For example, a heterogeneous sample, with respect to age of healthy normally menstruating women, was studied by Carroll and colleagues (Carroll et al., 1984). For half of the women, the follicular session was completed first and for the other half the luteal session was scheduled first. Baseline resting HR levels were comparable across phases, in contrast to the other studies where HR was elevated in the luteal phase (Little & Zahn, 1974; Stoney et al., 1986). Overall, there were no reliable phase differences in video game challenge-induced HR changes over resting levels.

Vaginal smears have been used to index ovarian function in healthy normally menstruating women (von Eiff et al., 1971). Women were monitored twice before ovulation and twice after ovulation. Physiological parameters were monitored during math stress and rest. Resting values were comparable across phase. Although stress differences between the two phases were not directly compared, and stress levels were not reported, the degree of estrogenic activity was negatively correlated with DBP, HR, and respiration rate, during the post-ovulatory (luteal) phase only. These findings suggest decreased reactivity during the luteal phase, when estrogen levels would be relatively high.

The results of a recent report, where women underwent a reactivity assessment during either their follicular or luteal phase, provides further evidence for decreased BP reactivity to challenge during the luteal phase (Polefrone & Manuck, 1988). Women evaluated during the follicular phase exhibited greater SBP reactivity to a mental arithmetic task and a concept formation task than women evaluated during the luteal phase. Follicular and luteal phase women displayed comparable DBP and HR responses to stress.

In sum, the neuroendocrine and cardiovascular menstrual cycle reactivity literature yields a varied picture. Urinary catecholamine responses to stress were evaluated in two studies (Collins et al., 1985; Wasilewska et al., 1980). In one study, elevated NE stress responses occurred during the ovulatory phase and increased E responses emerged during ovulatory and premenstrual phases (Wasilewska et al., 1980). The findings from the Collins study (Collins et al., 1985) suggested that the greatest stress-induced catecholamine response was associated with the luteal phase, though the response habituated with repeated exposure. In contrast, stress-induced cortisol was not found to be related to menstrual cycle phase whether evaluated once (Abplanalp et al., 1977) or repeatedly in the same subjects (Collins et al., 1985).

It is noteworthy that there were no menstrual phase effects on stress-induced cardiovascular responses in four of the five studies that involved repeated assessment across phase (Carroll et al., 1984; Collins et al., 1985; Little & Zahn, 1974; Stoney et al., 1986). Even when neuroendocrine responsivity was affected by menstrual cycle phase, no effects on cardiovascular parameters were observed (Collins et al., 1985). In the fifth study (von Eiff et al., 1971), comparisons were not made between phase-related responses, though DBP and HR responses were negatively related to mucosal estrogen during the luteal phase. The only studies that reported cycle-related differences in

cardiovascular responses were two studies that used between-subject designs whereby participants were evaluated with stress procedures only once (Hastrup & Light, 1984; Polefrone & Manuck, 1988). Heightened SBP responding was characteristic of the follicular phase (Polefrone & Manuck, 1988) and luteal phase (Hastrup & Light, 1984), respectively.

The pattern of results implies that potential cardiovascular differences in reactivity associated with menstrual cycle phase are obscured by multiple exposure to the same stressors in studies that employ within-subject designs. This situation suggests the value of developing laboratory challenges that do not habituate with repeated presentation. In studies that employ between-subject designs, cycle-related differences in reactivity emerge for SBP, but are not phase-specific (Hastrup & Light, 1984; Polefrone & Manuck, 1988). The conflicting findings may be attributable to different challenges and procedures used across studies.

Noteworthy methodological characteristics of this body of research include control for daily scheduling of evaluation, especially when repeated assessments were involved (e.g., Carroll et al., 1984; Collins et al., 1985; Little & Zahn, 1974). Information about consumption of substances that affect physiological responding, however, was unavailable in numerous cases (Abplanalp et al., 1977; Carroll et al., 1984; Little & Zahn, 1974; von Eiff et al., 1971; Wasilewska et al., 1980).

The variability in indexing menstrual cycle phase, across studies, also needs to be underscored. Self-report was most commonly used to determine menstrual cycle phase (Abplanalp et al., 1977; Carroll et al., 1984; Hastrup & Light, 1984; Polefrone & Manuck, 1988; Stoney et al., 1986) with hormonal markers and/or temperatures being used less frequently (Abplanalp et al., 1977; Collins et al., 1985; Little & Zahn, 1974; von Eiff et al., 1971; Wasilewska et al., 1980). Even when dates of subsequent periods are confirmed (e.g., Hastrup & Light, 1984; Polefrone & Manuck, 1988), self-reported designation may be erroneous. For example, in one study, self-report was not in accord with hormonal indexes in a substantial number of cases (Abplanalp et al., 1977). Furthermore, standardization in designation of the phases is also requisite. For example, the follicular phase has been defined as narrowly as days 5–7 (e.g., Collins *et al.*, 1985) and as broadly as days 5–11 (e.g., Stoney *et al.*, 1986). In those same studies, luteal phases did not even overlap: days 15–20 (Stoney *et al.*, 1986) and days 22–25 (Collins *et al.*, 1980), respectively.

In the present section, hormonal influences associated with the menstrual cycle were explored. In the subsequent section, the influence of exogenous hormones in menstruating and menopausal women is discussed. In addition, the impact of menopausal status, which is accompanied by major hormonal change, is examined.

Hormonal Status and Physiological Responsivity

The impact of exogenous hormones on physiological responses to challenge is of considerable interest given the risk of cardiovascular and cerebrovascular disease and hypertension associated with their usage. In younger women, the use of oral contraceptives has been extensive. Hormones used in oral contraceptives are synthetic and typically are prescribed in estrogen–progesterone combination (Bush & Barrett-Conner, 1985). The possibility that oral contraceptives might be implicated in future disease seemed to be unanticipated when it was first evidenced in the early 1960s. Several studies reported a relationship between oral contraceptive usage and stroke (e.g., Jick, Dinan, & Rothman, 1978; Royal College of General Practitioners, 1981; Vessey, Doll, Peto, Johnson, & Wiggins, 1976), hypertension (e.g., Stern, Brown, Haskell, Farquhar, Wehrle, & Wood, 1976), and MI (e.g., Jick *et al.*, 1978; Mann & Inman, 1975; Mann, Inman, & Thorogood, 1976; Royal College of General Practitioners, 1981). Across studies the relative risk of MI for users, relative to nonusers, ranged from 2.7 to 15.0. Overall, case-control, cohort, and prospective studies demonstrate that healthy women under the age of 45 are at increased risk for cardiovascular disease as a result of oral contraceptive usage. This presentation is exacerbated when other risk factors

are present, such as diabetes and hypertension (Mann & Inman, 1975; Mann *et al.*, 1976). Furthermore, smoking conferred substantial risk, independent of any relationship to other established risk factors such as hypertension or diabetes (e.g., Royal College of General Practitioners, 1981).

Hormones and Menstruating Women

The relationship between hormone replacement and cardiovascular disease has also been examined. Although some studies report a substantial risk of MI to menopausal estrogen therapy users below the age of 45 years (Jick *et al.*, 1978), other studies show little or no relationship in young and older women (e.g., Adams, Williams, & Vessey, 1981; Bain *et al.*, 1981; Rosenberg, Armstrong, & Jick, 1976; Stampfer *et al.*, 1985) of cardiovascular risk. Typically, natural conjugated estrogens (e.g., Premarin) are prescribed, though synthetic substances (e.g., piperazine estrone sulfate) are also used. Estrogen in hormone replacement is prescribed at lower dosages than that available in oral contraceptives (Bush & Barrett-Connor, 1985). Conjugated estrogens appeared to have no effect or increased BP, while certain synthetic hormones have been associated with a substantial decrease in BP in postmenopausal women (Wren & Routledge, 1981). It is noteworthy that in secondary prevention studies, conjugated estrogens given to men at high risk for cardiovascular disease were associated with excess mortality (Coronary Drug Project Research Group, 1973). The weight of the evidence leads to the conclusion that exogenous estrogens offer no protection to men at risk for cardiovascular disease by virtue of a past history of MI.

The study of the impact of hormonal status on physiological reactivity to challenge has been accomplished in two ways. The influence of exogenous hormones on reactivity has been evaluated in menstruating women (Garrett & Elder, 1984; Ladisich, 1977; Marinari *et al.*, 1976; Neus & von Eiff, 1985). The effect of menopausal status on reactivity has been examined in women receiving exogenous hormones (Collins *et al.*, 1982; von Eiff *et al.*, 1971), in women who have undergone bilateral oopherectomy (Hastrup, Kraemer, &

Phillips, 1986), and in women who had a natural menopause, free of hormone replacement (Saab, Matthews, Stoney, & McDonald, in press).

The influence of exogenous hormones on physiological responses to stress in menstruating women has been compared at different points of the menstrual cycle. Ladisich (1977) examined the influence of Provera (progesterone) on HR and respiration before, during, and after a word learning task with shock. Young healthy women who had not used oral contraceptives for at least 4 months, participated in two stress sessions: (1) 6 days before expected menses, when progesterone was expected to be high; and (2) 1 day before expected menses, when progesterone was expected to be low. The order of sessions was counterbalanced across women. In a double-blind manner, half of the women received a 1-week supply of Provera (10 mg/day), and the other half were given placebo. Medication began 8 days before the onset of the next expected menstrual period. Heart rate increase during stress was significantly greater the day before expected menstruation relative to 8 days before for the women in the Provera condition only. Stress-induced HR change for the session 1 day before menses was greatest during the first stress session. This finding suggests that experience with the stressor influenced the physiological response.

The effects of oral contraceptives on stress-induced responses were also studied by comparing oral contraceptive users to nonusers (Garrett & Elder, 1984; Marinari et al., 1976; Neus & von Eiff, 1985). Garrett and Elder (1984) evaluated matched groups of young women: (1) oral contraceptive users and (2) women with no history of contraceptive use. Women were evaluated four times during two menstrual cycles. The groups reportedly did not differ on HR and BP responses to simple RT or mental arithmetic challenges. However, HR differences were significant at $p < 0.06$. Since only four subjects in each group completed the study, this finding is relevant. Unfortunately, HR means were not reported, though differences could likely be large, given the sample size. In fact, others have reported that contraceptive users display increased stroke volume and vasodilation and decreased stress-induced SBP relative to nonusers

(Neus & von Eiff, 1985). These findings suggest that oral contraceptives may modulate cardiovascular response to stress.

Attenuated cortisol responding was also detected in oral contraceptive users (Marinari et al., 1976). Young women comprised the following groups: (1) users tested premenstrually, (2) users tested midcycle, (3) nonusers tested premenstrually, and (4) nonusers tested midcycle. Cortisol was sampled after an interpersonal-evaluative challenge during which the subject discussed self-perceptions. Oral contraceptive users had substantially higher baseline cortisol than nonusers. Nonusers, studied premenstrually, had greater weight-adjusted cortisol stress increases than other groups. The findings suggest that women, who are free from exogenous hormones, display enhanced adrenal-cortical reactivity to psychological stress during specific menstrual phases.

Across studies, subject characteristics of exogenous hormone-present and hormone-absent groups tended to be underreported (Ladisich, 1977; Garrett & Elder, 1984; Marinari et al., 1976; Neus & von Eiff, 1985). Important subject characteristics such as weight and age were used to match groups in only one study (Garrett & Elder, 1984). Also, as observed in other research, no information about other factors that might influence physiological reaction to stress was provided.

In sum, the available data suggest that exogenous hormones may indeed influence stress-induced responses in menstruating women. One study suggested that progesterone may augment HR reactions to challenge (Ladisich, 1977). This finding, however, is limited to acute progesterone usage. Other research indicates that relative to no hormones, oral contraceptives are associated with attenuated cortisol and cardiovascular responses to challenge (Marinari et al., 1976; Neus & von Eiff, 1985).

Hormones and Menopausal Women

The influence of exogenous and endogenous hormones on reactivity has been studied in women who are no longer menstruating (Collins et al., 1982; von Eiff et al., 1971). The effect of endogenous hormones has been examined in women who underwent a surgical menopause (Hastrup, Krae-mer, & Phillips, 1986) and in women who have undergone a natural menopause (Saab *et al.,* in press). von Eiff and his associates (von Eiff *et al.,* 1971) attempted to test the hypothesis that ovarian hormones protect women against hypertension, an established risk factor for coronary heart disease. Normotensive women who had a natural meno-pause were compared with normally menstruating women. No reactivity differences to a math stressor were observed. Only SBP baseline dif-ferences were obtained, favoring premenopausal women. In the same report, bilateral oopherec-tomy women were also monitored. The oopherec-tomized women were injected with either long-acting estrogen, combination estrogen/progester-one, or placebo. Both hormone groups had signifi-cantly lower SBP reactivity during stress, com-pared to the placebo group.

Although the authors (von Eiff *et al.,* 1971) in-terpreted these findings as supportive of a protec-tive effect for estrogen on blood pressure, the base-line results in the first comparison (natural menopause versus premenopause) may be due to substantial age difference between the two groups. Even the second comparison did not directly sup-port their hypothesis. The differences among oopherectomized groups were not due to ovarian function, but due to acute exogenous influences that do not mimic the use of such hormones in everyday life.

The influence of hormone replacement therapy on neuroendocrine and cardiovascular responses to stress was investigated in healthy menopausal women (Collins *et al.,* 1982). Middle-aged women were exposed to three stressors (visual search, SCWT, and mental arithmetic) on three separate occasions over 12 weeks. Half of the sample start-ed hormone replacement after session 1 and the remainder began treatment after session 2. Signifi-cant stress-induced HR changes from baseline occurred during all sessions. There were no stress-induced changes on BP taken immediately follow-ing the stressors. In addition, BP, catecholamine, and cortisol responses were not significantly af-fected by the hormone replacement. It was noted, however, that the magnitude of the E response be-fore and after hormone replacement was somewhat

higher than what had typically been observed in younger samples of women that had been pre-viously studied. This observation suggests that menopausal women might be approximating an E response that is more characteristic of a high-risk group for cardiovascular disease, i.e., males.'

Recently, a project has been completed that sys-tematically compared the stress-induced car-diovascular and plasma neuroendocrine responses of healthy normotensive age-matched middle-aged premenopausal and postmenopausal women who were free from exogenous hormones (Saab *et al.,* in press). Women were considered premenopausal if they reported menstruating regularly. Women were classified as postmenopausal if they had not menstruated for at least 12 months, did not have a hysterectomy, and did have serum FSH levels in criterion ranges. Demographic and baseline physi-ological characteristics of the two groups were similar. Premenopausal women were assessed only during days 6–13 of their cycle. Women were monitored during rest and four stressors: (1) psy-chomotor, (2) cognitive, (3) social-evaluative, and (4) physical. Postmenopausal women had substan-tially greater stress-induced HR change across all tasks. Postmenopausal women also exhibited greater increases in HR, SBP, and E than pre-menopausal women during the social-evaluative task.

The social-evaluative task distinguished itself as a potent stressor in the above study. This task focuses on evaluation of factors of particular con-cern to women in midlife: appearance and commu-nication skills. Thus, it was a conceptually rele-vant task. In contrast, the cognitive and psychomotor stressors require skills on which women are relatively less adequate: sequential arithmetic and visual-spatial integration. The fact that the postmenopausal and premenopausal wom-en did not differ in responses to all stressors sug-gests that hormonal factors interact with environ-mental variables in determining the stress responses of middle-aged women.

The stress-induced cardiovascular responses of comparably aged premenopausal women and sur-gical menopausal women (who had had hysterec-tomies with bilateral oopherectomy) were also stud-ied (Hastrup *et al.,* 1986). The complete surgical menopausal group was unique since it was comprised of women whose ovarian and uterine sources of hormones were eliminated more completely than women who undergo a natural menopause. The HR, SBP, and DBP stress-induced increases to mental arithmetic, spelling, and RT did not differentiate the premenopausal and surgical menopausal women. Family history of hypertension was associated with heightened SBP responding and DBP responding (covarying age) in surgical menopausal women relative to premenopausal women, with or without a family history of hypertension.

The BP findings (Hastrup *et al.*, 1986) are intriguing and suggest that the absence of major sources of endogenous hormones is associated with augmented BP responding in women with a genetic predisposition for hypertension. It is noteworthy, however, that natural postmenopausal women and oopherectomized women are reported to have similar levels of estrogen, hydroxyprogesterone, and progesterone but differ in androgen levels (e.g., Vermeulen, 1976). While these results (Hastrup *et al.*, 1986) are interesting, they must be viewed with caution as they were based on group sizes of five subjects each.

Taken together, the findings from the four menopause studies (Collins *et al.*, 1982; Hastrup *et al.*, 1986; Saab *et al.*, in press; von Eiff *et al.*, 1971) are only suggestive that there may be a change in physiological reactivity that accompanies menopausal status. It is necessary to note that menopausal groups in the aforementioned studies were heterogeneous with respect to time since last menstrual period. This is particularly relevant in natural menopausal women since it is well established that there may be ovarian function in some women well after menstruation has ceased (e.g., Lucisano *et al.*, 1984). Nonetheless, premenopausal women responded with substantially less HR reactivity to a variety of challenges relative to age-matched women who had undergone a natural menopause and were free from exogenous sources of hormones (Saab *et al.*, in press). In contrast, premenopausal women did not differ in cardiovascular responsivity to a challenge compared to older postmenopausal women (von Eiff *et al.*, 1971) or to similarly aged women who had had a hysterectomy with bilateral oopherectomy.

Treatment with hormone replacement had no apparent effect on stress-induced cardiovascular and neuroendocrine responses in natural menopausal women (Collins *et al.*, 1982). von Eiff's finding (von Eiff *et al.*, 1971) was contrary to the aforementioned, as acute exposure to exogenous hormones was associated with attenuated systolic responsivity in bilateral oopherectomized women. It is unclear from the results of the von Eiff study whether responsivity would be reduced in oopherectomized women receiving typical hormone replacement therapy.

Summary and Implications for Future Work

Certain consistencies have emerged in the reactivity literature pertinent to the issue of sex differences. Sex differences are apparent in resting BP and HR, but equivocal for neuroendocrine functioning. Heart rate tends to be higher in women while BP is greater in men prior to their 60s. As such, consideration should be given to controlling baseline differences when examining sex differences in physiological responses to challenge, as they may contribute to apparent sex differences.

The majority of data examining neuroendocrine responses to challenge support augmented E responding in males. The conflicting evidence for NE and cortisol responding does not substantiate that a sex difference exists. The cardiovascular reactivity literature evaluating sex differences (independent of TABP) reveals that men are more systolically reactive than women, but identical in diastolic responding. In contrast, the evidence for a sex difference in HR responding was quite mixed. In the literature reviewed, males and females are comparable in their likelihood of displaying augmented HR responding (see the sections Neuroendocrine Responses to Stress in Males and Females, and Cardiovascular Responses to Stress in Males and Females).

The TABP reactivity literature germane to sex differences and women was also presented. Interactions for sex and TABP were present in the majority of research, though findings were inconsistent across studies. The vast majority of the literature comparing Type A and B women did not find differences in reactivity. This may be a function of the manner by which TABP status was determined and the types of challenges used (see the section Type A, Sex, and Physiological Responsivity).

Reactivity was also evaluated across the menstrual cycle. There is some minimal evidence of increased stress-induced catecholamine responses in the second half of the menstrual cycle. Most consistent is the absence of phase-related cardiovascular effects in studies that involve repeated assessment across phase. The lack of effects may be accounted for, in part, by habituation to the stressors, after repeated exposure (see the section Menstrual Phase and Physiological Responsivity).

Hormonal influences on reactivity were also examined by determining the impact of exogenous and endogenous hormones in menstruating and menopausal women. Acute exposure to progesterone was associated with heightened HR responses. Oral contraceptive users, relative to nonusers, reacted with attenuated stress-induced cortisol and cardiovascular responses, suggesting that oral contraceptives might decrease reactivity in young women. These findings are in contrast to epidemiological data that indicate that oral contraceptives are associated with excess cardiovascular risk, in somewhat older women. Similarly, acute exposure to estrogen and/or progesterone in bilateral oopherectomized women was associated with decreased systolic responding to challenge. Hormone replacement therapy, however, appears to have no effect on cardiovascular and neuroendocrine responding in natural menopausal women. There is some suggestion that enhanced physiological responsivity is related to menopausal status when menopausal women (natural menopause or complete surgical menopause with a positive family history of hypertension) are compared to age-matched premenopausal women (see the section Hormonal Status and Physiological Responsivity).

Despite the large amount of research that has been accomplished, additional work is requisite. Areas that warrant attention include, but are not limited to, the following: (1) development of stressor/challenges; (2) menstruation-related responses; (3) menopause-related responses; (4) interaction of cardiovascular risk factors with sex, menstrual cycle, menopausal status, and hormonal status; and (5) exploring mechanisms that may account for reactivity differences.

With regard to stressors, a plethora have been used in the research reviewed above. The vast majority of tasks were cognitive or neuropsychologically oriented. As a consequence, such challenges may, by their nature, be more relevant for males than for females, given the expectancies for performance that are likely to vary for males and females in such situations (Lenney, 1977). It is of paramount importance to develop challenges that are equally engaging and involving to males and females. This would permit more equivalent comparisons between the sexes in terms of their physiological responses. Studies using interpersonal-evaluative or social-evaluative stressors with women and men have been promising in elucidating within-sex or between-sex differences (e.g., Baldwin & Clevenger, 1980; MacDougall *et al.*, 1981; Saab *et al.*, in press). Effort needs to be devoted to the development of stressors that maintain potency with repeated exposure. This necessity was underscored by the within-subject designs used to study menstrual phase. It is likely that increased familiarity with tasks obscures any potential phase-related differences. In general, increased standardization of procedures would be beneficial. Development of collaborative protocols or consentual criterion for procedures, such as the type of stressors employed and the timing of, and the type of, sampling of physiological responses is needed. At present, stressors vary from a maximum of 2 h to a minimum of 30 s. In addition, parameters considered to be stress-related were obtained before, during, and after stressors. Parameters sampled following stressors (particularly cardiovascular) would more appropriately be regarded as recovery samples. Clearly, this makes it difficult to compare and generalize across studies. By refining techniques and methods, and standardizing procedures, researchers will be better able to explore the influence of sex on reactivity.

A particular area of research that would benefit from refinement of techniques and standardization of methods is the literature that considers menstrual phase effects. Across studies, a variety of methods were employed to identify menstrual cycle phase. In the reactivity literature, determination by self-report for one or more cycles was used most frequently, while physiological markers such as vaginal mucosal indices and serum hormone levels were used infrequently. Validity differs for these parameters. Physiological markers are preferable, though frequently unavailable to many researchers. Researchers must be aware of the limitations of indexing phase by self-report. Specifically, reactivity assessments will not necessarily occur in the intended phase. It is unclear what contribution this situation has made to the mixed results in the literature (see the section Menstrual Phase and Physiological Responsivity).

Given the suggestive evidence of menstrual phase effects in between-subject designs, consideration should be given to controlling potential effects for menstrual cycle phase on reactivity, especially if only one reactivity assessment is to be made. For example, when comparing men and women, evaluation of women could occur during a common phase. This might be accomplished by studying women in the menses phase, or the early follicular phase, as those times appear to be more reliably indexed from self-report in regularly menstruating women. Or, if available, hormonal markers would be optimal. At a minimum, information should be collected regarding date of last period and date of next expected period, as well as medication usage, particularly estrogens and progesterones (e.g., oral contraceptives).

Menopausal status also requires evaluation, even when dealing with relatively young samples. First, it should not be assumed that the menopause groups, i.e., natural menopause, hysterectomy only, unilateral oopherectomy, bilateral oopherectomy, and complete hysterectomy, are equivalent in their physiological responses to challenge. There is some evidence, albeit mixed, that cardiovascular risk may differ across these groups (e.g., Centerwall, 1981; Kannel *et al.,* 1976; Stampfer *et al., 1985)*. Second, menopause studies using natural menopausal women accepted participants who had ammenorrhea for a minimum of either 6 or 12 months. Since hormonal changes

associated with menopause can occur over several years, recruiting women with a longer history of ammenorrhea is preferable. Status verification can be accomplished with hormonal determinations. Furthermore, the interaction of menopausal status and hormone replacement on physiological responses needs additional exploration in each of the menopausal groups. Given the equivocal findings for hormone replacement and cardiovascular disease risk, investigation of responses to challenge may be informative.

Another important avenue to pursue involves examining the interaction of cardiovascular risk factors with sex, menstrual cycle, menopausal status, as well as hormonal status. For example, little research considering the interaction of lipids, smoking, obesity, or diabetes with the above factors has been reported. Again, valuable information about the contribution that hyperreactivity to challenge may make to cardiovascular disease risk might be ascertained. In addition, preliminary hypotheses regarding mechanisms that might account for reactivity differences are likely to be generated.

Hypotheses pertaining to socialization factors and hormonal influences have been offered to explain reactivity differences with respect to sex. Nonetheless, additional work investigating physiological mechanisms is necessary. Continued research exploring sex differences in sympathetic receptor sensitivity (e.g., Freedman *et al.,* 1986) might help explain sex differences in reactivity. Similarly, examination of the effects of exogenous hormones (natural as well as synthetic) or changes in fluid retention and the renin–angiotensin system (Bush & Barrett-Connor, 1985) or E and NE release (Lobo, Shoupe, Roy, & Wellington, 1984) would make a significant contribution to understanding reactivity differences.

In conclusion, certain sex differences in reactivity emerge that parallel the sex differential for cardiovascular disease observed in the United States and other Western industrialized nations. This literature as well as the literature that explores the influences of TABP, menstrual and menopausal status, and endogenous hormones does not provide an entirely consistent picture. Nonetheless, continued exploration, especially using more standardized procedures, is warranted. Furthermore, investigation into the possible mechanisms for reactivity differences should be pursued.

References

Abplanalp, J. M., Livingston, L., Rose, R. M., & Sandwisch, D. (1977). Cortisol and growth hormone responses to psychological stress during the menstrual cycle. *Psychosomatic Medicine, 39,* 158–177.

Adams, S., Williams, V., & Vessey, M.P. (1981). Cardiovascular disease and hormone replacement treatment. A pilot case control study. *British Medical Journal, 282,* 1277–1278.

Anderson, N. B., Williams, R. B., & Lane, J. D. (1984). Cardiovascular responses to mental arithmetic and interpersonal challenge among black female adults. *Psychophysiology, 21,* 568 (Abstract).

Aslan, S., Nelson, L., Carruthers, M., & Lader, M. (1981). Stress and age effects on catecholamines in normal subjects. *Journal of Psychosomatic Research, 25,* 33–41.

Awaritefe, A., & Kadiri, A. U. (1982). The state–trait anxiety inventory and sex. *Physiology and Behavior, 29,* 211–213.

Bain, C., Willet, W., Hennekens, S. C., Rosner, B., Belanger, C., & Speizer, F. E. (1981). Use of postmenopausal hormones and risk of myocardial infarction. *Circulation, 64,* 42–46.

Baldwin, S. F., & Clevenger, T. (1980). Effect of speakers' sex and size of audience on heart rate changes during short impromptu speeches. *Psychological Reports, 46,* 131–134.

Bell, G. H., Davidson, J. N., & Scarborough, H. (1968). *Textbook of physiology and biochemistry.* London: Livingstone.

Berkson, D. M., Stamler, J., & Cohen, D. B. (1964). Ovarian function and coronary atherosclerosis. *Clinical Obstetrics and Gynecology, 7,* 504–530.

Bush, T. L., & Barrett-Connor, E. (1985). Noncontraceptive estrogen use and cardiovascular disease. *Epidemiologic Reviews, 7,* 80–104.

Carroll, D., Turner, J. R., Lee, H. J., & Stephenson, J. (1984). Temporal consistency of individual differences in cardiac response to a video game. *Biological Psychology, 19,* 81–93.

Centerwall, B. A. (1981). Premenopausal hysterectomy and cardiovascular disease. *American Journal of Obstetrics and Gynecology, 139,* 58–61.

Collins, A., Eneroth, P., & Landgren, B. (1985). Psychoneuroendocrine stress responses and mood as related to the menstrual cycle. *Psychosomatic Medicine, 47,* 512–526.

Collins, A., & Frankenhaeuser, M. (1978). Stress response in male and female engineering students. *Journal of Human Stress, 4,* 43–48.

Collins, A., Hanson, V., Eneroth, P., Hagenfeldt, K., Lundberg, U., & Frankenhaeuser, M. (1982). Psycho-

physiological stress responses in postmenopausal women before and after hormonal replacement therapy. *Human Neurobiology, 1,* 153–159.

Coronary Drug Project Research Group (1973). The Coronary Drug Project findings leading to discontinuation of the 2.5 mg/day estrogen group. *Journal of the American Medical Association, 226,* 652–657.

Cuche, J. L., Kuchel, O., Barbeau, A., & Genest, J. (1975). Sex differences in the urinary catecholamines. *Endocrine Research Communications, 2,* 549–559.

Dalmaz, Y., & Peyrin, L. (1982). Sex-differences in catecholamine metabolites in human urine during development and at adulthood. *Journal of Neural Transmission, 54,* 193–207.

Davidson, L., Vandongen, R., Rouse, I. L., Beilin, L. J., & Tunney, A. (1984). Sex-related differences in resting stimulated plasma noradrenaline and adrenaline. *Clinical Science, 67,* 347–352.

Emmens, C. W., & Martin, L. (1964). Estrogens. *Methods in Hormone Research, 3,* 1–8.

Forsman, L., & Lindblad, L. E. (1983). Effect of mental stress on baroreceptor-mediated changes in blood pressure and heart rate and on plasma catecholamines and subjective responses in healthy men and women. *Psychosomatic Medicine, 45,* 435–445.

Frankenhaeuser, M. (1983). The sympathetic-adrenal and pituitary adrenal response to challenge: Comparison between the sexes. In T. M. Dembroski, T. H. Schmidt, & G. Blumchen (Eds.), *Biobehavioral bases of coronary heart disease* (pp. 91–105). Basel: Karger.

Frankenhaeuser, M., Dunne, E., & Lundberg, U. (1976). Sex differences in sympathetic-adrenal medullary reactions induced by different stressors. *Psychopharmacology, 47,* 1–5.

Frankenhaeuser, M., Lundberg, U., & Forsman, L. (1980). Dissociation between sympathetic-adrenal and pituitary-adrenal response to an achievement situation characterized by high controllability: Comparison between Type A and Type B males and females. *Biological Psychology, 10,* 79–91.

Frankenhaeuser, M., von Wright, M. J., Collins, A., von Wright, J., Sedvall, G., & Swahn, C. G. (1978). Sex differences in psychoendocrine reactions to examination stress. *Psychosomatic Medicine, 40,* 334–343.

Freedman, R. R., Sabharwal, S. C., & Desai, N. (1987). *Sex differences in peripheral vascular adrenergic receptors.* *Circulation Research, 61,* 581–585.

Frey, M. A., & Siervogel, R. M. (1983). Cardiovascular response to a mentally stressful stimulus. *Japan Heart Journal, 24,* 315–323.

Gackenbach, J. (1982). Collegiate swimmers: Sex differences in self-reports and indices of physiological stress. *Perceptual and Motor Skills, 55,* 555–558.

Garrett, K. F., & Elder, S. T. (1984). The menstrual cycle from a bio-behavioral approach: A comparison of oral contraceptive and non-contraceptive users. *International Journal of Psychophysiology, 1,* 209–214.

Gasul, B. M., Arcilla, R. A., & Lev, M. (Eds.). (1966). *Heart disease in children: Diagnosis and treatment*. Philadelphia: Lippincott.

Goldstein, D. S., Levinson, P., & Keiser, H. R. (1983). Plasma and urinary catecholamines during the human ovulatory cycle. *American Journal of Obstetrics, 146*, 824–829.

Graham, L. A., Cohen, S. I., & Shavonian, B. M. (1966). Sex differences in autonomic responses during instrumental conditioning. *Psychosomatic Medicine, 28*, 264–271.

Hastrup, J. L., Kraemer, D. L., & Phillips, S. M. (1986, October). *Blood pressure and heart rate of women under 45 with total hysterectomy: Effects and stress and family history of hypertension*. Presentation at the annual meeting of the Society for Psychophysiological Research, Montreal.

Hastrup, J. L., & Light, K. C. (1984). Sex differences in cardiovascular stress responses: Modulation as a function of menstrual cycle phases. *Journal of Psychosomatic Research, 28*, 475–483.

Hjortland, M. C., McNamara, P. M., & Kannel, W. B. (1976). Some atherogenic concomitants of menopause: The Framingham study. *American Journal of Epidemiology, 103*, 304–311.

Holmes, D. S., Solomon, S., & Rump, B. S. (1982). Cardiac and subjective response to cognitive challenge and to controlled physical exercise by male and female coronary prone (Type A) and noncoronary prone persons. *Journal of Psychosomatic Research, 26*, 309–316.

Houston, B. K. (1986). Psychological variables and cardiovascular and neuroendocrine reactivity. In K. A. Matthews, S. M. Weiss, T. Detre, T. M. Dembroski, B. Falkner, S. B. Manuck, & R. B. Williams, Jr. (Eds.), *Handbook of stress, reactivity, and cardiovascular disease* (pp. 207–230). New York: Wiley.

Jick, H., Dinan, B., & Rothman, K. J. (1978). Oral contraceptive, and nonfatal myocardial infarction. *Journal of the American Medical Association, 239*, 1403–1406.

Johansson, G. (1972). Sex differences in the catecholamine output of children. *Acta Physiologica Scandinavia, 85*, 569–572.

Johansson, G., Frankenhaeuser, M., & Magnussen, J. (1973). Catecholamine output in school children as related to performance and adjustment. *Scandinavian Journal of Psychology, 14*, 20–28.

Johansson, G., & Post, B. (1974). Catecholamine output of males and females over a year period. *Acta Physiologica Scandinavia, 92*, 557–565.

Jorgensen, R. S., & Houston, B. K. (1981). Family history of hypertension, gender, and cardiovascular reactivity and stereotypy during stress. *Journal of Behavioral Medicine, 4*, 175–189.

Kannel, W. B., Hjortland, M. C., McNamara, P. M., & Gordon, T. (1976). Menopause and risk of cardiovascular disease. *Annals of Internal Medicine, 85*, 447–452.

Klaiber, E. L., Broverman, D. M., Haffajee, L. I., Hochman, J. S., Sacks, G. M., & Dalen, D. J. E. (1982). Serum estrogen levels in men with acute myocardial infarction. *American Medical Journal, 73*, 872–880.

Krantz, D. S., & Manuck, S. B. (1984). Acute psycho-physiological reactivity and risk of cardiovascular disease: A review and methodologic critique. *Psychological Bulletin, 96*, 435–464.

Ladisich, W. (1977). Influence of progesterone on serotonin metabolism: A possible causal factor for mood changes. *Psychoneuroendocrinology, 2*, 257–266.

Lamprecht, L., Matta, R. J., Little, B., & Zahn, T. P. (1974). Plasma dopamine-beta-hydroxylase (DBH) activity during the menstrual cycle. *Psychosomatic Medicine, 36*, 304–310.

Lane, J. D., White, A. D., & Williams, R. B., Jr. (1984). Cardiovascular effects of mental arithmetic in Type A and Type B females. *Psychophysiology, 21*, 39–46.

Lawler, K. A., Allen, M. T., Critcher, E. C., & Standard, B. A. (1981). The relationship of physiological responses to coronary-prone behavior pattern in children. *Journal of Behavioral Medicine, 4*, 203–216.

Lawler, K. A., Rixse, A., & Allen, M. T. (1983). Type A behavior and psychophysiological responses in adult women. *Psychophysiology, 20*, 343–350.

Lawler, K. A., & Schmied, L. A. (1986). Cardiovascular responsivity, Type A behavior and parental history of heart disease in young women. *Psychophysiology, 23*, 28–32.

Lawler, K. A., Schmied, L., Mitchell, V. P., & Rixse, A. (1984). Type A behavior and physiological responsivity in young women. *Journal of Psychosomatic Research, 28*, 197–204.

Lenney, E. (1977). Women's self-confidence in achievement settings. *Psychological Bulletin, 84*, 1–13.

Liberson, C. W., & Liberson, W. T. (1975). Sex differences in autonomic responses to electric shock. *Psychophysiology, 12*, 182–186.

Little, B. C., & Zahn, T. P. (1974). Changes in mood and autonomic functioning during menstrual cycle. *Psychophysiology, 11*, 579–590.

Lobo, R., Shoupe, D., Roy, S., & Wellington, P. (1984). Central and peripheral metabolites of norepinephrine and dopamine in postmenopausal women. *American Journal of Obstetrics and Gynecology, 149*, 548–552.

Lucisano, A. A., Campora, M. E., Russo, N., Maniccia, E., Montemurro, A., & Dell'Acqua, S. (1984). Ovarian and peripheral plasma levels of progestins, androgens and estrogens in post-menopausal women. *Maturitas, 6*, 45–53.

Lundberg, E., & Frankenhaeuser, M. (1980). Pituitary-adrenal and sympathetic-adrenal correlates of distress and effort. *Journal of Psychosomatic Research, 24*, 125–130.

MacDougall, J. M., Dembroski, T. M., & Krantz, D. S. (1981). Effects of types of challenge on pressor and heart rate responses in Type A and B women. *Psychophysiology, 18*, 1–9.

Mann, J. I., & Inman, W. H. W. (1975). Oral contraceptives and death from myocardial infarction. *British Medical Journal, 2*, 245–248.

Mann, J. I., Inman, W. H. W., & Thorogood, M. (1976). Oral contraceptive use in older women and fatal myocardial infarction. *British Medical Journal, 2*, 445–449.

Manuck, S. B., Craft, S., & Gold, K. J. (1978). Coronary-prone behavior pattern and cardiovascular response. *Psychophysiology, 15*, 403–411.

Marinari, K. T., Leshner, A. I., & Doyle, M. P. (1976). Menstrual cycle status and adrenocortical reactivity to psychological stress. *Psychoneuroendocrinology, 1,* 213–218.

Matthews, K. A. (1982). Psychological perspectives on the Type A behavioral pattern. *Psychological Bulletin, 91,* 293–323.

Matthews, K. A., Weiss, S. M., Detre, T., Dembroski, T. M., Falkner, B., Manuck, S. B., & Williams, R. B., Jr. (Eds.). (1986). *Handbook of stress, reactivity and cardiovascular disease.* New York: Wiley.

McConathy, W. J., & Alaupovic, P. (1981). Effects of estrogens on the plasma lipoprotein system in menopausal and postmenopausal women. In R. M. Greenshalgh (Ed.), *Hormones and vascular disease* (pp. 319–330). London: Pitman Press.

Myrstern, A. L., Lundberg, U., Frankenhaeuser, M., Ryan, G., Dolphin, C., & Cullen, J. (1984). Sex-role orientation as related to psychological and physiological responses during achievement and orthostatic stress. *Motivation and Emotion, 8,* 243–258.

National Center for Health Statistics (1977). Blood pressure levels of persons 6–74 years of age. United States 1971–1974. *Vital and Health Statistics, 11,* 203.

Neus, H., & von Eiff, A. W. (1985). Selected topics in the methodology of stress testing: Time course, gender and adaptation. In A. Steptoe, H. Ruddel, & H. Neus (Eds.), *Clinical and methodological issues in cardiovascular psychophysiology* (pp. 78–92). Berlin: Springer-Verlag.

Patkai, P., Johansson, G., & Post, B. (1974). Mood alertness and sympathetic-adrenal medullary activity during the menstrual cycle. *Psychosomatic Medicine, 36,* 503–512.

Phillips, G. B. (1978). Sex, hormones, risk factors and car-11.

Polefrone, J. M., & Manuck, S. B. (1988). Effects of menstrual phase and parental history of hypertension on cardiovascular response to cognitive challenge. *Psychosomatic Medicine, 50,* 23–36.

Prosser, C. L. (1973). *Comparative animal physiology* (3rd ed.). Philadelphia: Saunders.

Rauste-von Wright, M., von Wright, J., & Frankenhaeuser, M. (1981). Relationships between sex-related psychological characteristics during adolescence and catecholamine excretion during achievement stress. *Psychophysiology, 18,* 362–370.

Rosenberg, L., Armstrong, B., & Jick, H. (1976). Myocardial infarction and estrogen therapy in post-menopausal women. *New England Journal of Medicine, 294,* 1256–1259.

Royal College of General Practioners' Oral Contraception Study (1981). Further analyses of mortality in oral contraceptive users. *Lancet, 1,* 541–546.

Saab, P. G., Matthews, K. A., Stoney, C. M., McDonald, R. H. (in press). Premenopausal and postmenopausal women differ in their cardiovascular and neuroendocrine responses to behavioral stressors. *Psychophysiology.*

Schlaadt, R. G., & Shannon, P. T. (1986). *Drugs of choice.* Englewood Cliffs, NJ: Prentice–Hall.

Stamfer, M. J., Willett, W. C., Colditz, G. A., Rosner, B., Speizer, F. E., & Hennekens, C. H. (1985). A prospective study of postmenopausal estrogen therapy and coronary heart disease. *The New England Journal of Medicine, 313,* 1044–1049.

Stamler, J. (1975). Epidemiology of hypertension: Achievements and challenges. In M. Moser (Ed.), *Hypertension: A practical approach* (pp. 1–43). Boston: Little, Brown.

Stern, M. P., Brown, B. W., Haskell, W. L., Farquhar, J. W., Wehrle, C. L., & Wood, D. S. (1976). Cardiovascular risk and use of estrogens or estrogen/progesteron combinations. *Journal of the American Medical Association, 235,* 811–815.

Stoney, C. M., Langer, A. W., & Gelling, P. D. (1986). The effects of menstrual cycle phase on cardiovascular and pulmonary responses to behavioral and exercise stress. *Psychology, 23,* 393–402.

Stout, R. (1982). *Hormones and atherosclerosis.* Lancaster: MTP Press.

Tennes, K., & Kreye, M. (1985). Children's adrenocortical responses to classroom activities and tests in elementary school. *Psychosomatic Medicine, 47,* 451–460.

Tracy, R. E. (1966). Sex difference in coronary disease: Two opposing views. *Journal of Chronic Diseases, 19,* 1245–1251.

Van Egeren, L. F. (1979). Cardiovascular changes during social competition in a mixed motive game. *Journal of Personality and Social Psychology, 37,* 858–864.

Vermeulen, A. (1976). The hormonal activity of the post menopausal ovary. *Journal of Clinical Endocrinology and Metabolism, 42,* 247–253.

Vessey, M., Doll, R., Peto, R., Johnson, B., & Wiggins, P. (1976). A long-term follow-up study of women using different methods of contraception—An interim report. *Journal of Biosocial Sciences, 8,* 373–427.

von Eiff, A. W., Plotz, E. J., Beck, K. J., & Czernik, A. (1971). The effect of estrogens and progestins on blood pressure regulation of normotensive women. *American Journal of Obstetrics and Gynecology, 109,* 887–892.

Wasilewska, E., Kobus, E., & Bargiel, Z. (1980). Urinary catecholamine excretion and plasma dopamine-beta-hydroxylase activity in mental work performed in two periods of menstrual cycle in women. In E. Usdin, R. Kvetansky, & I. J. Kopin (Eds.), *Stress and catecholamines: Recent advances* (pp. 549–554). Amsterdam: Elsevier/North-Holland.

Williams, R. B., Lane, J. D., Kuhn, C. M., Melosh, W., White, A. R., & Schanberg, S. M. (1982). Type A behavior and elevated physiological and neuroendocrine response to cognitive tasks. *Science, 218,* 483–485.

Wren, B. G., & Routledge, A. D. (1981). Blood pressure changes: Oestrogens in climacteric women. *Medical Journal of Australia, 2,* 528–531.

Zacur, H. A., Tyson, J. E., Ziegler, M. G., & Lake, C. R. (1978). Plasma dopamine-β-hydroxylase activity and norepinephrine levels during the human menstrual cycle. *American Journal of Obstetrics and Gynecology, 130,* 148–151.

Zuspan, F. P., & Zuspan, K. J. (1973). Ovulatory plasma amine (epinephrine and norepinephrine) surge in the woman. *American Journal of Obstetrics and Gynecology, 117,* 654–660.

Psychometric Assessment

Section Editors: Charles S. Carver and Karen A. Matthews

The assumption that underlies this section of the handbook is that one or more "psychological variables" may play a role in producing sustained or transient physiological and pathophysiological activity, and may thereby influence eventual development of cardiovascular disease. If the role of these psychological variables is to be studied, they must be measured. To study psychological variables adequately requires much more than measuring personality and chronic levels of stress. It also requires measuring how research subjects perceive the situations in which they find themselves, and their motivational and affective reactions to those situations. None of these acts of measurement is as easy as it sounds. Rather, each sort of psychological assessment requires a careful and rigorous consideration of complex methodological and conceptual issues.

The six chapters in this section identify and discuss issues that arise in measuring psychological variables of various types. Chapter 30 by Carver and Matthews addresses the topic of "psychological variables" by outlining a model of the several ways in which psychological qualities are involved when people react to stress. This model serves as a heuristic device for thinking about the role of psychological variables in cardiovascular behavioral

Charles S. Carver • Department of Psychology, University of Miami, Coral Gables, Florida 33124.   *Karen A. Matthews* • Department of Psychiatry, Western Psychiatric Institute and Clinic, Pittsburgh, Pennsylvania 15213.

medicine. This chapter also addresses several issues that are sufficiently broad that they apply to all of the areas of assessment described in later chapters.

In Chapter 31 Houston describes issues that arise in considering research on how relatively stable personality differences may be determinants of exaggerated physiological responses to stress, and of eventual cardiovascular disease. As a conceptual guide to reviewing an enormously large literature, this chapter offers a cognitive model of processes leading to affective arousal, and relates major personality dimensions to three aspects of the model: perceptual and cognitive styles, affective arousal itself, and processes of coping with and altering the environment.

In Chapter 32 Monroe focuses on the assessment of acute stress, chronic stress, and social support. The first part of this chapter summarizes the major theoretical dimensions of these constructs; the second part outlines current assessment techniques and comments on their adequacy. This review indicates that we do have ways to measure these constructs, but it also suggests that the fit between the conceptual and operational definitions of the constructs often leaves a good deal to be desired.

Two chapters focus specifically on assessment in laboratory situations. In Chapter 33 Strube examines issues that arise when one uses self-reports to find out how subjects construe the laboratory situations in which they have been placed. The use of such situational assessment is based on the assumption that subjects' actions and reactions are based at least in part on how they understand and view their behavioral context. If interpretation of the situation *does* have a major influence on people's behavior, it is important to determine how the experimental context is being interpreted by the people whose reactions are being measured. Strube presents a detailed account of several key issues that arise in virtually every type of experimental setting.

Though self-reports are the most common way to measure subjects' temporary states, not all situational assessment relies on self-report. Chapter 34 by Tennenbaum and Jacob reviews techniques for determining the affective states of research subjects by analyzing their verbal and nonverbal behavior. Several systems have been established for coding expressive qualities into preestablished categories, which are both reliable and valid. Although these techniques have not been widely used in research in behavioral medicine, they offer cer-

tain advantages over self-report procedures, and appear to be worthy of wider consideration than they have yet received. This chapter highlights observational techniques currently in use and describes their advantages and disadvantages.

The final chapter of this section, Chapter 35, by Dembroski and Williams, addresses the assessment of coronary-prone behavior. Because of the unique role that research on Type A behavior has played in the evolution of cardiovascular behavioral medicine, this chapter has a more specific focus than do the other chapters in this section. Dembroski and Williams describe how examination of the Type A pattern has led researchers down a somewhat twisting path, in search of the answer to the question of what exactly constitutes coronary-prone behavior. The tentative answer that Dembroski and Williams provide to that question is interesting and itself raises important assessment issues.

CHAPTER **30**

An Overview of Issues in Psychometric Assessment

Charles S. Carver and Karen A. Matthews

The notion that psychological variables influence physiological processes and cardiovascular disease (CVD) seems simple and straightforward, at first. Upon closer examination, however, this idea turns out to be substantially more complex. Indeed, it has several rather distinct facets, each of which warrants examination in its own right.

What Are "Psychological Variables"?

What do we mean when we use the phrase "psychological variables"? When people who work in cardiovascular behavioral medicine hear this phrase, they probably think first of aspects of personality.* These are the psychological variables that have been given the most attention thus far by these researchers. The clearest illustration of

---

*We will ignore here the fact that there is a wide range of theoretical approaches to the concept of personality. Personality variables, for present purposes, are any dimensions of enduring individual differences that are at least partly psychological or behavioral.

Charles S. Carver • Department of Psychology, University of Miami, Coral Gables, Florida 33124. *Karen A. Matthews* • Department of Psychiatry, Western Psychiatric Institute and Clinic, Pittsburgh, Pennsylvania 15213.

this is the well-known search for a traitlike coronary-prone personality. Personality is an age-old construct, but the process of assessing it has always been controversial. If researchers in cardiovascular behavioral medicine are to benefit from assessing dispositional individual differences, they must be aware of some of the dimensions of the controversy, so as to make reasoned decisions about how to measure those individual differences (see Houston, this volume).

Personality is not, however, the only meaningful category of psychological variables that is important to consider when undertaking psychophysiological research. Another relevant category is people's momentary, transient shifts in motivation, cognition, or affect. If these states influence physiological reactions (which they seem to do), then it is important to assess changes in these transitory psychological states, in order to better understand the mediation of the physiological reactions.

How are these transient states to be measured? One approach to this assessment process focuses on the person's subjective experience. Repeated measures of that subjective experience should in principle allow you to determine changes that occur as a function of various experimental procedures. Yet, even rigorously collecting such self-reports of states may not be good enough (see Strube, this volume), for a variety of reasons. For example, some of the changes in people's motivation and affect are not prominently represented in consciousness. This raises questions about how well self-reports actually reflect what is happening in the research situation, whenever the experiences are not focal in consciousness. Accordingly, it is important to consider the possible utility of other methods of assessing transient psychological states.

Personality dispositions and transient states may be viewed as two opposite extremes on a dimension of permanence or stability among "psychological variables." There is also a gray area of psychological experience that lies somewhere between these two. Specifically, it sometimes is the case that shifts in motivation or affect are sustained over fairly extended periods of time, as a product of the person's life circumstances. As an example, some people live under a chronically high degree of stress, and may be responding to it continuously. Sustained changes such as this may have effects that are quite different from the effects of short-term changes.

As this brief sketch indicates, the phrase "psychological variable" has several rather distinct categories of meaning. Each of these categories of psychological variables has its own implications for research in cardiovascular behavioral medicine, and each of these implications deserves the careful attention of researchers planning psychophysiological research.

The Rocky Road from Planning the Study to Measuring Reactivity

Let's stop for a moment, and look at these sets of variables in a slightly different way. Consider the typical research project in which the influence of psychological variables on reactivity is being studied. Most of this research involves subjecting people to one or more experimental manipulations, or having people work at one or more experimental tasks in a laboratory setting. The situation created in the laboratory is expected to reveal differences in reactivity, as a function of the psychological variables under study.

It may be instructive to examine this research strategy, and to consider what issues arise when

looking at it carefully (see also Strube, this volume). Some of the issues that emerge serve to highlight places (and ways) in which psychological variables may become important in producing reactivity. Other issues highlight sources of potential error in attempting to link the hypothetically important psychological variable to reactivity.

The influence of a laboratory situation on subjects' reactivity is exerted across what might be thought of as a series of "filters" or "transformations." The impact of the situation on the subject does not, in fact, begin in the laboratory at all. It begins in the mind of the researcher, and in the translation of the researcher's intentions into an operationalization (see Figure 1). This translation is the first filter, or the first transformation.

The step represented by this translation is by no means trivial. You may, as a researcher, intend to cause subjects to experience a particular psychological state in your research setting. In order to induce that state, you choose an experimental task and embed it in a social context (the research protocol). If this operationalization does not match up well with your intention, however, you have already introduced a major source of error into the matrix of influences you are studying.

Creating the desired operationalization is, in fact, a more difficult task than is commonly acknowledged to be. Relatively small differences in how a procedure is carried out can have dramatic effects on the psychological climate that is created in the laboratory. It is important to realize this, and to keep this point in mind while you develop and standardize your laboratory procedures. It is also highly desirable to gather information on the validity of the operationalization before proceeding to collecting the data that are of primary interest (see Strube, this volume).

The situation as it is created in the laboratory constitutes an objective reality. It is not, however, experienced directly by the subject as such. Rather, the situation is interpreted and construed by the person who is placed into it (Figure 1). A great many factors can influence this construal process. The more carefully focused is the operationalization, the more likely are subjects to be led to one particular construal. The more ambiguous is the operationalization, the more likely are subjects

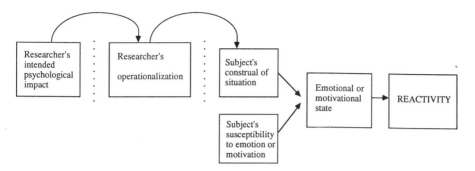

Figure 1. Four steps between the researcher's conceptualization of a laboratory situation and observing its effect on reactivity. The researcher intends to create a psychological state in subjects, and translates that intent into an operationalization. Subjects construe the operationalization, rather than assimilate it directly. A given construal can have an impact on emotional or motivational states, but the impact is moderated by other psychological variables. These changes in emotional or motivational state presumably influence reactivity.

to differ from each other in how they interpret the situation. Individual differences can also influence construals in a systematic way, particularly when the situation is ambiguous (see Houston, this volume). These systematic differences in construing situations have not typically been considered important in cardiovascular behavioral medicine. Perhaps they should be.

The subject's interpretation of the situation may include the perception of some element that constitutes a potential cause for emotional or motivational change—for example, a threat or challenge of some sort (see Lazarus & Folkman, 1984). The resulting emotional or motivational change does not occur to a uniform degree among all persons, however. The degree to which the change occurs depends in part on the degree to which the person is *susceptible* to its occurrence (Figure 1). To continue with this example, some people are more susceptible than others to reacting emotionally when experiencing a threat. To put it differently, some people get upset more readily than others, even if they have identical interpretations of the objective nature of the situation they are in. These differences in emotional reaction may be dispositional, or they may reflect differences in such contextual variables as availability of social support resources.

To be thorough psychometrically, one must consider the possible need to assess each of the layers of experience of the subject—the construal of the situation, the state of affect or motivation that is being experienced, and other variables (e.g., personality dispositions, social support) that may mediate the generation of an affective or motivational state from the construal. These various aspects of psychological assessment, and the issues that emerge from thinking about them, constitute the basis for the other chapters that make up this section of the handbook.

Broad Issues in Psychometric Assessment

In the remainder of this overview chapter, we address several issues that appear to transcend any one of the specific topics taken up in the other chapters of this section. Some of the issues to be addressed here apply to assessment of each type of psychological variable that we have just outlined. Other issues arise in considering the various psychological variables in conjunction with each other.

What Kinds of Psychological States Shall We Create?

Much recent attention has been given to the physiological changes that occur when people work on a variety of laboratory tasks. It should be noted, however, that associated with every task that yields a change in physiological state is a psychological state (or states) that may add to, suppress, or interact with physiological requirements of the tasks. A very fundamental question that receives less attention than it deserves is just what kind of psychological state we really want to produce in people in reactivity studies. When we study reactivity, are we interested simply in creating reactivity of *any* sort (see Manuck, this volume)? Are anger arousal, fear arousal, and task involvement functionally equivalent for purposes of examining the effect of psychological variables on reactivity? Or are these affective and motivational states sufficiently different from each other that we should study one and not the others, or study several and contrast them with each other?

A related question is whether it is sensible, or even possible, to study any specific one of these states in a meaningful fashion unless the experimental manipulation is aimed at producing that specific psychological state. For example, does it make any sense to study how hostility affects reactivity during achievement tasks that are devoid of any clear instigation to anger? Or is it necessary to use tasks that elicit annoyance in most people?

If it is necessary to create a specific psychological state, then we need to think carefully about what psychological state we are most interested in, before choosing the experimental tasks for the research. This, in turn, may mean thinking carefully about what personality dimensions (or life-situation dimensions) we want to use to predict responses, and tailoring the task to these dimensions. The result should be a planned integration of individual difference predictors, intended psychological state, and target task.

External Validity versus Experimental Control

Assume for the moment that it is best to try to create some *particular* type of psychological state through an experimental manipulation. (This seems to be the position that is usually taken, at least by implication.) Most reactivity research in laboratory settings thus uses carefully controlled behavioral manipulations to experimentally create changes in psychological state. The desire for close control over these manipulations has led to extensive reliance on such laboratory tasks as video games, interviews, reaction time tasks, impromptu speeches, and the like.

Reliance on this sort of task leads to another general question (which also comes up in Section III of the handbook). Do these tasks really produce the kinds of psychological states that we want to produce? Suppose that you know that the task elicits an increase in anger or frustration, but you also know that the task has little or nothing in common with anger-eliciting situations in the real world. How confident can we be that the anger experienced in this task is telling us anything about how anger occurs in the world outside the laboratory (see Strube, this volume)?

Perhaps it would be better to use tasks in which people interact with people they know, in situations that bring out naturalistic and meaningful anger (see Tennenbaum & Jacob, this volume), even though these interactions are based on an idiosyncratic and largely unknown history. One may also ask a more general question in this context. In studies of important human emotions, is it better to have subjects interact with strangers or with people they know well? If one is interested in maximizing external validity, the answer depends partly on the extent to which intense emotions can be elicited by strangers, and on the extent to which these emotions are more frequently elicited in people's lives by strangers or friends.

There is an inherent trade-off between exercising close experimental control and maintaining ecological or external validity. The kinds of tasks now commonly used allow a great deal of control, but they may provide little ecological validity. Engaging people in real-life interactions in the laboratory, or using ambulatory monitoring techniques, promotes greater ecological validity. On the other hand, one usually has little control over the objective nature of the events that occur while the subjects are being monitored.

Recognition of the trade-off between external validity and experimental control has led some researchers to attempt to collect both laboratory data (controlled) and ambulatory data (naturalistic) on the same subjects. This allows one to examine the similarity between findings from the two settings, provided that the laboratory tasks have been chosen on the basis of their conceptual relevance to the naturalistic phenomena under investigation. This sort of research should, in the long run, provide information about the magnitude of the problem that is introduced by relying exclusively on one or the other technique.

Social Desirability in Responding

The issue of ecological validity versus experimental control is a very general one, applying to all aspects of research, not just psychological variables. An issue that is more specific to the measurement of psychological qualities in research concerns the tendency of people to portray themselves in socially desirable ways. The issue here is the degree to which this tendency contaminates and thereby invalidates self-reports and overt behavior. Some investigators (e.g., Hogan, 1983) have come to believe that self-reports are not accurate reflections of what people are like, but rather are reports of how people would like to be viewed. This issue is one that can be raised with respect to all areas of psychological assessment. It bears on personality assessment, on self-reports of such variables as current life events and levels of social support, and on self-reports of such situational variables as state anger or state anxiety. It is also relevant to the question of how people choose their actions in the research setting.

The social desirability issue sometimes is not important, in that many of the variables that one might measure have no good or bad connotations. Unfortunately, many of the psychological variables that are coming to be seen as focal in research in cardiovascular behavioral medicine are variables that tend to have negative connotations—variables such as anger and hostility. One has to be somewhat concerned about the natural tendency of people to minimize the presence of these qualities in themselves, either as personality dispositions or as transient emotional experiences.

There is no simple answer to this problem. One way to approach it is to determine the degree to which a given personality measure typically correlates with social desirability tendencies [measured

by such indices as the Crowne and Marlowe (1964) social desirability scale]. This provides an indication of the magnitude of the potential problem, but unfortunately does little more than that.

Another possibility is that one may assess levels of social desirability displayed by the subjects in the study in which contamination from this variable is a concern. The anger or hostility (or whatever) measure could then be adjusted statistically for this variable in any further computations. This solution is less than wholly satisfactory, for at least two reasons. First, existing measures of social desirability are not pure measures of distortion in self-portrayal. The items that make up these scales are written so that a person who endorses them is "too good to be true." Some portion of the variance in these responses, however, clearly *must* be attributable to individual differences in actual behavior, as opposed to differences in social desirability as a self-report response bias.

Another reason why this solution is less than wholly satisfactory is that it may result in the masking of potentially interesting and important associations, because of the fact that social desirability as a conceptual quality is related to other psychological variables that are of interest in cardiovascular behavioral medicine. For example, people who score high on the Cook–Medley hostility scale (see Dembroski & Williams, this volume) are low in the tendency to distort their responses in socially desirable ways. If one were to adjust Cook–Medley scores to control for social desirability, one might thereby obscure any actual association that exists between Cook–Medley scores and the dependent variable under study.

Another approach to the social desirability problem is to take steps to create the perception that the investigator already has access to the true attitudes and feelings of the subject—even unacceptable feelings—through some physiological channel (see Sigall & Page, 1971). This makes it easier for the subject to admit to having negative feelings, because of the belief that those feelings are already exposed. The subject's primary motivation shifts from a social desirability concern to a desire not to look foolish by contradicting the responses read out by the physiograph.

As an example of how such a technique might

be implemented, in a "warm-up" phase of the experiment an investigator can ostensibly "predict" from the patterns of physiological responses a participant's preferences for food. In reality, the prediction is based on a previously administered questionnaire to which the subject should not anticipate the investigator to have had access. Having thereby "validated" the equipment's ability to provide direct information about positive and negative reactions, the investigator can then expect the subject to be more forthright than would otherwise be the case. Though it can be effective, this approach has the disadvantage of being quite cumbersome to implement.

Another approach to the social desirability problem is to attempt to create a situation in which subjects feel relatively free to report feelings and personal qualities that may be somewhat undesirable. Creating such a situation is partly a matter of developing orienting instructions that convey to subjects the fact that people experience a lot of different feelings, that having these feelings is not a bad thing, that it just a matter of people being different from each other and differing from time to time. In many ways, this seems to be the most satisfactory of the available alternatives, and it is doubtlessly the most common approach to this issue among personality and social psychologists. Clearly, situations can vary substantially in the degree to which they create evaluative concerns for the subject. One can easily create unintended influences on subjects' responses—and thereby the outcomes of the research—by maintaining a highly evaluative atmosphere in the research setting (for discussion of a specific case in which this may have occurred, see Dembroski & Williams, this volume). Diminishing such pressures should be one goal of the researcher unless there is a specific reason for wanting to create them.

How Accurate Can Self-Reports Be Expected to Be?

A question that is increasingly being asked in personality and social psychology is what information a person can reasonably be expected to provide via self-reports (e.g., Nisbett & Wilson,

1977). It seems obvious that some sorts of qualities are especially difficult to introspect. Measuring these qualities thus can be expected to be problematic for researchers who are interested in them.

For example, if you are interested in measuring the degree to which a laboratory task or an experimental manipulation produces anger, you must confront the question of how *aware* people are of their transient states of anger. If you measure their state anger levels retrospectively, 30 s after the completion of the task, are the measurements meaningful? What if you measure the anger levels 5 min, or 30 min afterward? The problem can also be put in individual difference terms. Is anger experienced by some people so frequently that they are no longer aware of their anger when it is present? Has it become for these people a highly automatic, "scripted" response that is unavailable to recall?

A somewhat different aspect of the introspection problem arises when a researcher wishes to measure qualities that are conceptualized as being distinct from each other, but which the subject may have difficulty in distinguishing from each other. For example, consider the experience of anger. This experience clearly is multidimensional (see Siegel, 1986). For example, the subjective experience of anger may be primarily physiological or primarily mental. The ease with which people can become angry (given a relatively standard stimulus) is different from the frequency with which they become angry in day-to-day life, and both of these are different from the typical intensity of the anger response (when it does occur), the typical duration of the anger, and whether the anger typically is expressed or suppressed.

These dimensions are all distinct from each other conceptually. It is an open (and interesting) question how distinct they are empirically. But in order to study these dimensions, we need to be able to assess them, and assess them separately from each other. Can people distinguish, introspectively, among the dimensions? Can they even introspect meaningfully about *one* dimension—for example, the frequency with which they become angry? (Ask yourself: How often do *you* become angry? How confident are you that your answer is accurate?)

Questionnaire Formats to Measure Dispositions

A question that is related to the matter of accuracy in introspections is how best to ask people about their dispositional psychological characteristics. When we ask people to report on traitlike qualities, the format of the question often focuses on a "typical" way of acting or feeling—for example, "Do you get angry easily?" One hopes that people responding to such a question engage in a brief mental review of a range of opportunities for anger to occur, and derive their answer from how they feel they respond across those various opportunities. This is an elaborate and somewhat difficult process. Most people probably are not very efficient at it.

It is possible, of course, that this characterization of how respondents go about answering these questions is quite wrong. Perhaps when responding to such a question people sample an anger opportunity at random from whatever set of situations is represented in memory, and make their judgment on that basis. This would not seem to be an especially reliable process, inasmuch as the situation sampled at random may or may not reflect the full range of variability.

There are several possible alternatives to the "typical" response format, which may get around this potential problem, and which thus may deserve some consideration. One alternative is to ask people to indicate their "maximal" response in the domain. One might ask, for example, given a particular (described) situation, ". . . what is the *most* angry you could become?" A possible advantage to this procedure is that it allows the respondent to focus on one end of the potential response continuum, which may make the mental consolidation process easier. There is some evidence that "maximal" self-reports do better at predicting both maximal *and* typical levels of the target behavior than do "typical" self-reports, though the mechanism by which this occurs is far from clear (Turner, 1978; Willerman, Turner, & Peterson, 1976).

A second alternative strategy to personality assessment focuses on a different facet of whatever quality of personality is under examination—the frequency with which the person has engaged in disposition-relevant acts in the relatively recent past (Buss & Craik, 1984). As a concrete example, one could compile a set of relatively common actions that imply hostility or aggression. Subjects would indicate whether they had done any of these actions in the past 3 months, and if so how often. This strategy requires the subject only to recall occurrences of acts, not to integrate or consolidate them in any way. It seems likely that memory for specific acts (or act categories) is better than memory for one's typical way of acting, or one's personality qualities in the abstract, which should enhance accuracy. The act frequencies reported then are combined into an index of a disposition by the researcher (rather than by the respondent). There is evidence that act frequency accounts represent a useful strategy for studying consistency in behavior (Buss, 1985), though whether this approach has greater predictive validity than alternative strategies remains to be tested.

However you choose to proceed in assessment, you should keep in mind that the format used in the scale dictates what information is obtained from the person. Consider the example just used, concerning assessment of the frequency of engaging in actions that imply hostility or aggressiveness. This measurement technique inherently assumes that what is really important about this dimension of personality is the *frequency* of engaging in hostile behavior. This technique completely ignores differences in the magnitude or intensity of the hostile act, and it completely ignores differences in the type of anger or aggression that is taking place (see Siegel, 1986). These alternative dimensions may, however, be as important as the frequency dimension, or even more important.

Our point here is not that one or another approach to personality assessment is intrinsically better or worse than another approach. Which type of scale is better for *you* depends on what hypothesis you want to examine. Our point, rather, is that every scale is devised from some particular point of view, and that that viewpoint influences the form of the scale's items. As you design your research, you should carefully examine the items of the scale, to determine whether it will permit you to find out what you really want to know. The title of the scale (and even a description of the scale) will not answer this question for you.

One last point should also be made in this context. It is a simple point, but one that is all too often overlooked. In choosing an assessment device (or in developing one), it is important that the items be worded in a manner that is appropriate to the vocabulary and linguistic competence of the subject population for which it is intended. Research subjects will often answer items that they do not understand with a random response, rather than ask for clarification. If subjects answer items without understanding them, the result is increased measurement error.

Need to Equate Level of Generality of Assessment Device and Situation Examined

Another issue that has received considerable attention in personality and social psychology in recent years concerns the level of generality or specificity with which psychological variables are assessed. The clearest case of how this issue can be important in prediction is a body of research on associations between attitudes and actions. This research makes the case that attitudes predict overt behaviors better when the two are assessed at an equivalent level of generality. An attitude that is very general is not likely to be a good predictor of a specific behavior, even if that behavior falls within the domain of the attitude. If, on the other hand, a set of four different behaviors are combined into an index, the attitude predicts the index quite well (Fishbein & Ajzen, 1974; McGowan & Gormly, 1976; Weigel & Newman, 1976). The complementary pattern also emerges, with a very specific attitude being a good predictor of a very specific behavior, but poorer at predicting a multiple-act index (Heberlein & Black, 1976; Weigel, Vernon, & Tognacci, 1974).

This issue of equating level of generality of assessment may also have implications for research in cardiovascular behavioral medicine. If one is interested in predicting reactivity to a specific type of task, one may wish to focus assessment more explicitly on that domain. For example, if your task is making an impromptu speech before an evaluative audience, you are probably better off assessing speech anxiety than using an overall index of trait anxiety. If you wish to assess reactivity across a range of anxiety-provoking situations, you may be better off assessing a generalized propensity toward anxiety, rather than a person's tendency toward anxiety in any specific domain of life. If you wish to predict the occurrence or progression of disease over time, rather than situational reactivity, it would seem more appropriate to use a general assessment device, rather than a specific one.

Comparability of Manipulated States and Parallel Personality Dimension

We often assume an equivalence between a manipulated state (e.g., anger) and a personality disposition (e.g., anger proneness). That is, if a manipulation of anger creates a physiological response, we often infer that a person who is prone to anger will experience such physiological responses more frequently than will a person less prone to anger. Is this true? We do not really know.

At least a partial answer to this question will come through the use of ambulatory monitoring techniques. Ambulatory techniques will permit the determination of actual anger frequency (assuming that the appropriate self-report questions are asked, and that people are able to respond to them effectively). In order for such research to be informative on this question, however, the studies must incorporate relevant personality measures of anger proneness. Otherwise, the data will reveal the presence of different anger frequencies, but not the link between this outcome and self-reported anger proneness.

The case of anger and anger proneness is useful for illustrating the parallel between personality dimensions and situational states. It is also a case, however, in which there seems little difficulty in inferring a direct link between the two. The implicit link between personality dimension and situational state is not always this clear. It is desirable to conduct experimental research with situational manipulations, in order to verify causality. But it sometimes is hard to be sure that the same process as is created by an experimental manipulation is what causes the personalities of two sets of people to differ from each other.

As another illustration, experimental manipulations of situational expectancies for favorable versus unfavorable outcomes establish that variations in expectancy *cause* variations in behavior (and other dependent measures). These expectancies are analogous to dispositional optimism versus pessimism (Scheier & Carver, 1985). But is it sensible to equate the two variables in drawing more extended conclusions? Not, in our view, without additional research.

Interactions of Dispositions with Transient versus Recurrent Stress

Laboratory investigations of reactivity expose people to short-term stress, whereas ambulatory studies can measure reactivity to both short-term and repeated stress. A question with practical implications is whether the people who are reactive to discrete short-term stressors are the same people who are reactive to recurrent stress. In principle, it is reactivity to *recurrent* or long-term stress that is most important. Studies doubtlessly will be conducted eventually to identify people who continue to react to recurrent stress, and to follow them across long periods of time. If laboratory stressors can be used to identify these people, then a brief laboratory session can be substituted for a more elaborate assessment procedure, when one wishes to identify highly reactive subjects for longitudinal research.

Are the people who are especially reactive in the laboratory the same people who are especially reactive to long-term stress? We do not know. The only way to answer this question is to observe the same subjects reacting both to laboratory stressors and to chronic stress outside the laboratory (i.e., with ambulatory measurement of reactivity).

Summary

Informed measurement of psychological variables in psychophysiological research requires addressing a series of questions: What are the conceptually relevant variables for manipulation

and measurement? What tasks should be selected to operationalize those variables? Are the tasks perceived by subjects as intended? Do the tasks induce the desired motivational and mood states under investigation? What are the dispositions that influence reactions to those manipulated variables?

To begin to address those questions (and to complement more focused discussions in the following chapters), we have raised several issues that are shared across domains of psychological assessment. These issues are the relative advantage of external validity versus experimental control; how to avoid problems of social desirability in responding; the accuracy of self-reports of states that may not be easily introspected; relationships between transient states and enduring dispositions; specificity versus generality of behavioral assessment; and the relation between reactivity to short-term and reactivity to long-term stress. In most cases we have provided no complete resolution to these issues, but rather indicated avenues by which progress can potentially be made toward their resolution. Closer examination of additional issues arising in studying psychological influences on physiological reactivity is elaborated in the succeeding chapters.

References

Buss, D. M. (1985). The temporal stability of acts, trends, and patterns. In C. D. Spielberger & J. N. Butcher (Eds.), *Advances in personality assessment* (Vol. 5, pp. 165–196). Hillsdale, NJ: Erlbaum.

Buss, D. M., & Craik, K. (1984). Acts, dispositions, and personality. In B. A. Maher & W. B. Maher (Eds.), *Progress in experimental personality research* (Vol. 13, pp. 241–301). New York: Academic Press.

Crowne, D. P., & Marlowe, D. (1964). *The approval motive: Studies in evaluative dependence.* New York: Wiley.

Fishbein, M., & Ajzen, I. (1974). Attitudes toward objects as predictors of single and multiple behavioral criteria. *Psychological Review, 81,* 59–74.

Heberlein, T. A., & Black, J. S. (1976). Attitudinal specificity and the prediction of behavior in a field setting. *Journal of Personality and Social Psychology, 33,* 474–479.

Hogan, R. (1983). A socioanalytic theory of personality. In M. Page (Ed.), *Nebraska symposium on motivation* (pp. 55–89). Lincoln: University of Nebraska Press.

Lazarus, R. S., & Folkman, S. (1984). *Stress, appraisal, and coping.* New York: Springer.

McGowan, J., & Gormly, J. (1976). Validation of personality traits: A multicriterion approach. *Journal of Personality and Social Psychology, 34,* 791–795.

Nisbett, R. E., & Wilson, T. D. (1977). Telling more than we can know: Verbal reports on mental processes. *Psychological Review, 84,* 231–259.

Scheier, M. F., & Carver, C. S. (1985). Optimism, coping, and health: Assessment and implications of generalized outcome expectancies. *Health Psychology, 4,* 219–247.

Siegel, J. M. (1986). The multidimensional anger inventory. *Journal of Personality and Social Psychology, 51,* 191–200.

Sigall, H., & Page, R. (1971). Current stereotypes: A little fading, a little faking. *Journal of Personality and Social Psychology, 18,* 247–255.

Turner, R. G. (1978).Consistency, self-consciousness, and the

predictive validity of typical and maximal personality measures. *Journal of Research in Personality, 12,* 117–132.

Weigel, R. H., & Newman, L. S. (1976). Increasing attitude–behavior correspondence by broadening the scope of the behavioral measure. *Journal of Personality and Social Psychology, 33,* 793–802.

Weigel, R. H., Vernon, D. T. A., & Tognacci, L. N. (1974). Specificity of the attitude as a determinant of attitude–behavior congruence. *Journal of Personality and Social Psychology, 30,* 724–728.

Willerman, L., Turner, R. G., & Peterson, M. (1976). A comparison of the predictive validity of typical and maximal personality measures. *Journal of Research in Personality, 10,* 482–492.

CHAPTER 31

Personality Dimensions in Reactivity and Cardiovascular Disease

B. Kent Houston

Model of Affective Arousal

The purposes of the present chapter are to discuss personality dimensions that have been or might be related to reactivity and cardiovascular disease (CVD), and to point out some of the issues that need to be considered by researchers who are interested in the possible link between personality, reactivity, and CVD. A personality dimension does not influence reactivity or the development of CVD in some isolated fashion but in a framework of other variables and processes. One approach for considering the psychological influence of personality dimensions on reactivity and CVD is in the context of a model of affective arousal. Consequently, a cognitive model of affective arousal will be briefly outlined here that emphasizes process, interaction between variables, and transaction with the environment.

This particular approach, including the model, is helpful for several reasons, which will become more apparent in subsequent portions of this chapter. (1) It helps to integrate consideration of what might otherwise be isolated and fragmented associations between personality dimensions and reactivity or CVD. (2) It serves to stimulate thought about further personality dimensions that might be fruitful to investigate. (3) It makes explicit certain assumptions that are frequently overlooked or unarticulated in studies of reactivity, e.g., the individuals whose reactions are being studied have thoughts and feelings which influence their reactivity. Thus, investigators need to assess whether subjects think about or perceive the experimental situation as was intended. How this may be assessed is elaborated in subsequent chapters by Strube, and Tennenbaum and Jacob. Moreover, investigators should measure the kind(s) of affect(s) that their subjects experience. This should be done because different affects may be associated with different patterns of physiological response (Henry & Meehan, 1981; Schwartz, Weinberger, & Singer, 1981). For example, it has been suggested that anger, relative to other affects, is related to greater norepinephrine secretion while anxiety is related to greater secretion of epinephrine (Henry & Meehan, 1981). Drawing inferences about a study or a group of studies solely on the basis of physiological measures may be clouded by not knowing what kind(s) of affect(s) was/were involved. (4) It highlights certain issues that need to be routinely considered, e.g., whether the situation engages the personality dimension, or in other words, the issue of person by situation interaction (noted in the preceding chapter by Carver and Matthews). (5) It serves as a reminder

B. Kent Houston • Department of Psychology, University of Kansas, Lawrence, Kansas 66045.

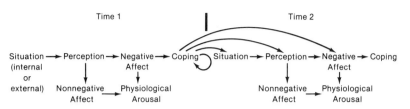

Figure 1. Model of affective arousal.

that individuals' physiological responses to the objectively same stimulus situation may well change over time. (6) It provides a vehicle for pointing out that individuals are not merely passive respondents to arousing situations, but rather that some individuals seek or create situations that are arousing.

While personality has been defined in a variety of ways, it is defined here as those thoughts, feelings, motives, and behaviors that characterize a person. This definition is used because it accords well with the model of affective arousal that is presented here. While transient aspects of personality (i.e., transient thoughts, feelings, desires, and behavior) are important for a broader description and understanding of individuals, the focus of the present chapter is on enduring aspects of personality. This is the case because CVD takes time to develop, and if personality variables are going to influence this process, they need to persist for a certain period of time. [See Conley (1984) and Costa and McCrae (1986) concerning temporal stability of personality dimensions.]

The cognitive model of affective arousal is depicted in Figure 1. A situation may be perceived in such a way to lead to positive, negative, or neutral affect. Each affect, whatever its valence, has a physiological arousal component. In general terms, the more intense the affect, the greater is the physiological arousal. The relation between affective intensity and physiological arousal is probably more readily observed from within than between subject comparisons. The physiological arousal associated with affective response(s) will combine with the physiological responses associated with the physical requirements of the situation or task (e.g., active versus passive responding, sensory intake versus mental work, effortfulness of responding, and so forth; see Krantz, Manuck, & Wing, 1986)

to produce the physiological responses that are measured in studies of reactivity. Chronic physiological responses associated with affective arousal and the physical requirements of naturalistic situations probably contribute to the chronic physiological arousal that has been hypothesized to contribute to CVD (see Herd, 1983; Williams, 1985). Because it is negative affect that has been suggested as contributing to CVD, e.g., anger and anxiety, the focus of the following presentation will be on this kind of affect.

Perception has been defined in various ways, but it is regarded here as a cognitive process whereby sensory input is transformed and meaning is assigned to it. Moreover, the basic meaning concerning the positivity/negativity of specific elements of the sensory input can be arrayed on a continuum varying in the extent to which the meaning is unlearned (or ''hard-wired''; see Zajonc, 1984) to the extent to which it is influenced by prior learning and experience.*

Clearly, any one situation may evoke multiple meanings and hence multiple affects. Take, for example, a person's undertaking the cold pressor test. The relatively hard-wired meaning of the cold sensations may lead to the experience of pain while the meaning of being subjected to a pain-inducing situation may, through prior learning, also lead to the experience of anger and/or fear. Thus, psychological factors including personality dimensions may influence individuals' reactions to what may

---

*Viewed in this manner, the debate between Zajonc (1984) and Lazarus (1984) concerning the roles that unlearned and cognitive factors play in affect is reconciled by suggesting that Zajonc and Lazarus are each focusing on a separate portion of the aforementioned continuum.

be regarded as "physical" as well as "psychological" stressors.

Additionally, the perception of a stimulus situation is influenced by other situational factors (for instance, other sensory inputs from the situation, e.g., the social stimulus value of an experimenter) and personality factors (e.g., the extent to which the situation may engage some motive on the individual's part, the extent to which the individual thinks he or she can effectively deal with the situation, the individual's mood, and so forth; see Lazarus, 1966; Lazarus & Folkman, 1984).

The model depicted in Figure 1 also indicates that negative affect leads to coping, which is defined here simply as a response or responses whose purpose is to reduce or avoid negative affect. The arrows in Figure 1 indicate that coping responses can be targeted on different parts of the model. [See Houston (1987) for elaboration.] The choice of coping responses is influenced by both situational and personality factors (see Lazarus, 1966).

The inclusion of the time dimension in the model (illustrated by Time 1 and Time 2) indicates that affective arousal to a situation is not a static event but is a process that changes with time. This is the case whether the situation remains objectively the same or changes as a function of an individual's coping responses. Because of the changing nature of this process, it is not surprising that when measures of reactivity to the objectively same task are obtained at periods removed in time from one another, they are not more highly correlated. For example, correlations between different indices of reactivity to the same task that range from 0.24 to 0.81 have been reported by Manuck and Garland (1980). However, the magnitude of these correlations, even though attenuated by the changing process of affective response to a situation, indicates that there is a fair degree of temporal consistency or stability of reactivity.

Various personality dimensions will now be considered under four headings that relate to the major components of the model of affective arousal. Thus, personality dimensions are discussed that: (1) affect the perceptual process, (2) modulate affective arousal, (3) influence coping responses, as well as (4) are unclear as to whether they affect perceptual processes, kind of affective

response, and/or coping responses. A personality dimension is considered under the heading that seems most appropriate in terms of its original conceptualization. In doing so, however, it is recognized that any one personality dimension could be considered under other headings because the dimension may be correlated with dimensions that are relevant to other headings.

It should be kept in mind from the outset that not all personality dimensions that are associated with reactivity may in fact contribute to or be a marker for a pathogenic process for CVD, e.g., Type A as measured by the Jenkins Activity Survey (JAS) (see Matthews & Haynes, 1986), trait anxiety (see below), and so forth. Thus, a proper evaluation of the contribution to CVD of the personality dimensions that are discussed here depends on further research on the pathophysiology of CVD and, ultimately, on epidemiological research that includes measures of the personality dimensions.

Personality Dimensions Affecting the Perceptual Process

There are at least three categories of personality dimensions that may affect the perceptual process: (1) beliefs about interactions with the physical and/or interpersonal environment; (2) strength of motive engaged by the situation; and (3) perceptual or cognitive styles.

Beliefs about Interpersonal or Physical Environment

As mentioned earlier, the perception of a situation is influenced by the extent to which individuals believe they can effectively deal with it (see Lazarus, 1966; Lazarus & Folkman, 1984). Locus of control is a personality dimension that is relevant in this regard. Locus of control (Rotter, 1966) refers to differences in people's beliefs that what happens to them is the result of their own behavior and attitudes (internal control) versus the result of luck, fate, chance, or powerful others (external control). Beliefs concerning control should be distinguished from a desire for control, which is discussed in the next section.

A measure of locus of control has been related to cardiovascular reactivity in several studies (Houston, 1972; Manuck, Craft, & Gold, 1978; DeGood, 1975). Generally, internal locus of control individuals exhibit greater systolic blood pressure (SBP) and heart rate (HR) reactivity in various situations although external locus of control individuals may exhibit greater diastolic blood pressure (DBP) reactivity when they are given control over an aversive situation (see DeGood, 1975).

Another dimension, similar in some respects to locus of control, that deserves consideration here is dispositional optimism–pessimism (Scheier & Carver, 1985). This dimension refers to the extent to which people have generalized expectations that their desired outcomes are or are not attainable. Although this dimension has not been related to reactivity, it has been found to relate to development of physical symptoms and recovery from coronary artery bypass surgery (Scheier & Carver, 1987).

Individuals' perceptions of situations will be influenced by their general beliefs about the goodness or badness of the world and the people in it. In this connection, hostility is important because it has been defined as an enduring attitude of ill will and a negative view of others (see Matthews, 1985).

A number of studies in reactivity and/or CVD have been conducted in which measures of hostility were employed. In several studies, ratings of hostility derived from the structured interview (SI) assessment of Type A have been investigated for their possible relations to cardiovascular reactivity and CVD. One rating procedure, referred to either as a ''clinical rating'' of hostility or ''potential for hostility,'' focuses on the content and intensity of the interviewee's responses as well as the interviewee's style of interacting with the interviewer (Dembroski, 1978). Ratings for potential for hostility have been found to be associated with severity of coronary atherosclerosis and incidence for coronary heart disease (CHD; see chapter by Dembroski and Williams). In studies conducted by Dembroski, MacDougall, and colleagues, ratings of potential for hostility have generally been found to be positively and significantly related to cardiovascular reactivity to various task situations

(Dembroski, MacDougall, Shields, Petitto, & Lushene, 1978; MacDougall, Dembroski, & Krantz, 1981). However, opposite results were obtained in a study by Glass, Lake, Contrada, Kehoe, and Erlanger (1983). Ratings of potential for hostility were found to be negatively related to cardiovascular responses to a mental arithmetic task (serial subtraction) and a modified Stroop task. It is unclear why these conflicting results were obtained by Glass et al., though perhaps they were due to problems with the method for rating potential for hostility and/or the experimental procedure.

The hostility scale (Ho) developed by Cook and Medley (1954) from the MMPI has been investigated in regard to its association with CVD and reactivity. The Ho scale has been found to be significantly related to the incidence of CHD and to the severity of coronary atherosclerosis (see chapter by Dembroski and Williams). Yet, in neither of two studies were Ho scores found to be related to cardiovascular reactivity to laboratory tasks (Anderson, Williams, Lane, & Monou, 1984; Smith & Houston, 1987). However, it is possible that neither of these studies engaged the cynicism and suspiciousness which are major characteristics of subjects with high Ho scale scores (see Smith & Frohm, 1985). Perhaps aggressing against or frustrating subjects in what appeared to be a devious or malicious manner would evoke greater reactivity in high compared to low Ho score subjects. This possibility underscores the necessity for carefully considering the notion of person by situation interaction when investigating personality dimensions and reactivity. This notion is highlighted when one considers personality and reactivity in the context of a model of affective arousal.

There are other dispositional beliefs that have been hypothesized to influence people's affective arousal via their perception of situations which, however, have received little attention in regard to reactivity. For instance, Ellis (1962) proposed that emotional distress results from various irrational or unreasonable beliefs, e.g., ''The idea that one should be thoroughly competent, adequate, and achieving in all possible respects, if one is to consider oneself worthwhile'' (p. 63). It would seem worthwhile to investigate the relation between reactivity and valid and reliable measures of Ellis's

(1962) notions concerning such beliefs. [See, in this regard, Malouff and Schutte (1986) and Smith, Houston, and Zurawski (1984).]

Strength of Motive Engaged by Situation

It was mentioned earlier that the strength of a motive which is engaged by a situation influences the perception of the stimulus situation. There are several personality dimensions associated with motives that have been related in some fashion to reactivity and/or CVD: aggression, dominance, competition, power, and achievement.

Aggression, as a personality dimension, may be defined as a characteristic impulse or motive to inflict harm on animate or inanimate objects. Few studies with humans have related reactivity or CVD to measures of aggression (as distinct from anger). However, in a study of cynomolgus monkeys by Manuck, Kaplan, and Clarkson (1983), it was found that monkeys that were high in HR reactivity to threatened capture and physical handling were rated as more behaviorally aggressive and were found to have more extensive coronary atherosclerosis at autopsy.

In regard to dominance, again working within an animal model, Kaplan, Manuck, Clarkson, Lusso, and Taub (1982) found that dominant monkeys in unstable social environments exhibited more atherosclerosis than submissive monkeys in the same environments or dominant monkeys in stable social environments. However, a significant relation was not found between dominance/submission and HR responses to threatened capture and physical handling (Manuck et al., 1983). It is possible, though, that the stressor employed in this study was not sufficiently relevant to dominance/submission vis-à-vis other members of the same species to evoke differential HR responses.

Self-reported competitiveness (in particular with peers) was found to be associated with the incidence of CHD in a reanalysis of data from the Western Collaborative Group Study (WCGS; Matthews, Glass, Rosenman, & Bortner, 1977). Moreover, several studies have been conducted in which ratings of verbal competitiveness in the SI were related to cardiovascular reactivity. Positive results were obtained in a study of males by Dembroski et al.

(1978), but a trend toward a negative relation was found by Glass et al. (1983) in a study of males, and null results were found in two studies of females by MacDougall et al. (1981). The reason for these discrepant results is unclear.

McClelland (1979) reported that a measure of inhibited power motivation significantly predicted signs of hypertensive pathology in a group of men 20 years later. Individuals characterized by inhibited power motivation are described as desiring to affect others by aggressive or other means but to inhibit overt expression of aggression. Inhibited power motivation was not found to be related to reactivity in studies by Glass et al. (1983) or Blumenthal, Lane, and Williams (1985). The latter authors, however, did find a relation between reactivity and power motivation independent of the inhibition factor.

A very strong desire for achievement ("overachievement") in boys was found to be positively associated with epinephrine levels in an achievement situation by Bergman and Magnusson (1979). Moreover, in a prospective study by Bonami and Rime (1972), men who developed CHD exhibited a greater need for achievement as assessed by a projective test than men who remained free of CHD.

Another motive that merits consideration is desire for control. Stemming from Glass's (1977) suggestion that a strong need for control is an important dimension underlying Type A behavior, Dembroski, MacDougall, and Musante (1984) found that Type As, defined by both the SI and the JAS, got significantly higher scores on a measure of desire for control (Burger & Cooper, 1979) than Type Bs. Although a measure of desire for control has not been related to either reactivity or CVD, it would seem worthwhile to investigate such relations.

Perceptual and Cognitive Styles

Personality dimensions that reflect differences in characteristic ways in which people perceive and/or conceptualize the world should also be considered in regard to reactivity and CVD. Field dependence/independence is one such dimension. Field dependence/independence refers to the kinds of orientations or frameworks people employ in making perceptual judgments. People at one extreme (field dependent) rely more on external frames of reference in making perceptual judgments while people at the other extreme (field independent) rely more on internal frames of reference in making perceptual judgments (Goodenough, 1978). In relation to risk for CVD, field-dependent individuals have been found to have higher levels of serum cholesterol than field-independent individuals (Flemenbaum & Anderson, 1978; Flemenbaum & Flemenbaum, 1975). Whether field dependence/independence relates to reactivity and/or CVD awaits exploration.

Personality Dimensions Modulating Affective Arousal

There are personality dimensions that can be conceptualized as modulating intensity of affective experience, and hence the reactivity of individuals in stimulus situations. Two of the dimensions of personality promoted by Eysenck (1967), namely, introversion/extraversion and neuroticism, are relevant in this regard.

Briefly, introversion/extraversion (Eysenck, 1967) reflects the extent to which individuals are oriented toward their own private experiences (introversion) or toward the external environment and the people and objects around them (extraversion). Eysenck hypothesized that, because of possible innate biological differences, introverts, relative to extraverts, are more cortically aroused and thus have lower thresholds for response to sensory stimulation. If introverts do have lower sensory thresholds, one might expect that introverts would exhibit greater reactivity. Geen (1984; Study II) found that introverts relative to extraverts, measured by the Eysenck Personality Inventory (Eysenck & Eysenck, 1964), exhibited greater HR responses to noise of intermediate levels, but introverts and extraverts did not differ in HR responses to the most and least intense levels of noise. In contrast, in a study by Glass et al. (1983), no relation was found between introversion/extraversion as measured by the 16 PF and measures of cardiovascular reactivity to a mental arithmetic task and a modified Stroop task. Perhaps the discrepancy in the results

of the two studies was due to differences in the measures of introversion/extraversion that were employed.

Eysenck (1967) hypothesized that, again because of possible innate differences, individuals high in neuroticism are characterized by an overactive autonomic nervous system, which one might anticipate would lead them to be more affectively aroused or reactive in situations that engaged this personality dimension. This notion, however, has received little empirical test. Neuroticism has been associated with the development of chest pains (Jenkins, 1976), although it appears unlikely that these symptoms reflect true CHD (Costa & McCrae, 1985).

Emotionality is a dimension, similar to Eysenck's conceptualization of neuroticism, that would be expected to influence affective arousal (Buss & Plomin, 1975). However, little research has been done relating a measure of emotionality per se to reactivity or CVD. Tangentially relevant are the findings from studies (Bakker, 1967; Lebovits, Shekelle, & Ostfeld, 1967) of a relation between emotional instability as measured by the 16 PF and angina.

Another dimension, similar to that of emotionality, that is relevant here is affect intensity. A self-report measure of affect intensity has been found to relate to the intensity of self-reported affective responses to both positive and negative life events (Larsen, Diener, & Emmons, 1986). Although a measure of affect intensity has not been related to reactivity, a measure of intensity of positive and negative affective response that was obtained from a structured interview has been found to predict recurrent myocardial infarction (MI) (Powell & Thoresen, 1985).

Activity level is another dimension that might be expected to influence reactivity because whatever factor (perhaps heredity; Buss & Plomin, 1975) that energizes some individuals more than others may contribute to greater responsivity to stimulus situations. Relevant to this, the Activity subscale of the Thurstone Temperament Schedule (1949) (sometimes, however, regarded as a measure of Type A) has been found to be related to both reactivity (Pittner, Houston, & Spiridigliozzi, 1983) and premature CHD (Brozek, Keys, & Blackburn, 1966).

Personality Dimensions Affecting Coping

There are various personality dimensions that may affect the coping responses which people employ. One such dimension that may be conceptualized as affecting the perceptual process is denial. In a study by Houston (1973), subjects who got high scores on the Little–Fisher Denial scale were found to evidence significantly less HR reactivity across both avoidable and unavoidable shock conditions than subjects who got low trait denial scores.

Two other dimensions of this kind that appear promising are monitoring and blunting (Miller, 1987). Individuals who are high on the monitoring dimension seek threat-relevant information, while individuals who are high on the blunting dimension avoid threat-relevant information. The measures of these dimensions (from the Miller Behavior Style Scale) have been demonstrated to have a certain amount of construct validity (Miller, 1987). As yet, however, these dimensions have not been directly related to reactivity or CVD (see Miller, 1979).

The aforementioned dimensions are focused on the perceptual process. As mentioned earlier, coping may be focused on various elements within the stress model. Thus, coping may be focused on the affect generated, including the expression of the affect.

Relevant to this, the inhibition or suppression of anger expression has been related to both reactivity and CVD. In a study by Holroyd and Gorkin (1983), subjects who scored low on the Novaco scale (1975) (interpreted by the authors as reflecting inhibition of anger expression) manifested greater SBP and HR responses to role-played social interactions than subjects who scored high on the Novaco scale.

In a study by Haynes, Feinleib, and Kannel (1980), scores reflecting the inhibition of anger expression, viz., low self-reports of expressing anger outwardly, were found to predict CHD for male white-collar workers, and low self-reports of discussing anger with others, were found to predict angina for women. In addition, scores reflecting the inhibition of anger expression derived from subjects' self-reported responses to five hypothetical provoking situations were found to be associated with greater risk of essential hypertension (EH) in a study by Gentry, Chesney, Gary, Hall, and Harburg (1982). Inhibition of anger expression was operationalized in this study both in terms of not reporting feelings of anger to the provoking situations and reporting feeling anger but not showing it.

Across studies, suppression or inhibition of anger has been defined in heterogeneous ways, viz., via low self-reports of anger (e.g., Holroyd & Gorkin, 1983), low self-reports of anger expression (e.g., Haynes et al., 1980), and/or self-reports of not expressing angry feelings (Gentry et al., 1982). Considering this, it would seem that the conceptualization and measurement of anger suppression or inhibition would benefit from clarification.

Dimensions Affecting Perception, Affective Response, and/or Coping

There are several personality dimensions of interest in regard to reactivity and CVD, but it is theoretically unclear whether they involve dispositions for perceiving particular situations in certain ways, dispositions for responding with specific affective responses following more general perceptions of situations, and/or dispositions for particular coping responses. Personality dimensions of this kind can be distinguished in terms of being either single-faceted constructs (e.g., trait anxiety, trait anger) or multifaceted constructs (e.g., Type A).

Single-Faceted Constructs

Anxiety

Anxiety has been associated with the development of angina (Jenkins, 1976), although Costa and McCrae (1985) have questioned whether these symptoms reflect true CHD. The results of several studies indicate limited evidence for a direct relation between various measures of anxiety and cardiovascular reactivity (Glass et al., 1983; Hodges, 1968; Holroyd, Westbrook, Wolf, & Badhorn, 1978; Houston, 1977; Knight & Borden, 1979;

Smith, Houston, & Zurawski, 1984). However, when defensive underreporting of anxiety, as measured by the Marlowe–Crowne social desirability scale, is taken into consideration, a more consistent and stronger relation between anxiety and cardiovascular reactivity is found (Asendorpf & Scherer, 1983; Weinberger, Schwartz, & Davidson, 1979).

Anger

To distinguish it from such similar concepts as hostility and aggression, anger has been defined as an emotional state that involves displeasure, ranging in intensity from mild irritation to rage, and which frequently is accompanied by the impulse to inflict harm (Izard, 1977; Kaufmann, 1970; Spielberger, Jacobs, Russell, & Crane, 1983). In a study by Matthews *et al.* (1977), self-report items reflecting irritation, frequency of anger, and directing anger outward were found to be significantly related to incidence of CHD. In contrast to research relating hostility or anger inhibition to reactivity, few studies have examined the relation between measures of characteristic anger and reactivity.

Recently, two measures of anger have been developed that deserve consideration in future studies of reactivity and CVD. One is the Trait Anger Inventory (Spielberger *et al.*, 1983) which measures anger susceptibility, and the second is the Multidimensional Anger Inventory (Siegel, 1985) which measures multiple aspects of the anger experience.

Multifaceted Constructs

The Type A behavior pattern is a multifaceted personality construct about which there is uncertainty concerning the ways it influences affective arousal. However, it is foremost among this kind of variable in being related to reactivity and CVD. Type As are characterized by impatience, chronic time urgency, enhanced competitiveness, aggressive drive, and an inclination for hostility (Rosenman, 1978). The evidence concerning the relation between Type A and CVD has been thor-

oughly reviewed recently by Matthews and Haynes (1986; see also Dembroski and Williams, this volume).

Numerous studies have been conducted in which the relation between Type A behavior and subjects' neuroendocrine and/or cardiovascular responses to various situations have been examined. [Extensive recent reviews of this area may be found in Houston (1988) and Wright, Contrada, and Glass (1985).] In these studies, Type A is most commonly measured by means of the SI (Rosenman, 1978), the JAS (both the adult version: Jenkins, Rosenman, & Zyzanski, 1974; and the student version: Krantz, Glass, and Snyder, 1974), and the Framingham Type A Scale (FTAS; Haynes, Levine, Scotch, Feinleib, & Kannel, 1978). It should be noted that these measures are only weakly interrelated, which indicates that they are measuring somewhat different characteristics (Matthews, 1982).

A review of the reactivity studies in which global Type A was measured by the SI suggests the following. For males, SI-defined Type A is most likely to be related to reactivity in situations in which the individual is annoyed or harassed (see Glass *et al.*, 1980, Study I; Lake, Suarez, Schneiderman, & Tocci, 1985) or in situations in which there is moderate incentive to accomplish something that is viewed as difficult, but not highly difficult. The reason for using the adjective "moderate" with "incentive" in the foregoing statement is that in situations in which there is high incentive to accomplish something, Type Bs appear to become as aroused as Type As (see Blumenthal *et al.*, 1983). Further, the reason for characterizing the situations in the foregoing statement as "difficult, but not highly difficult" is that in situations that are viewed as highly difficult, Type As typically do not become more aroused than Type Bs (e.g., see Ward *et al.*, 1986), perhaps because the perceived probability of success, or avoidance of failure, is so low.

SI-defined Type A is most likely to be related to reactivity in verbal exchanges such as the SI for middle-class, white females (see MacDougall *et al.*, 1981, Study II), but perhaps not for lower-class and/or black females (Smyth, Call, Hansell, Sparacino, & Strodtbeck, 1978). Moreover, SI-defined Type A for females is not related to reactivity to the kinds of tasks for which Type A/B reactivity differences have been found for males (see Lawler, Schmied, Mitchell, & Rixse, 1984; MacDougall *et al.,* 1981, Study I and II; Mayes, Sime, & Ganster, 1984).

A review of the reactivity studies in which global Type A was measured by the JAS suggests the following. For males, JAS-defined Type As relative to Type Bs are more likely to exhibit greater reactivity to tasks that require speed of response, are difficult but not extremely difficult (e.g., see Jorgensen & Houston, 1981), and involve a moderate degree of incentive for performance (see Manuck & Garland, 1979). Unlike what was said about SI-defined Type A for males, however, JAS-defined Type A does not appear to be related to reactivity in situations in which the individual is annoyed or harassed (see Holmes & Will, 1985; Zurawski & Houston, 1983).

For college females, there is little evidence that JAS-defined Type A is related to reactivity (see Lane, White, & Williams, 1984; Lawler & Schmied, 1986; Lawler *et al.,* 1984; MacDougall *et al.,* 1981, Study I and II). For noncollege females, there is some evidence that JAS-defined Type A is related to reactivity for the same kinds of tasks as those for males (Lawler, Rixse, & Allen, 1983; Mayes *et al.,* 1984).

The FTAS has been related to reactivity in very few studies. FTAS-defined Type As relative to Type Bs were found to exhibit significantly greater SBP reactivity in a study by Smith, Houston, and Zurawski (1985). In a study of college males by Dembroski, MacDougall, Herd, and Shields (1979), FTAS-defined Type As relative to Type Bs responded to a reaction-time task in a low-challenge condition with significantly less finger pulse volume (FPV; indicating greater arousal) but not greater SBP, DBP, or HR. However, there were no differences between FTAS-defined Type As and Bs in cardiovascular response in a high-challenge condition or either high- or low-challenge conditions for a cold pressor test. And in two studies of college females, no differences in cardiovascular reactivity were found between FTAS-defined Type As and Bs to a reaction-time task, the cold pressor test, or the SI (MacDougall *et al.,* 1981). At present, it seems reasonable to

conclude that the relation between FTAS-defined A/B Type and reactivity is weak at best.

Implications of Model for Person by Situation Interaction

The affective arousal model outlined here helps to highlight or make explicit that a person by situation interaction is involved whenever one considers the relation between personality dimensions and reactivity or CVD. The nature of the situation determines whether a particular personality dimension may contribute to affective arousal, hence reactivity and/or possible CVD.

The notion of a person by situation interaction is quite apparent when some aspect of a situation or task is experimentally manipulated with the intention of examining the combined effect of the manipulation and a personality dimension. The literature on JAS-defined Type A illustrates this. In three studies of males, JAS-defined Type As relative to Type Bs were found to exhibit significantly greater cardiovascular responses to tasks that subjects had been told were difficult or that subjects found through their own experience to be difficult, but no differences in reactivity between JAS-defined Type As and Bs were found for moderately difficult or easy tasks (Gastorf, 1982; Holmes, McGilley, & Houston, 1984; Contrada, Wright, & Glass, 1984). These studies consistently show that the difficulty of experimental tasks is important in influencing whether reactivity differences between JAS-defined Type A and B males are obtained in experimental situations.

A person by situation interaction also is involved in the choice of single situations or tasks with which subjects are confronted in reactivity studies. Considering the conceptualization of Type A, one would not expect physical threats, e.g., exposure to painful stimuli, snakes, and so forth, to evoke differences in reactivity between As and Bs, but one would expect events that involve harassment, threats to control of important events, and so forth, would evoke differences in reactivity. Indeed, this is what is typically found, at least for males (see Houston, 1988; Wright *et al.,* 1985).

In discussing person by situation interactions, consideration should be given to two kinds of situations that may engage a personality dimension. One kind is that which is congruent with the essential characteristic(s) of the disposition, e.g., a situation that elicits striving for leadership in an individual with a high need for power. Another kind of situation is that which is incongruent with or frustrates the essential characteristic(s) of the disposition, e.g., a situation that blocks a person from striving for power. It is important to consider what personality dimensions are susceptible to which kind of engagement, and what the implications for arousal are of acute versus chronic engagement of the two different kinds of potential engagement. For example, acute frustration may lead to substantial short-term arousal but chronic frustration may lead to apathy. In contrast, chronic exposure to engaging situations that are congruent with the essential characteristic(s) of a disposition may lead to long-term arousal.

Interaction between Personality Dimensions

In the foregoing discussion, personality dimensions were considered singly in regard to their relations to affective arousal, reactivity, and CVD. However, whenever a phenomenon is influenced by two or more variables, consideration should be given to whether they do so in an additive or interactive fashion. Rarely have interactions between personality dimensions been examined in regard to reactivity and/or possible CVD.

A prominent exception to this has been research that has examined interactions between Type A and other personality dimensions. McCranie, Simpson, and Stevens (1981) studied the interaction of field dependence/independence and Type A. It was found that JAS-defined Type As who are field dependent had the highest levels of cholesterol and low-density lipoproteins. However, whether field dependence/independence interacts with Type A in predicting reactivity or eventual CVD awaits further investigation.

Haynes reported that FTAS-defined Type A interacted with a measure of anger expression in predicting CHD in women and white-collar men (Matthews & Haynes, 1986). CHD was primarily found in FTAS-defined Type As who were also characterized by low self-report of expressing anger outward (which was interpreted as inhibition of anger expression).

If interactions between personality dimensions are examined, an expanded person by situation framework needs to be considered. In other words, it is important to consider whether all the dimensions will be engaged by the situation under consideration, e.g., whether, as intended, a situation evokes propensities for both anger and the desire to compete. Moreover, personality dimensions should not be chosen for study haphazardly but on the basis of some conceptualization as to how they fit together, as for instance the model of affective arousal proposed here.

Finally, while the focus of this chapter is on personality dimensions, possible interactions should not be overlooked between personality dimensions and biological variables (e.g., family history of hypertension; see Jorgensen & Houston, 1986), age and socioeconomic class (see Haynes et al., 1980), and so forth.

Personality Dimensions and Transactions with Environment

Most models of affective arousal, and most considerations of reactivity, assume that individuals are passive with regard to the occurrence and nature of the situation to which they react. This approach is congruent with laboratory research in which individuals are indeed passive in the sense that they are presented with situations by the experimenter and their response options are restricted by the experimenter.

The role that personality dimensions play in affective arousal, reactivity outside the laboratory, and CVD, is incomplete without the additional recognition that some personality dimensions may not only, or may not at all, influence affective arousal to certain kinds of situations, but they may influence the degree to which individuals seek or create arousing situations (see also Monroe, this volume).

Take, for example, individuals who are high in

need for achievement, high in need for power, high in the desire to compete, and so forth. It is reasonable to expect that such individuals will seek out situations congruent with their motives, or create situations that are congruent with their motives, e.g., set high standards for performance in accomplishment-oriented situations, turn an innocuous situation into a competitive one, and so forth. These situations in turn can be expected to be arousing, and thus these individuals are likely to experience more frequent, more intense, and/or more prolonged episodes of reactivity than other individuals. Such an analysis has been applied to Type As (Dembroski, MacDougall, Eliot, & Buell, 1983; Houston, 1981; Smith & Anderson, 1986; Smith & Rhodewalt, 1986). Moreover, there may be dimensions that are not particularly related to reactivity, but may be related to exposure to arousing situations and therefore may be of interest in the study of personality dimensions that relate to CVD. High sensation seeking, i.e., individuals who seek varied, stimulating experiences, may warrant attention in future studies of CVD (Zuckerman, 1978).

Personality Dimensions Associated with CVD Risk versus Resistance

Most of the personality dimensions reviewed above have been found to be, or are hypothesized to be, associated with reactivity and/or CVD, and to this extent are potential risk factors for CVD. Viewed in this manner, individuals who are low on these dimensions, e.g., low hostility, non Type A (i.e., Type B), and so forth, can be regarded as being relatively resistant to CVD.

However, there are at least two reasons for trying to identify personality dimensions that are something other than the converse of personality dimensions that are risk factors for CVD. One is that there may be dimensions the positive end of which may be associated with CVD risk, but the low end may be associated with average rather than low risk. In other words, there may be personality dimensions the ends of which are not anchored by high risk and high resistance. Such a possibility reinforces the desirability of identifying

personality dimensions specifically associated with low risk or high resistance. A second reason for trying to identify personality dimensions that are something other than the converse of dimensions associated with risk is that it accentuates the positive and may provide a positive model or positive instance of what people can be encouraged to strive for in contrast to merely encouraging people to avoid that which is negative or confers risk.

The notion of hardiness (Kobasa, 1982) that involves elements of control, commitment, and challenge certainly accentuates the positive. Unfortunately, hardiness is indexed by low scores on measures of negative attributes, viz., alienation from work and self, powerlessness, external locus of control, and so forth. Moreover, it is not clear that these scales are reasonable measures of the constructs intended. For example, conceptually the converse of alienation is a feeling of unity rather than a feeling of commitment. Perhaps measures of stress resilience or resistance will be developed that assess something other than the converse of negative attributes and which also will be related to resistance to CVD.

References

Anderson, N. B., Williams, R. B., Jr., Lane, J. D., & Monou, H. (1984). The relationship between hostility and cardiovascular responsivity following a mild harassment intervention. *Psychophysiology, 21,* 568 (Abstract).

Asendorpf, J. B., & Scherer, K. R. (1983). The discrepant repressor: Differentiation between low anxiety, high anxiety, and repression of anxiety by autonomic-facial-verbal patterns of behavior. *Journal of Personality and Social Psychology, 45,* 1334–1346.

Bakker, C. B. (1967). Psychological factors in angina pectoris. *Psychosomatics, 8,* 43–49.

Bergman, L. R., & Magnusson, D. (1979). Overachievement and catecholamine output in an achievement situation. *Psychosomatic Medicine, 51,* 181–188.

Blumenthal, J. A., Lane, J. D., & Williams, R. B., Jr. (1985). The inhibited power motive, Type A behavior, and patterns of cardiovascular response during the structured interview and Thematic Apperception Test. *Journal of Human Stress, 11*(2), 89–92.

Blumenthal, J. A., Lane, J. D., Williams, R. B., Jr., McKee, D. C., Haney, T., & White, A. (1983). Effects of task incentive on cardiovascular response in Type A and Type B individuals. *Psychophysiology, 20,* 63–70.

Bonami, M., & Rime, B. (1972). Approche exploratoire de la personalite pre-coronarienne par analyse standardisee de donnees projectives thematiques [Exploratory approaches to the precoronary personality through systematic analysis of themes of projective responses]. *Journal of Psychosomatic Research, 16,* 103–113.

Brozek, J., Keys, A., & Blackburn, H. (1966). Personality differences between potential coronary and noncoronary subjects. *Annals of the New York Academy of Sciences, 134,* 1057–1064.

Burger, J. M., & Cooper, H. M. (1979). The desirability of control. *Motivation and Emotion, 3,* 381–393.

Buss, A., & Plomin, R. (1975). *A temperament theory of personality.* New York: Wiley–Interscience.

Conley, J. J. (1984). Longitudinal consistency of adult personality: Self-reported psychological characteristics across 45 years. *Journal of Personality and Social Psychology, 47,* 1325–1333.

Contrada, R. J., Wright, R. A., & Glass, D. C. (1984). Task difficulty, Type A behavior pattern, and cardiovascular response. *Psychophysiology, 21,* 638–646.

Cook, W. W., & Medley, D. M. (1954). Proposed hostility and pharisaic-virtue scales for the MMPI. *Journal of Applied Psychology, 38,* 414–418.

Costa, P. T., Jr., & McCrae, R. R. (1985). Hypochondriasis, neuroticism, and aging. *American Psychologist, 40,* 19–28.

Costa, P. T., Jr., & McCrae, R. R. (1986). Personality stability and its implications for clinical psychology. *Clinical Psychology Review, 6,* 407–423.

DeGood, D. E. (1975). Cognitive control factors in vascular stress responses. *Psychophysiology, 12,* 399–401.

Dembroski, T. M. (1978). Reliability and validity of methods to assess coronary-prone behavior. In T. M. Dembroski, S. M. Weiss, J. L. Shields, S. G. Haynes, & M. Feinleib (Eds.), *Coronary-prone behavior* (pp. 95–106). Berlin: Springer-Verlag.

Dembroski, T. M., MacDougall, J. M., Eliot, R. S., & Buell, J. C. (1983). Stress, emotions, behavior, and cardiovascular disease. In L. Temoshok, C. Van Dyke, & L. S. Zegans (Eds.), *Emotions in health and illness: Theoretical and research foundations* (pp. 61–72). New York: Grune & Stratton.

Dembroski, T. M., MacDougall, J. M., Herd, J. A., & Shields, J. L. (1979). Effect of level of challenge on pressor and heart rate responses in Type A and B subjects. *Journal of Applied Social Psychology, 9,* 209–228.

Dembroski, T. M., MacDougall, J. M., & Musante, L. (1984). Desirability of control versus locus of control: Relationship to paralinguistics in the Type A interview. *Health Psychology, 3,* 15–26.

Dembroski, T. M., MacDougall, J. M., Shields, J. L., Petitto, J., & Lushene, R. (1978). Components of the Type A coronary-prone behavior pattern and cardiovascular responses to psychomotor performance challenge. *Journal of Behavioral Medicine, 1,* 159–175.

Ellis, A. (1962). *Reason and emotion in psychotherapy.* New York: Lyle Stuart.

Eysenck, H. J. (1967). *The biological bases of personality.* Springfield, IL: Thomas.

Eysenck, H. J., & Eysenck, S. B. G. (1964). *Manual of the Eysenck Personality Inventory.* London: University of London Press.

Flemenbaum, A., & Anderson, R. P. (1978). Field dependence and blood cholesterol: An expansion. *Perceptual and Motor Skills, 46,* 867–874.

Flemenbaum, A., & Flemenbaum, E. (1975). Field dependence, blood uric acid and cholesterol. *Perceptual and Motor Skills, 41,* 135–141.

Gastorf, J. W. (1982). Physiologic reaction of Type As to objective and subjective challenge. *Journal of Human Stress, 7*(1), 16–20.

Geen, R. G. (1984). Preferred stimulation levels in introverts and extraverts: Effects on arousal and performance. *Journal of Personality and Social Psychology, 46,* 1303–1312.

Gentry, W. D., Chesney, A. P., Gary, H. E., Jr., Hall, R. P., & Harburg, E. (1982). Habitual anger-coping styles. I. Effect on mean blood pressure and risk for essential hypertension. *Psychosomatic Medicine, 44,* 195–202.

Glass, D. C. (1977). *Behavior patterns, stress, and coronary disease.* Hillsdale, NJ: Erlbaum.

Glass, D. C., Krakoff, L. R., Contrada, R., Hilton, W. F., Kehoe, K., Mannucci, E. G., Collins, C., Snow, B., & Elting, E. (1980). Effect of harassment and competition upon cardiovascular and plasma catecholamine responses in Type A and Type B individuals. *Psychophysiology, 17,* 453–463.

Glass, D. C., Lake, C. R., Contrada, R. J., Kehoe, K., & Erlanger, L. R. (1983). Stability of individual differences in physiological responses to stress. *Health Psychology, 2,* 317–341.

Goodenough, D. R. (1978). Field dependence. In H. London & J. E. Exner, Jr. (Eds.), *Dimensions of personality* (pp. 165–216). New York: Wiley.

Haynes, S. G., Feinleib, M., & Kannel, W. B. (1980). The relationship of psychosocial factors to coronary heart disease in the Framingham Study. III. Eight-year incidence of coronary heart disease. *American Journal of Epidemiology, 111,* 37–58.

Haynes, S. G., Levine, S., Scotch, N., Feinleib, M., & Kannel, W. B. (1978). The relationship of psychosocial factors to coronary heart disease in the Framingham Study. I. Methods and risk factors. *American Journal of Epidemiology, 107,* 362–383.

Henry, J. P., & Meehan, J. P. (1981). Psychosocial stimuli, physiological specificity, and cardiovascular disease. In H. Weiner, M. A. Hofer, & A. J. Stunkard (Eds.), *Brain, behavior, and bodily disease* (pp. 305–333). New York: Raven Press.

Herd, J. A. (1983). Physiological basis for behavioral influences in atherosclerosis. In T. M. Dembroski, T. H. Schmidt, & G. Blumchen (Eds.), *Biobehavioral bases of coronary heart disease* (pp. 248–256). Basel: Karger.

Hodges, W. F. (1968). Effects of ego threat and threat of pain on state anxiety. *Journal of Personality and Social Psychology, 8,* 364–378.

Holmes, D. S., McGilley, B. M., & Houston, B. K. (1984). Task-related arousal of Type A and Type B persons: level of challenge and response specificity. *Journal of Personality and Social Psychology, 46,* 1322–1327.

Holmes, D. S., & Will, M. J. (1985). Expression of interpersonal aggression by angered and nonangered persons with the Type A and Type B behavior patterns. *Journal of Personality and Social Psychology, 48,* 723–727.

Holroyd, K. A., & Gorkin, L. (1983). Young adults at risk for hypertension: Effects of family history and anger management in determining responses to interpersonal conflict. *Journal of Psychosomatic Research, 27,* 131–138.

Holroyd, K. A., Westbrook, T., Wolf, M., & Badhorn, E. (1978). Performance, cognition, and physiological responding in test anxiety. *Journal of Abnormal Psychology, 87,* 442–451.

Houston, B. K. (1972). Control over stress, locus of control, and response to stress. *Journal of Personality and Social Psychology, 21,* 249–255.

Houston, B. K. (1973). Viability of coping strategies, denial, and response to stress. *Journal of Personality, 41,* 50–58.

Houston, B. K. (1977). Dispositional anxiety and the effectiveness of cognitive coping strategies in stressful laboratory and classroom situations. In C. D. Spielberger & I. G. Sarason (Eds.), *Stress and anxiety* (Vol. 4, pp. 205–226). Washington, DC: Hemisphere.

Houston, B. K. (1981, May). *What links the Type A behavior pattern and coronary heart disease?* Invited paper presented at the meeting of the Midwestern Psychological Association, Detroit.

Houston, B. K. (1987). Stress and coping. In C. R. Snyder & C. E. Ford (Eds.), *Coping with negative life events: Clinical and social psychological perspectives* (pp. 373–399). New York: Plenum Press.

Houston, B. K. (1988). Cardiovascular and neuroendocrine reactivity, global Type A, and components of Type A behavior. In B. K. Houston & C. R. Snyder (Eds.), *Type A behavior pattern: Research, theory, and intervention* (pp. 212–253). New York: Wiley.

Izard, C. E. (1977). *Human emotions.* New York: Plenum Press.

Jenkins, C. D. (1976). Recent evidence supporting psychologic and social risk factors for coronary disease. *New England Journal of Medicine, 294,* 987–994, 1033–1038.

Jenkins, C. D., Rosenman, R. H., & Zyzanski, S. J. (1974). Prediction of clinical coronary heart disease by a test for the coronary-prone behavior pattern. *New England Journal of Medicine, 290,* 1271–1275.

Jorgensen, R. S., & Houston, B. K. (1981). The Type A behavior pattern, sex differences, and cardiovascular response to and recovery from stress. *Motivation and Emotion, 5,* 201–214.

Jorgensen, R. S., & Houston, B. K. (1986). Family history of hypertension, personality patterns, and cardiovascular reactivity to stress. *Psychosomatic Medicine, 48,* 102–117.

Kaplan, J. R., Manuck, S. B., Clarkson, T. B., Lusso, F. M., & Taub, D. M. (1982). Social status, environment, and atherosclerosis in *Cynomolgus* monkeys. *Arteriosclerosis, 2,* 359–368.

Kaufmann, H. (1970). *Aggression and altruism.* New York: Holt, Rinehart, & Winston.

Knight, M. L., & Borden, R. J. (1979). Autonomic and affective reactions of high and low socially-anxious individuals awaiting public performance. *Psychophysiology, 16,* 209–213.

Kobasa, S. C. (1982). The hardy personality: Toward a social psychology of stress and health. In G. S. Sanders & J. Suls (Eds.), *Social psychology of health and illness* (pp. 3–32). Hillsdale, NJ: Erlbaum.

Krantz, D. S., Glass, D. C., & Snyder, M. L. (1974). Helplessness, stress level, and the coronary-prone behavior pattern. *Journal of Experimental Social Psychology, 10,* 284–300.

Krantz, D. S., Manuck, S. B., & Wing, R. R. (1986). Psychological stressors and task variables as elicitors of reactivity. In K. A. Matthews, S. M. Weiss, T. Detre, T. M. Dembroski, B. Falkner, S. B. Manuck, & R. B. Williams, Jr. (Eds.), *Handbook of stress, reactivity, and cardiovascular disease* (pp. 85–107). New York: Wiley.

Lake, B., Suarez, E. C., Schneiderman, N., & Tocci, N. (1985). The Type A behavior pattern, physical fitness, and psychophysiological reactivity. *Health Psychology, 4,* 169–187.

Lane, J. D., White, A. D., & Williams, R. B., Jr. (1984). Cardiovascular effects of mental arithmetic in Type A and Type B females. *Psychophysiology, 21,* 39–46.

Larsen, R. J., Diener, E., & Emmons, R. A. (1986). Affect intensity and reactions to daily life events. *Journal of Personality and Social Psychology, 51,* 803–814.

Lawler, K. A., Rixse, A., & Allen, M. T. (1983). Type A behavior and psychophysiological responses in adult women. *Psychophysiology, 20,* 343–350.

Lawler, K. A., & Schmied, L. A. (1986). Cardiovascular responsivity, Type A behavior, and parental history of heart disease in young women. *Psychophysiology, 23,* 28–32.

Lawler, K. A., Schmied, L., Mitchell, V. P., & Rixse, A. (1984). Type A behavior and physiological responsivity in young women. *Journal of Psychosomatic Research, 28,* 197–204.

Lazarus, R. S. (1966). *Psychological stress and the coping process.* New York: McGraw-Hill.

Lazarus, R. S. (1984). On the primacy of cognition. *American Psychologist, 39,* 124–129.

Lazarus, R. S., & Folkman, S. (1984). *Stress, appraisal, and coping.* Berlin: Springer.

Lebovits, B. Z., Shekelle, R. B., & Ostfeld, A. M. (1967). Prospective and retrospective studies of CHD. *Psychosomatic Medicine, 29,* 265–272.

MacDougall, J. M., Dembroski, T. M., & Krantz, D. S. (1981). Effects of types of challenge on pressor and heart rate response in Type A and B women. *Psychophysiology, 18,* 1–9.

Malouff, J. M., & Schutte, N. S. (1986). Development and validation of a measure of irrational belief. *Journal of Consulting and Clinical Psychology, 54,* 860–862.

Manuck, S. B., Craft, S., & Gold, K. J. (1978). Coronary-prone behavior pattern and cardiovascular response. *Psychophysiology, 15,* 403–411.

Manuck, S. B., & Garland, F. N. (1979). Coronary-prone behavior pattern, task incentive, and cardiovascular response. *Psychophysiology, 16,* 136–142.

Manuck, S. B., & Garland, F. N. (1980). Stability in individual differences in cardiovascular reactivity: A thirteen-month follow-up. *Physiology and Behavior, 21,* 621–624.

Manuck, S. B., Kaplan, J. R., & Clarkson, T. B. (1983). Behaviorally induced heart rate reactivity and atherosclerosis in *Cynomolgous* monkeys. *Psychosomatic Medicine, 45,* 95–108.

Matthews, K. A. (1982). Psychological perspectives on the Type A behavior pattern. *Psychological Bulletin, 91,* 292–323.

Matthews, K. A. (1985). Assessment of Type A behavior, anger, and hostility in epidemiological studies of cardiovascular disease. In A. M. Ostfeld & E. D. Eaker (Eds.), *Measuring psychosocial variables in epidemiological studies of cardiovascular disease: Proceedings of a workshop* (NIH Publication No. 85-2770, pp. 153–183). U.S. Department of Health and Human Services.

Matthews, K. A., Glass, D. C., Rosenman, R. H., & Bortner, R. W. (1977). Competitive drive, pattern A, and coronary heart disease: A further analysis of some data from the Western Collaborative Group Study. *Journal of Chronic Diseases, 30,* 489–498.

Matthews, K. A., & Haynes, S. G. (1986). Type A behavior pattern and coronary risk, update and critical evaluation. *American Journal of Epidemiology, 123,* 923–960.

Mayes, B. T., Sime, W. E., & Ganster, D. C. (1984). Convergent validity of Type A behavior pattern scales and their ability to predict physiological responsiveness in a sample of female public employees. *Journal of Behavioral Medicine, 7,* 83–108.

McClelland, D. C. (1979). Inhibited power motivation and high blood pressure in men. *Journal of Abnormal Psychology, 88,* 182–190.

McCranie, E. W., Simpson, M. E., & Stevens, J. S. (1981). Type A behavior, field dependence, and serum lipids. *Psychosomatic Medicine, 43,* 107–116.

Miller, S. M. (1979). Coping with impending stress: Psychophysiological and cognitive correlates of choice. *Psychophysiology, 16,* 572–581.

Miller, S. M. (1987). Monitoring and blunting: Validation of a questionnaire to assess styles of information-seeking under threat. *Journal of Personality and Social Psychology, 52,* 345–353.

Novaco, R. W. (1975). *Anger control: The development of an experimental treatment.* Lexington: Lexington Books.

Pittner, M. S., Houston, B. K., & Spiridigliozzi, G. (1983). Control over stress, Type A behavior pattern, and response to stress. *Journal of Personality and Social Psychology, 44,* 627–637.

Powell, L. H., & Thoresen, C. E. (1985). Behavioral and physiological determinants of long-term prognosis after myocardial infarction. *Journal of Chronic Diseases, 38,* 253–263.

Rosenman, R. H. (1978). The interview method of assessment of the coronary-prone behavior pattern. In T. M. Dembroski, S. M. Weiss, J. L. Shields, S. G. Haynes, & M. Feinleib (Eds.), *Coronary-prone behavior* (pp. 55–69). Berlin: Springer-Verlag.

Rotter, J. (1966). Generalized expectancies for internal versus external control of reinforcement. *Psychological Monographs, 80*(1, Whole No. 609).

Scheier, M. F., & Carver, C. S. (1985). Optimism, coping, and health: Assessment and implications of generalized outcome expectancies. *Health Psychology, 4,* 219–247.

Scheier, M. F., & Carver, C. S. (1987). Dispositional optimism and physical well-being: The influence of generalized outcome expectancies on health. *Journal of Personality, 55,* 169–210.

Schwartz, G. E., Weinberger, D., & Singer, J. A. (1981). Cardiovascular differentiation of happiness, sadness, anger, and fear following imagery and exercise. *Psychosomatic Medicine, 43,* 343–364.

Siegel, J. M. (1985). The measurement of anger as a multidimensional construct. In M. A. Chesney & R. H. Rosenman (Eds.), *Anger and hostility in cardiovascular and behavioral disorders* (pp. 59–82). Washington, DC: Hemisphere.

Smith, M. A., & Houston, B. K. (1987). Hostility, anger expression, cardiovascular responsivity, and social support. *Biological Psychology, 24,* 39–48.

Smith, T. W., & Anderson, N. B. (1986). Models of personality and disease: An interactional approach to Type A behavior and cardiovascular risk. *Journal of Personality and Social Psychology, 50,* 1163–1173.

Smith, T. W., & Frohm, K. D. (1985). What's so unhealthy about hostility? Construct validity and psychosocial correlates of the Cook–Medley Ho scale. *Health Psychology, 4,* 503–520.

Smith, T. W., Houston, B. K., & Zurawski, R. M. (1984). Irrational beliefs and the arousal of emotional distress. *Journal of Counseling Psychology, 31,* 190–201.

Smith, T. W., Houston, B. K., & Zurawski, R. M. (1985). The Framingham Type A Scale: Cardiovascular and cognitive–behavioral responses to interpersonal challenge. *Motivation and Emotion, 9,* 123–134.

Smith, T. W., & Rhodewalt, F. (1986). On states, traits, and processes: A transactional alternative to the individual difference assumptions in Type A behavior and physiological reactivity. *Journal of Research in Personality, 20,* 229–251.

Smyth, K., Call, J., Hansell, S., Sparacino, J., & Strodtbeck, F. L. (1978). Type A behavior pattern and hypertension among inner-city black women. *Nursing Research, 27,* 30–35.

Spielberger, C. D., Jacobs, G. A., Russell, S., & Crane, R. S. (1983). Assessment of anger: The state–trait anger scale. In J. N. Butcher & C. D. Spielberger (Eds.), *Advances in personality assessment* (Vol. 2, pp. 159–187). Hillsdale, NJ: Erlbaum.

Thurstone, L. L. (1949). *Thurstone Temperament Schedule.* Chicago: Science Research Associates.

Ward, M. M., Chesney, M. A., Swan, G. E., Black, G. W., Parker, S. D., & Rosenman, R. H. (1986). Cardiovascular responses of Type A and Type B men to a series of stressors. *Journal of Behavioral Medicine, 9,* 43–49.

Weinberger, D. A., Schwartz, G. E., & Davidson, R. J. (1979). Low-anxious, high-anxious, and repressive coping styles: Psychometric patterns and behavioral and physiological responses to stress. *Journal of Abnormal Psychology, 88,* 369–380.

Williams, R. B., Jr. (1985). Neuroendocrine response patterns and stress: Biobehavioral mechanisms of disease. In R. B. Williams, Jr. (Ed.), *Perspectives on behavioral medicine: Vol. 2. Neuroendocrine control and behavior* (pp. 71–101). New York: Academic Press.

Wright, R. A., Contrada, R. J., & Glass, D. C. (1985). Psychophysiologic correlates of Type A behavior. In E. S. Katkin & S. M. Manuck (Eds.), *Advances in behavioral medicine.* Greenwich, CT: Jai Press.

Zajonc, R. B. (1984). On the primacy of affect. *American Psychologist, 39,* 117–123.

Zuckerman, M. (1978). Sensation seeking. In H. London & J. E. Exner, Jr. (Eds.), *Dimensions of personality* (pp. 487–559). New York: Wiley.

Zurawski, R. M., & Houston, B. K. (1983). The Jenkins Activity Survey measure of Type A and frustration-induced anger. *Motivation and Emotion, 7,* 301–312.

CHAPTER 32

Stress and Social Support
Assessment Issues

Scott M. Monroe

Over the past several decades, there has been increasing interest in the concept of stress as a contributing factor to the development of physical and psychological disorders. In the context of incomplete explanations for numerous forms of disease, stress has assumed respect as a potentially important, widely applicable, explanatory construct. Consequently, many disciplines, and different laboratories within disciplines, study varied species and diverse disorders, all under this one common rubric. Stress appears to be an integrative concept, contributing to the progressive merging of biologic processes into eventual endpoints of pathology.

The simplicity, potency, and breadth of stress effects are a direct outgrowth of the early formulations of the idea (Cannon, 1932; Selye, 1976). Yet, as thinking and research on the topic progressed, unitary concepts fell to progressively more differentiated perspectives. The consequences of stress vary as a function of intensity, duration, or form of the particular stressor involved (Depue & Monroe, 1986; Depue, Monroe, & Shackman, 1979; Hinkle, 1977; Mason, 1975). As one would expect given the many resulting conceptualizations of stress, different measurement approaches proliferated, with considerable variability in quality.

The diversity of approaches to measuring stress becomes even more apparent when research on different disorders is considered. For instance, stress factors contributing to psychopathology may be very different from those contributing to physical diseases (Monroe, 1982b). Within psychopathologic disturbances, different types of stress have been found to predict different forms of disturbance (Monroe & Peterman, 1988). Such information suggests that, at least initially, modeling of stress effects should be relatively disorder specific (Depue *et al.*, 1979; Depue & Monroe, 1986; Hinkle, 1977). Furthermore, thinking on stress has been based upon disorders with relatively acute changes from baseline functioning—acute onset or episodic forms of disturbance. When the endpoint of interest involves more protracted developmental periods, or has multiple manifestations over time, the conceptualization of stress and its effects must be expanded. With specific reference to coronary heart disease (CHD), phenomena of interest include risk factors (e.g., hypertension, cholesterol levels, smoking), particular disease processes /endpoints (atherosclerosis, myocardial infarction, angina pectoris, stroke), and clinical course of the disease once known degrees of severity are attained (e.g., reinfarction, poststroke recovery). All of these aspects of the disease progression develop

Scott M. Monroe • Department of Psychology, University of Pittsburgh, Pittsburgh, Pennsylvania 15260.

over lengthy time periods, during which a variety of stress experiences (acute, chronic, or intermittent) could be related to their formation and/or expression.

Finally, in addition to the hypothesized direct contribution of stress to pathology, recent research has pointed to the importance of a variety of factors that may modify stress and/or its hypothesized impact. This has come about due to the appreciation of large individual differences in the response to stress: most individuals, even under severely stressful conditions, do not break down. The inclusion of these moderating variables in research may help to more fully explain the development and maintenance of disease. Particularly influential in current thinking on stress has been the research on social support (Cohen & Syme, 1985; Sarason & Sarason, 1985).

Given the foregoing considerations, where is one to begin in the measurement of stress and its modifiers? Since there is no "gold standard" against which to evaluate the existing procedures, it is necessary to be aware of many background considerations that place these assessment procedures within a broader perspective on multifactorial models of disease (Depue *et al.,* 1979). First, then, it is essential to have a firm grounding in the ideas behind the prevailing assessment methods. Accordingly, in the first section of this chapter the relevant conceptual and definitional issues will be discussed. The goal will be not only to convey what these terms are meant to represent, but also what they are *not* meant to represent. Second, both stress and social support measures are correlated with a wide variety of other psychosocial factors (as well as being possible consequences of disorder). If causal relationships are to be entertained, other predictors must be specified and studied in relation to stress, support, and disorder (Monroe & Steiner, 1986). This is a challenging yet extremely important task. In this section, then, pertinent design and statistical considerations for disentangling the effects of stress, support, and other psychosocial variables also will be covered.

The most salient assessment considerations, along with their implications for the particular measurement approaches adopted, will be covered in the second major section. This entails a brief

overview of the prerequisites that should be met by any assessment approach. Finally, the existing empirical literature on life stress and social support provides the core reference point of the review. This constitutes the third section of the chapter. Probably the majority of investigations on stress and social support have focused upon psychopathologic outcomes; we therefore will draw heavily from this area of study. However, especially given the premise of stressor–disorder specificity, the literature on stress and CHD is most relevant. When possible, we will attempt to include examples from the latter literature to provide conceptual and procedural bases for future inquiry.

Definitional and Conceptual Issues

Despite uniformity of opinion that "stress" and "social support" contribute in the development of pathology, there is little consensus on basic definitions for either term. In the absence of overall definitional clarity, though, there exist several perspectives that provide their own definitions. Since measures must follow from prevailing definitions and concepts, it is to a brief evaluation of the latter that we turn with respect to stress first, and then social support.

The review of current concepts will highlight the degree to which stress and social support are a fundamental part of the fabric of daily life. As such, they are difficult—if not impossible—to extract cleanly and measure in isolation from other features of the individual and the social environment. From a scientific perspective, this places considerable weight upon the research design and the control procedures for disentangling the many correlated variables potentially involved. Therefore, in the final portion of this section, these important concerns will be addressed.

Stress: Dimensions and Dynamics

Historically, stress has been viewed from a stimulus perspective (i.e., an objectively defined environmental demand, such as bereavement), a response perspective (i.e., changes in particular response domains, such as endocrine measures or psychological symptoms), and, more recently, from a transactional perspective (i.e., the interaction between environmental demands and individual responses as they develop over time) (Lazarus & Folkman, 1984; Mason, 1975). These viewpoints share a common basis in that stress represents some form of imbalance between the demands imposed upon an individual and the resources available to accommodate. Note, however, that such formulations are very general; "demands" or "stress" represent abstract summary concepts for a variety of specific circumstances (e.g., different forms of physical exertion, various dimensions of emotional distress, and so on). Although potentially powerful in an integrative sense, such generality also has possible limitations. At the extreme, almost any experience can be viewed as stressful. Greater specification of the particular aspects associated with the psychosocial conditions, particularly *before* tests of associations with disorder are undertaken, would help to avoid spurious findings.

At least in terms of research on the psychosocial antecedents of psychopathology, some progress has been made in clarifying the characteristics of the stressors involved. In contrast to the original idea that all environmental demands reflecting *either* desirable or undesirable requirements for readjustment may precipitate disorder (Holmes & Rahe, 1967), it is now generally accepted that adverse life experiences—perhaps especially those possessing attributes portending a protracted adverse impact—are most influential, at least for psychopathologic outcomes (Monroe & Peterman, 1988). Whether or not such characteristics are equally predictive for other forms of pathology (e.g., CHD) remains to be demonstrated.

Another important advance in definition and theory of stress over the past several years has been in the recognition of the temporal dynamics: the interplay over time between stress and the individual's adaptive (or maladaptive) responses. Rather than viewing stress in static terms, the unfolding interactions have become the target of assessment. This is illustrated in part by the identification of four broad types of stressors, differing primarily in their temporal characteristics: (1) acute, time-limited stressors (e.g., awaiting surgery, interviewing for an important job); (2) stressor sequences (e.g., a series of events that occur over time as a result of a major initiating event, such as job loss or marital separation; (3) chronic intermittent stressors (e.g., relatively time-limited events that happen with some degree of regularity over time, such as conflicted relations with an in-law that emerge during family gatherings); and (4) chronic stressors (e.g., ongoing difficulties that, although they may fluctuate in intensity, maintain an elevated degree of stress, such as ongoing marital conflict or permanent disabilities) (Elliot & Eisdorfer, 1982).

In summary, important developments in life stress theory concern the viewpoints on stress (stimulus, response, transaction perspectives), specific types of stressors individuals face, and the temporal aspects of stressful experiences.

Social Support: Networks and Functions

Initial ideas concerning social support came from findings from diverse literatures that socially integrated individuals faired better along a variety of psychologic and physical dimensions than individuals who were less well integrated. While the potential implications of social involvement had been highlighted in a general sense by others previously (Durkheim, 1951; House & Kahn, 1985), ideas concerning the various processes involved, along with approaches to measurement of the more specific components, only became prominent in the 1970s.

Historically, two perspectives on this topic may be discerned: the structural and the functional. The structural perspective focuses upon the existence and interconnections between individuals and their social ties—a mapping of the network of affiliations—and involves a variety of component dimensions (e.g., number of ties, interrelations between network members, homogeneity of network members). This is usually referred to as the study of social networks. The functional perspective concerns the *content* of the social ties—the actual provisions of social support and the processes involved. Specifically, what are the resources that are available to the individual and how are they accessed (particularly with respect to the potential for dealing with stress)? Again, a number of component dimensions have been discussed, including appraisal, emotional, and tangible support (Cohen & McKay, 1984).

The theme of specificity discussed previously now can be taken one step further, with the form of stressor being matched to the type of support provided, within the framework of studying particular disorders. For example, the negative psychologic effects of occupational stressors may be buffered most adequately through support provided by work affiliates (as opposed to family or friend support; Cohen & Wills, 1985; House & Kahn, 1985; Lieberman, 1986).

In summary, the two most important points concerning the concepts and definitions of social support concern the structural–functional perspectives (i.e., social networks versus social support), and, within the latter, the specificity of matching support functions with particular stress requirements.

Design Considerations and Control Procedures

A major point, but one that is consistently ignored, is that variability in stress and social support may be possible causes, concomitants, *and* consequences of disorder (Monroe & Steiner, 1986). This broadening of perspective opens up a host of very important considerations involving cause-and-effect issues. For example, the clinically depressed individual may create many stressful circumstances due to the disorder (e.g., work problems, marital problems, alienation of supportive ties); associations with disorder can represent clear artifact in such circumstances, owing to a reverse association between the two variables. These points appear to have equally compelling counterparts for the study of CHD, for aspects of the disease may influence stress levels (e.g., changes in life-style or work) or support (e.g., changes in relationships).

Perhaps even more important are other characteristics of the individual that could account for variability in *both* stress and social support, such as personality factors (Heller, 1979). For example, Type A individuals may create certain stressors (e.g., work stress); under such hypothetical conditions, stress could be artifactually related to subsequent CHD (Brown, 1974). Other personality features, and their influence upon stress or support in relation to CHD, can be easily envisioned. For example, hostility has been shown to be related to CHD (Dembroski & Williams, this volume); such a personality characteristic could contribute to a small support network, a lack of social support, and an increased level of stress (e.g., interpersonal conflicts).

Several strategies may be useful for disentangling these variables in relation to pathology. It should be emphasized, though, that this is one of the most delicate and demanding tasks facing the interested investigator. The suggestions that follow provide only general guidelines. First, and perhaps most important, is the use of prospective research designs. This means that the psychosocial variables are assessed initially and are used to predict *subsequent* development of disease. It is also necessary with these procedures to select individuals who are initially symptom-free (or individuals equated with respect to existing disease considerations or risk factors; e.g., MI survivors, smokers). This approach helps to eliminate the problem of reverse causation—the disease bringing about changes in the psychosocial factors. However, it does not by itself eliminate the possibility of other factors accounting for the associations (e.g., a hostile personality "creates" both heightened stress and decreased social support).

Since stress and social support have a variety of determinants, the most obvious and salient factors should be incorporated to clarify the meaning of the stress or support assessment (e.g., Type A behavior pattern, hostility). Control procedures are required to shed light upon whether or not the stress (or support) variables are (1) simply proxies for the underlying personality dimensions; (2) represent mechanisms via which the personality factor operates; or (3) are additional, independent contributors. Procedures for making such determinations include stratification procedures (e.g., studying the associations of stress and support at different levels of the personality factor), statistical controls (e.g., controlling for personality influence in multiple regression analyses; testing personality and stress or support interactions), or more sophisticated causal modeling procedures (Cook & Campbell, 1979; Kenny, 1979).

In summary, stress and social support represent

concepts that cannot be excised neatly from the personal and social contexts in which they arise, nor measured in an entirely discrete manner. Broader models, including the most relevant correlated parameters, are required to understand how stress and support operate within the context of the individual's life. Explicit design and data analytic techniques are required to clarify how the different variables fit into the causal picture.

Assessment Considerations

When undertaking any assessment, a number of basic considerations should be considered. One concern pertains to the psychometric qualifications of the assessment procedure. Although not unique to the study of stress or social support, this issue has been neglected with such frequency that it bears repetition. A second concern involves the information base on which stress or social support assessments are performed. In other words, who determines what qualifies as stress or social support?

Psychometric Considerations

Any assessment of stress or social support should provide information on the reliability and validity of the measure. Unfortunately, much of the research in the literature is based upon post hoc grouping of items loosely assembled to reflect the constructs. In surprisingly few of these investigations has there been any bother with psychometric prerequisites of the measures; instead, it is simply assumed that they perform their tasks consistently and with some true bearing upon the underlying concepts addressed.

Test–retest reliability (ensuring that the assessment provides the same measurement for the same time period on two separate occasions) is perhaps the most basic form of reliability. Care should be taken to ensure that the assessments cover the *same* time period (e.g., since stress and support vary over time, the reliability should reflect stability of the measure, not the construct). Internal consistency reliability, wherein the cohesion of the items in a scale is tested (i.e., how well all of the items correlate with each other, and represent a reliable

index of an underlying construct), is another form of reliability that may be necessary to include. It is important to note with this form of reliability that it is only required with particular conceptualizations of stress. For instance, in scales that purport to measure stress as a unidimensional construct (e.g., particularly response or interaction stress measures, such as perceived stress), internal consistency is a relevant consideration. However, some stress measures, particularly those that are stimulus-oriented, do not rely on the same assumption that the items should be reflections of underlying stress; rather, the items separately contribute to and essentially create the overall stress. For instance, life events reported on life event checklists should not correlate with one another across individuals (they should not necessarily show high internal consistency), yet when many events happen to a person, it is assumed that they combine to form stress.

Finally, it would be useful to demonstrate correlations between the measure of stress and other measures of the same construct, or other consequences of the construct, to provide an index of validity. Unfortunately, all too many assessment procedures appear to rely upon "face validity" (wherein item content appears appropriate for the construct assumed to be measured). As emphasized throughout this chapter, such optimism is unwarranted, for stress and support can be so broadly conceived as to connect virtually any array of disparate psychosocial conditions. A more precise theoretical and definitional approach, along with requisite psychometric evidence, is necessary.

Subjective and Objective Assessments: Implications and Caveats

Crucial to any assessment of stress or social support is the information base upon which measurement proceeds. Two general perspectives on this issue can be discerned. One—by far the most prevalent—is the subjective perspective. Most commonly, this involves the individual's self-report of perceptions of stress or support. Theoretically, this is justified (particularly for response or interactional stress models), for it seems reasonable to assume that the subject is "closest" to the information of importance and therefore the most appropriate informant. Practically, as well, it may be that the information of concern is not available via objective methods, but only via subjective ones (e.g., the subject's perception of the adequacy of support). However, although the information gathered is structured by the investigator through the wording and selection of particular questions, there can be large discrepancies between the investigator's intended meaning for a particular item and that inferred by the subject.

When the meaning attributed to items by the subject differs from the intended meaning of the investigator, the resulting assessment can reflect either idiosyncratic or systematic errors. Idiosyncratic errors are those that occur due to the unusual meanings attached to items by the individual. For example, one widely used form of stress assessment is the life event checklist (to be described more fully below). Owing to the brevity of description of each item, interpretations by the particular subject can vary considerably. For instance, for the event "serious illness in close family member," "serious" and "close family member" can be interpreted very loosely, ranging from a sister's bad cold to a husband's heart attack. Such misunderstanding between investigator and subject creates error variance and misclassification of individuals into high- and low-stress categories.

Perhaps more pernicious, however, are the systematic errors that can arise. In this circumstance, there are consistent biases in the subject's interpretation that influence the assessment and create spurious associations. For instance, individuals who suffered an MI may be more inclined to report heightened prior stress than healthy controls, in an attempt to "explain away" the episode by attributing it to stress. In this case, knowledge of the disorder can bias the subject to report increased stress (e.g., search harder in their memory to remember stressful events, or imbue existing events with higher stress qualities; Brown, 1974). Alternatively, subjective ratings may be in part determined by personality features, which may be related primarily to the disorder under study. (Here, once again, is further reason to follow the guidelines provided in the previous section, "Design Considerations and Control Procedures.")

Objective assessments attempt to keep the respondent's interpretation of the meaning of any item close to that intended by the developer of the item. In one approach, referred to as "investigator-based" procedures by Brown (1981), the developer structures the questioning and criteria such that variability (systematic or unsystematic) attributable to the subject's misinterpretation is minimized. For instance, again using the "serious illness in close family member" example, only certain relatives (e.g., first degree) or illnesses (e.g., life threatening and verified by a physician) are defined as meeting the criteria. Under such assessment conditions, there is a greater certainty that specific scores represent a standardized measure of stress that is replicable across different investigators and subjects. (This assessment approach will be described in greater detail below, under "Structured Interview" stress assessments.)

Summary and Conclusions

The issues raised in this section provide a framework within which the meaning of stress and social support assessments may be interpreted. Formal psychometric requirements, along with more subtle methodologic issues on the information base for deriving stress measures, reveal a variety of important considerations for the assessment of stress and social support. While there are many measures that will be reviewed for assessing stress and social moderators of stress next, the meaning of such approaches should not be elevated beyond the sophistication of the specific methods for assessing the construct and the procedures for controlling confounding factors.

The Assessment of Stress: Current Practices

We have established the foundation for reviewing existing procedures. Obviously, in light of the lack of a gold standard, no approach will escape criticism. The following overview is intended to provide a balanced perspective on the advantages and disadvantages of the various methods currently in use.

Most frequently, measures of stress do not distinguish between acute and chronic stress, let alone stressor sequences and intermittent stressors, although item composition suggests that all of these are tapped by different instruments to varying degrees. Yet, the bias has been toward interpreting virtually all assessment methods as measures of acute stress. Consequently, for convenience all types of stressors are dealt with in the next section in relation to the particular assessment procedures evaluated. Distinctions pertaining to the types of stress assessed will be discussed for specific procedures when relevant.

A range of approaches has been used to operationalize stress. These fall roughly within four classes: (1) single or multiple item indicators; (2) life event inventories; (3) perceived stress scales; and (4) structured interviews.

Single or Multiple Item Indicators

Many investigations have found single items, or a few items that at face value appear to tap aspects of stress, to be related to various forms of disorder. These assessments are distinguished from the other categories owing to (1) the small number of items included, and/or (2) the lack of an *a priori* rationale for the particular constellation of items. These forms of assessment, owing to their diversity, cannot be readily categorized into the "stimulus," "response," or "interactional" categories.

Two potential problems can develop from this form of measurement. The first involves the wedding of statistical artifact and post hoc reasoning. Put differently, in any study with many variables, some of the items will be significantly associated with the dependent variable owing to chance alone. As discussed previously, the breadth of the stress concept can accommodate a variety of disparate experiences under its heading, creating the temptation to include one or more variables that could be spurious correlates under one common descriptive theme.

Second, the association between the stress index and outcome variable may indeed be valid, yet the use of "stress" as an explanation can obscure rather than clarify the picture. For instance, "education" has been found to be associated with re-

currence of MI (Ruberman, Weinblatt, Goldberg, & Chaudhary, 1983); the assumed stress of life that can follow from such circumstances has been provided as an explanation (Jenkins, 1978). Yet there are many more specific correlates of education that could be responsible for the relationship (e.g., economic disadvantage, poor work conditions, access to medical resources, life-style characteristics, psychopathology). Again, such components may be united within the construct of stress, but with a potential loss of specificity and detail. Without a more precise approach to what is meant by the term, the generality of its use can trivialize its importance. What is required is a more detailed statement about what it is about the correlate and its specific implications for stress that may translate eventually into pathology.

Several instances of this approach to measuring and defining stress exist (e.g., Medalie & Goldbourt, 1976; Theorell, Lind, & Floderus, 1975). An interesting and important example, portraying both the advantages and potential disadvantages, is a recent study by Ruberman, Weinblatt, Goldberg, and Chaudhary (1984). As noted above, these investigators reported in an initial study that education was related to CHD; commendably, a follow-up investigation was undertaken to determine if stress and social support were responsible for the initial finding. In a subsequent prospective study, they found that high life stress was related to 3-year mortality risk (both total deaths and sudden cardiac death) for men following an initial MI. Importantly, this association was found to hold even when other variables (e.g., demographic and biologic) were accounted for statistically.

The stress measure in this study consisted of six items tapping very different aspects of psychosocial experience (ranging from dissatisfaction with work through low-status employment and "major financial difficulties in the previous year"; see Ruberman *et al.*, 1984). As a measure of stress, this approach is incomplete in covering relevant life areas (e.g., no questions concerning child problems, no specific questions about marital conflicts without divorce), confounds acute and chronic stressors (e.g., a violent event that upset the patient in the last year versus major financial difficulties during the past year), and does not provide explicit criteria to understand what actually happened (e.g., what qualifies as "major financial difficulty"?; an item on divorce/break-up is worded such that it could involve the patient, his or her relatives, or friends—distant or close—all of which could have very different implications for stress; and so forth). Furthermore, all but one of the items explicitly mentions negative psychologic responses by the patient (e.g., upset, dissatisfaction), thereby confounding stress and distress. Finally, endorsement of only one of the six items resulted in the individual being classified in the "high stress" group; the rationale for this cutoff criterion is not provided, and the "high stress" group is consequently composed of individuals with very different forms and severities of circumstances. Conversely, the "low stress" group could contain individuals with high stress levels that simply do not coincide with those included in the measure.

The basis for item selection and scale composition in this study is unclear (e.g., *a priori* designation of scale content versus post hoc reconstruction), as is the basis for cutoff criteria involving the classification in "high" or "low" stress groups. Without further validation of the measure (e.g., psychometric statistics on reliability, descriptive statistics on the breakdown of endorsed items for the "high stress" group, and correlations with other stress measures), it is impossible to know what it *means* to be included in either the high or low stress group. The Ruberman *et al.* (1984) report represents a potentially important finding, based on a study that included many highly desirable design features (e.g., prospective data, controls for a variety of other factors). Nonetheless, the limitations in conceptualization and measurement of stress are instructive for the development of assessments for future studies attempting to replicate and extend such interesting results.

Measures such as these are advantageous in terms of expediency, yet they do not do justice to the complexity of the stress construct. Such approaches to stress measurement are conceptually and psychometrically very weak. If, despite these caveats, such an approach is to be adopted owing to demands of economy and time, it would be most prudent to: (1) clearly designate the items *a priori*

for inclusion and exclusion, along with an appropriate rationale and criteria for such procedures; (2) provide supportive psychometric data (e.g., test–retest reliability; internal consistency when relevant; and so forth); (3) implement the appropriate procedures to control for other potentially correlated predictors (e.g., socioeconomic status; psychologic distress); and/or (4) for large samples, test the stress measure initially on one-half of the sample, and cross-validate it on the second half. Finally, any findings using such assessments, be they affirmative or negative, should be interpreted very cautiously.

Life Event Inventories

In the face of theoretical ambiguity and definitional difficulties surrounding stress, the development of life event checklists took a strong hold on the methodology of stress measurement for human research. As a procedure reflecting the stimulus orientation to stress theory, it possessed several desirable features. The basic premise was that diverse aspects of life experiences could be conceptualized and measured as relatively discrete events. These life events, in turn, were assumed to reflect the adaptational demands—or stress—in the life of the individual. Two aspects of this approach proved to be especially attractive. First, the events represented a core of experiences that were common and relevant for most people; consequently, studying life events could be viewed as a reasonably "standardized" approach to the measurement of stress. Second, owing to the focus on actual life changes, there was a lessened concern with the generalizability of findings (as opposed to laboratory paradigms). In fact, it seemed that the methodology provided the condensation of experiences that could define stress and could be most informative for future functioning. Such a seemingly straightforward method for operationalizing life changes also found grounding in the theoretical premises of Cannon (1932) and Selye (1976). Perhaps most importantly, at a broader level of conceptualization this development renewed an active interest in the consequences of environment, emotion, and mind for health and well-being (Monroe & Peterman, 1988).

The prototype life event checklist contains a variety of relatively common experiences, ranging from major events (e.g., death of child or spouse) to less dramatic experiences (e.g., a cut in wage or salary), and contains anywhere from 15 to over 100 events. The number of items included in a measure is less important than the representativeness of the items for the particular sample to be studied (i.e., the rationale for inclusion/exclusion of items depending upon the characteristics of the sample chosen for study). For example, if studying certain groups of individuals, the items should reflect experiences that are common and important (Hurst, 1979; Monroe, 1982a). (For general representative measures, see: Dohrenwend, Krasnoff, Askenasy, & Dohrenwend, 1978; Holmes & Rahe, 1967; Horowitz, Schaefer, Hiroto, Wilner, & Levin, 1977; Paykel, 1982; Rose, Jenkins, & Hurst, 1978; Sarason, Johnson, & Siegel, 1978.)

The time span covered by most life event inventories varies, but commonly encompasses a 6-month to 2-year retrospective period over which individuals are requested to indicate which events have happened to them. Often, study participants also may be asked to provide some form of subjective weight reflecting their perception of various dimensions associated with the experience (e.g., degree of unpleasantness, controllability). Finally, a variety of summary indices have been used, ranging from overall total scores for subjective weights, through simple counts of particular types of events. At least for the majority of studies investigating life events and psychologic symptoms, a simple total of undesirable events appears to be the most parsimonious and potent measure to be extracted (for more information on scoring procedures, see Monroe, 1982b).

One recent variation in the life events approach has been developed by Lazarus and colleagues (Kanner, Coyne, Schaefer, & Lazarus, 1981). Instead of studying the impact of major life events, these investigators suggested that the more minor daily experiences—collectively termed "daily hassles"—represent more proximal influences on psychologic well-being and health. They developed a self-report inventory with 118 items to assess such experiences, and it has been used in several studies predicting a variety of outcomes (DeLongis, Coyne, Dakof, Folkman, & Lazarus, 1982). This form of assessment is based upon the interactional model of stress, and has been criticized for the potential of confounding with psychiatric symptoms (see Dohrenwend & Shrout, 1985; Lazarus, DeLongis, Folkman, & Gruen, 1985; Monroe, 1983). Equally legitimate would be criticisms of potential confounding with personality variables (e.g., neuroticism). Nonetheless, in the majority of existing investigations, the measure of hassles has proven to be a stronger predictor of disorder than more traditional measures of life events (even when potential confounds have been controlled statistically).

Overall, the major advantage of the life events approach is the simplicity and relative ease of administration. A good deal of information can be gleaned quickly concerning the general picture of socioenvironmental stressors for the individual over the time period covered. Furthermore, as noted, several subscores can be derived to reflect more specific areas or dimensions of stress (e.g., negative events, job-related events). Finally, there is a very large empirical base substantiating the predictive validity of such measures for a wide range of psychologic and physical disorders (Monroe & Peterman, 1988; Rabkin & Struening, 1976; Thoits, 1983).

This approach also possesses limitations. Four problems are most relevant. First, such measures typically cover stressors associated with life changes; ongoing difficulties or chronic stressors (as well as stressor sequences and intermittent stressors) are not the focus of measurement. It should be pointed out, however, that many items more accurately represent chronic forms of stress (e.g., "work difficulties"), and that through appropriate calssification of items, indices of chronic stress could conceivably be developed (see Billings & Moos, 1982). (Interestingly, although the hassles scale was developed to assess relatively minor annoyances, test–retest reliability data suggest that the measure reflects a good deal of chronicity; either in the person's perception or social environment.) This issue may be especially applicable to the study of CHD development, wherein stress factors would be anticipated to operate over lengthy time periods.

Second, several studies have demonstrated that the accuracy and reliability of reporting past experience can be quite low, especially when long periods of recall are required (e.g., greater than 6 months; Jenkins, Hurst, & Rose, 1979; Monroe, 1982a; Paykel, 1982). Third, this approach is especially vulnerable to some of the problems noted above under "Assessment Considerations." Namely, given the self-report format, much idiosyncratic interpretation of what constitutes an event can take place; hence, the stress levels for different individuals can reflect very different "objective" conditions, rendering inferences concerning causality tenuous. Fourth, although the tendency is to view life events as being imposed on the individual, many of the circumstances commonly endorsed suggest some degree of involvement of the person in bringing the circumstances about; the design of the study again should provide for testing competing hypotheses of the event–disorder relationship.

In summary, if the life events approach is adopted for the assessment of stress, the following guidelines are recommended: (1) the retrospective interval for recall be at maximum 6 months; (2) a brief questioning with probes for each event follow the self-report administration, with *a priori* criteria established to define what qualifies as an event; (3) on the basis of the particular event and the additional information gleaned from the questioning, events be categorized as reflecting chronic or acute psychosocial conditions; and finally (4) events be distinguished with respect to those that are imposed on the individual versus those which the person has a role in bringing about.

Perceived Stress Scales

Relatively few measures have been developed explicitly to assess perceived stress. Such scales typically can be viewed either from the "stress as a response" perspective or, alternatively, from an interactional perspective. It should be noted that some measures of psychologic symptoms of distress have been used to reflect presumed levels of stress (e.g., Derogatis, 1982); as pointed out previously, however, it is important to keep stress and distress separate in the conceptualization and mea-

surement of these processes. Consequently, we will not review such pure response measures of stress presently. (The reader interested in further coverage of the latter issue is referred to Derogatis, 1982.)

The Perceived Stress Scale (PSS) is a 14-item measure based upon the transactional stress theory of Lazarus (Lazarus & Folkman, 1984), developed by Cohen, Kamarck, and Mermelstein (1983) to assess ". . . the degree to which situations in one's life are appraised as stressful" (p. 394). Cohen *et al.* (1983) present a series of studies providing supportive data for the psychometric characteristics of the instrument (i.e., test–retest reliability, internal consistency; see also Cohen, 1986). Recently, the scale has been criticized by Lazarus, DeLongis, Folkman, and Gruen (1985) based upon the apparent overlap of items reflecting both stress and distress [i.e., many of the items appear to be redundant with those typically used to assess psychologic symptoms; e.g., "In the last month, how often have you felt nervous or stressed?" (p. 394)]. In response to such criticism, Cohen (1986) has argued that although the PSS is not totally independent of psychopathology, several studies have demonstrated that the PSS is an independent and significant predictor of psychologic symptoms, physical symptoms, and health behaviors after controlling for any redundancy among the psychologic symptom measures (see also Cohen *et al.,* 1983). Interestingly, the PSS has been shown to be a significant inverse predictor of smoking cessation, even when psychologic distress was controlled for statistically (Cohen, 1986).

The Derogatis Stress Profile (DSP) is a recently developed instrument that ". . . explicitly incorporates stimulus, response, and interactional elements" (Derogatis, 1982; p. 285). The DSP is a 77-item instrument that contains 11 dimensions and two global scores. Of the 11 dimensions, 3 pertain to stimulus aspects of the individual's social environment (job, home, and health), 5 pertain to ". . . characteristic attributes and coping mechanisms that have been shown to have significant mediating effects regarding stress" (p. 285) (i.e., time pressure, driven behavior, attitude posture, relaxation potential, role definition), and 3 pertain to primary response-oriented measures of stress (aggression-hostility, tension-anxiety, depression). Although in a developmental phase (norms and psychometric characteristics were still being developed and studied; Derogatis, 1982), the measure holds promise for the assessment of stress.

These measures provide another route to the assessment of stress. They are easy to administer and require little subject time (e.g., the DSP—the longer of the two—can be completed in 10–15 min; Derogatis, 1982). Once again, if they are to be used, the guidelines outlined previously should be followed (i.e., control for alternative predictors).

Structured Interviews

A final approach to the assessment of stress has been developed by Brown and Harris over the past 15 years (Brown & Harris, 1978). Representing a significant departure from self-report measures of stress, the approach developed by these investigators—called the Bedford Life Events and Difficulties Scale (LEDS)—employs a lengthy, semistructured interview probing for both life events and ongoing difficulties (i.e., chronic stressors). A wide range of life areas are covered, with the respondent allowed (and encouraged) to provide detail concerning the specific events or situations, as well as other psychosocial factors that may moderate acute or chronic stressors. Elaborate records have been maintained to provide standard criteria for defining what does and does not constitute an event or chronic difficulty. Furthermore, a variety of dimensions of stress can be rated, again with a companion manual providing reference examples for standardizing the weighting procedure. There is strong supportive evidence for the adequacy of this approach in terms of the reliability of recall over at least 6-month intervals (see Brown & Harris, 1978).

Perhaps the most innovative aspect of this assessment approach is the concept of "contextual" measurement, wherein a particular event or difficulty is evaluated in the specific biographic context of the individual involved. Essentially, ratings are anchored in the view of what the average individual would experience under similar circumstances. For example, while the birth of a child is an event that is typically scored at a relatively low level of threat or unpleasantness (according to the standard criteria), the surrounding social circumstances, under appropriate conditions, can increase the stress level, such as when there is a recent separation from the mate and economic privation. According to these investigators, such procedures provide for the requisite control over definition and standardization of stress assessment, yet still provide sensitivity to the particular biographic circumstances of the individual involved. In other words, the sensitivity of the subjective approach can be retained without sacrificing the rigor of the objective approach (Brown & Harris, 1978).

The procedures developed by these investigators are unique, laborious, and time-consuming. The approach provides by far the most elaborate conceptualization of stress and its component dimensions, and the most rigorous and reliable procedures for defining and standardizing psychosocial experiences. As would be expected, extensive training is required in the methodology to achieve such results. At least for the study of depression, the investment in time and energy has proven to be impressively fruitful. In contrast to other life event studies that report weak but statistically significant associations (Rabkin & Struening, 1976), the work of Brown and Harris (1978) has documented much more compelling and robust associations between recent life stress and the onset of clinical depression. Obviously, not all research in which stress is not the primary issue of interest will adopt such extensive assessment procedures, but the merits should be considered most seriously.

Conclusions

The measurement approaches presented in this section are arranged roughly along a continuum of quality. All other factors considered equal, the LEDS of Brown and Harris (1978) is most highly recommended; the single or multiple item measures are least recommended. The perceived stress scales and life event inventories appear to be roughly comparable.

What is most important to reemphasize, however, is that none of these measures are adequate without attention to the other design and control considerations that have been outlined. The information gleaned from the least adequate scales in a study that incorporated a prospective design and other control procedures may be preferable to the information obtained from the best instruments without such design and method advantages. The measures are clearly important and of variable quality, yet they only convey part of the overall picture in life stress and disease.

The Assessment of Social Moderators: Current Practices

Procedures for assessing social networks and social support include a very diverse range of indicators. Consequently, it may be most productive to organize the discussion in this section according to: (1) social network measures; (2) social support measures; and (3) structured interview measures. (For an excellent, extensive review of specific social support measures and their associations with dysfunction, see Cohen & Wills, 1985.)

Social Network Measures

Many studies have used a small number of items assumed to assess the social network of the individual. A continuum of sophistication exists, with procedures ranging from single questions about the existence of specific relationships (e.g., the number of friends, marital status, or membership in religious or social groups; House, Robbins, & Metzner, 1982), through the combination of several of these features into a global index of the social network (e.g., Williams, Ware, & Donald, 1981).

Two criticisms can be made of such procedures. First, as we found with the assessment of stress, items are often naively assumed to be reliable, to be valid, and to cover the relevant domain of support. For instance, in the aforementioned Ruberman et al. (1984) study on psychosocial factors and reinfarction, social isolation was measured by three disparate items (reflecting few visits with family or friends prior to the MI; a lack of membership in clubs, social or religious groups; and not

talking with medical personnel about the need for life changes), two of which were employed as the criterion for defining "social isolation." Without a rationale for item inclusion/exclusion, the cutoff criterion, or supportive psychometric data, it is difficult to know what is being measured (and what may be overlooked of potential importance) with such an assessment, and consequently what it is about the measure that is related to eventual pathology.

A second general problem with network measures stems from an empirical perspective: recent reviews suggest that the functional dimensions—not structural ones—are the stronger predictors of changes in mental health under stress (House & Kahn, 1985; Kessler & McKleod, 1985). Structural measures appear to represent only very general relationships, and they often cannot distinguish between relationships of primary and secondary importance (e.g., close family members versus more distant family members). Delineating the ingredients that afford protection—the functional qualities of the structural tie—is the more meaningful focus (e.g., what is it about the married–not married dichotomy that predicts outcomes?).

In summary, assessments falling within this category provide expedient measures of social characteristics which have been shown to predict general well-being, and provide an overall summary of social imbeddedness (Cohen & Wills, 1985). However, owing to their generality and lack of detail, they are susceptible to being too diffuse to capture the relevant phenomena (e.g., the actual provisions supplied via such relationships), or to adequately weight the most important dimensions (e.g., ties with intimate other versus ties with neighbors).

Social Support Measures

Many different instruments are covered within this categorization of self-report measures. Some focus on specific relationships of importance, defining them on functional qualities (e.g., having a confidant—a close, confiding relationship—that provides emotional support; Brown & Harris, 1978). Other methods attempt to measure specific support functions that transcend specific relationships (e.g., self-esteem, tangible, appraisal, and belonging support; Cohen & Hoberman, 1983), or to measure perceived support from specific sources (e.g., family and friends; Procidano & Heller, 1983). An interesting distinction made recently within this broad class of measures concerns the differences between *perceived* and *enacted* support (Barrera, 1986; Tardy, 1985). Perceived social support refers to the individual's confidence in the availability, adequacy, or satisfaction with support resources (without necessarily using them; e.g., Sarason, Levine, Basham, & Sarason, 1983), whereas enacted support refers to recent transactions with individuals in which support may or may not have been received (e.g., Barrera, Sandler, & Ramsay, 1981).

The range of measures subsumed within this category defies summary appraisals. Some instruments have been developed on explicit theoretical grounds (assessing specific or general support functions), many of which have adequate psychometric qualifications. One such measure of perceived support is the Interpersonal Support Evaluation List (ISEL) by Cohen and Hoberman (1983). This is a 48-item inventory that assesses perceived availability of four separate functions of social support: tangible, appraisal, self-esteem, and belonging. A measure of enacted support is the Inventory of Socially Supportive Behaviors (ISSB; Barrera *et al.*, 1981), wherein individuals are requested to report the frequency of occurrence during the past month of a variety of specific supportive behaviors (e.g., given a ride to see a physician).

Certain limitations of these measures should be considered. Support reports may be distorted by colored perceptions as opposed to actual circumstances, owing to a variety of psychopathologic (e.g., depression) or personality (e.g., hostility) features. The control procedures advocated previously are again required. Nonetheless, several of these instruments are adequate for research purposes. Assuming psychometric adequacy of the scale, the selection of a measure should be based upon theoretical and/or empirical considerations. For instance, a scale might be chosen to represent a theoretical dimension of support that, although assessed in a different manner previously (and most

likely in a less than optimal manner), was found to be related to some aspect of CHD. Alternatively, particular dimensions of support might be selected on the basis of specific forms of stress to which the study participants are subjected (e.g., work stressors and work support; House & Kahn, 1985).

Structured Interviews

The fewest assessment approaches to the measurement of social support fall under this heading. Two groups of investigators are noteworthy. Once again, Brown and Harris (1978) have been instrumental in the conceptualization and measurement at this level of assessment. Based on their semistructured interview, these investigators developed a measure reflecting the degree to which the individual has a confidant (an individual, most often a spouse or opposite sex intimate relationship, with whom the individual can share innermost feelings and problems). This index proved to be a significant buffer of life events and difficulties in the prediction model for depression. Although unexplored in relation to CHD, it captures an important quality of a primary relationship; indeed, other research has suggested the general importance of the marital relationship in CHD (e.g., the development of angina pectoris; Medalie & Goldbourt, 1976).

The other methodology to be described within this category is the Interview Schedule for Social Interaction (ISSI), developed by Henderson, Byrne, and Duncan-Jones (1981). A clear theoretical rationale is presented by the authors for this measure, and an impressive amount of effort went into its development. Psychometric indices suggest adequate internal consistency and test–retest reliability. The major phenomena assessed include ". . . the existence of social relationships, the provisions obtained from them and the perceived adequacy or inadequacy of these . . ." (p. 52). Interestingly, owing to the temporal stability of many of these support qualities, along with their correlations with measures of personality, the authors point out the importance of the latter—personality—in accounting for potential support effects (see also Monroe & Steiner, 1986).

The advantages of these procedures are that they in general have firm conceptual bases and psychometric properties [although actual test–retest reliability of the confidant measure of Brown and Harris (1978) has yet to be demonstrated]. Unfortunately, they are time-consuming, and do not cover other areas of support that the current literature suggests may be of importance (e.g., different dimensions of support). Also, once again, controls for likely "third variables" and confounds are required.

Concluding Remarks

The goal of this chapter has been to provide an overview of the types of assessment procedures available for measuring both stress and social moderators. Since these approaches, however, can only be interpreted in the methodologic and conceptual context within which they are used, an equally important goal has been to provide a basic framework for understanding this important area of investigation. Without such considerations, little progress in unravelling the complex interrelations between stress, social moderators, and disease will be made.

The focus in this chapter on stress assessments has been on general measures that cover the different areas of an individual's life in which stress may exist. More specific scales have been developed to assess particular areas of life stress (e.g., family life—Moos & Moos, 1986; work situations—Moos, 1981). Most noteworthy in regard to CHD perhaps are the numerous scales developed to measure stress in the workplace. A variety of dimensions have been assessed, including physical properties, time factors, organizational features, changes, and so on (see Holt, 1982, for an extensive review of over 50 areas of work stress; also Cooper & Payne, 1980). Clearly, this area of study has been one of active investigation dealing with a variety of outcome variables (e.g., influences on health, well-being, productivity). Suggestions provided in the present chapter are applicable to these more specific stress indices, and should assist the interested investigator in research on this topic.

Recommendations for specific measures have been avoided. This has been intentional. It is un-

likely that any one measure will meet the need of different investigators, studying diverse aspects of CHD, within a variety of research designs and consequent measurement requirements. Also, the assessment of stress and social moderators is evolving rapidly, with new instruments emerging based on firmer theoretical and psychometric grounds. What has been provided is a current view of existing measures, their relative strengths and limitations, along with the background considerations applicable to the evaluation of any measurement device. It is hoped that this provides the potential investigator with an informed perspective on selecting the appropriate assessment procedures for any particular study, thereby facilitating the inclusion of such measures in studies on cardiovascular disorders.

ACKNOWLEDGMENTS. This work was supported in part by a National Institute of Mental Health New Investigator Research Award in Prevention, MH-39139, and BRSG Grant RR07084-20, awarded by the Biomedical Research Support Grant Program, Division of Resources, National Institutes of Health.

References

Barrera, M., Jr. (1986). Distinctions between social support concepts, measures, and models. *American Journal of Community Psychology, 14*, 413–445.

Barrera, M., Jr., Sandler, I. N., & Ramsay, T. B. (1981). Preliminary development of a scale of social support: Studies on college students. *American Journal of Community Psychology, 9*, 435–447.

Billings, A. C., & Moos, R. H. (1982). Stressful life events and symptoms: A longitudinal model. *Health Psychology, 1*, 99–117.

Brown, G. W. (1974). Meaning, measurement, and stress on life events. In B. S. Dohrenwend & B. P. Dohrenwend (Eds.), *Stressful life events: Their nature and effects*. New York: Wiley.

Brown, G. W. (1981). Life events, psychiatric disorder and physical illness. *Journal of Psychosomatic Research, 25*, 461–473.

Brown, G. W., & Harris, T. O. (1978). *Social origins of depression*. New York: Free Press.

Cannon, W. B. (1932). *The wisdom of the body*. New York: Norton.

Cohen, S. (1986). Contrasting the Hassles Scale and the Perceived Stress Scale: Who's really measuring appraised stress? *American Psychologist, 40,* 716–718.

Cohen, S., & Hoberman, H. (1983). Positive events and social supports as buffers of life change stress. *Journal of Applied Social Psychology, 13,* 99–125.

Cohen, S., Kamarck, T., & Mermelstein, R. (1983). A global measure of perceived stress. *Journal of Health and Social Behavior, 24,* 385–396.

Cohen, S., & McKay, G. (1984). Social support, stress and the buffering hypothesis: A theoretical analysis. In A. Baum, J. E. Singer, & S. F. Taylor (Eds.), *Handbook of psychology and health* (Vol. 4, pp. 253–267). Hillsdale, NJ: Erlbaum.

Cohen, S., & Syme, S. L. (Eds.). (1985). *Social support and health.* New York: Academic Press.

Cohen, S., & Wills, T. A. (1985). Stress, social support, and the buffering hypothesis. *Psychological Bulletin, 98,* 310–357.

Cook, T. D., & Campbell, D. T. (1979). *Quasi-experimentation: Design and analysis issues for field settings.* Boston: Houghton Mifflin.

Cooper, C. L., & Payne, R. (Eds.). (1980). *Current concerns in occupational stress.* New York: Wiley.

DeLongis, A., Coyne, J. C., Dakof, G., Folkman, S., & Lazarus, R. S. (1982). Relation of daily hassles, uplifts, and major life events to health status. *Health Psychology, 1,* 119–136.

Depue, R. A., & Monroe, S. M. (1986). Conceptualization and measurement of human disorder in life stress research: The problem of chronic disturbance. *Psychological Bulletin, 99,* 36–51.

Depue, R. A., Monroe, S. M., & Shackman, S. L. (1979). The psychobiology of human disease: Implications for conceptualizing the depressive disorders. In R. A. Depue (Ed.), *The psychobiology of the depressive disorders: Implications for the effects of stress.* New York: Academic Press.

Derogatis, L. R. (1982). Self-report measures of stress. In L. Goldberger & S. Breznitz (Eds.), *Handbook of stress.* New York: Free Press.

Dohrenwend, B. S., Krasnoff, L., Askenasy, A. R., & Dohrenwend, B. P. (1978). Exemplification of a method for scaling life events: The PERI Life Events Scale. *Journal of Health and Social Behavior, 19,* 205–229.

Dohrenwend, B. S., & Shrout, P. E. (1985). "Hassles" in the conceptualization and measurement of life stress variables. *American Psychologist, 40,* 780–785.

Durkheim, E. (1951). *Suicide.* New York: Free Press.

Elliot, G. R., & Eisdorfer, C. (Eds.). (1982). *Stress and human health.* Berlin: Springer.

Heller, K. (1979). The effects of social support: Prevention and treatment implications. In A. P. Goldstein & F. H. Kanfer (Eds.), *Maximizing treatment gains: Transfer-enhancement in psychotherapy.* New York: Academic Press.

Henderson, S., Byrne, D. G., & Duncan-Jones, P. (1981). *Neurosis and the social environment.* New York: Academic Press.

Hinkle, L. E., Jr. (1977). The concept of 'stress' in the biological and social sciences. *International Journal of Psychiatry in Medicine, 5,* 335–357.

Holmes, T. H., & Rahe, R. H. (1967). The social readjustment rating scale. *Journal of Psychosomatic Research, 11,* 213–218.

Holt, R. R. (1982). Occupational stress. In L. Goldberger and S. Breznitz (Eds.), *Handbook of stress.* New York: Free Press.

Horowitz, M., Schaefer, C., Hiroto, D., Wilner, N., & Levin, B. (1977). Life events questionnaires for measuring presumptive stress. *Psychosomatic Medicine, 39,* 413–431.

House, J. S., & Kahn, R. L. (1985). Measures and concepts of social support. In S. Cohen & S. L. Syme (Eds.), *Social support and health.* New York: Academic Press.

House, J. S., Robbins, C., & Metzner, H. L. (1982). The association of social relationships and activities with mortality: Prospective evidence from the Tecumseh Community Health Study. *American Journal of Epidemiology, 116,* 123–140.

Hurst, M. W. (1979). Life changes and psychiatric symptom development: Issues of content, scoring, and clustering. In J. E. Barrett (Ed.), *Stress and mental health.* New York: Raven Press.

Jenkins, C. D. (1978). Low education: A risk factor for death. *New England Journal of Medicine, 299,* 95–96.

Jenkins, C. D., Hurst, M. W., & Rose, R. M. (1979). Life changes: Do people really remember? *Archives of General Psychiatry, 36,* 379–384.

Kanner, A. D., Coyne, J. C., Schaefer, C., & Lazarus, R. S. (1981). Comparison of two modes of stress measurement: Daily hassles and uplifts versus major life events. *Journal of Behavioral Medicine, 4,* 1–39.

Kenny, D. A. (1979). *Correlation and causality.* New York: Wiley.

Kessler, R. C., & McKleod, J. D. (1985). Social support and mental health in community samples. In S. Cohen & S. L. Syme (Eds.), *Social support and health.* New York: Academic Press.

Lazarus, R. S., DeLongis, A., Folkman, S., & Gruen, R. (1985). Stress and adaptational outcomes: The problem of confounded measures. *American Psychologist, 40,* 770–779.

Lazarus, R. S., & Folkman, S. (1984). *Stress, appraisal, and coping.* Berlin: Springer.

Lieberman, M. A. (1986). Social supports—The consequences of psychologizing: A commentary. *Journal of Consulting and Clinical Psychology, 54,* 461–465.

Mason, J. (1975). A historical review of the stress field. Parts I and II. *Journal of Human Stress, 15,* 6–12, 22–36.

Medalie, J. H., & Goldbourt, U. (1976). Angina pectoris among 10,000 men: Psychosocial and other risk factors as evidenced by a multivariate analysis of a five year incidence study. *The American Journal of Medicine, 60,* 910–921.

Monroe, S. M. (1982a). Assessment of life events: Retrospective vs concurrent strategies. *Archives of General Psychiatry, 39,* 606–610.

Monroe, S. M. (1982b). Life events assessment: Current practices, emerging trends. *Clinical Psychology Review, 42,* 435–452.

Monroe, S. M. (1983). Major and minor life events as predictors of disorder: Further issues and findings. *Journal of Behavioral Medicine, 6,* 189–205.

Monroe, S. M., & Peterman, A. M. (1988). Life stress and psychopathology. In L. H. Cohen (Ed.), *Research on stressful life events: Theoretical and methodological issues* (pp. 31–63). New York: Sage.

Monroe, S. M., & Steiner, S. C. (1986). Social support and psychopathology: Interrelations with preexisting disorder, stress, and personality. *Journal of Abnormal Psychology, 95,* 29–39.

Moos, R. H. (1981). *Work environment scale.* Palo Alto, CA: Consulting Psychologists Press.

Moos, R. H., & Moos, B. S. (1986). *Family environment scale manual* (2nd ed.). Palo Alto, CA: Consulting Psychologists Press.

Paykel, E. S. (1982). Life events and early environment. In E. S. Paykel (Ed.), *Handbook of affective disorders.* New York: Guilford Press.

Procidano, M. E., & Heller, K. (1983). Measures of perceived social support from friends and from family: Three validation studies. *American Journal of Community Psychology, 11,* 1–24.

Rabkin, J. G., & Struening, E. L. (1976). Life events, stress, and illness. *Science, 194,* 1013–1020.

Rose, R. M., Jenkins, C. D., & Hurst, M. W. (1978). *Air traffic controller health change study* (edited by M. A. Levin). Boston: Boston University School of Medicine.

Ruberman, W., Weinblatt, E., Goldberg, J. D., & Chaudhary, B. S. (1983). Education, psychosocial stress and sudden cardiac death. *Journal of Chronic Diseases, 36,* 151–160.

Ruberman, W., Weinblatt, E., Goldberg, J. D., & Chaudhary, B. S. (1984). Psychosocial influences on mortality after myocardial infarction. *New England Journal of Medicine, 311,* 552–559.

Sarason, I. G., Johnson, J. H., & Siegel, J. M. (1978). Assessing the impact of life changes: Development of the Life Experiences Survey. *Journal of Consulting and Clinical Psychology, 46,* 932–946.

Sarason, I. G., Levine, H. M., Basham, R. B., & Sarason, B. R. (1983). Assessing social support: The social support questionnaire. *Journal of Personality and Social Psychology, 44,* 127–139.

Sarason, I. G., & Sarason, B. R. (Eds.). (1985). *Social support: Theory, research, and applications.* The Hague: Nijhoff.

Selye, H. (1976). *The stress of life* (2nd ed.). New York: McGraw–Hill.

Tardy, C. H. (1985). Social support measurement. *American Journal of Community Psychology, 13,* 187–202.

Theorell, T., Lind, E., & Floderus, B. (1975). The relationship of disturbing life-changes and emotions to the early development of myocardial infarction and other serious illnesses. *International Journal of Epidemiology, 4,* 281–293.

Thoits, P. A. (1983). Dimensions of life events that influence psychological distress: An evaluation and synthesis of the literature. In H. B. Kaplan (Ed.), *Psychosocial stress: Trends in theory and research.* New York: Academic Press.

Williams, A. W., Ware, J. E., & Donald, C. A. (1981). A model of mental health, life events, and social supports applicable to general populations. *Journal of Health and Social Behavior, 22,* 324–334.

CHAPTER 33

Assessing Subjects' Construal
of the Laboratory Situation

Michael J Strube

The manner in which subjects in laboratory research perceive, understand, and respond to the
situations created for them has been a topic of
widespread interest and great controversy throughout the history of psychology. One could argue, in
fact, that no serious examination of human behavior can escape considering the subjects' understanding of the situations in which they are studied:
Regardless of whether people have an accurate understanding of their world, they base their actions
(at least in part) on the world as they understand it
(see Heider, 1958; Kelley, 1967, 1973; Kelly,
1955; Jones & Davis, 1965). Laboratory research
is, of course, an attempt to create a highly controlled, well-specified situation in order to test
propositions about subjects' responses to that situation. This chapter will emphasize that a complete understanding of a subject's actions in the
laboratory requires a careful assessment of the subject's perceptions of that situation, and also that
careful attention be given to a number of potential
pitfalls.* Both the essential nature of assessing the

subject's psychological state, and the dangers lurk-
ing in such assessment, can be demonstrated by
considering as our starting point the role of the
manipulation check in experimental research.

The Manipulation Check in
Experimental Research

Consider again the purpose of a laboratory experiment. The researcher creates a highly controlled, well-specified situation for the subjects
through the manipulation of an independent variable. The intent is to create a psychological state in
the subject that is then expected to affect an outcome variable of interest.† This relationship is depicted in Figure 1. For example, a researcher
might be interested in testing the simple hypothesis
that initial exposure to noncontingent feedback induces perceived loss of control which in turn produces elevations in physiological arousal.

In order to make a valid inference about the
manipulation's effect on the outcome variable, it is
essential to demonstrate that the manipulation was

---

*Much of what will be said can be applied to nonlaboratory
research settings as well. Nonlaboratory settings, however,
raise additional issues about assessment due to the lesser control the researcher has over the situation and over assessment.
These issues will not be discussed here (but see Cook &
Campbell, 1979).

†This chapter will focus attention on assessment of the subjects'
psychological state before assessment of an outcome. This
reflects most researchers' emphasis on psychological state as a
mediator of outcome. However, most of what will be said can
be applied to assessment of psychological state after or concurrent with outcome assessment.

Michael J Strube • Department of Psychology, Washington
University, St. Louis, Missouri 63130.

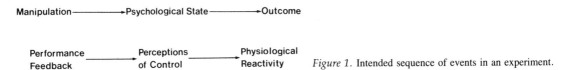

Figure 1. Intended sequence of events in an experiment.

carried out as intended and produced the desired psychological state. This is the purpose of the manipulation check. In fact, adequate demonstration of manipulation effectiveness requires attending to two distinct aspects of the manipulation: structural features and psychological features. Structural features of a manipulation refer to the mechanics of creating the distinct situations for the control and experimental groups. In many cases, the structural aspects of the manipulation are highly automated and are unlikely to vary within groups. This is the case, for example, when feedback is provided to subjects via computer-driven hardware. In such cases, there will be no variation in manipulation presentation within conditions (barring equipment failure). In other instances, the manipulation is delivered through less reliable means (e.g., experimenter or confederate) and needs to be checked. Unfortunately, attention to the structural features of the manipulation, which addresses the *reliability* of the manipulation, is ordinarily not given careful attention once the study has commenced. That is, although researchers may take great pains to train experimental personnel to deliver the manipulation in a standard fashion, there is often little effort made to ensure that such standardization is maintained throughout the study.* Consequently, many researchers may blame a "failed" manipulation on its invalidity rather than on its unreliable implementation. I will have little else to say about structural features of the manipulation because they do not

bear directly on assessing the subjects' construal of the situation, and because much has been written about constructing and implementing effective manipulations (e.g., Carlsmith, Ellsworth, & Aronson, 1976; Crano & Brewer, 1986; Kazdin, 1980; Kidder & Judd, 1986). It should suffice to emphasize that manipulations (i.e., independent variables) can be unreliable and introduce error into the inference process in the same way that measurement error produces problems in assessment of outcomes (i.e., dependent variables).

The psychological features are what are ordinarily assessed by a traditional "manipulation check." Here we are interested in validating that the manipulation produced the intended psychological state. Whereas assessing structural features of the manipulation allows a check on the *reliability* of the manipulation, assessing the intended psychological state addresses the *validity* of the manipulation (albeit only one part of validity). Ordinarily, the manipulation check is examined by comparing the control and experimental groups on the measure of psychological state (in our example, perceptions of control). When such a comparison is made, in combination with a comparison of groups on the outcome measure, four possible cases can arise and are depicted in Figure 2 (see Kazdin, 1980).†

Case 1 is typically considered to be sufficient evidence for claiming the validity of the set of relations indicated in Figure 1, provided the differences are in the predicted direction. In this case, the manipulation has produced reliable differences in the psychological state of interest (e.g., per-

---

*It can be argued that total, rigid standardization of procedure by experimenter (e.g., use of a standard script) may not be desired (Carlsmith, Ellsworth, & Aronson, 1976) in that it requires multiple experimenters to act in ways that may be unnatural to them. Consequently, this contrived behavior may tip subjects off to the fact that there are aspects of the study that are being concealed from them. Thus, natural variations in style, but not content, may be desirable. In these cases it is still crucial to check that the appropriate content of a script has been delivered consistently.

†The table in Figure 2 implies that manipulations work in an all-or-none fashion. Although this is not the case, researchers do tend to make inferences in this way (based on statistical significance; see Rosenthal & Gaito, 1963, 1964), and the oversimplification does allow for easier discussion of ideas. Note also that it is assumed that an obtained difference is in the predicted direction. Unexpected differences are problematic from an inferential standpoint.

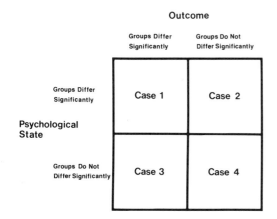

Figure 2. Possible study outcomes as a function of effectiveness of the manipulation and differences on the outcome measure.

ceived control loss), and has also produced differences in the outcome variable (e.g., physiological reactivity). In our example, we ordinarily would conclude that perceived loss of control produces elevations in physiological indicators. The remaining cases in Figure 2 create problems for drawing such inferences.

Cases 2 and 4 are usually dismissed as instances of null results, but usually with different implications for future empirical efforts. With Case 2, one might well abandon the problem given that the intended psychological state was created, but no outcome differences were detected. Case 4, on the other hand, typically leads to more empirical work because there is evidence that the intended psychological state was not created and thus it would be premature to infer no relation between manipulation and outcome. Any bias in the motivation to continue with more empirical work with Cases 2 and 4 may be unjustified, however. Researchers must bear in mind that different measures may be affected by the manipulation at different levels. That is, a manipulation may be strong enough to induce the psychological state, but may not be strong enough to alter outcome noticeably (i.e., different thresholds in the two variables; see Campbell, 1963; Kazdin, 1980). Thus, more empirical work may be equally justified in both cases.

Case 3 is a situation that is particularly problematic because it implies that, although the manipulation affects the outcome, the process in-

volved is not clear. This case highlights the important role that the subjects' perceptions play in the interpretation of a study's outcome. In the absence of information about the psychological state created by the manipulation, very little insight into the phenomenon under study is gained.

In discussing the four cases in Figure 2 it has been assumed that the measures used are both reliable and valid. Space does not permit a complete discussion of the construction of reliable and valid measures but several comments are pertinent (for more extensive discussions, see Anastasi, 1976; Crano & Brewer, 1986; Kazdin, 1980; Kidder & Judd, 1986; Nunnally, 1978). First, unreliable assessment can take a real instance of Case 1 and produce an apparent instance of Case 2, 3, or 4. Thus, validity of the inferences drawn from research is based on the assumption of reliable assessment of both the intended psychological state and the outcome. Where possible, multiple converging measures should be used. For example, in our hypothetical study we might ask subjects to report their perceptions of response–outcome contingency, competence, and confidence in future performance expectations. All of these measures should converge on the psychological state of perceived control loss, and the use of multiple measures should overcome the imperfect representation each bears to the underlying construct. Likewise, we might measure heart rate, systolic blood pressure, and diastolic pressure as indicators of physiological reactivity. Given high internal consistency among the individual items of these two "tests," we would have more confidence in the placement of our study within one of the cells in Figure 2.

Second, it is important to demonstrate the construct validity of the measures used. Researchers must recognize that their measures represent one of many possible operational definitions for the constructs being investigated. The degree to which a measure adequately represents the construct should be demonstrated, not assumed (e.g., see Stacy, Widaman, Hays, & DiMatteo, 1985). Often we can rely on past research to inform us as to the construct validity of our measures. All too often, however, we seem to rely on "face validity" or the idea that the measures appear to assess what they are intended to measure. As Kazdin (1980) put it, "Presumably, the reason this is called 'face validity' is to emphasize how difficult it is for us to *face* our colleagues after having established the validity of an assessment device in such a shoddy manner, especially when we know better" (p. 207). The danger in not adequately demonstrating the validity of our measures is that the interpretation of any of the cases in Figure 2 becomes ambiguous, if not quite misleading.

Finally, it is also vital to ensure that measures chosen or constructed are sensitive to the expected type and magnitude of change in psychological state. Again, we often rely on the results of past research to inform us on the sensitivity of potential measures. Where past research is silent on this issue, there is no substitute for careful pilot testing.

Throughout the rest of this chapter we will assume that care has been taken to construct reliable, valid, and sensitive measures. The relatively brief mention of reliability, validity, and sensitivity, however, should not be taken as an indicator of their importance. They are absolutely essential to the clear interpretation of any study.

Beyond the Manipulation Check

As noted previously, the measurement of the intended psychological state and the outcome resulting in an instance of Case 1 is typically considered to be sufficient evidence for the causal sequence depicted in Figure 1. Despite the traditional nature of this inference, it is seriously in error on both methodological and statistical grounds. The methodological inadequacy stems from the insufficiency of measuring only the intended psychological state.

Consider again the intent of an experimental manipulation. The purpose is to create a specific, well-defined psychological state in the subject, with the expectation that this state will largely, if not entirely, account for change in the outcome variable. This immediately suggests not only that it is important to validate that the intended psychological state was created, but that it is equally important to demonstrate that other psychological states have not also been created. In other words, a

manipulation may be multidimensional (i.e., may represent more than one construct) and all plausible dimensions must be assessed. Let us return to our hypothetical example for a moment. The exposure to noncontingent feedback would certainly be expected to produce a perceived loss of control. But it might produce other reactions as well. For example, subjects might believe that the task is impossible (rather than that they lack abilities) or that the task is rigged. Both perceptions could produce heightened physiological reactions because subjects might become angry. From a logical standpoint it is important to assess these psychological states. If the manipulation of feedback contingency produces differences in suspiciousness, for example, in addition to differences in loss of control, then it is less clear what is the mediating psychological process. Consequently, the failure to anticipate and assess other plausible mediating effects of the manipulation biases the inference process in favor of the preferred interpretation. Stated differently, the traditional manipulation check only addresses the *convergent validity* of the manipulation. In order to make truly valid inferences it is also necessary to assess the *discriminant validity* of the manipulation.

By considering the multidimensional nature of a manipulation, it becomes clear that assessing the subjects' construal of the situation is of paramount importance. The ability to make clear inferences from the data relies on such assessment. Unfortunately, even careful assessment of the multidimensional nature of the manipulation may not prevent inaccurate conclusions concerning the psychological state responsible for any outcome differences. These inaccuracies stem from limitations in the way statistical analyses of manipulation checks are conducted. Consider again the sequence of events and *possible paths of influence* present in our original example (see Figure 3).

We would like to argue that the manipulation produces changes in control perceptions that subsequently alter physiology, *and* that this sequence accounts in large part (if not entirely) for the observed differences in physiology. In other words, we would like to argue that Path 3 in Figure 3 is nonexistent. If the manipulation affects physiology independently of control perceptions, then we

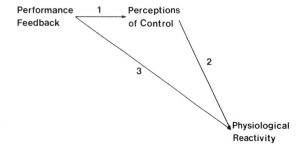

Figure 3. Possible paths of influence with an experimental manipulation.

know less about the process than we would like. The typical problem with traditional analyses of this process is that the alternative paths of influence are incompletely tested.

To demonstrate the inadequacy of traditional statistical analyses of manipulation checks, consider what evidence would be required to claim that the psychological state of perceived control loss mediates the effect of noncontingent feedback on physiological reactivity (see Baron & Kenny, 1986; Judd & Kenny, 1981a,b). First, the manipulation must produce changes in the outcome (physiology) and in the mediating variable (perceived control loss). In the absence of this information it makes no sense to talk about mediation (either because there is nothing to mediate or because the proposed mediator was not affected by the manipulation). Ordinarily this is all that is demonstrated in the typical experiment where significant F ratios may be reported for physiology and perceived control, respectively. It also is important, however, to demonstrate that the mediating variable and the outcome variable are related *independent of the manipulation.* This is rarely tested because it requires calculation of the correlation between perceived control loss and physiology with the manipulation statistically controlled. Stated differently, the mediating variable and the outcome variable should be correlated reliably within experimental conditions. This step validates that the outcome and mediator are related so that any induced variation in the mediator *can* be transmitted to the outcome variable. Satisfaction of this requirement indicates that perceived control loss is *a* mediator of physiology, but a further step is necessary. Lastly, to conclude that the mediation is complete, it should be demonstrated that the ma-

nipulation and the outcome are unrelated when the mediator (perceived control loss) is controlled statistically. If this last step is not satisfied, then one must conclude that perceived control loss is one mediator of physiology, but the manipulation also influences outcome independent of the intended mediator, possibly through other, unmeasured mediators. To underscore the above points, Figure 4 displays the pattern of data that would satisfy all three requirements for complete mediation. To further underscore these points, consider the three data patterns displayed in Figure 5, all of which are instances of Case 1 in Figure 2, and which ordinarily lead to a conclusion of mediation.

The first diagram indicates a case where the conclusion of mediation would be completely erroneous because perceived control loss bears no independent relation to physiology. That is, the manipulation clearly produces the intended psychological state, but this state bears no relation to

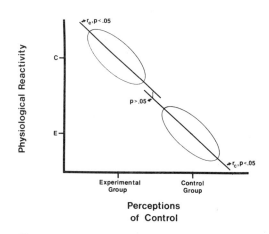

Figure 4. Data pattern representing complete mediation.

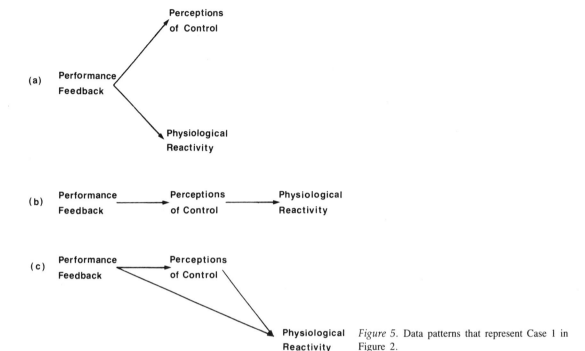

Figure 5. Data patterns that represent Case 1 in Figure 2.

the outcome variable. The second diagram represents a case of complete mediation, that is, all of the manipulation's influence on physiology acts through perceived control loss. The last diagram represents a case of partial mediation, where some of the manipulation's effect acts through perceived control loss, but not all. This diagram highlights again the need to examine the multidimensional nature of the manipulation; it is crucial to specify in advance and measure additional paths of influence. For example, had suspiciousness been assessed, its role as a mediator in addition to per-

ceived control loss could be examined (see Figure 6). Testing the magnitude of the additional paths might allow a decision to be made concerning the nature of any partial mediation (as in the third diagram in Figure 5).

It is useful to pause for a moment and consider the nature of the statistical analyses required and some problems inherent in them. The attempt to delineate the paths through which the manipulation affects the outcome requires the use of correlational analyses that can range in complexity from simple partial correlation to complex structural

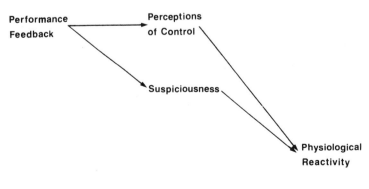

Figure 6. Additional effects of the manipulation.

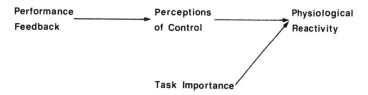

Figure 7. Additional variable of influence.

equation modeling (see Asher, 1963; Heise, 1975; Kenny, 1979; Judd & Kenny, 1981a,b; Jöreskog & Sörbom, 1984). Description of these procedures is beyond the scope of this chapter but some potential problems should be noted. First, measurement error can greatly distort the attempt to estimate the magnitude of path coefficients (i.e., standardized regression coefficients). However, if the measurement error can be estimated, it can be accounted for in the path model. This suggests another good reason to construct multiple measures of mediators and outcomes. Second, unaccounted-for sources of influence can also distort the estimation of path coefficients. This underscores the need for careful attention to possible multiple influences of the manipulation *before* the study is conducted.* Finally, researchers must also be alert to possible nonlinear relations.

Consideration of the requirements for demonstrating mediation emphasizes the need to assess carefully the multiple possible influences of the manipulation. There is yet a further complication: The manipulation may not influence all of the important characteristics of the situation, but these additional features may influence the process under study in important ways. Continuing with the loss of control example, one could very well imagine that the perceived importance of the task could

influence physiology. In fact, there are two major ways that this might occur. The first is through a direct effect on the outcome variable, independent of manipulation and mediator (see Figure 7). In this case, assessment of task importance is advantageous because it allows us to account for more of the variability in physiology.

There is a second, and equally important case that can also arise. In Figure 8, perceived task importance serves to alter the nature of the perceived control–physiology relationship. In other words, perceived task importance serves as a moderator variable (see Baron & Kenny, 1986). For example, it may be that for those individuals who find the task to be particularly unimportant, perceived control loss has no effect on physiology, but where task importance is perceived to be more important, the predicted relation is obtained (see Figure 9).†

To summarize, a complete account of the influence of a manipulation on an outcome variable necessarily requires a complete assessment of the subjects' construal of the environment created in the laboratory. This requires assessment of three basic types of subjective experience:

1. Those aspects presumed to mediate the effect of the manipulation on the outcome (i.e., the intended mediator).
2. Those additional consequences of the manipulation that need to be ruled out, or ac-

---

*The reader should be alerted to some caveats in carrying out the analysis of mediator variables. First, it is possible that a manipulation is so powerful that there is very little variability in responses within conditions (due perhaps to ceiling or floor effects). This lack of variability reduces the ability to detect within-condition correlations between mediator and outcome. Similarly, extremely powerful manipulations will produce a correlation between manipulation and mediator that is so high that detection of an independent mediator–outcome relation will be hampered (due to multicolinearity). Thus, it is possible to create a situation that does not allow testing of the mediator for statistical reasons and this should be distinguished from situations where mediation is testable but found to be untenable.

†Note that there are innumerable other possible path combinations that could be discussed. For example, it is possible for the mediator to influence another variable's effect on the outcome. That is, perceived control loss may increase the perceived importance of the task and lead to greater physiological response (i.e., two mediators). It is also possible for the mediator or the manipulation to influence another variable that then influences the mediator–outcome relation. The essential points regarding mediation and moderation apply to other combinations as well.

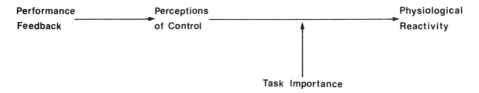

Figure 8. Moderator variable.

counted for, as intended mediators of the manipulation's effect on the outcome.

3. Those situational features that may affect the outcome directly, or that may moderate the effect of the mediating variable on the outcome.

Note that previous discussions of sources of artifact and bias in experiments (e.g., Kruglanski, 1975; Orne, 1962; Rosenthal & Rosnow, 1969) can be fit into the current conceptualization. Regardless of whether the problem is present in the experiment at large (e.g., evaluation apprehension) or is correlated with the manipulation (e.g., demand characteristics, experimenter bias), it represents part of the subjects' psychological state that can presumably be taken into account.

Levels versus Differences

Thus far, we have emphasized mediator and outcome *differences* between experimental and control

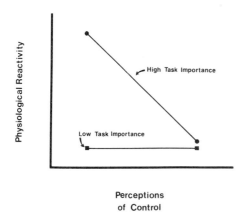

Figure 9. Data pattern for moderator variable.

groups as the information of primary importance. It is also important to consider the *absolute magnitude* of scores within conditions. This information provides additional insight into the nature of the psychological state created by the manipulation, and it places limits on the extent to which the results can be generalized. For instance, suppose that in the hypothetical example, perceived control loss had been measured with a 10-point scale (1 = no control, 10 = complete control). Suppose further that the groups differed in their physiological responses (experimental group more reactive) and that the means on the perceived control measure were 9 for the control group and 5 for the experimental group ($p < 0.05$). The interpretation necessarily must take into account the fact that the experimental group experienced "moderate" uncontrollability. There is no basis for generalizing the results to greater levels of uncontrollability in the absence of a strong theoretical model or empirical evidence indicating a linear relation between controllability and physiological reactivity. Researchers must attend to both the presence of a manipulation *and* its intensity.

In a similar fashion, researchers must attend to the magnitude of other psychological states present in the laboratory. Again, using the hypothetical example, it would be important to know what absolute levels of suspiciousness or perceived task importance subjects were experiencing. This information also places limits on the kinds of inferences that can be drawn by more completely defining the context in which the results are obtained.

These comments should not be taken as an endorsement for overinterpreting the scale values on the measures used to assess psychological states. Given the ordinal nature of most self-report measures, such overemphasis would be inappropriate. However, there is often a tendency to overemphasize group differences and ignore absolute scale values with a concomitant tendency to over-generalize results.

Objective versus Subjective Assessment

The previous sections have implicitly empha-sized the subjects' subjective experience but it is useful to consider this emphasis more explicitly and contrast subjective assessment with what might be called objective assessment. By subjec-tive assessment is meant the research participant's self-reported construal of the laboratory experi-ence. By contrast, objective assessment is taken to mean all other methods of gathering information about the laboratory experience. In some ways this latter term is a misnomer because some "objec-tive" methods rely on the judgments of observers (which are also impressionistic). Nonetheless, the terminology appears to be somewhat standard and is used here.

An obvious issue in the comparison of subjective and objective assessment is validity. Who is more accurate? This question has no easy answer. It depends on the kind of information desired. First, if there is a desire to validate the structural aspects of the manipulation, then objective assessment is usu-ally preferred, if not required. For example, mea-surement equipment can be used to validate sound, temperature, and light levels. External observers can be used to validate that the experimenters and confederates enacted their roles properly. These validations are critical, particularly the latter type where variability in the enactment of the manipula-tion can introduce error into the relation between the manipulation and other variables.

But, if the interest is in the experience of the subjects in the laboratory situation, then the sub-jects may represent the only source of information on that experience (see Tennenbaum & Jacob, this volume). Subjects will act on their perceptions, accurate or not, and so those are the perceptions that must be assessed. The use of judges to report on the meaning of subjects' behavior or self-report is necessarily one more step removed from the phenomenon of interest. Unfortunately, such prac-tice appears to be sufficiently common to require

emphasis. For example, a common practice in at-tribution research is to request an attribution from a group of subjects following a manipulation, but then to either assume, or have judges rate, the location of those causes along underlying dimen-sions. Thus, subjects may say they failed due to ability. Then, as has been true in the Type A liter-ature, the experimenter (or other external judge) may interpret this to mean that the subject made an internal and stable attribution (e.g., see Brunson & Matthews, 1981; Musante, MacDougall, & Dem-broski, 1984; Rhodewalt, 1984). This could be quite wrong. Subjects may vary considerably in their individual interpretations of where causal sources fall along underlying dimensions (see Krantz & Rude, 1984; Strube, 1986; Strube & Boland, 1986) and past research indicates that typ-ical assumptions about dimensional location of common causal sources are often in error (see Bet-ancourt & Weiner, 1982; Meyer & Koelbl, 1982; Ronis, Hansen, & O'Leary, 1983; Russell, 1982). For example, effort and task difficulty have been found to vary in their assumed stability (Elig & Frieze, 1979; Meyer, 1980; Ostrove, 1978; Valle & Frieze, 1976; Weiner, 1979) and luck has been found to shift along the internal–external dimen-sion (Meyer, 1980; Weiner, Nierenberg, & Gold-stein, 1976). This information would be lost if not assessed directly. Thus, whenever the subjects' in-terpretation of the situation is of interest, one should not rely on "objective" assessments of that interpretation (note, however, that external assess-ments of less "cognitive" reactions such as mood states may be advantageous; see Tennenbaum and Jacob, this volume).

Given this emphasis on subjective assessment, an issue of considerable importance is the degree to which subjects *can* validly report their experi-ences. A rather controversial but empirically justi-fiable position has been voiced by Nisbett and Wilson (1977; Wilson, 1985) who argue that under some conditions the cognitive processes that actu-ally guide behavior are not accessible to indi-viduals (they operate outside of awareness) and thus attempts to report on those processes are er-roneous (for empirical support of this proposition, see Nisbett & Bellows, 1977; Wilson, Dunn, By-bee, Hyman, & Rotondo, 1984; Wilson, Hull, &

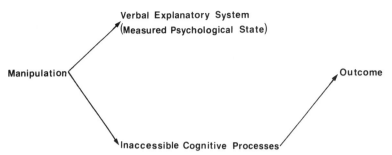

Figure 10. Paths of influence when the verbal explanatory system is engaged.

Johnson, 1981; for additional commentaries on this proposition, see Adair & Spinner, 1981; Ericsson & Simon, 1980; White, 1980). Instead, individuals provide plausible accounts of their behavior based on *a priori* theories about the causal links between stimuli and behavior. In other words, there is a conscious verbal explanatory system that may, under certain conditions, operate independently of the cognitive processes that guide behavior. Although Nisbett and Wilson emphasized a somewhat different situation (retrospective accounts of the causes of behavior) than that considered here (reports on the current psychological states that might influence later behavior), the implications are important to consider. In the present context, the Nisbett and Wilson proposition would argue that the subjects' interpretation of the situation may occur partly out of awareness and not be accessible to subjects in their self-reports. Consequently, the reports that are provided, although plausible, would not be the actual mediators of behavior (see Figure 10). Currently it is difficult to estimate when this problem is most likely to occur (Wilson, 1985) although behaviors that are highly automatic or "scripted" seem likely candidates because we have well-formed implicit theories about the causes of such behavior. Likewise, cognitive processes such as decisions or attributions seem less immune to this problem than intense immediate emotions. Furthermore, particularly salient situational features may prompt erroneous reporting. Until future research clarifies the conditions that induce independence between self-report and actual cognitive mediators, there does not appear to be any viable escape from this situation given the problems with external judges noted above (i.e., there is no guarantee that the judges

can report accurately on the process). Consequently, to the extent that subjects cannot accurately report experiences of importance, the ability to resolve the direct link between manipulation and outcome into some meaningful mediator is reduced.

A third problem related to subject self-report concerns the unwillingness, not the inability, to report accurately on one's perceptions. Biases in self-report have been a topic of considerable interest and debate, and a number of distinct distortions have been proposed. For example, Weber and Cook (1972) reviewed the literature on the roles that subjects may adopt in experimental settings and identified four major types: (1) "good" subjects (Orne, 1962), (2) negative subjects (Masling, 1966), (3) faithful subjects (Fillenbaum, 1966; Fillenbaum & Frey, 1970), and (4) apprehensive subjects (Rosenberg, 1965, 1969).* Good subjects attempt to uncover the experimenter's hypotheses and confirm them. Negative subjects also attempt to learn the experimenter's hypotheses, but with the intent of sabotaging the study (the "screw you" effect; Masling, 1966). Faithful subjects cooperate completely with the experimenter, carry out all instructions without question, and ignore all suspicions. Apprehensive subjects are concerned about the experimenter's evaluation of their abilities, personality, and so forth and react accordingly, such as by providing socially desirable responses (see also Edwards,

---

*Note that instigation of subject roles can arise as a function of the laboratory situation at large, as a function of subject characteristics, and as a function of the manipulation. This latter instance is particularly severe because then the role behavior is correlated or confounded with the manipulation.

1957; Crowne & Marlowe, 1964; Paulhus, 1984). Although there is debate about the independent influence of these roles, their prevalence, and the conditions that elicit them (e.g., Adair & Schachter, 1972; Adair, Spinner, Carlopio, & Lindsay, 1983; Carlston & Cohen, 1980, 1983; Christensen, 1977; Spinner, Adair, & Barnes, 1977), there is sufficient evidence that subjects do act in ways that deviate from their "natural" behavior (Kruglanski, 1975; Weber & Cook, 1972). This has led some to argue that because such role enactment represents a deviation from the subjects' "true" behavior, each role represents an artifact and a threat to the internal validity of the study (actually, this is only true if the enactment of a role is correlated with the manipulation). Others (e.g., Carlopio, Adair, Lindsay, & Spinner, 1983) have argued that all behavior is in some respects "role behavior," representing a person's response to the *perceived* situation. Consequently, measurement and understanding of the subjects' perceived role constraints becomes a topic of conceptual importance. Obviously there is no "correct" answer to this debate; one person's artifact is another person's conceptual variable of interest. Regardless of the side of the debate that a person prefers, the identification of artifact or valid response requires that the *subjects'* experiences be assessed.

Reactivity: The Heisenberg Principle in Social Research

Given that the laboratory researcher cannot escape the necessity of assessing the subjects' construal of the created situation, some additional problems must be recognized. Foremost among these is that the very act of requesting information from subjects may disrupt the phenomenon under study. This is analogous to the Heisenberg principle of uncertainty (Heisenberg, 1958) noted in physics whereby the act of measurement alters the object being measured. Three manifestations of this phenomenon may arise.

First, the mere act of measurement may disrupt the ongoing process by instigating the subject to engage in processing that ordinarily would not occur, and sensitizing the subject to crucial aspects of the study. For example, asking subjects to provide ratings of their perceptions of control, mood, or attributions necessarily prevents them from processing other potentially important aspects of the situation, and may induce them to process information they might ordinarily ignore. This has been a classic criticism of attributional research where it has been suggested that in many situations subjects do not spontaneously engage in attributional processing (see Pittman & D'Agostino, 1985; Wong & Weiner, 1981). Rather, they willingly do so when asked by experimenters. Similarly, both pretest sensitization (Lana, 1969) and posttest sensitization (Bracht & Glass, 1968) can cause problems in this regard. Subjects whose psychological state is assessed prior to the manipulation (for the purpose of examining change) are thus placed in a different psychological state due to measurement compared to nonpretested subjects. Likewise an overt self-report measure of outcome or mediation creates, as well as assesses, a psychological state. The danger is that the phenomenon under study will not readily generalize to situations where the subject is not probed for subjective impressions. Furthermore, there is a danger that the content of the questions will reveal some or all of the experimenter's true purpose and open the study up to a "demand characteristics" criticism (embedding key questions in a lengthier questionnaire composed of extraneous filler items may help reduce this problem).

A second, and related problem is that the nature of the questions asked of the subjects may induce them to make distinctions that they might not ordinarily make. For example, do people make attributions along the various dimensions that have been proposed (e.g., internality, stability, controllability) or is it the case that they *can* do so if asked? Again, it is entirely possible that researchers are investigating theories about constructed realities that bear little resemblance to the real world. This is not to say that such conditions do not exist or could not exist outside the laboratory (Henshel, 1980); they might. But laboratory researchers must be constantly aware of the many ways they channel the experiences of subjects and predetermine what they will find. It would appear that a better balance between confirmatory and exploratory methods in subjective assessment is needed.

A final problem that stems from obtrusive measurement is that repeated assessment (either over time, or multiple variables) either may produce less careful responding due to boredom or fatigue, or may produce more careful responding due to sensitization (see Lana, 1969). Although our previous discussion indicates the need for a complete assessment of the subjects' experiences in the laboratory, a cost is that such comprehensive assessment can be overdone and may distort or destroy the validity and reliability of the data.

Some Solutions for Reactive Responding

The problems of reactive responding discussed in the previous section are potentially serious threats to valid inference. There are several possible solutions to the problem that should be noted, some of which should be avoided. We will assume that the mediating psychological state is of sufficient importance that some assessment is desired, ruling out omission of all measures of the subjects' construal of the laboratory situation.

One solution that clearly should be avoided is to assess the mediating psychological state at the conclusion of the study, after the outcome has been assessed (in an attempt to avoid outcome contamination). This tactic provides very little useful information in that no conclusions concerning mediation can be made (the temporal ordering obviates such a conclusion) and there is no guarantee that the assessment has not been contaminated by the outcome. Furthermore, it may not be possible for subjects to recall accurately their prior psychological states (see Carlsmith *et al.*, 1976; Nisbett & Wilson, 1977; Wilson, 1985).

A second solution is to rely on other indirect assessments that are presumed to correlate with the psychological state. Thus, nonverbal and behavioral assessments might be used as proxies for the direct self-report (see Tennenbaum & Jacob, this volume; see also Webb, Campbell, Schwartz, & Sechrest, 1966; Webb, Campbell, Schwartz, Sech-

rest, & Grove, 1981). The use of this approach carries with it problems related to the validity of such measures in relation to the construct assessed by self-report. Researchers should have strong prior evidence that indirect measures provide suitable substitutes for the direct self-report of the intended psychological state.

There is a third approach that can be used that is characterized by a two-stage procedure. In the first stage, all that is attempted is to demonstrate that the manipulation produces the intended psychological state. The manipulation is carried out and the groups are assessed to determine if they report differences in the predicted direction and of the expected magnitude. No outcome measure is administered because severe reactivity effects are expected. This stage is used to demonstrate the convergent and discriminant validity of the manipulation and should be carried out with the same care as in an actual study (despite its usual classification as a pilot study). The second stage includes the manipulation and the outcome, but no intervening assessment (and thus no contamination); it is assumed that the appropriate intervening psychological stage mediates outcome. This type of procedure can be made somewhat more powerful by including indirect measures in both phases, thus providing a crucial point of contact. The procedure is, however, an imperfect solution because mediation cannot be assessed directly and there is no guarantee that the assessment itself does not induce, at least in part, the psychological state. The only solution to this problem is to conduct two complete studies (outcome assessed in both) but where the assessment of psychological state is omitted in one study. Comparability of outcome differences would allow the argument that reactivity was not a problem.

When Manipulations Fail: The Role of Internal Analyses

Despite the researcher's best efforts, manipulations can and do fail. That is, analyses may indicate an instance of Case 4 (Figure 2) where the manipulation has no discernible effect on the proposed mediator nor the outcome variable. From a logical standpoint, the experiment has failed and no causal inferences can be made. Yet it is still possible to obtain valuable information from the study through the use of internal analyses of subjects' perceptions. Using our previous example, the question to be asked is: "Given that the manipulation did not produce changes in perceived control loss or physiology, is perceived control loss *related* to physiology?" Essentially, one is interested in whether individuals who differ in perceived control loss (for whatever reason) also differ in physiology. As can be seen, this is one of the crucial pieces of information that is required to infer the existence of a mediator. If the internal analyses indicate that the mediator and outcome are correlated significantly, then there is justification for attempting to construct a more reliable and powerful manipulation. It is critical to realize, however, that the internal analysis provides little guidance as to what form that new manipulation might take, nor does it allow the inference that the mediator is causally linked to the outcome.

Measurement Scales: An Old Problem Revisited

One final topic to be discussed is the issue of measurement scales. Measurement scales are a topic familiar to most researchers who early in their training learn the essential differences between nominal, ordinal, interval, and ratio assessments (Stevens, 1946, 1968). Discussing all the ramifications of scale choice is well beyond the scope of this chapter. It will suffice to point out that the choice of measurement scale is not as trivial as most researchers think, and the controversy over appropriate scaling continues to rage (e.g., Gaito, 1980; Lodge, 1981; Maxwell & Delaney, 1985; Michell, 1986; Townsend & Ashby, 1984; Wegener, 1982). Its importance in the present context follows from our previous discussion of mediators. Thus far, we have discussed the mediator–outcome relation as though the shape of that relation did not matter. But as knowledge and theory advance we are often in a position to specify precisely the "shape" of the relation. The ability to accurately test such hypotheses requires that measurement scales be used that

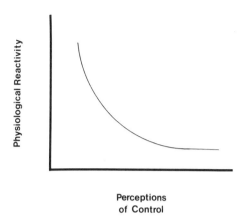

Figure 11. Spurious relationship arising from scaling artifact.

are equal to the task. Consider again our example of perceived control loss and physiological response and assume that we assess subjects' perceived control loss using a typical ordinal five-point scale (1 = no control, 2 = slight control, 3 = some control, 4 = moderate control, 5 = complete control). Assume also that we hypothesize a nonlinear relation between perceived control loss and physiological reactivity (see Figure 11).

Given that our perceived control scale is only ordinal in nature it is entirely possible to achieve such results artifactually (if, for example, the scale is less sensitive in the upper region). The point is that although we are not likely to do much damage by ignoring measurement scales in the sense of detecting the presence of a relation, we might err considerably in determining the shape of that relation. It is not as difficult as once thought to construct interval and ratio scales of social attitudes and opinions (Lodge, 1981). Thus, whenever the shape of the relation is of importance (some would say regardless of its importance), researchers should use measurement scales that can achieve the results predicted without artifact.

Conclusion

This chapter began with the statement that measurement of the subjects' construal of the laboratory experience is central to understanding the processes under investigation. It was argued that rather than being of secondary importance as manipulation checks and ancillary evidence (see Kazdin, 1980), the subjects' reported experiences are central to both the logic and interpretation of the experiment. Regardless of the situation that the experimenter has created, the subjects' view of that situation *is* the situation of interest and great care must be taken to ensure that situation is assessed completely. We must resist the egocentric temptation to interpret the laboratory experience from our standpoint as researchers and instead be willing to "get inside the head" of our subjects and view the situation from their perspectives (see Orne, 1973). It is, after all, our subjects' behavior, not our own, that we wish to explain.

References

Adair, J. G., & Schachter, B. S. (1972). To cooperate or to look good? The subjects' and experimenters' perceptions of each others' intentions. *Journal of Experimental Social Psychology, 8,* 74–85.

Adair, J. G., & Spinner, B. (1981). Subjects' access to cognitive processes: Demand characteristics and verbal report. *Journal for the Theory of Social Behavior, 11,* 31–52.

Adair, J. G., Spinner, B., Carlopio, J., & Lindsay, R. (1983). Where is the source of artifact? Subject roles or hypothesis learning. *Journal of Personality and Social Psychology, 45,* 1229–1231.

Anastasi, A. (1976). *Psychological testing* (4th ed.). New York: Macmillan Co.

Asher, H. B. (1963). *Causal modeling* (2nd ed.). Beverly Hills, CA: Sage.

Baron, R. M., & Kenny, D. A. (1986). The moderator-mediator variable distinction in social psychological research: Conceptual, strategic, and statistical considerations. *Journal of Personality and Social Psychology, 51,* 1173–1182.

Betancourt, H., & Weiner, B. (1982). Attributions for achievement-related events, expectancy, and sentiments: A study of success and failure in Chile and the United States. *Journal of Cross-Cultural Psychology, 13,* 362–374.

Bracht, G. H., & Glass, G. V. (1968). The external validity of experiments. *American Educational Research Journal, 5,* 437–474.

Brunson, B. I., & Matthews, K. A. (1981). The Type A coronary-prone behavior pattern and reactions to uncontrollable stress: An analysis of performance strategies, affect, and attributions during failure. *Journal of Personality and Social Psychology, 40,* 906–918.

Campbell, D. T. (1963). From description to experimentation: Interpreting trends as quasi-experiments. In C. W. Harris

(Ed.), *Problems in measuring change.* Madison: University of Wisconsin Press.

Carlopio, J., Adair, J. G., Lindsay, R. C. L., & Spinner, B. (1983). Avoiding artifact in the search for bias: The importance of assessing subjects' perceptions of the experiment. *Journal of Personality and Social Psychology, 44,* 693–701.

Carlsmith, J. M., Ellsworth, P. C., & Aronson, E. (1976). *Methods of research in social psychology.* Reading, MA: Addison–Wesley.

Carlston, D. E., & Cohen, J. L. (1980). A closer examination of subject roles. *Journal of Personality and Social Psychology, 38,* 857–870.

Carlston, D. E., & Cohen, J. L. (1983). Avoiding bias in the search for artifact: A reply to Carlopio, Adair, Lindsay, and Spinner. *Journal of Personality and Social Psychology, 45,* 1225–1228.

Christensen, L. (1977). The negative subject: Myth, reality, or a prior experimental experience effect? *Journal of Personality and Social Psychology, 35,* 392–400.

Cook, T. D., & Campbell, D. T. (1979). *Quasi-experimentation: Design & analysis issues for field settings.* Chicago: Rand McNally.

Crano, W. D., & Brewer, M. B. (1986). *Principles and methods of social research.* Boston: Allyn & Bacon.

Crowne, D. P., & Marlowe, D. (1964). *The approval motive: Studies in evaluation dependence.* New York: Wiley.

Edwards, A. L. (1957). *Techniques of attitude scale construction.* New York: Appleton–Century–Crofts.

Elig, T. W., & Frieze, I. H. (1979). Measuring causal attributions for success and failure. *Journal of Personality and Social Psychology, 37,* 621–634.

Ericsson, K. A., & Simon, H. A. (1980). Verbal reports as data. *Psychological Review, 87,* 215–251.

Fillenbaum, S. (1966). Prior description and subsequent experimental performance: The "faithful" subject. *Journal of Personality and Social Psychology, 4,* 532–537.

Fillenbaum, S., & Frey, R. (1970). More on the "faithful" behavior of suspicious subjects. *Journal of Personality, 38,* 43–51.

Gaito, J. (1980). Measurement scales and statistics: Resurgence of an old misconception. *Psychological Bulletin, 87,* 564–567.

Heider, F. (1958). *The psychology of interpersonal relations.* New York: Wiley.

Heise, D. R. (1975). *Causal analysis.* New York: Wiley.

Heisenberg, W. (1958). *Physics and philosophy.* New York: Harper & Row.

Henshel, R. L. (1980). The purposes of laboratory experimentation and the virtues of deliberate artificiality. *Journal of Experimental Social Psychology, 16,* 466–478.

Jones, E. E., & Davis, K. E. (1965). From acts to dispositions: The attribution process in person perception. In L. Berkowitz (Ed.), *Advances in experimental social psychology* (Vol. 2, pp. 219–266). New York: Academic Press.

Jöreskog, K. G., & Sörbom, D. (1984). *LISREL VI: Analysis of linear structural relationships by the method of maximum likelihood.* Mooresville, IN: Scientific Software, Inc.

Judd, C. M., & Kenny, D. A. (1981a). *Estimating the effects of social interventions.* Cambridge: Cambridge University Press.

Judd, C. M., & Kenny, D. A. (1981b). Process analysis: Estimating mediation in treatment evaluations. *Evaluation Review, 5,* 602–619.

Kazdin, A. E. (1980). *Research design in clinical psychology.* New York: Harper & Row.

Kelley, H. H. (1967). Attribution theory in social psychology. In D. Levine (Ed.), *Nebraska symposium on motivation* (Vol. 15, pp. 192–240). Lincoln: University of Nebraska Press.

Kelley, H. H. (1973). The process of causal attribution. *American Psychologist, 28,* 107–128.

Kelly, G. A. (1955). *The psychology of personal constructs.* New York: Norton.

Kenny, D. A. (1979). *Correlation and causality.* New York: Wiley.

Kidder, L. H., & Judd, C. M. (1986). *Research methods in social relations* (5th ed.). New York: Holt, Rinehart, & Winston.

Krantz, S. E., & Rude, S. (1984). Depressive attributions: Selection of different causes or assignment of dimensional meanings? *Journal of Personality and Social Psychology, 47,* 193–203.

Kruglanski, A. W. (1975). The human subject in the psychology experiment: Fact and artifact. In L. Berkowitz (Ed.), *Advances in experimental social psychology* (Vol. 8, pp. 101–147). New York: Academic Press.

Lana, R. E. (1969). Pretest sensitization. In R. Rosenthal & R. Rosnow (Eds.), *Artifact in behavioral research* (pp. 119–141). New York: Academic Press.

Lodge, M. (1981). *Magnitude scaling: Quantitative measurement of opinions.* Beverly Hills, CA: Sage.

Masling, J. (1966). Role-related behavior of the subject and psychologist and its effects upon psychological data. In D. Levine (Ed.), *Nebraska symposium on motivation* (Vol. 14, pp. 67–103). Lincoln: University of Nebraska Press.

Maxwell, S. E., & Delaney, H. D. (1985). Measurement scales and statistics: An examination of construct validity. *Psychological Bulletin, 97,* 85–93.

Meyer, J. P. (1980). Causal attributions for success and failure: A multivariate investigation of dimensionality, formation, and consequences. *Journal of Personality and Social Psychology, 38,* 704–718.

Meyer, J. P., & Koelbl, S. L. M. (1982). Students' test performance: Dimensionality of causal attributions. *Personality and Social Psychology Bulletin, 8,* 31–36.

Michell, J. (1986). Measurement scales and statistics: A clash of paradigms. *Psychological Bulletin, 100,* 398–407.

Musante, L., MacDougall, J. M., & Dembroski, T. M. (1984). The Type A behavior pattern and attributions for success and failure. *Personality and Social Psychology Bulletin, 10,* 544–553.

Nisbett, R. E., & Bellows, N. (1977). Verbal reports about causal influences on social judgments: Private access versus public theories. *Journal of Personality and Social Psychology, 35,* 613–624.

Nisbett, R. E., & Wilson, T. D. (1977). Telling more than we can know: Verbal reports on mental processes. *Psychological Review, 84,* 231–259.

Nunnally, J. C. (1978). *Psychometric theory* (2nd ed.). New York: McGraw-Hill.

Orne, M. T. (1962). On the social psychology of the psychological experiment: With particular reference to demand characteristics and their implications. *American Psychologist, 17,* 776–783.

Orne, M. T. (1973). Communication by the total experimental situation: Why it is important, how it is evaluated, and its significance for the ecological validity of findings. In P. Pliner, L. Krames, & T. Alloway (Eds.), *Communication and affect.* New York: Academic Press.

Ostrove, N. (1978). Expectations for success on effort-determined tasks as a function of incentive and performance feedback. *Journal of Personality and Social Psychology, 36,* 909–916.

Paulhus, D. L. (1984). Two-component models of socially desirable responding. *Journal of Personality and Social Psychology, 46,* 598–609.

Pittman, T. S., & D'Agostino, P. R. (1985). Motivation and attribution: The effects of control deprivation on subsequent information processing. In J. H. Harvey & G. Weary (Eds.), *Attribution: Basic issues and applications* (pp. 117–141). New York: Academic Press.

Rhodewalt, F. (1984). Self-attribution, self-involvement, and the Type A coronary-prone behavior pattern. *Journal of Personality and Social Psychology, 47,* 662–670.

Ronis, D. L., Hansen, R. D., & O'Leary, V. E. (1983). Understanding the meaning of achievement attributions: A test of derived locus and stability scores. *Journal of Personality and Social Psychology, 44,* 702–711.

Rosenberg, M. (1965). When dissonance fails: On eliminating evaluation apprehension from attitude measurement. *Journal of Personality and Social Psychology, 1,* 28–42.

Rosenberg, M. (1969). The conditions and consequences of evaluation apprehension. In R. Rosenthal & R. Rosnow (Eds.), *Artifact in behavioral research* (pp. 279–349). New York: Academic Press.

Rosenthal, R., & Gaito, J. (1963). The interpretation of levels of significance by psychological researchers. *Journal of Psychology, 55,* 33–38.

Rosenthal, R., & Gaito, J. (1964). Further evidence for the cliff effect in the interpretation of levels of significance. *Psychological Reports, 15,* 570.

Rosenthal, R., & Rosnow, R. L. (Eds.). (1969). *Artifact in behavioral research.* New York: Academic Press.

Russell, D. (1982). The causal dimension scale: A measure of how individuals perceive causes. *Journal of Personality and Social Psychology, 42,* 1137–1145.

Spinner, B., Adair, J. G., & Barnes, G. E. (1977). A reexamination of the faithful subject role. *Journal of Experimental Social Psychology, 13,* 543–551.

Stacy, A. W., Widaman, K. F., Hays, R., & DiMatteo, M. R. (1985). Validity of self-reports of alcohol and other drug use:

A multitrait–multimethod assessment. *Journal of Personality and Social Psychology, 49,* 219–232.

Stevens, S. S. (1946). On the theory of scales of measurement. *Science, 103,* 677–680.

Stevens, S. S. (1968). Measurement, statistics, and the schemapiric view. *Science, 161,* 849–856.

Strube, M. J. (1986, August). *Type A behavior and post-performance attributions.* Presented at the 94th meeting of the American Psychological Association, Washington, DC.

Strube, M. J., & Boland, S. M. (1986). Post-performance attributions and task persistence among Type A and B individuals: A clarification. *Journal of Personality and Social Psychology, 50,* 413–420.

Townsend, J. T., & Ashby, F. G. (1984). Measurement scales and statistics: The misconception misconceived. *Psychological Bulletin, 96,* 394–401.

Valle, V. A., & Frieze, I. H. (1976). Stability of causal attributions as a mediator in changing expectations for success. *Journal of Personality and Social Psychology, 33,* 579–587.

Webb, E. J., Campbell, D. T., Schwartz, R. D., & Sechrest, L. (1966). *Unobtrusive measures: Nonreactive research in the social sciences.* Chicago: Rand McNally.

Webb, E. J., Campbell, D. T., Schwartz, R. D., Sechrest, L., & Grove, L. (1981). *Nonreactive measures in the social sciences.* Boston: Houghton Mifflin.

Weber, S. J., & Cook, T. D. (1972). Subject effects in laboratory research: An examination of subject roles, demand characteristics, and valid inference. *Psychological Bulletin, 77,* 273–295.

Wegener, B. (Ed.). (1982). *Social attitudes and psychophysical measurement.* Hillsdale, NJ: Erlbaum.

Weiner, B. (1979). A theory of motivation for some classroom experiences. *Journal of Educational Psychology, 71,* 3–25.

Weiner, B., Nierenberg, R., & Goldstein, M. (1976). Social learning (locus of control) versus attribution (causal stability) interpretations of expectancy of success. *Journal of Personality, 44,* 52–68.

White, P. (1980). Limitations on verbal reports of internal events: A refutation of Nisbett and Wilson and of Bem. *Psychological Review, 87,* 105–112.

Wilson, T. D. (1985). Strangers to ourselves: The origins and accuracy of beliefs about one's own mental states. In J. H. Harvey & G. Weary (Eds.), *Attribution: Basic issues and applications* (pp. 9–36). New York: Academic Press.

Wilson, T. D., Dunn, D. S., Bybee, J. A., Hyman, D. B., & Rotondo, J. A. (1984). Effects of analyzing reasons on attitude–behavior consistency. *Journal of Personality and Social Psychology, 47,* 5–16.

Wilson, T. D., Hull, J. G., & Johnson, J. (1981). Awareness and self-perception: Verbal reports on internal states. *Journal of Personality and Social Psychology, 40,* 53–71.

Wong, P. T. P., & Weiner, B. (1981). When people ask "why" questions, and the heuristics of attributional search. *Journal of Personality and Social Psychology, 40,* 650–663.

CHAPTER 34

Observational Methods for Assessing Psychological State

Daniel L. Tennenbaum and Theodore Jacob

Psychological States of Interest

Interest in the emotional responding of subjects has a well-established and important role in many sectors of the behavioral and biological sciences. As such, methods for describing the current psychological state of subjects need to be given careful attention. Investigators have become increasingly aware of problems associated with requesting immediate self-reports from subjects regarding their emotional state. An important and potentially effective alternative to self-report approaches is to gather data on emotional state through observational procedures. The purpose of this chapter is to review some of the better alternatives available for conducting such assessments both with individual subjects and during dyadic interactions.

Although the expression ''psychological state'' has many possible meanings, readers probably will have the most interest in assessing the various emotional responses exhibited by subjects. Possible reasons for conducting such assessments include attempting to confirm that experimental procedures have actually induced intended emotional

states, or determining whether specific emotions are differentially elicited from groups divided on theoretically interesting variables (e.g., hypertensive fathers compared to normotensive fathers). Hopefully, a more sophisticated understanding of cardiovascular reactivity will result from the use of concurrent assessments of emotion and psychophysiology.

The programmatic work of Ekman and Friesen (1982) will figure prominently in the following discussion because their work is so closely related to the concerns of this chapter and because they have greatly stimulated the field. Additional focus will be on the development of coding systems designed to describe ongoing behavior: Ekman and Friesen (1978) with a molecular focus on the expression of affect in the face and Weiss (Hops, Wills, Weiss, & Patterson, 1972; Weiss & Summers, 1983) and Gottman (1979, 1983) with their attempts to describe dyadic interactions. Additionally, paralinguistic indexes of speech will be briefly covered.

Although our vocabulary includes words for describing many emotional states and their various gradations, both theoretical (Tomkins, 1962, 1963, 1982) and practical considerations suggest that only a relatively small group of emotional expressions are of value to investigate. At the most general level, coding systems have categorized behaviors

Daniel L. Tennenbaum • Department of Psychology, Kent State University, Kent, Ohio 44242. *Theodore Jacob* • Division of Family Studies, University of Arizona, Tucson, Arizona 85721.

into positive emotional expressions, negative emotional expressions, or neutral ones. Even when more discrete emotions are originally coded, they may be grouped into these three categories for the purposes of analysis (e.g., Gottman & Levenson, 1985). Ekman and Friesen (1975), building on the theoretical work of Tomkins and their own empirical efforts, have identified six primary emotions: happiness, sadness, disgust, anger, fear, and surprise. These emotions have become the focus of their work.

Justification for Use of Observational Procedures

Whether we actually can determine the emotional experience of another person is an important issue to address prior to discussing relevant coding systems. At a personal level, all of us frequently make predictions about what people around us are feeling. This is necessary in order for us to respond appropriately to our families, friends, and associates. Our survival in a socially complex world is evidence that our predictions are often accurate. Our personal experiences, therefore, suggest that we can assess psychological state through observational procedures. However, to qualify this conclusion, all people are not equally good at perceiving affective expressions accurately. Some people either are better observers, or are better able to integrate and interpret what they observe, or a combination of both of these factors (Zuroff & Colussy, 1986).

Clearly, this intuitively based argument needs to be supported by empirical evidence. An initial question concerning whether individuals can recognize the same emotion from the same stimuli has already been addressed. Judgment studies have been conducted in which subjects are asked to describe particular stimuli, for example, photographs of faces with posed emotional expressions. Although conceptual problems exist with the use of such stimuli, adults appear able to identify and differentiate a small group of emotional expressions (Izard, 1971).

Although individuals recognize the facial expressions of certain emotions, it does not necessarily follow that they actually use these behaviors themselves when expressing emotion. Ekman and Friesen (1975) suggest that although facial behaviors may be universal, each culture develops "display rules" which govern when and in what way individuals will modify their emotional expressions. For example, they compared American and Japanese subjects watching emotion-eliciting films under two conditions: one when the subjects were alone, and another when an authority figure was present in the room. As expected, similar emotional expressions were observed across groups during the "alone" condition but different emotional responses were observed when the authority figure was present (Friesen, 1972). Awareness of the potential impact of display rules is helpful for designing experiments because it explicitly encourages the use of procedures that do not lead to subjects managing their emotional expression.

Overall, there appears to be some justification for assessing emotional states using observational procedures. Various procedures will now be described which do just that. As an organizational aid, the contexts within which assessments will take place will be described first.

Contexts of Assessment

The need to assess emotional states arises in investigations which use quite different procedures. Each procedure, however, constrains in some way the type of data gathered. A primary consideration is who is present in the experimental context. Often, studies involve the assessment of individual subjects being conducted through a laboratory procedure. Another possibility involves strangers interacting with one another. Finally, the importance of assessing behavior in relevant social contexts has led to an increasing interest in the observational study of family interaction (Jacob & Tennenbaum, 1988). Within the family, marital interaction has been an important focus of observational study. Additionally, investigators have assessed various combinations of parent–child groupings (Baer, Vincent, Williams, Bourianoff, & Bartlett, 1980).

Another context-related issue is whether observable emotional expressions are elicited by a particular experimental procedure. Investigators will always need to determine, at the very onset, whether subjects are influenced enough by a particular procedure for visible responses to be observed. The coding systems to be described all assume a minimal visible level of emotional expression.

Individual Subject Assessments

Before discussing specific coding systems, the general process followed by most coding systems will be presented. A coding system usually contains a series of well-specified rules that allow independent raters to make similar decisions with regard to the occurrence of specific behaviors. Coders use a permanent record of subjects behavior, usually a videotape, which they watch until they can correctly describe the observed behaviors. This is a time-consuming activity which usually involves the repetition of small segments of tape because of the detail that is required. The use of a time-date generator or other visual or audible signal on the tape allows raters to locate observed behaviors in time. Although variations exist (e.g., some coding systems described in subsequent sections require transcripts of interactions in addition to the videotape), the coding systems to be described follow this pattern.

Face

Although various nonverbal and verbal cues have been investigated (Harper, Wiens, & Matarazzo, 1978), including body movements and voice tone, a major emphasis has been placed on the role of the face in emotional expression. Theoretical positions originally advanced by Darwin (1872) and more recently by Tomkins (1962, 1982) encouraged this choice of assessment target. Ekman and Friesen (1982) have argued that a focus on specific facial behaviors (movements of facial muscles) is necessary so that precise descriptions of emotional expressions can be documented. Stimulated by Tomkins' (1962, 1963, 1982) theory of emotion, Ekman and Friesen, as well as Izard

(1979) have developed coding systems designed to capture emotional expression in the face. [See Ekman (1982) for a review of facial action coding systems.] Increasing sophistication in this area, gained by having conducted programmatic research since the late 1960s, has led to the development of a series of coding systems for assessing the face.

An early version, the Facial Affect Scoring Technique (FAST; Ekman, Friesen, & Tomkins, 1971), was designed to assess facial behavior relevant to six basic emotions: happiness, sadness, anger, surprise, fear, and disgust. The FAST requires raters to make judgments concerning the presence of specific facial features in three areas of the face: brow and forehead, eyes and lids, lower face. Raters use a catalogue containing relevant pictures of specific types of facial features that were to be assessed. Rather than using written descriptions, coders match particular features in a target face with those in the FAST catalogue. Coders, therefore, made judgments about the presence or absence of facial features and not about particular emotions. Specification of which emotion is being expressed is accomplished by the use of formulas which integrate the ratings across these three facial zones.

Building on the FAST, Ekman and Friesen developed a new coding system, the Facial Action Coding System (FACS; Ekman & Freisen, 1978), which, as its name implies, explicitly codes all possible facial movements. Rather than focusing on facial features in three arbitrary regions of the face as was done in the FAST, the FACS is used to assess changes in facial features using more natural units of behavior. That is, it attempts to describe the movements of facial muscles acting alone and in combination. With all facial movements coded (assigned the appropriate facial action number) an expanded amount of material is available for integration which, in turn, allows for a more thorough understanding of facial behavior. The comprehensiveness of the FACS broadens the potential scope of research so that facial movements correlated with emotions can be identified in a more sophisticated manner, and so that other functions of facial movements can be studied.

The FACS is applied to videotapes of subjects

because the focus is on actions rather than on static features. The start and end points of each movement are recorded so that the duration of behaviors can be determined. As a more comprehensive system, it takes considerable time (approximately 100 h) to train coders to use the FACS. Reported reliability for the FACS is high (above 70% agreement between coders). Reports of facial actions are integrated using formulas which characterize the meaning of a particular combination of facial movements.

Using the FACS, Ekman and Friesen (1982) have been able to differentiate different types of smiles: true happy smiles, smiles which were intended to deceive the observer, and smiles conveying sadness. The FACS has also been used in an investigation of the venerable question concerning whether specific emotions, in this case happiness, sadness, anger, disgust, fear, and surprise, can be differentiated by autonomic nervous system activity (Ekman, Levenson, & Friesen, 1982). Subjects were asked to both pose and relive these six emotions while various measures of autonomic activity were recorded. They used the FACS to determine when subjects were experiencing the particular emotions of interest. The emotions were differentiable physiologically only during the periods of time identified by the FACS as containing the appropriate emotion. These strong results, in answering a historically difficult question, lend support to the value of the FACS in describing facial behaviors relevant to the description of particular emotional states.

The frequent interest in assessing emotional expression, rather than other facial behaviors, led the authors of the FACS to develop a modified version which only includes facial movements believed to be related to emotion. This Emotional FACS (EMFACS; Ekman & Friesen, 1982) includes other modifications; e.g., only requiring coders to identify the occurrence of a behavior rather than its duration which decreases the amount of time needed for its application. Although EMFACS coders still need to be trained on the FACS, time is saved during the application of the system. As a new coding system, the EMFACS has not been extensively used as yet. The quality of its predecessor, however, suggests that it will become a reasonable

choice for the assessment of emotions when the additional material contained in the FACS is not needed.

Paralinguistic Measures

In addition to facial movements, other features of subjects' behaviors have been investigated with respect to their relationship to emotional state. Paralinguistic measures of speech, including speech dysfluency, speech rate, and talk time (or silence), have all been related to a particular emotional state—anxiety. Mahl, the major influence on the use of speech disfluencies, was interested in indicators of anxiety to be found in the content-free aspects of speech of clients during psychotherapy interviews (Kasl & Mahl, 1965; Mahl, 1956, 1959). He developed a speech disturbance ratio (SDR) which was divided into an "ah" ratio, which is not strongly related to anxiety, and a "non ah" ratio (e.g., stutters, word repetitions). The "non ah" ratio has been shown to be higher in subjects who are experiencing anxiety (Horowitz, Weckler, Saxon, Lirandais, & Boutacoff, 1977; Jurich & Jurich, 1974; Kasl & Mahl, 1965). Decreased total talk time and an increasing duration of silent pauses between speeches have also been related to increased levels of anxiety (Murray, 1971).

The advantages of these paralinguistic measures are that rater training is relatively simple and only limited equipment is needed. A limitation is that the majority of studies using these indices have involved somewhat artificial contexts. For example, subjects have often been assessed while giving a speech or during a conversation. How appropriate these measures are for assessing relative anxiety in other contexts is not well documented. Another problem with these paralinguistic measures is that although they are procedurally simple, they can still take considerable time to apply. Whether the investment is worth it depends on whether anxiety is a primary psychological state of interest to the investigator. Finally, these measures provide summary statistics for entire observational periods rather than continuous measures of affect, which makes them inappropriate for assessing affect at specific moments in time.

Voice Characteristics

Voice characteristics are also features of speech that convey emotional meaning. Similar to our personal experience with interpreting facial expressions, we are sensitive to the emotional aspects of voice qualities. However, both methodological and technological problems have hindered gathering the necessary support for the validity of these features as appropriate for identifying specific emotional states (Scherer, 1979). Guided by new theories (Scherer, 1986), advances in the interpretation of emotion from voice qualities are currently taking place, but more research still needs to be conducted before such assessments can be productively used in the assessment of emotional state.

Dyadic Assessments

Problem Solving, Affect Combinations

The preceding assessment tools all evolved out of an interest in determining various psychological states primarily of subjects assessed individually in a laboratory context. Another stream of research, interested in marital and family interaction, has led to the development of observational coding systems aimed at assessing dyadic and small group interaction. As the importance of understanding behavior in naturalistic contexts gains further support, the value of these instruments to investigators interested in family influences on cardiovascular functioning will increase. A current study being conducted by Karen Mathews—involving the relationship between physiological measures of reactivity and concurrent emotional expression in family members—exemplifies this trend. The instruments to be discussed next were developed to assess interactions in family contexts although their use for the assessment of the interactions of strangers is also appropriate.

The Marital Interaction Coding System (MICS; Hops *et al.*, 1972), now in its third version (Weiss & Summers, 1983), has played a very influential role in marital interaction research and is probably

the most frequently used coding system in this area of research. The MICS was developed to describe the behavior of couples as they engaged in videotaped problem-solving discussions in a laboratory setting. The 30 MICS codes provide a minimally inferential behavioral description of couples communication during a problem-solving interaction. The MICS-III provides seven summary categories for grouping the 30 codes: Problem Description, Blame, Proposal for Change, Validation, Invalidation, Facilitation, and Irrelevant. Behavior is coded sequentially so that patterns of interaction can be described. The most recent version also has provisions for making a simultaneous record of both speaker and listener behavior, again to allow for a more complete interpretation of observed patterns.

Notwithstanding the many strengths of the MICS, there is an important limitation in using this procedure to describe emotional state. Although certain code categories are often accompanied by the expected positive or negative affect, neither the molecular codes nor the summary codes explicitly describe affective behavior. When applied to the MICS, various multivariate procedures do identify a factor which falls along a positive–negative dimension (Jacob & Krahn, 1987). Although labeled as positive or negative, however, the codes that load on this factor include an unspecified mixture of content and affect rather than solely a description of observed affect.

The MICS has led to one interesting finding related to research on cardiovascular disorders. When comparing normotensive to hypertensive families during conflict discussions involving the parents and one child, differences in the rates of nonverbal-negative behaviors were found (Baer *et al.*, 1980). This effect was attributable to differences in only one code—Not Tracking—a listener code which occurred more frequently in hypertensive families, particularly when the speaker was making a negative comment. This finding was followed up by another study (Baer *et al.*, 1983) that directly rated ''gaze aversion'' and confirmed the original result.

A more recent study from a different laboratory, which assessed communication behavior using the MICS and compared the occurrence of MICS behaviors with gaze aversion coded separately, was unable to replicate the previous findings (Woodall, 1986). This study included additional control groups containing families with an alcoholic or depressed father. Gaze aversion was found to be related to psychopathology rather than to hypertension in normal families. Although the validity of the gaze aversion hypothesis in hypertensive families remains in doubt, the MICS has already played a stimulating role in this area of research.

Building on work from several research areas, Gottman and his colleagues created the Couples Interaction Scoring System (CISS; Gottman, 1979). The CISS, like the MICS, was also developed to describe marital interaction during problem-solving discussions. Each behavior described using the CISS, however, receives two types of codes: a problem-solving or content code and an affect rating. The problem-solving codes were derived from the MICS codes, a coding system developed by Olson and Ryder (1970), and Gottman's own experiences in observing couples. In addition to developing new content codes, such as Summarizing Self and Summarizing Other, an important innovation in the CISS is the separate coding of affect.

The affect rating system requires raters to identify behavior as positive, negative, or neutral. The instructions for determining the affect rating are an integration of the cues identified by Ekman and Friesen as being related to the expression of specific positive and negative emotions. This dual coding of content and affect allowed for a more differentiated view of the resulting codes. Gottman reported that Disagree (which is usually collapsed into a negative summary category) was sometimes spoken in a neutral tone and sometimes in a negative tone. Greater differences were obtained between maritally distressed and nondistressed couples when the more homogeneous negative Disagree codes were analyzed. The CISS, therefore, offers a more informative description of the behavior being engaged in by each spouse and one more directly related to emotional state.

Affect

Continuing with the direction begun by the CISS affect rating system, Gottman then developed a coding system, the Coding System for Specific Affect (SPAFF; 1983), that is focused entirely on emotional expression observable during marital interaction. Previous marital research had documented the importance of negative behaviors in the differentiation of distressed and nondistressed couples as well as cycles of negative affect reciprocity which have been found to be more common in distressed couples (Gottman, 1979; Margolin & Wampold, 1981). However, since the majority of this work had utilized coding systems that did not specifically code for affect, but rather captured some combination of affect and content within their codes, such a coding system was a logical next step. As a newer coding system, its use has been limited, but it appears to be a very promising approach.

The development of the SPAFF began as an attempt to extend the affect rating section of the CISS by integrating the advances found in the FACS (Ekman & Friesen, 1978). Rather than a simple extension of the FACS, however, Gottman found that a new approach was required for adequately capturing affective expression in this complex interactional situation. His experience in observing marital behavior led him to conceptualize two types of coding systems—the "physical specimen" and "cultural informant" approaches. Traditional behavioral coding systems, such as the MICS and FACS, fall into the physical specimen variety because they attempt to carefully define the exact behavior described by each code. He found that as he expanded his affect coding system to include rules for describing how every spouse expressed a particular emotion, his code definitions became increasingly complex and burdensome. As a solution, he adopted an alternative approach which was to focus on using coders who were naturally good and experienced at recognizing emotional expression. Initially he used actors because of their skills and training. He then guided their natural ability with systematic knowledge derived from the FACS and other standard criteria for interpreting emotional expression so that coding could still be conducted in a reliable manner. Because it ultimately relies on the expert knowledge of coders, the SPAFF is an example of what he would call a cultural informant coding system.

Coders work with a videotape and a verbatim

transcript of the interaction when applying SPAFF codes. The ten SPAFF codes include four positive codes, broadly suggested by the following code category names: P1—Humor, P2—Affection, Caring, P3—Interest, Curiosity, and P4—Anticipation, Surprise, Excitement, Enjoyment, Joy. The five negative codes are broadly suggested by the following category names: N1—Anger, N2—Disgust, Scorn, Contempt, N3—Whining, N4—Sadness, and N5—Anxiety, Stress, Worry, Fear. The tenth code is for Neutral expressions.

The SPAFF has been used to compare the ratings of husbands' and wives' reports of their own feelings to those of outside observers (Gottman & Levenson, 1985). In this study, spouses were asked to return to the laboratory to rate their own videotapes using a dial ranging from 1, very negative, to 9, very positive. Among other interesting findings, they found a positive relationship between spouse ratings of their feelings and summary codes of positive, negative, and neutral, obtained from the SPAFF. This result needs to be replicated so that its strength can be clarified.

Although a new and time-consuming instrument, the SPAFF has considerable potential for being a valuable tool for identifying psychological state during complex dyadic interactions. While continued investigation of the psychometric properties of this instrument is needed, it is the primary interest for assessing emotional expression during marital discussions. Since the level of differentiation offered by the ten code categories covers many of the important emotions of interest, the use of this instrument needs to be strongly considered in laboratory investigations of dyadic behavior.

Another nonintrusive approach to assessing psychological state, suggested by the study in the SPAFF description, is to have subjects rate their own behavior. Although stopping in the middle of a laboratory procedure and asking subjects how they feel is intrusive and creates methodological confounds, potentially interesting self-report data may still be gathered in other ways; specifically, by having spouses rate their own videotapes after the laboratory procedure is complete.

The only study in the marital literature which has assessed spouses' reports of their own feelings during an interaction with trained coders also explicitly assessing affect is the previously mentioned study by Gottman and Levenson (1985) using the SPAFF. In that study they did find some agreement between spouses' and observers' reports of emotional expression. This initial support for the validity of such a procedure needs to be supplemented so that the experimental contexts and characteristics of subjects that optimize this strategy can be identified.

Compatibility with Concurrent Psychophysiological Measurements

Since the James–Lange (James, 1884) theory of emotion was popularized, which stated that emotions occurred as a response to specific physiological changes, theories of emotion and the assessment of emotion have been inextricably intertwined with physiological assessments. Even though other theories have arisen (Schachter & Singer, 1962), interest in the relationship of psychological phenomenon to physiological phenomenon has remained high. Regardless of one's perspective, the physiological concomitants of psychological states can be assessed with the hope that the resulting information will extend our knowledge of the relationship between these two aspects of individuals. At present, no physiological index can be used as a direct measure of specific emotions as has been done with coding systems. A more complete description of emotional state will be afforded, however, by such joint assessments.

Within the marital interaction literature, Levenson and Gottman (1983, 1985) have conducted one of the few studies that has reported both spouse behavior and physiological assessments. In fact, they were able to predict marital satisfaction 3 years after initial assessment using physiological assessments (heart rate, pulse transmission time, skin conductance, and general somatic activity) obtained during the baseline period just prior to an interaction. Clearly, valuable complementary information is available from physiological assessments.

Every additional assessment procedure, however, expands the technical and methodological difficulties attendant to a study. The synchronism of physiological and behavioral data, the reduction in movement often required by physiological recorders, and the influence of attaching gadgets to subjects are practical and methodological issues that investigators need to address.

Statistics

The use of coding systems to assess dyadic interactions results in data that are ordered in time. Interesting questions can therefore be answered regarding the sequential pattern of particular behaviors. For example, distressed couples have been found to have longer cycles of negative affect following negative affect than nondistressed couples. The statistical analysis of behavioral patterns only has a brief history. Currently the approaches being used include the application of log-linear models (Bishop, Fienberg, & Holland, 1975) and the "z" statistic (Bakeman & Gottman, 1986) to categorical data, and the application of time series analysis (McCleary & Hay, 1980) to continuous data. Developing an appreciation for these statistical approaches would increase the richness of results that are available from the complex coding procedures described in this chapter.

Expenses

All current methods for describing psychological/emotional states by external observers are very expensive. All of the procedures discussed require extensive training of raters, and systematic supervision of raters to ensure high levels of reliability and to protect against observer drift. Another important factor to consider is that most observational coding systems take an extensive amount of time to apply, resulting in very large labor costs if raters are paid a reasonable salary. As the unit of behavior assessed gets smaller, as in the FACS or EMFACS, the time to code expands as well. Additionally, the purchase of videotape equipment, although declining in price, both for initial recording and for subsequent rating needs to be considered. Obtaining training materials themselves requires an initial investment. Finally, extensive software is needed for almost all of these procedures for storage and analysis of data. With the increasing availability of better methods for assessing psychological state in an unobtrusive manner, such as those described in this chapter, there will hopefully be an accompanying increase in their use. Investigators need to realize, however, that the present level of sophistication in coding individual and interactional behavior unfortunately is accompanied by a high price in terms of time and money.

In addition to the various costs, the use of observational assessment procedures requires an awareness and concern for certain methodological problems. The importance of establishing and maintaining reliability has already been mentioned. A related problem is the need to keep coders blind to the hypothesis of the study so that their work will not be influenced by the experimenter's beliefs. It is probably the case that as the unit of behavior observed gets smaller, coders need to make very specific decisions and therefore blindness may be less of an issue. However, this has not been well documented yet. Hopefully, future studies will offer more support for this point.

Another potentially important methodological issue is whether the assessment procedure itself influences the observed behavior. Are subjects' facial movements the same, for example, when they are being videotaped as when they are not being recorded? Researchers may take some solace in the fact that across a variety of research contexts, the influence of observers on behavior has been hard to consistently document (Harris & Lahey, 1982, Jacob, Tennenbaum, & Krahn, 1987). Furthermore, subjects appear to habituate to observation if given enough time, although how much time is required will vary depending on the context. Ekman and Friesen (e.g., Ekman and Friesen, 1974) usually report that when they videotape a subject they do it surreptitiously and request consent for this aspect of the experimental procedure after the subject's participation has been completed. This strategy does minimize observer effects but it raises issues concerning the use of deception. Another approach that is frequently followed is to give subjects time to become comfortable in the laboratory setting. Having subjects practice in front of video cameras with warm-up tasks similar to the tasks of interest should greatly reduce the impact of observation on their behavior. In general, for all new contexts that are utilized, the investigator using observational procedures should make an attempt to address this issue.

Conclusion

Researchers now have available for use a variety of procedures for unobtrusively assessing psychological/emotional state. As befits the complexity of the task, the procedures are also complex, and require the large investments of time and money that have already been amply described. For studies using individual subjects, the FACS and the EMFACS can be recommended as excellent assessment tools. As with all of these procedures, further research will continue to expand the interpretive meaning of these instruments, but they are certainly ready for use at present. For researchers interested in the assessment of emotional state during dyadic interactions, the SPAFF, although still relatively new, offers great promise for coding psychological state. If particular segments of these interactions turn out to be of interest, then they could be recorded with a more molecular system like the EMFACS. In this way an effective utilization of resources would be accomplished. As these coding systems become applied in new contexts, the gathered data will contribute to the evidence for their validity as measures of emotional state. This information will benefit researchers with substantive questions who need to assess emotional state and also expand our ability to interpret the measurements themselves.

References

Baer, P. E., Reed, J., Bartlett, P. L., Vincent, J. P., Williams, B. J., & Bourianoff, G. G. (1983). Studies of gaze during induced conflict in families with a hypertensive father. *Psychosomatic Medicine, 45*(3), 233–242.

Baer, P., Vincent, J., Williams, B., Bourianoff, G., & Bartlett, P. (1980). Behavioral response to induced conflict in families with a hypertensive father. *Hypertension, 2,* 170–177.

Bakeman, R., & Gottman, J. M. (1986). *Observing interaction: An introduction to sequential analysis.* London: Cambridge University Press.

Bishop, Y. M. M., Fienberg, S. E., & Holland, P. W. (1975). *Discrete multivariate analysis: Theory and practice.* Cambridge, MA: MIT Press.

Darwin, C. (1872). *The expression of the emotions in man and animals.* London: John Murray.

Ekman, P. (1982). Methods for measuring facial action. In K. R. Scherer & P. Ekman (Eds.), *Handbook for methods in nonverbal behavior research.* London: Cambridge University Press.

Ekman, P., & Friesen, W. V. (1974). Detecting deception from the body or face. *Journal of Personality and Social Psychology, 29,* 288–298.

Ekman, P., & Friesen, W. V. (1975). *Unmasking the face: A guide to recognizing emotions from facial clues.* Englewood Cliffs, NJ: Prentice–Hall.

Ekman, P., & Friesen, W. V. (1978). *Facial Action Coding System (FACS): A technique for the measurement of facial action.* Palo Alto, CA: Consulting Psychologists Press.

Ekman, P., & Friesen, W. V. (1982). Felt, false and miserable smiles. *Journal of Nonverbal Behavior, 6,* 238–252.

Ekman, P., Friesen, W. V., & Tomkins, S. S. (1971). Facial Affect Scoring Technique (FAST): A first validity study. *Semiotica, 3*(1), 37–58.

Ekman, P., Levenson, R. W., & Friesen, W. V. (1983). Nervous system activity distinguishes among emotions. *Science, 221,* 1208–1210.

Friesen, W. V. (1972). *Cultural differences in facial expression in a social situation: An experimental test of the concept of display rules.* Unpublished doctoral dissertation, University of California, San Francisco.

Gottman, J. M. (1979). *Marital interaction: Experimental investigations.* New York: Academic Press.

Gottman, J. M. (1983). *Rapid coding of specific affects.* Unpublished manuscript, University of Illinois, Urbana–Champagne.

Gottman, J. M., & Levenson, R. W. (1985). A valid procedure for obtaining self report of affect in marital interaction. *Journal of Consulting and Clinical Psychology, 53,* 151–160.

Harper, R. G., Wiens, A. N., & Matarazzo, J. D. (1978). *Nonverbal communication: The state of the art.* New York: Wiley.

Harris, F. C., & Lahey, B. B. (1982). Subject reactivity in direct observational assessment: A review and critical analysis. *Clinical Psychology Review, 2,* 523–538.

Hops, H., Wills, T. A., Weiss, R. L., & Patterson, G. R. (1972). *Marital Interaction Coding System.* Eugene: University of Oregon and Oregon Research Institute.

Horowitz, L. M., Weckler, D., Saxon, A., Lirandais, J. D., & Boutacoff, L. I. (1977). Discomforting talk and speech disruptions. *Journal of Consulting and Clinical Psychology, 45,* 1036–1042.

Izard, C. E. (1971). *The face of emotion.* New York: Appleton–Century–Crofts.

Izard, C. (1979). *The maximally discriminative facial movement coding system.* Unpublished manuscript. Available from Instructional Resources Center, University of Delaware, Newark.

Jacob, T., & Krahn, G. (1987). The classification of behavioral observation codes in studies of family interaction. *Journal of Marriage and the Family, 49,* 677–687.

Jacob, T., Tennenbaum, D. L., & Krahn, G. (1987). Factors influencing the reliability and validity of observation data. In T. Jacob (Ed.), *Family interaction and psychopathology: Theories, methods and findings* (pp. 297–328). New York: Plenum Press.

Jacob, T., & Tennenbaum, D. (1988). *Family assessment: Rationale, methods and future directions.* New York: Plenum Press.

James, W. (1986). What is an emotion? In M. Arnold (Ed.), *The nature of emotion.* Baltimore: Penguin. (Originally published in 1884)

Jurich, A. P., & Jurich, J. A. (1974). Correlation among nonverbal expressions of anxiety. *Psychological Reports, 38,* 199–208.

Kasl, S. V., & Mahl, G. F. (1965). The relationship of disturbances and hesitations in spontaneous speech to anxiety. *Journal of Personality and Social Psychology, 1,* 425–433.

Levenson, R. W., & Gottman, J. M. (1983). Marital interaction: Physiological linkage and affective exchange. *Journal of Personality and Social Psychology, 45,* 587–597.

Levenson, R. W., & Gottman, J. M. (1985). Physiological and affective predictors of change in relationship satisfaction. *Journal of Personality and Social Psychology, 49,* 85–94.

Mahl, G. F. (1959). Exploring emotional states by content analysis. In I. C. Pool (Ed.), *Trends in content analysis.* Urbana: University of Illinois Press.

Mahl, G. F. (1956). Disturbances and silences in the patients' speech in psychotherapy. *Journal of Abnormal Social Psychology, 53,* 1–15.

Margolin, G., & Wampold, B. E. (1981). Sequential analysis of conflict and accord in distressed and nondistressed marital partners. *Journal of Consulting and Clinical Psychology, 49*(4), 554–567.

McCleary, R., & Hay, R. (1980). *Applied time-series analysis for the social sciences.* Beverly Hills, CA: Sage.

Murray, D. C. (1971). Talk, silence and anxiety. *Psychological Bulletin, 75,* 244–260.

Olson, D. H., & Ryder, R. G. (1970). Inventory of Marital Conflicts (IMC): An experimental interaction procedure. *Journal of Marriage and the Family, 32,* 443–448.

Schachter, S., & Singer, J. E. (1962). Cognitive, social and physiological determinants of emotional state. *Psychological Review, 69,* 379–399.

Scherer, K. R. (1979). Nonlinguistic vocal indicators of emotion and psychopathology. In C. E. Izard (Ed.), *Emotions in personality and psychopathology.* New York: Plenum Press.

Scherer, K. R. (1986). Vocal affect expression: A review and model for future research. *Psychological Bulletin, 99,* 143–165.

Scherer, K. R., & Ekman, P. (1982). *Handbook of methods in nonverbal behavior research.* London: Cambridge University Press.

Tomkins, S. S. (1962). *Affect, imagery, consciousness: Vol. 1. The positive affects.* Berlin: Springer.

Tomkins, S. S. (1963). *Affect, imagery, consciousness: Vol. 2. The negative affects.* Berlin: Springer.

Tomkins, S. S. (1982). *Affect, imagery, consciousness: Vol. 3. Cognition and affect.* Berlin: Springer.

Weiss, R. L., & Summers, K. J. (1983). Marital Interaction Coding System-III. In E. Filsinger (Ed.), *Marriage and family assessment.* Beverly Hills, CA: Sage.

Woodall, K. L. (1986). *Gaze behavior during induced conflict interaction in families with hypertensive, alcoholic, or depressed parents.* Unpublished master's thesis, University of Pittsburgh.

Zuroff, D. C., & Colussy, S. A. (1986). Emotion recognition in schizophrenic and depressed inpatients. *Journal of Clinical Psychology, 42*(3), 411–417.

CHAPTER 35

Definition and Assessment of Coronary-Prone Behavior

Theodore M. Dembroski and Redford B. Williams

Introduction

Any consideration of assessment issues regarding coronary-prone behavior must begin with a review and evaluation of the evidence that certain psychological/behavioral constructs are "coronary-prone," i.e., that certain psychological/behavioral characteristics are associated with and/or predictive of such manifestations of coronary heart disease (CHD) as myocardial infarction, cardiac death, angina, and coronary atherosclerosis (coronary artery disease, CAD). On the basis of such evidence it will be possible to draw conclusions regarding the best available means of assessing coronary-prone characteristics, as well as what further research is needed to improve our ability to assess such characteristics.

To be considered of comparable importance to the traditional risk factors (habitual cigarette smoking, high blood pressure, and hyperlipidemia), any psychological/behavioral characteristic should predict a two- to sixfold increase in CHD risk, and 5–14% of persons with that char-

acteristic should develop clinical CHD during a follow-up period of 5–10 years (see Pooling Project Research Group, 1978). At the same time, nonspecificity should not necessarily be viewed as evidence against risk factor status. If increased lipids and frequent cigarette smoking can be risk factors for both CHD and cancer, similar nonspecificity should not be advanced as evidence against CHD risk factor status for psychological/behavioral factors.

In addition to refinements of known risk factors (e.g., consideration of HDL as well as total cholesterol), the identification of additional, new risk factors could help to increase our potential understanding of CHD etiology, and thus possibly lead to improved prevention, treatment, and rehabilitation of CHD. Major research efforts over the past three decades have focused on the role of psychological/behavioral characteristics as potential new risk factors for CHD. In the remainder of this chapter, we shall: (1) review the research that identified the Type A behavior pattern (TABP) as a useful construct in the search for new CHD risk factors; (2) review the recent research that has identified hostility and anger as the critical toxic aspects of the TABP, and thus helped to refine our understanding of coronary-prone behavior; and (3) review evidence concerning the relationship of other psychological factors, especially neurot-

Theodore M. Dembroski • Department of Psychology, University of Maryland Baltimore County, Catonsville, Maryland 21228.   *Redford B. Williams* • Department of Psychiatry, Duke University Medical Center, Durham, North Carolina 27710.

icism, to CHD endpoints. In the context of this review of the evidence relating psychological/behavioral factors to CHD risk and pathogenesis, issues regarding the assessment of coronary-prone behavior will be addressed in some depth.

The Emergence of the TABP

During the 1950s, two pioneering cardiologists collaborated in the formulation of a coherent definition of a behavior pattern which they considered coronary-prone, and in the development of a reliable method for its assessment (Friedman & Rosenman, 1974). This behavior pattern they labeled Type A for descriptive purposes (Rosenman, 1986). Based on their research, Friedman and Rosenman consolidated several attributes into a single construct, which they called the Type A coronary-prone behavior pattern (TABP). TABP was defined as ''an action–emotion complex that can be observed in any person who is aggressively involved in a chronic, incessant struggle to achieve more and more in less and less time, and, if required to do so, against the opposing efforts of the other things or other persons'' (Friedman & Rosenman, 1974; Rosenman & Friedman, 1974). At this point they were ready to undertake the crucial next step in establishing the relationship between TABP and CHD: a prospective epidemiological study called the Western Collaborative Group Study (WCGS).

Initial attempts to develop questionnaires to measure TABP in the WCGS were deemed failures because Friedman and Rosenman's clinical experience suggested to them that the Type A individual lacked insight into his or her own behavior. According to Rosenman (1986), paper-and-pencil methods could not reveal the emotional overtones or pronounced psychomotor mannerisms and vigorous voice stylistics which they considered key indices of the TABP. They did not conceptualize TABP to be a personality trait, but rather as overt patterns of behavior that are evoked by certain environmental challenges in susceptible individuals. Therefore, the Structured Interview (SI) was developed to assess the TABP (Rosenman, 1978).

The SI was used in the prospective WCGS to assess TABP in 3154 men, aged 39–59, who were then followed for 8.5 years. SIs were tape-recorded and preserved for later auditing by Rosenman. A repeated and explicit principle was that the *manner* in which the subject responded, rather than the content of the responses, was the primary criterion used to identify Type A and B status (Rosenman, 1978). Therefore, subjects' descriptions of their own hard-driving behavior, impatience, competitiveness, speed of activity, and the like, which are the principal attributes emphasized in the conceptual definition of TABP, are actually given minor or secondary consideration in the SI assessment procedure. Friedman, Brown, and Rosenman (1969) and a large number of other research groups have verified that the major criteria used in the TABP designation reflect emphatic and pronounced voice stylistics, primarily loud, explosive, and rapid-accelerated speech (Dembroski & MacDougall, 1985; Howland & Siegman, 1982; Glass, Ross, Isecke, & Rosenman, 1982; MacDougall, Dembroski, & Musante, 1979; Matthews, Krantz, Dembroski, & MacDougall, 1982; Musante, MacDougall, Dembroski, & Van Horn, 1983; Scherwitz, Berton, & Leventhal, 1977; Schucker & Jacobs, 1977). The use of electronic devices as well as subjective judgments has consistently confirmed that enhanced voice stylistics are clearly the main criteria used in designating TABP status. As will become relevant later in this chapter, it is important to note that indices of hostility are also seriously considered in making TABP judgments, but in the final analysis, the voice stylistics prevail as the principal set of criteria for assigning Type A and Type B designations.

Approximately one-half of the WCGS subjects were classified as Type A at intake. Reports of the 8.5-year follow-up disclosed that Type A subjects relative to Type Bs were slightly more than twice as likely to show clinical manifestations of CHD (Brand, 1978; Rosenman et al., 1975). The approximate two-to-one risk ratio remained significant after multivariate statistical adjustment for the traditional risk factors. The amount of risk associated with the TABP was about the same as that of any other risk factor. Moreover, TABP ratings predicted the incidence of CHD regardless of the presence or absence of any combination of the traditional risk factors.

Results of the multivariate analyses in the

WCGS offered the first clear prospective demonstration that TABP is an independent risk factor for CHD. Other research revealed that the TABP was related to the severity of coronary artery disease (CAD) documented by autopsy in the WCGS (Friedman, Rosenman, Strauss, Wurm, & Kositchek, 1968), and through cardiac catheterization by independent investigative groups (Blumenthal, Williams, Kong, Schanberg, & Thompson, 1978; Frank, Heller, Kornfeld, Sporn, & Weiss, 1978; Zyzanski, Jenkins, Ryan, Flessas, & Everist, 1976).

The evidence linking TABP to CHD was strong enough by the late 1970s to stimulate two major conferences supported by the National Heart, Lung and Blood Institute (NHLBI). The first, held in June 1977, addressed evidence for the following issues regarding TABP: (1) epidemiological association with CHD; (2) psychometric assessment procedures; (3) underlying physiological and pathophysiological mechanisms; (4) socialization, behavioral etiology, and cultural influences; and (5) intervention methods (Dembroski, Weiss, Shields, Haynes, & Feinleib, 1978). The first conference set the agenda for the second, which was held in December 1978. The second conference, held under the auspices of both the American Heart Association and the NHLBI, assembled a distinguished panel of scientists to evaluate the evidence consolidated by the first conference. After extensive evaluation of the evidence, the Panel concluded that the TABP was associated with increased risk for CHD ". . . over and above that imposed by age, systolic blood pressure, serum cholesterol and smoking and [that increased risk due to TABP] appears to be of the same order of magnitude as the relative risk associated with any of these factors" (Review Panel on Coronary-Prone Behavior and Coronary Heart Disease, 1981).

Emergence of Contradictory Findings

By the late 1970s and early 1980s, it appeared that the medical community for the first time was prepared to formally accept a psychosocial factor as a bona fide risk factor for CHD. Unfortunately, about the same time, research results that began to emerge from a series of studies caused many to question whether the Panel's conclusions were premature. These new studies suggested that (1) questionnaire approaches to assessment of the global TABP may not be very useful in evaluating the relationship between TABP and CHD endpoints, and (2) that globally defined TABP itself may not be the best possible measure of coronary-prone behavior.

Since the Panel met in 1978, an expanding body of epidemiological research has failed to find a significant relationship between the globally defined TABP, however assessed, and either incidence of CHD or angiographically documented CAD. With respect to questionnaire measures, in research involving many thousands of subjects, several prospective epidemiological studies and studies of patients undergoing coronary angiography have failed to demonstrate a positive association between CHD endpoints and scores on the Jenkins Activity Survey (JAS), a questionnaire-based measure of TABP (see Matthews & Haynes, 1986, for a comprehensive review). Of particular importance, when appropriate statistical analyses were used to examine the association between JAS scores and CHD incidence in the WCGS, no significant relationship appeared (Brand, 1978).

Another questionnaire measure of TABP was derived from a 300-item inventory administered to participants in the Framingham Heart Study during the 1960s (Haynes, Feinleib, & Kannel, 1980). Ten items were selected from the total inventory on the basis of face validity and the advice of experts. At present, it is unknown whether the brief Framingham Type A scale is predictive of CHD events in other samples. Inspection of the items contained in the scale reveals close similarities to what is measured in the Hard Driving and Speed/Impatience scales of the JAS, which have had no success in predicting CHD outcomes. In addition, like the JAS, the Framingham scale correlates but weakly with the SI method of assessment of global TABP (MacDougall et al., 1979). It remains to be demonstrated what is being captured by the Framingham scale that is not assessed by the JAS. In any case, this 10-item Framingham Type A scale cannot by itself qualify as a valid measure of coronary-prone behavior until it can be demonstrated that it can successfully stand on its own in independent cross-validation studies. More important, its relationship to neuroticism and prediction primarily of angina pectoris raises questions (see below) regarding its prediction of other CHD endpoints.

Finally, there is now ample evidence that the SI, the currently preferred means of assessing TABP, and the various questionnaire-based TABP assessment tools are essentially measuring different constructs (Chesney, Black, Chadwick, & Rosenman, 1981; MacDougall *et al.*, 1979; Matthews *et al.*, 1982; Matthews, 1982; Musante *et al.*, 1983). Based on the considerations just noted, it appears unwise to use *only a questionnaire method* to assess TABP itself. As will be seen below, however, there is now emerging evidence that questionnaire-based approaches to assessment of certain aspects of the global TABP may provide useful methods to assess *coronary-prone behavior per se.*

An irony here is that, although the JAS does not appear to be a particularly useful measure of coronary-prone behavior, it is probably the best available measure of many of the key defining attributes contained in the *conceptual* definition of TABP. For example, in a large body of personality and social psychology research, JAS-defined Type As relative to Type Bs consistently showed more hard-driving, more time-urgent, more job-involved, and more productive and achievement-oriented behaviors (see Matthews, 1982, for a review of the construct validity of JAS-defined TABP). The failure of the JAS to predict or correlate with various indices of CHD, despite its generally good construct validity, may contain an important clue regarding which aspects of the global TABP are coronary-prone: conspicuously absent from the above list of TABP attributes that are assessed by the JAS is any mention of hostility or anger.

Far fewer studies have addressed the construct validity issue using the SI method of TABP assessment, although as noted above, it is plain that vigorous voice mannerisms are the principal criteria used for TABP classification. SI-defined TABP correlates with few other psychological or personality measures (Chesney *et al.*, 1981; Matthews, 1982; Musante *et al.*, 1983). Here, significant but generally weak correlations have been reported between SI-defined TABP and measures of extraversion, dominance, activity level, and the like, but measures of the latter attributes cannot be considered substitutes for SI assessment of TABP. It is important to note that, unlike the JAS, the SI does contain information regarding subjects' hostility and anger levels. As will be described below, this may account for its superiority to questionnaire-based TABP measures, as well as point the way to identification of those aspects of the global TABP which are, in fact, coronary-prone.

Turning now to consideration of the epidemiological evidence with respect to the global TABP, it is important to recognize that consistency of association with disease endpoints is a major criterion that must be satisfied in the establishment of any risk factor, especially for CHD (Matthews & Haynes, 1986). Using the modest criteria of one study implicating TABP through multivariate analyses in new incidence of CHD and at least one study showing a positive relationship between TABP and angiographically documented CAD severity, it is possible to conclude that TABP is a risk factor for CHD in the United States, but only when TABP is assessed by the SI method. However, if the criteria for risk factor status include the requirement that positive findings outweigh the negative results in studies designed to examine the relationship between global TABP and CHD outcomes, the situation is much less encouraging.

Considering first the findings from studies of angiographic samples, the evidential basis for a significant relationship between CAD and TABP, even if limited to studies employing the preferred SI assessment, is primarily confined to data from Columbia University (Frank *et al.*, 1978) and Duke University (Blumenthal *et al.*, 1978; Williams *et al.*, 1980). Since the latter studies were conducted, at least seven angiographic studies have failed to find a significant association between SI-defined global TABP and CAD severity at the time of coronary angiography (see Dembroski & MacDougall, 1985, and Matthews & Haynes, 1986, for reviews). Even with the Duke patient sample, it was not possible to demonstrate a significant global TABP effect in a random sample of 131 patients drawn from the total population of over 2000 Duke patients with behavioral data (Dembroski, Mac-Dougall, Williams, Haney, & Blumenthal, 1985).

Some clarification of this paucity of positive findings in angiographic samples is provided by a recent comprehensive multivariable analysis of the association between SI-defined TABP and CAD severity in the entire population of 2289 patients with SI data at Duke University (Williams *et al.*, 1986). Confirming the limitations of question-naire-based measures of global TABP, JAS scores were unrelated to CAD severity. A significant TABP–CAD relationship was found, but only using SI assessments and only among the younger patients. Among the older patients there was actu-ally a reversal, with Type Bs showing more severe CAD. This reversal of the positive relationship be-tween Type A behavior and CAD in the older pa-tients was interpreted as showing a survival effect. The assumption here is that among the older pa-tients, the Type As with more severe CAD are missing due to death or development of disease at an earlier age. Since none of the negative studies of TABP–CAD relationships in angiographic sam-ples took age into account, this could, in part, account for their failure to detect a TABP–CAD relationship.

An even more likely explanation is that TABP effect revealed among the younger Duke patients is so small that the negative studies lacked adequate statistical power to detect it. Among the Duke pa-tients, both smoking and hyperlipidemia showed interactions with age similar to that just described for TABP: smoking and hyperlipidemia were both associated with more severe CAD among only the younger patients; among the older patients, these risk factors were uncorrelated with CAD severity. The effect size for both smoking and hyper-lipidemia among the younger patients was much stronger, however, than that for TABP.

Based upon the TABP effect size in the younger Duke patients, a power analysis indicated that with sample sizes of 150 or less, the statistical power to detect that effect would be no more than 17%. Since all of the negative studies of SI-defined TABP–CAD relationships in angiographic sam-ples had sample sizes of 150 or less, it is not sur-prising that they failed to detect a TABP effect. Indeed, the negative finding with respect to global

TABP in the Duke data (Dembroski *et al.*, 1985) now becomes more understandable. Given the small size of the TABP effect, with a sample size of 131, there may not have been adequate power to detect it.

Taken as a whole, the findings leave the impres-sion that SI-defined TABP *is associated* with more severe CAD among younger angiographic pa-tients, but the size of this association is so small that its clinical significance must be seriously questioned. More importantly for research pur-poses, the small effect size indicates that investiga-tions of global TABP in convenience samples will be of limited use. Finally, one is left with the con-clusion that we can probably do much better than global TABP in defining coronary-prone behavior. In fact, it is possible that the earlier studies found a positive association between TABP and severity of CAD because auditors may have weighted some attributes (e.g., hostility) more than others (e.g., rapid speech) in making a Type A and B designa-tion (Dembroski & MacDougall, 1985).

This conclusion is strengthened still further by a consideration of post-WCGS research on prospec-tive prediction of clinical CHD events by TABP in epidemiological studies. The decision by the Re-view Panel (1981) to accept TABP as a CHD risk factor was most heavily influenced by the prospec-tive findings from the WCGS. Now, however, there are contradictory data available from another large-scale prospective study of the relationship between SI-defined global TABP and incidence of documented clinical manifestations of CHD.

The Multiple Risk Factor Intervention Trial (MRFIT) was a large-scale clinical trial designed to alter behaviors associated with the traditional risk factors in many thousands of people across the United States to determine whether incidence of CHD could be reduced by such interventions (MRFIT Group, 1979). A subset of MRFIT par-ticipants ($N = 3110$) was recruited for a special prospective study to determine whether the CHD incidence findings for global TABP in the WCGS could be replicated in a different sample (Shekelle *et al.*, 1985). MRFIT investigators recognized that assessment was critical, so they saw to it that Dr. Rosenman trained and certified those who ad-ministered and/or audited the MRFIT SIs. He also adjudicated all disagreements between auditors in TABP designation. Eight centers from diverse localities in the United States followed standardized methods in both the assessment and average 7-year follow-up phases of the study. Cause of death was designated by a Mortality Review Committee, whereas nonfatal myocardial infarction (MI) was defined by ECGs analyzed by an expert committee. All endpoint assessments were made blind to TABP status. These stringent procedures decreased the number of CHD events available for inclusion, but in the process many possible sources of bias were eliminated. Final results indicated no relationship between SI-defined global TABP (or JAS-defined TABP) and any clinical manifestation of CHD (Shekelle *et al.*, 1985). While the MRFIT study differed from the WCGS in that subjects were selected on the basis of having one or more risk factors, it should be recalled that in the WCGS, TABP predicted CHD at all levels of risk; in fact, the increment in risk associated with TABP was greater among WCGS subjects with increased levels of traditional risk factors (Brand, 1978).

Accumulation of evidence indicating that TABP effects are either weak, as in the angiographic studies, or absent, as in the MRFIT study, suggests that assessment of *only* global TABP, however defined, at present is not the most profitable research strategy to pursue in attempting to understand the nature of coronary-prone behavior.

In addition to the growing body of weak or negative findings, there is another bothersome trend: many studies report that between 70 and 90% of subjects are categorized as Type A (Chesney *et al.*, 1981; Friedman *et al.*, 1982). In the MRFIT study, 74% were designated Type A (Shekelle *et al.*, 1985); and recently, 70% of adult males aged 39–59 in a large-scale community probability sample not selected for risk factor status were also classified as Type A (Gordon Moss, personal communication, April 1986). Dembroski and MacDougall (1983) found in two separate studies that 85 and 90% of top-level business executives and senior-level military officers, respectively, were classified as Type A by the SI. Placing such large proportions of groups under study in an at-risk category is not

consistent with sound epidemiological or clinical practice.

How can this confusing state of affairs be resolved? A first step is to appreciate the distinction between the concepts of TABP and coronary-prone behavior (Dembroski *et al.*, 1978). Thus, it may be that not all components of the multidimensional global TABP are coronary-prone; in fact, some may even be protective (e.g., job involvement), just as some components—i.e., HDL-cholesterol—of the total serum cholesterol are protective rather than coronary-prone. If only certain aspects of the multidimensional TABP are "toxic," then assessment of the global TABP will provide a measure which contains a considerable amount of "noise" in addition to the coronary-prone "signal." That such is indeed the case, and that we can improve over global TABP in defining coronary-prone behavior, is suggested by a growing body of recent research in which different attributes contained in both the conceptual and operational definitions of TABP have been assessed, using various means, and related to CHD indices.

Recent Refinements: The Role of Hostility and Anger

That some aspects of the global TABP are more predictive of the incidence of CHD than others was first suggested in a study of 62 new cases of clinical CHD under the age of 50 that occurred during the first 4 years of the WCGS (Matthews, Glass, Rosenman, & Bortner, 1977). These cases were compared with 124 symptom-free participants who were matched for age and place of work. Comparisons were made with respect to over 40 different attributes in the SI that were rated separately by the late Dr. Bortner. Results revealed that the best discriminator between cases and controls was the SI-defined potential for hostility dimension followed by anger directed outward, competitiveness, experience of anger more than once a week, vigorous answers, irritation at waiting in lines, and explosive voice modulation. Most of the attributes characteristic of the cases reflected the hostility/anger dimension and were probably significantly intercorrelated. No multivariate analyses were performed on these data, however, so it is impossible to say now whether all the variance in psychological differences between cases and controls could be attributed to the hostility/anger dimension.

Based on these findings, as well as the long-standing interest in hostility and anger-expression in the pathogenesis of CHD (Diamond, 1982) and the repeated conceptual emphasis Friedman and Rosenman have placed on the hostility component of the TABP, there has been considerable research emphasis in the past several years on the hostility/anger dimension of TABP. This research focus also has been stimulated by the evidence, reviewed above, that the global TABP by itself may not provide an adequate measure of coronary-prone behavior. As will become evident in the following review, this research provides strong support for the hypothesis that the hostility/anger dimension is the major, if not the only, aspect of the TABP which is coronary-prone.

The research linking aspects of the hostility/anger dimension with various indices of CHD can be grouped into two broad categories, based on the assessment tools used to assess hostility/anger: (1) questionnaire-based instruments, especially the Cook–Medley (1954) Hostility (Ho) scale from the MMPI; and (2) SI-based approaches to the measurement of Potential for Hostility (PoHo), components of hostility, and mode of anger expression.

Evidence Based on the Cook–Medley Ho Scale

Beginning in 1976, the research group at Duke University began to collect, in addition to SI- and JAS-based measures of TABP, MMPI and other psychosocial data on patients referred for diagnostic coronary angiography. Guided by the considerations reviewed above, as well as by preliminary indications (Blumenthal & Williams, unpublished data) that Ho scores were positively correlated with CAD severity, they evaluated the relationship of both SI-defined TABP and MMPI-based Ho scores to CAD severity (Williams *et al.*, 1980) and found both to be significantly associated with

increased CAD severity in a sample of 424 male and female patients. The effect size for Ho scores was larger, however, than that for TABP: Type As were about 1.3 times more likely than non-As to have a clinically significant arterial occlusion, while patients with higher Ho scores were about 1.5 times more likely to have significant disease than those with low Ho scores. Multivariate analysis showed that with control for gender and TABP, the significance of the Ho–CAD relationship increased from a univariate level of $p = 0.02$ to $p = 0.008$; in contrast, with control for gender and Ho, the significance level for the TABP–CAD association decreased from a univariate level of $p < 0.01$ to $p = 0.05$.

These findings have several noteworthy implications. It will be recalled that the evidence reviewed above indicated that questionnaire-based measures of *TABP* perform less well than the SI-based measure in correlating with CHD indices. Yet, here is a questionnaire-based measure of the *hostility/anger* dimension that showed a stronger effect size in relating to CAD severity than the SI-based TABP categorization (Williams *et al.*, 1980). Since it is unlikely that any questionnaire could capture as well as direct observation during the SI the intensity of emotional responses, exaggerated psychomotor mannerisms, and vigorous voice stylistics considered essential features of the TABP (Rosenman, 1986), the finding of a stronger effect size for Ho scores in the Williams *et al.* (1980) study suggests that these motor behaviors may not be crucial aspects of coronary-proneness. More specifically, if even a questionnaire-based measure of the hostility dimension is a better index of coronary-prone behavior than SI-based measures of global TABP, then the hostility attribute may be the only aspect of TABP which is coronary-prone.

The case that the Ho scale is measuring an aspect of the hostility domain that is coronary-prone is strengthened by the findings in two prospective epidemiological studies that were stimulated by the Ho–CAD link described above. Shekelle, Gale, Ostfeld, and Paul (1983) reported a significant prediction of increased 10-year CHD event rates as a function of higher Ho scores among the 1877 middle-aged men who originally completed the MMPI in the Western Electric Study over 20 years ago. Similarly, Barefoot, Dahlstrom, and Williams (1983) found a four- to fivefold higher CHD event rate over a 25-year follow-up period among 255 physicians who had completed the MMPI during a medical school clerkship 25 years previously.

Thus, not only were higher Ho scores correlated with more severe CAD in a cross-sectional study, they were also predictive of increased CHD rates in both young and middle-aged men over follow-up periods of 10–25 years. The larger effect size (risk ratio of 4–5) among the physicians aged 25 at intake suggests the action of survival effects in determining the smaller risk ratio (about 1.5) among the older (mean age = 45) Western Electric Study participants: if those with high Ho scores are dying or developing chronic disease at a younger age, then surviving older men with high Ho scores may represent a biologically hardier (or at least not genetically "cursed") group than young men with high Ho scores.

That survival effects are operating is suggested even more strongly by consideration of the relationship between Ho scores and all-cause mortality in both the Shekelle *et al.* (1983) and Barefoot *et al.* (1983) studies. Among the middle-aged men at intake in the Western Electric Study, those with higher Ho scores were approximately 1.5 times (29 versus 18%) more likely to die over a 20-year follow-up period than those with lower Ho scores. In contrast, among the men in the physician study, who were aged 25 at intake, the risk ratio for all-cause mortality was approximately sixfold (2.2% in low Ho scorers versus 14% in high scorers). It should be noted that in both studies neither the Ho–CHD nor Ho–mortality relationships appeared due to associations with any of the traditional risk factors.

That survival effects are also acting with respect to the TABP is suggested by findings from a recently reported analysis of data from the WCGS (Ragland, Brand, & Rosenman, 1986). In contrast to the significant prediction of CHD morbidity by TABP during the original 8.5 years of follow-up in the WCGS (Rosenman *et al.*, 1975), during subsequent years TABP did not predict CHD mortality. In fact, more detailed analyses showed that the size of the TABP effect diminished across the later years of follow-up. This diminution of the TABP effect is consistent with the survival interpretation that surviving Type A men are biologically hardier due to drop out of more biologically vulnerable Type A men during the earlier years of follow-up.

In both the studies described above, the relationship of Ho scores to both CHD and mortality outcomes was nonlinear, with no further increase in risk once an apparent "threshold" Ho score of 13 was exceeded. In yet a third prospective study, however, a significant linear relationship has been found between Ho scores and all-cause mortality in a sample of 115 law students followed up 25 years after completing the MMPI while in law school (Barefoot, Williams, Dahlstrom, & Dodge, 1987). Interestingly, the all-cause mortality risk ratio in this study of a much smaller sample was comparable (fivefold) to that observed in the earlier physician study. While the apparent absence of a dose–response relationship between Ho scores and health outcomes in all but one study may be a cause for some concern, it is important to recall that TABP did not show a dose–response effect in the WCGS. Perhaps with better definition of just which aspects of what the Ho scale is measuring are coronary-prone, a more linear effect will be uncovered.

There has been one study, comparable to the Barefoot *et al.* (1983) study, in which Ho scores did not predict CHD or mortality in a sample of 478 physicians who were followed up 25 years after completing the MMPI *prior* to medical school admission (McCranie, Watkins, Brandsma, & Sisson, 1986). An important methodological difference between these two studies may account for the failure of the latter study to replicate the earlier results. In the Barefoot *et al.* (1983) study, the students completed the MMPI as a class exercise during their psychiatry clerkship and were told that the results would have no bearing on their grades, but would be used for research purposes only. In the McCranie *et al.* (1986) study, however, the students completed the MMPI as part of the application process during their visit for admission interviews. Not surprisingly, both Ho scores and validity scale scores were significantly different in the two samples, consistent with the interpretation that social desirability and evaluation apprehension factors were operating to affect MMPI scale scores in the McCranie *et al.* (1986) subjects (see Carver & Matthews, this volume). Thus, the failure to replicate the earlier Ho findings cannot be accepted as a fully valid test of the effects of Ho scores on health outcomes, because bias associated with the testing situation was probably influencing responses.

Of course, replication of findings is essential and must proceed. However, in connection with this process, the McCranie *et al.* (1986) study does make the important point that the conditions under which any psychological assessment tool is employed can exert profound effects upon its validity. When evaluation apprehension is aroused, for example, responses on a self-report instrument can be so affected as to render them useless in measuring the construct for which the tool was intended. Indeed, we cannot be certain that even SI-based assessments would not be flawed if administered in such an evaluative setting in which demand characteristics are made so salient. This problem is not unique to psychobehavioral assessments, however. A glucose tolerance test or a lipid panel performed after the ingestion of a large fatty meal would be no more valid measures of carbohydrate or lipid metabolism than the MMPI is of psychological traits when given to medical school applicants.

What is the nature of the factor measured by the Ho scale? A growing body of research suggests that rather than overt aggressiveness (i.e., behaviors intended to inflict harm on others), the Ho scale might more accurately be described as a "cynicism" scale, since most of its items reflect a general distrust of human nature and motives. This description is supported by the derivation of a major cynicism factor from factor analyses of the Ho scale (Costa, Zonderman, McCrae, & Williams, 1986), as well as of the entire MMPI item set (Johnson, Butcher, Null, & Johnson, 1984; Costa, Zonderman, McCrae, & Williams, 1985). In a large-scale study of the construct validity of the Ho scale, Smith and Frohm (1985) concluded that "the scale primarily assesses suspiciousness, resentment, frequent anger and cynical distrust of others rather than overtly aggressive behavior or general emotional distress." Smith and Frohm (1985) also report that persons with high Ho scores

also display more anger, less hardiness, more frequent and severe hassles, and fewer and less satisfactory social supports. Thus, the terms "cynical mistrust" (Costa *et al.*, 1986) and "cynical hostility" (Smith & Frohm, 1985) have been proposed to describe at least one psychological construct measured by the Ho scale.

Recent research by Barefoot *et al.* (1987) suggests that a subset of 24 items on the Ho scale reflecting a cynical attitude toward humankind in general, frequent experience of anger, and a tendency to respond to frustration with aggressive behavior are responsible for the prediction of all-cause mortality by the overall Ho scale.

Taken together, the findings for the Ho scale appear rather consistent and suggest that it is measuring a stable trait (test–retest correlations in several studies have been in the range of 0.8–0.9) that has "a broad effect on survival" (Shekelle *et al.*, 1983). While it has consistently predicted increased CHD risk, suggesting that the Ho scale is measuring an important aspect of coronary-prone behavior, it has proven an even stronger predictor of mortality due to all causes. It shall remain a task for further research to determine whether combination of Ho scores with other measures, or refinements of the Ho item set will produce a more specific assessment of coronary-prone behavior. If such efforts are unavailing, we will be left with the conclusion that the trait measured by the Ho scale is a general risk factor for a wide variety of adverse health outcomes, just, it might be added, as is the case with smoking and high serum cholesterol levels at the present time.

Whatever the outcome, the prediction of health outcomes by the Ho scale has now been firmly established in several prospective studies, and the effect size in younger subjects (sixfold higher risk of dying, absolute mortality of 14%) is comparable to that for all three traditional risk factors combined. Thus, it is quite likely that further research to uncover the psychological and physiological mechanisms underlying the Ho scale's predictive capacity will prove useful in efforts to understand better the nature of coronary-prone behavior, and, ultimately, to do something about it.

Before considering SI-based assessment approaches, one other questionnaire measure of hostility deserves comment. Friedman *et al.* (1982) found that a self-report measure of hostility and anger was predictive of CHD morbidity during the first year's follow-up in the Recurrent Coronary Prevention Project, even though measures of global TABP were not significant predictors in the same analyses.

Evidence from SI-Based Assessment of PoHo and Its Components

Another approach that has proven fruitful in moving beyond global TABP has been to use the SI as a means of assessing separately the various attributes contained in both the conceptual and operational definitions of TABP (Dembroski & Mac-Dougall, 1985). This approach is derived from the original components scoring approach developed by Dr. Bortner and applied in the Matthews *et al.* (1977) study of a subsample of cases and controls in the WCGS. This scoring system has been developed further (see Dembroski *et al.,* 1978; Dembroski & MacDougall, 1983, 1985; Dembroski & Costa, 1987, for more detail on the component scoring system) and provides for ratings of speech stylistics including loud, explosive, rapid/accelerated speech, and short response latency. The system was also designed to capture a conceptual definition of hostility as the relatively stable tendency to react to a broad range of frustration-inducing events with responses indicative of anger, irritation, disgust, contempt, resentment, and the like, and/or actually to express antagonism, criticalness, uncooperativeness, and other disagreeable behaviors in similar situations (Dembroski *et al.,* 1985; Dembroski & Costa, 1987).

SI-defined PoHo is scored on a five-point scale as are other components in this assessment system. Attention is devoted to three primary categories of responses in assigning a PoHo score. First, *content* of the answer is considered. Here, frequent reports of experiencing or expressing annoyance, irritation, resentment, anger, and similar negative affects during the common frustrating circumstances of everyday life contribute to a high hostility score. Second, *intensity* of response is also heavily weighted in the PoHo score, including the use of emotionally laden words (e.g., hate), profanity,

and voice emphasis. Third, *style* of interaction with the interviewer contributes markedly to a high hostility score when such attributes as rudeness, condescension, disagreeableness, contempt, and the like are discerned. Until recently, all three categories were collapsed into one PoHo score (Dembroski & MacDougall, 1983). In current practice, each category is scored separately in addition to a final judgment of PoHo in order to examine the possibility that some components of hostility may be more coronary-prone than others. This further refinement of the SI-based hostility scoring system also allows for the probability that the hostility construct is no less multidimensional than the global TABP (Dembroski & Costa, 1987).

It is important for the reader to realize that assessment of PoHo and its components, while easy to describe in words as above, is not a simple matter. Anyone wishing to employ the assessment of these measures using SI data is strongly advised to obtain extensive supervised training in their use before attempting to employ this approach in research. Even with such training, it is essential to have at least two raters audit the SI tapes, to ensure adequate reliability of the measurements in terms of good interrater agreement.

Another important aspect of the hostility/anger dimension which can be assessed in the SI is mode of anger expression. The key construct here is Anger-In, which is indexed by content responses indicative of an inability or unwillingness to express negative affect toward the source of a frustration (Dembroski *et al.,* 1985).

Support for the utility of the components scoring approach using the SI is provided by two recent studies in which components related to the hostility/anger dimension were found correlated with CAD severity in angiographic samples. In a reanalysis of 131 taped SIs from the Duke sample, Dembroski *et al.* (1985) found that both PoHo and Anger-In were significantly and positively correlated with CAD severity, even when the traditional risk factors and age and sex were controlled. There was a significant interaction between these variables, such that CAD severity increased as a function of hostility scores only among those patients who were high on Anger-In. Another intriguing finding was that, although insignificantly and positively correlated with CAD severity in univariate analyses, a measure of Type A speech stylistics, explosiveness, became significantly *negatively* correlated with CAD in multivariate analysis controlling for PoHo and Anger-In.

In a similar reanalysis of SI data from a sample of patients from Massachusetts General Hospital (Dimsdale, Hackett, Hutter, Block, & Cantanzano, 1979), MacDougall, Dembroski, Dimsdale, and Hackett (1985) also found both PoHo and Anger-In to be positively correlated with CAD severity. In contrast to the Dembroski *et al.* (1985) study, however, these two components did not show a significant interaction in this study. Explosive speech was also negatively correlated, though with marginal significance ($r = -0.14$, $p = 0.10$), with CAD severity after statistical control for PoHo and Anger-In. Another component reflecting the time urgency aspects of TABP— time pressure—was also significantly *negatively* correlated with CAD severity.

While it may be tempting to interpret these negative associations between other TABP aspects and CAD severity when hostility is controlled as reflecting a protective effect of these attributes, it is important to keep in mind that these negative relationships could just as easily result from the effect of more severe disease, with the attendant symptoms, to cause patients to slow down in a variety of behavioral areas. Only with results from prospective studies, such as the reanalyses of the MRFIT SI data now being conducted by the first author (T. M. D.), can we resolve which of the above interpretations is correct.

These two studies have several important implications for understanding the nature of coronary-prone behavior, as well as devising better assessment approaches to it. First of all, in both the Duke and Massachusetts General Hospital samples, globally defined TABP was not significantly related to CAD severity, though in the Duke sample there was a marginally significant positive relationship when only the extreme TABP groups were examined. In light of the small effect size for TABP noted above (Williams *et al.,* 1986), this failure to detect a TABP effect in these small samples—both less than 150 patients—is not surprising. The fact that components of the hostility/anger dimension do relate significantly to CAD severity, despite the small sample sizes, is clear evidence that this dimension is far more strongly related to CAD severity than is global TABP itself.

Another important finding in both studies is the negative association between CAD severity and measures of non-hostility/anger dimension components. Even if prospective studies show these negative relationships to be effects of more severe disease, rather than causes of less severe disease, the fact remains that, other than measures of the hostility dimension, no other aspects of the global TABP were associated with more severe CAD. Thus, the failure of SI measures of global TABP to predict CHD events, e.g., in the MRFIT data, could result from the focus in the SI-based assessment of TABP on the speech stylistics, which appear unrelated to disease.

Work currently in progress will determine whether assessment of PoHo and other hostility components in the MRFIT data set will show that, whereas global TABP failed to predict cases, measures of the hostility/anger dimension will succeed. Such a finding would constitute yet more strong evidence, beyond that already cited with respect to the Ho measure, that the hostility/anger dimension is the only aspect of TABP which is coronary-prone.

The significant finding for Anger-In in the angiographic studies appears to contradict the earlier report of Matthews *et al.* (1977) that SI ratings of potential for hostility and *Anger-Out* were prospectively associated with CHD in the WCGS. Moreover, frequent reports of the outward expression of anger significantly contribute to a high SI-defined PoHo score (see above and Dembroski *et al.,* 1978). Thus, the very procedures used to assess hostility in the SI suggest that there should be an inverse relationship between PoHo and Anger-In. In the angiographic studies, it appears that *both* PoHo and Anger-In could be significantly related to CAD severity only if they were *positively* correlated or uncorrelated. This is borne out by correlation of zero between PoHo and Anger-In in the random sample of 131 angiography patients from the Duke University patient population of more than 2000 patients (Dembroski *et al.,* 1985). Yet, in a normal, nonpatient sample, the predicted inverse correlation between SI-defined PoHo and Anger-In was, in fact, significantly negative ($r = -0.47, p < 0.01$) (Musante *et al.*, 1986). The apparent contradiction may be resolved by considering the interesting hypothesis (see above) that Anger-In may well be a *consequence* of disease rather than an etiological factor. The Duke sample provides an ideal data base to permit at least initial exploration of this hypothesis because patients with no significant disease were compared with patients suffering from extremely severe coronary occlusions.

Among those patients in the Duke sample employed in the Dembroski *et al.* (1985) study, there was a significant negative correlation ($r = -0.48$, $p < 0.01$) between PoHo and Anger-In in patients *without* severe disease or symptoms. This negative correlation was nearly identical to that obtained in the normal nonpatient sample (Musante, MacDougall, Dembroski, & Costa, unpublished data). On the other hand, the correlation between PoHo and Anger-In in the patients with symptoms (e.g., past MI) *and* severe disease was positive though nonsignificant ($r = 0.13$, n.s.). It is thus possible that atherosclerosis and associated symptoms increase the likelihood that overt anger expression may cause pain. This could lead to a change from Anger-Out to Anger-In as the preferred mode of anger expression. Such would be especially likely in an individual who had suffered an MI and who would be urged to "avoid emotional upsets" by both cardiologists and significant others. This hypothesis could receive a definitive test, however, only from a prospective study designed to determine whether low suppression of anger changes to high suppression as signs and symptoms of CHD emerge (Dembroski & Costa, 1987). If our hypothesis is correct, Anger-In should *not* be related prospectively to clinical CHD in the MRFIT study.

In another study employing component scoring techniques with SI data, Hecker, Frautschi, Chesney, Black, and Rosenman (1985) compared component scores of all available CHD cases ($N = 250$) in the WCGS with those of 500 matched controls free of CHD during the entire 8.5-year follow-up. Again, a measure of potential for hostility emerged as the best significant predictor of incident cases relative to matched controls. Even more important, multivariate analyses showed that no other measure from the extensive battery of components that were

scored in this study added significantly to the explained CHD event variance beyond that accounted for by the PoHo measure.

Taken altogether, the results from both questionnaire-based and SI-based studies make a compelling case that the hostility/anger dimension is the major, and probably the only, aspect of the global TABP that is coronary-prone. The large body of evidence available from studies of the Cook–Medley Ho scale suggest that a cynical mistrust of others is one aspect of the hostility/anger dimension that is coronary-prone. The large body of evidence from studies employing components scoring of the SI suggest that coronary-proneness is not only characterized by a cynical mistrust (and dislike) of others; it also may be reflected by a relatively low threshold for the expression of this negative regard for others.

Recently, Dembroski filled out an adjective checklist instrument for subsets of SIs derived from both the WCGS and MRFIT (Dembroski & Costa, 1987). The results revealed that ratings of PoHo from these SIs were primarily associated with descriptors of antagonism: uncooperative, rude, disagreeable, callous, and the like. Secondarily, however, PoHo ratings were also related to hostility facets of neuroticism, which, along with antagonism, is one of five factors contained in a comprehensive mapping of established dimensions of individual differences (Costa & McCrae, 1987). Examples of descriptors here included irritable versus good-natured, impatient versus patient, temperamental versus even-tempered, and the like. Interestingly, PoHo was not strongly correlated with dimensions reflecting the anxious, vulnerable, and self-pitying attributes often found in individuals scoring high on neuroticism scales (Dembroski & Costa, 1987).

Before concluding this survey of means useful to assess behavioral and psychological factors that are coronary-prone, it is important to consider briefly the possible effects of neuroticism.

Neuroticism and Other Psychological Factors

Neuroticism may be defined as the dimension of personality underlying the expression of consistently high levels of chronic negative affects, the tendency to express distress, and to complain about many things, including chest pains (Costa, 1986). It is not surprising that many investigators have studied the relationship between measures of neuroticism and CHD endpoints, given the plethora of negative affects reflected in the construct.

Somewhat surprisingly, these studies have failed to find any positive association between neuroticism measures [usually questionnaire-based; examples of measures of neuroticism are the Depression (D), Hypochondriasis (Hs), and Hysteria (Hy) scales of the MMPI, the Spielberger State–Trait Anxiety Inventory, and the like] and "hard" CHD endpoints, such as MI and cardiac death. What has been consistently found, however, is an association, in both cross-sectional and prospective studies, between neuroticism indices and an increased tendency to complain of anginalike chest pain (Costa, 1986). Ostfeld, Lebovits, Shekelle, and Paul (1964) reported that high scores on the MMPI Hs scale significantly predicted the risk of developing new angina, but not MI, in the Western Electric Study. Williams *et al.* (1986) found that high Hs scores were the best single predictor of failure to obtain angina relief with medical management among patients with documented CAD in the Duke angiographic sample.

Several studies show how measures that appear to assess the hostility/anger dimension may be confounded by associations with neuroticism. The Spielberger Trait Anger Scale (STAS) appears to be a measure of the hostility/anger dimension, yet it correlates heavily with indices of neuroticism (Costa & McCrae, 1987). Not surprisingly, therefore, STAS scores were not related to CAD severity in two recent studies (Smith, Follick, & Korr, 1984; Schocken, Worden, Green, Harrison, & Spielberger, 1985) and were negatively related to CAD severity in a third study (Spielberger, personal communication). Noteworthy in this context is that of all the extant measures of the TABP, only the Framingham Type A scale consistently shows significant relationships with various measures of neuroticism (Chesney *et al.,* 1981; Haynes *et al.,* 1980). Therefore, it should not be surprising to learn that analyses of the Framingham data (Haynes *et al.,* 1980) suggest that the prediction of "CHD" by the Framingham Type A scale is mainly due to

prediction of angina complaints, especially in the women.

The importance of the relationship between some measures of hostility and indices of neuroticism was underlined in a recently completed study in which the Buss Durkee Hostility Inventory (BDHI; Buss & Durkee, 1957) was used to examine the association between level of hostility and CAD severity (Siegman, Dembroski, & Ringel, 1987). A factor analysis of the BDHI scales revealed two factors. One reflected primarily the experience of anger and was labeled "neurotic hostility" because it significantly correlated with anxiety scores. The other factor was labeled reactive or "expressive hostility" and was unrelated to indices of anxiety. The first factor, neurotic hostility, was significantly related to CAD severity in an *inverse* direction, whereas the expressive hostility factor was significantly related to CAD severity in a *positive* direction. As might be expected, total BDHI scores were unrelated to extent of CAD because the negative relationship of the first factor to CAD canceled the positive association of the second factor.

Recent analyses of the CAD–neuroticism link in the Duke angiographic data set (Barefoot & Williams, unpublished data) confirmed the inverse association between neuroticism measures and CAD severity: high MMPI Hs scores were negatively correlated with CAD severity.

The clinical significance of neuroticism for CAD research has been comprehensively reviewed by Costa (1986). He makes the important observation that the tendency of neurotic individuals to complain more frequently and demandingly of anginalike chest pain will result, if reported to a physician, in an increased likelihood of referral for coronary angiographic testing—the "therapeutic coronary angiogram." However, since the symptoms are neurotic rather than disease-based in origin, the probability of discovering significant CAD at the time of cardiac catheterization is diminished.

Inspection of the items reflecting the BDHI neurotic hostility factor revealed individuals who mistrust the motives of other people, feel resentment with their life in general, and believe they often have been mistreated. Such people are prone to experience anxiety, depression, and somatic symptoms, all markers of neuroticism. On the other hand, persons scoring high on the expressive hostility factor, which is not correlated with neuroticism, endorse items indicating that they frequently argue with others who disagree with them and do so with a loud voice; and are capable of physical assault if sufficiently provoked.

The latter profile appears much more conceptually consistent with the sort of hostility assessed by the SI-based PoHo construct than it does with the resentment and suspiciousness reflected by the neurotic hostility factor. Indeed, a recent study showed that the SI-derived PoHo ratings were significantly correlated with expressive hostility (Musante *et al.*, in press).

It may be readily appreciated that the Cook–Medley Ho scale contains items which reflect both the neurotic hostility and expressive hostility factors which emerged from the Siegman *et al.* (1987) study—e.g., ''No one cares much what happens to you'' (neurotic hostility) versus ''I have at times had to be rough with people who were rude or annoying'' (expressive hostility). Smith and Frohm (1985) found the Ho scale to correlate significantly with trait anxiety, albeit more weakly than with cynicism/anger measures. It may well be the case that its striking success in correlating with CAD and predicting CHD and mortality outcomes is attributable less to its association with neuroticism than to its ability to provide a valid index of nonneurotic aspects of the hostility/anger dimension. As mentioned earlier, support for this interpretation is provided by the recent finding (Barefoot *et al.*, 1987) that Ho items reflecting cynicism, anger, and aggression are predictors of mortality, while items reflecting paranoid attributions and other more neurotically tinged items are not.

Similarly, and as noted above, overall SI-defined PoHo contains some elements of neuroticism, particularly those attributes reflecting irritability, impatience, and the like. It will be interesting to determine whether these neurotic aspects of PoHo, relative to the antagonistic facets, are differentially related to clinical CHD (Dembroski & Costa, 1987).

Conclusions

Progress in science proceeds in a characteristic series of steps, from early, often accidental or anec-

dotal observations, to ideas about the meaning of those observations, to tests of those ideas in planned research, to refinements of those ideas based on the research findings. Such was the case with the CHD–lipid hypothesis: first, Virchow found yellow deposits in the coronary arteries of persons who died suddenly; second, chemists determined that cholesterol was a prominent constituent of those deposits; third, the idea was formed that cholesterol in blood may cause heart disease; fourth, prospective epidemiological studies demonstrated that persons with higher levels of cholesterol in blood were more likely to develop CHD; fifth, more sophisticated biochemical studies showed that the total serum cholesterol was made up of many components, some of which are coronary-prone and some of which are actually coronary-protective; and sixth, massive public health efforts have been mounted to reduce blood levels of LDL cholesterol and raise levels of HDL cholesterol with the goal of reducing the massive toll exacted by CHD.

As we have attempted to review in this chapter, a similar process has been under way with respect to coronary-prone behavior. Attempts to move beyond and refine the global TABP construct have led to the conclusion that not all aspects of TABP are coronary-prone; just as with cholesterol, some TABP components may even be coronary-protective, while only a few—apparently those related to hostility/anger—are coronary-prone. Mainly due to the availability of prospective data on cohorts followed over several years with respect to health outcomes, most of the research attempting to achieve a better definition of coronary-prone behavior has concentrated on the SI and the MMPI-based Ho scale. This does not mean these will prove ultimately to be the best measures of coronary-prone behavior, however.

As conceptual clarification—e.g., the distinction of cynical mistrust and expressive hostility from neurotic hostility—proceeds, objective assessment can be expected to replace many of the more subjective techniques that by necessity are presently being used. Present and future consistency of findings will profitably guide research to develop more effective means of prevention, treatment, and rehabilitation with respect to CHD, once validated coronary-prone behaviors and psychological traits can be targeted with more precision.

Specificity of coronary-prone behaviors will enable more efficient and effective identification of psychophysiological and basic pathophysiological mechanisms whereby such behaviors and traits are translated into CAD and contribute to the precipitation of acute CHD events. Parallel research can then explore genetic, socialization, and cultural variables associated with particular coronary-prone behaviors. Finally, more sophisticated epidemiological research can be launched to examine prediction of a variety of disease endpoints.

References

Barefoot, J. C., Dahlstrom, W. B., & Williams, R. B. (1983). Hostility, CHD incidence and total mortality: A 25-year follow-up study of 255 physicians. *Psychosomatic Medicine, 45,* 59–63.

Barefoot, J. C., Williams, R. B., Dahlstrom, W. G., & Dodge, K. A. (1987). Predicting mortality from scores on the Cook–Medley scale: A follow-up study of 118 lawyers. *Psychosomatic Medicine, 49,* 210 (Abstract).

Blumenthal, J. A., Williams, R. B., Kong, Y., Schanberg, S. M., & Thompson, L. W. (1978). Type A behavior pattern and coronary atherosclerosis. *Circulation, 258,* 634–639.

Brand, R. (1978). Coronary-prone behavior as an independent risk factor for coronary heart disease. In T. M. Dembroski, S. M. Weiss, J. L. Shields, S. G. Haynes, & M. Feinlieb (Eds.), *Coronary-prone behavior.* Berlin: Springer-Verlag.

Buss, A. H., & Durkee, A. (1957). An inventory for assessing different kinds of hostility. *Journal of Consulting Psychology, 21,* 343–349.

Chesney, M. A., Black, G. W., Chadwick, J. H., & Rosenman, R. H. (1981). Psychological correlates of the Type A behavior pattern. *Journal of Behavioral Medicine, 4,* 217–229.

Cook, W., & Medley, D. (1954). Proposed hostility and pharisaic-virtue scales for the MMPI. *Journal of Applied Psychology, 238,* 414–418.

Costa, P. T. (1986). Is neuroticism a risk factor for CAD? Is Type A a measure of neuroticism? In T. H. Schmidt, T. M. Dembroski, & G. Blumchen (Eds.), *Biological and psychological factors in cardiovascular disease.* Berlin: Springer-Verlag.

Costa, P. T., & McCrae, R. R. (1987). Neuroticism, somatic complaints, and disease: Is the bark worse than the bite? *Journal of Personality, 55,* 299–316.

Costa, P. T., Zonderman, A. B., McCrae, R. R., & Williams, R. B. (1985). Content and comprehensiveness in the MMPI: An item factor analysis of a normal adult sample. *Journal of Personality and Social Psychology, 48,* 925–933.

Costa, P. T., Zonderman, A. B., McCrae, R. R., & Williams, R. B. (1986). Cynicism paranoid alienation in the Cook and Medley Ho scale. *Psychosomatic Medicine, 48,* 283–285.

Dembroski, T. M., & Costa, P. T. (1987). Coronary-prone behavior: Components of the Type A pattern and hostility. *Journal of Personality, 55,* 211–235.

Dembroski, T. M., & MacDougall, J. M. (1983). Behavioral and psychophysiological perspectives on coronary-prone behavior. In T. M. Dembroski, T. H. Schmidt, & G. Blumchen (Eds.), *Biobehavioral bases of coronary heart disease.* Basel: Karger.

Dembroski, T. M., & MacDougall, J. M. (1985). Beyond global Type A: Relationships of paralinguistic attributes, hostility, and anger-in coronary heart disease. In T. Field, P. McCabe, & N. Schneiderman (Eds.), *Stress and coping.* Hillsdale, NJ: Erlbaum.

Dembroski, T. M., MacDougall, J. M., Williams, R. B., Haney, T. L., & Blumenthal, J. A. (1985). Components of Type A, hostility, and anger-in: Relationship to angiographic findings. *Psychosomatic Medicine, 47,* 219–233.

Dembroski, T. M., Weiss, S., Shields, J. L., Haynes, S., & Feinlieb, M. (1978). *Coronary-prone behavior.* Berlin: Springer-Verlag.

Diamond, E. L. (1982). The role of anger and hostility in essential hypertension and coronary heart disease. *Psychological Bulletin, 244,* 413–420.

Dimsdale, J. E., Hackett, T. P., Hutter, A. M., Block, P. C., Cantanzano, D., & White, P. J. (1979). Type A behavior pattern and coronary angiographic findings. *Journal of Psychosomatic Research, 23,* 273–276.

Frank, K. A., Heller, S. S., Kornfeld, D. S., Sporn, A. A., & Weiss, M. B. (1978). Type A behavior pattern and coronary angiographic findings. *Journal of the American Medical Association, 240,* 761–763.

Friedman, M., & Rosenman, R. H. (1974). *Type A behavior and your heart.* New York: Knopf.

Friedman, M., Rosenman, R. H., Strauss, R., Wurm, M., & Kositchek, R. (1968). The relationship of behavior pattern to the state of the coronary vasculature. A study of 51 autopsy subjects. *American Journal of Medicine, 244,* 525–538.

Friedman, M., Brown, M. A., & Rosenman, R. H. (1969). Voice analysis test for detection of behavior pattern. *Journal of the American Medical Association, 208,* 828–836.

Friedman, M., Thoresen, C., Gil, J., Ulmer, D., Thompson, L., Powell, L., Prince, V., Elex, S. R., Rabin, D. D., Breel, W. S., & Pigget, G. (1982). Feasibility of altering Type A behavior pattern after myocardial infarction. Recurrent coronary prevention project study: Methods, baseline results, and preliminary findings. *Circulation, 266,* 83–92.

Glass, D. C., Ross, D. T., Isecke, W., & Rosenman, R. H. (1982). Relative importance of speech characteristics and content of answers in the assessment of behavior pattern A by the structured interview. *Basic and Applied Social Psychology, 23,* 161–168.

Haynes, S. G., Feinlieb, M., & Kannel, W. B. (1980). Psychosocial factors and CHD incidence in Framingham: Results from an 8-year follow-up study. *American Journal of Epidemiology, 108,* 229.

Hecker, M., Frautschi, N., Chesney, M., Black, G., & Rosenman, R. (1985). *Components of Type A behavior and coro-*

nary heart disease. Paper presented at the annual meeting of the Society of Behavioral Medicine, New Orleans.

Howland, E. W., & Siegman, A. W. (1982). Toward the automated measurement of the Type A behavior pattern. *Journal of Behavioral Medicine, 5*, 37–53.

Johnson, J. H., Butcher, J. N., Null, C., & Johnson, K. N. (1984). Replicated item level factor analysis of the full MMPI. *Journal of Personality and Social Psychology, 49*, 105–114.

MacDougall, J. M., Dembroski, T. M., Dimsdale, J. E., & Hackett, T. (1985). Components of Type A, hostility, and anger-in: Further relationships to angiographic findings. *Health Psychology, 4*, 137–152.

MacDougall, J. M., Dembroski, T. M., & Musante, L. (1979). The structured interview and questionnaire methods of assessing coronary-prone behavior in male and female college students. *Journal of Behavioral Medicine, 2*, 71–83.

Matthews, K. A. (1982). Psychological perspectives on the Type A behavior pattern. *Psychological Bulletin, 91*(2), 293–323.

Matthews, K. A., Glass, D. C., Rosenman, R. H., & Bortner, R. W. (1977). Competitive drive, pattern A, and coronary heart disease: A further analysis of some data from the Western Collaborative Group Study. *Journal of Chronic Diseases, 30*, 489–498.

Matthews, K. A., & Haynes, S. G. (1986). Type A behavior pattern and coronary risk: Update and critical evaluation. *American Journal of Epidemiology, 123*, 923–960.

Matthews, K. A., Krantz, D. S., Dembroski, T. M., & MacDougall, J. M. (1982). The unique and common variance in the structured interview and the Jenkins Activity Survey measures of the Type A behavior pattern. *Journal of Personality and Social Psychology, 42*, 303–313.

McCranie, E. W., Watkins, L., Brandsma, J., & Sisson, B. (1986). Hostility, coronary heart disease (CHD) incidence, and total mortality: Lack of association in a 25-year follow-up study of 478 physicians. *Journal of Behavioral Medicine, 9*, 119–125.

Multiple Risk Factor Intervention Trial Group (1979). The MRFIT Behavior Pattern Study. 1. Study design, procedures, and the reproducibility of behavior pattern judgments. *Journal of Chronic Diseases, 32*, 293–305.

Musante, L., MacDougall, J. M., Dembroski, T. M., & Costa, P. T. (in press). Potential for hostility the dimensions of anger. *Health Psychology,*

Musante, L., MacDougall, J. M., Dembroski, T. M., & Van Horn, A. E. (1983). Component analysis of the Type A coronary-prone behavior pattern in male and female college students. *Journal of Personality and Social Psychology, 245*, 1104–1117.

Ostfeld, A. M., Lebovits, B. Z., Shekelle, R. B., & Paul, O. (1964). A prospective study of the relationship between personality and coronary heart disease. *Journal of Chronic Diseases, 17*, 265–276.

Pooling Project Research Group (1978). Relationship of blood pressure, serum cholesterol, smoking habits, relative weight, and ECG abnormalities to incidence of major coronary

events: Final report of the pooling project. *Journal of Chronic Diseases, 31*, 201–306.

Ragland, D. R., Brand, R. J., & Rosenman, R. H. (1986). Coronary heart disease in the Western Collaborative Group Study. *American Journal of Epidemiology, 124*, 522.

Review Panel on Coronary-Prone Behavior and Coronary Heart Disease (1981). Coronary-prone behavior and coronary heart disease: A critical review. *Circulation, 63*, 1199–1215.

Rosenman, R. H. (1978). The interview method of assessment of the coronary-prone behavior pattern. In T. M. Dembroski, S. M. Weiss, J. L. Shields, S. G. Haynes, & M. Feinlieb (Eds.), *Coronary-prone behavior*. Berlin: Springer-Verlag.

Rosenman, R. H. (1986). Current and past history of Type A behavior pattern. In T. H. Schmidt, T. M. Dembroski, & G. Blumchen (Eds.), *Biological and psychological factors in cardiovascular disease*. Berlin: Springer-Verlag.

Rosenman, R. H., Brand, R. J., Jenkins, C. D., Friedman, M., Strauss, R., & Wurm, M. (1975). Coronary heart disease in the Western Collaborative Group Study: Final follow-up experience of 8½ years. *Journal of the American Medical Association, 223*, 872–877.

Rosenman, R. H., & Friedman, M. (1974). Neurogenic factors in pathogenesis of coronary heart disease. *Medical Clinics of North America, 58*, 269–279.

Scherwitz, L., Berton, K., & Leventhal, H. (1977). Type A assessment and interaction in the behavior pattern interview. *Psychosomatic Medicine, 39*, 229–240.

Schocken, D. D., Worden, T., Green, A. F., Harrison, E. F., & Spielberger, C. D. (1985). Age differences in the relationship between coronary artery disease, anxiety, and anger. *Gerontologist, 225*, 36.

Schucker, B., & Jacobs, D. R. (1977). Assessment of behavioral risk of coronary disease by voice characteristics. *Psychosomatic Medicine, 39*, 219–228.

Shekelle, R. B., Gale, M., Ostfeld, A. M., & Paul, P. (1983). Hostility, risk of coronary disease, and mortality. *Psychosomatic Medicine, 45*, 109–114.

Shekelle, R. B., Hulley, S., Neaton, J., Billings, J., Borhani, N., Gerace, T., Jacobs, D., Lasser, N., Mittlemark, M., Stamler, J., & the MRFIT Research Group (1985). The MRFIT behavior pattern study. II. Type A behavior pattern and incidence of coronary heart disease. *American Journal of Epidemiology, 122*, 559–570.

Siegman, A. W., Dembroski, T. M., & Ringel, N. (1987). Components of hostility and the severity of coronary artery disease. *Psychosomatic Medicine, 48*, 127–135.

Smith, T. W., & Frohm, K. D. (1985). What's so unhealthy about hostility? Construct validity and psychosocial correlates of the Cook and Medley Ho scale. *Health Psychology, 4*, 503–520.

Smith, T. W., Follick, M. L., & Korr, K. S. (1984). Anger, neuroticism, Type A behavior, and the experience of angina. *British Journal of Medical Psychology, 257*, 249–252.

Williams, R. B., Barefoot, J. C., Haney, T. L., Harrell, F. E., Blumenthal, J. A., Pryor, D., & Peterson, B. (1986). Type A behavior and angiographically documented coronary atherosclerosis in a sample of 2,289 patients. *Psychosomatic Medicine, 48*, 302 (Abstract).

Williams, R. B., Haney, T. L., Lee, K. L., Kong, Y., Blumenthal, J. A., & Whalen, R. (1980). Type A behavior, hostility, and coronary atherosclerosis. *Psychosomatic Medicine, 42,* 539–549.

Zyzanski, S. J., Jenkins, C. D., Ryan, T. J., Flessas, A., & Everist, M. (1976). Psychological correlates of coronary angiographic findings. *Archives of Internal Medicine, 136,* 1234–1237.

Research Design and Statistics

Section Editor: Stephen B. Manuck

By its interdisciplinary nature, cardiovascular behavioral medicine exploits the expertise of individuals having diverse professional backgrounds. One result of such diversity is that the methodological and quantitative sophistication of investigators who work in this field also varies substantially, owing to different levels of prior training received in such areas as experimental methods and statistics. It is not surprising that persons trained in clinical medicine frequently have had little exposure to techniques of multivariate statistical analysis, whereas experimental psychologists must often take five or more courses devoted to quantitative methods as a part of their predoctoral curriculum. (Needless to say, the psychologist's curriculum usually entails little exposure to circulatory physiology, much less to diseases of the heart and vasculature.) Many areas of cardiovascular investigation also involve research designs (e.g., clinical trials, pooling projects) that are rarely covered in traditional courses on experimental methodology. Hence, the purpose of the following section of this handbook is to provide an introduction and general background to issues of research design and statistical analysis that are pertinent to cardiovascular behavioral medicine. Because these issues are equally applicable to other areas of experimental and clinical investigation,

much of the material that follows is necessarily of a "generic" nature. Most of the specific examples presented, however, relate directly to cardiovascular research. In addition, each of the following chapters should prove accessible to a wide range of interested readers, including those who have had only limited formal training in experimental design and inferential statistics.

Chapter 36 by Ray provides an introduction to the logic of experimental inference, as well as an overview of the principal experimental, quasi-experimental, and correlational research designs. Also discussed is the "validity" of conclusions drawn from research studies and the common threats to such validity that arise from flaws in data collection or interpretive constraints of the investigational strategy employed. In Chapter 37 Van Egeren outlines the process of the data analysis and selection of primary statistical tests for the examination of data sets. Considered specifically are the analysis of variance, multiple regression analysis, multivariate statistical procedures, time series analysis, and causal modeling. Van Egeren also addresses many practical questions that confront the investigator; these range from the formulation of an explicit plan of analysis to the treatment of "outliers" and missing data.

The next four chapters address topics that have assumed increasing importance in recent years—statistical power, experimental studies in the field, techniques of metaanalysis, and the pooling of data from multiple sites or investigations. As Muenz

Stephen B. Manuck • Department of Psychology, University of Pittsburgh, Pittsburgh, Pennsylvania 15260.

writes in the introduction to Chapter 38, "Power is the probability that a statistical analysis of experimental data will detect a true effect." This probability is determined by decisions made at the time an investigation is conceived and designed, and typically reflects an interplay between the magnitude of an expected outcome (effect) and the size of the sample recruited into the study. Power analysis offers a rational foundation on which to make these decisions. Muenz's chapter provides a basis for understanding statistical power and its calculation, as well as its application to different forms of experimental design.

In Chapter 39 Singer addresses the problems and issues associated with doing biobehavioral research in field settings. The emphases in this chapter are upon the appropriate selection of control groups, issues concerning subject recruitment and retention, and the modification of laboratory procedure necessitated by the field setting.

Metaanalysis refers to statistical procedures that permit combining evidence from similar research studies. This is a particularly valuable tool where a large number of investigations address the same or related questions. The pooling of results from published reports and their statistical analysis in aggregate allows quantitative inferences to be applied to entire literatures. In Chapter 40 Hedges discusses the various models of metaanalysis, their utilities, areas of application, assumptions, and quantitative features. In addition to combining the results of reported studies, one can also combine the raw data collected in multiple investigations. Such pooling of data enhances the power to detect significant treatment effects and may permit an examination of hypotheses that are not testable within the scope of the individual studies. Kaufmann presents an overview of pooling procedures in Chapter 41, focusing on pragmatic issues such as the formulation of objectives, the selection of studies and data to be included, the mechanics of pooling, and considerations pertinent to data analysis.

The final chapter in this section addresses methodological aspects of epidemiological investigations and, specifically, of randomized clinical trials. In Chapter 42, Kuller discusses the experimental rationale underlying clinical trials and describes the many design considerations that clinical trials entail. The latter include the blinding of interventions, recruitment of participants, problems in adherence to the study protocol, and the measurement of appropriate endpoints. Also considered are community intervention trials (where communities, rather than individuals, are the targets of treatment) and points germane to the statistical analysis of clinical trial data.

CHAPTER 36

Research Designs in Behavioral Cardiovascular Research

William J. Ray

Introduction

Science is a human activity in which we attempt to establish knowledge within particular domains of interest. There have been a number of attempts to specify how science works although no satisfactory solution has yet been achieved. Understanding science in a complete sense is a difficult if not impossible task since to specify science we would also need to specify the important parameters of those performing science which we lack at this time. However, the utility of science is assumed and stands as the major way of developing and establishing knowledge. In the development of knowledge we can begin to articulate the goals in which the scientific enterprise is directed. In science we attempt to articulate at least three different types of relationships or representations. First, there are theoretical representations. Second, there are research representations. And third, there exist quantitative representations.

The first type of representation is analytic in nature. In this approach to understanding a domain, we attempt to represent a process (e.g., the development of hypertension) by decomposing the overall process into its constituent parts. In this manner we seek to specify particular mechanisms and the causal or probabilistic sequence which leads to the process under study. It is rare that we see or even can see the entire mechanism in process. Thus, we must analytically reconstruct the process in the form of a theoretical representation or mathematical representation. Logic (including mathematical proof and manipulation) and rhetoric are the most commonly used means for the presentation and verification of theoretical ideas.

The second type of representation is one in which we seek to understand our ideas (i.e., constructs) by mapping them onto some particular domain by which we can achieve a quantitative representation. For example, we might seek an analogous empirical situation which we assume to reflect the conceptual one. In such empirical situations, constructs are represented in terms of quantitative processes. Measurement becomes the important aspect of this process and statistics the means by which a relationship is established. Once a statistical relationship can be stated, then the task is to map this relationship in an analogous fashion back onto the conceptual domain and to consider the logic underlying this representation. Traditionally, the goal has been the establishment of causal inferences between one variable (the independent variable) and another (the dependent vari-

William J. Ray • Department of Psychology, Pennsylvania State University, University Park, Pennsylvania 16802.

able) in a study. The completion of a causal inference is thus both a statistical consideration and a validity problem.

The third type of representation is that in which one set of quantitative measures is related to another set of quantitative measures without an attempt to create a conceptually analogous setting or specify causal relationships. This third approach is more mechanical in nature and seeks to present a more direct understanding of the processes under study in some descriptive manner (e.g., correlation, time series analysis, differential equations) whether they be differential analysis of blood flow, Newtonian mechanics, or time series analysis of stock market changes. The main criteria for using these more mechanical procedures are pragmatic ones. That which works is adopted.

In this chapter we will review these three procedures for scientific understanding with the greatest emphasis being placed on the second type of representation. In order to facilitate this discussion, we will consider the structure of research designs as well as questions of validity within the context of cardiovascular research. We will not discuss in depth questions of statistical inference, field study approaches, clinical trials, or meta-analysis since these topics will be covered in later chapters. Other methodological presentations have focused on aging (see Nesselroade & Labouvie, 1985), and clinical research (Maher, 1978) and should be consulted for research involving these special populations and topics.

One of the major jobs of cardiovascular research is to bridge the gap between these three levels of representation. This process is not difficult when one is able to specify the necessary dimensions of an area under study. For example, if one was able to say that a particular drug at a particular dosage for a particular population increased heart rate by 4.7 beats/min, then the task would be to make a measurement within a certain error of measurement. Questions of validity are relatively easy in such situations since there exists an established standard of measurement specified by the appropriate parameters. Mark (1986) rephrases the question of valid inference into a more genetic statement concerning what causes what for whom under what conditions. He recognizes that a more

complete statement would also include the temporal dimension as well as effect size (Reichardt, 1986). Thus, a more complete statement would ask, what causes what for whom and when, under what conditions and with what magnitude. However, it is rare that the behavioral cardiovascular researchers are able to make such point predictions. They usually find themselves faced with a less exact theoretical statement in which many of the parameters are not known. Thus, it is initially a judgment decision to determine the appropriate point to perform the research since one cannot simultaneously study the important parameters of subjects, conditions, treatments, effects, and magnitudes. It is for this reason that specifying a mechanism becomes so important. But, how does one go about making valid statements concerning important processes? For example, if theory states that increasing heart rate and blood pressure causes baroreceptor activation which inhibits cortical functioning through a particular mechanism in a particular situation, then one must determine how to evaluate such a statement. To say the least, one would not only want to demonstrate that this effect does indeed take place and under what conditions, but more important, one would also want to show if one of the mediational factors was not present, then the event would not happen. It cannot be stressed enough that although it is our human nature to want to ''prove'' things and seek confirmatory evidence, the logic of science requires the ability to disconfirm theoretical statements. In order to accomplish this goal, it is necessary to create an idealized situation in which the important factors can be controlled and a logical statement made. Laboratory research offers such an opportunity. One purpose of research design is to aid in this presentation. Numerous theoretical presentations have been addressed toward one's ability to make valid statements given a particular research approach (Campbell & Stanley, 1966; Cook & Campbell, 1979; Cochran, 1983; Trochim, 1986). As has been clearly pointed out in these presentations, there is no one research design that answers all the questions one wishes to answer. Neither are research designs developed in isolation. Good research is always conceived within a particular research domain since this dictates which validity considerations are relevant in a given study. In this sense, research is always a unique blending of methodology, knowledge of a particular research domain, and judgment.

Examples from Cardiovascular Research

There are a variety of types of research that cardiovascular researchers perform. These range from highly controlled laboratory studies to the less well-controlled field studies. Said in other terms, these types of studies range from those in which the researcher is able to create a closed system and thus simplify and control the process under study to that of an environmental open system in which the researcher has little control or design over the factors that influence the processes. In this section five studies will be presented which draw from both laboratory and field studies although none could be considered a "true experiment" in the strict sense which we will discuss later. Following the presentation of these studies, we will use these as examplars for the presentation of particular types of designs and inferential problems with each.

Study 1—Barefoot, Dahlstrom, and Williams (1983) reported a retrospective study in which medical graduates from the University of North Carolina in the years 1954–1959 were asked to complete a qustionnaire concerning their current health status. Of a possible 343 subjects, 255 were used in the final sample. Since the MMPI has been given as part of medical training, it was possible to use this instrument to construct a derived hostility subscale. Subjects were divided into four groups based on the hostility score, and incidence of coronary heart disease was examined in terms of these groups.

Study 2—Dembroski, MacDougall, Williams, Haney, and Blumenthal (1985) sought to determine which aspects of Type A patterning would be most predictive of cardiovascular disease severity. From a larger population of 2000 patients who underwent diagnostic coronary angiography, 131 patients were randomly selected from each of two severity categories (not severe or very severe coronary artery disease). The primary data for the study consisted of audiotapes of the Type A structured interview. The Type A components were used as predictor variables for relative presence of signs of coronary artery disease and related factors. Risk factors such as age, sex, smoking, family history, and so forth were used as control variables. Initial data analysis consisted of specifying the relationship between the predictors and endpoint measures using correlational procedures followed by a stepwise multiple regression analysis for the coronary index rating and the number of vessels occluded and a stepwise discriminant function analysis for angina measure and the number of previous myocardial infarctions.

Study 3—Corse, Manuck, Cantwell, Giordani, and Mathews (1982) studied Type A and B individuals with and without coronary heart disease. The subjects were selected after a review of the records from a preventive cardiology clinic in order to create two groups of subjects (those with and those without a history of coronary heart disease). Type A behavior was assessed by two different instruments: the Structured Interview and the Jenkins Activity Survey. During the experimental session three difficult cognitive tasks (concepts, mental arithmetic, and picture completion) were administered with heart rate and blood pressure being taken. The psychophysiological reactivity to these tasks was measured.

Study 4—Scher, Hartman, Furedy, and Heslegrave (1986) suggested that T-wave amplitude is a more sensitive measure of sympathetic myocardial influences than heart rate. Using this measure, they sought to determine the cardiovascular responses of Type As and Bs to mental effort. Subjects for the experiment were 15 Type A and 15 Type B males with a mean age in the 30s. Heart rate and T-wave amplitude measures were taken during a series of subtraction tasks as well as baseline periods.

Study 5—Friedman et al. (1984) sought to determine if Type A behavior patients could be modified and if this modification would be associated with a reduced rate of myocardial infarctions. The subjects were 862 individuals who had suffered myocardial infarctions at least 6 months earlier.

They were randomly divided into a control and experimental group both of which received cardiologic counseling (i.e., information concerning diet, exercise, medical information) but only the experimental group received Type A behavioral counseling. Both groups continued to be seen by their local physicians. Measures taken during the study included both physiological processes (e.g., ECG, serum cholesterol, and urine analysis) and measures of Type A behavior (questionnaires completed by patient, spouse, and work colleague as well as a Type A interview). These measures were taken at regular intervals during the 3 years, and included initial baseline measurements.

Types of Research Designs

Researchers interested in cardiovascular processes are drawn from a variety of fields, each with its own terminology for referring to research designs. Most design designations attempt to specify the quality of inferences that can be made. The strongest inferences can be made with those designs which best limit alternative interpretations of the results. Those studies which limit alternative interpretations through random sampling, random assignment to groups, and appropriate experimental control are referred to as "true experiments" by Campbell and Stanley (1966). On the other extreme are those studies which the experimenter has no control over and may even involve events that have already taken place as in a retrospective study. These types of studies are referred to as "correlational" in psychology and as a special case of "observational" referred to as "analytic surveys" by such authors as Cochran (1983). One difficulty is that these terms have very different meanings throughout the sciences. Although not without its problems, we will use the term "natural associational research" to refer to this type of study. Thus, one could imagine a spectrum which runs from the "true experiment" on one end to the "natural associational experiment" on the other. In between are research designs also referred to as "observational" and as "quasi-experimental." In this chapter we use the term "quasi-experimental" for such studies. Quasi-experimental designs may include such measures as control groups, timing of measurement, and other such devices for strengthening inferences. In the following sections, we will discuss these three types of designs.

Experimental Design

In this section the formal principles that have evolved in discussions of experimental design will be discussed. These principles establish the structures that require consideration across topic domains in general. However, it should be remembered that particular theoretical domains contain within themselves a statement of which variables are to be measured and how they are to be measured as well as which factors need to be controlled and which can be safely ignored without losing definition of experimental results. For example, Krantz and Manuck (1984) outline those factors that must be considered when performing psychophysiological reactivity studies in relation to risk of cardiovascular disease. This type of information allows the experimenter to gain experimental control in the experimental situation. Implicit in the traditional understanding of experimental design is the idea that the experimenter has achieved an important degree of control over the experimental situation and thus is able to make valid inferences concerning the results of the research. In general, we wish to be able to make a statement of the form that one variable (said to be independent since it is set before the experiment begins) had some form of influence on another (said to be dependent since its values depend on the experimental situation through the action of the independent variable). The task of the researcher is to statistically demonstrate that numerical differences were present that could only infrequently be attributed to chance and to logically present the case that it is valid to conclude that any changes observed in the experiment were the resultant of the independent variable.

The traditional means to increase inferential validity is through experimental control. There are a variety of ways in which a researcher is able to gain control. For the present we will emphasize experimental design as a means of achieving control. For presentational purposes let us use Figure 1

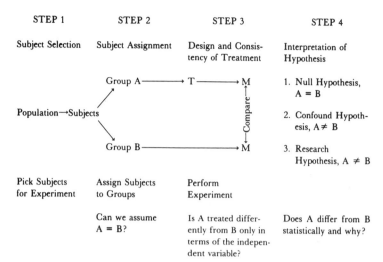

Figure 1. Conceptual steps in experimentation. Adapted from Ray and Ravizza (1988) with permission.

to aid in understanding the traditional experiment as a four-step process with different types of control being required at each step. Steps 1 and 2 focus on subject selection and assignment. The classical method for subject selection and assignment emphasizes the experimenter's ability to randomly sample from a larger population and to assign this sample randomly to two or more groups. The main purpose of random assignment is to ensure that before the experiment begins the subject groups are equal. Although this sounds straightforward, it is not uncommon for researchers to adopt procedures unknowingly which invalidate the claim of initially equal groups. Suppose, for example, someone chose mice for a drug study by simply reaching into a group cage and making the first ten mice picked out the group that would receive a drug and the second ten the group that would not. Such a procedure would lead to the quicker mice (i.e., those that moved away from the experimenter's hand) being in the second group and the slower or less afraid mice being in the drug group. Similarly, consider an experimenter who ran an ad in the paper for subjects with certain symptoms (e.g., angina) and assigned the subjects to groups as they responded. Here there are two separate types of problems. The first problem relates to the question of representativeness and asks if a particular type of angina subject would respond to ads whereas others would not (e.g., those people who

were afraid to find out if they really had a heart problem). Although this would not hurt the logic of the experiment *per se,* it would present difficulties if the experimenter sought to make a statement concerning all angina patients and not just those who seek help. The second type of problem would hurt the logic of the experiment since like the mice example, one group would be composed of subjects who responded to the ad quickly and the other group would be composed of those who put off responding but called after some delay. There are, of course, easy procedures to prevent these problems such as random assignment or control through alternative assignment to subject groups, but the point remains that in the traditional experimental design all procedures must lead to the knowledge that subject groups are equal before the experimental procedure begins.

Moving to step 3 of Figure 1 we ask the question, is the independent variable (i.e., the treatment) the only manner in which the groups in the experiment are treated differently? If indeed this is the case, we are in a stronger position to claim that the differences between the groups in the experiment were indeed the resultant of our treatment variable. If this was not the case, then one's logic is greatly weakened. Again, one must consider in some detail the actual experimental protocol, for both subtle and not so subtle procedures are often inadvertently included. For example, imagine a treatment comparison study which compares traditional psychotherapy with an educational program alone. The educational program is presented by a clinician who is knowledgeable and has been in practice for 20 years whereas the psychotherapy is offered by beginning interns. In such a study it would be difficult if not impossible to differentiate the effects of the specific treatments from that of clinical experience and patient acceptance, and the logic of the experiment would be greatly compromised.

At point four, the question of interpretation becomes the major focus. In essence, we ask three separate but related questions. First, we ask if there exists a statistical difference between the groups in the experiment. Conceptually, in the Analysis of Variance model, we are asking the question, are the differences (i.e., variance) between groups greater than those found between individuals within each group? In the ideal case, the between- and within-groups variance should be the same. Thus, the ratio of between-group variance divided by within-group variance should equal 1 if no treatment (i.e., independent variable) has been applied. After treatment, this statistical ratio should reflect the treatment procedure such that the ratio is greater than 1. How large a number is required to conclude that the outcome did not result from chance and the factors that influence these statistical considerations will be presented in Chapters 37 and 38. Second, we ask the question, are the different levels of the independent variable (i.e., the treatments) the only way in which the groups in the experiment have been treated differently? That is, are there confounds which would not allow one to logically conclude that the independent variable affected the dependent variable? For example, what if during a cross-sectional study of stress and cardiovascular processes in physicians, it was announced that recent graduates would be drafted? Such an event would confound such an experiment in that younger male physicians (those who could be drafted) would be differentially affected in comparison to older ones. After questions one and two of step four have been answered successfully, one is then able with greater certainty to conclude that the findings of an experi-

ment were indeed the resultant of the treatment variable.

To summarize, subject selection and assignment as well as a well-thought-out experimental design are the traditional means by which control is achieved. These procedures allow one to make valid statements concerning the relationships under study in an experiment. The ideal experimental design is also referred to as a "true experiment" and represents the case when subjects can be randomly assigned to groups and the experimental design contains the proper comparison groups which allow for valid inferences. Because such a situation is an idealized closed system, questions concerning the influence of one variable on another are generally clear within the experimental context. Within this context, we can present the traditionally noted conditions for causality:

1. Covariation between the variables should be present.
2. There should exist a temporal priority in which the variable seen to be the cause precedes that variable seen to be the effect.
3. Influences other than those being examined should be ruled out or controlled.
4. It should be possible to replicate the observed relationship.

There are two major types of designs that have been used for establishing causal inference. These are between-subjects designs and within-subjects designs.

Between-Subjects Designs

Between-subjects designs are a general class of designs in which different subjects are used in each group. The statistical comparison is between different groups of subjects. One important characteristic of the between-subjects design is that any given subject receives only one level of the independent variable. An example of such a design is one in which one group, the experimental group, receives a treatment and is compared with another group, the control group, which receives a zero level of the treatment. Given a study in which the effect of a certain drug on heart rate was the question of interest, one could compare the heart rates found in the group that took a certain level of the drug with those of a control group that received none of the drug. Such a design would appear as follows:

Assignment	Group	Independent variable	Dependent variable
R	Experiment group	Drug	Heart rate
R	Control group	No drug	Heart rate

"R" indicates that the subjects were randomly assigned to each group. Such a design is referred to under a variety of names including the "completely randomized design," the "simple randomized design," or the "simple random subjects design." A commonly used variation is to include a pretest measure to aid in the demonstration that the groups were equal before the administration of the independent variable. This is referred to as the pretest–posttest control group design and is diagrammed as follows:

$$R \quad M1 \quad T \quad M2$$
$$R \quad M1 \quad \quad M2$$

Subjects are assigned randomly (R) to each group. Both groups would receive the pretest measure (M1) and the posttest measure (M2) with only the experimental group receiving the treatment (T). An advantage of this design is that if random assignment breaks down through attrition, it is possible to establish the manner in which the resulting groups are similar to the original groups. The incorporation of pretreatment baselines is thus imperative in studies in which attrition may be expected. The treatment study by Friedman *et al.* (1984) followed this basic design with the time frame being spread over 3 years.

A common design in the psychological literature utilizes the logic of the between-subjects design with more than one independent variable. Such a factorial design allows not only for the determination of the effects of each independent variable but also any type of interaction among these. For ex-

ample, one might study the effects of sodium in the diet as one factor and amount of exercise as another. Such a factorial design would not only allow the researcher to make statements concerning the effects of sodium and statements concerning the effects of exercise, but also any interactions that might result. For example, it might be the case that high sodium causes cardiovascular risk only when there is low exercise.

Within-Subjects Designs

The second approach is referred to as within-subjects designs. In this type of design, one uses subjects (i.e., the group of subjects) as the basis of comparison such that each subject receives all levels of the treatment. In this manner each subject serves as his or her own control, rather than there being a separate control group. In the example of the effects of a particular drug on heart rate, the design might consist of two levels (level 1 = no drug; level 2 = drug) and be diagrammed as follows:

	Level 1 (no drug)	Level 2 (drug)
Subject 1		
Subject 2	Measure heart rate	Measure heart rate
$\vdots$		
Subject n		

There are a number of advantages of within-subjects designs, three of these advantages being the equation of groups before the presentation of the independent variable, the ability to use a smaller number of subjects in an experiment, and the reduction of within-group (error) variance. That is to say, first, since the same set of subjects receive both treatments, we know before the experiment that the results of the different treatments are not due to subject characteristics and thus may be related to the treatment effects. Second, since all subjects receive all treatment levels, fewer subjects are required than would be the case if each treatment level was given to a separate group of subjects. This is a particularly important point when special subjects such as individuals having a rare disorder are the focus of the research. Third, the within-group variance is reduced because we would expect someone's behavior in a series of different conditions to be more similar than the behavior of different individuals in different conditions (as in a between-subjects design). The statistical advantage of this third point is that since the error term of the F-ratio is smaller (than with a between-subjects design), smaller treatment differences are required for rejection of the null hypothesis and thus the sensitivity of the treatment is increased.

There are also important disadvantages of within-subjects designs. The category of problems results from the design being temporally sensitive. This may be manifested in a variety of ways including practice effects (in which subjects become better at a task over the course of the experiment), fatigue effects (in which subjects become worse at a task over the course of the experiment), and carryover effects (in which the effects of a treatment such as a drug or even information carry over into the next treatment condition). As a general rule, if a treatment influences or changes the subject in any way, then within-subjects designs are usually not appropriate. However, if the carryover effects are unknown or thought to be slight, an alternative is to counterbalance the presentation such that each subject receives a different order of presentation. In a study of emotional valence, for example, half of the subjects could receive positive stimuli first and the other half, negative ones.

Mixed Designs

It is possible to combine within- and between-subjects designs to utilize the advantages of both approaches. One popular variation of such mixed designs, referred to as a repeated measures design, is to utilize time as one factor in a factor design and in this way measure any changes (e.g., learning) over time. Such a design might study level of exercise (high, medium, low) with cardiovascular fitness over time. The design would be diagrammed as shown at the bottom of the page.

Subject Designs

A common variation of the previous design is to use types of subjects as the between factor and the various tasks as the within factor. For example, Scher et al. (1986) gave Type A and Type B individuals (the between factor) subtraction problems over 20 trials (the within factor). T-wave amplitude was then measured. In a more complex study, Corse et al. (1982) used coronary status (no presence of coronary disease versus presence of disease) as one between factor, Type A/B as a second between factor, and three difficult cognitive tasks as the within factor. Although the between-subjects design which uses subject variables as one of the factors is a common and important design, it must be noted that the logic of the experiment is greatly weakened since it is impossible to control for the previous history of the subjects and thus would not be considered a "true experiment." For example, as Corse et al. pointed out, if one compared coronary patients with noncoronary ones in terms of blood pressure responses to various tasks, one potential problem or confound would result from the possible differential usage of β-adrenergic blocking medications by the coronary group, since under certain stressful conditions β-adrenergic blockade may potentiate rather than reduce pressor responses. Thus, care must be taken

		Within factor Week								
		1	2	3	4	5	6	7	8	9
Between factor (amount of exercise)	Low exercise Medium exercise High exercise									

in the design and interpretation of such experiments.

It should be remembered that even the best design can be eroded through differential dropout rates, inadequate compliance, and other such problems. Thus, it is best to consider the worst case situation that might happen, and to design for such a possibility through additional baselines, measurements, and other experimental checks.

When random assignment is not possible, or the experimenter knows that a particular factor is of great importance, groups can be equated by means other than random selection and assignment. One important method is through matching of subjects such that one of each matched pair of subjects is in the experimental group and the other the control.

Quasi-experimental Designs

Many of the important questions the cardiovascular researcher is called upon to answer are within the domain of real-world settings. In such situations it is usually impossible to have exact experimental control over all the major variables, much less to be able to randomly select and assign subjects to experimental treatments and groups. The context of such research is thus removed from the closed system of the laboratory with total control and moves to the less controlled open system in which the researcher can specify only a few of the important factors. Still, the question of what causes what and how remains the focus of much of our research but becomes difficult if not impossible to specify. In the experience of less control over the experimental processes, we seek guidelines for inferring how one variable influenced another. Unfortunately, there are few universally accepted guidelines for performing such research and in relation to such studies. Even when one turns to philosophy of science, Cook and Campbell (1979) remind us that the current state of epistemological thinking in terms of causality approaches near chaos. However, there do exist a number of pragmatic approaches which, although they do not satisfy the formal requirements of causality, are able to clarify better the relationships of one variable with another. One of these approaches emphasizes design and logic and is referred to as quasi-experi-

mental designs. Another approach emphasizes statistical procedures and is referred to as causal modeling (Bentler, 1980).

Quasi-experimental designs are a class of designs that lacks the necessary controls of the experimental situations to be able to rule out alternative hypotheses as a way of understanding the factors that influenced the dependent variables. In such a situation it is necessary to replace direct control of the experiment including the structure of the experimental design as a means of exerting control on the situation. Logic, reasoning, and knowledge of the experimental domain become even more important as the main tools with which one works. For example, in an applied psychology study, Voevodsky (1974) sought to determine if adding a third light to the back of taxis would reduce the accident rate. Although having a control of taxis without lights would help evaluate such a light, it would still not give one complete information. In order to present a compelling case for the effects of the warning light, one would need to question what factors should influence such a study. Even when the warning light was shown to reduce accident rates, it was still necessary to rule out alternative explanations. One such factor might be that the taxi drivers would drive more carefully since they knew themselves to be part of the study. This alternative explanation could be ruled out by comparing accident rates in the experimental and control groups with those from previous years. A more compelling case for warning lights could be made if it could be shown that the overall accident rate did not decrease but that the accident rate involving rear-end accidents in which someone ran into a taxi from behind did. From such data, it could be reasoned that the warning light did not affect the driving patterns *per se* as demonstrated by the number of accidents in which the taxi ran into someone else. Given a similar accident expectation for rear-end accidents, then it would be more compelling to argue that warning lights played an important role in reducing accidents through affecting the driving patterns of those who follow rear light-equipped cars. This type of applied research parallels the experience of the cardiovascular researcher in that most studies cannot be run in a highly controlled laboratory nor can the researcher specify the important variables beforehand.

One of the most common means of control in quasi-experimental approaches is through the use of multiple baselines (pre- and posttreatment measurements). For example, one might measure (M) blood pressure over a number of weeks, introduce a new treatment (T) procedure, and continue to measure blood pressure for the weeks that followed. Such a design would be diagrammed as follows:

M   M   M   M   M T M   M   M   M   M

The inferential strength of this simple design could also be increased by including a number of alternative strategies such as a control group which received no treatment or a variety of groups that received the treatments at different times in the multiple baseline procedures. Thus, one group would receive the treatment after two baselines, another after four, a third after six, and a fourth after eight.

In the case where there is more than one treatment and the treatments do not have a long-term effect, it is possible to use a reversal design and present a logical argument to suggest differential effects of treatments. Such a design would be as follows:

T1 M   T2 M   T1 M   T2 M

If one also included a second group which received the treatments in the reverse order, then the design would increase in strength of inference.

Natural Associational Research

At times we may want to ask if there exists a relationship between two variables which we cannot easily manipulate in a laboratory setting. For example, we might want to know if certain characteristics such as playing sports in high school or drinking at an early age are associated with greater risk factors for later cardiovascular problems. The study by Barefoot *et al.* (1983) presented earlier is such a design. In a retrospective manner, they compared hostility scores taken during medical school with self-reported health status some 25 years later. From these data the authors determined the relationship between the MMPI hostility score and later coronary heart disease as well as calculating the differential survival rates for individuals with high and low hostility scores. Initially, the goal of this study could not be that of establishing a causal link of one variable (hostility) with another (coronary heart disease) since there exists a plethora of alternative explanations which could account for such an association. However, the presence of this association would not allow one to rule out the existence of such a causal link and thus suggests the value of future research. Further analysis of these data also showed that hostility was not associated with health problems other than cardiovascular ones ruling out the possibility that hostility causes major health problems in general. In this manner a study such as this is invaluable for ruling out potential causal inferences but is in no manner useful for inferring causal relationships between two variables.

The statistic commonly used for establishing a degree of association is that of the correlation coefficient (e.g., Pearson product moment). An extension of the correlation analysis is a regression formulation in which one variable is used to predict the other. This type of analysis was used by Dembroski *et al.* (1985). In this study, 131 patients were randomly selected from 2000 patients who underwent diagnostic coronary angiography to form two severity categories (not severe or very severe coronary artery disease). The study sought to predict coronary artery disease factors (endpoints in the regression) from a Type A structured interview session (predictors). Risk factors such as age, sex, smoking, family history, and so forth were used as control variables. Initial data analysis consisted of specifying the relationship between the predictors and endpoint measures using correlational procedures followed by a stepwise multiple regression analysis for the coronary index rating and the number of vessels occluded and a stepwise discriminant function analysis for an angina measure and the number of previous myocardial infarctions. The particulars of these techniques are discussed in the statistical chapter by Van Egeren.

When considering results based on the correlational statistic, there are a number of important points to remember. One is that there are some cases where such a design would be more appropriate than using more factorial designs in which the subjects are placed into arbitrary groups. For example, if a researcher was interested in the relationship of a variable such as IQ and performance, more information would be gained by using a correlational study than by placing subjects into high- and low-IQ groups as in the traditional factorial design. Another point to remember is that correlational procedures are not useful when the range is restricted. For example, when doing research with individuals in college, test scores such as SATs are a good predictor of academic performance since the range of SAT scores is large. However, if one performed similar research on graduate students, such test scores will have little predictive value since the majority of graduate students have high SAT scores (thus, the range is restricted). It should also be noted that correlational procedures are totally empirical techniques (e.g., stepwise multiple regression) and may capitalize on a specific event and not replicate. Another point to remember is that correlational procedures are based on the idea of a linear relationship and thus give erroneous data if the underlying distribution is U shaped or representative of a sine function. Finally, correlational procedures are not useful when ranks change consistently with treatment. For example, if one were to determine the association between amount of exercise and self-reported well-being both before and after an exercise treatment program, the degree of association would probably remain the same. That is to say, although the overall amount of exercise might have increased, it would still be the case that those who exercised the most would also report feeling better about themselves.

Validity of Inferences

In the experimental situation validity asks the overriding question as to the correctness or truth of a claim. Technically, validity (or invalidity) refers to the best available approximation to the truth (or falsity) of propositions (Cook & Campbell, 1979)

or seen in a slightly different light, the plausibility of the conclusion (Cronbach, 1982). An excellent discussion combining these approaches with other validity typologies is that by Mark (1986). However, regardless of the approach taken, the major questions rest with the researcher's ability to make and communicate inferences. The following presentation will broaden the definitions and include additional material such that the discussions will be useful for cardiovascular research.

Originally, Campbell (1957) suggested two types of validity, internal and external, which Campbell and Stanley (1966) popularized. It should be pointed out that the Campbell approach emphasizes an ideal laboratory situation in which the experimenter has total control over the important variables. Thus, questions of internal and external validity should be seen from this position. In a nutshell, questions of internal validity ask if a study was performed well such that valid inferences can be drawn concerning the manner in which one variable is responsible for observed effects on a second variable. In this manner a study may be internally valid but have no implications for other times, settings, or subjects. Thus, questions of internal validity are a historical exercise in logic. Questions of external validity, on the other hand, look beyond the experimental situation and ask if the results of a particular study can be generalized beyond that particular study to other persons, situations, and times.

The focus of the Campbell and Stanley discussion centers around the ability to make valid inferences concerning research. Problems or conditions which would prevent valid inferences from being drawn are referred to as "threats to validity." Thus, what we seek to discover are alternative explanations that would explain the observed results and thus decrease one's certainty that a particular conclusion was valid. In this sense, we become like a defense attorney who constantly seeks alternative explanations to that of the prosecutor to account for the observed data.

More recently, Cook and Campbell (1979) extended the discussion of validity further by dividing the two validity types into what they consider to be four practical questions that researchers ask. The first question asks if there exists a relationship between the variables in one's experiment. As you remember from the brief presentation of causation, the first of the four conditions for causation required that the variables covary together. For example, one might ask if giving a particular drug reduces blood pressure. If blood pressure did not change in the presence of the drug, then the demonstration of causation would not be possible. The exact nature of the covariation required is an important question and there exist numerous statistical procedures to answer such a question. However, from a validity standpoint, it must be asked if there exist alternative explanations that may account for the observed results. For example, if one had collected a number of paper-and-pencil personality measures and correlated these with a number of biochemical measures from the experimental subjects, traditional statistical procedures would suggest that approximately 5% of these correlations would be significant by chance. This situation could lead one to assume that real relationships existed that were in actuality the resultant of statistical probability (i.e., chance). In such a situation any inference that concluded that two variables were related one to another would be weakened by the working of chance. These types of problems as well as a general discussion of statistics is presented in Chapters 37 and 38.

The second question posed by Cook and Campbell begins with the demonstration of a covariation. This question asks, given that there exists a relationship between the variables in a study, is it valid to assume that the observed numbers related to one variable are in some way affected by the other variable? In terms of validity we ask if we can consider reasons or an alternative explanation that would allow for the results seen in an experiment. If we could find such exceptions, then the logic of the proposition that one variable affected the other would be weakened. In Campbell and Stanley's terms, we would have discovered a "threat to the internal validity" of the experiment.

Campbell and Stanley (1966) suggested some general possible threats to internal validity (also called sources of invalidity) which include history, maturation, testing, instrumentation, statistical regression, selection, mortality, selection–maturation interaction, and diffusion or imitation of treat-

ments. However, it would be to no one's advantage to control for a potential threat when that threat was not appropriate to the domain of the topic under study. Thus, these potential threats are best seen for a checklist in order for researchers to better clarify their designs. For example, a cardiovascular researcher might ask how his or her present design could allow for the effects of history to play a role. History, in this technical sense, refers to the possibility that events which are not related to the independent variable have taken place between measurements in an experiment. One way in which history could play a role in a cardiovascular study would be for one group differentially to have exercised more, changed their diets, and/or reordered their lives during the period in which they received the treatment procedure.

Let us now briefly present the major Campbell and Stanley sources of invalidity. Maturation refers to the possibility that subjects grow wiser, stronger, and healthier as well as more tired, more bored, and so forth as an experiment continues. For example, in a study looking at emotional responsiveness to various tasks, giving a subject too many tasks to accomplish could confound the emotional responding with fatigue or anxiety. Testing refers to the problems that result from repeated measurement of the same subject. For example, if one group has had blood drawn a number of times, their initial blood pressure and biochemical response to the procedure itself would be less reactive than a control group that was having blood drawn for the first time. Instrumentation refers to problems related to change in the person or device that is making a measurement. For example, new researchers will become much more adept at making an observational rating over the life of the study. In such a situation, the initial baseline rating would have been made with less precision than the posttreatment ratings. Statistical regression refers to the situation in which subjects' scores become less extreme (regress to the mean) over time. A related problem is found with some clinical disorders (e.g., headaches, colds) with which patients seek treatment when the disorder is at its worst and/or ignore treatment when it is at its best. This confounds any conclusions concerning the effects of treatment. Selection problems relate to the condition when one group differs initially from the subjects in another group. There are a variety of conditions that produce such problems. However, most can be overcome when all subjects come from the same population. Mortality problems come about when subjects drop out or refuse to take part in an experiment, especially when it occurs differentially from one group compared to another. At times, this may result from the experiment itself. For example, one group may be given a drug that has negative side effects and show a larger dropout rate than another. The problem is compounded since those subjects who do not drop out in such a study may represent a special population (e.g., different physiology, different temperament). Selection–maturation interaction refers to the condition in which one group of subjects changes along a given dimension faster than another. For example, because lower- and middle-class children develop cognitive abilities at different rates, this would confound treatment changes found with such groups. More recently, Cook and Campbell have added additional threats including diffusion or imitation of treatments. This refers to the condition in which subjects communicate with each other concerning the experiment and this communication affects the differences between groups. This last consideration moves us to the next topic, the experimental context considered in a broad sense.

In considerations of internal validity it should be remembered that the level on which one is operating is fairly concrete. Yet, the level on which we wish to speak is often more abstract. For example, one might perform a study that relates stressing an animal (dropping it in water) with a measure of intelligence (time to complete a maze). It may, for example, be valid to make the inference that dropping an animal in water increases how quickly an animal goes through a maze. However, the question still remains as to whether it is valid to infer that stress increases intelligence. The relationship between experimental measures and their mapping onto theoretical constructs has been referred to as construct validity (Cronbach & Meehl, 1955) and is included in the present conception of external validity. One approach to the question of measuring a construct is to use a variety of measures in

such a way that one has a convergence across different measures or manipulations of the construct. Likewise, one should be able to demonstrate a different pattern of responses to different constructs even if related. For example, anxiety and depression can be measured on a variety of levels (e.g., biochemical, self-report, observation, psychophysiological), yet for the constructs to be meaningful, it would be necessary to be able to differentiate between the two. For the interested reader, Cook and Campbell suggest a number of threats to valid inferences in terms of construct validation. All of these threats center around the question, do one's research operations reflect one's research constructs and reflect the discussion presented in this section?

The third question of Cook and Campbell moves beyond the level of internal validity to that of external validity. This question asks, given that one variable affects another, what valid inferences can one draw on the level of the construct? In discussing questions of external validity in this third question, Cook and Campbell are referring to overall questions of confounding. For example, in an experiment that seeks to study a particular blood pressure medication, any procedure (e.g., the certainty of the physician that the drug will work which is communicated to the patient, the expectancy on the part of the patient that he or she will improve, the physical environment if it influences how the person feels) other than the medication itself would be considered a confound and pose a threat to the external validity of the experiment. To reduce these types of problems, double-blind experiments with placebo control have been developed in which the patient is given a substance or procedure which is identical in every manner to the one under test but lacks the active ingredient by individuals who do not know whether they are dispensing the active or placebo substance. Outside of medication experiments, such procedures are also important, but it is difficult with behavioral procedures (such as psychotherapy) to know what should be considered the active ingredient. Likewise, when one treatment is compared with another (e.g., medication versus exercise for reducing blood pressure), it is important to ensure that the person offering the treatment presents both procedures in an equal manner and in no way suggests that one is better and in this manner does not confound the actual treatment under consideration with subject expectations.

What Cook and Campbell refer to as confounding requires consideration in a broader context including overall relationships experienced by the subject and experimenter both inside and outside of the research setting. This might be referred to as the ecology of the experiment since we wish to emphasize the relationship of subjects and experimenters with each other and with their internal and external environments. This type of consideration is a necessary part of drug research which we have just discussed in the form of placebo designs. But, in a variety of other situations it may be equally the case that subject and experimenter expectations enter greatly into treatment results and thus must be considered in the interpretation of the data. However, it is also important to realize that subjects respond not only to the experiment but to the greater context of their life. For example, let us imagine a study in which patients in a reduced fee setting (e.g., VA hospital, social medicine) were asked to respond to a questionnaire of well-being after being part of an exercise program. The initial conclusion would be that the reports would be related to the exercise program. However, given the larger context of the particular system, it would also be necessary to consider the possibility that subjects would see their reports of well-being as related to future compensation. That is, in spite of the exercise program, subjects could report lesser well-being believing that this would maintain or increase their disability payments. Thus, it is important to note that research is always performed within a particular environmental context which cannot be ignored. Another commonly noted process is the so-called Hawthorne effect in which subjects who are part of an experiment feel special and respond more in terms of this feeling than in terms of the independent variable. For example, subjects who are first ''to be allowed'' to be part of a study for a new treatment may work harder and seek means other than the treatment under examination to ensure that they improve. In this sense, a researcher must always question what demands are being placed on the subjects (and also the experimenters) both in terms of the experiment itself and the broader context of the subjects' environment.

The fourth question of Campbell and Stanley lies at the heart of traditional external validity considerations. It asks the questions, given that one construct is responsible for the effect observed in another, is this relationship generalizable (1) to particular persons, settings, and times, and (2) across persons, settings, and times? In consideration of the threats to external validity, Campbell and Cook list three. First, the interaction of selection and treatment refers to the situation in which the subjects in the group are a specialized subsample of the target population. For example, an experiment involving clinicians which examined their treatment of cardiovascular problems would be more generalizable if the procedure required a minimal amount of time rather than all day since the latter procedure would exclude clinicians who had a busy practice and little free time. Likewise, a volunteer study of cardiovascular process which required repeated return to the laboratory might exclude certain types of individuals (e.g., Type As) who would not give up the time. Second, the interaction of setting and treatments refers to the condition in which one setting is more available and thus overrepresented in the data from which generalizations are made. For example, in a behavioral medicine experiment, it might be difficult to get access to hospitals with low morale, bad labor relations, or inadequate staffing whereas hospitals more available for use in research would reflect other factors (interest in new programs, more progressive, and so forth). In such a situation, the validity of the generalization of research results could be limited. And third, the interaction of history and treatment refers to the possibility that a unique situation exists during the time in which the experiment was conducted. For example, during a period in which a particular cardiovascular problem is portrayed by a popular movie or experienced by a major political figure, subject awareness including subjective reports of occurrence, generalized anxiety, and life-style can be greatly influenced. Any generalization from these periods could be invalid. The answer to the question of external validity is to clearly note to which particular settings, persons, and tasks one is seeking to generalize the results and to design the studies around such considerations. Likewise, replication of results strengthens the inferential considerations although we are always faced with the impossibility of logically concluding the future will be like the past. Additionally, a difficulty exists in cardiovascular research when one seeks to identify a potential member of a population (e.g., heart attack patients) before the actual event has occurred.

To summarize, in the discussion of internal and external validity it should be noted that the emphasis is on that of analysis and drawing valid inferences. Internal validity refers to the experimental situation itself and the various processes that take place during an experiment. External validity, on the other hand, looks at the experiment within a larger context and asks broader questions. On a practical side, Cook and Campbell (1979) suggest that there are four stages. The first asks if there exists a relationship between two variables. The second asks if given that there exists a relationship between two variables, can one of the variables be said to be responsible for the effects observed on the second. Third, given that one variable can be said to be responsible for the effects observed, then what construct can be regarded to be involved. And fourth, given that there is a relationship between constructs, how generalizable is this relationship across persons, places, and times.

Performing Efficient Research

Since no one is able to consider all possible parameters of a topic domain nor is one able to predict all possible alternative explanations before a research study is performed, we must accept that our science is based on our reasoning ability as human beings as well as motivational factors that shape our world. In this sense it behooves us to not only understand how we reason (e.g., how our reasoning reflects our nervous system) as well as how this may limit us (e.g., our tendency to seek confirmatory evidence) but also to seek more efficient means of conducting research. We have some hints of which types of research approaches increase the possibility that research will produce

beneficial results. Lakatos (1978) has suggested that important advances in science are made through the adherence to research programs in which a series of research questions are considered within a broad structure. With a better articulated theory and greater specificity, the study of the relationship of personality and cardiovascular processes as exemplified by Type A studies might be one such research program. However, the question for Lakatos remains that of distinguishing when a research program is progressive and thus leads to novel discoveries (i.e., predicts new facts) and when it is degenerative and only reinterprets known facts within the context of its theory. Another approach to research is suggested by Platt (1964). Platt suggested that certain fields within science have developed rapidly because they adopted a particular approach to research which he called strong inference. Strong inference is based on two ideas. The first is to consistently ask what experiment would be necessary to disprove a particular hypothesis. The second idea is to state alternative hypotheses with alternative possible outcomes within the context of research such that each outcome would disprove the other. Of course, such an approach also requires a greater level of specificity than is commonly observed in behavioral cardiovascular research but it is not an impossible task to be clearer concerning what causes what for whom, under what conditions, with what magnitude, and by what mechanism.

References

Barefoot, J., Dahlstrom, G., & Williams, R. (1983). Hostility, CHD incidence, and total mortality: A 25-year follow-up study of 255 physicians. *Psychosomatic Medicine, 45,* 59–63.

Bentler, P. (1980). Multivariate analysis with latent variables: Causal modeling. *Annual Review of Psychology, 31,* 419–456.

Campbell, D. (1957). Factors relevant to the validity of experiments in social settings. *Psychological Bulletin, 54,* 297–312.

Campbell, D., & Stanley, J. (1966). *Experimental and quasi-experimental designs for research.* Chicago: Rand McNally.

Cochran, W. G. (1983). *Planning and analysis of observational studies.* New York: Wiley.

Cook, T., & Campbell, D. (1979). *Quasi-experimentation: De-*

signs and analysis issues for field settings. Chicago: Rand McNally.

Corse, C., Manuck, S., Cantwell, J., Giordani, B., & Mathews, K. (1982). Coronary-prone behavior pattern and cardiovascular response in persons with and without coronary heart disease. Psychosomatic Medicine, 44, 449–459.

Cronbach, L. J. (1982). Designing evaluations of educational and social programs. San Francisco: Jossey–Bass.

Cronbach, L. J., & Meehl, P. E. (1955). Construct validity in psychological tests. Psychological Bulletin, 52, 281–302.

Dembroski, T., MacDougall, J., Williams, R., Haney, T., & Blumenthal, J. (1985). Components of type A, hostility, and anger-in: Relationship to angiographic findings. Psychosomatic Medicine, 47, 219–233.

Friedman, M., Thoresen, C., Gill, J., Powell, L., Ulmer, D., Thompson, L., Price, V., Rabin, D., Breall, W., Dicon, T., Levy, R., & Bourg, E. (1984). Alteration of type A behavior and reduction in cardiac recurrences in postmyocardial infarction patients. American Heart Journal, 108, 237–248.

Krantz, D., & Manuck, S. (1984). Acute psychophysiologic reactivity and risk of cardiovascular disease: A review and methodologic critique. Psychological Bulletin, 96, 435–464.

Lakatos, I. (1978). The methodology of scientific research programmes. London: Cambridge University Press.

Maher, B. (Ed.). (1978). Special issue: Methodology in clinical research. Journal of Consulting and Clinical Psychology 46, 595–838.

Mark, M. (1986). Validity typologies and the logic and practice of quasi-experimentation. In W. M. Trochim (Ed.), Advances in quasi-experimental design and analysis. San Francisco: Jossey–Bass.

Nesselroade, J., & Labouvie, E. (1985). Experimental design in research on aging. In J. Birren & W. Schaie (Eds.), Handbook of the psychology of aging (2nd ed.). Princeton, NJ: Van Nostrand.

Platt, J. R. (1964). Strong inference. Science, 146, 347–353.

Ray, W., & Ravizza, R. (1988). Methods toward a science of behavior and experience (3rd ed.). Belmont, CA: Wadsworth.

Reichardt, C. (1986). Estimating effects. Unpublished manuscript, University of Denver.

Scher, H., Hartman, L., Furedy, J., & Heslegrave, R. (1986). Electrocardiographic T-wave changes are more pronounced in type A than in type B men during mental work. Psychosomatic Medicine, 48, 159–166.

Trochim, W. M. (Ed.). (1986). Advances in quasi-experimental design and analysis. San Francisco: Jossey–Bass.

Voevodsky, J. (1974). Evaluation of deceleration warning light for reducing rear-end automobile collisions. Journal of Applied Psychology, 59, 270–273.

CHAPTER 37

The Analysis of Continuous Data

Lawrence F. Van Egeren

Introduction

Primary Questions

After tackling the problems of gathering a batch of observations according to some systematic plan, the scientist faces the problem Eve brought Adam—the troubling fact of choice. What treatments should be applied to the data, arithmetically or graphically? Why these treatments rather than some others? What principles can aid in making the choices? How can we organize our thinking about the overall process of data analysis?

Harvesting the information implicit in a body of data involves answering two basic questions. First, what happened? What is here in the sample? Second, what *might* have happened? What is out there in the parent population, and is likely to appear if the study is repeated? Stated differently, what are the experimental effects and the reliability of those effects?

This chapter is limited to the analysis of continuous variables. We will focus on certain general ideas underlying the use of the analysis of variance (ANOVA), multiple regression analysis (MRA), and path analysis (PA). The ideas behind these methods of analysis rather than specific tests and procedures will be emphasized. For greater detail

the reader should consult the many excellent sources available (e.g., Mosteller & Tukey, 1977; Winer, 1971) as well as the chapters on experimental design (Chapter 36) and power analysis (Chapter 38) in this volume.

Shifting Emphases

The present chapter was written from the point of view that data analytic practice has been shifting toward greater:

- Use of ad hoc exploratory procedures to augment confirmatory hypothesis testing procedures
- Emphasis on fitting models to data in contrast to testing effects
- Attention to "misfits" in a body of observations (residuals and outliers)
- Use of diagnostic procedures to explore how formal models fail and what remedies might be applied
- Recognition that MRA and ANOVA satisfy the same general linear model
- Emphasis on explicit causal modeling

Confirmatory statistical procedures are employed to test hypotheses that are selected in advance of the data. Following their arrival, one can ask the data one question at a time, pass them through a preplanned statistical test, and retrieve at the other end two numbers, one (the value of the

Lawrence F. Van Egeren • Department of Psychiatry, Michigan State University, East Lansing, Michigan 48824.

statistic) giving an answer to the question, and the other (usually a significance level) indicating the degree of confidence in the answer. The output is a "yes" or "no" answer and an error rate for the answer.

Data analysis is typically more iterative, branching, and recursive in nature than the formal testing of a fixed set of preselected questions implies. Questions are raised, data are analyzed, the results give rise to new questions, the data are rearranged and reanalyzed, and so on. Alongside the pursuit of preselected questions, questions raised by the data themselves are pursued, with some uncertainty about where the process will end. Unexpected and unusual events are welcome because they may express or lead to important discoveries.

Welcoming the "unexpected" places the residuals of a formal statistical model in a new perspective. The residuals are the parts of the dependent response that the formal model cannot explain. We can approach them, as we can approach unexpected guests, with mere tolerance or active curiosity. Curiosity is justified because the residuals are more than "error" sullying a theory. The residuals are potentially valuable (1) clues to the next step to take to advance understanding, (2) diagnostic information about the validity of statistical assumptions, and (3) signs of instability in the data that provide a yardstick for estimating the reproducibility of experimental results.

The process of fitting formal models to data, as opposed to testing effects, shifts attention from yes–no answers to the *precision* of results. The size of effects and the exact amount of information contained in experimental results acquire new importance. A model and a body of data, like a hat and a head, fit together in degrees, and often fail to fit in limited and specific ways. The residuals of the model can aid in determining not only "whether" ideas are false, but also "how" they are false. After all, what we need are not safe yes–no answers but accurate answers (Mosteller & Tukey, 1977). Accuracy implies not only correctness but also precision.

The rules of confirmatory hypothesis testing have the salutary effect of limiting the rate at which scientists make false claims of knowledge to some acceptable value, usually 5% of all deci-

sions. There is a danger, however, that rigid use of confirmatory procedures will suppress much of the adventure and creativity upon which breakthroughs in science depend. Surprises and unusual events in the data may be impatiently dismissed as chance intrusions into the preplanned search for expected truths.

A statistical procedure is an exploratory procedure when the purpose is to inspect or examine something rather than to confirm or disconfirm a preselected hypothesis. Exploratory approaches guided by the data themselves have many valuable applications but also have some common shortcomings. The promiscuous use of ad hoc analyses can lead to undisciplined fishing expeditions, "milking" or "praying over" data, capitalization on chance, selective reporting of findings, and loss of control over the Type I error rate.

Advancing a field of study, not only safely but also opportunistically and efficiently, requires a rational balance between confirming old ideas and remaining open to new ideas. A successful balance will result in an acceptable trade-off between Type I and Type II errors. To preserve flexibility and creativity in data analysis, Tukey (1962) advises the subject matter specialist to regard statistical rules as guides, not commands, and to prefer an approximate answer to the right question over an exact answer to the wrong question.

Managing the Data Analytic Process

An explicit plan for data collection and analysis can help avoid blunders and confusion. In the plan one can define the problem, select key variables, establish goals, and set up checkpoints for evaluating and revising the data analytic process itself. Are the important variables included in the study? Are they pruned down to a reasonable number? Are they reliably and validly measurable? How will the quality of the data be checked before they are analyzed? What graphical procedures will be used to inspect the data? How will initial variables for statistical models be selected? How will residuals be examined and the possibility of abnormalities in statistical models checked and, if present, corrected? What procedures will be used to revise models? How will the results be checked to see whether research objectives have been met? What will happen if the original goals cannot be met?

Preparing Data for Analysis

Graphical Procedures

No method brings detailed information to the mind more efficiently than a good graph or diagram. Scatterplots, histograms, stem-and-leaf displays, and box plots can provide a bird's-eye view of what is present in the sample. They can be helpful aids in uncovering surprises in the data, spotting problems caused by blunders or missing data, suggesting ad hoc analyses, and offering quick checks on statistical assumptions and the need to transform scales. When observations are standardized (centered at 0, scaled to 1.0), a stem-and-leaf value reflects the probability of an observation, which makes it easy to spot outliers, and box plots reflect the significance of differences between groups.

Dealing with Outliers

In any batch of data there can be a number of wildly deviant (unrepresentative, rogue, outlying) observations that capture unanticipated, and often unwanted, events or sources of variance. These outliers can seriously contaminate the data, or point to unexpected, useful phenomena.

It is important to thoughtfully consider why the data are misbehaving in the tails of the distribution before deciding what to do about outliers. Is chance playing tricks or is something else at work? Extreme observations can occur because:

- Many small causes randomly coincide to produce one large effect (chance is playing tricks, and one will have to live with the outlier).
- A single potent cause of rare occurrence in fact occurs (one would like to identify this

cause, viz., disease processes often operate at the margins of the normal range of controls).
- A blunder, an error of measurement, or the like has occurred (the population under study has been invaded by a foreign population one has no interest in studying; remove or replace the outlier).

The presence of outliers can ruin an otherwise good model of the data by increasing the error variance and abnormally influencing the fit of the regression surface to the observations. When a sample of observations contains 10% outliers, which have a standard deviation equal to 3σ, the outliers contribute a variance equal to the variance contributed by the remaining 90% of the observations, which have a standard deviation equal to 1σ (Mosteller & Tukey, 1977).

There are different opinions about how extreme a value should be before it is considered an outlier (it is sometimes defined as a value three or more standard deviations from the mean) and what, if anything, should be done about it (Barnett & Lewis, 1978). One can ignore the outlier, accommodate the outlier by using robust procedures that are relatively insensitive to outliers (e.g., statistics based on medians rather than on means), toss out the outlier while adjusting statistical tests for the fact that it is being tossed out, or toss out the outlier without making any adjustment at all, a practice that is not recommended.

When the extreme value is likely to have been caused by a blunder, equipment failure, or the like, which distorts the sample information, there are some simple remedies available. One is to "trim" the data, and another is to "Winsorize" them. Trimming means setting aside some fraction of the measurements from each tail of the distribution, say the lowest 5% and highest 5% of the observations, and accepting the remaining observations, the middle 90%, as the sample data that are analyzed.

When data are Winsorized, observations are replaced rather than discarded. First, a decision is made about how many deviant measurements to replace. Let us suppose that there are two outliers. These two observations, and the two smallest observations, are then replaced by the observations that are closest to those being replaced. If there are 42 observations ranked from the lowest to the highest, as $Y_1, Y_2, \ldots, Y_{42}$, then Y_1 and Y_2 are replaced by Y_3, and Y_{41} and Y_{42} are replaced by Y_{40}.

Work has been done on obtaining the sampling distributions of statistics computed on trimmed and Winsorized data (Barnett & Lewis, 1978). For example, if g observations have been replaced in each tail of the sample by Winsorization, then $N - 2g = h$ observations remain, and Student's t can be adjusted by $(N - 1)/(h - 1)$ to obtain a value to apply to the Winsorized data. In the example above, Student's $t_{05} = 1.68$. The t value computed on the Winsorized data that would approximate this point in the Student t distribution is $t = (42 - 1)/(38 - 1)t_{05} = 1.11(1.68) = 1.87$. The t statistic computed on the Winsorized data will have to reach a value of 1.87 or larger to be significant at the 0.05 level.

Missing Data

What to do when observations are missing depends on how many are missing, where they occur, and why they are missing. The missing values can sometimes be estimated from other values. At other times it is better to analyze the incomplete data. When observations are missing from the tails of the distribution, it may be better to Winsorize the data and adjust significance values accordingly. When many observations are missing, it is sometimes informative to create a "missing data" variable, scored "1" when observations are missing and "0" otherwise. By correlating the "missing data" variable with other variables it may be possible to better understand why observations were lost.

General Linear Model

It is not always appreciated that many procedures for analysis of continuous variables—correlation analysis, regression analysis, analyses of variance, with and without covariates—satisfy a single general linear model. The model can be expressed as

$$Y = b_0 + b_1X_1 + \cdots + b_pX_p + e \quad (1)$$

where Y is the dependent variable one wishes to understand, the X's are independent variables that are thought in some sense to explain the variability in Y, the b's are fitted constants (unknowns that must be solved for), and e is an expression of error in the model (the residuals, unexplained variability in Y).

The X's might be continuous variables in an MRA problem or nominal "dummy" variables in an ANOVA model. Dummy variables are numerical tags (e.g., an array of 1's and 0's) indicating whether or not an individual in a study did or did not receive a particular treatment (e.g., "1" might mean that the individual was given drug A and "0" that the individual was not given drug A), or does or does not belong to a particular group (e.g., "0" might stand for males and "1" for females). Interactions in ANOVA can be included in the general linear model as dummy variables that are products of the dummy variables for the factors entering into the interaction.

The right side of equation (1) describes a predictable part of Y, $(b_0 + b_1X_1 + \cdots + b_pX_p)$, designated $\hat{Y}$, plus a measurement of the error of prediction, e. Equation (1) can also be written as

$$Y = \hat{Y} + e$$

or

Actual measurement = explainable measurement + residual

Equation (1) describes a linear curve (regression surface) that is offered as a simple summary of the data. Its small number of terms may summarize thousands of data values. Whether it provides a good (accurate) summary is what the data analytic procedure must determine.

In order to evaluate the model, the sample observations must be analyzed to determine values for the b's. This requires adopting some criterion, such as the least-squares optimization criterion, for deciding when b values are good values, i.e., values that produce accurate predictions of Y. With the least-squares method, the goal is to choose b's so that the errors of prediction, $Y - \hat{Y}$, are a minimum. We wish to minimize the sum of the squares of the errors of prediction,

$$\Sigma(Y - \hat{Y})^2 = \Sigma[Y - (b_0 + b_1X_1 + \cdots + b_pX_p)]^2$$
$$= \Sigma(Y - b_0 - b_1X_1 - \cdots - b_pX_p)^2 \quad (2)$$

The expression on the right side of equation (2) can be minimized by taking the partial derivatives with respect to the b's, setting what results equal to zero, and solving the equations for the b's. With values for the b's, a value for e can also be determined.

So far, equation (1) merely describes a batch of numbers, the sample of observations. The sample b values can transcend themselves to describe parameters of the parent population. To do so, we must be able to assume that the Y values are randomly sampled for each value of the X's and that the errors of prediction, e_i, are distributed normally at each value of the X's with mean 0 and a common variance, σ^2, in the population. In order to acquire this transcendent quality, the sample b values must be dependably related to a set of probability values, i.e., they must satisfy a probability model. The sample-to-sample stability of the b values, as experimental results, can then be evaluated. We can ask of these values what we ask of the mean difference between two groups or any other experimental outcome: can we count on them, do they represent a reliable experimental result?

Several key assumptions and constraints are implied in the general linear model. Some constraints are mathematical in nature. When one X is a linear combination of other X's, the system of normal equations will have more unknowns (b's) than equations and will lack a unique solution. Highly correlated independent variables should not be included in the same theoretical model of Y, e.g., a total test score plus its component scores should not appear together.

Independent variables that are highly correlated cause many statistical problems. The ANOVA model assumes that the various main effects and their interactions are additive, independent sources of variability in Y. Independent variables that start

out uncorrelated, e.g., as factors in a randomized block design, can become correlated when data are lost and cell n's become unequal and disproportional. When independent variables are highly intercorrelated in multiple regression problems, the regression coefficients become unstable and more difficult to interpret in physiological or behavioral terms.

The Additive–Decomposition Philosophy

Additivity is the hallmark of the MRA and ANOVA methods of analyzing data. These procedures divide the entire variability of a dependent response into its major claimant classes, the independent variables and error. They are variance partitioning procedures based on additive-decomposition operations. Information is added up across influences, and can be subtracted out as well. Breaking down data in a two-way table by taking out row and column means illustrates decomposition operations in ANOVA nicely (Mosteller & Tukey, 1977). What is left in the table are the residuals of the original measurements, numerical debris remaining after the effects have been removed.

A measurement can be regarded as a composite that can be split into separate and independent parts. For example, arterial blood pressure (BP) is the result of many different causes and mechanisms of regulation. We might think of a single BP reading as an average BP (the grand mean for many individuals) plus increments or decrements, according to whether the person is awake or asleep, angry or calm, obese or thin, diseased or healthy, and so forth. It is then possible to perform "accounting" operations on the measurement. It is as though a measured systolic BP of 146 mm Hg can be broken down into separate parts and added up again as follows:

104 mm Hg of pressure for basal metabolic demands
12 mm Hg of pressure for walking
9 mm Hg of pressure for anger

5 mm Hg of pressure for joint effect of walking and anger

10 mm Hg of pressure for arterial rigidity due to disease

6 mm Hg of pressure for error (hidden causes, etc.)

_____

146 mm Hg

BP mechanisms may not regulate BP additively but may have effects that accumulate additively. Ambulatory monitoring may reveal that a person when walking has a slightly higher BP than a person not walking, a person angry has a slightly higher BP than a person not angry, and walking when angry adds an increment beyond that due to walking and anger alone. From known values of BP, activity, and mood, one might want to estimate the importance of the influences on BP illustrated by the numbers 104, . . . , 12 in the example above by dividing the total BP variability into its various source components.

The ability to partition response variability into constituent components is a powerful tool. Selected influences operating on the response can be separated and removed, somewhat like pulling leaves off an onion. What is left is an internal core of error. This internal randomness in the dependent response, the response scrubbed free of the external independent influences, is a valuable reference standard for evaluating the dependability of the independent influences (reliability of experimental results).

The ability to estimate what will happen when an experiment is repeated, without ever actually repeating the experiment, is an amazing tour de force of inferential statistics. Within-experiment instability of observations is used to estimate across-experiment stability of experimental outcomes. The common F ratio combines internal variability in the response with variability induced by an external independent influence to form bilayers of variance. The top layer indicates the strength of the influence and the bottom layer the sample-to-sample instability of the influence.

The F ratio expresses the variability in a dependent response due to independent variables (treatments in ANOVA, predictors in MRA) as a multi-ple of the inherent instability of the system in the absence of the independent variables. In the ANOVA fixed effects model, the denominator of the F ratio is the within-cell variability, i.e., the variability in the response when the treatments do *not* vary and therefore do not exist as variables. In MRA the denominator is the response variability about the regression surface (the variability of the residuals), i.e., the response variability when the predictors do *not* vary and therefore do not exist as variables. Variability in a response due to some influence ordinarily must be several times the variability in the response in the absence of the influence before the influence can be regarded as stable or dependable (statistically significant).

Constraints on the Correlation Coefficient

The correlation coefficient is a measure of the strength of association of two variables. A number of other statistics, e.g., regression coefficients, can be derived from correlation coefficients. Consequently, the correlation coefficient serves as a foundation for a number of statistical procedures. It is important that this foundation be as solid as possible. Many conditions exist that can cause the nominal value of the correlation coefficient to be very different from the actual strength of association between two variables. This in turn can lead to incorrect interpretations of research results.

Common factors that cause the correlation coefficient to be smaller than it should be are restricted range, unreliability, and skewness in the distributions of the variables (particularly when the two variables are skewed in the opposite direction). Continuous variables are often dichotomized to form factors in ANOVA, e.g., subjects over a wide age range will be stratified into "young" and "old." This is rarely good practice because dichotomization reduces the range of variables and the information available. Correlation coefficients for normally distributed variables are usually reduced by dichotomization, sometimes drastically. The reduction is likely to be greater as the proportions depart from a median (50–50) split. The correlation between a continuous variable and a rare disease state may be small or insignificant simply due to the small variance of the disease state in the population.

Measurement error reduces the size of the correlation coefficient. For example, a correlation between two variables measured without error of 0.60 drops to 0.48 when the reliability of each variable is 0.80. What a correlation would have been had errorless measures been used can be estimated as

$$r'_{xy} = r_{xy}/(r_{xx}r_{yy})^{1/2}$$

where r_{xy} is the observed correlation and r_{xx} and r_{yy} are the reliability coefficients for the two variables. The formula can be used to estimate the correlation between true scores (errorless measures), a process known as correcting for attenuation. When the focus is on causation, it is essential to correct relationships for attenuation so as not to confuse lack of causation with lack of reliability of measurement.

A large table of correlations often has some moderately large values simply due to chance. When a correlation table has many small values, it is often valuable to know whether it is possible to reject the hypothesis that the entire set of correlations are zero in the population. An omnibus test that can be used for this purpose is:

$$\chi^2 = [N - 1 - (2p + 5)/6] \Sigma r_{ij}^2$$

where N is the number of subjects, p is the number of variables, and the summation extends over the $p(p-1)/2$ correlations of the table (above or below the principal diagonal). The test values are distributed as chi square with $df = p(p-1)/2$.

ANOVA

Specifying ANOVA Models

Any ANOVA situation can be represented by a general linear regression model [equation (1)], provided certain precautions and constraints are applied. Consequently, some of the material on

MRA discussed below applies to ANOVA as well. We will consider a few special topics. An extensive treatment of ANOVA is available in Winer (1971).

When approaching an ANOVA data analysis it is useful to take a number of simple steps to organize one's thinking, such as:

1. List the important influences (independent variables) thought to be operating in the data; call these major ways of classifying the data the "main effects."
2. Write a linear equation to represent the dependent response in terms of the main effects and their interactions.
3. Indicate for each main effect whether observations at the different levels of the factor are correlated (repeated within each subject) or uncorrelated, i.e., indicate whether the effect is a "within-subject" or "between-subject" effect.
4. Indicate whether each main effect is a random variable (i.e., levels of the factor are randomly sampled) or a fixed variable (levels are selected by investigator, not sampled).

As an example, suppose that we have applied two different treatments to two different diseases and have some measure of treatment effectiveness (Y) on each patient. The important influences are treatments and diseases, and we can write the following breakdown of the dependent measure Y:

$$Y_{jki} = \bar{Y} + A_j + B_k + AB_{jk} + e_{jki} \quad (3)$$

Equation (3) indicates that the observed treatment response for patient i, Y_{jki}, is a sum of five parts: (1) an overall mean for the group of patients ($\bar{Y}$), (2) the effect of possessing disease j (one level of disease factor A), (3) the effect of receiving treatment k (one level of treatment factor B), (4) the joint effects of disease j and treatment k, AB_{jk}, and (5) a random element e_{jki}. It is assumed that the random element is sampled from a population that is normally distributed with mean zero and variance σ^2. If each patient received only one treatment and different patients occupied the four cells of the model, all Y observations would be uncorrelated and the two main effects would be between-subject effects. The treatments and diseases were not randomly sampled from a population of treatments and diseases, so the main effects would be fixed effects.

ANOVA models can be divided into the fixed effects model (Model I), the random effects model (Model II), and the mixed effects model (Model III), according to whether levels of the factors are "fixed" (selected) by the experimenter, randomly sampled from a population, or a mixture of the two, respectively. True examples of Model II and Model III are relatively rare. The practical significance of the three types of models is that they have different error terms for the F ratio.

Constructing F Ratios

The goal in ANOVA, as in inferential statistics generally, is to find answers to questions and to assign a confidence statement to each answer. The confidence statement indicates the sample-to-sample stability of the answer, i.e., the reproducibility of the experimental result. It is usually expressed as a significance level or a confidence limit. Validity is identified with intersample stability and error with intersample instability. Concerning the effect of treatment A, we seek an answer that is lasting, which holds for *all* samples. In the fixed effects model, everything in an experimental result that varies from sample to sample is error. Error, and the denominator of the F ratio, have definite meaning, namely, sample-to-sample variability.

In the most general terms, an F ratio can be written as:

$$F = \frac{\text{an answer}}{\text{instability of the answer}}$$

$$= \frac{\text{stability} + \text{instability}}{\text{instability}}$$

The F ratio contains a calculation of response variability in two different ways: once with the experimental effect (representing an answer to some experimental question) figured in and another time with it omitted. The former is placed in the numerator and the latter in the denominator.

The general rule for constructing an F ratio for some effect A is that the numerator should equal the denominator when the null hypothesis (H_0) is true; F = 1.0 when $\sigma^2_a = 0$. Specifically, the same expected population variances should appear in the numerator and the denominator when H_0 is true. A second rule is that the denominator should contain sample estimates of all sources of sample-to-sample variability of the effect (σ^2_a) being tested. We should ask, "What are all the things that can cause the effect to vary from one sample to the next?", and make sure all those sources of variability are included in the denominator. The numerator should contain everything put in the denominator plus σ^2_a, the effect being tested.

In the fixed effects model, the denominator of the F ratio is the variability in Y computed *within* each level of the independent factors (within-cell variance). It is variability in the dependent variable when the independent variables do *not* vary and therefore do not exist as variables. It is a measure of inherent instability in Y as a carrier of information about the independent variables. This inherent instability is unshakable and will be part of the Y measure as it moves from level to level of the factor where it acquires additional variability due to the effect of the factor or manipulated influence.

Consider a two-factor experiment with p levels of factor A and q levels of factor B. Variability in the dependent response (Y) as it moves from level to level on factor A is expected to have two sources of variability in the population, as well as in new samples, namely:

$$E(MS_a) = \sigma^2_e + nq\sigma^2_a$$

where $E(MS_a)$ is the expected total variability of Y in the population, σ^2_e is the expected within-cell (error) variability of Y in the population, $nq\sigma^2_a$ is the expected variability in Y due to the influence of factor A in the population, and n is the (equal) number of subjects in each cell.

Sample variances are estimates of composite population variances. The sample MS_a is an estimate of the population effect A, which will contain sources of error variance σ^2_e as well as σ^2_a. The sample MS_e is an estimate of the population error variance σ^2_e. Consequently, the F ratio for the fixed effects model is:

$$F = MS_a/MS_e$$

The F ratio for testing the A main effect when the ANOVA model is a random effects model is:

$$F = MS_a/MS_{ab}$$

For the random effects model, the relationship between sample variances (mean squares) and population variances are such that $E(MS_a)/E(MS_{ab}) = (\sigma^2_e + n\sigma^2_{ab} + nq\sigma^2_a)/(\sigma^2_e + n\sigma^2_{ab})$. When the null hypothesis is true, the $nq\sigma^2_a$ term will equal zero and the F ratio will equal 1.0, as the rule for constructing F ratios requires.

While it is intuitively reasonable that MS_e (within-cell variability in Y) is the proper error term in the fixed effects model, it is not immediately obvious that MS_{ab} is the proper error term in the random effects model. As indicated above, the random effects model has an additional source of expected sample-to-sample variability in the A main effect, namely σ^2_{ab}, variability due to the AB interaction. This additional source of variability in Y arises for the following reason. When there is an AB interaction the A effect is different at different levels of factor B. There are as many A "simple" effects as there are levels of B, and the A main effect is a composite of the simple effects. When the study is repeated, levels of B will be randomly sampled, with some variability in the distribution of levels possible. Variability in the levels of B upon resampling will produce a different mix of simple A effects and, consequently, a different A main effect. The expected change in the A main effect due to a change in the levels of B, upon resampling, must be allowed for in the F ratio by including σ^2_{ab} in the denominator.

The general logic in constructing F ratios is to include in the denominator all sources of variance that can influence the effect (main effect or interaction) being tested upon resampling, keeping in mind that when the effect contains a random factor, other random factors interacting with the effect can influence the variability of the effect and therefore must be included in the F ratio. When an effect contains only fixed factors, it will not be affected by variability in other effects when a fresh sample is drawn, and therefore the other effects need not appear in the F ratio.

Multiple Comparisons of Means

After the general structure of the data has been specified in a linear model, and its separate components evaluated through ANOVA, it is often valuable to compare pairs of means that are embedded in the overall effects. For example, an overall drug effect may indicate that three antihypertensive drugs differed in their effects on BP. It is then reasonable to ask whether drug A differed from drug B, drug A differed from drug C, and drug B differed from drug C.

When the number of levels of a factor is large and many means are compared via individual t tests, Type I error may balloon out of control. The "individual" error rate, say 5%, for each t test will be accurate, but the "family" error rate for the entire set of t tests (i.e., the chances of at least one Type I error) can become considerably greater than 5%. The family error rate for *all* the tests will be unknown unless some allowance is made for the fact that multiple individual comparisons are being made, with an opportunity for unwittingly capitalizing on chance. The extravagant use of t tests while looking for significant differences among a large group of means is one of the most common abuses of statistics.

There are many procedures for controlling Type I error while making multiple comparisons between means (Winer, 1971). A simple approach offered by Bonferonni and R. A. Fisher is to divide the alpha level by the number of comparisons and use the new alpha level as the critical value for rejecting the null hypothesis. To keep the protection level for k comparisons at alpha, use alpha/k to reject H_0 for each comparison. This is a safe and somewhat conservative approach.

Fisher also proposed testing the overall main effect in ANOVA first, and then proceeding to test individual pairs of means by the usual t test (with the significance level set at alpha) *if and only if* the F test for the overall effect is statistically significant at the level of alpha. It is sometimes recommended that when this procedure is used the number of comparisons not exceed the degrees of freedom for the effect. Suppose that the number of levels (j) for a main effect is seven. Then the degrees of freedom for the effect is $df = j - 1 = 6$. The maximum number of comparisons between the means that is possible is $j(j - 1)/2 = 21$. If the number of comparisons is confined to six, by deciding what really matters instead of making all 21 comparisons, the family error rate for the set of tests will be better protected, i.e., closer to the level of alpha.

There are procedures such as the Newman–Keuls, Scheffe, and Tukey HSD that rank order a set of means according to size and adjust the level of alpha when comparing two means on the basis of how many steps apart they are in the rank order. This approach takes account of the fact that large differences between means are more likely to capitalize on chance than are small differences.

The many tests available for multiple comparisons differ in power and do not necessarily give the same result when applied to the same data.

Robustness of F and t Tests

Studies of the behavior of the t statistic and F ratio, such as the famous studies of Box (1954), indicate that these tests are "robust" in the sense that violations of the normality and homogeneity of variance assumptions of the test do not significantly increase the likelihood of Type I error. An illustration is Box's demonstration that when the F ratio was used to test the means of three sets of observations having variances in a ratio of 1:1:3 instead of being equal, alpha was raised merely from 0.050 to 0.059.

Knowledge that the t and F tests are robust can easily lead to a false sense of security and a casual attitude toward violating assumptions. There is little to justify this attitude. Violations of normality and homogeneity assumptions may not seriously alter Type I error. But they can significantly increase Type II (false negative) error and decrease the power of a test, and have other undesirable side effects.

Heterogeneity of variance introduces uncertainty into the interpretation of experimental results. Within-cell variance in ANOVA and residual vari-

ance in MRA are a measure of the precision of the data. Error variance provides a "ruler" with which to gauge the significance and sample-to-sample reliability of experimental results. When different portions of the data differ in error variance, we in effect are using different rulers to evaluate the significance of an experimental result. There is little reason to be complacent about this state of affairs. A physicist would not feel comfortable knowing that two balances differing in accuracy give significantly different answers to a critical research question.

When within-cell variances differ, one should think hard about what may be causing the difference. Can the difference be reduced by expanding the ANOVA model to include the causal variable as a factor (or covariate) or by transforming the scale of measurement? Consider the common situation in which response variability is proportional to mean response, e.g., variability in BP is greater for obese people than for thin people. Then some, but not all, obese people have high BP. Something must be interacting with body weight to affect BP. What might the interacting condition be? We might look for the factor among observations already in hand. If it cannot be found and included in the ANOVA model, its effects can be mitigated by transforming BP into the square root of BP and analyzing the square root measure.

MRA

A major purpose of science is to cut ideas to fit facts. Building a regression model of a dependent response is one way to achieve this purpose. The regression model may serve to summarize data, to make predictions and practical recommendations, and to attempt causal analysis of the dependent response. It is a powerful technique but has some pitfalls.

The MRA Model

The regression model is described in equation (1). The coefficients (b's) constituting some empirical model are related, or in data analytic jargon, "fitted," to the observations. The coefficients act to weight, or tailor, the independent variables so that the variables fit the dependent response better than they would unweighted. Geometrically, the coefficients define a regression surface in the sample space. The model fits the data well if the observations in sample space are close to the regression surface.

Fitting a model to data by weighting independent variables is like fitting a coat to the body by remodeling it, trimming off a little here, adding a little there. In this case, however, the tailored coat (fitted Y values, $\hat{Y}$'s) should fit the body (observed Y's) as tightly as possible rather than being comfortably loose. The least-squares criterion leads to b's that minimize $\Sigma(Y - \text{fitted } Y)^2$, the space between the body and the coat in our "tailoring" metaphor.

The tailoring metaphor can aid in raising some basic questions about MRA. How big a coat should we make, how much of the body should the coat cover (how many X's should be in the model, how much variability in Y should be explained)? Who should make this decision, a tailor or a machine (should the X's be selected by the investigator's judgment or by a formal automated procedure such as stepwise regression)? What should be the criterion of a "good fit" when the goal is to cover the most body with the least material (what should be the criterion for the goodness of fit when the goal is to maximize the amount of data fitted per parameter in the model)? Will a good fit today be a good fit tomorrow (can the regression coefficients stand up to cross-validation)? Just as tailors' measurements vary and the body changes, so there is sample-to-sample variability in the b's and the Y values, and a fine regression equation may fit fresh data shabbily, and often does.

The least-squares method for obtaining regression coefficients or weights that minimize $\Sigma(Y - \text{fitted } Y)^2$ yields *partial* coefficients. The coefficients are "partial" in the sense that they reflect only part of the variability of X and Y, namely, the part that remains after the other X's are taken out of both X and Y. Only the parts of the independent variables that are free of each other are related to Y. Correlated X's are transformed into uncorrelated parts of X's that are related to the part of Y that is unique to each X.

Suppose that there are three X variables in the equation. The b_2 coefficient will be the slope for

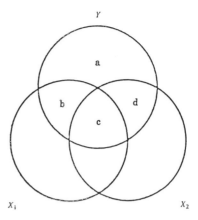

Figure 1. Relationship between variances (circles) and covariances (overlap of circles) of a dependent variable (Y) and two independent variables (X_1 and X_2). Covariances related to regression coefficients are represented by area "b" (X_1) and area "d" (X_2).

the straight-line regression of a Y residual ($Y - \text{fitted } Y'$) on an X_2 residual ($X - \text{fitted } X'$). The fitted Y' results from regressing Y on X_1 and X_3, and the fitted X' results from regressing X_2 on X_1 and X_3. The b_2 coefficient is the slope of the regression of the Y residual on the X_2 residual after removing X_1 and X_3 from both. The b_1 and b_3 coefficients are defined and determined likewise.

Figure 1 illustrates the partialling process. Each circle represents the variance of X_1, X_2, and Y variables; areas of overlap represent covariances. The partialling process produces a regression coefficient that represents the covariance that X_1 and X_2 uniquely share with Y, areas b and d, respectively, in the diagram.

Steps in Building a Regression Equation

There are a number of logical steps that can be taken to build and evaluate a regression equation:

- Construct an initial equation between Y and a subset of X's, using either an automated (program-driven) procedure or a manual (investigator-driven) procedure.
- Check the goodness of fit of the equation.
- Compare the equation to competitive equations.
- Revise the equation as needed.

- Perform diagnostics as a final check.
- Validate the equation on a fresh batch of data.

Procedures for Finding the "Best" Equation

The least-squares method produces the "best" equation in the sense that the regression coefficients will minimize prediction errors. But which predictor variables belong in the model? Selecting predictors from a large set without a rational plan is like sticking a pitchfork into a haystack in the hope of hitting something, anything, solid. There are many approaches to building regression equations. One approach, the "all variables" method, throws in the whole haystack.

One question that arises in constructing regression models is whether to include a constant (b_0) in the model. The b_0 is the Y intercept. When a constant is omitted, b_0 is set equal to zero, and the regression surface is forced through the origin of the observation space because that is where the Y intercept is zero. When the Y and the X's are standardized, omitting the constant is appropriate. The observations are centered at zero, so the best fit line will pass through the origin. There are other cases in which, empirically or logically, there is an expectation that whenever the independent influences are zero the dependent response will also be zero. One may require the model of the response to satisfy this expectation by omitting the constant from the model and forcing the regression surface through the origin. Unless there is a specific reason to omit a constant, regression models should ordinarily include a constant. It is rare, the above exceptions notwithstanding, that a regression surface passing through the origin will just happen to fit the observations better than a regression surface cutting through the Y axis at any other point.

The *stepwise forward inclusion* approach (Draper & Smith, 1981) to building regression models inserts X variables, one at a time, until the regression equation satisfies some stop criterion. At each step, partial correlation coefficients determine which of the X's outside the equation, if any, to select. Suppose that of ten X variables X_6 is chosen on the first step because it has the highest simple correlation with Y. At step two, Y and the nine X's

outside the equation are adjusted for their linear relationships with X_6, in the manner described above. The nine adjusted X's are then correlated with the adjusted Y, yielding nine partial correlation coefficients. Of the nine, the X with the highest partial correlation with Y (say X_2) is entered next. The process is then repeated, now adjusting Y and the eight outside X's for their relationships with X_6 and X_2, etc., until the addition of an X to the equation fails to pass the stop test, usually some criterion p value for the significance of the reduction in the residual sum of squares (SS).

Significance tests at each step are based on the increment in the squared multiple correlation (R^2) or the increase in the ratio of the regression mean square (MS) to the residual MS (the partial F ratio) associated with the step. Significance tests for the entire final equation are based on the final R^2 or the ratio of the regression MS to the residual MS for the equation as a whole.

The *backward elimination* procedure for calculating the "best" regression equation works in the opposite direction. It first fits Y to all the X's and then begins tossing out X's one at a time until some stop criterion is reached. At each step, the partial F test value is computed for each X in the equation and the X with the lowest F value is removed, until the lowest F exceeds the criterion F for retaining X's, say the F for which $p = 0.05$.

The *all possible regressions* procedure looks at everything (Draper & Smith, 1981). All possible regressions of Y on the X's are formed and tested. In any regression equation, each X variable does or does not appear, two possibilities, resulting in 2^p equations for p predictor variables. Significance tests are applied to each equation. Nothing will be missed by this procedure, but the volume of results can swamp the mind. For 10 X's, $2^{10} = 1024$ equations will be calculated!

It is sometimes valuable to regress the dependent variable on *all* the independent variables in order to determine the unique contribution each makes when the broadest network of influences is operating. This might be called the *all variables* regression procedure.

There are other regression procedures such as robust procedures that are recommended when assumptions for standard regression are seriously violated (Draper & Smith, 1981). Different procedures applied to the same data will not necessarily produce the same "best" regression equation.

Checking the Goodness of Fit

The "best" equation found by an automated computer routine may not be a good equation. The equation should be tentatively entertained, not accepted blindly. Are the right number of X's in the equation? The stop rule for adding or eliminating variables in automated procedures is arbitrary and does not really indicate when enough is enough.

There are a number of indices that indicate how well a regression model fits the data, such as the residual MS (Draper & Smith, 1981). Specialized statistics like Mallow's C_p take into account the residual SS, p, and N, where N is the number of subjects and p the number of parameters in the model. These measures provide an objective basis for checking the fit of a model and comparing the fit for different combinations of X's.

As variables are added, the residual MS typically drops and eventually stabilizes at an asymptote. Adding variables beyond this point would be unnecessary overfitting. One way to check the change in fit as each independent variable is added to the equation is to plot the residual MS against the number of variables in the equation.

The residuals themselves contain more detailed information about the nature of the fit of a regression model than can be expressed in a quantitative measure of the degree of fit. A quantitative measure such as the residual MS will not reveal that a particular equation fits 90% of the individuals well and only a few individuals poorly. In this case, the "misfits" should be checked. What makes these people different from the others? Do they have something in common we can add to the model to improve the fit?

Curve-fitting is nonegalitarian. Some observations influence the size of the regression coefficients, i.e., the position of the regression surface in sample space, more than others. Some, but not necessarily all, outlying observations are likely to be disproportionately influential. When a few ob-

servations have great influence on the mathematical solution, the regression equation will be shaky, as any change in these observations upon resampling can change the equation dramatically. A good fit is not only a tight fit (small residual MS) but also a stable fit. Influential observations affect the stability of the regression equation.

The Cook statistic (Draper & Smith, 1981) is an aid in locating influential observations. It compares regression coefficients with and without the ith observation in the equation. If deletion of the ith observation changes the b's substantially, the observation is highly influential and should be flagged. It may be better to remove the observation or to collect more data.

Revising and Comparing Equations

Correlations between residuals and variables outside the model can indicate how to expand the model. The residuals are the errors of prediction. Which of the X's outside the equation can best predict the errors and therefore remove them? The F ratio (regression MS/residual MS) for the equation with and without the new candidate variable can be compared to determine whether the new variable is a statistically significant addition.

A new addition to an equation may be statistically significant but unimportant in practical terms. Plotting the mean absolute residual against the number of predictors in the model can aid in determining how much gain in knowledge of the response each predictor contributes. While constructing models of 24-h average BP recently we found a statistically significant predictor that increased the average precision of the model, i.e., decreased the mean absolute residual, by only 0.4 mm Hg. BP readings within 5 mm Hg are typically regarded as equivalent within the expected error of measurement. Consequently, we decided that a gain in knowledge of BP of 0.4 mm Hg was too small to justify adding the predictor to the model.

Quite often a decision hinges on whether an equation is better than some other equation representing a competing model. The goodness of fit of two models can be compared by examining the difference between their residuals. A simple $X-Y$ plot of residuals, in which one axis represents the residuals for one model and the other axis the residuals for the competing model, can aid in comparing models.

The X–Y plot of absolute residuals in Figure 2 compares two models of ambulatory BP. Thirty-two working adults were monitored for 24 h. Model 1 fitted the individual's gender, behavior type (Type A versus Type B), and the joint effects of gender and behavior type to the average systolic BP. Model 2 added body weight to Model 1. Points on the diagonal represent individuals whose BP was described (predicted) equally well by Model 1 and Model 2. Points above the diagonal represent individuals whose BP was described better by Model 2. Points below the diagonal represent an advantage for Model 1. Figure 2 shows that there were four people whose blood pressure was not well represented by either model (residuals > 10 mm Hg). Model 2 is clearly superior to Model 1 for only one person, a 270-lb man with elevated BP, and marginally superior for three others. Should we include the body weight parameter in our model in order to more accurately represent the BP of only 1 of 32 people? We must still make a subjective choice, but at least the issue is clear.

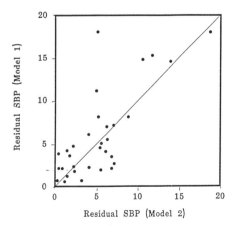

Figure 2. An X–Y plot of the absolute value of residuals for two models of average 24-h systolic blood pressure (SBP). Model 1 fitted SBP to a constant, the Type A behavior pattern (A), gender (B), and the AB interaction. Model 2 added body weight to Model 1.

Performing Diagnostics

A plot of residual $(Y - \hat{Y})$ values against fitted $(\hat{Y})$ values can indicate whether something is seriously wrong with a regression model and point to possible remedies. A normal plot will form a uniform horizontal band of points, indicating that the equation is equally accurate for different predicted Y values. Curvilinearity in the plot will indicate curvilinearity in relationships between variables, perhaps removable by a transformation of scale or requiring linear and quadratic terms in the model. A fan-shaped band of points, wider at one end than at the other end, will indicate the presence of heteroscedasticity of variance, perhaps requiring a transformation of scale or a weighted least-squares analysis. Outliers will appear as points lying outside an otherwise uniform horizontal band.

Most models assume that errors (residuals) are independent random variables distributed $N(0, \sigma^2)$. When the assumption is met, serial correlations between residuals will equal zero within sampling and measurement error. Subject-to-subject dependency or serial correlation in the observations can creep into the data inadvertently. Male or female subjects may be bunched together in a BP study, creating a "run" of high BPs or low BPs. Patients with the most severe disease may be tested first in a drug study, creating an early run of large treatment effects. The existence of long runs in the residuals indicates that some important variable such as gender or severity of disease has been omitted from the model. Subject-to-subject independency will be indicated by many short runs in the residuals.

The Durbin–Watson statistic (Draper & Smith, 1981) tests whether there is serial correlation in the residuals of a model. If the residuals are significantly correlated, one should try to find an assignable cause (such as gender and severity of illness in the aforementioned examples) and include a measure of the cause or a simple time variable in the model. If the observation–observation dependency cannot be removed, it may be necessary to adjust the degrees of freedom for the dependency. A formula for estimating the actual degrees of freedom in a time series of sequentially dependent paired observations is presented below.

Validation Procedures

Regression models become less reliable, and therefore less trustworthy, in proportion to the number of independent variables in the model, their unreliability, and the magnitude of their intercorrelation. Attempting to estimate the population regression coefficient for a variable embedded in a large network of interdependent, unreliable variables is like trying to measure the effects of a delicate force applied to the node of a spider web that is jiggling erratically in the wind. Random noise in other variables (nodes) will be transmitted by way of relationships (filaments) to the variable in question, causing major flux and making it very difficult to detect the true relationship between the variable and the dependent response.

The optimization process of the least-squares procedure is opportunistic and will pull into the calculation of regression coefficients all the wiggles and idiosyncrasies in the data. Many of the wiggles and idiosyncrasies may not be reproducible. Consequently, a regression equation should be validated before it is taken seriously. Validating the equation requires determining whether it can make accurate predictions in a fresh batch of data. Validation methods proceed by first splitting a total set of observations into two parts, then constructing the regression equation on one part (the "construction sample"), and finally testing its ability to make accurate predictions on the second part (the "test sample") (Draper & Smith, 1981). Cross-validating an equation from one study to another is a familiar example.

The "construction sample" multiple correlation will always be larger than the "test sample" multiple correlation, the difference reflecting capitalization on chance. The smaller R^2, sometimes called the "shrunken" or "adjusted" R^2, will better estimate the population R^2. It can be estimated as:

$$R_s^2 = 1 - (1 - R^2)(N - 1)/(N - p) \quad (4)$$

where p is the number of parameters in the model including the constant. The equation indicates that upon cross-validation the R^2 is expected to shrink in direct proportion to the number of parameters in the model and in inverse proportion to the number of subjects. Consequently, it is a good strategy to make N as large and p as small as possible, consistent with budget constraints and theoretical interests.

Interpreting Regression Models

Interpretation concerns how much faith to put in significance statements for the whole equation and for individual coefficients, what substantive meaning to give coefficients, and when to recommend practical action based on predictions of the equation.

One reason, besides unreliability, to view coefficients from a single study cautiously is that a coefficient indicates the relationship between an independent variable and a dependent variable *when the other independent variables are in the equation.* All other variables in the equation are "side conditions" for the relationship of each variable to the response. Change the other variables and the regression coefficient for X_j may change radically; it may even change sign. Because coefficients are context-dependent, a coefficient may have a sign opposite that of the variable's simple correlation with the dependent response. What firm meaning, in physiological or behavioral terms, can we give an "independent" variable that is highly context-dependent? This question becomes of central concern in causal analysis.

Because of context-dependency, it is misleading to remove a single predictor X_j from a larger equation and predict b_j units of change in Y (say, incidence of disease) for each unit change in X_j (say, a specific risk factor). The size of b_j depends entirely on the presence of the other independent variables in the model. It is better to keep the equation intact when making predictions.

Caution is warranted when considering practical recommendations based on regression results. Estimating the reduction in disease from a given reduction in risk factors without a controlled trial is very hazardous. The MRFIT controlled trial study to reduce coronary heart disease (MRFIT, 1982) illustrated how variables omitted from the original risk factor equation can alter the results of recommended actions.

The quantity $1 - R^2$ indicates the proportion of response variance that is unexplainable by the regression equation. It is a measurement of the unassignable causes of the response. The set of variables we are working with is never the complete set, so this figure is often large. When it is large, many unmeasured causes *outside* the regression equation that are correlated with variables *inside* the equation can sabotage causal models and practical recommendations. There are important statistical and conceptual advantages to be gained from reducing $1 - R^2$ as much as possible by including in the regression model all major measurable antecedents of the response, even though a particular antecedent (e.g., body weight in a model of BP) may be of little theoretical interest. The reduction of the residuals can lead to correct detection of weak relationships in the population that would otherwise be (falsely) interpreted as null relationships.

Multivariate Statistical Procedures

Few data analyses take into account explicitly the essential multiplicity of the response system under study. What has been discussed thus far are procedures for constructing and testing models of a single response (dependent variable). There are multiple-response analogues for these single-response procedures. Hotelling's T^2 statistic is a multivariate analogue of Student's t statistic and multivariate ANOVA is an analogue of univariate ANOVA. Canonical correlation analysis has some similarities to multiple correlation analysis.

Multiple-response procedures are useful for studying the effects of independent variables on a *system* of dependent variables rather than on a single variable. A multivariate model of an integrated behavioral or physiological system may provide a more comprehensive and less fragmented picture of research results. When a set of variables constitutes different facets of an integrated system, as is often the case, multivariate procedures are usually more appropriate than univariate procedures.

A key idea in multivariate procedures is that the aggregate properties of a set of dependent measures are studied by joining the dependent measures into one (composite) measure. By linearly transforming multiple dependent variables into a single composite variable, *a multivariate situation is essentially converted into a univariate situation.* The linear transformation is accomplished in such manner as to concentrate in the new (composite) dependent variable in maximum amount some familiar statistical property of the observation system, its variance [in factor analysis (FA)], the covariance between two distinct sets of measures [in canonical analysis (CA)], or the differences between groups [in multivariate analysis of variance (MANOVA) and discriminant function analysis].

We seek linear transformations of (standardized) Y scores of the form

$$Z_i = w_1 Y_{i1} + w_2 Y_{i2} + \cdots + w_p Y_{ip} \qquad (5)$$

where Z_i is the composite variable score of individual i, Y_{i1} his or her score on dependent measure 1, and w_1 the weight that is applied to measure 1 when computing the composite score. Optimal weights must be determined such that some mathematical function of Z_i is maximized: s^2_z, the variance of Z_i in FA, $r_{z_1 z_2}$, the Pearson product moment correlation between two different Z variates (sets of weighted Y dependent variables) in CA, and $s^2_{z_h}/s^2_{z_e}$, the ratio of hypothesis variance (i.e., variance due to some hypothesized "effect") to error variance, the multivariate F ratio, in MANOVA and discriminant function analysis.

The fundamental mathematical problem in multivariate analysis is to find the optimal linear weights (coefficients) shown in equation (5). Since both the w's and Z's are unknown, the w's cannot be found by a straightforward application of differential calculus to the linear equations. A unique nontrivial solution for the equations exists only when some constraint is placed on the coefficients. The convention is to require that the coefficients be normalized, i.e., require that $\Sigma w^2_j = 1.0$ ($j = 1, 2, \ldots, p$). Finding the first derivative of a function with a restriction condition imposed on it can be handled through an application of the method of Lagrange multipliers. Lagrange multipliers are the ever-present eigenvalues of multivariate procedures. The key statistical quantities in multivariate analyses are derivatives of eigenvalues.

It can be shown (Anderson, 1958) that the

eigenvalues (λ) can be obtained by solving the general determinantal equation:

$$|G - \lambda I| = 0$$

where G is a correlation matrix (R) in factor analysis, a product matrix of correlation matrices and their inverses $(R_{22}{}^{-1}R_{21}R_{11}{}^{-1}R_{12})$ in canonical correlation analysis, and the product of an inverse error mean products matrix and hypothesis mean products matrix $(M_e{}^{-1}M_h)$ in the multivariate analysis of variance. The linear weights (w_j) sought are eigenvectors associated with the eigenvalues or derivatives of the eigenvectors. Elsewhere (Van Egeren, 1973) I have compared these three basic multivariate procedures and have illustrated the calculation of the matrices and the determinantal equation shown above on problems that are small enough to be worked out on a desk calculator.

Much of the mystery of multivariate analyses can be removed by keeping in mind that the key quantity, as in univariate analyses, is variance (and the related quantity, covariance). Only now, the quantity refers to the variance of a *set* of dependent variables instead of a single variable. The variance of the sum of two variables X and Y is:

$$\begin{aligned} s^2{}_{X+Y} &= 1/N \; \Sigma(x + y)^2 \\ &= 1/N(\Sigma x^2 + \Sigma y^2 + 2 \; \Sigma xy) \\ &= s^2{}_X + s^2{}_Y + 2s_{XY} \end{aligned}$$

where x and y are the deviation scores for variables X and Y. That is, the variance of the sum of X and Y is the sum of the variance of X plus the variance of Y plus twice the covariance of X and Y. These quantities are the elements of the so-called "dispersion matrix" (variance–covariance matrix) for the two variables. The variances are the diagonal elements and the covariance is the off-diagonal element. The sum of the elements of the dispersion matrix is a multivariate variance, i.e., the variance of the multivariate quantity, or linear composite variable, $X + Y$.

Multivariate variance is the fundamental building block of multivariate procedures, just as univariate variance is the fundamental building block of univariate procedures. The matrices that appear in the key determinantal equation above are disper-sion matrices or transformations of dispersion matrices. The solutions to the determinantal equation yield eigenvalues, the key statistical quantity in multivariate procedures, which in turn lead to eigenvectors, a transformation of which are the w's of equation (5) that are sought.

Just as the two basic univariate procedures, MRA and ANOVA, are variations of a single linear model, the three basic multivariate procedures, FA, CA, and MANOVA, are variations of a single model. Different matrices appear in the model that lead to the concentration in maximum amount in the derived dependent variable (factor variate, canonical variate, or discriminant variate) different fundamental aspects of the observation system.

The factor variate can be represented geometrically as the axis that maximally separates individuals in the multivariate sample space. FA is ideally suited to the study of individual differences because it produces the measurement dimensions (factor variates) on which individuals are maximally different. FA can be used to examine the linear organization of variables (an exploratory procedure) or to test a hypothesized organization of variables (a confirmatory procedure).

Confirmatory FA can be used to test an explicit measurement model of a theoretical variable. Many theoretical variables in cardiovascular behavioral medicine are too complex to be operationally defined by a single measure. Multiple measures or indicators are required. When the multiple indicators are caused by the same underlying (latent) process, as hypothesized, a single factor should account for their organization and be extractable from their intercorrelations. This critical assumption should be tested more often than it is in practice.

Paired canonical variates are the two axes in the multivariate sample space that have a maximum cosine, indicating a maximum correlation between the two composite variates. The canonical correlation is the Pearson product–moment correlation between the two composite canonical variates. The correlation represents a channel of maximum association between two sets of variables or domains of measurement. The two domains might be cardiovascular variables and behavioral variables, or risk variables and disease variables. One may be interested in the independent linkages that connect the two sets of variables. The linkages may indicate paths of causal influence functionally connecting the two domains of phenomena.

CA is like a double-sided regression analysis. MRA is univariate–multivariate (univariate on the dependent variable side of the equation and multivariate on the independent variable side). CA is multivariate–multivariate (multivariate on both sides of the equation).

The discriminant variate resulting from MANOVA is the unique dimension in sample space on which point-locations of subjects belonging to one group have a minimum overlap with subjects belonging to the other groups in the analysis. It maximally separates *groups* of individuals, in contrast to FA, which maximally separates *individuals*. MANOVA is valuable for answering the broad question, "Do these groups (or treatments) differ with respect to the *entire system* of response measures?" MANOVA is less piecemeal than performing a series of ANOVAs on a set of measures treated as single measures. It is sometimes a good alternative to the repeated measures ANOVA model. MANOVA allows the investigator to examine the influence of independent variables on response variables treated as an integrated system.

Time-Series Data Analysis

A time series is a set of observations that occur in a temporal order. When an observation is made repeatedly on the same individual or individuals are tested at different points in time, time can become an important ordering variable and sequential dependency in the observations can occur. Time-series analysis is a set of exploratory and confirmatory procedures for examining the internal organization of a set of observations ordered in time. The observations may represent an organized process. One may wish to examine a time trend in the process (observations), or smooth the process by calculating moving averages, or decompose the process into a small number of sine and cosine components, which are thought to represent underlying cyclical functions (Fourier analysis), or represent observations as functions of other observations occurring earlier or later in the same series

(autocorrelations and autoregressions) (Kendall, 1973).

Sequential dependency is often undesirable. Temporal dependency of observations *within* variables can distort relationships *between* variables that are of primary interest. We often assume that observations made at different points in time are made independently of one another. If so, the residuals will lack temporal systematization. As illustrated earlier, temporal systematization can creep into the data unwittingly. The Durbin–Watson test provides an index of the extent to which sequential order is present in the residuals (Draper & Smith, 1981).

The extent to which a given observation is dependent on the observations preceding it can be estimated by calculating the autocorrelation in the series of observations. Given the observations X_1, $X_2, \ldots, X_n$, the $(n - 1)$ pairs $(X_1, X_2), (X_2, X_3)$, $\ldots, (X_{n-1}, X_n)$ constitute a set of bivariate values that can be correlated in a standard way (Kendall, 1973). Such a correlation is called an "autocorrelation" or a "serial correlation" because it is a correlation between paired observations within the same variable or time series. A correlation between observations two units apart, i.e., the correlation between the $(n - 2)$ pairs of observations $(X_1, X_3), (X_2, X_4), \ldots, (X_{n-2}, X_n)$, is called an autocorrelation of "lag two," instead of "lag one," as above. Autocorrelations, and partial autocorrelations, between observations more and more remote in time can be calculated. A partial autocorrelation denotes interdependency between observations after observations located between them in time have been partialled out of the relationship.

The degrees of freedom for the mean of sequentially dependent observations made on the same individual is less than $N - 1$. Consequently, it is important to remove sequential dependency or to adjust the degrees of freedom for its presence before applying standard statistics. The effective number of independent paired observations in a bivariate time series can be estimated as:

$$N' = N/(1 + 2r_{1y}r_{1x} + 2r_{2y}r_{2x} + \cdots)$$

where N is the number of observations on which

r_{xy} is based, r_{1y} and r_{1x} are the serial correlations of lag one for the Y variable and the X variable, respectively, and r_{2y} and r_{2x} are the serial correlations of lag two (Holtzman, 1963).

When repeated observations on each of a number of variables are available, it is often desirable to calculate intercorrelations between the variables within each individual separately. A significance test of the correlation coefficient computed on a single subject can be applied, using $N' - 2$ as the estimated degrees of freedom, where N' is the effective number of paired observations computed as shown above.

Estimating the number of degrees of freedom in interdependent observations has a number of practical applications, such as the use of standard confirmatory statistics for N of 1 data and determining how far apart to space observations (e.g., sequential ambulatory BP readings) for maximum gain in information. Many other useful and interesting applications of the analysis of time series data can be found in primary sources on the subject (e.g., Kendall, 1973).

Causal Modeling

Causal Relations

The ideal method of science is the study of the direct influence of one variable on another in a controlled experiment. Often this approach is not possible. We are forced to settle for indirect evidence of influence in the form of the correlation coefficient. The correlation coefficient describes an association without explaining the underlying causation. There may be little difficulty in suggesting a plausible explanation of a single correlation on experimental grounds. It is more difficult to interpret an *entire system* of correlations and be sure there is logical and factual consistency throughout (Wright, 1921).

Causal relations can be represented conveniently in a diagram like that in Figure 3, in which paths of influence are shown by arrows. Some relationships between variables are *directly* causal, as when variation in X directly determines variation in Y (Figure 3a). Other pairs of variables may be connected *indirectly* through an intermediary variable, e.g., variable Y is determined by variable Z and Z is determined by a more remote cause X (Figure 3c). Some variables are related as effects of a common cause (Figure 3b). Such relationships are *spurious* causal relationships, because neither variable directly or indirectly causes the other.

A path of influence in a complex network of causes and effects can be difficult to trace. Sewall Wright (1921) offers advice on how to trace a path. A causal path cannot pass through a variable more than once. A path connecting two variables via a common cause (spurious factor) must move from

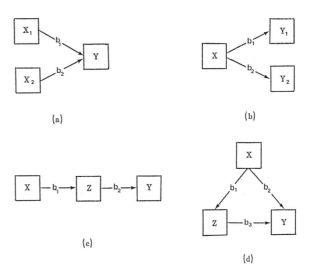

Figure 3. Arrow diagrams illustrating (a) direct causal influence of variables X_1 and X_2 on variable Y, (b) spurious influence of X on relationship between Y_1 and Y_2, (c) indirect causal influence of X on Y via Z, and (d) direct causal influence of X on Y (b_2 link) and indirect causal influence of X on Y via Z (b_1b_3 linkage).

one variable to the cause continuously against arrows (from effects to causes), and from the cause to the other variable continuously with arrows (from causes to effects).

Two variables are often linked through more than one path of influence (Figure 3d). Some paths may be directly causal, others indirectly causal, and still others spurious. The correlation coefficient gives merely the resultant effect of all paths of influence connecting the two variables. It would often be desirable to be able to determine the type (direct, indirect, or spurious) of each particular path connecting two variables. Linear structural equation ("path analysis") models aim at providing this information. The goal is to answer the following kinds of questions. How many causal paths connect X and Y? What are the relative strengths of the paths? How are the causal influences connecting two variables divided into direct effects, indirect effects, and spurious effects?

Path Analysis

Path analysis employs systems of simultaneous linear equations to examine causal processes underlying a limited set of variables. Current theory and practice owe much to seminal papers by Sewall Wright (1921) and Herbert Simon (1954), and work on linear structural equations in econometrics and statistics. Detailed treatments are available in Asher (1976), Duncan (1975), and Hunter and Gerbing (1982).

Correlation does not imply causation (as every student of introductory statistics learns), but causation *does* imply correlation. Path analysis begins with this fact. One starts with the most satisfactory causal "hypothesis" about a given subject and then considers the covariation consequences that follow from it. Can the hypothesis (causal ordering of variables) generate the facts (correlations between variables)? Observed correlations can be compared with correlations implied (reproduced, predicted) by the causal model, both to determine the satisfactoriness of the model and to revise it.

Suppose that variation in X is the sole cause of variation in Z which is the sole cause of variation in Y. Then removing the influence of Z from the

$X–Z–Y$ sequence should cause the $X–Y$ relationship to vanish. Given that the causal relations are specified correctly, it will follow that, within sampling and measurement error, the partial correlation $r_{xy.z}$ will equal zero. It will also follow that the correlation between the end variables of the causal chain will be reproducible from the correlations between the end variables and the intermediate variable Z, i.e., $r_{xy} = r_{xz}r_{zy}$. This consequence of the causal ordering of the three variables can be demonstrated by setting the equation for the appropriate partial correlation coefficient equal to zero, dividing through the equation by the denominator, and rearranging terms:

$$r_{xy.z} = (r_{xy} - r_{xz}r_{zy})/[(1 - r^2_{xz})(1 - r^2_{zy})]^{1/2}$$
$$= 0$$
$$r_{xy} - r_{xz}r_{zy} = 0$$
$$r_{xy} = r_{xz}r_{zy}$$

The result above illustrates a key to path analysis, the "product rule" for calculating the causal impact of variables along a path connecting any two variables X and Y. The net causal impact of the entire path is the product of the links between all variables along the path from variable X to variable Y. The quantitative measurement of a link is called a "path coefficient," symbolized p_{zx} for the causal impact of X on Z.

The main steps in path analysis can be summarized as follows: (1) list the important variables defining some system, (2) draw arrows to indicate hypothesized causal links between the variables (construct a qualitative diagram of relations), (3) obtain a quantitative estimate of the strength of each causal link by solving a system of linear equations (each equation expressing the relationship between a dependent variable and the independent variables that impinge on it) for unknown path coefficients (thus converting the qualitative diagram into a quantitative diagram), (4) using the product rule, calculate the net causal effect of each path connecting any two variables as the product of the path coefficients on the path, (5) express the correlation between any two variables as equal to the sum of the contributions of all paths connecting them, (6) compare correlations reproduced by the causal model with the observed correlations in order to evaluate the goodness of fit of the model to the data, and (7) revise the model as needed.

There are a number of ways to estimate the basic parameters of the model, the path coefficients. For linear relations and "recursive" postulated causes, the path coefficients can be conveniently obtained as ordinary regression coefficients, using a standard computer routine. If only X has a causal impact on Y, then $p_{yx} = b_x = r_{yx}$, where b_x is a regression coefficient. If both X and Z causally impinge on Y, then $p_{yx} = b_{x.z}$ and $p_{yz} = b_{z.x}$, where $b_{x.z}$ and $b_{z.x}$ are the two coefficients for the regression of Y on X and Z. It is helpful to use *standardized* regression coefficients as path coefficients when comparing the strengths of two or more paths, as the coefficients on different paths will then be expressed in the same standardized unit.

A causal model is "recursive" when no path returns, or "feeds back," on itself. A model that postulates bidirectional causation, e.g., X is both cause and effect of Y simultaneously, is nonrecursive. Nonrecursive models are sometimes more realistic than recursive models but also are mathematically more complicated.

"Missing" links in models (pairs of variables that do not have an arrow connecting them) are essential to statistical evaluation of the model. Regression coefficients can be mathematically derived from correlation coefficients. Without missing links in a causal model, path coefficients would be derived completely from the very information needed to evaluate the accuracy of the model. The process of extracting path coefficients from the correlations and then arithmetically combining the coefficients to predict the quantities from which they originated would be tautological. The coefficients would not be "free" to be wrong; the reproduced correlations and the observed correlations would be numerically identical. Omitting causal links from the diagram (essentially setting path coefficients for the pairs of variables equal to zero) omits the corresponding path coefficients and correlation coefficients from the system of linear equations and creates the degrees of freedom necessary to evaluate the model. Path coefficients that

successfully predict an omitted link are reproducing a datum from which they did not originate. Consequently, they have an opportunity (degree of freedom) to be wrong.

Illustrative Examples

A concrete example will illustrate how path analysis can expose and test the implications of a causal hypothesis. Consider the putative association between hostility and blood pressure. The "commonsense" explanation for the association is that hostile (H) people have frequent anger (A) flare-ups that cause surges in blood pressure (P). Applying the product rule of path analysis to the hypothesized causal sequence H–A–P, implies $r_{hp} = p_{ah}p_{pa}$. The H–P correlation will equal the product of the H–A and A–P links in the chain if the causal hypothesis is correct.

We were able to test the commonsense hypothesis in a sample of working adults who were assessed for trait hostility (via an interview) and reported anger episodes in a diary during 24-h ambulatory BP monitoring. The correlation between hostility and average systolic BP was 0.29. The correlations for the two links of the causal chain were 0.24 for the H–A link and 0.18 for the A–P link, resulting in a reproduced H–P correlation of $0.24 \times 0.18 = 0.04$. The commonsense path linking together hostile traits, anger states, and BP accounted for only a small fraction of the observed correlation. A second path connecting hostility and BP through body weight accounted for most (0.24) of the correlation (0.29). The correlation predicted by the two-path model was 0.04 (indirect anger effect) + 0.24 (spurious weight effect) = 0.28.

A more complex example will furnish a more complete illustration of path analysis. Figure 4 presents a hypothesized causal ordering of 14 putative antecedents and consequences of hypertension. Three variables serve as "starter" variables to initiate causal processes: (a) stress, (b) heritable risk factors for hypertension (e.g., as estimated by documented family history of hypertension), and (c) sodium intake. The exogenous or starter variables are hypothesized to directly

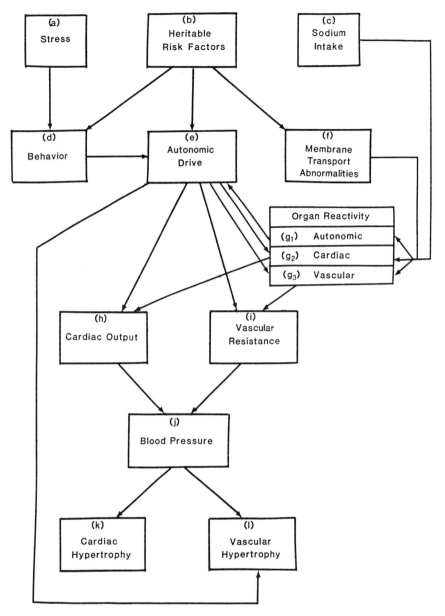

Figure 4. Hypothesized causal model of hypertension. Arrows indicate the direction of causal influences.

causally influence (d) behavior (e.g., hostility, anger suppression), (e) autonomic drive (e.g., plasma norepinephrine), (f) membrane transport abnormalities (e.g., inadequate lithium–sodium countertransport), and (g) organ reactivity, which is subdivided into reactivity of (g_1) the autonomic nerves, (g_2) the heart (e.g., response of cardiac output to a dose of isoproterenol), and (g_3) the blood vessels. The model states that behavior and autonomic reactivity directly influence autonomic drive. Variables (e) and (g) are hypothesized to have a direct causal impact on (h) cardiac output (β

effect) and (i) vascular resistance (α effect), which determine (j) blood pressure level, which eventually determines target organ damage in the form of (k) cardiac hypertrophy and (l) vascular hypertrophy.

The present analysis will require that we possess measures on all variables, the measures have been standardized, and relations are linear. Relations between some variables in the model are nonlinear over the long period of time in which there is a transition from hyperkinetic normotension to normokinetic hypertension. This transition is accompanied by a shift from β-adrenergic drive, high cardiac output, and normal vascular resistance to α-adrenergic drive, normal cardiac output, and high vascular resistance (Julius, Weder, & Hinderliter, 1986). However, the relationships can be linear over the short term covered by a cross-sectional study of the kind represented by the present example. A dynamic model of causation for the pathophysiological transition from a healthy state to a diseased state would require additional considerations.

We will assume that any bidirectional causation, e.g., between cardiac output and vascular resistance, can be converted into unidirectional causation by lagging one of the variables (Duncan, 1975), so that the causal model will be "recursive." The interaction between cardiac output and vascular resistance is not represented in Figure 4 and will be ignored in this illustration.

The causal diagram does not show residual variables for the endogenous dependent variables (variables d through l). Residual variables are measures of all unexplained (error) variability. With residual variables implicitly included in the model, we can proceed *as if* the system of variables is causally complete and ask, "What pattern of empirical relations (correlations) will such a causal system produce?"

The model implies that autonomic function has a number of influences on cardiac output and vascular resistance: a *direct* causal impact, an *indirect* impact through the effect of enhanced autonomic drive on the reactivity of the heart and the blood vessels, and *spurious* effects due to the common antecedent causes of heredity, membrane abnor-

malities, and sodium intake. Heredity affects autonomic state, as well as cardiac output and vascular resistance, via membrane transport abnormalities and organ reactivity. The correlation between autonomic drive (e.g., plasma norepinephrine) and vascular resistance predicted by the model is:

$$r_{ei} = p_{ie} \text{ (direct effect)} +$$
$$p_{g_3e}p_{ig_3} \text{ (indirect reactivity effect)} +$$
$$p_{eb}p_{fb}p_{g_3f}p_{ig_3} \text{ (spurious heredity effect)} +$$
$$p_{eg_1}p_{g_1f}p_{g_3f}p_{ig_3} \text{ (spurious membrane effect)} +$$
$$p_{eg_1}p_{g_3c}p_{g_3c}p_{ig_3} \text{ (spurious sodium effect)}$$

The required path coefficients could be obtained by appropriate regression analyses. Specifically, $p_{ie} = b_{e.g_3}$ and $p_{ig_3} = b_{g_3.e}$ (where $b_{e.g_3}$ and $b_{g_3.e}$ are the coefficients for the regression of a measure of vascular resistance on the measures of plasma norepinephrine and blood vessel reactivity), $p_{fb} = r_{bf}$, $p_{g_3c} = b_{c.ef}$, $p_{g_3f} = b_{f.ec}$, and $p_{g_3e} = b_{e.fc}$ (where $b_{c.ef}$, $b_{f.ec}$, and $b_{e.fc}$ are the coefficients for the regression of blood vessel reactivity on the measures of norepinephrine, membrane transport abnormalities, and sodium intake), and $p_{eb} = b_{b.dg_1}$ for the regression of norepinephrine on behavior, familial risk, and autonomic reactivity. The remaining path coefficients for the spurious membrane and sodium effects would be obtained similarly.

A correlation between plasma norepinephrine and forearm vascular resistance of 0.48 in a group of borderline hypertension patients has been reported (Egan, Fitzpatrick, Schneider, & Julius, 1985). The causal model would allow us to split that correlation into direct, indirect, and spurious parts as illustrated above.

The present model indicates that even in a simplified scheme the relationship between antecedent causes and harmful target organ effects can be quite complex. For example, the model specifies ten linkages between enhanced autonomic function and cardiac hypertrophy, five by way of the "β path" (cardiac output) and five by way of the "α path" (vascular resistance). There are: (1) the direct influence of autonomic drive on cardiac output and vascular resistance, (2) the long-term influence of autonomic drive on the "reactivity" of the heart and blood vessels, which also affects cardiac output and vascular resistance, and (3) the spurious connections linking autonomic function to cardiac output and vascular resistance through the common antecedent causes of heredity, membrane abnormalities, and sodium intake.

A correlation between plasma norepinephrine and cardiac hypertrophy (left ventricular wall mass) of 0.56 has been reported (Egan *et al.,* 1985). The causal model would split that correlation into the ten parts (paths) listed above.

The report (Egan *et al.,* 1985) of a stronger correlation between plasma norepinephrine and vascular hypertrophy than between blood pressure and vascular hypertrophy ($r_{el} > r_{jl}$) indicates that the causal diagram in Figure 4 requires a direct causal path between autonomic drive and vascular hypertrophy, in addition to the paths for the two indirect effects and the two spurious effects. The model without the direct path implies $r_{el} < r_{jl}$, since the relationship between the end members of a compound linkage must be smaller than the relationship between the members constituting the weakest link.

There are many other implications of the model that could be checked against empirical data. For example, the model does not specify a direct causal path from autonomic drive to cardiac hypertrophy. The entire effect of long-term autonomic hyperactivity on enlargement of the heart is assumed to act through BP elevation. The model predicts that the partial correlation between plasma norepinephrine and ventricular wall thickness with BP held constant, $r_{ek \cdot j}$, will equal zero within sampling and measurement error.

Evaluating the hypothesized hypertension model would require (1) computing intercorrelations between the 12 variables in the model, (2) estimating path coefficients by solving the appropriate regression equations, (3) calculating correlations implied by the model as illustrated above, and (4) subtracting the reproduced correlations from the observed correlations to obtain the errors of prediction (residual correlations). Entries in the residual correlation matrix might suggest how the model could be changed to provide a better fit of the data. One might also apply the chi square test presented earlier to determine whether it is possible to reject the hypothesis that the entire set of residual correlations is zero in the population. Failure to reject the hypothesis would offer evidence that the causal model successfully explains the observed correlations among the 12 variables.

Interpreting Causal Models

The assumptions underlying regression analysis apply to path analysis as well. It is also necessary to assume, if we wish to take the path coefficients seriously, that variables have been measures without error. When errors of measurement are too large to ignore, correlation and regression coefficients should be corrected for attenuation. Without the correction, path coefficients can easily give a false picture of causation. Two paths can differ in path estimates, and presumed causal strength, merely because the variables on one path were measured more reliably. Worse yet, false coefficients can be created through "incomplete partialling" caused by measurement error. For example, when the hypothesized X–Z–Y causal chain is correct, $r_{xy \cdot z}$ should equal zero, but will be nonzero if Z is incompletely removed (partialled) from X and Y.

Path analysis cannot provide proof that a causal model is correct. It can only indicate that a causal model is *consistent* with the data. This is true even when the model successfully reproduces the observed relations between the variables. The reason is that other causal models may also reproduce the correlations as satisfactorily. A successful causal model is a set of plausible, but not proven, causal hypotheses. Plausibility is of less value than proof, but can still be of considerable worth, which it would be imprudent to ignore. Plausibility is the most any statistical methodology can provide. Proof cannot be obtained by statistical arguments alone.

Scientists rarely spell out their assumptions and the conclusions that follow from them. Path analysis is a valuable aid to help them translate an implicit vision into an explicit, testable theory. It is useful for putting the meaning of a proposed hypothesis forcibly and clearly before the mind. Implications that are easy to overlook are exposed. Causal influences can be untangled and clarified, even though there is inescapable uncertainty because the system of variables being studied is never a closed system. Outside influences can always seep in to contaminate the results. Experimental controls can reduce but never totally eliminate the uncertainty.

Data Analysis Issues Revisited

The statistical procedures discussed above examine data from different perspectives and deal with different issues. More detailed information about the data is obtained as we move from ANOVA to MRA to PA. ANOVA emphasizes testing of specific effects. The key issue here is: Is this hypothesis right or wrong—for the whole group of subjects (entire population)? MRA focuses more on building and testing models of the dependent response. The key issues become: To what degree is the hypothesis (model) right or wrong, by how much does it miss the mark (how far are the data points from the regression surface), for which subjects does the hypothesis fit well, for which does it fit poorly?

ANOVA and MRA are concerned with the direct relationships between the independent variables and the dependent variable. PA is concerned with the relationships between the independent variables, as well as the relationships between the independent variables and the dependent variable. For PA, the key question is: By what causal mechanisms (direct, indirect, spurious) do the independent variables interact to produce some resultant effect on the dependent variable?

We can also contrast the methodologies by the following questions they raise. Is a direct cause of the dependent response present or absent (ANOVA)? How much information about the dependent response does a particular cause, in the context of other causes, provide (MRA)? Are there multiple independent causal paths connecting variables (MANOVA, CA, FA)? What is the nature of the causal paths (direct, indirect, spurious) connecting variables (PA)?

Facing Up to Real Complexity

Ideally, we would like to know the causal mechanisms operating in a working system, not as the mechanisms *can* operate in the laboratory but as they *actually do* operate in the intact individual under natural conditions. Smith, Astley, Hohimer, and Stephenson (1980) put the question this way: "What are the regulatory mechanisms actually used by the organism in adjusting its circulatory responses to the stresses imposed by the environment and the organism's behavior?" (p. 4).

To deal with this question, we need data analytic techniques that can aid in unraveling the great variety and complexity of relations that can exist in even simple natural systems. In short, we need tools for systems analysis. All the procedures reviewed above, with the exception of path analysis, deal with direct causation only, even though indirect causation and often spurious factors are present. This is a serious limitation. Reality does not limit itself to direct causal influences.

There is a major gap between what can be done and what is done in the analysis of data in cardiovascular behavioral medicine. Formal causal modeling is a promising and innovative approach to the analysis of natural systems. I believe that a more explicit causal approach can help us face up to some of the complexities of the real world outside the controlled conditions of the laboratory.

ACKNOWLEDGMENTS. I wish to thank Drs. Larry Hedges, John Hunter, Ernest Johnson, Stevo Julius, William Ray, and James Stapleton for their helpful comments on a draft of this chapter.

References

Anderson, T. W. (1958). *An introduction to multivariate statistical analysis*. New York: Wiley.

Asher, H. (1976). *Causal modeling*. Beverly Hills, CA: Sage.

Barnett, V., & Lewis, T. (1978). *Outliners in statistical data*. New York: Wiley.

Box, G. E. P. (1954). Some theorems on quadratic forms applied in the study of analysis of variance problems. *The Annals of Mathematical Statistics, 25,* 290–302, 484–498.

Draper, N. R., & Smith, H. (1981). *Applied regression analysis.* New York: Wiley.

Duncan, O. (1975). *Introduction to structural equation models.* New York: Academic Press.

Egan, B., Fitzpatrick, M., Schneider, R., & Julius, S. (1985). Vascular hypertrophy in borderline hypertension: Relationship to blood pressure and sympathetic drive. *Clinical and Experimental Hypertension, 7,* 243–250.

Holtzman, W. H. (1963). Statistical models for the study of change in the single case. In C. H. Harris (Ed.), *Problems in measuring change.* Madison: University of Wisconsin Press.

Hunter, J., & Gerbing, D. (1982). Unidimensional measurement, second order factor analysis, and causal models. *Research in Organizational Behavior, 4,* 267–320.

Julius, S., Weder, A., & Hinderliter, A. (1986). Does behaviorally induced blood pressure variability lead to hypertension? In K. Matthews, S. Weiss, T. Detre, T. Dembroski, B. Falkner, S. Manuck, & R. Williams (Eds.), *Handbook of stress, reactivity, and cardiovascular disease.* New York: Wiley.

Kendall, M. G. (1973). *Time-series.* New York: Hafner.

Mosteller, F., & Tukey, J. W. (1977). *Data analysis and regression.* Reading, MA: Addison–Wesley.

Multiple Risk Factor Intervention Trial Research Group. (1982). Multiple risk factor intervention trial. *Journal of the American Medical Association, 248,* 1465–1477.

Simon, H. (1954). Spurious correlation: A causal interpretation. *Journal of the American Statistical Association, 49,* 467–479.

Smith, O., Astley, C., Hohimer, A., & Stephenson, R. (1980). Behavioral and cerebral control of cardiovascular function. In M. Hughes & C. Baines (Eds.), *Neural control of circulation.* New York: Academic Press.

Tukey, J. W. (1962). The future of data analysis. *The Annals of Mathematical Statistics, 33,* 1–67.

Van Egeren, L. F. (1973). Multivariate statistical analysis. *Psychophysiology, 10*(5), 517–532.

Winer, B. J. (1971). *Statistical principles in experimental design.* New York: McGraw–Hill.

Wright, S. (1921). Correlation and causation. *Journal of Agricultural Research, 20,* 557–585.

CHAPTER 38

Power Calculations for Statistical Design

Larry R. Muenz

Introduction

What Is Power?

Power is the probability that a statistical analysis of experimental data will detect a true effect. Experiments have high or low power owing to decisions made at the planning stage. Although a carefully chosen method of analysis is more likely to find interesting results than routine or thoughtlessly chosen methods, nothing can be done to increase power for a particular analysis once the data have already been collected. High enough values of power—there is no universal definition of "enough"—give the experimenter good reason to hope that when the data are analyzed, if an experimental effect exists it will be found. Contrarily, low power means that negative results will be impossible to interpret. Was no effect found because none exists or because the experiment is unlikely to find an effect? Because this question cannot be answered in low-power studies, statisticians believe that such experiments should not be conducted.

Medical experiments, particularly behavioral ones, depend strongly for their success upon statistical planning with an emphasis on the interplay

This chapter is dedicated to the memory of Professor Rupert G. Miller, Jr.

Larry R. Muenz • SRA Technologies, Inc., 4700 King Street, Alexandria, Virginia 22302.

between power and sample size. Often in behavioral studies, sought-for effects are small, there is great variation between and within subjects, and data collection is tedious and expensive. The costs and delay associated with careful statistical design are modest compared with the costs and disappointment due to a study that did not and could not detect anything. For studies with little or no precedent it may be worthwhile to conduct a pilot study not only to debug operating procedures but also to provide preliminary estimates of quantities (e.g., variances) needed in power calculations.

The Intended Audience for This Chapter

The reader is imagined to be a sophisticated experimental practitioner who is comfortable with algebra and elementary statistics, particularly the properties of the normal distribution and the distinction between sample-based estimates and population parameters. Practical prerequisites are a desire and a need to *do* power computations as opposed to merely hearing of them from a consulting statistician. This is not intended to minimize the importance of working with a consulting statistician when one is available. Scant attention is given in this chapter to practical problems arising from subjects dropping in or out of studies, from missing data, and from designs more complex than the small selection found in the section entitled "Power Calculations for Specific Designs." For those purposes, collaboration with a professional statistician is a necessity.

Four Basic Design Factors

Power is but one of the four quantities that, in many practical cases, suffice to describe the statistical aspects of an experimental design. Recalling that power is the probability of detecting a true effect, these four quantities are

- α: the probability of asserting that an effect exists when this is false, i.e., when there is no effect. This false assertion is called a "type I error" and so α is the probability of a type I error.
- β: the probability of asserting there is no effect when an effect does exist (this is one minus the power). This false assertion is called a "type II error."
- δ: the minimal true effect perceived as worth detecting; any smaller effect is of no practical import, any larger effect is even more important than the effect of magnitude δ.
- N: the sample size. Depending upon the mathematical formulation relating the four quantities, N might be the size per group or the total sample size for all groups.

The type I and type II error probabilities, α and β, are often assigned easy-to-remember values such as 0.10, 0.05, or 0.01 but this still leaves many possible combinations, even before considering the wealth of choices for δ and N. Exploring the trade-offs between these four quantities is a critical planning task which must precede the choice of particular numerical values. Example 1 begins this chapter with a brief, qualitative exploration of these trade-offs. A detailed numerical example then illustrates some of the major facets of a power calculation. Since power is but one feature of design, Example 2 concerns the design of a hypothetical experiment.

Example 1: We boldly propose that, among persons with mild to moderate hypertension, a behavioral therapy may permit a reduction in drug levels as well as induce a decrease in blood pressure (BP)

from baseline. An exploratory (as opposed to confirmatory) investigation is a randomized comparison of conventional pharmacotherapy to a stepped reduction of drug levels combined with the behavioral intervention. The purpose of the example is to discuss qualitatively how one might choose α, β, δ, and N.

Suppose that, as is realistic, treatments are compared using the change in diastolic blood pressure (DBP) from baseline. The outcome is then defined as (standard treatment final pressure − standard treatment baseline pressure) − (new treatment final pressure − new treatment baseline pressure).

Positive values of this quantity would indicate superiority for the new treatment. We begin by choosing δ, the minimal "difference of differences" which is worth detecting, to be quite small, say 2 mm Hg DBP. Any change less than 2 mm has, presumably, no medical importance and any larger change is even more important. We insist that the new therapy be better than, not merely equivalent to, the standard because dosage reduction can be risky, possibly leading to sudden pressure spikes. Furthermore, no more than 100 subjects can be accrued in each group in the available time (i.e., $N = 100$). In the context of this experiment, α is the probability of asserting that the new, combined therapy will induce a drop in DBP that is at least 2 mm Hg more than the drop among persons receiving the standard treatment *when this is false*. This erroneous assertion would suggest to clinicians that the standard method can be replaced by a new therapy which is less than 2 mm Hg better than the standard. To avoid an ineffective and risky therapy, we might therefore wish to choose α to be quite small, perhaps 0.01 or even less.

The opposite error would occur if we failed to recognize that the new, combined therapy really is superior to the standard regimen. We might argue that an exploratory experiment is the ideal format for showing that the new method can replace the old. It would follow that we must maximize power, the chance of finding an effect if one exists, lest a promising therapy be abandoned. To avoid this error, we might choose power of 0.95 or even 0.99 ($\beta = 0.05$ or 0.01).

But, with fixed choices of δ and *N,* an experiment which is very likely to detect a true difference is also likely to find differences which do not exist: smaller β means larger α and vice versa. This might mean, and often does, that with the given δ and *N* (2 mm Hg and 100/group) it is impossible to have α and β both equal to 0.01.

How can we compromise? One possibility is to raise δ to 5 mm Hg since it is easier to find this larger difference (more power). Or we could admit that, while lowering the chances of finding a new treatment would be regrettable, other opportunities will come along so that β of 0.10 or even 0.20 (power of 0.90 or 0.80) would be adequate and permit α to be as small as 0.01. Or perhaps we could raise α from 0.01 to 0.05 or even find a few extra experimental subjects (larger *N*). //*

Type I and type II errors arise because of the random variation inherent in samples from a population. Even if the treatment for hypertension is "truly" effective, Nature is under no obligation to show this effectiveness in a sample of subjects. But the experimenter can exercise some control via a choice of *N,* α, β, and δ. So what is the right choice? Without more substance, the previous example is purely qualitative. But in the "real world" the experimenter must understand that each selection favors a different set of interests:

- Decreasing β enhances the discovery of new treatments
- Decreasing α or raising δ helps to avoid ineffective treatments
- Decreasing N economizes on patient and monetary resources

But none of the four quantities can be changed without some impact upon the others; calculations which permit this interplay to be explored are the theme of this chapter. Using a simple experiment, the next example provides a more careful presentation of the relations among the four design features.

Example 2: An experiment is conducted to compare serum cholesterol level in smokers and non-

*The end of each example is marked by "//."

smokers. The design calculations in this example concern sample size and power. We will find

- the sample size, *N* per group, needed to ensure that, should it exist, a true difference δ of at least one standard deviation between groups will be found with type II error probability β = 0.10 while retaining type I error probability α = 0.05, and
- the observed difference needed between mean cholesterol levels in the two groups in order to infer that there is a population difference of at least δ.

Our hypothetical study design and analysis are simple to the point of naiveté: choose *N* smokers and *N* nonsmokers so that the two groups have similar distributions of factors such as sex, age, health status, and smoking history. Take serum measurements and compare the observed group means. If the smokers' mean is sufficiently larger than the nonsmokers', there is evidence of a smoking effect. We assume that before the experiment began, cardiologists advised the experimenter of two major points:

- If smoking status is unrelated to cholesterol level, then both experimental groups are representative of a general population with mean cholesterol level 200. More formally, the *null hypothesis* that both groups are samples from a common population is written as

$$H_0: \mu_s = \mu_{ns} = 200$$

where the μ's are the population mean serum levels and "s" and "ns" denote "smoker" and "nonsmoker."
- Historical precedent has shown that the between-subject standard deviation of cholesterol levels in either group, σ, is about 10.
- But if smoking is associated with increased cholesterol, then it is clinically important to find any effect greater than 10 points. In the natural units of this experiment, that is relative to the standard deviation σ, the *alternative hypothesis* is

$$H_1: (\mu_s - \mu_{ns})/\sigma = \delta > 0$$

and, in particular, it is important to detect δ of 1.0 or more, i.e., the change in cholesterol of 10 divided by standard deviation of 10.

Besides δ, two other aspects of the experimental design are relevant to the choice of N.

α: This is the probability of committing a type I error by falsely asserting that the data are consistent with hypothesis H_1 of a smoking effect when, in fact, the two samples are drawn from a population described by hypothesis H_0 of no smoking effect. This quantity is almost invariably chosen by the experimenter and not implied by other design choices.

β: This is the probability of committing a type II error by falsely asserting that the data are consistent with H_0 when, in fact, the samples arise from two distinct populations consistent with H_1. Correctly asserting H_1 when H_1 is true is the complementary event and so power is $1 - \beta$. Power is often chosen by the experimenter or may be implied by other design choices.

This experiment is now described by four features: N, α, β, and δ. Planning the experiment is equivalent to knowing the values of all four but there is a relationship between them that implies a variety of trade-offs. In fact, we can choose values of any three of the quantities and calculate the fourth. For this example, we will choose α, β, and δ and calculate the needed N. The actual equation that links the four symbols,

$$N = 2[z(\alpha/2) + z(\beta)]^2/\delta^2$$

where $z(\alpha/2)$ and $z(\beta)$ are the upper $100\alpha/2\%$ and $100\beta\%$ points of the normal distribution, follows from the famous Central Limit Theorem which asserts that sample averages have a normal distribution regardless of the underlying distribution of the data. In particular, we suppose that

1. The N observed smokers' cholesterol levels have a distribution with mean μ_s and variance σ^2. The mean of these smokers' data is written as $\bar{x}_s$.

2. The N observed nonsmokers' cholesterol levels are a sample from a distribution with mean μ_{ns} and variance σ^2. The nonsmokers' observed mean is written as $\bar{x}_{ns}$.

We will infer that H_1 is more nearly consistent with the data than is H_0 if $\bar{x}_s - \bar{x}_{ns} > c > 0$. That is, we select H_1 over H_0 if the smokers' mean level sufficiently exceeds the nonsmokers' mean by at least c. Suppose (as is conventional) we choose $\alpha = 0.05$ and $\beta = 0.10$.

The steps in the design calculation are now:

Step 1. Choose c so that if H_0 is true, the probability of a type I error will be 0.05.

If $H_0: \mu_s = \mu_{ns} = 200$ is true, then $\bar{x}_s - \bar{x}_{ns}$ has a normal distribution with mean 0 and variance $2\sigma^2/N$. [This is written more succinctly as $N(0, 2\sigma^2/N)$; the N outside the parentheses comes from the first letter of *normal*.] That such a quantity exceeds c is equivalent to a standard (mean 0, variance 1) normal variable exceeding $\sqrt{(N/2)}\, c/\sigma$. But we can consult a table of the cumulative standard normal distribution to find that the upper 5% point is 1.645. Solving $\sqrt{(N/2)}\, c/\sigma = 1.645$ yields $c = 2.326\sigma/\sqrt{N}$.

Step 2. For the c from step 1, choose N so that, if H_1 is true, the probability of a type II error is 0.10.

If H_1 is true, the event $\{\bar{x}_s - \bar{x}_{ns} < c\}$ causes a type II error which the experimenter wishes to occur with probability $\beta = 0.10$. Furthermore, when H_1 holds, $\bar{x}_s - \bar{x}_{ns}$ has a normal distribution with mean $\mu_s - \mu_{ns} = \delta\sigma$ and variance $2\sigma^2/N$. The probability that such a quantity is less than c is again available from the table of the cumulative standard normal distribution: the standardized (mean 0, variance 1) normal variate exceeds $1.645 - \delta\sqrt{(N/2)}$ with probability 0.10. Since the upper 10% point of the standard normal distribution is 1.28, we can solve $1.28 = 1.645 - \delta\sqrt{(N/2)}$ for N to find $N = 17.13/\delta^2$.

So with $\delta = 1$, to distinguish between H_0 and H_1 with $\alpha = 0.05$ and $\beta = 0.10$, the experimenter needs 18 smokers and 18 nonsmokers after rounding N up to the next integer. In fact, the rounding causes β to be 0.088 at $N = 18$ compared to 0.102 at $N = 17$. //

Contents of This Chapter

The next section considers the theory of hypothesis testing and the role of power. Section three defines the notion of experimental design and presents and classifies particular designs that might be encountered in a behavioral cardiology study (or in many other subjects). For several of these designs, detailed power calculations are given in section four. That section, the chapter's longest, presents power calculations in cookbook fashion but it is a cookbook for those who want something more creative than TV dinners but less complex than haute cuisine. Section five discusses the consequences of choosing specific alternatives to equality such as an increasing trend compared to the more general alternative of inequality. Finally, section six cites some published papers on power and useful tables and charts.

Theory of Hypothesis Testing and Power

Experiments and Experimental Effects

Experiments are efforts to understand nature by using observations taken from an underlying population to detect the presence or absence of a population effect or to estimate its magnitude. Examples of an effect are a true difference between groups or a true association between two quantities. Hypotheses are assertions about effects, often phrased in terms of the numerical value of parameters which describe the underlying population. In Example 2, the sought-for effect is a serologic difference between smokers and nonsmokers expressed as the inequality of the parameters μ_s and μ_{ns}, both of which are population means.

As with any feature of a population, it is impossible to know whether $\mu_s = \mu_{ns}$ or $\mu_s > \mu_{ns}$ but an experiment permits an informed assertion to be made; the probability of correctly asserting that $\mu_s > \mu_{ns}$ is the power of the experiment. If there is no effect but we assert that one exists, we are committing a type I error; the letter α is used to denote the probability of this error. If there is an effect and we assert there is none, we are committing a type II error and the probability is denoted by $\beta = 1 -$ power.

Two Steps in Calculating Power

Step 1. The statistician specifies what experimental evidence will be necessary to infer that the effect exists. Such evidence always consists of specifying observations that would occur with small probability (α, in fact) if there were no effect.

Example 3: Evidence for a smoking effect is an observed mean smokers' cholesterol $\bar{x}_s$ sufficiently greater than the observed mean nonsmokers' cholesterol $\bar{x}_{ns}$. In particular, we want the constant c so that the event $\{\bar{x}_s - \bar{x}_{ns} > c > 0\}$ occurs with probability α when $\mu_s = \mu_{ns}$. This is a straightforward calculation based upon the properties of the normal distribution and appears in Step 1 of Example 2.

Suppose, however, that for slightly greater generality the two sample sizes are not equal and take values N_s and N_{ns}. If H_0: $\mu_s = \mu_{ns}$ holds, the quantity $\bar{x}_s - \bar{x}_{ns}$ has the distribution $N(0, \sigma^2(1/N_s + 1/N_{ns}))$. The probability that such a quantity exceeds a constant c is $1 - \Phi(\sqrt{\{N_s N_{ns}/(N_s + N_{ns})\}}\, c/\sigma)$ where Φ is the tabled normal cumulative distribution for mean 0 and variance 1. It is this probability we set to α. Doing so, and solving for c, we find $c = z(\alpha)\sigma\sqrt{\{(N_s + N_{ns})/(N_s N_{ns})\}}$ where $z(\alpha)$ is the upper $100\alpha\%$ point of the normal distribution. If $\sigma = 10$, $N_s = 15$, $N_{ns} = 30$, and $\alpha = 0.10$, we have $c = 10 \times 1.282\sqrt{\{45/450\}} = 4.05$. //

Step 2. The statistician finds the probability of detecting this evidence, i.e., power, if a specified true effect exists so that μ_s is not equal to μ_{ns}.

Example 4: Let $(\mu_s - \mu_{ns})/\sigma = \delta > 0$; for a given δ, power is the probability that $\bar{x}_s - \bar{x}_{ns} > c$. This is also a simple calculation and appears in Step 2 of Example 2.

Again generalizing that example, $\bar{x}_s - \bar{x}_{ns}$ has distribution $N(\mu_s - \mu_{ns}, \sigma^2(1/N_s + 1/N_{ns}))$ if H_1: $\mu_s > \mu_{ns}$ holds. The probability that such a quantity exceeds the c calculated in Example 3 is

$\Phi(\delta\sqrt{\{N_sN_{ns}/(N_s + N_{ns})\}} - z(\alpha))$. If $\delta = 1$, $N_s = 15$, $N_{ns} = 30$, $\alpha = 0.10$, and $c = 4.05$, this is $\Phi(\sqrt{10} - 1.282) = 0.97$. //

Theoretical Notions

The critical steps in this process are the choice of α and the specification of the evidence as embodied by c. The evidence must be unlikely if H_0 holds and likely if H_1 holds. We now proceed with a more general presentation of these notions by surveying the landscape of concepts and notation. Those with greater interest in the solution of practical problems and lesser interest in the underlying theory ought to skip the rest of this section and turn to section three.

H_0 and H_1 are the null and alternative hypotheses which describe the population from which the data $\underline{x}$ are a sample.

F is the probability distribution of the sample $\underline{x}$, denoting the list of observed values; the exact form of F depends upon a parameter θ which might be a list of more than one item.

θ_0 and θ_1 are two possible values of θ; the former holds if H_0 describes the data and the latter if H_1 describes the data. The problem is to find if F makes use of θ_0 or θ_1.

There are two collections of values of $\underline{x}$, the rejection and the acceptance regions. (It is H_0 that is being accepted or rejected.) That $\underline{x}$ landed in the rejection region is the evidence for H_1; that $\underline{x}$ landed in the acceptance region is the evidence for H_0.

Example 5: We string out the entire set of $2N$ observations from Example 2 so that $\underline{x} =$ (all smokers' data, all nonsmokers' data). Then, $\theta = (\mu_s, \mu_{ns}, \sigma^2)$ and F is the normal distribution. Population mean μ_s refers to the first N observations and population mean μ_{ns} refers to the second N. If the underlying population satisfies H_0, then the list $\theta = \theta_0$ in which $\mu_s = \mu_{ns}$, but if H_1 holds, then $\theta = \theta_1$ in which $\mu_s > \mu_{ns}$. //

Example 6: Again using Example 2, the test to distinguish between H_0 and H_1 took the form "choose H_0 if $\bar{x}_s - \bar{x}_{ns} < 2.533\sigma/\sqrt{N}$, otherwise choose H_1." Hence, the acceptance region is all possible values of the $2N$ numbers in $\underline{x}$ satisfying the above inequality. The rejection region is the collection of all $\underline{x}$ values for which the inequality is reversed. //

A false assertion will be made if, due to random variation, the data land in the rejection region when $\theta = \theta_0$ or vice versa. In particular,

- a type I error occurs when $\underline{x}$ is in the rejection region if $\theta = \theta_0$ and
- a type II error occurs when $\underline{x}$ is in the acceptance region if $\theta = \theta_1$.

So power is the probability that $\underline{x}$ is in the rejection region when the distribution of $\underline{x}$ is F with parameter θ_1. Operationally, a power calculation can require complex calculations including numerical integration but, fortunately, for most practical cases the computations are available either in tables or from package computer programs.

Example 7: Assessment of distances between "3-D" images on a computer screen is used to test visual perception of a single subject. According to whether the subject sees the screen as flat ("2-D") or makes use of the third dimension, standardized distance ("SD") has a chi-square distribution with either two or three degrees of freedom. Thus, F is the chi-square distribution with θ being the degrees of freedom, θ is either $\theta_0 = 2$ or $\theta_1 = 3$. How should we distinguish between H_0: perception is in 2-D and H_1: perception is in 3-D?

Large distances are more consistent with H_1 than with H_0, i.e., the rejection region consists of sufficiently large values of SD. If H_0 is true and the SD has a 2 d.f. chi-square distribution we expect to see an SD > 5.991 with probability $0.05 = \alpha$. (The rejection region is thus all values of SD greater than the upper 5% point of the 2 d.f. chi-square.) But if H_1 is true and the SD has a 3 d.f. chi-square distribution, it will exceed 5.991 with probability 0.11. (The probability that the SD is in the rejection region if $\theta = \theta_1 = 3$ is the "upper-tail" probability beyond 5.991 of the 3 d.f. chi-square distribution.) This is a very low power and we conclude that an experiment to discriminate between H_0 and H_1 for individual subjects is a poor idea. //

Trade-offs between the Four Design Factors

For many practical problems the full generality of the θ's is not necessary and a simple numerical measure of the "distance" between H_0 and H_1 appears in the power calculation. In Example 2, θ has three elements $(\mu_s, \mu_{ns}, \sigma^2)$; when $\theta = \theta_0$, $\mu_s = \mu_{ns}$, but when $\theta = \theta_1$, $\mu_s > \mu_{ns}$. But the example shows that only $\delta = (\mu_s - \mu_{ns})/\sigma$ is actually needed for the power calculation. In the discussion that follows we consider what else can be done when the distance between H_0 and H_1 is capable of such simplification. We repeatedly use the example of a two-group comparison, but the principle of algebraically manipulating one equation to isolate the term—N, α, β, or δ—of interest is valid for other designs.

When four numbers (N, α, β, δ) suffice to specify major features of the experimental design, as mentioned, knowledge of any three of these fixes the fourth. There are, of course, four possibilities for the omitted item, but α is not often computed as a function of N, β, and δ. The other three cases follow:

Fix σ, β, and δ; compute N. What sample size is needed so that, with a specified type I error, there is probability $1 - \beta$ of finding a difference of δ? This is the basis of the common sample size calculation for a comparison between groups. For example, with two equal-sized groups and a continuous response, when H_0 is the equality of population means and H_1 is their inequality in either direction: $N = 2(z(\alpha/2) + z(\beta))^2/\delta^2$.

Fix N, α, and β; compute δ. We choose power as well as the type I error and have a fixed sample size which might be, for example, the consequence of a constrained budget. What is the smallest δ to which the experiment will be sensitive? If that difference is so large that some meaningful distinctions may be missed, perhaps the experiment should not be run. For the same two-group experiment, reworking the previous equation, we find that $|\delta| = \sqrt{(2/N)} \, (z(\alpha/2) + z(\beta))$.

Fix N, α, and δ; compute β. For a fixed budget and type I error, how likely is the experiment to detect a difference of δ? Again reworking the same equation, we find that power $= 1 - \beta = \Phi[\sqrt{(N/2)}|\delta| - z(\alpha/2)]$.

Because all four of N, α, β, and δ cannot be varied simultaneously, there are trade-offs to be made between them. For example, suppose we fix N and δ, vary α, and compute β. We will find an

inverse relation: as one increases, the other decreases. Recalling that increased α means a greater chance of falsely asserting an effect exists, it is only sensible that this is accompanied by a decreased chance β of falsely asserting an effect does not exist.

If α decreases, β will increase and so power will drop. In section five of this chapter, we consider the consequences of decreasing α not for a single hypothesis but rather because many hypotheses are tested on a single data set.

For a given design, all versions of the formulas that relate the four design components are equivalent. But tables and charts which display the omitted element as a function of the others can be extremely helpful in designing experiments in which some features are constrained (e.g., cost, δ, and α) and the remaining one must be selected.

An important case is the computation of power as a function of the other three terms. A common display uses the vertical axis to show the result of the power computation, the horizontal axis to display δ, and a curve is drawn for each of a few α values such as 0.01, 0.05, and 0.10. The resulting picture is a collection of "power curves." Examples of power curves and the related curves for δ as a function of N appear in the text by Friedman, Furberg, and DeMets (1980). When $\delta = 0$ and H_0 is actually true (more generally, when $\theta_0 = \theta_1$), power formulas reduce to α. Consequently, power curves begin at α and then rise as δ increases.

Types of Designs and Their Impact upon Power

Classifying Designs

In principle, experimental data can be collected in an endless variety of ways. But the complexity of working with human subjects leads to a relatively modest number of designs for realistic medical experiments. In addition, statistical theories rarely contain the detail needed for complete depiction of all that happens between experimenter and subjects and so designs are often further simplified for purposes of power calculation. In particular, three dimensions suffice to classify the design of many medical studies. These are

- the type of response variable,
- the dependence, if any, between responses, and
- the hypothesis being tested.

Table 1 shows some examples of each of the three dimensions. Hypothetical studies can be created that use combinations of these design features such as the ones appearing below.

- Measure serum cholesterol to compare smokers and nonsmokers (continuous, independent responses; hypothesis concerns difference between two groups).
- Measure depression levels over time and compare by type of medication (multilevel, ordered response, serially correlated; hypothesis concerns differences between > 2 groups).
- Compare cardiovascular morbidity between reactive Type A males and nonreactive Type A males (binary responses; hypothesis compares proportion between two groups).
- Relate therapist contact hours to dietary weight loss (trend linking continuous response and predictor).
- Confirm that a previous study's compliance rate can be matched using a more difficult regimen (binary response; hypotheses concern a mean rate equal or not equal to a known value).

Table 1. Examples of the Three Major Dimensions Used to Classify Experimental Designs

I. Major hypothesis	II. Response variable	III. Dependence of responses
1. Single mean is known	1. Continuous	1. Independent
2. Group difference	2. Binary	2. Correlated
3. Correlation	3. Ordered	
4. Association Trend	4. Nominal	
	5. Survival	
	6. Multivariate Simultaneous Repeated	

The entries in Table 1 are numbered so that any included design can be indexed by three integers. For example, design 1.1.1 concerns the comparison of a single mean of a continuous quantity with a standard using independent observations. Only a few of the possible combinations of features in the three columns actually make sense and only some of these are considered in section four which contains the power calculations for particular designs. Calculations for many more designs are found in the References.

Event Time as an Outcome

A major design feature which appears in the above list but which is not considered further in this chapter is the use of survival as a response variable. Power computations for studies which use time-to-death or, more generally, time-to-an-event as a response are complex for two reasons. First, a group's survival experience is summarized not by a single number but by an entire curve which depicts, as a function of time "t," the probability of surviving at least t years after study entry. The infinite flexibility of curves makes it more difficult to specify the meaning of the hypothesis: Persons in group A will live longer than those in group B. Second, the survival time of persons still alive at the time of data analysis is not directly observable; it is said to be "censored" and is only known to be at least as great as the interval from study entry to the present. Such times are informative even if not as much so as directly observed times of death. But the inclusion of censored times in the power calculation raises the technical difficulty above the level of the rest of this chapter. The paper by Donner (1984) and, for a general view of survival studies, the book by Lee (1980) are particularly recommended.

Stratification and Matching

Critical design choices such as the use of a binary rather than a quantitative outcome measure or the choice of two study groups rather than three are major determinants of power. But other features such as stratification and matching may also be important. The former refers to the assignment of subjects to groups of persons similar to themselves. The latter refers to the selection of one or more "mates" for each study subject, again chosen from similar persons. The stratification or matching "factors" are those subject characteristics—age, sex, and disease features are examples—used to define these groups. Generally, we can say that an analysis that makes use of a meaningful stratification or matching is more likely to find an effect than one that does not. But stratification and matching are both irrelevant unless the factors which define the strata and the matched pairs (or triplets, etc.) are related to the study outcome.

Suppose we are comparing two interventions. Stratification or matching can increase power because the variability in the outcome measure between individuals in the same stratum or in the same matched pair is less than between arbitrarily chosen persons. This lowers the σ that appears in the ratio $\delta = (\mu_A - \mu_B)/\sigma$ and so increases the chance that a difference will be found. But data analyses that fail to make explicit use of these aspects of design can gain no advantage from them. Nor does there appear to be any substantial advantage, in terms of power, to stratification or matching unless the factors used to define the groups are strongly related to the outcome.

The Consequences of Testing Many Hypotheses

Another design feature which, inadvertently, has an impact upon study power is the ease with which dozens or hundreds of hypotheses on many different response variables are tested in one data set. The attraction of using cheap and powerful computation to perform every conceivable hypothesis test is nearly irresistible but the cost is an increased likelihood that many of the inferences that some effect exists will be false. Exploratory Data Analysis (Tukey, 1977) deals with this by avoiding p values altogether. But suppose that we do make use of p values and that α is the probability that any one null hypothesis is falsely rejected. If k tests are independent of one another, then the probability of at least one type I error is $1 - (1 - \alpha)^k$ which can be alarmingly large for even

moderate values of k (for $\alpha = 0.05$, this is > 0.40 for $k = 10$). Such independent tests arise in the examination of subsets of the same data, e.g., all possible categories of gender, race, socioeconomic status, and so forth.

A possible response to this is to test each hypothesis at a very small type I error probability. If each test uses type I error probability α' so that $1 - (1 - \alpha')^k = \alpha$, then the overall probability of at least one type I error is still α. The approximate solution is $\alpha' = \alpha/k$ or 0.005 when $\alpha = 0.05$ and $k = 10$. But the impact on power of such small α' can be devastating. Imagine a one-sided hypothesis of equal normal means with $N = 50/\text{group}$, an α of 0.05, and a power of 0.90. If ten such hypotheses were to be tested and α were correspondingly adjusted to 0.005, the power for each would decrease to 0.62; if the cautious experimenter testing 100 hypotheses set $\alpha' = 0.0005$, the power would be 0.33 for each test. Thus, in the laudable effort to control false inferences, we have made it virtually impossible to detect anything. Moral of the story: if you must test many hypotheses, do not believe the p values.

A similar phenomenon occurs if the tests are not independent, e.g., if many hypotheses are tested on the same data. Consider a comparative study with three groups rather than the more common two. One may test for the existence of *some* difference between the three possible pairs of groups and such a single test may be only slightly less powerful than a comparison between two groups. But if the results are significant, which of the three pairs is the source of the difference? The simplest expedient for keeping at α the probability of a type I error for any of the three comparisons of pairs of interventions is to perform each at $\alpha/3$. But a test using $\alpha = 0.05/3 = 0.0167$ rather than $\alpha = 0.05$ suffers a degradation in power similar to, although less severe than, the examples described immediately above.

Human frailty also leads to missing data, to subjects failing to comply with experimental regimens, and to subjects dropping out altogether or switching to another study group, to name a few of the practical problems facing the study designer. There is some controversy as to how, or whether, to consider these issues in data analysis but there is little disagreement that they ought to be considered at the design stage. All lead to lowered power and so, if power is to be retained at the desired level, some combination of α, δ, and N must be adjusted.

Deficient Sample Size

Suppose, for example, that at the time of data analysis, we have fewer subjects than planned for in the design stage. How sensitive is power to this failure to achieve sample size goals?

Example 8: Serum levels are to be compared in two groups using a sample size of $N/$group. What happens if we can only find $n < N$ subjects? It follows from the calculations appearing below for Design 2.1.1 that, for a two-sided test, the *change in power* is

$$\Phi(\sqrt{N}\,\delta - z(\alpha/2)) - \Phi(\sqrt{n}\,\delta - z(\alpha/2))$$

where Φ is the cumulative normal distribution and δ is the difference of group population means relative to their common standard deviation. For a few choices of α and δ, we have computed this quantity as a function of $n < N$ (Table 2).

A more complete version of Table 2 would be lengthy, but the calculations are simple enough that they could be done for any combination of α, N, and n relevant to the problem at hand. Perhaps the most striking conclusion from this brief tabulation is that moderate decreases in sample size do

not have a very dramatic effect on power. Particularly in the second case, where power is good, it remains that way until the sample size is hardly more than half its desired value. //

An approach in the case of noncompliance, dropouts, and "dropins" is to compute the effective δ that results from these problems. Suppose the alternative hypothesis is that at the end of the experiment two study groups will have unequal means μ_A and μ_B. But if a proportion p_1 of subjects assigned to group A actually received intervention B and a proportion p_2 of subjects assigned to group B actually received intervention A, the group A and B means will be $(1 - p_1)\mu_A + p_1\mu_B$ and $p_2\mu_A + (1 - p_2)\mu_B$, respectively. The standardized difference of these two groups means (δ) is smaller by a factor of $(1 - p_1 - p_2)$ than it would have been in the absence of crossovers and the sample size must be divided by the square of this factor to compensate. For $p_1 = p_2 = 0.05$, 5% of subjects switching in either direction, a 23% increase in sample size is needed to maintain power.

These sorts of calculations have been pursued in much more detail in the case of studies that involve long-term follow-up of subjects. Imaginative scenarios are created that show what might happen in each year of follow-up to compromise N and δ. The results are estimates of the effective N and effective δ which then may be used in the standard calculations. Two recent papers on this subject are

Table 2. Some Examples of the Change in Power as the Desired Sample Size per Group Is Not Achieved for a Two-Sample Comparison of Means

$\alpha = 0.10$, desired $N = 50$, $\delta = 0.4$, power $= 0.639$

n	45	40	35	30	25	20	15	10		
Decrease in power	0.04	0.08	0.13	0.18	0.23	0.29	0.35	0.41		

$\alpha = 0.10$, desired $N = 30$, $\delta = 0.8$, power $= 0.927$

n	27	24	21	18	15	12	9			
Decrease in power	0.03	0.06	0.10	0.15	0.22	0.30	0.41			

$\alpha = 0.05$, desired $N = 80$, $\delta = 0.4$, power $= 0.716$

n	75	70	65	60	55	50	45	40	35	30	25
Decrease in power	0.03	0.06	0.09	0.12	0.16	0.20	0.24	0.28	0.33	0.37	0.42

Lakatos (1986) and Lachin and Foulkes (1986), the latter particularly relevant to studies using patient survival as an endpoint.

Power Calculations for Specific Designs

This section contains notes and comments, at varying levels of detail, for some of the designs classified in the previous section. For some of the sensible combinations there is no well-developed theory; for others the theory is quite elaborate and only references are given. Some designs (particularly 1.1.1 and 2.1.1 from Table 1) appear more than once in this section because of the variety of assumptions that can be made about the experimenter's *a priori* knowledge. For example, the number of groups to be compared may be two or more than two, or the variance σ^2 may or may not have been adequately estimated in previous experiments.

Continuous Outcomes

Design 1.1.1: Comparison of a mean with a standard, one sample, standard deviation *known.*
The hypotheses are

$$H_0: \mu = \mu_0, \sigma = \sigma_0 \text{ and } H_1: \mu \neq \mu_0, \sigma = \sigma_0$$

where μ_0 and σ_0 are known constants. (The hypotheses are often written without noting that the σ's are the same under H_0 and H_1.) We have N observations in one sample and wish a two-sided test with type I error α and power $1 - \beta$.

If $\bar{x}$ is the observed mean, the test rejects H_0 if $\sqrt{N}(x - \mu_0)/\sigma$ is outside the interval $[-z(\alpha/2), +z(\alpha/2)]$ and the power is the probability of this event when the mean is actually μ. This is seen to be

$$\text{Power} = 2 - \Phi(z(\alpha/2) + \delta\sqrt{N}) - \Phi(z(\alpha/2) - \delta\sqrt{N})$$

for $\delta = (\mu - \mu_0)/\sigma$.

Example 9: Using a large survey data base, the mean ponderal index [weight (lb)/height (ft)^3] for 60-year-old men is reported to be $\mu = 0.93$. We anticipate a study with 50 men and historical data indicate that the standard deviation of the ponderal index is 0.22; with what probability can we detect an increase in the ponderal index of 7.5% from the standard using a two-sided test with $\alpha = 0.10$?

The hypothesis H_0 is that the 50 men come from a population with mean index 0.93 and known standard deviation 0.22. Under H_1 the index is 7.5% (0.07) more or less than 0.93. We reject H_0 with $\alpha = 0.10$ if $\sqrt{50}(x - 0.93)/0.22$ is outside the range $[-z(0.05), +z(0.05)] = [-1.645, +1.645]$. If the true mean μ is 7.5% greater than 0.93 (i.e., 1.00), then the observed mean x has a normal distribution $N(1.00, 0.22^2/50)$ and the power is the probability that $\sqrt{50}(x - 0.93)/0.22$ is outside $[-1.645, +1.645]$. But this is the probability that a $N(0, 1)$ variable is outside the range $[-3.89, -0.611]$ which is about 0.73. Or applying the formula directly, the power is $2 - \Phi(1.645 + 0.32\sqrt{50}) - \Phi(1.645 - 0.32\sqrt{50}) = 2 - \Phi(3.89) - \Phi(-0.61) = 0.73$ using $\delta = (1.00 - 0.93)/0.22 = 0.32$.

Thus, with $N = 50$, $\sigma = 0.22$, and $\alpha = 0.10$, there is a 73% chance of detecting that the true ponderal index is 7.5% more than 0.93 using a two-sided test. //

For a one-sided alternative $H_1: \mu > \mu_0, \sigma = \sigma_0$, a similar calculation gives

$$\text{Power} = \Phi(\delta\sqrt{N} - z(\alpha))$$

In the above example we might be sure that $\delta > 0$ and calculate the power to detect an increase in the ponderal index 7.5% above the survey value using a one-sided test. This is $\Phi(0.968) = 0.83$, 10% better than the power of the two-sided test. //

For the two-sided case, we cannot easily solve the power equation for N in terms of β and numerical trial and error is needed. But for the one-sided case, we have that $N = (z(\alpha) + z(\beta))^2/\delta^2$ rounded up to the next highest integer.

The basic assumption underlying this power computation is that a description of the data in terms of a single mean is useful. By the Central Limit Theorem, so fundamental to statistics, for large sample size the observed mean will have a normal distribution under a wide variety of circumstances, including highly asymmetric or multimodal distributions of the observations. ". . . hence the inferences about the mean μ . . . must be correct for large n regardless of the form of the population" (Scheffe, 1959, p. 335). But if the distribution of the observations is not unimodal (one peak for the histogram) and reasonably symmetric, the mean loses much of its value as a descriptor.

Also, we assume that the variance from the standard population is known to be the same variance as found in the experimental group. If this is wrong and the true variance of the experimental data is greater, we will overestimate the power or underestimate the sample size for a given power. The result will be to infer there is a difference between μ and μ_0 when none exists.

Design 1.1.1: Comparison of a mean with a standard, one sample, standard deviation *unknown*.

Power for this problem is computed in terms of the ratio $(\mu - \mu_0)/\sigma$ where μ is the unknown population mean, μ_0 is the standard mean, and σ is the unknown standard deviation; the ratio is the deviation of the mean from the standard in units of the unknown parameter σ. That is, the calculation cannot be done in the units of the observations, but only in the units of the unknown σ. An alternative approach (Stein, 1945) uses two samples, one to estimate σ and one to use for the test. For a discussion of such multistage procedures see Bishop and Dudewicz (1978).

The hypothesis H_0: $\mu = \mu_0$ is rejected in favor of H_1: $\mu \neq \mu_0$ if the test statistic $\sqrt{N}(\bar{x} - \mu_0)/s$ is outside the interval $[-t(N - 1, \alpha/2), +t(N - 1, \alpha/2)]$ where $\bar{x}$ is the observed mean, s is the observed standard deviation, the first argument in the Student's t is the degrees of freedom and the second is the significance level of the test. For true population mean μ, the probability of not being in the interval is the probability that a *noncentral Student's* $t = \sqrt{N}(\bar{x} - \mu_0)/s$ with *noncentrality parameter* $\sqrt{N}(\mu - \mu_0)/\sigma$ is outside that interval. H_0 is rejected in favor of H_1: $\mu > \mu_0$ if the same noncentral t exceeds $t(N - 1, \alpha)$.

Example 10: Suppose that the problem is similar to Example 9 except that σ of the experimental population is no longer assumed known. We measure the ponderal indices for a sample of 50. What

is the power of the two-sided test, $\alpha = 0.10$, that the mean index is actually 0.32 standard deviation larger than the survey value of 0.93? This is the probability that a noncentral t with 49 d.f. and noncentrality parameter $\sqrt{50}(1.00 - 0.93)/0.22 = 2.26$ will be outside the range $[-t(49, 0.05), +t(49, 0.05)] = [-1.678, +1.678]$. To two digits, 0.73, this is the same value as in Example 9. //

Example 10 illustrates that, if the sample size is at least moderate, failure to know the population standard deviation has minimal impact on power. Of course, we do not know σ and so 0.32 standard deviation may not be 0.07 as it was in Example 9.

Designs 2.1.1 and 2.1.2: Comparison of two means, standard deviations known, responses correlated or not.

For this problem, the data may have a natural pairing, or not. Test–retest studies provide an example of the former situation; comparing two groups of persons under the same conditions gives an example of the latter case.

In either case, the hypothesis test, and hence the power analysis, are based upon comparing the difference of the two means to zero. Suppose that the hypotheses are

$$H_0: \mu_A = \mu_B \text{ and } H_1: \mu_A \neq \mu_B$$

and that σ_A and σ_B are known. Furthermore, suppose that the two sample sizes are N_A and N_B. If the samples are paired, necessarily $N_A = N_B = N$ and, for any subject, the before–after difference has a normal distribution with population mean $\mu = \mu_A - \mu_B$ and variance $\sigma^2 = \sigma_A^2 + \sigma_B^2 - 2\sigma_A\sigma_B\tau$ where τ is the correlation between the two measurements. Without a natural pairing, e.g., if the data come from two distinct groups, $\tau = 0$ and σ^2 simplifies to $\sigma_A^2 + \sigma_B^2$.

In this format, the problem is the same as that described in Design 1.1.1 and the power calculations can be obtained by setting $\mu_0 = 0$.

Example 11: We compare psychological test scores before and after an intervention with a sample size of $N = 30$ and a before–after correlation of $\tau = 0.5$. The scores are standardized relative to a large sample so that, both before and after the intervention, the scores have standard deviations $\sigma_A = \sigma_B = 10$. (Equality of the known standard deviations is not a necessary feature of the example.)

What is the power of a two-sided test with $\alpha = 0.05$, to detect a difference of 5 between "before" and "after"?

The standard deviation of the observed before–after difference for a given subject is $\sqrt{(10^2 + 10^2 - 2 \times 10 \times 10 \times 0.5)} = 10$, 29% smaller than it would have been if the data were not paired. Using the formula from Design 1.1.1, the power is $2 - \Phi(1.96 + 5\sqrt{30}/10) - \Phi(1.96 - 5\sqrt{30}/10) = 2 - \Phi(4.7) - \Phi(-0.78) = 0.78$. //

Design 2.1.1: Comparison of two means, standard deviation unknown but assumed equal.

A test of the equality of population means is based upon a comparison of the two sample means. The hypothesis $H_0: \mu_A = \mu_B$ is rejected in favor of $H_1: \mu_A \neq \mu_B$ if the quantity $(\bar{x}_A - \bar{x}_B)/s\sqrt{\{(1/N_A) + (1/N_B)\}}$ is outside the interval $[-t(N_A + N_B - 2, \alpha/2), t(N_A + N_B - 2, \alpha/2)]$, $\bar{x}_A$ and $\bar{x}_B$ denote the group means, and s^2 is the usual pooled variance estimate. H_0 is rejected in favor of $H_1: \mu_A > \mu_B$ if the same quantity is larger than $t(N_A + N_B - 2, \alpha)$. These are, respectively, two-sided and one-sided tests.

The power of the test is the probability that a noncentral t with $N_A + N_B - 2$ d.f. and non-centrality parameter $(\mu_A - \mu_B)/\sigma\sqrt{\{(1/N_A) + (1/N_B)\}} = \delta \sqrt{\{N_A N_B/(N_A + N_B)\}}$ is outside the specified interval.

Example 12: We redo Example 2, but without assuming σ to be known. Suppose we have $N_A = 18$ smokers and $N_B = 18$ nonsmokers, and $\alpha = 0.05$. What is the power of a one-sided test if $\delta = 1$? This is the probability that a noncentral t with $18 + 18 - 2 = 34$ d.f. and noncentrality parameter $\sqrt{7.5} = 2.73$ will exceed the upper 5% point of a central t-distribution with 34 d.f. which is 1.691. Performing the computation (see section six for reference to computer programs) we find that this probability is 0.902, which is only 0.01 less than the power if we knew σ. //

Design 2.1.1: Comparison of samples from more than two groups, standard deviations unknown but assumed equal.

The generalization of the t test to more than two samples is the F test as it is used in the analysis of variance (ANOVA). When the group means are not all equal, the F statistic no longer has the familiar (central) F distribution; instead its distribution is called the *noncentral F distribution*. The power

of the F test is the probability that a quantity with the noncentral F distribution will exceed a point chosen from the central F distribution.

The choice of population means under the alternative hypothesis is difficult. Suppose that the means for k groups are $\mu(1), \ldots, \mu(k)$. It can be shown that the power of the test depends only upon the quantity $\sqrt{(n\Sigma(\mu(i) - \bar{\mu})^2)}/\sigma$ where the sum is over i, the group index (Fleiss, 1986, p. 371). Merely specifying that some of the $\mu(i)$'s are unequal to one another gives no value for this quantity, so how do we choose it?

One possible choice arises from assuming that all the $\mu(i)$'s except for one are equal, i.e., $\mu(1) = \mu(2) = \ldots = \mu(k - 1)$ and $\mu(k) = \mu(1) + \theta$. Under the null hypothesis, $\theta = 0$ and we wish a test to detect values of θ other than zero. Another alternative is $\mu(i) = \mu(1) + (i - 1)\theta$ for $i = 2, \ldots, k$. If θ is not zero, the population means show a linear trend according to the index i; the F test distinguishes between equality, when $\theta = 0$, or a trend line. The F test here is equivalent to testing the hypothesis that the slope $b = 0$ in the model $y_{ij} = a + bi + \text{error}$ which relates the jth observation from the ith group to the group index, i. Thus, the power computation for this design includes simple linear regression as a special case. Some further discussion of the power computation for this problem appears in section five on the choice of alternative hypotheses.

Binary Outcomes

Design 2.2.1: Comparison of two proportions.

Suppose we compare the proportion of successes between two methods, A and B, of carrying out an experiment. A useful format is that of a 2×2 table: where s is a constant > 0 which permits the two sample sizes to be unequal.

Observed counts of successes and failures

	Method A	Method B
Failure	a	b
Success	c	d
Total number of trials	$a + c = N$	$b + d = sN$

The above table contains the results of the proposed experiment. It corresponds to an unknown (and unknowable) table of population probabilities:

Population probabilities of success and failure

	Method A	Method B
Failure	$1 - p_A$	$1 - p_B$
Success	p_A	p_B

We observe samples of N and sN for the two methods; of these, c succeeded using method A and d succeeded using method B. Comparison of the methods is equivalent to asking if the observed probabilities of success, $c/N = c/(a + c)$ and $d/sN = d/(b + d)$, might have arisen from populations with the same underlying probability of success, $p_A = p_B$.

Thus, the null hypothesis is $H_0: p_A = p_B$ and the alternative hypothesis is $H_1: p_A - p_B = \delta$ which is not $= 0$ (nor to be confused with the δ used in the analysis for normally distributed data). An approximate, although already quite complicated, formula that relates sample size, α, β, and δ (the difference of the success probabilities if hypothesis H_1 holds) is

$$N = \{z(\alpha)\sqrt{[(s + 1) P(1 - P)]} + z(\beta)\sqrt{[sp_A(1 - p_A) + p_B(1 - p_B)]}\}^2/(s\delta^2)$$

where $P = (p_A + sp_B)/(s + 1)$. The formula is due to Fleiss, Tytun, and Ury (1980). When $s = 1$, there are equal numbers of subjects receiving methods A and B. A simpler and reasonably accurate version of the more general formula is then given by

$$N = (z(\alpha) + z(\beta))^2[2P(1 - P)]/\delta^2$$

(only for $s = 1$)

These design formulas for an experiment that compares two proportions are substantially more complicated than those that used a standardized measure of difference $(\mu_A - \mu_B)/\sigma$ for the comparison of two means from continuous data. In particular, the formulas now depend upon the values of p_A and p_B and so tabled results become bulkier.

The added complexity is mainly due to the dependence of the variability of a proportion upon the true response probability when that true probability is outside the range [0.25, 0.75]. Recall that in Gaussian data we can write that a variable has mean μ and variance σ^2 and the choice of these two quantities is quite arbitrary aside from $\sigma^2 > 0$. But for data on proportions, the variance of an estimate of p_A is $p_A(1 - p_A)/N$ and terms of this sort can be seen in the above formulas for N. There is, of course, still a dependence of the variance upon the probability for p inside [0.25, 0.75] but it seems not to be very important numerically.

What about β or $\delta = p_A - p_B$ as a function of the other parameters? Either the very complicated $(s \neq 1)$ or less complex $(s = 1)$ formula for N can be solved for β yielding power results that an exact theory indicates are adequate. But because p_A and p_B appear individually, as well as in their difference, δ, there is no simple algebraic manipulation to extract δ as a function of the other parameters. An alternative theory is based upon the estimation of arcsin $\sqrt{p}$ rather than p. The variance of an estimate of this (somewhat odd-looking) quantity does *not* depend upon p for p outside the range [0.25, 0.75], precisely the region in which estimation of p is most difficult.

Example 13: Suppose that $\alpha = 0.01$, $\beta = 0.20$. The null hypothesis is that the probabilities p_A and p_B are equal. The alternative hypothesis is that $p_A = 0.8$ and $p_B = 0.9$. What is the necessary sample size if the two groups are to be equal $(s = 1)$? We apply the two sample size formulas given above using $z(0.01) = 2.32$, $z(0.20) = 0.842$, $s = 1$, $\delta = 0.1$, and $P = 0.85$. Rounding up, $N = 254$ (longer formula) or 255 (shorter formula) per group. //

Example 14: We have 100 observations in each group. If $\alpha = 0.05$, with what probability can a difference between $p_A = 0.2$ and $p_B = 0.4$ be detected? We now solve the two sample size formulas for $z(\beta)$ using $z(0.05) = 1.645$ and $\delta = 0.2$. Then $z(\beta) = 1.477$ and power $= 0.929$ (longer formula) or $z(\beta) = 1.441$ and power $= 0.925$ (shorter formula). //

There is another power calculation that is commonly encountered. Suppose that the proportions p_A and p_B are extreme (e.g., 0.001, 0.03, 0.97, or 0.999). Then the Gaussian approximations used above are no longer accurate and a Poisson approximation is needed. Two excellent and accessible references for this problem of experimental design when faced with very large or small proportions are Gail (1974) and Brown and Green (1982).

Correlation between Two Continuous Outcomes

Design 3.1.1: Test of correlation between two Gaussian variables.

Once more, this problem takes a standard format which, at this point, the reader should recognize. What is the probability that a sample correlation coefficient from a two-dimensional normal distribution with nonzero population correlation will exceed a specified constant? The constant is chosen from the distribution of the sample correlation coefficient when the population correlation is zero.

The theory is based upon Fisher's z transformation $z(r) = 0.5 \ln((1 + r)/(1 - r))$ where r is the sample Pearson correlation coefficient and ln is the logarithm to the base e. The transformed correlation has an approximate normal distribution $N(z(\tau), 1/(N - 3))$ when there are N data pairs, τ is the true correlation, and $z(\tau)$ is the same function of τ as $z(r)$ is of r.

Example 15: What is the power for detecting a population correlation of 0.4, with $\alpha = 0.05$, using a sample size of 50? Assuming the null hypothesis is H_0: $\tau = 0$, this is the same as the probability, using a one-sided test, of rejecting the null hypothesis H_0: $z(\tau) = z(0) = 0$ and accepting the alternative hypothesis H_1: $z(\tau) \neq 0$ when, in fact, $\tau = 0.4$ so that $z(\tau) = 0.424$. Under both H_0 and H_1, the standard deviation of $z(r)$ is approximately $\sqrt{1/47} = 0.146$.

A one-sided test with $\alpha = 0.05$ will reject H_0 when $z(r)$ exceeds $z(0) + 1.645 \times 0.146 = 0.240$. The power is the probability that a normally distributed variable with mean 0.424 and standard deviation 0.146 will exceed 0.240. This is $\Phi((0.424 - 0.240)/0.146) = 0.90$. //

Association between Two Binary Outcomes

Design 4.1.2: Test of association between two binary variables.

The hypothesis refers to the association between two, two-level variables and the test uses a chi-square statistic. Suppose that the four observed counts in the table are

a	b	with population probabilities	$p(1)$ $p(2)$
c	d	that add to 1	$p(3)$ $p(4)$

We assume that $N = a + b + c + d$ individuals are sampled and then put into one of the four cells. Despite the similarity of the display to that used for Design 2.2.1, this is not the same problem as that one. Now only N, the grand total, is fixed and four proportions add to 1.0. In Design 2.2.1, the columns of the table had sample sizes of N and sN and the proportions summed to 1.0 for each column. A useful discussion of the difference between various designs used to estimate proportions is found in Guenther (1977).

The test of the hypothesis of association uses the continuity-corrected test statistic

$$X^2 = N(|ad - bc| - N/2)^2/\{(a + b)(c + d) \\ (a + c)(b + c)\}$$

This has a chi-square distribution with 1 d.f. under the hypothesis that the row and column variables of the observed table are not associated. But under the alternative hypothesis that there is an association, X^2 has a *noncentral chi-square distribution* with 1 d.f. and *noncentrality parameter* $= N \times$

$$\{(p(1)p(4) - p(2)p(3))^2/ \\ ((p(1) + p(2))(p(3) + p(4))(p(1) + p(3))(p(2) + p(4))\}$$

which we simplify by writing $N \times H$, where H is the complicated term in brackets. The noncentral chi-square distribution is a generalization of the more familiar chi square so that when the noncentrality parameter is 0, the two distributions are the same.

As always, the form of the test is determined by the distribution of the test statistic under H_0 but the power is determined by the distribution under H_1. So the power of a chi-square test with type I error probability α is the probability that the appropriate noncentral chi square exceeds the upper α point of an ordinary (central) chi square with the same degrees of freedom.

Until relatively recently, the computation of

probabilities from the noncentral chi-square distribution was a formidable task. Two options available to the experimenter were to use numerical approximations or to use routine MDCHN in the IMSL package (IMSL, Inc., 1984). Now, however, various computer packages have the noncentral chi-square computation available; for example, it may be found in SAS, which is a powerful tool for statistical design and analysis (SAS Institute, 1985, p. 261).

Example 16: Suppose that under the null hypothesis, all four p's are $1/4$. But under the alternative hypothesis, $p(2) = 1/4 - a$ and $p(4) = 1/4 + a$ for $0 < a < \frac{1}{4}$. Such probabilities might arise from an educational experiment in which half the subjects are evenly split regarding their opinion of some subject but the other half express a strong preference in one direction. Using the formula above for the noncentrality parameter, it is easy to show that $H = 4a^2/(1 - 4a^2)$. We can now calculate the power of an experiment with sample size N to detect various size a's:

$\alpha = 0.10$, $N = 100$, $a = 0.15$, power $= 0.933$
$\alpha = 0.10$, $N = 50$, $a = 0.20$, power $= 0.925$
$\alpha = 0.01$, $N = 50$, $a = 0.20$, power $= 0.695$

Choice of the Alternative in Power Calculations

Why the Choice Matters

A strongly focused beam of light will help find something if we already know where to look, but a broader, paler beam may be better if we are less sure of the quarry. This metaphor refers to the choice of alternative in power calculations. If the only reasonable departure from the equality of population means, μ_A and μ_B, is H_1: $\mu_A > \mu_B$, we should take advantage of this knowledge and use a test sensitive only to departures in this direction, i.e., a one-sided test. If, for several means, it is known that a trend is the only reasonable alternative to equality, a test should be used that is particularly suited to the detection of trends.

In both these cases, a test that is sensitive only to the anticipated alternative has more power to detect that alternative than a test sensitive to a wider range of possibilities. But if neither the null nor the alternative hypothesis is correct, the choice of test may backfire. For example, suppose that, for two groups, the hypotheses are H_0: $\mu_A = \mu_B$ and H_1: $\mu_A > \mu_B$ but that the observed mean for group A is smaller than that for group B. Strictly speaking, the data are more consistent with H_0 than with H_1 but, in fact, neither equality nor the selected alternative is reasonable. We should have chosen H_1: $\mu_A \neq \mu_B$ as the alternative.

But if the data were consistent with the one-sided alternative, we would have a better chance to detect this by the appropriate one-sided test. It is particularly simple to show the increase in power for one-sided versus two-sided tests (again, supposing we choose the correct side) since it corresponds to increasing the type I error probability from $\alpha/2$ to α.

Example 17: With an equal sample size in each group, we perform an $\alpha = 0.10$ test on two samples to choose between H_0: $\mu_A = \mu_B$ and H_1: $\mu_A \neq \mu_B$. (The standard deviations for the two groups are assumed equal and known.) Now we learn that the only reasonable alternative to H_0 is H_1: $\mu_A > \mu_B$. How much has the power increased?

For this special case of Design 2.1.1 (special because $\sigma_A = \sigma_B$) we have the following relation between the sample size N in each group, α, β, the two population means, and σ:

$$N = 2 \times (z(\alpha) + z(\beta))^2/\delta^2$$

where δ is the standardized difference of the two group means $(\mu_A - \mu_B)/\sigma$. Suppose that β_1 is the type II error probability $(1 - \text{power})$ in the one-sided case and β_2 is the same quantity in the two-sided case. Solving the above equation for $z(\beta)$ and subtracting the results for the two cases we find that $z(\beta_1) - z(\beta_2) = z(\alpha/2) - z(\alpha)$. With $\alpha = 0.10$, $z(\alpha/2) - z(\alpha) = 0.363$. So if $\beta_2 = 0.20$ (power $= 80\%$), we find that $\beta_1 = 0.114$. Switching to a one-sided test has increased power from 0.80 to 0.886 or, put more encouragingly, nearly halved the type II error probability.

Testing for Group Difference versus Testing for Trend

A similar calculation can be performed for regression using the F test as the basis of the analysis. From an earlier discussion in this chapter, we know that, if the populations means are not equal, the F statistic has a *noncentral F distribution* with the appropriate degrees of freedom and *noncentrality parameter* $(\sqrt{n}\Sigma(\mu(i) - \bar{\mu})^2)/\sigma$.

Suppose, however, similar to the discussion for Design 2.1.1, that the means are linearly increasing so that $\mu(i) = \mu(1) + (i - 1)\theta/(k - 1)$ for $i = 1, \ldots, k$; some algebra shows that the noncentrality parameter is $\theta/\sigma \times \sqrt{\{Nk(k + 1)/12\}}$. This model causes $\mu(i)$ to show a trend with the index i such that the spread from smallest to largest population mean does not increase as the number of categories grows. This facilitates the comparison of power for various choices of k. For a test of trend the F statistic has a noncentral F distribution with 1 and $N - 1$ d.f. and the indicated noncentrality parameter. Now suppose that we do not look for a trend but just perform a one-way analysis of variance (ANOVA). Then the F statistic has the same noncentrality parameter but with $k - 1$ and $N - 1$ d.f.

For $N = 50$ and $\theta/\sigma = 0.33$, we tabulate the noncentrality parameter ("NC") and power in Table 3 as a function of the number of groups. This computation can also be done using SAS (SAS Institute, 1985, p. 262).

For two groups, the ANOVA and test of trend must be equivalent. With more groups, both tests become more powerful. But the trend test always has higher power—because there really is a trend—although the advantage must shrink when both tests have high power.

Table 3. Power for ANOVA versus Test of Trend Using a Model in Which the Population Means Increase Linearly

k	2	3	4	5	8
NC	1.67	2.36	3.04	3.73	5.77
ANOVA	0.373	0.522	0.755	0.909	>0.99
Trend	0.373	0.637	0.846	0.955	>0.99

Similar principles hold for the analysis of count data which can be displayed as a $2 \times k$ table. Consider a binary response, e.g., "success" or "failure" and a predictor taking a few levels. An example of such a predictor might be a laboratory procedure with values $(-)$, (0), $(+)$, $(++)$; $k = 4$ for this example. The competitive methods of data analysis are the ordinary chi-square test (ignores the ordering) and procedures which make use of the sequence such as the Mantel-Haenszel 1-d.f. chi-square test (Mantel, 1963). Unfortunately, the guidance concerning how to maximize power is not as clear as in the case of a continuous response (Moses, 1985).

Texts, Software, and Articles

A convenient source for power and sample size calculations in designs with two groups (either normal or binary outcomes) is a PC program available at cost from the author. The program is "user-friendly" and requires an MS/DOS operating system.

Another relevant microcomputer program is PC-SIZE, written by Gerard E. Dallal (53 Beltran Street, Malden, MA 02148) and sold by him at a modest price. PC-SIZE is harder to use than the author's program, can only compute sample size for given values of the other design factors, but can do so for a much wider range of designs than the author's program. Quoting Dallal,

> PC-SIZE determines the sample size requirements for single factor experiments, two factor experiments, randomized blocks designs, and paired t-tests. . . . PC-SIZE can determine the sample size needed to detect a non-zero population correlation coefficient when sampling from a bivariate normal distribution. It can also be used to obtain the common sample size required to test the equality of two proportions.

As mentioned previously, SAS also has the capacity to perform a wide variety of power calculations using the noncentral t, chi square, and F distributions but the user must first compute the noncentrality parameter rather than being able to specify more natural features such as sample size and group means.

Every journal article about the calculation of

sample size, and there are hundreds, is also about power and must include the relations between power $(1 - \beta)$, sample size (N), type 1 error probability (α), and the smallest difference, δ, perceived as worth detecting. And power is but one aspect of the process of experimental design which requires answers to questions such as

- What is the underlying scientific question addressed by the experiment?
- What would I do if I already knew the answer to the scientific question?
- Do I have the resources (e.g., staff, equipment, data, time, money) to do the experiment properly?

There is a substantial scholarly literature on the subject of experimental design and in particular the relations among the design parameters α, β, N, and δ for various sorts of design.

The journal *Technometrics* specializes in applied experimental design. *Biometrics,* a journal of biostatistical methods, has frequent articles on aspects of design including power. Two particularly accessible review papers which consider power and sample size calculations in a broad variety of designs for medical studies are Donner (1984) and Lachin (1981). In addition, there are many textbooks; the following collection of citations and brief descriptions contains some of the more accessible, elementary and/or famous of the 48 books described in Volume 2, pp. 359–366, of *The Encyclopedia of Statistics* (Kotz & Johnson, 1982).

Box, G. E. P., Hunter, W. G., & Hunter, J. S. (1978). *Statistics for experimenters: An introduction to design, data analysis, and model building.* New York: Wiley.

> . . . is an introduction to the philosophy of experimentation and the part that statistics plays in experimentation. . . . it provides a practically motivated introduction to basic concepts and methods of experimental design. Readers are assumed to have no previous knowledge of the subject. The book includes numerous examples and case studies and provides appreciable detail about many elementary and a few more advanced designs.

Cohen, J. (1977). *Statistical power analysis for the behavioral sciences* (rev. ed.). New York: Academic Press.

> This extremely practical book provides recipes for calculating power in many common designs. Cohen defines the notion of a small, medium or large experimental effect and provides extensive sample size tables to achieve desired power in each of these cases.

Cox, D. R. (1958). *Planning of experiments.* New York: Wiley.

> This book provides a simple survey of the principles of experimental design and of some of the most useful experimental schemes. . . . emphasizes basic concepts rather than calculations or technical details.

Fleiss, J. L. (1986). *The design and analysis of clinical experiments.* New York: Wiley.

> This very recent work uses medical examples to give detailed, relatively advanced analyses of a variety of experimental designs including parallel groups, Latin squares, repeated measures, and factorial designs. The emphasis is on the analysis of designed studies rather than the design process.

Kempthorne, O. (1952). *Design and analysis of experiments.* New York: Wiley. (Reprinted by Krieger, Huntington, NY, 1975).

> This book is directed principally at readers with some background and interest in statistical theory. . . . uses matrix notation. Factorial experiments are discussed in detail. Chapters are devoted to fractional replication and split plot experiments.

Winer, B. J. (1971). *Statistical principles in experimental design* (2nd ed.). New York: McGraw–Hill.

> . . . written primarily for . . . the behavioral and biologic sciences . . . is meant to provide a text as well as a comprehensive reference on statistical principles underlying experimental design. Chapters are devoted to single-factor and multi-factor experiments with repeated measures on the same elements (or subjects).

A more general introduction to the design, conduct, and analysis of medical studies—including a review of power calculations—also appears in two books on clinical trials: Buyse, Staquet, and Sylvester (1984) and Friedman *et al.* (1981); the latter has a particularly cardiovascular perspective.

ACKNOWLEDGMENTS. Dr. Peter Kaufmann of the National Heart, Lung, and Blood Institute invited me to write this chapter and so helped me learn more about power. Professor Larry Hedges of the University of Chicago carefully reviewed an earlier version of the chapter; of course I am responsible for any remaining mistakes.

References

Bishop, T. A., & Dudewicz, E. J. (1978). Exact analysis of variance with unequal variances: Test procedures and tables. *Technometrics, 20,* 419–430.

Box, G. E. P., Hunter, W. G., & Hunter, J. S. (1978). *Statistics for experimenters: An introduction to design, data analysis, and model building.* New York: Wiley.

Brown, C. C., & Green, S. B. (1982). Additional power computations for designing comparative Poisson trials. *American Journal of Epidemiology, 115,* 752–758.

Buyse, M. E., Staquet, M. J., & Sylvester, R. J. (Eds.). (1984). *Cancer clinical trials.* London: Oxford University Press.

Cohen, J. (1977). *Statistical power analysis for the behavioral sciences* (rev. ed.). New York: Academic Press.

Cox, D. R. (1958). *Planning of experiments.* New York: Wiley.

Donner, A. (1984). Approaches to sample size estimation in the design of clinical trials—A review. *Statistics in Medicine, 3,* 199–214.

Fleiss, J. L. (1986). *The design and analysis of clinical experiments.* New York: Wiley.

Fleiss, J. L., Tytun, A., & Ury, H. K. (1980). A simple approximation for calculating sample size for comparing independent proportions. *Biometrics, 36,* 343–346.

Friedman, L. M., Furberg, C. D., & DeMets, D. L. (1981). *Fundamentals of clinical trials.* Boston: John Wright.

Gail, M. (1974). Power computations for designing comparative Poisson trials. *Biometrics, 30,* 231–237.

Guenther, W. C. (1977). Power and sample size for approximate chi-square tests. *American Statistician, 31*(2), 83–85.

Johnson, N. L., & Kotz, S. (1970). *Continuous univariate distributions* (Vol. 2). New York: Wiley.

IMSL, Inc. User's Manual (1984). *FORTRAN subroutines for mathematics and statistics* (Vol. 3, Edition 9.2). Houston: IMSL.

Kempthorne, O. (1952). *Design and analysis of experiments.* New York: Wiley. (Reprinted by Krieger, Huntington, NY, 1975).

Kotz, S., & Johnson, N. L. (Eds.). (1982). *The encyclopedia of statistics* (Vol. 2). New York: Wiley.

Lachin, J. M. (1981). Introduction to sample size determination and power analysis for clinical trials. *Controlled Clinical Trials, 2,* 93–113.

Lachin, J. M., & Foulkes, M. A. (1986). Evaluation of sample size and power for analyses of survival with allowance for nonuniform patient entry, losses to follow-up, noncompliance, and stratification. *Biometrics, 42,* 507–519.

Lakatos, E. (1986). Sample size determination in clinical trials with time-dependent rates of losses and noncompliance. *Controlled Clinical Trials, 7,* 189–199.

Lee, E. T. (1980). *Statistical methods for survival data analysis.* Belmont, CA: Lifetime Learning.

Mantel, N. (1963). Chi-square tests with one degree of freedom; extensions of the Mantel–Haenszel procedure. *Journal of the American Statistical Association, 58,* 690–700.

Moses, L. (1985). *The $2 \times k$ contingency table with ordered columns: How important to take account of the order?* Technical Report No. 109, Stanford University Division of Biostatistics.

SAS Institute (1985). *SAS user's guide: Basics* (Version 5). Cary, NC: Author.

Scheffe, H. (1959). *The analysis of variance.* New York: Wiley.

Stein, C. M. (1945). A two-sample test for a linear hypothesis whose power is independent of the variance. *Annals of Mathematical Statistics, 16,* 243–258.

Tukey, J. W. (1977). *Exploratory data analysis.* Reading, MA: Addison–Wesley.

Winer, B. J. (1971). *Statistical principles in experimental design* (2nd ed.). New York: McGraw–Hill.

CHAPTER 39

Experimental Studies in the Field
Some Pragmatic Considerations

Jerome E. Singer

Research is an activity that has grown and prospered in the laboratory. Until recently, studies in the field were concentrated in a number of well-defined areas, such as clinical trials, agricultural experiments, and epidemiological studies. Each of these fields has generated its own methodologies and textbook. As investigators have moved toward planning other types of biomedical investigation in the field, new problems and issues have arisen. There are few systematic treatises on the methods and procedures for these field studies.

There are many ways in which the issues and problems associated with doing biomedical research in field settings can be addressed. Each of the issues and problems is in part reflected in the consideration of other disciplines. Statistics, laboratory methodology, behavioral experimentation, and survey research all have a legitimate claim to contribute to this general area. Obviously, not all of these areas can be discussed in a single essay. In this chapter, discussion will be focused on three topics: the use of control groups, subject recruit-

ment and retention, and modification of laboratory procedure. There are many general references covering various aspects of general research design, e.g., Carlsmith, Ellsworth, and Aronson (1976), Cochran and Cox (1957), Hays (1981), Jones (1985), and Kidder (1981).

Although the field of experimental design is usually regarded as a subbranch of statistics, there is much more to experimental design than just the statistical arrangement of subjects into groups and the procedures for data analysis. Appropriate statistics are still necessary for efficient experimental design, but the conceptual requirements of the study of the topic at issue must take precedence over the statistical aspects of the design. Often, the rote application of one or another element of statistical design shifts the focus of the study from the question of interest to the investigator to the question that can be answered most precisely. There is no great virtue obtaining precise answers to questions in which one has no real interest.

This is not to encourage bizarre experimental designs that lead to uninterpretable research and the avoidance of sound statistical design practice, but rather to stress that proper and adequate research designs, necessary for the testing of the hypotheses and questions of interest in the field, can quickly outstrip the compendia of prepared research designs.

The reason for this is simple. Most of the re-

Jerome E. Singer • Department of Medical Psychology, Uniformed Services University of the Health Sciences, Bethesda, Maryland 20814. The opinions or assertions contained herein are the private ones of the author and are not to be construed as official or reflecting the views of the Department of Defense or the Uniformed Services University of the Health Sciences.

search designs available in experimental design books have a background of laboratory or agriculturally developed procedures as their progenitors. These procedures rely on the ability of the experimenter to exert an enormous amount of experimental control over the variables and subjects in the study. Such control is often not the case when human field research is done. With the best of intentions, prearranged statistical designs such as Latin squares and the like, often are not appropriate for field research; the requirements of the research pose problems that standard designs usually cannot handle. In general, the most sophisticated statistical designs possible should be used, provided they do not interfere with, confound, or make the investigator study a problem other than the one in which he or she is interested.

With that caveat as a general principle, there are a number of specific areas in which lessons learned from experience can aid the investigator in preparing or conducting experimental field studies.

Control Groups

1. Control groups are so named because they control for alternative explanations. In contradistinction, experimental groups are groups whose members have been subjected to an experimental procedure. In order to clarify that for a particular group the experimental procedure under test is the only thing that has produced whatever changes or responses are obtained, control groups are used. Although for expository convenience textbooks frequently describe studies with many experimental factors contrasted with a single control, it is not always the case that there is one control group and many experimental groups. Rather there are as many experimental groups as there are treatments, or treatment variations, and as many control groups as need be, in order to account for or rule out alternative explanations.

2. There is no fixed procedure for determining how many control groups are needed for the investigator to advance an unequivocal experimental explanation for an effect. If the investigator can conceive a plausible alternative explanation, then control groups, if available, can be used to dis-

credit these plausible alternatives as operating factors, and strengthen the support for the experimental effects. The word ''plausibility'' used to modify the alternative explanation is a vague one. To one investigator, a particular alternative will be so implausible as to not need discrediting while another investigator will decide that it is plausible enough to need a control group. Different investigators will have different criteria for deciding when additional control groups are to be used. Investigators will have different strategies for confirming an experimental effect. One will build a large number of control groups into an initial experiment, another will discredit alternatives with a series of experiments, after first demonstrating that some effect has occurred. These sorts of variations in the use of control groups are perfectly reasonable as long as the major plausibility of the alternative explanation is discredited via comparison with an appropriate control group somewhere along the line.

3. As in most other areas of research, Occam's razor prevails. That is, the simpler explanation is always preferred to the more complicated one. One application of this principle is that if an effect is discovered in an experimental group, that it not be attributed to the experimental factor until the alternatives with fewer assumptions are first ruled out. Ordinarily, the alternative with the fewest assumptions will be the statistical null hypothesis. In one form or another, this states that there really were no experimental effects; differences between the experimental groups were just a function of random variation in sampling from a population that was homogeneous in regard to the measure being analyzed as the dependent variable. Consequently, a test that sampling variation produced the ostensible effect is usually always appropriate and germane.

4. The usual control group discussed in statistical texts and employed in most experiments is that of ''no treatment.'' This controls for some aspects of random sampling. By having a group that receives no treatment compared to a group, or groups, that have had a treatment(s), one can estimate how much variation could have occurred under the null hypothesis that all groups, including the experimental one, were random samples drawn

from the same population. If the differences between the randomly sampled control group and the experimental groups are so large as to be improbable at some conventional significance level, then the experimental group is reported as having a true difference from the control group, and random sampling as a null hypothesis, the application of Occam's razor, is ruled out.

5. Many experiments, however, have more than a single control group. In some fields, for instance, the use of several controls is standard. In some biochemical assays where substances are first prepared and then put in some sort of assay machine (e.g., a gamma counter, a beta counter, HPLC), several controls are routinely used. One is a blank sample that just gives an estimate of the background radiation, for example, of what the assay machine is counting. Another control group consists of the vehicle in which the experimental samples are transported to estimate the effect of reagents on the counts obtained by the machine. There are also standards—measures of fixed amounts of the substances to be measured in the experimental groups—which are used to standardize and calibrate the machine. In the real sense, all of these—blanks, vehicles, and standards—are control groups and their use rules out alternative explanations. They guard against the experimenter accepting as a result of an experimental manipulation that which is a result of the quality of the machine, the spectrum, the emission rate of the standard, the effects of the vehicle, and so forth. Similar types of multiple control groups are often equally or of greater necessity in the field because of the difficulty of finding any one group that will serve to rule out several different plausible alternative explanations.

6. Controls are easier to operationalize, to obtain, and to match in the laboratory than in the field because of the greater ease and precision with which laboratory experiments can be designed. In the lab, controls can be tailored precisely to the null hypothesis, and both experimental treatments and control conditions are under greater experimenter control and manipulation. There is a greater potential need for multiple groups in the field because the subjects are not as likely to be randomly assigned to conditions as they are in the lab.

They either self-select themselves or nature assigns them one or another condition. For example, one does not assign cancer and normal physiology at random to homogeneous groups of subjects. One rather takes subjects with cancer and seeks appropriate matched control groups in order to study the effect of an intervention.

Problems arise in many cases in finding any control group that is satisfactory for a particular experimental group, precisely because the experimental group has not been randomly assembled. What, for instance, would be a control group for men who volunteer for vasectomies? It is unclear what the basis of the volunteering is; it is, therefore, unclear as to what plausible explanation should be ruled out. In the absence of identifying a critical factor, it is impossible to locate a single control group that matches the experimental group in all but this unknown critical factor. Multiple different control groups have to be used in effect to triangulate on a plausible or possible set of factors that could have confounded the experimental effect with other factors related to the nonrandom selection or self-selection process.

7. The use of multiple control groups and the search for different ways to rule out different alternative explanations puts researchers in a double bind. Adding control groups makes interpretation of the experimental groups' findings easier and places them on a sounder logical footing. Nevertheless, to add control groups may—and in general does—lower the overall probability for concluding that the factor being studied is statistically significant. That is, if there is one experimental group and five control groups and if, in fact, the experimental factor is the only one producing an effect, of the six groups in the study five will be equal and one will be different. It will be harder to find that difference than if only one control group were used under the same circumstances. And, in fact, since many statistics books recommend that a t test between the experimental groups and any of the control groups be protected (i.e., be done only if the factor has a significant effect), the lowering of the ability to find an overall F test might lead one to ignore follow-up t tests, treating them as protected (e.g., see Harris, 1985). In general, this is a sound policy as it lowers experimentwise error and pro-

tects the experimenter from capitalizing on chance. But the policy cannot be followed blindly; judicious common sense must be employed. If the control groups are added to make a multi-control group study, the restriction to use only protected *t* tests should be relaxed when required by the logic of the studies. That is, the investigator should be selective in comparing experimental groups to control groups even if the overall *F* fails to reach conventional significance.

8. Good statisticians and good statistics tests permit such comparisons when done *a priori*. However, the general injunction against such comparisons when done *a posteriori*, and the stringency with which many statistics texts approach this issue mean that the ability to run *t* tests after nonsignificant *F* tests (or the equivalent for other data analytic strategies such as multiple regression/correlation; Cohen & Cohen, 1983) has not filtered down to all investigators. Once again, the question asked by the experimenter and the general logic of the investigation must take precedence over textbook situations that are ill-advised in particular cases.

9. The use of multiple control groups involves a number of issues, one of which is cost. If one is studying an experimental effect, how many subjects and how much effort should be allocated to control groups? Using multiple control groups may mean that more resources are used in processing controls than are expended for experimentals. The relative allocation of resources is a complicated problem. Some aspects of this issue are discussed by Gail, Williams, Byar, and Brown (1976). They provide an analytic treatment of the case of one experimental group and one control group. They conclude that larger control groups are appropriate when experimental treatments are in limited supply, costly, or hazardous, and discuss the optimal size of control groups to limit costs without sacrificing power. Their analytic treatment is limited to the case of a single experimental group compared to a single control group, but the general principles can be applied to more complex designs.

In general, this is not a well-organized topic. There are not any really hard-and-fast rules; the investigator must use judgment about how important it is to rule out particular alternative explanations by including yet another control group. With respect to the multiple comparison errors—i.e., having several control groups escalates both the possible number of experimental–control group comparisons and the likelihood that some will be called significant although merely a result of sampling variation. There are rules for adjusting the alpha levels for each individual comparison so that the total alpha for the study does not exceed a specified level—experimentwise error. One can guard against such experimentwise error by using the Bonferroni inequalities (see Hays, 1981).

For sampling, if there is one experimental group and five control groups, the experimenter may wish to do five two-way comparisons (i.e., the experimental group contrasted with each of the control groups). If the experimenter wishes to keep the five independent comparisons at an overall alpha level of 0.05, the experimenter may partition the alpha of 0.05 in any of several ways, so long as the sum of the alpha levels of the five comparisons does not exceed 0.05. If the experimenter is making the five comparisons discussed above, he or she could treat each of the comparisons at an alpha level of 0.01 so that all five of them total up to 0.05 and still be at an experimentwise error rate of 0.05. Alternatively, however, the experimenter could compare the experimental groups versus all control groups together at an alpha level of 0.03 and make four other independent comparisons, either intercontrol comparisons or experimental group versus a particular control, each at an alpha level of 0.005, for a total, five comparison alpha, of 0.05. The use of the Bonferroni inequalities to split the alpha levels among all comparisons equally is rather standard, but the use of the procedures to split alphas at different levels among different comparisons to weight them for their importance is not yet as common as it should be.

The issue involves more than just protecting the alpha level from experimentwise error, because as the Bonferroni inequality splits an alpha level along many comparisons, it, perforce, reduces the alpha level for any single comparison. Therefore, it also increases the beta error of each comparison, making it more difficult to find an effect when one exists. The use of different levels of alpha within the Bonferroni comparisons enables an experimenter to judiciously decide where he or she wishes to maximize the finding of effects (reduced beta error) and where he or she wishes to guard against spurious effects (reduced alpha level). The experimenter can correspondingly adjust the alpha levels within the Bonferroni specifications to take advantage of his or her own bets on where these important aspects of the comparisons might be.

Subject Recruitment and Attention

1. The problems of recruiting and retaining subjects tend to be greater in field studies than in laboratory studies. This stricture applies to the expense of recruiting, of maintaining contact, and of keeping subjects involved in multisession, or longitudinal studies. The costs of subject recruitment, retention, and replacement in those cases where subjects drop out of the design should be factored into the planning of a field study. Quite often, designers of field studies do not plan on the large costs of either oversampling to make the field sample size appropriate, or midstudy replacement expenses to cover attrition. It is not unusual to see investigators engage in sophisticated power analyses to determine optimal sample sizes—costs balanced against power—and then casually assume that subjects, once recruited, will all remain in the study.

2. Random assignment is easily accomplished if one has a pool of subjects who merely have to be divided into two or more treatment categories. This is often possible and realistic in a laboratory setting, but is difficult when in the field. What are needed are some sophisticated quasi-random ways to sample not only particular subjects but those other factors that could influence outcomes. For instance, one should consider the time of day in which subjects are measured or run in the experiment to ensure that different aspects or characteristics of subjects that covary with time of day are not differentially represented in the experimental and the control groups.

In some cases, subjects are selected, not from a directory of names, but rather from a quasi-random sample of housing units. In such cases, the pattern of requests—time of day, the person in the household who is at home—may produce distortions in the representativeness of the sample and its generalizability to the population of concern. In addition, sometimes subjects are recruited by telephone or telephone sampling, such as random digit dialing within a particular set of telephone exchanges. The sex of the person answering the phone will vary as a function of interaction of work patterns, life-style, and time of day. If one does telephone sampling during the day, the sample will be overrepresented with women or men who do not work out of the house or who work on nonstandard shifts. If one were to sample the same household in the early evening, one might find that a greater proportion of men answered the phone than did at midday. The issue is not so much one of experimental versus control group differences, but one of biases in generalizing to a population given that different elements of the population are differentially sampled by procedures that *appear* to be appropriately random.

Randomly digit dialing within a telephone exchange is often touted as a technique for getting a random cross section of the population within field study restrictions. That it does. The point is that the population of which it is getting a cross section (i.e., the population at home and available to answer the phone) varies from neighborhood to neighborhood, from time of day to time of day, and from life-style to life-style. This particular population is a subset of a broader population and is not necessarily representative of the entire one. The population from which the sample is drawn may not be the one the experimenter intended to sample and to which the experimenter wishes to generalize. Reliance on what looks to be a perfectly valid randomization technique may in fact still result in a biased sample with the source of bias overlooked.

3. The survey research community has been active in developing procedures and designs for selection and sampling of subjects. They are very sophisticated in issues of sampling in the field and have a number of techniques which could apply very well to experimentalists doing work in the field (Tanur, 1981, 1985; Turner & Martin, 1981). But because the survey research community are not composed of the same people as the field ex-

perimental community, quite often their techniques are unknown and unappreciated by the field experimental researchers. Ways in which these survey techniques can be developed and modified are needed in order to alert field researchers not only to the existence of problems, but also to give them the lead on possible ways to solve the problems or avoid those particular difficulties.

4. As mentioned earlier, longitudinal or multisession experiments conducted in the field will almost certainly experience an attrition of subjects over time. The experimenter must make an early decision as to how large the sample should be initially so that even with attrition, at the end the groups will be appropriately large enough for reasonable analyses to be made and for conclusions to be drawn. The larger the sample at the start, the greater will be the expense of maintaining the sample. Issues such as the ability to replace subjects in midstudy should be considered at the beginning, but to plan a study with minimal sample sizes under the expectation of no attrition is to guarantee having groups that are too small at the end to be useful for the purpose at hand. A common error is to consider only main effects when estimating needed sample sizes. If samples are to be cross-classified, or split for internal analyses, sufficiently large samples are needed for the main groupings so that subgroups are likely to remain large enough for subanalyses to be feasible.

5. Investigators may attempt to avoid the difficulties of longitudinal studies by doing multiple cross-section studies, i.e., taking different samples at different times instead of following groups over time with multiple measurements. Multiple cross-section studies have their own difficulties, problems, and ways of proceeding. These are discussed in some detail in the chapter by Kuller. The use of multiple cross sections instead of a longitudinal design does make a study cheaper to run. However, it also adds variance, as the use of different groups at different times adds subject variance to the time and treatment variance. Although there may be a cost advantage to the cross-sectional procedures, the result of having groups with more variance may make the effects one is looking for more difficult to detect. Consequently, larger multiple cross-section designs would be needed than longitudinal ones, in light of the additional vari-

ance, in order to have the same power of finding an effect.

6. It is often possible for experimenters to design compound studies (i.e., in which some longitudinal components are interspersed in a cross-sectional design). Thus, if one does not have the resources to follow a longitudinal sample over a period of time, one can take a small longitudinal sample (e.g., 20% of the total) and follow them through each session over time, while taking the remaining 80% of the subjects as a different cross-sectional sample each time. The use of such a design enables long-term, longitudinal comparisons to determine what changes within subjects are occurring over time, and also enables one to estimate experimental effects with the cheaper cross sections at each time point. It also enables estimates of various components. Also to be encouraged, or considered, are the use of panel designs—adding subjects as each section progresses. These enable separate consideration of age effects, cohort effects, and time effects. The use of panel designs is standard in many fields, such as voting, epidemiology, and consumer behavior, but is all too infrequently considered as a possibility in behavioral biomedical field research studies.

7. Given that all studies will have attrition over time, the one sure thing is that attrition cannot be assumed to be random. There are usually selective factors in attrition that produce dropouts and these will occur for both experimental and control groups. For almost any conceivable scenario of artifacts that could occur to produce selective attrition, the only guarantee is that no matter how absurd they seem, some of them will probably be operating.

8. One way to reduce the effects of the attrition is to get some measure specific to the dropouts and to the refusers (i.e., those who decline to participate) so that they may be compared to those who do participate and remain in the study. For example, at the time of recruitment, it is possible to give anonymous demographic questionnaires to those who decline to participate. The straightforward explanation, ''We would like to know characteristics of those who do not participate so that we can compare them to those who do choose to volunteer,'' is sufficient most of the time to get people to fill them out. The absence of identifying material

reinforces to the refusers that no follow-ups will occur. Under these circumstances, people are not usually reluctant to give this information. The demographic characteristics of the refusers can be compared to those of the participants to get some gross index of how similar they are. Also, questionnaires—anonymous or otherwise—can be prepared for participants who choose to drop out. Although anonymity cannot as easily be provided as for subjects who refuse to participate, often many people who drop out just leave the study. While they have the right to do this, they can be questioned, and most often do not refuse, as to why they do not wish to continue. Those reasons can be used to selectively infer what biases may be operating or what factors, if any, may be producing selective rather than random dropout.

9. Statistical analyses of groups with dropouts can often be facilitated by using analytic designs that enable the dropout effects to be studied. For example, Cohen and Cohen (1983) devote a chapter to exploring multiple regression/correlation designs that use dropout as a dummy variable; the procedures can examine predropout effects in an analogous manner to what is done for missing survey data. For example, many surveys have questions that partition a sample, such as, "Are you married?" If the answer is yes, a branch goes to one set of questions; if the answer is no, the survey skips to a different point. Those questions answered only, for example, by married subjects are then coded and the effects of marriage can be analyzed, without the lack of response from the unmarried subjects treated as missing data. It is equally possible to take subjects who drop out, code dropout or nondropout as a dummy variable in a regression design, and examine what effect dropping out has had on questions previously answered. One can do this in a number of ways depending on the questions to be asked [i.e., an experimenter can check whether background variables have an effect on who dropped out using dropout as a dependent (obviously, one entered after the fact) variable, or one can examine dropout first and see what effect that status has had on what the experimental results were up to the time of dropout].

10. A particular problem that often crops up in a field study is that subjects voluntarily change from one group to another. This is often detectable only if checks on the experimental variable are built into the study at several time periods and repeated. For example, imagine that one is studying smoking cessation and assembles groups of those who have decided to stop smoking under experimental manipulation and a control group which is allowed to continue to smoke. Over a period of time, there are bound to be crossovers—experimental subjects who resume smoking and control subjects who voluntarily quit smoking. When an experimenter discovers such people, it is often a problem as to how the data collected from these crossover subjects are to be treated.

There are several ways of handling such data. First, one could eliminate all of those subjects who crossed over. The remaining subjects are all correctly classified in their groups. The difficulties with this solution are: (1) there is a selective bias in who elects to engage in crossover behavior and (2) there is loss of power from having fewer subjects. Second, one can keep the crossover subjects, treat them as though they had remained in the group to which they were assigned, and say that this matches the extent to which these effects occur within the population. This increases beta error by making the experimental effect harder to find and increases the error variance in each group. By analyzing the study as if there had been no crossover, one does not void those randomization processes that assigned subjects to one or the other groups. Third, one could run an internal analysis, changing the classification of the crossover subjects after-the-fact. This procedure loses randomization and thereby increases selectivity errors and bias, although it does sharpen the contrast between the correctly classified subjects: in this case those who actually continued smoking versus those who actually stopped.

None of these procedures dominates the other. That is, no one is much better than the other in so many instances that the other should be discarded. There is, in fact, no really good way to uniformly handle this problem. It is probably best to consider all three analyses, do them all, and see if they all point to a common set of inferences. That is, an experimenter should analyze the data three ways: analyze the data with the crossover subjects eliminated; analyze the data with the subjects left in their original groups despite their crossover; and do an internal analysis. If the three analyses disagree, then experimenter judgment and hints and clues from other aspects of the data must be employed to make intelligent judgments about what has occurred. But if all three give the same sort of picture, then there can be some confidence that, despite the crossover, the effects observed were reasonable reflections of the population.

11. There is often a great deal of confusion in experimental studies taken from the lab to the field as to whether the interpretation of the samples should be done on a fixed or random basis. That is, does the study examine the effects of a group in the abstract or the effects of a group in proportion to their influence in the population? In laboratory studies, experimental groups (e.g., Protestants, Catholics) are usually sampled in equal, or perhaps proportional, numbers, and the abstract effects of being Protestant or Catholic on the dependent variable are inferred. If, in the population, the Protestants number four times the Catholics, experimental results do not directly generalize. This is a fixed effect design. Alternatively, a random sample of the population can be obtained in which the sample proportions of Protestants and Catholics mirror their proportions in the population, and the relative effects of being Protestant or Catholic within that sample assessed. These results will generalize directly to the population, but because of their different sample sizes, the abstract effects of Protestant or Catholic on the dependent variable will not be directly assessable. This is a random effect design. (The problem is discussed in Cohen and Cohen in the context of interpreting multiple regression effects.)

To illustrate the issue, let us imagine that an experimental effect is to be analyzed as a function of the religion of the subjects. There are two broad strategies for accomplishing this. One can do a random sample of the population and assume that the sample proportions of different religions mirror the population proportions. The interpretation of the result will be that what had happened in the sample would be what would happen in the population. However, for minority religions the size of the sample will be very small and it may be that religious effects will go undetected. Alternatively,

one could decide what religions are of experimental interest and sample for equal numbers of people from each religion to participate in the study. The interpretation will, in fact, then show the contribution of religion to the effects under consideration. It will not, however, be an accurate picture of religion's different effects in the population because the sample proportions of each religion being made equal (artificially, by forced sampling) will not mirror the population proportions of each religion. Consider the question, for instance, of prayer in the public schools. A sample randomly drawn from the population will differ from a sample composed of equal members of each denomination. There is no right or wrong answer as to which sample procedure should be used. Clarity on the part of the experimenter is needed concerning what is of primary importance, e.g., the abstract effect of religion versus mirroring of the population.

Modification of Laboratory Procedures

1. There are many studies which use techniques adapted from and developed in the laboratory. To take such studies and procedures into the field often requires some modification. The modification may result in some changes in experimental design. The basic point to keep in mind is that despite all advances in technology, Murphy's law still rules—things will go wrong. For example, there are research studies requiring that automated blood pressure measurements be taken in the field, often from ambulatory patients. Measurement of blood pressure is fairly standardized in the laboratory and clinic. Many companies market devices that are claimed to work unfailingly in field situations. Despite these claims, it is not clear that anyone has developed the perfect blood pressure monitor. Difficulties and malfunctions do occur. When they occur in the laboratory, it may be easy enough to switch to another means of blood pressure recording, such as hand recording via a stethoscope and sphygmomanometer. In the field, this is not always possible.

It is necessary to a greater extent in field studies

to have available backups, both for the individual case and on an experimentwise basis. Otherwise, one will find the study to be technologically advanced in its early stages but progressively more primitive with respect to the quantity, the quality, and even the type of data, as the study proceeds. Attention must be paid to the quality and condition of apparatus to avoid a time-related drift in data quality.

2. When studies are conducted in the laboratory, potential noncompliance with experimental procedures can be managed on an acute basis. These same problems cannot so easily be managed in the field. For example, if one is studying a biochemical process in which it is necessary to control the subject's smoking or eating, it is often possible to get somebody to come into the laboratory not having smoked or eaten for a fixed period of time before. Or, at the very least, the extent of noncompliance can be checked and noted. The monitoring of such smoking and eating activities in the field is much more difficult and unreliable, and the propensities for subjects to cheat while in the field are great. And, unfortunately, the experimenter may not even be aware of it. When a subject is sitting in the experimenter's laboratory, the surveillance by the experimenter and the reduced availability of the means to cheat (very few people would smoke or eat in a laboratory if explicitly asked to refrain) virtually eliminate the problem. In the field, ancillary questions and measures must be incorporated to check on noncompliance and to help maintain data quality.

3. There are many ways in which circadian rhythms or other rhythms can influence subjects' responses. In laboratory studies, there is a better control of the schedule of the study and a clearer idea of the scheduling of the subjects. One can ensure that experiments are not run such that the experimental groups are all in the afternoon and control groups are all in the morning. In field studies, quite often, where technicians or experimenters go out among the subjects to record the data, or the subjects record their own data at some fixed point or time and scheduling is at the mutual convenience of subjects and experimenters, such potential circadian rhythm biases often go undetected because times are unrecorded or seem unable to be controlled. Nevertheless, systematic biases owing to scheduling that confounds experimental conditions with time of day, or week, or other temporal variables, may often interfere with the validity of many measures.

4. When biological samples, such as blood or urine, are collected for later analysis, these need to be preserved from degradation. In the field, it is not always possible, for example, to spin blood samples in a centrifuge and freeze them. Therefore, between collection in the field and return to the laboratory, preservatives must be added of one sort or another to most of the samples. Often, preservatives for a particular assay may interfere with the assay for a different constituent or element. The handling of samples and the selection of preservatives is crucial and must be considered in great detail. In addition to having chemical imperatives about which preservatives not to use, there are also logistical limitations. Both common sense and liability considerations suggest that chemicals such as caustics or hazardous substances not be used in the home. For example, although hydrochloric acid may be a useful preservative in the laboratory, one does not give a subject a urine collection container partially filled hydrochloric acid. The unthinking application of laboratory procedures to handling samples in the field can result in loss of data or damage to the study.

5. Consideration should be given to inexpensive extensions of an experiment. If one is collecting blood in the field, a variety of assays can be performed after-the-fact. An extra 10-ml Vacutainer can be extracted from each subject. If one guesses right on the preservative or can spin and freeze the samples at a low temperature early enough, then at a later date one can do a prospective retrospective study cheaply. If someone later proposes a hypothesis that under the conditions previously used in a study, some biochemical product will be affected, a new study need not be conducted. The Vacutainers of blood can be removed from the ultralow freezer and assayed without the expense of having to mount another experiment to re-create the original conditions. The likelihood of getting something very useful out of this procedure is not extremely great, but the cost of an extra Vacutainer of blood—given the ex-

penses of a field study to begin with—is so minimal that it is worth the gamble and investment so that when a new neuropeptide or hormone becomes the focus of research speculation, some insight into whether it is plausible or at all relevant can be gained very quickly.

6. It is possible in field studies to request that subjects collect their own urine samples. On an acute basis, this is not overly difficult, and even on a continued basis, subjects can be requested to, and usually comply in providing 15- or 24-h urine samples. The problems that occur usually are concerned with the subjects' folkloristic beliefs about the nature of urine, their unwillingness to put the sample container in the refrigerator to keep it cool, and their general aversion to excretory products. Nevertheless, with reasonable precautions, such as a clear common language description of the procedures and amenities, providing an opaque bag into which the collection container can be placed so that the subject does not see the urine container, many long-term urine collections are possible.

7. The cost of many assay procedures in field studies is high, both for collecting samples and for assaying them. Collecting is often expensive because of the cost of personnel in the field. For blood draws, for example, some trained personnel—phlebotomist, nurse, or even physician—may be necessary. These specially trained people may be in shorter supply and may have a higher cost than the personnel necessary to administer other aspects of the study. In addition, although it is possible to assay one sample for several components by dividing it into aliquots and testing each aliquot for a number of different biochemical products, the cost of such procedures is usually high. To run an affordable study, when many such assays are necessary, may result in too few subjects for the study to have sufficient statistical power. One answer is to run the inexpensive part of the study with as large a sample as possible or necessary, and subsample within each condition for the expensive procedures. This is very analogous to the procedure, suggested earlier, of running some longitudinal subjects while the others are run cross-sectionally. At the very least, this type of procedure of subsampling for the expensive aspects of the study will yield variability estimates for accurate power analyses so that a follow-up study can employ optimal sample sizes for the expensive data, i.e., optimal in balancing cost against power.

8. Often the set of procedures and tasks for a field study is too long a battery to administer at one session. Since the expense of sending personnel out to test a subject in the field is high, investigators pack each session with materials to be administered or samples to collect. That is, given the fixed costs of sending an investigator into the field, one would like to obtain as much information as possible. Nevertheless, practical and logistical reasons suggest that subjects are not going to participate in 4-, 6-, or 8-h sessions very readily. One good solution, which now has a theoretical base (Tanur, 1981, 1985), is to purposely confound measures so that certain interactions cannot be tested, although main effects can be assessed. This sort of purposive confounding is a standard procedure in much of human factors' research and is well documented in experiment design tests (e.g., Winer, 1971). The basic principle is that if each subject receives a partially overlapping set of materials, most of the power of the total sample size can be applied to the analysis of each partially sampled variable.

For example, in a large study, each subset of subjects can get a different subbattery of tasks, as long as the subbatteries are distributed across the experimental conditions in a carefully balanced confound. That is, no subsample receives all the tasks; each subsample is tested in a limited time span.

By judiciously arranging the tasks with confounding, the experimenter sacrifices the higher-order interactions—the third- or fourth-order interaction between four or five tasks, for example—in order to have full-power evaluation of the main effects and the first-order interaction effects. The loss is not really great at all, as most of the higher-order interactions would be uninterpretable if found, and of limited theoretical interest at best.

Other Issues

In recent years, investigators in laboratories have become sensitized to such things as demand characteristics, Hawthorne effects, and subject expectancies (Cook & Campbell, 1979). The Hawthorne effect is the well-known phenomenon that subjects singled out for research often behave in unnatural ways, and the mere singling out of a person to participate in a research study will often generate different behaviors and responses than would be obtained under more routine circumstances. Demand characteristics refer to those subtle views, hints, and pressures placed by the experimenter on the subject as to what the experimenter wants and expects from the participants. Subjects may either complacently comply with what they think the experimenter wants and modify their behaviors accordingly, or become reactive and give the experimenter behaviors opposite to what they think the experimenter wants. In any event, normal behavior will change in response to perceived experimenter demands. Even if the experimenter manages not to be demanding—as would occur, for example, in some aspect of double-blind studies—subjects have expectancies about the experiment and bring their own set of self-generated demands. Again, this results in a distortion of response and its consequent effects on the data. Although these issues have been discussed in the context of the laboratory, there is every reason to believe that they are equally operative in the field. Whereas the laboratory puts a great emphasis on standardization of experimenter interaction with subjects so that many of these effects are minimized or controlled, quite often, because of the nonstandard nature of the field, when people interviewed or tested at different sites, at different times of the day, under different conditions, by different experimenters, these potential effects are often overlooked. Investigators would be well advised to be sensitized to these artifacts and make sure that appropriate control groups, operating instructions, and training of experimenters are all carefully designed to minimize extra experimental influences on the data.

Conclusion

Experiments in the laboratory require a number of specialized techniques and procedures. Methodologists and statisticians have been successful in developing them and disseminating them to researchers. When behavioral biomedical research is conducted in field situations, additional problems and issues often arise. While there are no special treatises that address the collection of field data, a number of the problems can be ameliorated with a combination of common sense and the application of some pragmatic adjustments. As more of this research is conducted, the more useful and successful of these design interventions will be routinely incorporated into field research methodology.

References

Carlsmith, J. M., Ellsworth, P. C., & Aronson, E. (1976). *Methods of research in social psychology.* Reading, MA: Addison–Wesley.

Cochran, W. G., & Cox, G. M. (1957). *Experimental designs* (2nd ed.). New York: Wiley.

Cohen, J., & Cohen, P. (1983). *Applied multiple regression/correlation analysis for the behavioral sciences.* Hillsdale, NJ: Erlbaum.

Cook, T., & Campbell, D. T. (1979). *Quasi-experimentation: Design and analysis issues for field settings.* Chicago: Rand McNally.

Gail, M., Williams, R., Byar, D. P., & Brown, C. (1976). How many controls? *Journal of Chronic Diseases, 29,* 723–731.

Harris, R. J. (1985). *A primer of multivariate statistics* (2nd ed.). New York: Academic Press.

Hays, W. L. (1981). *Statistics* (3rd ed.). New York: Holt, Rinehart, & Winston.

Jones, R. A. (1985). *Research methods in the social and behavioral sciences.* Sunderland, MA: Sinauer.

Kidder, L. H. (1981). *Research methods in social relations* (4th ed.). New York: Holt, Rinehart, & Winston.

Tanur, J. M. (1981). Advances in methods for large-scale surveys and experiments. In *The 5-year outlook on science and technology 1981: Source materials* (Vol. 2). Washington, DC: National Science Foundation.

Tanur, J. M. (1985). Survey research methods in environmental psychology. In A. Baum & J. E. Singer (Eds.), *Advances in environmental psychology* (Vol. 5). Hillsdale, NJ: Erlbaum.

Turner, C. F., & Martin, E. (Eds.). (1981). *Surveys of subjective phenomena: Summary report.* Panel on survey measurement of subjective phenomena, Committee on National Statistics, Assembly of Behavioral and Social Sciences, National Research Council. Washington, DC: National Academy Press.

Winer, B. J. (1971). *Statistical principles in experimental design.* New York: McGraw–Hill.

CHAPTER 40

Metaanalysis of Related Research

Larry V. Hedges

The research literature of behavioral medicine, along with that of many other areas of scientific research, is experiencing dramatic growth. Many important research areas now have several or even dozens of research studies or clinical trials that address similar questions. These circumstances pose new problems in the appraisal, evaluation, and use of the collective body of research evidence on important questions. The use of quantitative procedures for combining research results has become important as a response to increasingly complex research literatures in biostatistics as well as in the social, behavioral, and physical sciences. Such procedures can make the synthesis of research findings more rigorous and potentially more valid, while providing feasible means for addressing ever larger and more complex collections of research findings.

The purpose of this chapter is to provide an introduction to statistical methodology for combining evidence from related research studies. The use of statistical methods in the process of combining evidence is often called metaanalysis. The terms *overview, pooling of results, research review,* or *research synthesis* are also used as synonyms for *metaanalysis*. Whatever term is used, the general outline of the procedures are the same. Each study in a collection of studies is believed to provide evidence about a relationship of interest (e.g., a treatment effect). The problem of metaanalysis is how to extract information from each study in a comparable form and combine that evidence across studies in a meaningful way. In simple cases this may involve combining across studies estimates of a parameter representing the relationship or effect size of interest. In more complex situations this may involve studying the variability of the effect or relationship across studies.

Metaanalysis has several advantages. First, the pooling of evidence from several studies yields statistical tests that have greater power than those in any individual research study. Second, utilizing evidence from many studies makes it possible to examine the variation between studies (and between strata within studies) which is impossible in any single study. Third, metaanalysis makes use of data that already exist and are summarized in the results of existing studies. Finally, carefully conducted metaanalyses may utilize all (or nearly all) of the existing empirical data to provide summary conclusions with the greatest possible base of empirical support.

Conceptualizing Metaanalysis

Metaanalyses are in many ways similar to original research projects. They involve most of the procedures that are part of original research, including

Larry V. Hedges • Department of Education, University of Chicago, Chicago, Illinois 60637.

- problem formulation—defining precise questions,
- data collection—obtaining a sample of possibly relevant studies and extracting summary information from each of them,
- data evaluation—deciding what possibly relevant studies are of high enough quality to provide reliable evidence,
- data analysis and interpretation—using the evidence from many studies to draw conclusions, and
- reporting results—presenting procedures and conclusions.

Since each of these procedures involves a considerable amount of subjectivity, variations in procedure are inevitable. Some variations in procedure lead to biases that render research results invalid or at least uninterpretable. Methodological standards are designed to help ensure that variations in procedure are constrained to help ensure the validity of research by reducing the possibility of biases due to procedural variation.

Perhaps the most crucial methodological standard in clinical trials research is the requirement of protocols for clinical trials (Chalmers, 1982). Protocols constrain procedural variation by specifying the details of procedure. Protocols are equally important in metaanalysis (if somewhat different in content) as they are in clinical trials. The protocol for a metaanalysis or pooling project should specify fundamental aspects of procedure in each of the procedural areas listed above. It should be a detailed plan for the metaanalysis. The remainder of this chapter addresses each of the procedural areas in detail, suggests important aspects of procedure which must be decided, and suggests considerations that should be weighed in each case.

Problem Formulation

Problem formulation is often conceptualized as the first step in any original research study or research review (Cooper, 1984; Light & Pillemer, 1984). It involves formulating the precise questions to be answered by the review. One aspect of formulating questions is deciding whether the purpose of the review is confirmatory (e.g., to test a few specific hypotheses about treatment effects) or exploratory (e.g., to generate hypotheses about conditions under which a treatment works best). In this chapter the primary purpose of reviews is assumed to be confirmatory rather than exploratory.

A second aspect of problem formulation concerns decisions about when studies are similar enough to combine. That is, deciding whether treatments, controls, experimental procedure, and study outcome measure are comparable enough to be considered "the same" for the purposes of pooling. It is helpful in thinking about this problem to distinguish the *theoretical* or *conceptual* variables about which knowledge is sought (called *constructs*) from the actual *examples* of these variables that appear in studies (called *operations*). For example, the construct of morbidity might be defined conceptually as the presence of any debilitating symptoms in the patient but the corresponding operations in a study might be the presence of angina and a few other *specific* symptoms.

Thus, defining questions precisely in a research review involves deciding on the constructs of independent variables, study characteristics, and outcomes that are appropriate for the questions addressed by the review and deciding on the operations that will be regarded as corresponding to the constructs. That is, the reviewer must develop both construct definitions and a set of rules for deciding which concrete instances (of treatments, controls, or measures) correspond to those constructs.

Although the questions (and constructs) of interest might seem completely self-evident in a review of related clinical trials, a little reflection may convince the reader that there are subtleties in formulating precise questions. For example, consider clinical trials in which the outcome construct is the death rate. At first the situation seems completely clear-cut, but there are subtleties. Should deaths from all causes be included in the death rate or only deaths related to the disease under treatment? If the latter approach is used, how are deaths related to side effects of the treatment to be counted? If there is follow-up after different intervals, which intervals should be used? Should unanticipated or data-defined variables (such as "sudden death") be used? Careful thinking about the problem under review usually leads to similar issues of construct definition that require consideration.

Selecting Constructs and Operations

The reviewer, of course, has no control over the constructs or operations chosen by the primary researcher. Different studies will use different operations and constructs and the reviewer inevitably must face the task of organizing this variety into meaningful categories. It is usually helpful to start by proposing an *a priori* set of categories of independent variables, dependent variables, subject characteristics, and study procedures. Such an organization should specify the various types of independent and dependent variables that are of interest, the subject characteristics that are of primary interest, and the types of study design or procedure that are expected. This organization is then refined by pilot testing: attempting to classify a selection of studies. This empirical procedure usually tests the original classification scheme, provides concrete examples for the development of coding protocols, and reveals something about the variety of operations that correspond to each of the constructs. The *a priori* categories are usually modified somewhat and a concrete set of guidelines are then developed for deciding which particular operations that appear in studies correspond to which constructs. Often, such guidelines are formalized into a coding form or instrument which is used to represent the important characteristics of a study (i.e., what constructs are included in the study).

An inevitable tension in the development of construct definitions is between inclusion or breadth and exclusion or specificity. It is easy to develop construct definitions that are so precise that they apply to virtually none of the available studies. Excessively narrow constructs suggest that studies are too different to be combined. Although this may be an accurate reflection of the state of research in an area, it may also suggest that the reviewer has framed the summary question in too narrow a fashion. Summary questions should usually be broader than questions addressed in specific studies to benefit from the evidence of at least

several studies. Moreover, broad constructs have the characteristic that they admit evidence from different studies which operationalize these constructs in a slightly different fashion. The use of evidence from multiple operations has the advantage that each different operation probably incorporates slightly different irrelevances. Multiple operations can enhance the confidence in relationships between constructs if the analogous relationships between operations hold under a variety of different (and each imperfect) operations. However, increased confidence comes from multiple operations only when the different operations are in fact more related to the desired construct than to some other construct (see Webb, Campbell, Schwartz, Sechrest, & Grove, 1981, for a discussion of multiple operationism). Thus, although multiple operations can lead to increased confidence through "triangulation" of evidence, the indiscriminate use of broad operations can also contribute to invalidity of results via confoundings of one construct with another (see Cooper, 1984).

Perhaps the most successful applications of broad or multiple constructs in metaanalysis are those that may *include* broad constructs in the review but *distinguish* narrower constructs in the data analysis and presentation of results. This permits the reviewer to examine variations in the pattern of results as a function of construct definition. It also permits separate analyses to be carried out for each narrow construct. A combined analysis across constructs may be carried out where appropriate or distinct analyses for the separate constructs may be presented.

Data Collection

Data collection in metaanalysis consists of assembling a collection of research studies and extracting quantitative indices of study characteristics and of effect magnitude (or relationship between variables). The former is largely a problem of selecting studies that may contain information relevant to the specific questions addressed in the review. It is largely a sampling process. The latter is a problem of obtaining quantitative representations of the measures of effect magnitude and the other characteristics of studies that are relevant to the specific questions addressed by the review. This is essentially a measurement process similar to complex tasks in other research contexts. The standard psychological measurement procedures for ensuring the reliability and validity of ratings or judgments are as appropriate in metaanalysis as in original research (Rosenthal, 1984; Stock *et al.,* 1982).

Sampling in Metaanalysis

The problem of assembling a collection of studies in metaanalysis is often viewed as a sampling problem: the problem of obtaining a representative sample of all studies that have actually been conducted. Because the adequacy of samples necessarily determines the range of valid generalizations that are possible, the procedures used to locate studies in metaanalysis have been regarded as crucially important. Much of the discussion on sampling in metaanalysis concentrates on the problem of obtaining a representative or exhaustive sample of the studies that have actually been conducted. Although large-scale studies in an area will usually be known to the reviewer, a variety of techniques are usually necessary to come close to obtaining an exhaustive sample (including smaller or more obscure) of studies.

Searches for relevant studies using indexing or abstracting services such as *Index Medicus, Psychological Abstracts,* or *Dissertation Abstracts International* (for doctoral dissertations) are usually a first step. Such searches can be conducted via computerized data bases and often yield a surprising number of unexpected studies. Searches of the bibliographies of studies already identified or published reviews of research are also helpful. References provided by prominent researchers or hand searches of relevant journals are also sometimes useful. Reference librarians can help with the details of searches for relevant studies (see also Cooper, 1984, or Glass, McGaw, & Smith, 1981).

Missing Data in Metaanalysis

Missing data are a problem that plagues many forms of applied research. Survey researchers are

well aware that the best sampling design is ineffective if the information sought cannot be extracted from the units that are sampled. Of course, missing data are not a substantial problem if they are "missing at random," that is, if the missing information is essentially a random sample of all the information available (Rubin, 1976). Unfortunately, there is usually very little reason to believe that missing data in metaanalysis are missing at random. On the contrary, it is often easier to argue that the causes of the missing data are systematically related to the study outcome or to important characteristics of studies. When this is true, missing data pose a serious threat to the validity of conclusions in metaanalysis.

Studies (such as single case studies) that do not use statistical analyses are one source of missing data on study outcome. Other studies use statistics but do not provide enough statistical information to allow the calculation of an estimate of the appropriate outcome parameter. Sometimes this is a consequence of failure to report relevant statistics. More often it is a consequence of the researcher's use of a design or analysis that makes difficult or impossible the construction of a parameter estimate that is completely comparable to those of other studies. Perhaps the most pernicious sources of missing data are studies which *selectively* report statistical information. Such studies sometimes report only information on effects that are statistically significant, exhibiting what has been called reporting bias (Hedges, 1984). Missing effects can lead to very serious biases, identical to those caused by selective publication, which are discussed in the section on publication bias.

One strategy for dealing with incomplete effect size data is to ignore the problem. This is almost certainly a bad strategy. If nothing else, such a strategy reduces the credibility of the metaanlaysis because the presence of at least some missing data is obvious to knowledgeable readers. A better strategy is to extract from the study any available information about the outcome of the study. The direction (sign) of the effect can often be deduced even when an effect size cannot be calculated. A tabulation of these directions of effects can therefore be used to supplement the effect size analysis. In some cases such a tabulation can even be used to derive a parametric estimate of effect (Hedges & Olkin, 1985).

Publication Bias

An important axiom of survey sample design is that an excellent sample design cannot guarantee a representative sample if it is drawn from an incomplete enumeration of the population. The analogue in metaanalysis is that an apparently good sampling plan may be thwarted by applying the plan to an incomplete and unrepresentative subset of the studies that were actually conducted.

The published literature is particularly susceptible to the claim that it is unrepresentative of all studies that may have been conducted (the so-called publication bias problem). There is empirical evidence that the published literature contains fewer statistically insignificant results than would be expected from the complete collection of all studies actually conducted (Bozarth & Roberts, 1972; Hedges, 1984; Sterling, 1959). The tendency of the published literature to overrepresent statistically significant findings can lead to biased overestimates of effect magnitudes from published literature (Lane & Dunlap, 1978; Hedges, 1984).

Publication or reporting bias may not always be severe enough to invalidate metaanalyses based solely on published articles, however (see Light & Pillemer, 1984). Theoretical analysis of the potential effects of publication bias showed that even when nonsignificant results are never published (the most severe form of publication bias), the effect on estimation of effect size may not be large unless both the within-study sample sizes and the underlying effect size are small. However, if either the sample size in the studies or the underlying effect sizes are small, the effect on estimation can be substantial (Hedges, 1984).

The possibility that publication or reporting bias may inflate effect size estimates suggests that reviewers may want to consider investigating its possible impact. One method is to compare effect size estimates derived from published (e.g., books, journal articles) and unpublished sources (e.g., conference presentations, contract reports, or doctoral dissertations). An alternative procedure is to use statistical corrections for estimation of effects

under publication bias (see Hedges & Olkin, 1985).

Data Evaluation

Data evaluation in metaanalysis is the process of critical examination of the corpus of information collected, to determine which study results are expected to yield reliable information. This process is crucial to the validity of conclusions in metaanalysis since the validity of overall conclusions depends strongly on the validity of the study results incorporated. Judgments of study quality are the principal method of data evaluation. A second aspect of data evaluation is the use of empirical methods to detect outliers or influential data points. When properly applied, empirical methods have uses both in metaanalysis (see Hedges & Olkin, 1985) and in primary research (Barnett & Lewis, 1978; Hawkins, 1980).

Metaanalysts and other reviewers of research have sometimes used a single binary (high/low) judgment which may be useful for some purposes such as deciding which studies to exclude from the review, but it is seldom advisable to make such judgments directly. The reason is that different researchers do *not* always agree on which studies are of high quality. Empirical research suggests that direct ratings of study quality have very low reliability (see Orwin & Cordray, 1985). Consequently, most metaanalysts at least initially characterize study quality by using multiple criteria. One approach to criteria for study quality is the threats-to-validity approach, in which each study is rated according to its susceptibility to some general sources of bias such as those on the lists presented by Sackett (1979) or Cook and Campbell (1979). A second approach is the methods-description approach (Cooper, 1984) in which the reviewer exhaustively codes the stated characteristics of each study's method. A third approach to assessing study quality is a combination of the first two approaches involving coding of the characteristics of study methodology and assessing threats to validity that may not be reflected in the characteristics of study methods (Cooper, 1984).

Because decisions about study quality lead to

decisions about which studies should be included in the analysis, this process can be the source of serious biases in the review process. Consequently, some experts recommend that all ratings of study quality should be carried out in blinded fashion, meaning that the raters of study quality should not have access to the results of the studies that they rate. Such blinding is designed to ensure that a study's results do not influence decisions about inclusion of the study in the review.

Data Analysis and Interpretation

Data analysis and interpretation are the heart of metaanalysis and have a long history in statistics and the physical sciences. In the early part of this century, modern statistical methods were constructed for the analysis of individual agricultural experiments, and shortly thereafter statistical methods for combining the results of such experiments were developed.

Two distinctly different directions have been taken for combining evidence from different studies in agriculture almost from the very beginning of statistical analysis in that area. One approach relies on testing for statistical significance of combined results across studies. The other approach involves combining estimates of treatment effects across studies. Both methods date from as early as the 1930s (and perhaps earlier) and continue to generate interest among the statistical research community to the present day (see Hedges & Olkin, 1985).

Testing for the statistical significance of the combined results of agricultural experiments is perhaps the older of the two traditions. One of the first proposals for a test of the statistical significance of combined results (now called testing the minimum p or the Tippett method) was given by L. H. C. Tippett in 1931. Soon afterwards, R. A. Fisher (1932) proposed a method for combining statistical significance, or p values, across studies. Karl Pearson (1933) independently derived the same method shortly thereafter, and the method variously called Fisher's method or Pearson's method was established. Research on tests of the significance of combined results has flourished since that time, and now well over 100 papers in

the statistical literature have been devoted to such tests.

Tests of the significance of combined results are sometimes called omnibus or nonparametric tests because these tests do not depend on the type of data or the statistical distribution of those data. Instead, tests of the statistical significance of combined results rely only on the fact that p values are uniformly distributed between zero and one when the null hypothesis is true. Although omnibus tests have a strong appeal in that they can be applied universally, they suffer from an inability to provide estimates of the magnitude of the effects being considered. Thus, omnibus tests do not tell the experimenter how much of an effect a treatment has.

In order to determine the magnitude of the effect of an agricultural treatment, a second approach was developed which involved combining numerical estimates of treatment effects. One of the early papers on the subject (Cochran, 1937) appeared a few years after the first papers on omnibus procedures. Additional work in this tradition appeared shortly thereafter (e.g., Yates & Cochran, 1938; Cochran, 1943). It is also interesting to note that work on statistical methods for combining estimates from different experiments in physics dates from the same era (Birge, 1932).

Combined Significance Tests

Suppose that k independent studies are assembled and that each study tests essentially the same substantive hypothesis. (Note that the condition that studies are independent requires that studies are based on different samples of individuals.) The hypothesis tested in the ith study can be stated formally as a null hypothesis

$$H_{0i} : \theta_i = 0$$

about a parameter θ_i that represents the substantive effect or relationship of interest. For example, in studies that assess a relationship via an odds ratio between one group and another, θ_i might be one minus the odds ratio so that $\theta_i = 0$ when the odds ratio is one. Alternatively, in studies that measure the effect of group membership via a logistic regression, θ_i might be the regression coefficient for group membership. Denote by T_i the test statistic used to actually test H_{0i} in the ith study.

The hypotheses $H_{01}, \ldots, H_{0k}$ need not have the same substantive meaning, and similarly, the statistics $T_1, \ldots, T_k$ need not be of related form. The omnibus null hypothesis H_0 is that the null hypothesis is true in every study, i.e., that all the θ_i's are zero:

$$H_0: \theta_1 = \theta_2 = \ldots = \theta_k = 0$$

Note that the composite hypothesis H_0 holds only if each of the subhypotheses $H_{01}, \ldots, H_{0k}$ holds.

The one-tailed p value p_i for the ith study is the probability that the test statistic T_i exceeds the obtained value t_{io} given that the null hypothesis is true. That is,

$$p_i = \text{Prob}\{T_i \geq t_{i0} | H_o\}$$

where t_{i0} is the value of the test statistic actually obtained (the sample realization of T_i) in the ith study. The one-tailed p value is the raw material for all omnibus tests of the statistical significance of combined results. Hence, the first step in combined significance testing is calculating a one-tailed p value for each study. Note that a statistically one-tailed p value should be computed regardless of whether the hypothesis in the individual studies are one- or two-tailed. One-tailed p values are used in metaanalysis so that small p values will have a consistent interpretation. The direction (tail) chosen should reflect the direction in which the preponderance of effects is expected to lie. The direction used should in principle be picked prior to examination of the data, and not as a reaction to it.

Many tests of the statistical significance of combined results have been proposed. It can be shown mathematically that no one combined significance test is the best (most powerful) in all situations, but the three tests discussed below have been shown to have generally good properties in many situations.

The Minimum p Method

The first combined significance test, proposed by Tippett (1931), is also the simplest. This method uses the minimum p value as a combined test

statistic. The logic of this test is that if any one p is small enough, H_0 should be rejected. If $p_1, \ldots, p_k$ are the one-tailed p values for k independent studies, the minimum p method rejects the combined null hypothesis at significance level α if

$$
\begin{aligned}
p_{\min} &= \text{minimum } \{p_1, \ldots, p_k\} < \alpha^* \\
&= 1 - (1 - \alpha)^{1/k}
\end{aligned}
\tag{1}
$$

One advantage of the minimum p method is that it is very easy to use, involving almost no computation. Its primary disadvantage is that it can reject H_0 only if at least one p value is already significant at level α. It is insensitive to situations in which several studies have small p values, but none is quite small enough to be significant by itself.

The Inverse Chi-Square Method

The most widely used combination procedure is that proposed by Fisher (1932) and independently by Pearson (1933). The method is usually called Fisher's method but is occasionally identified as a method due to Pearson. Given the one-tailed p values $p_1, \ldots, p_k$ from k independent studies, this method uses the product $p_1 p_2 \cdots p_k$ to combine the p values. The method is called the inverse chi-square method because when the null hypothesis H_0 is true,

$$P = -2 \log (p_i \cdots p_k) = -2 \sum_{i=1}^{k} \log p_i \tag{2}$$

has a chi-square distribution with $2k$ degrees of freedom. Thus, the inverse chi-square test rejects H_0 at significance level α if the statistic P exceeds the $100(1 - \alpha)$ percentile point of the chi-square distribution with $2k$ degrees of freedom.

The Inverse Normal Procedure

Another procedure for combining p values is the inverse normal method proposed by Stouffer, Suchman, DeVinney, Star, and Williams (1949). This procedure involves transforming each p value to the corresponding normal score, and then "averaging." More specifically, define z_i by $p_i =$

$\Phi(z_i)$, where $\Phi(x)$ is the standard normal cumulative distribution function. That is, z_i is the z score corresponding to the probability p_i. When H_0 is true, the statistic

$$Z = \frac{z_1 + \cdots + z_k}{\sqrt{k}}$$
$$= \frac{\Phi^{-1}(p_1) + \cdots + \Phi^{-1}(p_k)}{\sqrt{k}} \quad (3)$$

has the standard normal distribution. Thus, the inverse normal test rejects H_0 whenever Z exceeds the appropriate critical value of the standard normal distribution.

Example

Data from four studies of the relationship between Type A behavior and the incidence of coronary heart disease (CHD) are given in Table 1. The measure of Type A behavior, the definition of CHD, the covariates used, and the results reported are listed for each study. Note that two of the studies (Framingham and the Western Collaborative Study) reported data on two different samples of individuals which are treated as independent in this analysis. The one-tailed p value, the log of p and $z = \Phi^{-1}(p)$ are also given for each study. These values are used to compute the inverse normal and inverse chi-square summary statistics. The overall null hypothesis, in each study, is that the risk of CHD for individuals who are classified as Type A is the same as that for individuals who are not classified as Type A. The three combined significance tests will now be used to test this omnibus null hypothesis at the $\alpha = 0.01$ level of significance.

The test using the minimum p method consists of comparing 0.001, the minimum p value, with $0.0017 = 1 - (1 - 0.01)^{1/6}$, the value of α^* given in equation (1). Since the minimum p value is less than α^*, we reject H_0 using the minimum p method. Hence we conclude that there is a relationship between Type A behavior and CHD in at least one study.

The test of H_0 using the inverse chi-square method involves first calculating the combined test statistic P given in (2). In these data, $P = -2 \Sigma$

Table 1. Examples for Application of Combined Significance Tests: Studies of the Relationship between Type A Behavior and CHD

	Measure of Type A behavior	Outcome	Covariates[a]	Result reported	p	log p	z
French–Belgian Collaborative Group (1982)	Bortner Scale	MI	A, S, C, SBP, N	$p < 0.05$	0.050	−3.0	1.64
MRFIT (Shekelle *et al.*, 1985)	JAS	MI, CHD death	A, S, C, DBP, Al, E	$b = -0.006$ $SE = 0.005$	0.885	−0.12	−1.20
Framingham Study (Haynes *et al.*, 1980)	Framingham Scale	MI, CI angina, CHD death	A, S, C, SBP, P, Al				
Males aged 45–64				$t = 2.59$	0.005	−5.30	2.59
Females aged 45–64				$t = 2.83$	0.002	−6.21	2.83
Western Collaborative Study (Rosenman *et al.*, 1975)	SI	CHD	S, C, SBP, DBP, ST, SL, H				
Males aged 30–39				$p < 0.001$	0.001	−6.91	3.09
Males aged 50–59				$p < 0.001$	0.001	−6.91	3.09

[a]A, age; S, smoking; C, serum cholesterol; SBP, systolic blood pressure; DBP, diastolic blood pressure; N, neuroticism; Al, alcohol consumption; E, education; P, number of promotions; ST, serum triglycerides; SL, serum β/α lipoprotein ratio; H, family history of CHD.

$\log p_i = -2 (28.45) = 56.90$. Because 56.90 exceeds 26.2, the 99% point of the chi-square distribution with $2(6) = 12$ degrees of freedom, we also reject H_0 using the minimum p method.

The test of H_0 using the inverse normal method involves first calculating the combined test statistic Z given in (3). In these data $Z = \Sigma z_i/\sqrt{k} = 12.04/\sqrt{6} = 4.92$. Since 4.92 exceeds 2.33, the 99% critical value of the standard normal distribution, we also reject H_0 using the inverse normal procedure.

Limitations of Combined Significance Tests

In spite of the intuitive appeal of using combined test procedures to combine tests of treatment effects, there frequently are problems in the interpretation of results of such a test of the significance of combined results (e.g., see Adcock, 1960; Hedges & Olkin, 1985; Wallis, 1942). Just what can be concluded from the results of an omnibus test of the significance of combined results? Recall that the null hypothesis of the combined test procedure is

$$H_0: \theta_1 = \theta_2 = \ldots = \theta_k = 0$$

i.e., H_0 states that the treatment effect is zero in every study. If we reject H_0 using a combined test procedure, we may safely conclude that H_0 is false. However, H_0 is false if at least one of θ_1, $\ldots, \theta_k$ is different from zero. Therefore, H_0 could be false when $\theta_1 > 0$ and $\theta_2 = \ldots = \theta_k = 0$. It is doubtful if a researcher would regard such a situation as persuasive evidence of the efficacy of a treatment.

The difficulty in the interpretation of omnibus tests of the significance of combined results stems from the nonparametric nature of the tests. Rejection of the combined null hypothesis allows the investigator to conclude only that the omnibus null hypothesis is false. Errors of interpretation usually involve attempts to attach a parametric interpretation to the rejection of H_0. For example, an investigator might incorrectly conclude that because H_0 is rejected, the treatment effects are greater than zero (Adcock, 1960). Alternatively, an investigator might incorrectly conclude that the average treatment effect $\bar{\theta}$ is positive. Neither parametric interpretation of the rejection of H_0 is warranted without additional *a priori* assumptions.

An additional assumption that is sometimes made is that there is "no qualitative interaction." This assumption is that if the treatment effect in any study is positive, then no other treatment effect is negative. That is, all of the treatment effects are of the same sign but not necessarily of the same magnitude. If there is no qualitative interaction, then rejection of the omnibus null hypothesis does provide the basis for concluding that the average treatment effect $\bar{\theta}$ is positive. However, it is important to recognize that although the assumption of no qualitative interaction may seem innocuous, it is an assumption which must (in principle) be made independent of the data. There is often reason to believe that this assumption may be false. Consider the example of studies of the efficacy of a drug treatment. If a drug that actually has a positive effect on a specific disease also has toxic side effects, it might actually increase the death rate among some (e.g., older or sicker) patients. If some studies have more older or sicker patients, it is plausible that they might obtain negative treatment effects while other studies with younger or healthier patients found positive treatment effects.

The strength of combined significance tests is that they can be used to combine evidence on related hypotheses from studies with very different designs and using very different statistical analyses. Situations frequently arise where the differences between studies do not permit the description of study results in terms of any common index of treatment effect, yet the studies all test the efficacy of the same treatment. For example, different studies of the relationship between Type A behavior mortality due to CHD use quite different designs. Some studies report (and test the statistical significance of) relative risks, others report odds ratios, still others report the covariate adjusted difference in risk between Type A and Type B individuals. It may be difficult or impossible to derive a common index of effect magnitude given the summary statistics reported in the various studies. A combined significance test is possible, however, and can give some indication of whether the collection of results obtained in the various studies is likely to have occurred due to chance if there is no effect of Type A behavior.

An important application of omnibus test procedures is to combine the results of dissimilar studies to screen for any treatment effect. For example, combined test procedures can be used to test whether a treatment has an effect on any of a series of different outcome variables. Alternatively, combined test procedures can be used to combine the results of effect size analyses based on different outcome variables. Combined test procedures can even be used to combine the results of related analyses computed using different parameters such as correlation coefficients and effect sizes.

Omnibus tests of the statistical significance of combined results are poorly suited to the task of drawing general conclusions about the magnitude, direction, and consistency of treatment effects across studies. On the other hand, techniques based on combination of estimates of effect magnitude do support inferences about magnitude, direction, and consistency of effects. Therefore, statistical analyses based on effect sizes are preferable for most applications of metaanalysis.

Combined Estimation

When all of the studies have similar designs and measure the outcome construct in a similar (but not necessarily identical) manner, the combined estimation approach is probably the preferred method of metaanalysis (Hedges & Olkin, 1985). The first step in combined estimation is the selection of an index of effect magnitude. Many different indices of effect magnitude have been used in metaanalysis including the raw mean difference between the treatment and control groups (e.g., Cochran, 1937), the standardized difference between treatment and control group means (e.g., Smith & Glass, 1977), the observed minus expected frequency of some outcome like death (e.g., Yusuf, Peto, Lewis, Collins, & Sleight, 1985), the risk ratio between treatment and control groups (Canner, 1983), or the simple difference between proportions of some outcome in the treatment and control groups (e.g., Devine & Cook, 1983).

Statistical analysis procedures for metaanalysis using any of these indices of effect magnitude are analogous (Elashoff, 1978; Fleiss, 1973; Gilbert, McPeek, & Mosteller, 1977; Hedges, 1983; Hedges & Olkin, 1985; Mantel & Haenszel, 1959; Sheele, 1966). All involve large-sample theory and differ mainly in the details of calculation of standard errors and bias corrections.

Fixed, Random, and Mixed Models in Metaanalysis

Just as there are three statistical models for the analysis of variance, there are three somewhat analogous conceptualizations of statistical methods in metaanalysis: fixed-, random-, and mixed-effects models. Procedures for data analyses in these models are similar but the details and interpretation of statistical tests are somewhat different (see Hedges & Olkin, 1985).

In the fixed-effects analysis conceptualization, the true or population values of the treatment effects in the study are an (unknown) function of study characteristics. This is analogous to fixed-effects analysis of variance where the treatment effects are fixed, but unknown constants related to levels of the design factors. Fixed-effects models involve the assumption that stable relationships between study characteristics and treatment effects explain essentially all of the variability in study results except for that attributable to within-study sampling variability. In some cases, models for between-study variation are proposed and evaluated. However, fixed-effects models are not the only way to conceptualize data analysis in metaanalysis.

The random-effects conception arises from a model in which the treatment effects are *not* functions of known study characteristics. In this model (as in random-effect analysis of variance), the true or population values of treatment effects vary randomly from study to study, as if they were sampled from a universe of possible treatment effects (see Cronbach, 1980). Between study variation is conceived to be unsystematic in random-effects models and consequently explanation of this variance is not possible. Instead the data analyst usually seeks to quantify this variation by estimating a treatment by studies interaction "variance component": an index of the variability of population treatment effects across studies. Random-effects models have been used extensively in the study of validity generalization (see Schmidt & Hunter, 1977, or Hunter, Schmidt, & Jackson, 1982).

Mixed models involve a combination of the ideas involved in fixed- and in random-effects models. In these models, some of the variation between treatment effects is fixed (i.e., explainable) and some is random. Consequently, the data analyst seeks to explain some of the variation between study results and quantify the remainder by estimating the variance component (Raudenbush & Bryk, 1985). Such models have considerable promise as data analytic tools for situations in which it is useful to treat some but not all of the variability between study results as random.

The most important difference in the outcomes produced by the three types of statistical analyses lies in the standard errors that they associate with the overall (combined) estimates of the treatment effect. Fixed-effects analyses incorporate only within-study variability into the estimate of the standard error of the combined treatment effect. Fixed-effects analyses produce the smallest standard error estimates because they are, in fact, conditional on the known and unknown characteristics of the particular studies that have been done. Random-effects analyses include the between-study variance component in estimates of the standard error of the overall (combined) estimate of the treatment effect. Random-effects analyses typ-

ically produce larger standard errors because they incorporate the uncertainty associated with sampling from a superpopulation of studies. Mixed-effects analyses incorporate only unexplained between-study variation into the estimate of the standard error of the overall (combined) estimate of the treatment effect, and hence produce standard errors between those of fixed- and random-effects analyses.

Effect Size Estimates and Their Standard Errors

Suppose that $T_1, \ldots, T_k$ are independent estimates of effect magnitude from k studies with treatment and control group sample sizes n_1^T, $n_1^C, \ldots, n_k^T, n_k^C$ and unknown population effect magnitude parameters $\theta_1, \ldots, \theta_k$. Denote the sample estimated standard errors of $T_1, \ldots, T_k$ by $S_1, \ldots, S_k$. The procedures usually used in metaanalysis depend on the assumption that each T_i has a normal distribution when n_i^T and n_i^C are large. That is, we assume that in large samples

$$T_i \sim N(\theta_i, S_i^2) \qquad (4)$$

Fortunately, many indices of effect magnitude satisfy this assumption. A listing of indices of effect size and the formulas for their standard errors in large samples is given in Table 2. The description of statistical methods that follows describes the statistical analyses generally in terms of $T_1, \ldots, T_k$ and $S_1, \ldots, S_k$.

Table 2. Examples of Indices of Effect Magnitude and Their Standard Errors[a]

	T	S^2
Standardized mean difference	$(\bar{x}^T - \bar{x}^C)/s$	$(n^T + n^C)/n^T n^C + T^2/2(n^T + n^C)$
z-Transformed correlation	$0.5 ln[(1 + r)/(1 - r)]$	$1/(n - 3)$
Log odds ratio	$ln[p^T(1 - p^C)/p^C(1 - p^T)]$	$[n^T p^T(1 - p^T)]^{-1} + [n^C p^C(1 - p^C)]^{-1}$
Difference in proportions	$(p^T - p^C)/\bar{p}\bar{q}$	$(n^T + n^C)/(n^T n^C \bar{p}\bar{q})$
Mantel–Haenszel statistic	$(p^T - p^C)(n. - 1)/(n. \bar{p}\bar{q})$	$(n. - 1)/(\bar{p}\bar{q}n^T n^C)$

[a] $\bar{p}, \bar{q}$, and $n.$ are defined as follows: $\bar{p} = (n^T p^T + n^C p^C)/(n^T + n^C)$, $\bar{q} = 1 - \bar{p}$, and $n. = n^T + n^C$. For further details see Hedges and Olkin (1985) or Fleiss (1973).

Statistical Methods for Fixed-Effects
Metaanalysis

Estimating the Overall Average Treatment

One of the first statistical questions that arises is how to estimate the overall average treatment effect when it is believed that $\theta_1, \ldots, \theta_k$ are very similar. One way of combining the estimates is obviously to take the simple average of $T_1, \ldots, T_k$. The most precise combination (i.e., the most efficient estimator of θ when $\theta_1 = \ldots = \theta_k = \theta$) is a weighted average that takes the standard errors $S_1, \ldots, S_k$ into account. This weighted average is

$$T. = \sum_{i=1}^{k} \omega_i T_i \Big/ \sum_{i=1}^{k} \omega_i \qquad (5)$$

where $\omega_i = 1/S_i^2$. When all of the studies have reasonably large samples, the combined estimator $T.$ of θ has approximately a normal distribution given by

$$T. \sim N(\theta, S_.^2) \qquad (6)$$

where

$$S.^{-2} = \sum_{i=1}^{k} S_i^{-2} \qquad (7)$$

This result can be used to compute tests of significance and confidence intervals for θ based on $T.$. For example, a $100(1 - \alpha)$ percent confidence interval for θ is given by

$$T. - z_{\alpha/2} S. \leq \theta \leq T. + z_{\alpha/2} S. \qquad (8)$$

where $z_{\alpha/2}$ is the two-tailed critical value of the standard normal distribution. Alternatively, a test of the hypothesis that $\theta = \theta_0$ uses the statistic

$$Z = (T. - \theta_0)/S. \qquad (9)$$

which is compared to the critical values of the standard normal distribution.

Testing Homogeneity of Treatment Effects

Combining estimates of effect magnitude across studies is reasonable if the studies have a common population effect magnitude θ. In this case, the estimates of effect size differ only by unsystematic sampling error. However, if the studies have very different underlying treatment effects, it can be misleading to combine estimates of treatment effect across studies. For example, if half of the studies have a large positive population treatment effect and half of the studies have a large negative effect of equal magnitude, then the average— zero—is not representative of the treatment effects in any of the studies. The obvious question is, how is it possible to determine whether population treatment effects are relatively constant across studies? That is, how do we test for treatment-by-study interactions?

A simple test for homogeneity of treatment effects uses the statistic

$$H_T = \sum_{i=1}^{k} \omega_i (T_i - T.)^2 \qquad (10)$$

where $\omega_i = 1/S_i^2$ is the weight used in (5) and $T.$ is the weighted mean given by (5). The H_T statistic is simply the weighted sum of squares of the effect size estimates $T_1, \ldots, T_k$ about the weighted mean $T.$. If all studies share a common treatment effect θ, then H_T has approximately a chi-square distribution with $(k - 1)$ degrees of freedom. Thus, the test for treatment-by-study interaction rejects homogeneity of effect size for large values of H_T.

Although (10) helps to illustrate the intuitive nature of the H_T statistic, a computational formula is more useful in actually computing values of H_T. It can be shown that (10) is algebraically equivalent to the computational formula

$$H_T = \sum_{i=1}^{k} \omega_i T_i^2 - \left(\sum_{i=1}^{k} \omega_i T_i \right)^2 \Big/ \left(\sum_{i=1}^{k} \omega_i \right)$$

$$(11)$$

The advantage of (11) is that H_T can be computed from the sums across studies of three variables: ω_i, $\omega_i T_i$, $\omega_i T_i^2$. The weighted mean T. and its standard error S. can also be computed from the sums of ω_i and $\omega_i d_i$ values.

Partitioning Between-Study Variation

When effect magnitudes are not homogeneous across studies—i.e., when study-by-treatment interactions are present—it may be desirable to try to explain variations in effect magnitudes by variations in the characteristics of studies. One way of proceeding is to group studies that share characteristics than can influence effect size. Thus, the metaanalyst would seek to create groupings in which the variability of effect sizes was small.

A statistical procedure that permits this kind of analysis for effect magnitudes is an analogue to analysis of variance for effect sizes (see Hedges & Olkin, 1985). The analysis permits the testing of the effects of grouping and also permits the investigator to test whether the remaining variation within groups of effect sizes is significant. Thus, the metaanalyst can determine whether the explanatory grouping variable adequately explains the treatment-by-study interaction.

The analysis of variance for effect sizes involves a partitioning of the overall homogeneity statistic H_T given in (10) into two independent homogeneity statistics: H_B, reflecting between-group homogeneity, and H_W, reflecting within-group homogeneity. These homogeneity statistics are related by the algebraic identity $H_T = H_B + H_W$, which is analogous to the partitioning of sums of squares in analysis of variance.

The between-group homogeneity statistic H_B is a weighted sum of squares of weighted group mean effect size estimates about the overall weighted mean effect size. If there are L groups,

$$H_B = \sum_{j=1}^{L} \omega_{j.} (T_{j.} - T..)^2 \quad (12)$$

where $T..$ is the overall weighted mean across all studies ignoring groupings, $T_{j.}$ is the weighted

mean of the effect size estimates in the jth group, and $\omega_{j.} = 1/S_{j.}^2$ is the reciprocal of the variance of $T_{j.}$. Here the weighted means and their variances are calculated using (6) and (7).

When there are L groups, H_B has approximately a chi-square distribution with $(L - 1)$ degrees of freedom when there is no variation between group mean effect sizes. Thus, the test for variation in effect sizes between groups compares H_B with the $100(1 - \alpha)$ percent critical value of the chi-square distribution with $(L - 1)$ degrees of freedom. If H_B exceeds the critical value, the variation between group mean effect sizes is significant at level α.

The within-group homogeneity statistic is the sum of the homogeneity statistics calculated for each of the L groups separately. That is,

$$H_W = H_{W1} + \cdots + H_{WL} \quad (13)$$

where $H_{W1}, \ldots, H_{WL}$ are the homogeneity statistics (10) calculated as if each group were an entire collection of studies. Whenever a group contains more than one study, the within-group homogeneity statistic for the group can be used to test the homogeneity of effect sizes within that group. If there is only one effect size estimate in a group, then $H_{Wi} = 0$ for that group. The total H_W provides an overall test of homogeneity of effect size within the groups of studies.

If a total of k studies is divided into L groups, then H_W has a chi-square distribution with $(k - L)$ degrees of freedom when the effect sizes are homogeneous within groups. The test for homogeneity of effect size within groups at significance level α consists of comparing H_W with the $100(1 - \alpha)$ percent critical value of the chi-square distribution with $(k - L)$ degrees of freedom. The homogeneity of effect sizes within groups is rejected if H_W exceeds the critical value.

Let us suppose that the metaanalyst "explains" the variations in effect sizes by finding that effect sizes are reasonably homogeneous within groups but that they differ between groups. If there are only two groups of studies, then a significant H_B statistic indicates that there is a significant difference between their population effect sizes. If there are more than two groups, then the meta-analyst may want to use comparisons or contrasts analogous to those in analysis of variance to explore the differences among effect sizes for the different groups. Procedures for testing comparisons among the effect sizes of different groups follow from the properties of T; they have been discussed by Hedges and Olkin (1985).

The easiest way to compute the partitioning of between-study variation is to compute three variables for each study: $\omega_i = 1/S_i^2$, $\omega_i T_i$, and $\omega_i T_i^2$. The sums of these three variables across all studies can be used with (11) to compute H_T. The sums of ω_i, $\omega_i T_i$, and $\omega_i T_i^2$ for each group (of studies) separately permit H_{Wi} to be computed for each group using (11). Then, H_W is calculated as $H_W = H_{W1} + \cdots = H_{WL}$. Finally, H_B is computed as $H_B = H_T - H_W$. Note that the sums of ω_i and $\omega_i T_i$ for each group can also be used to compute the weighted mean effect size $T_{j.}$ and its standard error $S_{j.}$.

Statistical Methods for Random-Effects Metaanalysis

Again suppose that T_1, ...,T_k are independent estimates of treatment effects from k experiments with (unknown) population treatment effects θ_1, ...,θ_k. Again denote the estimated standard error of T_i given θ_i by S_i. Assume as before that the T_i are approximately normally distributed. Now, however, introduce the random-effects model that $\theta_1, \ldots ,\theta_k$ are sampled from a hyperpopulation of treatment effects. Often the θ_i are assumed to be normally distributed. The object of the analysis is to estimate the mean $\bar{\theta}$ and variance σ_θ^2 (the hyperparameters) of the distribution of population treatment effects, and to test the hypothesis that $\bar{\theta} = 0$.

A distribution-free approach to estimating σ_θ^2 is analogous to the procedure used to estimate the variance component in the one-factor random-effects analysis of variance. The estimate $\hat{\sigma}_\theta^2$ is given by

$$\hat{\sigma}_\theta^2 = S_T^2 - \sum_{i=1}^{k} S_i^2 / k \qquad (14)$$

where S_T^2 is the usual sample variance of $T_1, \ldots ,$ T_k (see Hedges & Olkin, 1985). More complex

procedures for estimating σ_θ^2 under various distributional assumptions on the θ_i are given in Champney (1983), Raudenbush and Bryk (1985), and Hedges and Olkin (1985).

A test of the hypothesis that $\sigma_\theta^2 = 0$ is exactly the same as the test of homogeneity of effect magnitude given in the section on fixed-effects analyses. Note, however, that the estimate $\hat{\sigma}_\theta^2$ of σ_θ^2 can differ substantially from zero even when it is not large enough to be statistically significant.

The usual estimate of $\bar{\theta}$ is the weighted mean

$$T^*_. = \sum_{i=1}^{k} \omega_i^* T_i \bigg/ \sum_{i=1}^{k} \omega_i^* \qquad (15)$$

where $\omega_i^* = 1/[\hat{\sigma}^2 + S_i^2]$. The weighted mean $T^*_.$ is approximately distributed

$$T^*_. \sim \mathrm{N}(\bar{\theta}, \sigma_*^2) \qquad (16)$$

where

$$\sigma_*^{-2} = \sum_{i=1}^{k} \omega_i^*$$

Consequently, an approximate confidence interval for $\bar{\theta}$ is given by

$$T^*_. - z_{\alpha/2}\sigma_* \leq \theta \leq T^*_. + z_{\alpha/2}\,\sigma_* \qquad (17)$$

where $z_{\alpha/2}$ is defined as in (8). Note that the weights ω_i^* used in (15) are not the same as the weights ω_i used in (5) unless $\hat{\sigma}_\theta^2$ is exactly zero. Usually $\hat{\sigma}_\theta^2$ is larger than zero and consequently $T^*_.$ differs from $T_.$. Moreover, the standard error σ_* of $T^*_.$ is usually larger (often much larger) than the standard error $\sigma_.$ of $T_.$. As a result, overall treatment effects that are significantly different from zero in a fixed-effects analysis may not be significant in random-effects analysis. The difference, of course, results from differences in the conceptualization of the model, and in what counts as sampling error.

Statistical Methods for Mixed-Effects Metaanalysis

Statistical methods for mixed-effects meta-analyses have received less complete treatment in the literature than have fixed- and random-effects models. There is a great deal of work in progress on metaanalysis with mixed-effects models. This work shows a great deal of potential for resolving differences between fixed- and random-effects approaches. One useful treatment of mixed-effects metaanalyses in the context of educational research is Raudenbush and Bryk (1985).

Example

Data from three studies of the relationship between Type A behavior patterns and the incidence of CHD are presented in Table 3. The general characteristics of these studies were summarized in Table 1. Note, however, that two samples (of males aged 45–64 and females aged 45–64, respectively) in the Framingham Study and two samples (of males aged 30–39 and males aged 50–59, respectively) in the Western Collaborative Study are treated as independent in this analysis. Table 3 presents the number of individuals at risk in the Type A and Type B classifications as well as the proportion who developed CHD. Using the log odds ratio as the estimator T, the square of the standard error is computed via the formula given in Table 2. The statistics $\omega_i = 1/S_i^2$, $\omega_i T_i$, and $\omega_i T_i^2$ used in the analysis are also given in Table 3.

The pooled estimate $T.$ of the log odds ratio is given by (5) as

$$T. = 56.60/99.98 = 0.567$$

and the standard error of $T.$ is given by (7) as

$$S(T.) = [1/99.98]^{-1/2} = 0.100$$

Hence, a 95% confidence interval for the pooled log odds ratio θ is

$$0.371 = 0.567 - 1.96(0.100) \le \theta \le 0.567 + (1.96)\,0.100 = 0.763$$

Because this confidence interval does not contain 1 [or alternately because $Z = (1.0-0.567)/0.100 = 4.33$ exceeds 1.96], the hypothesis that $\theta = 1$ is easily rejected at the $\alpha = 0.05$ level of significance.

To test the homogeneity of the log odds ratios, compute the statistic H_T given in (10) using the computational formula (11), which yields

$$H_T = 46.10 - (56.60)^2/99.98 = 14.03$$

Because 14.03, the obtained value of H_T, exceeds the 95% point of the chi-square distribution with

Table 3. Example of Data for Combined Estimation Studies of the Relationship between Type A Behavior and CHD

	Type A		Type B						
	n	$p(\%)$	n	$p(\%)$	T^a	S^2	ω	ωT	ωT^2
MRFIT (Shekelle et al., 1985)	2314	4.06	796	4.40	−0.083	0.041	24.42	−2.05	0.17
Framingham (Haynes et al., 1980)									
Males aged 45–64	276	16.7	294	9.52	0.645	0.66	15.26	9.84	6.34
Females aged 45–64	348	9.19	372	4.30	0.812	0.i00	10.02	8.14	6.61
Western Collaborative Study (Rosenman et al., 1975)									
Males aged 30–39	1067	8.9	1182	4.23	0.794	0.032	30.82	24.47	19.42
Males aged 50–59	522	15.9	383	7.57	0.837	0.052	19.36	16.20	13.55
Sums							99.98	56.60	46.10

^{a}Note: Here T is the log odds ratio.

$4 = 5 - 1$ degrees of freedom, we reject the hypothesis that all of the studies have the same log odds ratio. Hence, at least one study has a log odds ratio that differs from those of other studies. Therefore, the studies as a whole support the relationship between Type A behavior and CHD but do not agree on magnitude of the relationship expressed by the log odds ratio.

References

Adcock, C. J. (1960). A note on combining probabilities. *Psychometrika, 25,* 303–305.

Barnett, V., & Lewis, T. (1978). *Outliers in statistical data.* New York: Wiley.

Birge, R. T. (1932). The calculation of errors by the method of least squares. *Physical Review, 16,* 1–32.

Bozarth, J. D., & Roberts, R. R. (1972). Signifying significant significance. *American Psychologist, 27,* 774–775.

Canner, P. L. (1983). Aspirin in coronary heart disease: A comparison of six clinical trials. *Israel Journal of Medical Sciences, 19,* 413–423.

Chalmers, T. C. (1982). The randomized controlled trial as a basis for therapeutic decisions. In J. M. Lachin, N. Tygstrup, & E. Juhl (Eds.), *The randomized clinical trial and therapeutic decisions.* New York: Dekker.

Champney, T. F. (1983). *Adjustments for selection: Publication bias in quantitative research synthesis.* Unpublished doctoral dissertation, University of Chicago.

Cochran, W. C. (1937). Problems arising in the analysis of a series of similar experiments. *Journal of the Royal Statistical Society (Supplement), 4,* 102–118.

Cochran, W. C. (1943). The comparison of different scales of measurement for experimental results. *Annals of Mathematical Statistics, 14,* 205–216.

Cook, T. D., & Campbell, D. T. (1979). *Quasi-experimentation.* Chicago: Rand McNally.

Cooper, H. M. (1984). *The integrative research review: A systematic approach.* Beverly Hills, CA: Sage.

Cronbach, L. J. (1980). *Toward reform of program evaluation.* San Francisco: Jossey–Bass.

Devine, E. C., & Cook, T. D. (1983). Effects of psychoeducational interventions on length of hospital stay: A meta-analytic review of 34 studies. In R. J. Light (Ed.), *Evaluation studies review annual* (Vol. 8.) Beverly Hills, CA: Sage.

Elashoff, J. D. (1978). Combining the results of clinical trials. *Gastroenterology, 28,* 1170–1172.

Fisher, R. A. (1932). *Statistical methods for research workers* (4th ed.). London: Oliver & Boyd.

Fleiss, J. L. (1973). *Statistical methods for rates and proportions.* New York: Wiley.

French–Belgian Collaborative Group (1982). Ischemic heart disease and psychological patterns. *Advances in Cardiology. 29,* 25–31.

Gilbert, J. P., McPeek, B., & Mosteller, F. (1977). Progress in surgery and anesthesia: Benefits and risks of innovation therapy. In J. Bunker, B. Barnes, & F. Mosteller (Eds.), *Costs, risks, and benefits of surgery.* London: Oxford University Press.

Glass, G. V., McGaw, B., & Smith, M. L. (1981). *Meta-analysis in social research.* Beverly Hills, CA: Sage.

Hawkins, D. M. (1980). *Identification of outliers.* London: Chapman & Hall.

Haynes, S. G., Feinleib, M., & Kannel, W. B. (1980). The relationship of psychosocial factors to coronary heart disease in the Framingham study. *American Journal of Epidemiology, 111,* 37–58.

Hedges, L. V. (1983). Combining independent estimators in research synthesis. *British Journal of Mathematical and Statistical Psychology, 36,* 123–131.

Hedges, L. V. (1984). Estimation of effect size under nonrandom sampling: The effects of censoring studies yielding statistically insignificant mean differences. *Journal of Educational Statistics, 9,* 61–85.

Hedges, L. V., & Olkin, I. (1985). *Statistical methods for meta-analysis.* New York: Academic Press.

Hunter, J. E., Schmidt, F. L., & Jackson, G. B. (1982). *Meta-analysis: Cumulating research findings across studies.* Beverly Hills, CA: Sage.

Lane, D. M., & Dunlap, W. P. (1978). Estimating effect size: Bias resulting from the significance criterion in editorial decisions. *British Journal of Mathematical and Statistical Psychology, 31,* 107–112.

Light, R. J., & Pillemer, D. B. (1984). *Summing up: The science of reviewing research.* Cambridge, MA: Harvard University Press.

Mantel, N., & Haenszel, W. (1959). Statistical aspects of the analysis of data from retrospective studies. *Journal of the National Cancer Institute, 22,* 719–748.

Orwin, R. G., & Cordray, D. S. (1985). Effects of deficient reporting on meta-analysis: A conceptual framework. *Psychological Bulletin, 97,* 134–147.

Pearson, K. (1933). On a method of determining whether a sample of given size n supposed to have been drawn from a parent population having a known probability integral has probably been drawn at random. *Biometrika, 25,* 379–410.

Raudenbush, S. W., & Bryk, A. S. (1985). Empirical Bayes meta-analysis. *Journal of Educational Statistics, 10,* 75–98.

Rosenman, R. H., Brand, R. J., Jenkins, C. D., Friedman, M., Straus, R., & Wurm, M. (1975). Coronary heart disease in the Western Collaborative Group Study. *Journal of the American Medical Association, 233,* 872–877.

Rosenthal, R. (1984). *Meta-analytic procedures for social research.* Beverly Hills, CA: Sage.

Rubin, D. B. (1976). Inference and missing data. *Biometrika, 63,* 581–592.

Sackett, D. L. (1979). Bias in analytic research. *Journal of Chronic Diseases, 32,* 51–63.

Schmidt, F. L., & Hunter, J. E. (1977). Development of a general solution to the problem of validity generalization. *Journal of Applied Psychology, 62,* 529–540.

Sheele, P. R. (1966). Combination of log-relative risks in retrospective studies of disease. *American Journal of Public Health, 56,* 1745–1750.

Shekelle, R. B., Hulley, S. B., Neaton, J. D., Billings, J. H., Borhani, N. O., Gerace, T. A., Jacobs, D. R., Tasser, N. L., Mittlemark, M. B., & Stamler, J. (1985). The MRFIT Behavior Pattern Study. *American Journal of Epidemiology, 122,* 559–570.

Smith, M. L., & Glass, G. V. (1977). Meta-analysis of psychotherapy outcome studies. *American Psychologist, 32,* 752–760.

Sterling, T. C. (1959). Publication decisions and their possible effects on inferences drawn from tests of significance—or vice versa. *Journal of the American Statistical Association, 54,* 30–34.

Stock, W. A., Okun, M. A., Haring, M. J., Miller, W., Kinney, C., & Cuervorst, R. W. (1982). Rigor in data synthesis: A case study of reliability in meta-analysis. *Educational Researcher, 11,* 10–14, 20.

Stouffer, S. A., Suchman, E. A., DeVinney, L. C., Star, S. A., & Williams, R. M., Jr. (1949). *The American soldier: Vol. I. Adjustment during Army life.* Princeton, NJ: Princeton University Press.

Tippett, L. H. C. (1931). *The method of statistics.* London: Williams & Norgate.

Wallis, W. A. (1942). Compounding probabilities from independent significance tests. *Econometrica, 10,* 229–248.

Webb, E., Campbell, D. T., Schwartz, R., Sechrest, L., & Grove, J. (1981). *Nonreactive measures in the social sciences.* Boston: Houghton Mifflin.

Yates, F., & Cochran, W. G. (1938). The analysis of groups of experiments. *Journal of Agricultural Research, 28,* 556–580.

Yusuf, S., Peto, R., Lewis, J., Collins, R., & Sleight, P. (1985). Beta blockade during and after myocardial infarction: An overview of the randomized trials. *Progress in Cardiovascular Diseases, 27,* 335–371.

CHAPTER **41**

Pooling of Data from Independent Studies

Peter G. Kaufmann

Introduction

The large-scale, randomized clinical trial is generally regarded as a standard against which the credibility of other clinical investigations is evaluated. This is especially true if the effects to be studied are small or occur infrequently, and the trial has been conducted with a sample size sufficient to determine unequivocally the presence or absence of an effect. Increased sample size, or power, is therefore one immediately apparent reason for pooling data from several independent studies. This was the case in a study of several randomized trials comparing streptokinase therapy and heparin anticoagulation for the treatment of deep venous thrombosis (Goldhaber, Buring, Lipnick, & Hennikens, 1984). Pooling of results from several studies indicated a significant advantage of streptokinase treatment over heparin, but also revealed a significantly higher incidence of major bleeding complications for that treatment. Although the results of pooling could not resolve these questions of efficacy and safety, they did succeed in demonstrating a likelihood that a large-scale clinical trial would be able to do so. Pooling has also been used to extend the interpretation of data beyond the original aims of the individual studies, such as in explicating the relationship of risk factors to the incidence of coronary heart disease (Pooling Project Research Group, 1978), or to resolve ambiguous outcomes, as in evaluating the prophylactic efficacy of β-blockers after myocardial infarction (Bassan, Shalev, & Eliakim, 1984). However, because of the statistical nature of the benefits of pooling, it is not possible to use this approach to resolve truly conflicting results. That is, when several studies show statistically opposite outcomes, it is unlikely that these were caused by chance variations in the data, and the source of disagreement cannot be resolved by statistical techniques. These studies must be examined in detail to identify possible differences in experimental design, subject population, or other factors which may have affected the dynamics of the system under study. Finally, pooling can serve as an excellent vehicle for the detailed review of existing empirical or clinical procedures. The process of pooling data from independent studies can be a worthwhile and scholarly effort, likely to lead to new insights as well as the formulation of new hypotheses, provided appropriate cautions and limitations are kept in mind.

At least one attempt has been made to examine the possibility of establishing a psychophysiological data base which would be accessible via computer networks to allow drawing standardized information from a pool of documented data (Dolan, 1981). One advantage of such a data base is to decrease the need for repeated creation of control group data for basic psychophysiological

---

Peter G. Kaufmann • Behavioral Medicine Branch, National Heart, Lung, and Blood Institute, Bethesda, Maryland 20892.

665

research. A second is the opportunity for more extensive modeling and statistical inference as the size of the data base grows. The possibility of such an application was correctly seen as dependent on standardized methods of collecting and managing data, which may, however, restrict creativity in research. Another consideration is the limited utility of using historical controls, since characteristics of patients as well as clinical practice may be affected by changes in the cultural and social spheres, and by rapid evolution and refinements in traditional therapy and instrumentation.

Pooling of data is a tool which should be used with caution. In particular, due consideration must be given to the level of pooling that may be appropriate, with the objectives of the pooling subservient to the limits imposed by the available data and experimental designs. In general, there seem to be four levels at which data can be combined:

a. Data sets can be "seamlessly" joined, as if originating from the same experiment. To be eligible, protocols, procedures, eligibility criteria, and other aspects of experimental design and execution must be identical. This is an ideal rarely, if ever, achievable in biobehavioral studies.

b. Data sets can be joined, but the original source must be retained as a stratification variable to preserve the original randomization. This results in increased analytical complexity, but a necessary one. For example, two studies comparing the efficacy of alternate treatments for a disease may have been identical with respect to all aspects of experimental design. If one has been conducted in a primary care facility, and the other in a tertiary care facility, any observed differences in the relative success of the treatments under study may be entirely due to differences in the relative severity or progression of the disease. Breaking the original randomization would only serve to obscure important differences stemming from perhaps unintended, but real differences in the sample of patients.

c. The original data sets cannot be joined, but the same summary measures can be calculated, and it is these measures that can be

presented in a unified manner. The simplest of these is the pooling of z values, rather than actual test scores, from tests which measure the same attribute on different scales.

d. At the lowest level, not even the same measures can be computed for each of the diverse data sets, but statistical summaries, such as chi-square or p values, are accessible. This would be the only way to summarize results if some studies reported quantitative, others qualitative outcomes. For example, some studies comparing treatments for hypertension have used the change in blood pressure achieved by the participants as an objective measure of success, while others have employed a count of the number of participants who succeeded in reducing, or eliminating, medications. These results cannot be combined directly.

Thus, the degree of uniformity in experimental design and execution decreases from (a) to (d), influencing the level at which results can be pooled. Similarly, the degree of confidence in, and the definitiveness of the conclusions possible become progressively weaker in the same direction. Most metaanalytical studies are performed at levels (c) and (d).

Although no formal boundary has been defined, the difference between pooling and metaanalysis is that the latter can be thought of as the statistical analysis of the *summarized* data from a number of studies while pooling consists of the collection and analysis of the actual raw data. In the absence of identical protocols, a circumstance which is best regarded with much skepticism, the outcome of pooling data from several independent studies can never be regarded as equivalent to that of a single study which was conducted with an identical sample size, or to that of a coordinated trial in which several sites carried out identical protocols independently. Differences among the populations from which the samples are drawn, entry or disease criteria, methods employed, and even unknown influences of secular trends when studies were conducted at different points in time will make it difficult to justify combining data directly. In behavioral studies, analysis of methodological differences should be conducted with special care, since subtleties of instructions, therapist style, or expectation of the subject are more powerful influences in these studies than in studies comparing, for example, the efficacy of two medications delivered in pill form. Finally, many of the associations of behavioral factors with disease, and the mechanisms through which they exert their positive or negative influences, are very complex and poorly understood. Behavioral interventions are often less specific than interventions through medications or surgery, and their success is perceived to depend on a greater number of incidental variables. For these reasons, lack of vigilance in assessing experimental design issues is likely to result in errors of interpretation.

In this chapter, we will discuss some practical considerations for the pooling of data from independent studies, beginning with the formulation of objectives of the project, and going on to selection of studies and data, the mechanics of pooling, and additional considerations in data analysis. Technical issues of data analysis are treated in other chapters of this handbook, especially Chapter 40.

Planning Phase

Defining the Objectives

Design of pooled data analysis should not differ from that of *de novo* research in most respects. Experimental designs must be responsive to the questions to be asked and the issues to be addressed. Questions that can be addressed by pooling of data are not in any way unique. Feasibility will still be based on the basic mechanisms believed to underlie the processes to be examined, the present state of knowledge in the field, the experience of clinical practice, and so forth. It is useful to consider from the outset whether the goals are to (1) determine clinical efficacy or safety, (2) examine mechanisms, (3) test hypotheses, or (4) generate new hypotheses, as the answers to these questions will influence the choice of studies and type of data to be collected. For example, the question "Is relaxation therapy effective for reducing blood pressure?" requires different data than the question "Is cardiovascular reactivity affected by β-blockers?" In the first instance, success of a study would depend on strict definitions of eligibility, randomized group assignment, and detailed procedures for treatment and follow-up. However, the clinical application of relaxation therapy is probably practiced with some degree of individual differences among therapists, depending to some extent on the skills and style of the practitioner. A certain amount of variability among different sites of a multicenter clinical trial in carrying out the protocol would probably not be surprising and, in spite of the added statistical noise, perhaps even be regarded as desirable, as it would reflect the range of results that could be expected to occur in everyday clinical practice.

The question of cardiovascular reactivity, on the other hand, deals with physiological mechanisms. Attention is concentrated on obtaining data by a consistent technique under specific, controlled circumstances to assure that identical processes are measured. On the other hand, since much of the data might consist of biochemical determinations such as serum glucose, catecholamine, or electrolyte concentrations, whose measures exhibit relatively low variability, and each subject serves as his or her own control, a much smaller sample size might suffice to answer the question posed.

Testing of hypotheses requires a different degree of similarity of experimental design than is required for generating new hypotheses. The greater the differences in experimental design between different studies, the greater is the likelihood that the data will contain biases that do not allow comparability. However, pooling of data on a large number of variables from several small trials may allow for possibly important associations to emerge which, even though not statistically significant and derived from post hoc subgroup analysis, may suggest fruitful new avenues of research in the context of other knowledge at the disposal of the researcher. This is also the reason that involvement of individuals with expertise in the substantive issues addressed by the studies is essential for pooled data analysis to be maximally productive.

Choosing an Experimental Design

A useful strategy for establishing the design criteria for studies to be included in the pooled data is to determine the design of a *de novo* experiment or experiments which would best address the questions posed. There may be several possible alternative designs that would be equally acceptable, and it may not be necessary to choose only one of these. Inclusion criteria should consider, among other factors, criteria used in screening, the time of randomization, characteristics of patients, diagnostic criteria, stage of the disease at which patients are entered into the study, and duration, type of intervention, and length of follow-up. In behavioral studies, insufficient attention is frequently given to the effects of varying the duration of interventions, which can be regarded as analogous to drug dosage. Pooling of data from trials with treatment of different durations may require some consideration of that fact. This is especially true if the intervention is delivered "to effect," rather than for a specified period of time.

The context in which behavioral interventions are provided may also be important. For example, interventions for hypertension are frequently provided against a background of pharmacotherapy. Patients who need the support of behavioral interventions in addition to drugs (or vice versa) may be different from those for whom a single treatment modality is sufficient, not only because drugs fail to control their hypertension adequately, but because they may want to withdraw from drugs because of side effects. In either case, these groups may not be representative of the hypertensive populations as a whole, and even more unrepresentative of persons who are not yet hypertensive, but for whom behavioral interventions are advised as a preventive measure. Conclusions regarding the effectiveness of behavioral approaches based on data obtained from one of these groups may not be generalizable to the others. It would therefore be prudent to separate studies which used different inclusion criteria, especially those in which some disease-related inclusion criteria were used.

In contrast to the medical characteristics of the patients, it is often desirable that the demographic characteristics be allowed to vary as much as possible, including patients of diverse socioeconomic background, age, sex, employment status, and so forth, thus making the conclusions more generalizable, and enhancing the possibility of subgroup analysis. Hypotheses with respect to these sub-

groups should be formulated before the outcome of the main analysis is known.

In addition to establishing the desirable characteristics of studies to be included, it is useful to lay out beforehand the data and information that will be necessary to answer the questions posed. Before beginning the literature search, the desirable attributes of eligible designs should be tabulated and serve as a guide for analyzing candidate studies. Coding sheets can be prepared for this purpose to allow systematic recording of the information from each study and serve as a preliminary selection guide.

Selection of Studies

Literature Search

Although pooling does not involve obtaining new data, the amount of work involved in a thorough evaluation of the literature and analysis of published data is formidable. As much effort should be expended in this task as would go into design and conduct of an original research project. This process should fully utilize the search capabilities of bibliographic data bases such as *Medline, Biological, Psychological,* and *Dissertation Abstracts, Science Citation Index,* and *Social Science Citation Index.* Review of the literature will be made easier by the previously prepared model experimental designs regarded as suitable for inclusion. These decisions should be made on the basis of detailed evaluation of the methods in each study. For this purpose, it is very useful to interview the investigators from each study to verify details and clarify ambiguities in the published reports. Ideally, power analyses should be performed to determine the sample sizes necessary to adequately address all of the main and subsidiary questions which have been anticipated (see Chapter 38). This will help to determine in advance whether the number of studies available is sufficient for the purposes intended, or whether to expand the search. Different cell sizes will be necessary for different issues, and may serve as an additional guide for selecting studies to be included.

It is important to recognize that the outcome of pooling may well depend on the studies selected. Consequently, establishing the rules for inclusion or exclusion of studies, as discussed above, serves to make that selection process as unbiased as possible. Decisions are not to be regarded as irrevocable because, as detailed information becomes available at later stages of descriptive analysis, some of the studies may be found to be unsuited for inclusion. The pooling project for studying the relationship of blood pressure, serum cholesterol, smoking, and other risk factors to the incidence of coronary heart disease (Pooling Project Research Group, 1978) began with analysis of six studies, and two more were added at a later date. Finally, more detailed examination of the data revealed that only four of the original studies and one of the additional ones were sufficiently comparable to be combined. Data from the other three were presented separately.

Clearly, obtaining access to the raw data from a given study will require the cooperation of the owners of that data, who can also contribute substantially to its thoughtful analysis. They should be invited as full collaborators and included as coauthors of any reports to be published.

Selection of Data

When the studies have been selected and agreement secured from the contributing investigators, detailed arrangements have to be made for the selection and transfer of data to the center which will be responsible for compiling the data base. The type of arrangements necessary will depend on the size of the project, but in many instances it will be desirable, resources permitting, to convene a meeting of participants in order to clarify not only technical issues related to definitions of variables, data, or the mechanics of collection, but also administrative issues such as writing and publication of reports, allocation of resources, and so forth. The experience of clinical trials is very useful in this regard, as the conduct of a multicenter trial involves all of these issues (Friedman, Furberg, & DeMets, 1985). Thus, the participants may wish to meet periodically to review progress, deal with unexpected problems, or plan data analysis. Some of the data, such as a review of diagnoses based on consistent criteria, may require reinterpretation by an independent source. Thus, for large projects, a steering committee can serve the function of overseeing orderly review of those decisions that the organizers of the pooling project cannot or do not wish to make unilaterally. Such a committee can also participate from the outset in the decisions regarding the choice of data to be collected, since no one is as familiar with the methodological details as the investigators who conducted the original study.

Several committees were organized for the Hypertension Intervention Pooling Project (Kaufmann et al., 1988), which was organized to assess research in behavioral approaches for the treatment of hypertension: (1) Steering—to evaluate the aims of the project and act as an oversight committee; (2) Analysis—to examine in detail the experimental designs of the sites submitting data to the project, determine which data are suitable for inclusion, and participate in the design of the statistical analysis; and (3) Publications—to coordinate the writing of reports based on the findings, and to establish and oversee guidelines for their publication.

Additional, specialized committees evaluated endpoints, medications, and treatment variables. The organizational aspects of such an effort are formidable.

It is tempting to compile an exhaustive list of data to be collected in a pooling effort. This is a natural tendency for research scientists in any setting, but a balance must be struck between the known needs of the project, possibly interesting subgroup analyses that may be decided upon later, and the resources available to the project. The fact is that the workload grows very rapidly with the inclusion of each new variable, both in terms of the time required to retrieve and transcribe the data from the original, as well as to enter the data into the project files. Emphasis should be on data quality, rather than on quantity, both in the original and transcribed data.

The most important considerations in deciding whether a particular item should be included are whether a sufficient number of studies have collected it and whether it is likely to contribute to the analysis. A coding form that includes all of the candidate data should be constructed and used to tabulate available information. This can be compared with the requirements as determined by power analysis. In addition to information related to substantive issues of the project, collecting complete demographic and medical history may allow formulation of new hypotheses based on subgroup analyses. Information about age, sex, height and weight, race, marital status, occupation, education, smoking history, alcohol, coffee, and tea consumption, nutrition, exercise, coping styles, and other psychosocial attributes, is frequently collected. These attributes are of such frequent utility that their inclusion should not be the cause of much debate in larger projects. Medical files may also contain much information that is unlikely to be used, or has little overlap between studies. There are numerous laboratory values for blood chemistry, for example, only some of which may have been collected in different studies or which may be unrelated to questions of interest. Decisions on these should be a relatively simple matter. Data which have been collected repetitively and in large quantities should be carefully scrutinized. Consider, for example, the amount of blood pressure data that might have been recorded in a study on a particular treatment for hypertension. It is common to take blood pressure values for several consecutive cuffings, and not unusual for measurements to be duplicated in several different parts of a clinic during the same visit. Consequently, information may be available for readings obtained by any combination of physician, nurse, technician, medical student, or behavioral therapist. The readings may have been taken in a sitting, standing, or supine position, at rest or after exercise, prior to, during, or after a physical examination or relaxation therapy session. One or both arms may have been used, and measurements obtained on a mercury or aneroid manometer, a random zero or automatic device, and recorded with or without a scheme for rounding. Values at the disappearance of the fourth or fifth phase Korotkoff sounds may have been recorded.

Similar complexity may exist for psychosocial instruments. Data may have been collected by direct interview, self-administered questionnaire,

obtained from existing records or newly administered. Interviews or test administration may have been conducted by professionals, students, or technicians. It is not unusual for health habit or nutritional data to depend on recall. The accuracy of such information is a function of the time elapsed, and thus may vary from study to study. It will be necessary to decide whether scores were affected by the method of administration or time of data collection, selecting only those that are valid for the purpose of the project. Although there are only a limited number of variables in any one category of data that may be of interest, the cumulative effect of a large number of variables on the workload is easily underestimated. Making prudent choices early could save a lot of effort later in data entry, auditing, validating, editing the data files, and evaluating reams of summary statistics. The creation of a model experimental design as suggested earlier may serve as a resource for making such decisions.

Mechanics of Pooling

Missing Data and Exclusion of Subjects

Every clinical study has to contend with missing data because of noncompliance, dropouts, deaths, and other reasons. It is important that data be collected from all patients who were randomized in a study, regardless of the duration of their participation or the reasons for withdrawal. Randomization is carried out in order to minimize the possibility of selection bias. There is always the possibility that subjects who do not complete the protocol are a self-selected subset of the population. Regardless of what the rules of the original studies were, data should therefore be included on all subjects randomized. The greatest difficulty encountered in that regard is that considerable blocks of data may be unavailable for some individuals. If the number of subjects or amount of data missing is large, the analysis will be difficult and confidence in the outcome will be weakened. One method of dealing with this problem is to assign values for the missing data, based on estimates of the range of values that might have occurred (May, DeMets, Friedman, Furberg, & Passamani, 1981). Analyses are then carried out using projections of the worst and best case. If the objective of the project is the formulation of hypotheses, this kind of manipulation is not likely to affect the outcome of the conclusions. If the purpose is hypothesis testing, missing data will result in a need to qualify the conclusions because of the possibility that a selection bias has occurred.

Occasional missing data points are less problematic. If the sample size is large, and the effect robust, a missing value will simply have the effect of decreasing the sample size for that attribute and will not have a significant impact on the outcome. Alternatively, these values can also be interpolated based on data that are available. These issues are common and have been extensively discussed in the clinical trial literature, which should be consulted for additional thoughts on these issues (Friedman *et al.*, 1985; see also Hedges, this volume). It is important to recognize that there are not always "correct" solutions, but the implications of choosing one approach or another should be fully understood.

Transcription of Data

An important strategy decision is whether to use paper forms or enter the data directly into a computer. Clearly, the single most important objective at this stage is the compilation of accurate data files. Another consideration is to make the process less labor-intensive. Neither alternative is without disadvantages, and both have much in common. We will not consider the use of optical scanning methods, which require specialized equipment and are quite labor-intensive during design and when filling out data forms. In experienced hands they might, however, decrease errors of transcription.

For either approach, a comprehensive set of forms must be constructed which define and organize the data to be collected. If these forms have a simple structure, any item of information can be found quickly, without having to search the entire page. This also facilitates data entry and editing. The best structure is to have all data along one edge of the page, unless a tabular form is necessary. It is much easier to spend additional

time being thorough than to insert additional items after data collection has begun. If manual entry is chosen, numerous copies of the forms are printed and distributed to the participating sites, which will transcribe information from the existing records. If data are to be entered directly into a computer file, the forms will guide the design of a software program to enter information directly into a data base. The advantages of manual entry are that data entry can begin immediately while the software is being written and tested, no plans need to be made to assure compatibility of software with equipment available at each site, and little special training is required to fill out the forms correctly. However, one additional opportunity for error has been interpolated between the raw data files and the final data base. Although copying information from one file to another seems easy, it is a repetitive, boring task in which errors occur due to loss of vigilance over time. In the Hypertension Intervention Pooling Project (HIPP), the combined error rate for data entry was estimated at 0.05%. This was done by entering a 5% randomly chosen sample of the data twice, and comparing the resulting two files by a software program available for that purpose. Although an error rate of 0.05% seems small, the 20 Mbyte data base of the project was estimated to include ten thousand errors, many of which were significant and had to be corrected. Approximately two thirds of the errors were traced to the transcription of original data to the paper forms. Only one third was due to errors of keying while transferring information from the forms to the computer file. The forms did serve as a permanent record, or "paper trail," of the originally entered and corrected values, and could be compared with the medical records at the clinics.

Direct computer entry eliminates the intermediate step. In fact, an excellent method is to write an interactive program which displays, on a monitor, questions as they would appear on a paper form, and prompts the user for responses in the proper sequence. It is a simple matter to scroll back and forth within a record to edit or verify entries. Thus, although paper forms would not immediately be available to serve as a permanent record of the original transcribed data, a printed version of the records can be produced at will. In addition, the software can be designed to enter automatically the correct codes for data not collected at a given site, and permit only authorized personnel to change individual records after they are completed. Information identifying the clinic, subject, and key demographic characteristics need only be entered once, and can automatically be printed on every page of the report for a given subject. Although keying of data from the original files will be considerably slower than keying data from a uniform set of forms, the method will probably be more attractive to the person performing the work. The disadvantage is that much more advance planning and coordination is needed before data entry can begin. In the long run, it is likely that computer entry will save time and expense, as most of the software would be needed for either data entry method. Errors should be reduced substantially by eliminating one step in the compilation of data.

Whichever method is chosen, it is vital that a detailed data entry manual be written which anticipates any questions which may arise from the data entry personnel. Most uncertainties arise from ambiguities in interpretation of a given item. Although the interpretation is undoubtedly clear in the minds of those who conceived the question, it is not necessarily so in the minds of those having to translate medical records. For example, an item dealing with prescribed medications might request listing, for a given visit to a clinic, all medications the patient is taking. Should the response include medications newly prescribed at that visit, or only those already taken up to that time? The manual of procedures should be a complete rendition of the aims of the project, the study design, and, for each individual clinic, a section that deals with issues unique to that clinic. This should include a general description of the study design, specific inclusion and exclusion criteria for subjects, and the data to be expected from that particular study. A properly filled out sample form or, in the case of computer entry, copies of sample screens should be included in the manual. For computer entry, the data entry manual should include relevant sections from the software documentation manual.

Before data entry begins in earnest, it is a good idea to hold individual ''walk-throughs'' with each of the data entry personnel and review all data to be collected, item by item. This should be followed by detailed examination of several completed forms or computer records, and immediate feedback to clarify problems or confirm satisfaction with the product.

Finally, since most data are now processed by computer, the data from participating sites may be available for submission through a modem or on magnetic storage devices. Competent programmer-analysts would be able to extract the needed information in a format suitable for the data center.

Data Base Design and Data Entry

The value of early involvement of statistical and computer programming expertise cannot be overestimated. Computers have greatly facilitated data management and analysis, but also have amplified the distance of the investigator from the data and the magnitude of potential errors. There is nothing more frustrating than lack of access to one's data, lack of faith in the content or structure of data files, or a clumsy editing procedure. For large projects, a biostatistician with experience in clinical trials is a definite asset, and should be recruited at the time the objectives have been formulated. Computer programming expertise should be recruited as soon as the amount and type of data can be estimated so that the experience necessary can be matched to the needs of the project. The input of both the computer programmer-analyst and the statistician is essential for design of data entry procedures and the data base. Their assistance will only be as good as their understanding of the objectives. Their advice will also be needed to establish intermediate goals and timeliness, especially for the more mechanical tasks of data transfer and editing, which tend to be very labor-intensive and thus command the lion's share of the resources.

Editing and Cleaning of Data

Attention to data accuracy from the beginning will greatly reduce the work required to verify, edit, and correct the data files. Although the error rate is typically small in the absence of a systematic problem, for large studies even a small error rate can result in thousands of false entries. Many of these are noncritical. That is, they may reflect misspelling in a drug name or job description which need not necessarily be corrected. Others constitute errors in routine information such as subject or clinic identification, and can be easily traced. Most problematic are errors in numerical information such as laboratory or blood pressure values, for which no reliable editing scheme can be established.

A number of techniques can be applied to minimize errors at the time of data entry. One of the most important is to establish criteria for what may be considered as a valid entry for a given field. This includes defining a field as numeric, alphanumeric, or alphabetic. Thus, any alphabetic entry to a field which is to contain the year of birth would immediately be flagged. The entry would have to be edited before the program proceeds to the next field. Another is to tabulate the range of values that are valid for entries in a specific field. For example, it is very unlikely that LDL cholesterol concentrations fall outside of 75–300 mg/dl in Western industrial societies. Thus, entries that fall outside of this range are immediately suspect. Similar ''range check'' values can be established for virtually every numeric field in the data base. Another frequently used method is to compare mutually exclusive items. For example, it is unlikely that males would be taking oral contraceptives, and impossible that diastolic blood pressures would be higher than systolic. The first line of defense is therefore a thoughtfully constructed file editor which monitors values as they are entered. Make sure the data entry manual specifies procedures for dealing with problems that cannot be resolved by data entry personnel, who should not be relied upon to substitute a ''corrected'' value if the value they encounter falls outside of the specified range.

The next line of defense is to perform audits of data that can be checked according to some logic scheme, such as determining the chronological sequence of a series of clinic visits by a patient. Finally, summary statistics can be run to reveal discrepancies in group totals of various demographic characteristics, extreme values, or other anomalies. In almost all instances, it will be necessary to check the original records or the paper trail

to reveal the context of the problem and the possible solution. In clinical trials, it is not uncommon to deal with suspiciously high or low values by eliminating as much as 10–20% of the data at the extremes of the distribution. This may not be practical if one of the aims of the analysis is to reveal differences in variability of some characteristic as a function of an intervention, and a much more modest scheme may be applied to censor extreme values. It will never be possible to achieve an errorless data file, but systematic procedures during entry and editing can reduce errors to an insignificant level.

Data Analysis

Analysis of Individual Studies

If there is an analysis committee, the lead statistician and computer programmer should become members and attend all meetings. In any case, the analysis plan will have been outlined in good part at the time the study was designed, with substantial help from the statistician. The major difference between data pooling studies and an original research design, and its greatest weakness, is the lack of a single, coordinated research protocol. The results of the analysis will therefore be qualified by the degree to which the individual designs are dissimilar. Hence, it is important to document in some detail the methods and experimental design of the individual studies. This should be one of the first tasks undertaken following data entry, as that process will probably have revealed any subtle differences between studies that might have been missed during the initial evaluation. A complete rationale for excluding all studies whose participation was anticipated, or including substitute studies should be explicitly stated, and will contribute toward understanding the scope and delimiting parameters of the final data set.

Before beginning the pooled analysis, each study should be analyzed separately. It is likely that the results of the individual studies will already have been published independently. If not, the investigator nonetheless may have completed his or her own data analysis, whose outcome may be compared with that of the data set submitted for pooling as an additional check on the identity of the data sets, keeping in mind any differences in inclusion criteria between the original and pooled data.

Analysis of the Pooled Data Set

The investigators will have expended a lot of time and resources in arriving at an analysis file, and will want to reap a full harvest from the effort by conducting every comparison possible. Many of the statistical techniques appropriate for analysis of pooled data sets are discussed elsewhere in this volume (see Chapter 40), but a few principles with respect to direct comparison of subjects across studies, the relative contribution of individual studies to the pooled analysis, and analysis of subgroups are especially important to keep in mind.

Because of known as well as undetermined differences in design and subject population between studies, subjects from one study should never be compared directly with those from another for purposes of hypothesis testing (Goldhaber *et al.*, 1984). This would occur if, for example, all subjects receiving a specific intervention were combined to one group, and compared with all subjects receiving a different, or placebo intervention. In the extreme case, individuals from the control group of one study might be compared with the active intervention group from another. A statistically acceptable technique for estimating differences between groups with respect to event rates of, for example, death, myocardial infarctions, or hospitalizations, is the Mantel–Haenszel Procedure (Mantel & Haenszel, 1959; Friedman *et al.*, 1985). This comparison is accomplished by treating each study as a stratum, and examining whether the distribution of observed versus expected events from the strata differs randomly from zero. Stratified analysis can also be applied to subgroups from each study, and when comparing continuous variables.

When it is suspected that highly significant results from one or two studies determine the outcome of a pooled analysis, it may be useful to perform an additional analysis based on separate pooling of the studies whose results failed to reach statistical significance. This was done in the pooled analysis of seven trials to determine whether prophylactic treatment with β-blockers improves the prognosis of post-myocardial infarction patients (Pooling Project Research Group, 1978). Only two of the seven trials which met the inclusion criteria for pooling had found a significant reduction in mortality in the β-blocker group. The pooled analysis of all seven studies also showed a statistically significant advantage for the treated group, but it was possible that this outcome was driven by the two successful studies. However, pooling of results from the five trials which, individually, failed to find a significant advantage for β-blocker therapy also confirmed this outcome, greatly bolstering confidence in the results.

Analysis of data by subgroups which were not specified at the time the trial was designed has been a source of controversy because, as the number of statistical tests increases, so does the likelihood of type I error (see Chapter 37). It is especially viewed with suspicion when the main hypothesis has not been supported or even contradicted. Conceivably, the pooling project itself may have been motivated by the belief that even though a given study or series of studies failed to uncover the benefit of an intervention, such a benefit exists for some undefined segment of the population.

It would be unfortunate, however, not to attempt to uncover information which may be either especially advantageous or harmful for certain groups of patients. In pooling data from several studies, certain subgroup analyses may become possible because sample sizes for given features will have increased to the point at which sufficient power exists to answer a particular question. Prudent clinical trial practice requires that the subsidiary questions to be answered by the pooled analysis be stated in advance, be based on characteristics which can be determined at randomization or baseline and, preferably, having a plausible explanatory mechanism with independent support in the scientific literature. Although subgroup analyses which are based on postrandomization variables are frowned upon (May *et al.*, 1981), it is difficult to ignore, for example, the influence of variations in adherence on efficacy of a treatment when a significant dose–response relationship exists (Lipid Research Clinics Program, 1984).

Subgroup analyses which were not specified in advance are to be interpreted with caution as it is always possible that the relationship is spurious. If, however, the outcomes of such analyses are regarded as hypotheses to be investigated, they will have fulfilled one of the prime purposes of data pooling.

Other Factors Influencing Data Analysis

Pooling of data from several independent trials has several inherent risks stemming from non-homogeneity of the experimental methods and populations from which the samples are drawn. Some of these have already been pointed out. They also have implications for data analysis and interpretation. Data may be gathered from studies with different screening methods, exclusion criteria, and baseline criteria. In HIPP, most designs stipulated a fixed length of time during which baseline data were collected. In one study the baseline period varied in duration from 6 weeks to 1 year, depending on whether or not blood pressure was stable for three consecutive weekly visits. Values of laboratory tests may vary in reliability depending on the methods used to perform the assays. Screening criteria may select patients with identical diagnoses, but in some of these, different disease processes may be operative. This is especially true for diseases whose diagnosis depends on the value of a continuous variable, such as blood pressure, which may be affected by pathology in any of the several physiological systems governing it. Older patients or those with more elevated blood pressures at entry may have more advanced disease, affecting a greater number or type of homeostatic processes, or have produced significantly different amounts of end-organ damage. Any of these might affect the outcome of a given therapy in unknown ways. If all patients are receiving behavioral interventions against a background of pharmacological treatment, termination or reduction of medications may either precede or follow success of the behavioral intervention to some criterion. In HIPP, plans were made for a single arbiter to evaluate the level of medications of patients in all trials, thus decreasing differences due to application of different criteria by several raters. Such independent audits could also be performed for medical or psychological diagnoses, causes of death, or interpretation of angiographic findings, CAT scans, or ECG tracings. Finally, because not all data are typically available from all sites participating in pooling, it may be that conclusions reached with respect to one dependent variable may be based on a different combination of samples than conclusions reached with respect to another variable. These conclusions may not be equally generalizable. It is therefore important that the written report emphasize the strengths as well as weaknesses of the data, point out differences between studies, and encourage independent thought with respect to the conclusions that have been reached.

Pooling of data has been discussed only with respect to independent studies. Most of the weaknesses of such an approach arise from differences in methodology which limit comparability of data. There is no reason that pooling could not be anticipated sufficiently in advance of the implementation or completion of a project so that experimental designs could be modified, or specific demographic or biobehavioral data included to enhance comparability with other trials. As investigators recognize the potential for increasing the power and generalizability of their research through pooling, collaborative activities are likely to be increased. The effort expended in such coordination would more than pay for itself in terms of scientific rigor and complexity of the questions that could be opened to systematic investigation.

ACKNOWLEDGMENT. This chapter is based on the experience of the Hypertension Intervention Pooling Project, an evaluation of research on behavioral interventions for hypertension. Review of the manuscript and helpful comments by Larry Muenz, the statistical consultant for that project, have been especially valuable.

References

Bassan, M. M., Shalev, O., & Eliakim, A. (1984). Improved prognosis during long-term treatment after myocardial infarction: Analysis of randomized trials and pooling of results. *Heart and Lung, 13,* 164–168.

Dolan, P. M. (1981). Invited editorial: Toward meeting the

scientific, technological and financial challenges of the 1980's. *Psychophysiology, 18,* 514–517.

Friedman, L. M., Furberg, C. D., & DeMets, D. L. (1985). *Fundamentals of clinical trials.* Littleton, MA: PSG Publishing.

Goldhaber, S. Z., Buring, J. E., Lipnick, R. J., & Hennikens, C. H. (1984). Pooled analyses of randomized trials of streptokinase and heparin in phlebographically documented acute deep venous thrombosis. *American Journal of Medicine, 76,* 393–397.

Kaufmann, P. G., Jacob, R. G., Ewart, C. K., Chesney, M. A., Muenz, L. R., Doub, N., Mercer, W., & HIPP Investigators (1988). Hypertension Intervention Pooling Project. *Health Psychology, 7* (Suppl.), 209–224.

Lipid Research Clinics Program (1984). The Lipid Research Clinics Coronary Primary Prevention Trial results. II. The relationship of reduction in incidence of coronary heart disease to cholesterol lowering. *Journal of the American Medical Association, 251,* 365–374.

Mantel, N., & Haenszel, W. (1959). Statistical aspects of the analysis of data from retrospective studies of disease. *Journal of the National Cancer Institute, 22,* 719–748.

May, G. S., DeMets, D. L., Friedman, L. M., Furberg, C., & Passamani, E. (1981). The randomized clinical trial: Bias in analysis. *Circulation, 64,* 669–673.

Pooling Project Research Group (1978). Relationship of blood pressure, serum cholesterol, smoking habit, relative weight and ECG abnormalities to incidence of major coronary events: Final report of the Pooling Project. *Journal of Chronic Diseases, 31,* 201–306.

CHAPTER 42

Clinical Trials

Lewis H. Kuller

Introduction

Epidemiological studies are classified into descriptive, analytical, and experimental or clinical trials. Descriptive studies quantify the distribution of disease or characteristics of individuals within defined populations such as a geographic area or an occupational group. This distribution is often related to the characteristics of both the individual such as age, race, and sex and the environment. Analytical studies are of two broad types, retrospective or case-control and longitudinal or prospective. The goal of analytical studies is to determine the relationship between a defined independent variable or a risk factor, and a disease or dependent variable, or certain other characteristics of the individual. The variables initially measured are called the independent variables and the outcome, dependent variables. The experimental or clinical trials modify the independent variables in order to determine the effects on a dependent variable or outcome. The science of epidemiology deals primarily with the determinants of epidemics and the evaluation of methods of their control and prevention. The epidemiological methods are useful for the study of most diseases whether traditional acute, usually

infectious diseases, or the longer-incubation-period, chronic diseases. The descriptive and analytical studies are of primary importance in determining the magnitude of the epidemic in relationship to time, place, and personal characteristics and the identification of probable risk factors of disease. Most of the interest in behavioral variables relates to diseases that have relatively long incubation periods, are difficult to accurately measure, and are often believed to have a "multifactorial" etiology. Often the estimated relative risk of any single variable is low and may be inconsistent from study to study. Many of these diseases have a relatively long incubation period prior to apparent clinical disease. Many also may have a relatively high prevalence of inapparent as compared to clinical disease. During the long incubation period, physiological changes may occur that result in modification of other risk factors for the disease. For example, weight loss and certain nutritional changes may occur years before the diagnosis of cancer. It is possible that metabolic changes at the cellular level may be the reasons for some of these early physiologic changes such as the weight loss. The subsequent weight loss as well as other nutritional changes and the cellular metabolic abnormalities then result in a substantial fall in the serum cholesterol levels. Measurement prospectively in a population study then is noted to have an inverse relationship with the subsequent risk of cancer (Sherwin *et al.*, 1987). The longer the time be-

Lewis H. Kuller • Department of Epidemiology, University of Pittsburgh, Graduate School of Public Health, Pittsburgh, Pennsylvania 15261.

tween cholesterol measurement and either the incidence or death from cancer, the weaker is the relationship between cholesterol and cancer.

Several of our recent studies have documented an association between various aspects of ion transport, obesity, serum insulin and triglyceride levels, and blood pressure (Bunker, 1987). It is possible that the determinants of the serum insulin levels are the primary factor that link these interrelationships. Insulin levels have effects on many metabolic processes including central nervous system function. Thus, behaviors supposedly related to blood pressure levels may only be a manifestation of insulin metabolism, or perhaps of the effects of insulin on cellular transport of sodium and potassium or divalent cations. Only experimental manipulation of these complex interrelationships will resolve some of these intriguing questions. Also, by the time the individual has developed clinical disease, e.g., hypertension, the initial metabolic abnormalities may have been substantially modified and do not appear to be important risk factors for the disease.

The concept that most of the chronic diseases are multifactorial may be an inappropriate approach to scientific investigation. The multiple origins of these diseases relate primarily to either a lack of understanding of the interrelationships between pathology, physiology, and clinical disease, or misclassification of several diseases with similar clinical characteristics as a single disease.

Clinical coronary heart disease is a good example of this multifactorial illusion. The clinical disease, i.c., myocardial infarction, sudden death, and angina pectoris, is determined by three unique pathophysiological events: one, the evolution of atherosclerosis; two, the formation of a thrombus; and three, changes predominately in left ventricular function secondary to the size of the myocardial infarction (Kuller, 1986).

Coronary atherosclerosis is primarily a disease of lipid metabolism (Stamler, 1980). The primary risk factor is the amount of cholesterol and saturated fat in the diet. Genetic factors contribute substantially to both the blood levels of the lipoproteins and the response of the arterial wall (Brown & Goldstein, 1976). Clearly, other variables may moderate the progression of the atherosclerosis,

but without high intake of dietary cholesterol and saturated fat, the evolution of atherosclerosis will be minimal.

The determinants of the thrombus are less well defined, related to factors that affect both platelet function and clotting. Cigarette smoking (U.S. Department of Health and Human Services, 1983), certain dietary factors such as the specific type of fat (Miller et al., 1986), and hormonal changes are all probably important in the development of the thrombus (Royal College of General Practitioners' Oral Contraception Study, 1981). Significant coronary thrombosis develops primarily only in the presence of coronary atherosclerosis.

The determinants of the evolution and size of a myocardial infarction are very poorly understood primarily because of the substantial difficulties of in vivo measurement of the size of the myocardial infarction. Most previous studies have depended on postmortem examination, measures of enzymes in the blood, or echocardiography. The effects of the size of the myocardial infarction and loss of left ventricular function are evaluated by such measures as history of congestive heart failure and decreased ejection fraction (Schulze, 1977; Moss, 1980).

The evolution of the clinical heart disease depends on these three steps. They are sequential in the sense that coronary atherosclerosis is generally required for thrombus to result in decreased oxygen supply to the myocardium and in the myocardial infarction, sudden death, and so forth. Clearly, other factors may injure the arterial intima and result in reparative processes that have similar characteristics to atherosclerosis. Certain vascular disorders may likewise result in an increased risk of thrombosis and even acute occlusions of a coronary artery. Various myocardiopathies may present with clinical stigmata of myocardial infarction, cardiac arrhythmias, and left ventricular dysfunction.

The probability of a clinical event rises as the extent of atherosclerosis increases in any individual (Pearson, 1984). There is substantial variability in the response. Occasionally, individuals will die suddenly with minimal coronary heart disease. It is unclear whether such deaths are due to a spasm of a coronary artery or to independent effects of the autonomic nervous system and cardiac arrhythmias. The behavioral precipitants of a "heart attack" may act either by modifying coronary blood flow by spasm, increasing the risk of thrombosis, or directly on ischemic vulnerable myocardium to increase the risk of a lethal cardiac arrhythmia (Verrier & Lown, 1982). It is extremely rare for such precipitants to "cause" clinical disease in the absence of severe atherosclerosis (Talbott, Kuller, Detre, & Perper, 1980).

Clinical coronary heart disease is multifactorial only when evaluated as a single event. It is more rational to consider each of the specific components as the sequential evolution to clinical disease. The incubation period of disease and the components of pathophysiology are important for understanding the design and implementation of clinical trials.

The experimental epidemiological studies or clinical trials should evolve from a clear understanding of the relationship between the specific risk factors and the defined end points. For example, the development of atherosclerosis in men is probably greatest from age 20 to 45. This is also the age span of greatest changes in risk factors such as lipoprotein cholesterol levels. Trials to prevent atherosclerosis, or at least progression of atherosclerosis, should more rationally focus on the younger age groups. Studies in older individuals will include subjects who have extensive atherosclerotic disease, and the rate of progression over time may be less steep. The reason for the selection of older individuals in many of the earlier studies was due to the fact that coronary angiography was the only objective, quantitative measure of atherosclerosis *in vivo* (Levy *et al.,* 1984), and therefore, limited studies to individuals who had evidence of clinical diseases or were at very high risk. New techniques to measure atherosclerosis may reduce the need for coronary angiography and may make it possible to test both the prevention and the progression of atherosclerosis.

Thrombosis, on the other hand, generally occurs in the presence of significant severe atherosclerosis. Thus, if there were good techniques to measure thrombosis *in vivo,* the experimental trials would necessarily focus on older aged populations in which the prevalence of severe atherosclerosis

was already substantial (Lewis *et al.,* 1983; Harker, 1986).

Finally, the evolution of clinical coronary artery disease and its complications is a function of both atherosclerosis and thrombosis. The incubation period from subclinical disease, i.e., extensive atherosclerosis or evolving thrombosis, to the acute clinical event may be extremely short as in the case of sudden and unexpected death, or over a relatively brief period of time as in unstable angina pectoris (Lewis *et al.,* 1983). The experimental approaches would, therefore, have to be in place prior to the onset of the acute event and would probably have to focus on high-risk populations, i.e., those who already have clinical disease, angina pectoris, or even prior myocardial infarction.

Experimental Epidemiology

Natural Experiments

Experimental epidemiological studies are of two types—natural experiments and clinical trials. Natural experiments include temporal changes in a population and unique geographic populations, and migrant studies.

Temporal Trends

The rise and then rapid fall of coronary heart disease and stroke mortality in the United States is an example of a natural experiment (Kuller, Perper, Dai, Rutan, & Traven, 1986). The specific reason for this decline has not been determined, but clearly the changes in the risk factors and incidence of disease are a response to certain social behavioral factors in the environment. The most interesting observations have been the greater decline in coronary heart disease in the better-educated and upper socioeconomic groups and the consequent striking change in socioeconomic gradient of disease over time. In the 1950s and early 1960s, there was a direct relationship between coronary heart disease incidence, mortality, and markers of socioeconomic status. Since that time, there has been a substantial reversal so that the rates are now much higher in the lower rather than the upper socioeconomic class (Ruberman, Weinblatt, Goldberg, & Chaudhary, 1984). Thus, any study that fails to include the potential confounding effects of education or other markers of social class is probably of limited utility.

Geographic Variations and Select Populations

The second example of natural experiments are the marked variations in coronary heart disease rates in geographic areas such as the United States as well as the differences among countries (Thom, Epstein, Feldman, & Leaverton, 1985). There are also striking ethnic and religious group variations in coronary heart disease. In a classical study, Kaplan, Cassel, Tyroler, Cornoni, Kleinbaum, and Hames (1971) evaluated the apparent increase in coronary heart disease in a rural North Carolina population exposed to rapid industrialization and urbanization. Several other studies have shown that certain religious groups such as Seventh Day Adventists (Phillips, Kuzma, Beeson, & Lotz, 1980), Mormons (Lyon, Wetzler, Gardner, Klauber, & Williams, 1978), and Orthodox Jews (Friedlander, Kark, & Stein, 1985) have lower coronary heart disease mortality rates than less observant individuals. The low rates of disease among religious groups, if consistent, might be a natural experimental model of the effect of social support or differential response to various environmental stimuli.

Migrant Studies

Migrant studies have provided us with an extremely important natural experiment. The most widely noted migrant studies are those of the Japanese Americans (Syme et al., 1975) and the migrants to Israel (Zahavi et al., 1987). The striking increase in coronary heart disease and decline in stroke among Japanese migrants to Hawaii and California have generally been attributed to changes in risk factors (Ueshima et al., 1982).

Another example of an important migrant study is currently being pilot tested. The high prevalence of hypertension and related disease among the black populations of the United States may be a function of the interaction of genetic and environ-

mental factors. Considerable interest has focused on various stress hypotheses related to poverty and discrimination (James, 1985). An alternative hypothesis is that dietary factors such as high salt or low potassium intake, or a high prevalence of obesity especially among black women in a genetically susceptible population is the primary cause of the high prevalence of hypertension and its complications (Dai, Kuller, & Miller, 1984). Three types of migrant studies of the black populations are currently being evaluated: a comparison of upwardly mobile black populations such as those in professional fields and college students; a comparison of changes in risk factors and disease among blacks living in areas of the United States with high rates such as the Southeast and migrants to areas with lower rates such as the Northeast or West; and a study of black populations in the United States and similar groups in West Africa, especially Nigeria. For example, black college students and various occupational groups in Nigeria and the United States may have similar educational levels and jobs, but strikingly different social behavioral situations and dietary practices. These natural experiments offer great opportunities to test various behavioral hypotheses in a real-world situation, and especially to test the consistency of hypotheses across different risk strata.

Randomized Trials

Introduction

The randomized clinical trial is the pinnacle of epidemiological research. The intervention trial provides the solid scientific evidence for a "causal" hypothesis. The randomized clinical trial is especially important for the evaluation of risk factors which are difficult to quantify in observational studies including many behavioral attributes. Most epidemiological and behavioral studies do poorly in attempting to quantify activities of normal everyday life especially in homogeneous populations. Thus, such activities as dietary intake, physical activity, social relationships, stress, attitudes, belief, and so forth are poorly quantified. Experimental manipulation of these behaviors probably offers the only way to evaluate the impact of most of the variables on risk factors and disease.

The technical aspects of implementing a clinical trial have been very well described in recent textbooks (Friedman, Furberg, & DeMets, 1982; Meinert, 1986). The major issues to be discussed in this chapter relate to some of the more important problems in successfully completing a clinical trial especially as related to behavioral factors and disease. The most critical issues to be considered are whether the intervention can be blinded or not, the recruitment of participants into a trial, adherence to specific intervention groups, measurements of end points, clinical trials in which the community is the unit of randomization, and subgroup analysis.

Blinded or Unblinded Trials

Most behavioral-type intervention trials are unblinded. The individuals are usually randomized into a specific type of behavioral intervention such as weight reduction, smoking cessation, increase physical activity, reduction of "stress," and a control group which is offered either no specific intervention or some alternative intervention which should have minimal effects on the dependent variable. Clinical trials that have been unblinded have either randomized individuals into an intervention group sometimes referred to as special care and either a comparison group, referred to their usual sources of health care, usual care, referred care (Sherwin *et al.,* 1981), or given some nonspecific intervention or health education program. In some randomized studies, the comparison group consists of individuals on a waiting list for a specific intervention such as a smoking cessation or a weight loss program. Another approach is to identify specific populations such as members of a health maintenance organization (HMO) (Shapiro, Venet, Strax, Venet, & Rosser, 1982). Individuals are then randomized to intervention and comparison group. The intervention group is provided with a specific treatment while the control group is not even advised of their participation in a study and followed through their medical records in the HMO. It is possible even to offer the intervention to the experimental group as part of their regular care without their knowledge of being participants in a clinical trial (Friedman, Collen, & Fireman, 1986). This approach has been particularly useful in studies of the effects of various early detection techniques for the diagnosis of disease and for the introduction of health education programs administered primarily by physicians or other health care providers.

The unblinded intervention in most behavioral studies creates very substantial methodological problems in clinical trial designs and interpretation of results. First is the problem of crossovers, individuals in the intervention group who do not adhere to the specific behavioral change such as weight loss or smoking cessation, or individuals in the comparison group who change their behavior to that of the intervention group. The sample size for an intervention trial is dependent on the estimated differences in the dependent variable such as disease between the experimental and control group, and the standard error of that difference. The success of the trial is based on the ability to maximize the differences in the independent variable such as weight loss or smoking cessation. The likelihood of a difference in dependent variables is a function of changes in dependent variables. Thus, the crossovers both from the intervention to the control and from the control to the intervention group present a very substantial problem. A major concern, therefore, in intervention trials that measure the effects of behavioral modification is the selection of the participants. Investigators in behavioral intervention trials often prefer to select participants who are at least willing to try and modify the specific intervention behavior, be it smoking cessation, exercise, weight loss, relaxation, dietary modification, or the like. Participants may also be attracted to the trial owing to the type of intervention proposed or even by the method of delivery of the intervention such as the type of weight reduction program, exercise, and so forth. The participants, therefore, prior to randomization are often highly motivated. Following randomization, the experimental group may respond favorably to the intervention, but the control group will also likely make similar behavioral changes so that the differences in the independent variable between the experimental and control group may be substantially less than planned prior to the beginning of the trial.

Another problem may be that the change in the behavior in the experimental group may not only be a function of the efficacy of the behavioral technique, but also the selection of the participants for the trial. Thus, the size of the effect in the experimental group may not be generalizable to the community, and the conclusion that the experimental intervention, at least in terms of modifying the independent variable, is highly successful, should be carefully tempered by the selection criteria for participation in the trial.

An example of some of the problems occurring in behavioral-type intervention trials can be seen in the Multiple Risk Factor Intervention Trial (Multiple Risk Factor Intervention Trial Research Group, 1982). The percentage of individuals quitting smoking in the intervention group was substantial and higher than that anticipated at the beginning of the trial. However, the percentage of men quitting smoking in the usual care was also much higher than anticipated. The usual care quit rate was a function of both the changes in behaviors occurring in the United States during the time of the trial, about 3–4% per year, and the fact that they had been selected for the trial because of their willingness to at least attempt to quit smoking. Only motivated individuals are likely to participate in a long-term behavioral intervention trial, and clearly only after randomization were advised of the fact that they were referred back to their usual source of medical care. Not only are such individuals most likely to be more highly motivated and perhaps health conscious, but also because of the selection criteria of such studies including their health status, a group of individuals at lower risk of disease is selected. The coronary heart disease mortality in the trial was a function of the differences in smoking cessation between the usual and special care and the anticipated reduction in coronary heart disease mortality associated with such changes in smoking habits. Briefly, the risk of coronary heart disease drops rapidly after smoking cessation because the effect of smoking is probably a precipitant of the heart attack such as a thrombus or changes in myocardial metabolism rather than on the evolution of atherosclerosis. The data from the MRFIT trial itself and other studies suggest that there might be a 50% decrease in risk associated with smoking cessation. Approximately 40% of the smokers quit in special intervention as compared to about 20% in usual care, a 20% difference. At the beginning of the trial, about 60% of the men were cigarette smokers. Thus, the overall estimated impact of smoking cessation in the trial would be a 50% reduction times a 20% difference among the 60% cigarette smokers or an overall 6% effect. This small difference in end-point coronary heart disease deaths, in spite of the remarkable success of the smoking cessation program, is due first to the fact that almost 60% of the smokers did not comply with the message to quit smoking in the special intervention, i.e., crossed-over to the usual care, and 20% of the usual care, quit smoking, crossed-over to the special intervention. This difficulty in evaluating the efficacy of smoking cessation to reduce coronary heart disease mortality or even lung cancer mortality in clinical trials is not unique to the MRFIT trial. Few, if any, clinical trials of smoking cessation have demonstrated a significant reduction in the mortality in the intervention as compared to the control group (Rose, Hamilton, Colwell, & Shipley, 1982).

There are several ways of dealing with this problem of crossovers. It is intuitively logical to assume that the more difficult it is to accomplish the intervention by the comparison group, the smaller will be the percentage of crossovers from control to experimental group. Thus, in studies that require a substantial reduction in dietary fat, let us say to 20% from the normal 40–45%, and therefore, major nutritional consultation and behavioral modifications, the crossovers from the control group will be substantially less than would be in a study of only a modest change in fat intake, to 30–35% of calories.

Selection of Participants

It is probable that the interventions would be more successful in the groups at highest risk. Such individuals may be both less amenable to behavioral changes on their own and also the effect of any behavioral change, i.e., the difference between experimental and intervention group may result in a greater change in the dependent variable, disease. The largest difference in smoking cessation in MRFIT and other studies was between those who smoked the most cigarettes at entry because few of the usual care quit smoking in these heavy smoking groups. In the MRFIT group, there was also a significant decrease in coronary heart disease mortality between special intervention and usual care among a subgroup of men who had a positive stress treadmill exercise test at entry to the trial (Rautaharju *et al.*, 1986). These men had evidence of some cardiac ischemia and were probably more responsive to the small differences in risk factor changes between usual care and special intervention. In the "Oslo Trial" (Hjermann, Holme, Velve-Byre, & Leren, 1981) of cholesterol lowering, the individuals selected had extremely high cholesterol levels at entry to the study. It is obvious, however, that selection of these high-risk individuals requires a substantial behavioral intervention effort in the experimental group in order to maximize the impact of the intervention. It is important also to stabilize the baseline measurements prior to randomization. Substantial regression to mean may markedly effect the high-risk levels prior to intervention.

Three simple rules for the selection of participants for unblinded trials may be helpful. First, select only interventions that are difficult to accomplish by the comparison group without substantial expert consultation and individual efforts. The success of the differences in the intervention between the treatment groups will, therefore, be primarily related to the efficacy of the intervention in the experimental group. Second, select individuals who have higher levels of the risk factors or who are more resistant to changes, those with higher levels of serum cholesterol, smoke more cigarettes, are very sedentary, or are more obese. Third, select high-risk individuals, those with positive exercise tests, history of angina, and so forth, so that more modest changes in the independent variable, i.e., changes in cholesterol, smoking, and weight, are more likely to have an effect on the dependent variable such as mortality and morbidity.

Adherence to Protocol

In the case of single- or double-blinded trials where the participants do not know whether they are receiving a placebo or an active treatment, the situation is quite different. The effect of crossovers is more likely a function of side effects of the active therapy and the impact of alternate medical care sources for the control participants. Selection of subjects should probably only include those who demonstrate evidence of willingness to adhere to the protocol and understand the implications of the trial. Participants in blinded trials are often better educated, from upper socioeconomic class, and tend to be at somewhat lower risk in order to reduce the likelihood of crossovers from placebos to active treatments due to an increase in the level of the independent variable beyond acceptable limits such as an increase in blood pressure above a certain predefined level where ethical considerations would require "open" treatment. Unfortunately, unblinded behavioral intervention trials often select the better educated, higher socioeconomic class because such individuals are more willing to participate in the experimental intervention. This results, as noted, in a substantial change in the control group as well as often smaller differences between the experimental and control group in the independent variable than anticipated. If one is going to opt for an unblinded behavioral intervention in the more compliant groups, then the control or comparison group should probably be offered some alternative intervention unlikely to either infringe on the change in the independent variable or affect the dependent variable, i.e., the change in disease. For example, in an unblinded intervention trial to reduce the risk of hypertension by dietary modification such as an increase in potassium or reduction of sodium in the diet, the comparison group would be offered a modified health education program which would include a modest reduction in fat intake without any substantial change in either the potassium or sodium in the diet. Weight in both groups would be held as constant as possible in order to avoid the confounding of weight change. The addition of this "sham" experimental intervention for the control group obviously substantially increases the cost of the study, but it is probably the best solution to this difficult situation.

It is apparent that the success of both the unblinded as well as the blinded intervention trials depends to a considerable degree on the ability to maximize the intervention in the experimental group and the differences in the independent variable between the experimental and control group. The ability of the experimental intervention to succeed in reaching its goal in reducing the independent variable is often lacking prior to the beginning of a major study. It is exceedingly important that pilot studies be done prior to the beginning of any behavioral intervention trials, and that such pilot studies clearly demonstrate the best approach to maximizing the interventions in the same type of populations that will be used in a full-scale trial.

A further problem in unblinded behavioral trials is the possibility that an intervention will result in a change in a risk factor for a disease other than the specific independent variable. For example, in the MRFIT study, individuals who quit smoking were more likely to gain weight and have a blunted reduction in their cholesterol levels. Individuals participating in an exercise trial may have a greater weight loss or a greater reduction in cigarette smoking. Similarly, those likely to exercise may have better pulmonary function or cardiac function, resulting in less breathlessness and fatigue following exercise. Increased social support by frequent visits to the clinics as part of an intervention can result in a modification of depression and anxiety. Such increase in social support and awareness of health status by itself may reduce the frequency of disease independent of the changes in the risk factors. There is probably no way of avoiding some type of multifactorial interventions. These changes in the other risk factors can be adjusted by various multivariant statistical techniques. However, a more scientific approach would be to include other interventions in both the experimental and control group to at least partially equalize the changes in the confounded risk factors. For example, weight reduction or weight modification might be considered part of the intervention for participants in a smoking cessation trial, those in both the experimental and control group. The goal would be to keep the amount of weight gain or weight loss similar in both groups. Caloric intake might be adjusted in an exercise trial in order to keep weight change to a minimum especially if the specific goal of the trial was to determine whether increasing exercise reduced morbidity and mortality independent of an effect on weight. Another alternative obviously would be to include another group in which weight loss occurred without any substantial increase in physical activity.

Specific End Points

The selection of a specific end point is crucial to the success of any of these intervention trials. As previously noted, the impact of any specific intervention on an independent variable should be predictable on the basis of the known pathophysiology of disease. The specific hypothesis of the clinical trial should include the evidence for the link between the independent risk factor, the pathophysiological changes expected, and the outcome measure. The closer the measure of the end point is to the anticipated pathophysiological change resulting from the modification of the independent variable, the more likely the trial will demonstrate the anticipated outcome. Also, it is important to attempt to identify end points that will change fairly rapidly in relation to modification of the independent variable. The ability to keep the participants in the trial over long periods of time and maintain the difference in the independent variable is difficult and very expensive. For example, trials to modify lipoprotein levels through dietary manipulation and drugs will probably be more valuable in the future when the end point is atherosclerosis and not just clinical coronary artery disease. Trials of blood pressure reduction are more powerful when the focus is on hypertensive complications such as stroke (especially intracranial disease and heart failure) than on cardiovascular disease or on clinical coronary artery disease. Smoking is a precipitant of a heart attack and the effects of cigarette smoking occur generally only in the presence of significant atherosclerosis. Thus, smoking cessation trials are more likely to show a positive effect in terms of reduction of coronary heart disease morbidity and mortality when the participants in the trial can be identified as already having existing coronary atherosclerosis or coronary heart disease. It is unlikely that behavioral intervention trials in which the end point is incident, i.e., first coronary heart disease, will be able to demonstrate a reduction in mortality and morbidity except in very unusual circumstances. Clinical trials of be-havioral interventions, and especially unblinded trials, would do much better to measure changes in an intermediate end point or a specific pathophysi-ological marker rather than attempt to measure changes in incident, myocardial infarction, or cor-onary heart disease deaths. For example, it will be possible to test whether increased physical activity raises HDL cholesterol or enhances weight loss, but not to be able to test a direct reduction in heart disease.

Community Intervention Trials

Community trials randomize groups of indi-viduals. Investigators who support community-based trials believe that the dissemination of infor-mation within the community, and especially the ability to utilize both media and various types of social networks, enhances the ability to do behav-ioral intervention studies. The community is the unit of behavioral change rather than the indi-vidual. These trials may select communities that either have high rates of disease or prevalence of risk factors that are to be modified (Puska, Sa-lonen, Tuomilehto, Nissinen, & Kottke, 1983), or have specific geographic characteristics that are suitable for the proposed community interventions (Blackburn & Leon, 1986; Lefebvre, Lasater, Carleton, & Peterson, 1987; Farquhar, 1978) such as access to television or radio, newspapers, com-munity groups willing to participate, and so forth. The control community may not be informed of participation in the study and evaluated in as pas-sive a way as possible in order to avoid changes in risk factors or disease outcomes. These community studies may also randomize occupational groups or other similar populations that can be clearly de-fined at the beginning and end of the trial (Re-search Group of the Rome Project of Coronary Heart Disease Prevention, 1986). There is also a strong belief that community intervention trials and subsequent programs are substantially cheaper than individual-type interventions. A community trial may combine individual interventions for high-risk individuals within the experimental com-munity with a more modest community health edu-cation approach. There are three unique meth-odological problems related to community intervention studies: (1) how to measure the inter-vention effect, (2) how to quantify the changes in the dependent variable such as a decrease in mor-bidity and mortality, and (3) how to determine what factors may have accounted for any changes in the dependent variable.

The unit of randomization in community studies is the community. The changes in the independent variable such as smoking, weight loss, exercise, blood pressure, or the like are evaluated in several ways. First, a comparison of the changes in levels between baseline prior to randomization of the communities, and some specific points in time after randomization can be done. It is necessary that the levels of these independent variables be measured prior to the determination of which of the communities is the experimental or control, for otherwise there is a substantial potential for bias ascertainment because of both the differential re-sponse rates to the baseline survey, and the impact on the individuals of being identified as part of the experimental community. Often, however, the ex-perimental and control communities are not se-lected randomly, but rather by convenience to the study investigators. Therefore, the experimental community may have been defined prior to the baseline surveys. Such approaches seriously limit, if not invalidate, the clinical trial design.

After the information is collected at the baseline survey, the changes in risk factors (independent variables) can be measured either by repeat cross-sectional surveys or by a longitudinal follow-up of the individuals originally sampled at baseline, the method usually done in individual randomized tri-als. If repeat cross-sectional surveys are used, then the changes in the independent variables are a function of both the variability of the point esti-mate in the two cross-sectional samples and the actual change in the independent variable over time. Since the sampling unit consists of the com-munity rather than individuals, the standard error of the point estimate is substantially larger and the sample sizes necessary for estimating effects must be larger than in individual trials. The variability of baseline effects of risk factor levels may be potentially reduced by repeat measurements over time prior to randomization and intervention. The statistical methods of community studies have been discussed by Cornfield (1978) and Jacobs *et al.* (1986). Differential migration in the communities as well as variations in response rates to the surveys may have profound effects on subsequent cross-sectional point estimates at different time perods, and could either mask the effects of interventions in the experimental community or overestimate them. It is also extremely important that the cross-sectional samples be drawn independent of the intervention effort in the experimental community. The cross-sectional sample should represent the status of the total experimental and control communities, not only those who are participating in the intervention process.

The longitudinal follow-up approach is similar to the individual-type intervention trial. However, there are substantial problems with these longitudinal surveys. First, individuals identified in the longitudinal samples may be preferentially included in the subsequent community intervention efforts. The noted risk factor changes in the longitudinal study may be much greater than those for the entire community. Just the identification of individuals in the longitudinal sample may affect the individuals' behavior with regard to specific risk factor modifications proposed in the experimental community health education program. If the studies continue over more than a few years, migration out of both the experimental and control communities may be substantial and present a serious problem of follow-up in these longitudinal samples. Individuals who migrate from the community or refuse to participate in follow-up surveys, may have very different risk factor changes than those who continue to be followed. Even the presumption that the characteristics of individuals lost to follow-up in the experimental and control groups are the same, may be incorrect. Migration from or nonparticipation in the experimental community are more likely for individuals who did not participate in the specific interventions as compared to those who remained or were resampled.

The dependent variable in some community studies is supposed to be a change in the incidence or mortality of a specific disease such as coronary artery disease or possibly total mortality. The measurement of these specific end points is complex.

The introduction of a community-based intervention program for the modification of a single or even group of risk factors in a community especially using a health education and social network approach may affect the medical care delivery system and other risk factors that can have a profound effect on the frequency of disease.

The experimental intervention may be engrafted in an existing decline in morbidity and mortality (Salonen, Kottke, Jacobs, & Hannan, 1986). The subsequent decline in morbidity and mortality may, therefore, be attributable to the intervention rather than the attributes of the community prior to the intervention. It is extremely important, therefore, that the trends in morbidity and mortality in a community be carefully monitored prior to the intervention. Communities in which the rates of disease have declined substantially prior to the intervention should probably not be selected for the study. Various regression models have been proposed to deal with change prior to randomization, but are of limited utility. It makes little sense to compare a community with declining rates prior to baseline with another with stable rates.

It is unlikely that community intervention programs will be able to replace individual-type clinical trials to measure the effects of specific interventions on morbidity and mortality for specific diseases. The only time that such community interventions can clearly replace individual-type intervention trials is when the entire community is affected by some common source such as a modification of the water supply by fluoridation, control of air pollution, or changes in the availability of the food supply. Community intervention-type trials in which the individuals themselves must actively participate in the behavioral change and in which there is a great likelihood of confounding with other changes, should probably be considered demonstration projects to provide further evidence for the most effective methods of applying known and acceptable risk factor modification strategies in the community. The primary end point in such studies becomes the risk factor change rather than the dependent variable or disease. The goal of the experimental design is primarily to compare various methods of maximizing modifications of risk factors in the population.

The end points can be quantified as a percentage of the population that had some predetermined modification in their risk factors such as the percentage of the population quitting smoking, or by mean change in risk factors such as mean cholesterol change, weight change, or the like. The use of mean changes as an end point is very risky and probably should be avoided. For example, an average 5-pound weight loss among 300 individuals in a community could be due to 30 individuals each losing 50 pounds and everybody else having no weight change, or to an average 5-pound loss among the 300 individuals. Obviously, some measure of the standard deviation of the weight loss would partially compensate for this variability. Likewise, changes in the mean number of cigarettes smoked are of little value. Since quit rates for cigarette smoking are so dependent on the initial dose, all quit percentages should be expressed in relation to the initial dose. At a minimum, the quit percentage should be expressed by pack(s) of cigarettes and possibly by objective measure of inhalation of tobacco products. Changes in dose of cigarettes are of little value. The use of some composite index of risk factor change should also be avoided. These "risk scores" are very suitable to relatively small changes in blood pressure and number of cigarettes smoked. Since the change in the number of cigarettes smoked is probably a weak, if not useless measure, risk measures dependent on such changes are also of very limited value.

Since the end point is usually the risk factor change rather than the distribution of disease, the accuracy and repeatability of the information should be carefully evaluated especially when nonobjective measures to quantify risk factor change are being utilized. Finally, as noted, the methods of quantifying the change in the community, the cross-sectional versus longitudinal sampling as well as the frequency of resampling in the community, should be carefully evaluated.

Subgroups

It is also important to recognize, especially in the individual intervention trials, but also to some degree in the community trials, that various subgroups of the population may respond quite differently to the specific behavioral interventions both in terms of changes in disease risk factors and end points. For example, the presumption that hypertension is one disease and that any specific intervention will affect all hypertensive individuals in the same way is probably incorrect. Weight reduction, for example, may be an effective way to reduce blood pressure levels among overweight hypertensive individuals. It is not necessarily true that such a reduction in blood pressure will have the same impact on reducing the risk of stroke or hypertensive complications as blood pressure reduction by drug therapy among relatively thin individuals who may have a different type of hypertensive disease. It is important prior to the beginning of a trial to define the subgroups and specific hypothesis related to subgroups. The approximate sample size for each subgroup should be considered in order to estimate the potential power to detect a defined difference in end point within each subgroup.

It is also important to note that any behavioral intervention or drug therapy may result in an unexpected adverse effect in at least a subgroup of the population. It is very unwise to attribute any excess disease in the experimental group to random variation without very careful review. All increased events in the experimental group should be evaluated as an adverse effect until proven otherwise. Comparison of adverse effects across studies should be evaluated carefully. Many of the cardiovascular trials have failed to note any decrease in total mortality in spite of decrease in coronary heart disease. This means that there must be an increase in noncardiovascular diseases. No specific pattern of excess mortality has emerged, but should be carefully evaluated in each study.

Discussion

Clinical trials, especially related to behavioral risk factors, are extremely difficult to do because the risk factor and its experimental modification are often unblinded. The crossovers from the experimental to control group and vice versa are usually very high, resulting in small differences in the risk factor change between the experimental and control group, and therefore, less than anticipated impact on the outcome or end point, usually morbidity and mortality from a disease, or change in some other major risk factor. At a minimum, all unblinded behavioral intervention trials should include an independent data collection and statistical analysis component in order to overcome at least some of the biases which clearly will creep into the studies owing to the unblinding of both participants and investigators. Results of unblinded intervention trials should be suspect until tested by other investigators using similar techniques, but in different populations.

The ability to maximize the differences in the independent risk factors between the experimental and control group is clearly the most important factor in the successful completion of these trials. At a minimum, a pilot study should be done first in order to determine the most successful intervention and the minimum loss-to-follow-up in the same type of population using the same approaches as will be used in a longer-term and larger-sample definitive trial. Participants for these clinical trials should be selected with great care so that nonadherence and crossovers from control to experimental groups are minimized. This requires that the proposed intervention techniques be at least reasonably unique so that it is unlikely that the control group can also accomplish the interventions by going to the corner store or picking up the local newspaper. The controls should require substantial help in order to complete the intervention.

Selection of the type of participants including their age, sex, education, and risk factor levels may also be a most important component of the trial. Recruitment for the trials is difficult and may be getting harder, especially in large single-center trials. Investigators may often be forced to accept less than the ideal participants for a specific trial, resulting in a smaller risk factor change and loss-to-follow-up. Multicenter trials with smaller samples from each of the centers are certainly more costly and difficult to manage, but may be preferable because of both better subject selection and the potential to test the intervention techniques across centers.

Objective measurements of the experimental variables and the outcome measures will certainly enhance the design of the trials. A pathophysiological model of the presumed relationship of the risk factor or behavioral variable to the outcome should be defined as part of the hypothesis at the beginning of the trial. The defined end point should then be clearly related to this pathophysiological model and be as specific as possible. The probability of identifying the end point will also determine to some degree the characteristics of the study population such as whether one conducts a primary or secondary prevention trial, uses younger or older age groups, and so forth. The testing of objective methods of measuring the end points of the trial should also be an important component.

It is extremely important in unblinded behavioral intervention trials that the experimental and control groups be treated in the same way with regard to all other confounding variables except the experimental manipulation. This especially includes such issues as the frequency of staff contacts, differences in social support between the experimental and control groups, education of participants about other risk factors such as smoking or alcohol, and especially about early detection of disease and symptomatology. Differential availability and utilization of medical care resources and technology between experimental and control group can also substantially bias the results of the study.

The measurement of the dependent variable should be as unbiased as possible. Clearly, the safest course is to have some objective measure which can be done independent of the intervention process itself. It is, therefore, also preferable to have the outcome measurements done by individuals not actively involved in the intervention or the experimental process and hopefully blinded to the specific intervention groups.

Many variables are sampled at only a few points such as measuring blood pressure at periodic intervals in a study. There is substantial biological variation in these measurements and it is possible for them to be influenced by the interaction of the observer and the subject, resulting in a spurious estimate of the intervention effect. Experimental subjects may learn to change their behavior positively with regard to a dependent variable especially at specific defined sampling times. For example, an individual may learn to relax when having his or her blood pressure measured at any one particular point in order to have a lower reading at sampling times. Individuals may change their diet or exercise habits immediately before a visit to the clinic. Objective measurements that integrate the behavior over a period of time, as well as measurements at random points within the study, and probably without specific feedback to the participants, i.e., blinding the participants to the results, may at least partially resolve these problems. On the other hand, some of these measurements are critical for the adequate success of the intervention program such as setting goals for weight reduction, cholesterol levels, and the like. Thus, the impact on the intervention process itself must be evaluated against the objective measurements of the end-point variables. Clearly, this is not a simple task and there are no specific rules that will resolve each issue.

Clinical trials which randomize communities rather than individuals present many unique problems in analysis and interpretation. The generally complex nature of these interventions often precludes any ability to test the efficacy of any specific intervention in relation to reduction in morbidity and mortality, or even changes in risk factors. The only situation in which this may not be true is in interventions related to some common source such as the water supply, air pollution, or in substantial modifications of available food sources at the production and supply end. Many of the risk behaviors of particular interest may be examples of common-source exposures such as high cholesterol and saturated fat intake for most individuals within a community. Interventions aimed at the production and supply of foods rather than specific health education of the individuals with regard to food selection may be the next generation of community intervention trials, and conceivably will have a bigger impact than current efforts through health education and information and even specific behavioral interventions for high-risk individuals. These so-called environmental manipulations so successful in control of waterborne disease, air pollution, and so forth, as well as in changing certain behaviors through increasing taxation and availability of various products, may also be applied to certain behavioral interventions.

Statistical Analysis

The methods of statistical analysis of clinical trials are very well presented in recent textbooks (Friedman *et al.*, 1982; Meinert, 1986). The analysis team should include a biostatistician experienced in clinical trials analysis. The biostatistician should be part of the initial team planning and designing the trial and not just as an "analyst consultant" at the end of the study.

Several points about the analysis of clinical trials are important:

1. There should be an independent verification of the results of the study. It is generally not advisable to have the investigators doing the experimental interventions also be responsible for the initial analysis. Clearly, further evaluation of the results and its interpretation is the responsibility of the investigators.
2. The results should always be presented in terms of a point estimate and confidence limits and not only p values.
3. The results should be compared in the context of other clinical trials. Thus, even if the confidence limits across the p values are not "significant," the consistency of the results in relation to previous studies may be strong evidence for the efficacy or lack of efficacy of an intervention.
4. The power of the trial to determine a specific end point should be evaluated carefully at the end of the trial. This should be done in relation to the observed change in the risk factor rather than the initial design criteria. For example, if a 50% reduction in smoking was hypothesized to lead to a 20% decrease in heart disease with a specific power for that sample size, then clearly the power is substantially reduced if only 20% of the individuals in the experimental group quit smoking.
5. The internal consistency of the trial results should be evaluated. In a study to determine

the effects of weight loss on the decrease in blood pressure levels, there should be a linear relationship between weight loss and blood pressure change within the experimental group.

6. The confounding variables should be carefully evaluated in the trial. In unblinded trials, the potential biases previously described should also be documented and included as part of the results.

7. It is important that all trial results be presented, even trials in which the null hypothesis, i.e., no effect, is accepted. Reporting of only "positive" studies may lead to a serious misinterpretation of the data.

References

Blackburn, H., & Leon, A. (1986). Preventive cardiology in practice: Minnesota studies of risk factor reduction. In M. Pollock & D. Schmidt (Eds.), *Heart disease and rehabilitation* (2nd ed., pp. 265–301). New York: Wiley.

Brown, M. S., & Goldstein, J. L. (1976). Receptor-mediated control of cholesterol metabolism. *Science, 191,* 150–154.

Bunker, C. H. (1987, March 19–21). *Are blood pressure and obesity related through salt transport and insulin?* Abstract prepared for the American Heart Association 27th Annual Conference on Cardiovascular Disease Epidemiology.

Cornfield, J. (1978). Randomization by group: A formal analysis. *American Journal of Epidemiology, 108*(2), 100–189.

Dai, W. S., Kuller, L. H., & Miller, G. (1984). Arterial blood pressure and urinary electrolytes. *Journal of Chronic Diseases, 37*(1), 75–84.

Farquhar, J. W. (1978). The community-based model of lifestyle intervention trials. *Journal of Epidemiology, 108*(2), 103–111.

Friedlander, Y., Kark, J. D., & Stein, Y. (1985). Religious orthodoxy and myocardial infarction in Jerusalem: A case-control study. *International Journal of Cardiology, 10,* 33–41.

Friedman, G. D., Collen, M. F., & Fireman, B. H. (1986). Multiphasic health check-up evaluation: A 16 year follow-up. *Journal of Chronic Diseases, 39*(6), 453–463.

Friedman, L. M., Furberg, C. D., & DeMets, D. L. (1982). Sample size. In *Fundamentals of clinical trials* (pp. 69–88). Boston: John Wright.

Harker, L. A. (1986). Clinical trials evaluating platelet-modifying drugs in patients with atherosclerotic cardiovascular disease and thrombosis. *Circulation, 73*(2), 206–223.

Hjermann, I., Holme, I., Velve-Byre, K., & Leren, P. (1981). Effect of diet and smoking intervention on the incidence of coronary heart disease: Report from the Oslo Study Group of a randomized trial in healthy men. *Lancet, 2,* 1303–1310.

Jacobs, D. R., Luepker, R. V., Mittlemark, M. B., Folsom, A. R., Pirie, P. L., Mascioli, S. R., Hannan, P. J., Pechacek, T. F., Bracht, N. F., Carlaw, R. W., Kline, F. G., & Blackburn, H. (1986). Community-wide prevention strategies: Evaluation of the Minnesota Heart Health Program. *Journal of Chronic Diseases, 39*(10), 775–788.

James, S. A. (1985). Psychosocial and environmental factors in black hypertension. In W. D. Hall, E. Saunders, & N. B. Shulman (Eds.), *Hypertension in blacks: Epidemiology, pathophysiology, and treatment* (pp. 132–143). Chicago: Year Book Medical.

Kaplan, B. H., Cassel, J. C., Tyroler, H. A., Cornoni, J. C., Kleinbaum, D. G., & Hames, C. G. (1971). Occupational mobility and coronary heart disease. *Archives of Internal Medicine, 128,* 938–948.

Kuller, L. H. (1986). Natural history of coronary heart disease. In M. Pollock & D. Schmidt (Eds.), *Heart disease and rehabilitation* (2nd ed., pp. 29–52). New York: Wiley.

Kuller, L. H., Perper, J. A., Dai, W. S., Rutan, G., & Traven, N. (1986). Sudden death and the decline in coronary heart disease mortality. *Journal of Chronic Diseases, 39*(12), 1001–1019.

Lefebvre, R. C., Lasater, T. M., Carleton, R. A., & Peterson, G. (1987). Theory and delivery of health programming in the community: The Pawtucket Heart Health Program. *Preventive Medicine, 16,* 80–95.

Levy, R. I., Brensike, J. F., Epstein, S. E., Kelsey, S. F., Passamani, E. R., Richardson, J. M., Loh, I. K., Stone, N. J., Aldrich, R. F., Battaglini, J. W., Moriarty, D. J., Fisher, M. L., Friedman, L., Friedewald, W., & Detre, K. M. (1984). The influence of changes in lipid values induced by cholestyramine and diet on progression of coronary artery disease: Results of the NHLBI Type II Coronary Intervention Study. *Circulation, 68,* 325–337.

Lewis, H. D., Davis, J. W., Archibald, D. G., Steinke, W. E., Smitherman, T. C., Doherty, J. E., III, Schnaper, H. W., LeWinter, M. M., Linares, E., Pouget, J. M., Sabharwal, S. C., Chesler, E., & DeMots, H. (1983). Protective effects of aspirin against acute myocardial infarction and death in men with unstable angina. Results of a Veterans Administration Cooperative Study. *New England Journal of Medicine, 309,* 396–403.

Lyon, J. L., Wetzler, H. P., Gardner, J. W., Klauber, M. R., & Williams, R. R. (1978). Cardiovascular mortality in Mormons and non-Mormons in Utah, 1969–1971. *American Journal of Epidemiology, 108*(5), 357–368.

Meinert, C. L. (1986). *Clinical trials: Design, conduct, and analysis.* London: Oxford University Press.

Miller, G. J., Martin, J. C., Webster, J., Wilkes, H., Miller, N. E., Wilkinson, W. H., & Meade, T. W. (1986). Association between dietary fat intake and plasma factor VII coagulant activity—a predictor of cardiovascular mortality. *Atherosclerosis, 60,* 269–277.

Moss, A. J. (1980). Prediction and prevention of sudden cardiac death. *Annual Review of Medicine, 31,* 1–14.

Multiple Risk Factor Intervention Trial Research Group (1982). Multiple Risk Factor Intervention Trial: Risk factor changes and mortality results. *Journal of the American Medical Association, 248*(12), 1465–1477.

Pearson, T. A. (1984). Coronary arteriography in the study of the epidemiology of coronary artery disease. *Epidemiology Review, 6,* 140–266.

Phillips, R. L., Kuzma, J. W., Beeson, W. L., & Lotz, T. (1980). Influence of selection versus lifestyle on risk of fatal cancer and cardiovascular disease among Seventh-Day Adventists. *American Journal of Epidemiology, 112*(2), 296–314.

Puska, P., Salonen, J. T., Tuomilehto, J., Nissinen, A., & Kottke, T. E. (1983). Evaluating community-based preventive cardiovascular programs: Problems and experiences from the North Karelia Project. *Journal of Community Health, 9*(1), 49–64.

Rautaharju, P. M., Prineas, R. J., Eifler, W. J., Furberg, C. D., Neaton, J. D., Crow, R. S., Stamler, J., & Cutler, J. A. (1986). Prognostic value of exercise electrocardiogram in men at high risk of future coronary heart disease: Multiple Risk Factor Intervention Trial experience. *Journal of the American College of Cardiology 8*(1), 1–10.

Research Group of the Rome Project of Coronary Heart Disease Prevention (1986). Eight year follow-up results from the Rome Project of Coronary Heart Disease Prevention. *Preventive Medicine, 15,* 176–191.

Rose, G., Hamilton, P. J. S., Colwell, L., & Shipley, M. J. (1982). A randomized controlled trial of anti-smoking behavior change among smokers in the Multiple Risk Factor Intervention Trial (MRFIT). *Preventive Medicine, 11,* 621–638.

Royal College of General Practitioners' Oral Contraception Study (1981). Further analysis of mortality in oral contraceptive users. *Lancet, 1,* 541–546.

Ruberman, W., Weinblatt, E., Goldberg, J. D., & Chaudhary, B. S. (1984). Psychosocial influences on mortality after myocardial infarction. *New England Journal of Medicine, 311,* 552–559.

Salonen, J. T., Kottke, T. E., Jacobs, D. R., & Hannan, P. J. (1986). Analysis of community-based cardiovascular disease prevention studies—Evaluation issues in the North Karelia Project and the Minnesota Heart Health Program. *International Journal of Epidemiology, 15*(2), 176–182.

Schulze, R. A., Humphries, J. D., Griffith, L. S. C., Ducci, H., Achuff, S., Baird, M. G., Mellits, E. D., & Pitt, B. (1977). Left ventricular and coronary angiographic anatomy: Relationship to ventricular irritability in the late hospital phase of acute myocardial infarction. *Circulation, 55,* 839–843.

Shapiro, S., Venet, W., Strax, P., Venet, L., & Rosser, R. (1982). Ten to fourteen year effect of screening on breast cancer mortality. *Journal of the National Cancer Institute, 69,* 349–355.

Sherwin, R. W., Kaelber, C. T., Kezdi, P., Kjelsberg, M. O., & Thomas, H. E., for MRFIT (1981). The Multiple Risk Factor Intervention Trial (MRFIT): The development of the protocol. *Preventive Medicine, 10,* 402–425.

Sherwin, R. W., Wentworth, D. N., Cutler, J. A., Hulley, S. B., Kuller, L. H., & Stamler, J., for the MRFIT Group (1987). Serum cholesterol and cancer mortality in the 361,662 men screened for the Multiple Risk Factor Intervention Trial. *Journal of the American Medical Association, 257,* 943–948.

Stamler, J. (1980). Data base on the major cardiovascular diseases in the United States. In R. Hegyeli (Ed.), *Atherosclerosis reviews: Vol. 7. Measurement and control of cardiovascular risk factors.* New York: Raven Press.

Syme, S. L., Marmot, M. G., Kagan, A., Kato, H., & Rhoads, G. (1975). Epidemiologic studies of coronary heart disease and stroke in Japanese men living in Japan, Hawaii, and California: Introduction. *American Journal of Epidemiology, 102*(6), 477–490.

Talbott, E., Kuller, L. H., Detre, K., & Perper, J. A. (1980). Sudden death due to arteriosclerotic disease: A study of women. In H. E. Kulbertus & H. J. J. Wellens (Eds.), *Sudden death.* Hingham, MA: Kluwer Boston.

Thom, T. J., Epstein, F. H., Feldman, J. J., & Leaverton, P. E. (1985). Trends in total morbidity and mortality from heart disease in 26 countries from 1950–1978. *International Journal of Epidemiology, 14,* 510–520.

Ueshima, H., Iida, M., Shimamoto, T., (1982). Dietary intake and serum total cholesterol level: Their relationship to different lifestyles in several Japanese populations. *Circulation, 66*(3), 519–526.

U.S. Department of Health and Human Services (1983). Cerebrovascular disease. In Cardiovascular Disease: The Health Consequences of Smoking (pp. 157–175). *Surgeon General Report.* Washington, DC: U.S. Government Printing Office.

Verrier, R. L., & Lown, B. (1982). Experimental studies of psychophysiological factors in sudden cardiac death. *Acta Medica Scandinavica Supplementum, 660,* 57–68.

Zahavi, I., Goldbourt, U., Cohen-Mandelzweig L., Katz, M., Appel, S., Harel, G., Sperling, Z., Lazarovici, M., Hart, J., & Neufeld, H. N. (1987). Distributions of total cholesterol, triglycerides, and high-density lipoprotein cholesterol in Israeli Jewish children of different geographic–ethnic origins ages 9–17 years. *Preventive Medicine, 16,* 35–51.

Glossary

Terms

Acceleration The rate of change of velocity (dV/dt)

Aldosterone A steroid hormone produced by the outer (glomerulosa) zona of the adrenal cortex which facilitates transport of sodium (in exchange for potassium and hydrogen) in the renal distal tubule and collecting duct and in other epithelial tissues (salivary and sweat glands, colonic mucosa). Its major function is to promote renal sodium reabsorption in the conservation of extracellular fluid volume

Adrenocorticotropic hormone (ACTH) A polypeptide hormone secreted by the anterior pituitary which regulates steroid production by the adrenal cortex, primarily mediating diurnal and stress-induced changes of glucocorticoid production by the inner zones and having lesser importance in the regulation of aldosterone

Alternative hypothesis The assertion that in a population there is a true effect

Aneroid sphygmomanometer A device for measuring blood pressure in which the cuff pressure is measured by a dial rather than a mercury column

Anger An emotional state that involves displeasure, ranging in intensity from mild irritation to rage, and which frequently is accompanied by the impulse to inflict harm

Anger-in The tendency to inhibit the overt expression of anger

Angina pectoris Chest pain due to inadequate blood supply to the heart muscle; can be due to increased demand for oxygen, as in exercise, or to decreased blood delivery, as in coronary artery spasm

Angiotensin I A decapeptide fragment cleaved from the *N*-terminus of angiotensinogen by the action of renin which is precursor of angiotensin II and is largely without significant physiologic actions of its own

Angiotensin II An octapeptide formed by the action of angiotensin-converting enzyme on angiotensin I, which is the active hormone of the renin–angiotensin system and which regulates blood pressure and extracellular volume by constricting arterioles, stimulating aldosterone production, and other direct actions on the kidney and central and peripheral nervous systems

Angiotensin-converting enzyme A peptidase present on vascular endothelium which is responsible for conversion of angiotensin I to II

Angiotensinogen A circulating globulin of hepatic origin which is the substrate of renin and the precursor of the angiotensin peptides

Atria Thin-walled reservoir chambers of the heart interposed between the central veins and the ventricle

Atrial natriuretic factor (ANF) A polypeptide hormone released by atrial myocytes in response to stretch which promotes sodium excretion and has diverse inhibitory effects on the renin–angiotensin–aldosterone system

Atropine A parasympatholytic agent often used to block effects of the vagus nerve on the heart

693

Auscultatory method   Blood pressure is measured by an observer with a stethoscope placed over the brachial artery, to detect the onset and cessation of Korotkoff sounds

Autonomic nervous system   (1) Involuntary central nervous centers and outflow systems through the sympathetic and vagus nerves, influencing viscereal function, particularly the heart and peripheral vascular system; (2) a division of the peripheral nervous system composed of sympathetic and parasympathetic nervous systems which innervates most visceral organs, glands, and cardiac muscle

Automaticity   The ability of specialized cardiac tissue to spontaneously initiate an action potential

Autonomic tone   The end product of interaction between the central autonomic drive, receptor properties, and organ responsiveness

Autoregulation   The innate tendency of vascular smooth muscle to change its contractile tension in response to stretch or to changing chemical environments in the tissues

Baroreceptor   A reflex arc involving a change in heart rate in response to a change in pressure at the baroreceptor

Baroreflex   A physiologic sensor located in aortic arch and carotid sinus of humans, responsive to changes in pressure

Blood pressure   Systolic, diastolic

Cardiopulmonary receptors   Specialized nerve endings located in the cardiac chambers, great veins, and pulmonary circulation which sense changes in stretch (*mechanoreceptors*) or chemical milieu (*chemoreceptors*) and reflexly alter autonomic nerve traffic

Cardiovascular reactivity   The amount of cardiovascular response to a standardized stimulus

Catecholamines   A group of sympathomimetic amines including epinephrine, norepinephrine, and dopamine

Circadian rhythm   An intrinsic biological rhythm (i.e., one that is independent of external cues) having a periodicity of approximately 24 h

Contractility   The force or vigor of cardiac contractions that cannot be ascribed to filling pressure or volume (preload) or outflow pressure (afterload); more discretely described in terms of the rates of change of flow, pressure, or dimensions during systolic ejection

Coronary angiography   A diagnostic technique in which radio opaque dye is injected directly into the coronary arteries while x-ray pictures are taken; used to determine the extent of coronary atherosclerosis

Cynicism   An attitude signaling basic mistrust of human nature and motives

Diastole   The period during which heart chambers are relaxed and fill with blood in preparation for the ensuing contraction or systole

Diffusion   The general tendency of substances in suspension or solution to migrate from regions of higher concentration to regions of lower concentration

Doppler   A type of echocardiography which utilizes the frequency shift that occurs when sound waves are reflected from moving interfaces

Doppler phase shift   Sound waves emitted or reflected by a moving object (e.g., red blood cells) show a change in pitch. This principle can be used instead of the auscultatory method, by focusing an ultrasound probe on the brachial artery just below the cuff

Excitability   The capacity of cardiac tissue to respond to a delivered electrical impulse by generating an action potential

Excitation   The process by which nerves and muscles are activated by changes in cell membrane permeability when the membrane potentials reach threshold levels

Extracellular volume   The volume of fluid outside of cells (i.e., plasma and interstitial fluid), which is predominantly regulated by the balance of sodium chloride intake and excretion by the kidneys

Glomerular filtration rate   The rate of filtration of plasma across the glomerular capillary loop

Hemodynamics   Studies of the blood flow and its determinants (pressure and resistance)

Hostility   (1) An enduring attitude of ill will and a negative view of others; (2) overtly antagonistic behavior

Hypothesis   An assertion that in a population a true effect does or doesn't exist; hypotheses are often phrased in terms of the value of one or more parameters

Impulse   A sudden, brief application of force (in physics, the rate of change of acceleration)

Isometric   Contraction of muscle at constant length, i.e., prevented from shortening

Isometric exercise   Exertion of force against an immovable object

Juxtaglomerular cells   Specialized granule-containing myoepithelial cells in the walls of renal vessels (predominantly the afferent arteriole of the glomerulus) which are the major site of renin biosynthesis and storage

Kallman's syndrome   An unusual medical condition characterized by the failure of sexual maturation combined with a markedly decreased sense of smell

Korotkoff signal   The mechanical vibrations that are recorded by a high-fidelity transducer over the brachial artery as the cuff just proximal to the stethoscope is deflated from above systolic to below diastolic. The Korotkoff sounds represent the audible part of the Korotkoff signal

Korotkoff sound   The sounds that are heard with a stethoscope over the brachial artery as the cuff just proximal to the stethoscope is deflated from above systolic to below diastolic pressure

Likert-style response scale   Subjects indicate their response to a statement in terms of ordered categories such as: strongly disagree, disagree, uncertain, agree, strongly agree. (Likert scale construction is also known as the method of summated ratings.)

Manipulation check   The attempt to validate that an experimentally controlled variable produced the intended state (e.g., psychological or physiological) in the organisms under investigation

Microcirculation   The terminal vascular networks comprised of arterioles, precapillary sphincters, capillaries, and venules

Mediating variable   A variable through which the causal influence of another variable or variables acts

Moderating variable   A variable, the level of which controls the magnitude and/or direction of the relation between two or more other variables

Myocardium   Specialized striated muscle arranged in a network or syncytium that is activated by an excitation process spreading rapidly through contiguous cells to activate the chambers of the heart

Neuroticism   Below-average emotional control, will-power, and capacity to exert self and a tendency to repress unpleasant facts

Null hypothesis   The assertion that in a population there is no true effect

Organ responsiveness   The degree to which an organ responds to a specific amount of autonomic stimulation; determined by the intrinsic properties of the organ cells and the structural (autonomic) properties of the whole organ

Oscillometric method   When a cuff over an artery is gradually deflated, the pulsation of the artery is transmitted to the air in the cuff. The maximal oscillation of pressure in the cuff occurs at mean arterial pressure

Parameter   A numerical description of the population from which an experimental sample is drawn

Parasympathetic nervous system   A portion of the autonomic nervous system which upon stimulation produces slowing of the heart and increased gastrointestinal motility

Personality   Those thoughts, feelings, motives, and behaviors that characterize a person

Pharmacologic probes   Agonists and antagonists of the autonomic nervous system utilized to investigate the overall autonomic tone in an individual

Phenylephrine   An alpha receptor stimulant which acts as a sympathomimetic vasoconstrictor

Photoplethysmograph   A device placed on a finger which detects arterial pulsation by changes in light transmitted through the artery

Placebo effect   A change in symptoms or a physiological variable (e.g., blood pressure) which depends more on the expectation of the subject or patient than on the intervention eliciting the change

Plasma renin activity (PRA)   A widely used measurement of renin levels in blood which measures the rate of angiostensin I formation from endogenous plasma angiotensinogen

Plasma renin concentration   A measure of renin activity in the presence of saturating concentrations of exogenous angiotensinogen

Population   The totality of subjects that might have been observed in an experiment; often presumed to be infinite in number

Power   The probability that statistical analysis of experimental data will detect a true effect

Prorenin (inactive renin)   The catalytically inactive biosynthetic precursor of renin which is the major circulating form in humans and which is to some extent regulated independently from active renin

Propranolol   A beta receptor blocker often used to block effects of the sympathetic nervous system on the heart

RR interval   One cardiac cycle as measured from one R peak to the next consecutive R peak

RR variation   The normal variation in heart rate which occurs primarily due to respiration; also referred to as sinus arrhythmia

Reactance   A potential effect of self-monitoring whereby the self-recording by individuals of their own behavior may change the behaviors under observation

Reactivity   (1) In social research, reactivity refers to the responses of research participants that arise from their awareness of their status as research participants. For example, research participants may respond in a more socially desirable fashion when they know their behavior is being examined. (2) Response to a specific environmental event, after adjusting for levels obtained during a controlled baseline period

Receptor properties   The overall state of autonomic receptors; determined by their number, affinity, and sensitivity

Reentry   The process by which a single impulse may travel repeatedly over a portion of cardiac tissue and thus give rise to cardiac arrhythmia

Reflex arc   A chain of neurons from sensor to end organ composing the path of an unconditioned reflex

Refractoriness   The property by which cardiac cells fail to respond to an oncoming stimulus because repolarization is incomplete and the voltage of the interior of the cell has not become sufficiently negative to initiate or propagate an action potential

Reliability   Consistency of measurement; the degree to which test scores are free from errors of measurement. Typical reliability evidence may include test/retest, internal consistency and/or parallel forms reliability

Renin   An aspartyl (acid) protease that is released into the circulation by the kidney (and which may also act locally in other organs) and that provides the principal physiologic regulation of angiotensin formation

Repetitive extrasystole threshold   The minimum stimulus intensity required to provoke a single ventricular depolarization following a previously stimulated beat

Response cost   The amount of time and effort a subject spends in answering questions (or recording diary information)

Self-monitoring   Individual's systematically recording aspects of their behavior and physical symptoms as well as events surrounding each instance of measurement

ST segment   The portion of the electrocardiographic signal between the S and T waves, which is an indicator of myocardial ischemia (e.g., ST segment depression)

Structured interview   A set of specific questions that is presented to a subject; analysis of the subject's overt responses is used to assess Type A behavior; developed by Rosenman and Friedman

Sympathetic nervous system   The portion of the autonomic nervous system which upon stimulation produces a functional state of preparation for flight or combat

Systole   The interval during which the walls of the cardiac chambers contract

Tonic hormonal activity   The prevailing hormonal level as opposed to the short-term pulse of hormonal activity

Type A behavior pattern   A set of overt behaviors that is displayed by Type A persons; consists of time urgency, competitive achievement striving, and free-floating hostility

Type I error   The assertion that an experimental effect exists when there is no true effect. The probability of this error is conventionally denoted by alpha (α)

Type II error   The assertion that no experimental effect exists when there is a true effect. The probability of this error is conventionally denoted by beta (β) and is one minus the power

Ultradian rhythm   An intrinsic biological rhythm having a periodicity of approximately 90 min

Ultrasound   High-frequency sound waves (above the audible range) that are transmitted by a probe placed over an artery and reflected by bodily tissues, including red blood cells

Vagus   The tenth cranial nerve, an important component of the parasympathetic nervous system

Validity   Whether a test or measure is measuring what it is supposed to be measuring; the appropriateness, meaningfulness, and usefulness of the specific inferences made from a measurement. Typically, validity evidence includes content, construct, and criterion-related validity

Ventricular fibrillation threshold   The lowest stimulus intensity current required to precipitate ventricular fibrillation when delivered in the vulnerable period

Ventricles   The right and left pumping chambers of the heart that eject blood into the pulmonary and systemic circulations, respectively

Vulnerable period   A zone of 10–20 msec during ventricular repolarization (the first half of the T wave on the surface ECG) during which a stimulus of sufficient energy can precipitate ventricular fibrillation

Zona fasciculata   The outermost zone of the adrenal cortex, which is responsible for the synthesis of aldosterone

Abbreviations

ANOVA   Analysis of variance
ANS   Autonomic nervous system
Ao   Aortic

BDHI   Buss–Durkee Hostility Inventory
BP   Blood pressure
BPM   Beats per minute
BSA   Body surface area, in m^2

CA   Canonical analysis
CAD   Coronary atherosclerosis

CI   Cardiac index, in liters min per m^2
CHD   Coronary heart disease
CO   Cardiac output, which equals HR $\times$ SV, in liters/min
CVD   Cardiovascular disease

DBH   Dopamine-beta-hydroxylase
DBP   Diastolic blood pressure
dD/dt   Rate of change of diameter (or dimension) as applied to contraction of cardiac chambers during systole
dP/dt   Rate of change or pressure as indicated by the upslope or downslope of a continuous pressure record, in mm Hg/sec
dV/dt   Rate of change of velocity (or acceleration) as applied to ejection of blood from the ventricular chambers
dZ/dt   First derivation of Z used to calculate cardiac stroke volume

E   Epinephrine
ECG   Electrocardiograph
EDV   End-diastolic volume, in ml
EH   Essential hypertension
E_{max} Maximum value of ventricular pressure/volume ratio during cardiac systole; a measure of myocardial contractility
EF   Ejection fraction, which equals SV/EDV, expressed as a fraction or percent
ESV   End-systolic volume, in ml

FA   Factor analysis
FTAS   Framingham Type A scale
FPV   Finger pulse volume

HDL   High-density lipoprotein
HI   Heather Index used to estimate contractility from the impedance cardiogram
Ho   Hostility Scale by Cook and Medley (hostility, as measured by the Cook–Medley scale from the MMPI)
HR   Heart rate; the number of ventricular contractions per unit time, expressed as beats/min

JAS   Jenkins Activity Survey

LDL   Low–density lipoprotein
LV, RV Left ventricle and right ventricle of the heart
LVET   Left ventricular ejection time, in sec or msec
LVH   Left ventricular hypertrophy

MANOVA Multivariate analysis of variance
M-mode Refers to echocardiography with a single probe signal set to record motion, e.g., one dimension versus time
MI   Myocardial infarction
MMPI   The Minnesota Multiphasic Personality Inventory
MRA   Multiple regression analysis
MRFIT   The Multiple Risk Factor Intervention Trial
MUGA   Multiple gated acquisition for nuclear ventriculogram

NE   Norepinephrine

PA   Path analysis
PCO$_2$ Partial pressure of carbon dioxide, in mm Hg
PEP   Preejection period, in seconds or milliseconds
PET   Positron emission tomography
PNS   Parasympathetic nervous system
PoHo   Potential for hostility, as assessed using the structured interview
PR   Peripheral resistance, in units of mm Hg liters per min

QRS complex   Wave of excitation (depolarization) through left and right ventricular myocardium recorded in the surface electrocardiogram

RE   Reaction time
R-R interval   One cardiac cycle measured by the electrocardiogram
rho   Resistivity, e.g., of blood which is a determinant of thoracic impedance

SBP   Systolic blood pressure, in mm HG
SBP/ESV   Systolic blood pressure divided by end-systolic volume; an estimate of myocardial contractility, which approximates E$_{max}$
SCWT   Stroop Color–Word Test
SI   Structured interview, by Rosenman and Friedman for assessing Type A behavior
SNS   Sympathetic nervous system
SPECT   Single photon emission computerized tomography
ST segment   The isoelectric interval between end of depolarization (QRS) and onset of repolarization (T wave) in the electrocardiogram
STAS   The Spielberger State–Trait Anger Scale
SV   Stroke volume, which equals LVEDV/LVESV, in ml
SVI   Stroke volume index, in ml/m^2

TABP   Type A behavior pattern
99mTc   The radionuclide (isotope) of technetium used to label the cardiac blood pool for nuclear ventriculograms
TEDMAC   Tridodecylmethylammonium chloride; a compound that binds heparin
Two-D   Refers to cross-sectional echocardiography to record two dimensions versus time

VLDL   Very-low-density lipoprotein
VPC   Ventricular premature contraction

WCGS   Western Collaborative Group Study

Zo   Basal thoracic impedance, in ohms
ΔZ   Change of impedance, in ohms/sec

Index